CORE CURRICULUM for ONCOLOGY NURSING

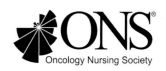

CORE CURRICULUM for ONCOLOGY NURSING

6TH EDITION

Editor

JEANNINE M. BRANT, PhD, APRN, AOCN®, FAAN

Oncology Clinical Nurse Specialist and Nurse Scientist
Collaborative Science and Innovation, Billings Clinic
Billings, Montana
Assistant Affiliate Professor
College of Nursing, Montana State University
Bozeman, Montana

Section Editors

DIANE G. COPE, PhD, APRN, BC, AOCNP®

Director of Nursing
Oncology Nurse Practitioner
Florida Cancer Specialists and Research Institute
Fort Myers, Florida

MARLON GARZO SARIA, PhD, RN, AOCNS®, FAAN

Tarble Foundation Oncology Clinical Nurse Specialist and Nurse Scientist
Providence Saint John's Health Center, Santa Monica, California
Assistant Professor
John Wayne Cancer Institute/Pacific Neuroscience Institute, Santa Monica, California
Clinical Nurse
US Air Force
March Air Reserve Base, California

ELSEVIER

Elsevier
3251 Riverport Lane
St. Louis, Missouri 63043

CORE CURRICULUM FOR ONCOLOGY NURSING, SIXTH EDITION   ISBN: 978-0-323-59545-2

Previous editions copyrighted 2016, 2005, 1998, 1992, 1987 by Oncology Nursing Society.

International Standard Book Number: 978-0-323-59545-2

Executive Content Strategist: Lee Henderson
Senior Content Development Specialist: Laura Goodrich
Publishing Services Manager: Julie Eddy
Senior Project Manager: Richard Barber
Book Designer: Renee Duenow

Printed in the United States of America

Last digit is the print number: 9 8 7 6 5 4 3 2 1

Working together
to grow libraries in
developing countries

www.elsevier.com • www.bookaid.org

CONTRIBUTORS

Kristine Deano Abueg, RN, MSN, OCN®, CBCN
Clinical Research Nurse
Oncology Clinical Trials
Kaiser Permanente
Roseville, California
Oncology Clinical Trials
Roseville, California

Suzanne Agarwal, RN, BS, BSN, MS
Interim Nursing Supervisor
Moores Cancer Center
UC San Diego Health System
La Jolla, California

Susan Weiss Behrend, RN, MSN, AOCN®
Clinical Nurse Specialist
Department of Nursing
Fox Chase Cancer Center
Philadelphia, Pennsylvania

Christine Boley, RN, MSN, ACNP-BC
Oncology Nurse Practitioner
Medical Oncology
Providence St. John's
Santa Monica, California

Roberta Bourgon, ND
Integrative Medicine
Billings Clinic
Billings, Montana

Christa Braun-Inglis, MS, APRN-Rx, FNP-BC, AOCNP®
Nurse Practitioner
Oncology
University of Hawaii Cancer Center
Assistant Researcher
Clinical Trials Office
University of Hawaii Cancer Center
Clinical Faculty
School of Nursing
University of Hawaii at Manoa
Honolulu, Hawaii

Dawn Camp-Sorrell, MSN, FNP, AOCN®
Oncology Nurse Practitioner
Oncology
Children's of Alabama
Birmingham, Alabama

Ellen Carr, RN, MSN, AOCN®
Clinical Educator
Multispecialty Clinic
UC San Diego Health System
Moores Cancer Center
La Jolla, California

Hana K. Choi, PhD, MSCP
Staff Psychologist
Comprehensive Pain Center
Minneapolis VA Health Care System
Minneapolis, Minnesota

Lani Kai Clinton, MD, PhD
Assistant Professor
Pathology
Duke University Health System
Durham, North Carolina

Kristi Coe, BSN, MS
Health Sciences Librarian/Assistant Professor of Library
    Science
Centennial Library
Cedarville University
Cedarville, Ohio

Stacie Corcoran, RN, MS, AOCNS®
Program Director, Adult Cancer Survivorship
Department of Medicine
Memorial Sloan Kettering Cancer Center
New York, New York

Gail W. Davidson, MS, NP-C
Nurse Practitioner
Hepatology
The Ohio State University
Columbus, Ohio

Marianne Davies, DNP, MSN, CNS, ACNP-BC, AOCNP®, RN
Associate Professor
Yale University School of Nursing
West Haven, Connecticut
Oncology Nurse Practitioner
Medical Oncology
Yale Comprehensive Cancer Center, Smilow Cancer Hospital
New Haven, Connecticut

Patty Davis, RN, BSN, OCN®
Manager of Nursing Operations
Infusion Center, Medical Oncology and
    Radiation Oncology
Frontier Cancer Center
Billings, Montana

Elizabeth Delaney, DNP, CNS, FNP-BC, OCN®, ACHPN
Nurse Practitioner
Medical Oncology
Dayton Physicians Network
Dayton, Ohio
Assistant Professor
School of Nursing
Cedarville University
Cedarville, Ohio

Julie Eggert, PhD, GNP BC, AGN-BC, AOCN®, FAAN
Professor Emerita
School of Nursing
Clemson University
Clemson, South Carolina
Advanced Practice Nurse Genetics Counselor
Oncology Services
Bon Secour-St. Francis Hospital System
Greenville, South Carolina

Jeanne Marie Erickson, PhD, MSN, BSN
Associate Professor
College of Nursing
University of Wisconsin-Milwaukee
Milwaukee, Wisconsin

Denise Falardeau, MSN, AGPCNP-BC, AOCNP®
Nurse Practitioner
Medical Oncology
City of Hope National Medical Center
Duarte, California

Regina M. Fink, PhD, APRN, CHPN, AOCN®, FAAN
Associate Professor
Co-Director Interprofessional Master of Science in Palliative
    Care Program
University of Colorado Anschutz Medical Campus School of
    Medicine and College of Nursing
Aurora, Colorado

Elizabeth Freitas, PhD, MS, BSN
Clinical Nurse Specialist
Pain & Palliative Care
The Queen's Medical Center
Honolulu, Hawaii

Eileen Galvin, MN, RN, OCN®
Oncology Nurse Educator
Oncology Unit
Boehringer Ingelheim
Ridgefield, Connecticut

Jaya M. Gill, MD, BSN, RN
Clinical Trials Supervisor
Neuro-Oncology
Providence Saint John's Health Center/John
    Wayne Cancer Institute
Santa Monica, California

Emily A. Haozous, PhD, RN, FAAN
Research Scientist
Behavioral Health Research Center of the Southwest
Pacific Institute of the Pacific
Albuquerque, New Mexico

Joshua B. Hardin, MSN, RN, CCRN, CPAN
Doctoral Student
College of Nursing
University of Wisconsin-Milwaukee
Milwaukee, Wisconsin

Anna Howard, PharmD, BCOP
Lead Oncology Clinical Pharmacist
Department of Pharmacy
Billings Clinic
Billings, Montana

Beverly Hudson, RN-BC, BSN
Nurse Case Manager
Head & Neck Surgical Oncology
UC San Diego Health System
Moores Cancer Center
La Jolla, California

Stephanie Jackson, MSN, RN, AOCNS®, BMTCN
Oncology Clinical Nurse Specialist
Hematology/Stem Cell Transplantation
Ronald Reagan UCLA Medical Center
Los Angeles, California

Catherine E. Jansen, PhD, RN, AOCNS®
Oncology Clinical Nurse Specialist
Department of Oncology and Hematology
The Permanente Medical Group
San Francisco, California
Clinical Professor
Department of Physiological Nursing
University of California, San Francisco
San Francisco, California

Pamela Katz, MSN
Staff RN
BMT/ Hematology
Rush University Medical Center
Chicago, Illinois

Brenda Keith, MN, RN, AOCNS®
Senior Oncology Clinical Coordinator III
Genentech, South San Francisco
San Francisco, California

Santosh Kesari, MD, PhD, FANA, FAAN
Chair and Professor
Translational Neurosciences and Neurotherapeutics
John Wayne Cancer Institute/Pacific Neuroscience
    Institute
Santa Monica, California

Barbara G. Lubejko, MS, RN
Oncology Clinical Specialist
Clinical Portfolio
Oncology Nursing Society
Pittsburgh, Pennsylvania

Sally Maliski, PhD, RN, FAAN
Dean and Franklin and Beverly Gaines Tipton
    Professor for Oncology Nursing
University of Kansas School of Nursing
Associate Director, Health Equity
University of Kansas Cancer Center
Kansas City, Kansas

Leslie Matthews, MS, ANP-BC, AOCNP®
Nurse Practitioner
Myeloma / Lymphoma Service
Memorial Sloan Kettering Cancer Center
Commack, New York

Tricia Montgomery, RN, BSN, OCN®
Clinical Coordinator
Cancer Research, Tumor Registry
Billings Clinic
Billings, Montana

Kathleen Murphy-Ende, PhD, PsyD, APNP, AOCNP®
Psychologist and Nurse Practitioner
Psychiatry
University of Wisconsin
Clinical Associate Professor
School of Nursing
University of Wisconsin
Madison, Wisconsin

Susie Newton, APRN, MS, AOCN®, AOCNS®
Oncology Advanced Practice Nurse
Palliative Care Consultant
Sr. Director, TMAC: The Medical Affairs Company
Dayton, Ohio

Carol Nikolai, DNP, APRN-CNP
Nurse Practitioner
Medical Oncology
Dayton Physicians Network
Dayton, Ohio
Assistant Professor
College of Nursing
The Ohio State University
Columbus, Ohio

Patricia W. Nishimoto, BSN, MPH, DNS
Adult Oncology Clinical Nurse Specialist
Department of Medicine
Tripler Army Medical Center
Honolulu, Hawaii

Judy Petersen, RN, MSN, AOCN®
Oncology Nurse Educator Consultant
Independent Practice
Seattle, Washington

Jan M. Petree, MSN, RN, FNP, AOCNP®
Nurse Practitioner, Medical Oncology
Infusion Treatment Center, Redwood City
Stanford Healthcare
Redwood City, California

Julie Ponto, PhD, APRN, CNS, AGCNS-BC, AOCNS®
Professor
Graduate Programs in Nursing
Winona State University-Rochester
Rochester, Minnesota

Nancy Robertson, MSN, ANP-BC, ACHPN
Assistant Professor
Palliative Care Nurse Practitioner
University of Colorado Anschutz
    Medical Campus
Aurora, Colorado

Krista M. Rubin, MS, FNP-BC
Nurse Practitioner, Center for Melanoma
Massachusetts General Hospital Cancer Center
Boston, Massachusetts

Rowena N. Schwartz, PharmD, BCOP, FHOPA
Associate Professor of Pharmacy Practice
University of Cincinnati, James L.
    Winkle College of Pharmacy
Oncology Clinical Pharmacy Specialist
UC Health
Cincinnati, Ohio

Jennifer Shamai, MS, RN, AOCNS®, BMTCN
Oncology Clinical Nurse Specialist
City of Hope National Medical Center
Duarte, California

Brenda K. Shelton, MS, RN, CCRN, AOCN®
Clinical Nurse Specialist
Sidney Kimmel Comprehensive Cancer
    Center at Johns Hopkins
Johns Hopkins Hospital
Associate Faculty
Nursing
Johns Hopkins School of Nursing
Baltimore, Maryland

Shama Shrestha, RN, BSN, OCN®
Nurse Case Manager
Palliative Care
UC San Diego Health System
Moores Cancer Center
La Jolla, California

Mady C. Stovall, MSN, ANP-BC
PhD Student
School of Nursing
Oregon Health & Science University
Portland, Oregon

Cathleen Sugarman, MSN, RN, AOCNS®, ACNS-BC
Nurse Manager
Comprehensive Breast Health Center
University of California, San Diego
La Jolla, California

Jazel Dolores Sugay, MSN, RN
Clinical Research Nurse
Robert H. Lurie Comprehensive Cancer Center
Northwestern University
Chicago, Illinois

Geline J. Tamayo, MSN, RN, ACNS-BC, OCN®
Cancer Center Clinical Nurse Specialist
Moores Cancer Center
UC San Diego Health System
La Jolla, California

Joseph D. Tariman, PhD, RN, ANP-BC, FAAN
Assistant Professor and Co-Director, DNP Program
Nursing
DePaul University
Nurse Practitioner
Hematology-Oncology
Northwest Oncology and Hematology, Hoffman Estates
Chicago, Illinois

Jennifer Alisangco Tschanz, RN, MSN, FNP, AOCNP®
Nurse Practitioner
Department of Hematology Oncology
Naval Medical Center San Diego
San Diego, California

Wendy Vogel, MSN, FNP, AOCNP®
Oncology Nurse Practitioner
Hematology/Oncology
Ballad Health
Kingsport, Tennessee

Kathy Waitman, DNP, FNP-BC, MSN, AOCNP®, BSN
Nurse Practitioner
Hematology/Oncology
Billings, Montana

Deborah Kirk Walker, DNP, FNP-BC, NP-C, AOCN®, FAANP
Associate Dean
Associate Professor
School of Nursing and Midwifery
Edith Cowan University
Joondalup, Western Australia

Joni L. Watson, DNP, MBA, RN, OCN®
Vice President, Patient Care
Baylor Scott & White Medical Center - Lake Pointe
Waco, Rowlett, Texas

Tia Wheatley, DNP, RN, AOCNS®, BMTCN, EBP-C
Oncology Clinical Nurse Specialist
Hematology & Stem Cell Transplantation
City of Hope National Medical Center
Duarte, California

Rita Wickham, BSN, MS, PhD
Adjunct Faculty
Adult Health Nursing
Rush University College of Nursing
Chicago, Illinois

Terry Wikle Shapiro, RN, MSN, CRNP
Nurse Practitioner
Pediatric Stem Cell Transplant
Penn State Children's Hospital
Hershey, Pennsylvania

Allison Winacoo, MSN, RN, CPNP, CPHON, BMTCN
Professional Practice Leader
Professional Practice and Education
City of Hope National Medical Center
Duarte, California

Brenda Blickhan, BSN, RN, OCN®
Director of Oncology Services
Quincy Medical Group
Ursa, Illinois

Marie Hartman Drewek, RN, MSN, M DIV
Formerly Northwestern Memorial Hospital—Retired
Swartz Creek, Michigan

Beth Faiman, PhD, MSN, AOCN®, CNP
Cleveland Clinic
Highland Heights, Ohio

Claudia Hepburn, RN, BSN, OCN®
Rex Hematology Oncology Associates
Garner, North Carolina

Pam S. Herena, MSN, RN, OCN®
Senior Director
Briskin Center for Clinical Research
City of Hope National Medical Center
Duarte, California

Patty Kormanik, RN, MS, NP-C, AOCNP®
UCSD Medical Center
Encinitas, California

Heather Mackey, MSN, RN, ANP-BC, AOCN®
Novant Health Derrick L. Davis Cancer Center
Kernersville, North Carolina

Jennifer Peterson, MSN, RN
Professional Practice Leader
City of Hope National Medical Center
Pasadena, California

Barb Rogers, CRNP, MN, AOCN®, ANP-BC
Fox Chase Cancer Center
Bensalem, Pennsylvania

Lisa Schulmeister, MN, RN, FAAN
Oncology Nursing Consultant
Self-Employed
New Orleans, Louisiana

Ruth VanGerpen, RN, MS, AOCNS®
Bryan Health
Lincoln, Nebraska

Adrienne Vazquez, MSN, ACNP-BC, AOCNP®
Sylvester Comprehensive Cancer Center
Survivorship Operations Leader
University of Miami Health System
Miami, Florida

Mary Ellyn Witt, MS, RN, AOCN®
University of Chicago Cancer Center at Silver
   Cross
La Grange, Illinois

Grace Wu, NP
City of Hope National Medical Center
Duarte, California

Vickie Yattaw, RN, BSN, OCN®
Oncology Education & Support Services Manager
C.R. Wood Cancer Center
Glens Falls Hospital
Glens Falls, New York

PREFACE

On behalf of the section editors, Diane Cope, Marlon Saria, and myself, we are pleased to bring you the sixth edition of the *Core Curriculum for Oncology Nursing*.

As in previous editions, the OCN® Test Blueprint is the organizing framework for the text. Sections and chapters reflect specific portions of the Test Blueprint. One of the major uses of this text is to prepare for the OCN® certification examination. The sixth edition features a more streamlined, clinically relevant application of the nursing process, which includes an overview of each problem, assessment, management, and expected patient outcomes. The easy-to-use outline format has been retained in this edition. An emphasis on QSEN competencies is included to alert clinicians of safety concerns, reduce errors in oncology nursing practice, and foster discussion on evidence-based strategies to improve both safety and quality care. Safety-related content has been highlighted using *Safety Alert* icons.

As cancer care is rapidly evolving, the book sections and content of the chapters have been updated to reflect the dynamic trends in cancer care delivery and cancer care. Section One of the book, "The Care Continuum," has two new chapters: "Navigation Across the Continuum" and "Advanced Care Planning, Communication, and Shared Decision Making." Section Two, "Scientific Basis for Practice" includes new discoveries in genetics, genomics, and molecular biology of cancer. "Precision Medicine" is a new chapter in this section. Section Three, "Treatment Modalities," includes updates in all modalities, with the most significant changes discussed in the "Biotherapy, Immunotherapy, and Targeted Therapy chapter." "Palliation of Symptoms" is the title of Section Four and adds two new chapters: "Cognitive Symptoms" and "Endocrine Symptoms." Section Six is "Psychosocial Dimensions" of care and includes updated content in cultural, spiritual, psychological, social, and sexual care.

Finally, Section Seven is "Professional Practice." Evidence-based practice, professional standards, and ethical issues are highlighted. A new chapter titled "Compassion Fatigue" is the final chapter of the book, reminding nurses about self-care and a balanced lifestyle.

In 2013, the Institute of Medicine (IOM) report, *Delivering High-Quality Cancer Care: Charting a New Course for a System in Crisis,* discussed the need for an adequately staffed, trained, and coordinated workforce. The report sets a goal that all individuals caring for cancer patients should have appropriate core competencies. The Oncology Nursing Society (ONS) has been a leader in the nursing profession in establishing certification programs that formally recognize oncology nurses' specialized knowledge, skills, and expertise. To meet this IOM goal, nursing should focus on increasing the number of oncology-certified nurses and promoting the role of institutions in requiring certification. We believe this textbook will help nurses with appropriate oncology experience prepare successfully for the OCN® certification examination.

Our thanks to ONS for providing us the opportunity to revise and update this text. Our special thanks to John Zaphyr from ONS press, who assisted with this edition of the *Core Curriculum.* Our special thanks to Lee Henderson and Laura Goodrich of Elsevier. As with any endeavor, it takes a village! It has been a pleasure to work with such an efficient and dedicated team. We also want to thank our families, who caught us editing at odd hours and were patient with us during those essential deadlines! Finally, we thank the contributors whose expertise and passion for oncology nursing is what makes this book a valuable resource for oncology nurses around the globe.

Jeannine M. Brant

CONTENTS

PART 5 Psychosocial Dimensions of Care

PART 6 Oncologic Emergencies

Epidemiology, Prevention, and Health Promotion

Joni L. Watson

OVERVIEW

I. Cancer epidemiology
   A. Definition
      1. Study of the distribution and determinants of cancer in population groups
      2. Assists in development of population-based risk profiles
   B. Global cancer statistics (International Agency for Research on Cancer and Cancer Research, 2018; World Cancer Research Fund International, 2018)
      1. Cancer incidence worldwide
         a. Approximately 14.1 million people were diagnosed with cancer in 2012.
         b. The cancer rate is projected to increase by 75% to 22 million new cases in 2030, primarily because of an increasing aging population; tobacco use; and reproductive, dietary, and hormonal risk factors (Stewart & Wild, 2014).
         c. The top five most commonly diagnosed cancers are lung (13%), breast (12%), colorectal (9.7%), prostate (7.8%), and stomach (6.8%).
            (1) Lung, breast, colorectal, stomach, and prostate cancers make up nearly 50% of all cases diagnosed.
            (2) Lung cancer is the most common cancer in men.
               (a) In 2012, approximately 58% of cancer cases occurred in less developed countries.
            (3) Breast cancer is the most common cancer in women.
               (a) Breast cancer incidence in North America is more than double that in Africa.
            (4) More than 68% of prostate cancer cases are diagnosed in more developed regions of the world.
      2. Cancer mortality worldwide (International Agency for Research on Cancer and Cancer Research, 2018)
         a. An estimated 8.2 million people died from the disease in 2012.
         b. The top five most common causes of death from cancer are lung (19%), liver (9.1%), stomach (8.8%), colorectal (8.5%), and breast (6.4%).
         c. About 48% of cancer-related deaths are seen in less developed regions of the world.
   C. Cancer statistics in the United States (U.S.) (American Cancer Society [ACS], 2018)
      1. Cancer incidence in U.S.
         a. Estimated 1,735,350 new cancer cases in 2018
         b. Approximately 4750 new cases every day
         c. Estimates exclude basal cell and squamous cell skin cancers and in situ carcinomas, except urinary bladder
         d. Estimates are not available for Puerto Rico
         e. For both sexes combined, the top five most commonly diagnosed cancers are breast, prostate, lung and bronchus, colorectal, and uterine corpus (Fig. 1.1).
         f. Among women, the five most common cancers are breast (30%), lung (13%), colorectal (7%), uterine (7%), and thyroid (5%).
         g. Among men, the five most common cancers are prostate (19%), lung (14%), colorectal (9%), urinary bladder (7%), and melanoma of the skin (6%).
      2. Trends in cancer incidence rates (Howlader et al., 2017)
         a. For all races, cancer incidence rates declined from 2005 to 2014
         b. Cancer site with increasing incidence trends from 2005 to 2014
            (1) Liver cancer incidence in women has been increasing approximately 2.6% each year

Top 10 Cancer Sites: 2014, Male and Female, United States–All Races

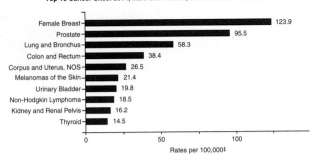

Fig. 1.1 Top 10 Cancer Sites: 2014, Male and Female, United States – All Races (From U.S. Cancer Statistics Working Group. (2017). *United States cancer statistics: 1999–2014, incidence and mortality web-based report.* Retrieved from https://nccd.cdc.gov/uscs/toptencancers.aspx? printfriendly¼1.)

since 2004. Still, less than 1% of men and women will be diagnosed with liver cancer in his or her lifetime.

(2) Cancers with increasing annual percentage changes of 1% or more per year include melanoma of the skin; cancer of the kidney; and thyroid, pancreas, and liver and intrahepatic bile duct cancers.

c. Cancer sites with decreasing incidence trends from 1975 to 2014

(1) Among men, the incidence rates declined 2% annually from 2005 to 2014.

(2) Among women, the cancer incidence rate significantly declined from 1998 to 2005 and was stable from 2005 to 2014.

(3) In addition to the four leading cancers (breast, prostate, lung, and colorectal cancer), incidence rates of other cancer sites are decreasing, including cancers of the ovary, stomach, uterine, cervix, and larynx.

3. Trends in cancer mortality rates (NCI, 2017a)

a. Estimated 609,640 deaths from cancer in 2018

b. About 1670 deaths per day

c. Cancer is the second leading cause of death in the U.S., second to heart disease.

d. One of every four deaths is caused by cancer.

e. Cancer is the leading cause of death for Hispanic and Asian Americans.

f. Cervical cancer is the second leading cause of death in women ages 20 to 39.

g. Among women, the five leading causes of cancer-related deaths are lung (25%), breast (15%), colorectal (9%), pancreas (7%), and ovary (5%).

h. Among men, the five leading causes of cancer-related deaths are lung (27%), prostate (9%), colorectal (9%), pancreas (6%), and liver/intrahepatic bile duct (6%).

i. For all cancers combined, cancer mortality rates steadily declined from 215 in 1991 to 159 per 100,000 in 2015.

j. For all races, cancer mortality rates declined from 1992 to 2015.

k. A reported 2.3 million fewer cancer deaths from 1991 to 2015, resulting from steady progress and advances in prevention, screening, treatment, and survivorship

4. Cancer survival statistics in the U.S. (ACS, 2018)

a. Between 2008 and 2015, the 5-year relative survival rate for all cancers was 68% in whites and 61% in blacks

b. As of January 1, 2016, the NCI estimated 15.5 million cancer survivors in U.S.

(1) Fifty-nine percent of cancer survivors are 65 years of age or older.

(2) For all stages combined, 5-year survival is highest for prostate (99%), melanoma of the skin (92%), and female breast cancer (90%).

(3) Survival is lowest for lung (18%), liver (18%), and pancreas (8%).

(4) The chronic myeloid leukemia relative survival rate has gone from 22% in the mid-1970s to 68% in 2013.

5. Cancer health disparities (NCI, 2017b)

a. Definition of "cancer health disparities"—adverse differences in incidence, prevalence, mortality, survivorship, and burden of cancer or related health conditions that exist among specific population groups in the U.S.

(1) Population groups may be characterized by age, disability, education, race/ethnicity, gender, income, poverty, lack of health insurance, geographic location, and medically underserved.

b. Statistics on race/ethnicity and cancer for 2014 (NCI, 2017b)

(1) African Americans have higher death rates for most cancers

(2) Historically for breast cancer, white women have had the highest incidence rate; however, African American women's rates have caught up. The highest mortality rate is seen among African American women.

(3) For cervical cancer, Hispanic/Latina women have the highest incidence rate; however, the highest mortality rate is seen among African American women.

(4) For prostate cancer, African American men have the highest incidence and mortality rates than other ethnic groups in the U.S.

(5) For both lung and colorectal cancers, African Americans have the highest incidence and mortality compared with other ethnic groups in the U.S.

(6) Asians/Pacific Islanders have the highest incidence and mortality rates of liver and stomach cancers compared with other ethnic groups in the U.S.

(7) American Indians/Alaska Natives have the highest incidence and mortality rates of kidney cancer in the U.S.

(8) African Americans have the highest cancer incidence rates, followed by whites, Hispanic/Latinos, Asian/Pacific Islanders, and American Indian/Alaskan Natives.

(9) African American men are more than twice as likely as white men to die of prostate cancer.

(10) American Indian/Alaska Native and Asian Pacific Islanders have the highest rates of liver and intrahepatic bile duct cancers.

(11) The lowest mortality rate is seen in Asian/Pacific Islander men.

6. Cancer mortality in U.S. (ACS, 2018)
   a. Age
      (1) The risk of developing cancer increases with age.
      (2) Approximately 87% of all cancers are diagnosed in persons 55 years or older.
   b. Gender
      (1) Women have a one in three lifetime risk of developing cancer.
      (2) Men have a one in two lifetime risk of developing cancer.
   c. Geography—significant incidence and mortality differences exist in different locations.
      (1) White women who live in Appalachia have a significantly higher risk of developing cervical cancer than other white women in the U.S. (NCI, 2017b).
      (2) Migratory data demonstrate adoption of the cancer pattern of the area to which migration occurs, suggesting lifestyle, behavioral, and environmental factors as causative or exacerbating.
   d. Socioeconomic status (SES)
      (1) Low SES is associated with increased risk of lung cancer, cervical cancer, stomach cancer, and cancer of the head and neck.
      (2) Tobacco use has increased among poorer populations.
      (3) More advanced disease at diagnosis is found among poor populations and those who live in rural areas.
      (4) High SES is associated with increased risk of breast, prostate, and colon cancers.
   e. Economic, social, and cultural factors may create barriers to accessing information and preventive services.

II. Cancer prevention
   A. Modifiable cancer risk factors
      1. Tobacco use (ACS, 2017)
         a. Single largest preventable cause of disease and premature death in the U.S.
            (1) Smoking responsible for approximately 480,000 premature deaths each year

(2) Twenty-one million deaths attributed to tobacco use since 1964, the first U.S. Surgeon General's report on smoking

(3) Accounts for at least 30% of all cancer deaths

(4) In 2012, accounted for $176 billion health care–related expenses

(5) Between 2005 and 2015, daily smoker prevalence decreased from 17% to 11%.

(6) Increases the risk of cancers of the lung, mouth, nasal cavities, larynx, pharynx, oral cavity, esophagus, stomach, colorectum, liver, pancreas, kidney, bladder, uterine cervix, ovary, and acute myeloid leukemia

b. Exposure to secondhand smoke is a risk factor for lung cancer and cardiovascular disease (U.S. Department of Health and Human Services, 2006).
   (1) Exposure causes 5% of lung cancers annually
   (2) About 43% of nonsmokers in the U.S. have detectable levels of cotinine, a biomarker used to measure exposure to tobacco smoke.
   (3) About 60% of children, aged 3 to 11 years, are exposed to secondhand smoke.

c. Smoking and gender
   (1) In 2015, 16.8% of adult men and 13.8% of adult women were current smokers.

d. Smoking and health disparities
   (1) Adults without a high school degree are two to four times more likely to be current smokers than those with a college degree.
   (2) Among current smokers, the highest percentage is found in American Indians/Alaska Natives.
   (3) Those who are uninsured are twice as likely to be current smokers than those who are insured.

e. Cigar smoking
   (1) Increases the risk of cancers of the lung, oral cavity, larynx, esophagus, and probably pancreas
   (2) Cigar smokers are 4 to 10 times more likely to die of laryngeal, oral, or esophageal cancers than nonsmokers
   (3) Estimated 10.4% of men and 3.1% of women currently smoke cigars
   (4) Cigar use highest among African Americans (9.2%), those with less than high school education (10%), and those with household income greater than $20,000 per year

f. Smokeless tobacco
   (1) Chewing tobacco and snuff not safe substitutes for smoking
   (2) Increases the risk of oral, pancreatic, and esophageal cancers
   (3) Electronic nicotine delivery systems (ENDS), also known as *e-cigarettes*

(a) Battery-operated devices in which the inhaled vapor is produced from cartridges that contain nicotine, flavor, and other chemicals

(b) Use may lead nonsmokers, especially children, to begin smoking

(c) As of 2016, the U.S. Food and Drug Administration (FDA) classified ENDS as a tobacco product, bringing them under FDA regulation

(d) The FDA has not approved any ENDS to date as a cessation aid

(e) As of 2016, more than 2 million middle and high school students were e-cigarette users, with appealing flavors as the primary reason for use

g. Healthy People 2020 goals regarding tobacco use (U.S. Department of Health and Human Services, 2013)

(1) Reduce the percentage of adults who currently smoke to 12%

(2) Reduce the percentage of adults who currently use smokeless tobacco to 0.3%

(3) Reduce the percentage of adults who currently smoke cigars to 0.2%

2. Obesity (ACS, 2017)

a. Definitions

(1) Obesity, physical inactivity, and poor nutrition major risk factors for cancer

(2) Overweight and obesity classification by body mass index (BMI) (Table 1.1)

(a) Overweight or preobese: BMI range between 25.0 and 29.9 kg/m^2

(b) Obese: BMI of 30.0 kg/m^2 or higher

b. Second only to tobacco use as a cancer risk factor

c. Responsible for about one quarter to one third of all cancers in the U.S.

d. Overweight/obesity contribute to an estimated 20% of all cancer-related deaths

(1) Increase the risk of 13 cancers: uterine corpus, esophagus (adenocarcinoma), liver, stomach (gastric cardia), kidney (renal cell), brain (meningioma), multiple myeloma, pancreas, colorectum, gallbladder, ovary, breast (postmenopausal), and thyroid

(2) May also be linked to risk of non-Hodgkin lymphoma (diffuse large B-cell lymphoma), male breast cancer, and fatal prostate cancer

e. Prevalence of obesity doubled from 1976 to 1980 (15%) and 2013 to 2014 (37.7%)

f. Obesity and gender

(1) Among men, overweight/obesity rate is 73.7%.

(2) Among women, overweight/obesity rate is 66.9%.

g. Obesity and race/ethnicity

(1) African American women (58%) have the highest rates of obesity compared with non-Hispanic white women (38%) and Hispanic women (47%).

h. Obesity and age

(1) Obesity prevalence tripled in adolescents (ages 12 to 19) from 5% in 1976% to 16% in 2002

i. Contributing factors

(1) Foods and beverages high in calories may contribute to altered amounts and distribution of body fat, insulin resistance, and higher concentrations of growth factors that promote cancer growth

(2) Processed and red meats

(a) Associated with increased risk of colorectal, prostate, and pancreatic cancers

(b) Nitrates or other substances used to preserve processed meats involved in carcinogenesis

(3) Decreased fruit and vegetable consumption

(a) Only 16% of adults reported eating three or more servings of vegetables daily in 2011.

(b) Increased consumption of fruits and vegetables associated with decreased risk of lung, esophageal, stomach, and colorectal cancers

(c) High intake of whole-grain foods associated with decreased risk of colorectal cancer

(4) Decreased physical activity

(a) In 2015, only about one half of adults reported meeting the recommended 150 minutes of moderate or 75 minutes of vigorous physical activity.

(b) Those with higher education levels were more likely to meet recommended physical activity levels.

3. Alcohol consumption

a. Alcohol is a known carcinogen, classified by the International Agency for Research on Cancer (IARC) similarly to tobacco and ultraviolet

TABLE 1.1 Classification of Overweight and Obesity by Body Mass Index (BMI)		
	Obesity Class	**BMI (kg/m^2)**
Underweight		<18.5
Normal		18.5–24.9
Overweight		25.0–29.9
Obesity	I	30.0–34.9
	II	35.0–39.9
Extreme obesity	III	>40

Data from National Institutes of Health, National Health, Lung, and Blood Institute. (n.d.). *Classification of overweight and obesity by body mass index.* Retrieved from https://www.nhlbi.nih.gov/health/educational/lose_wt/BMI/bmi_dis.htm.

(UV) radiation exposure in that there is no safe amount (Rehm & Shield, 2014).
   b. Risk factor for cancers of the mouth, pharynx, larynx, esophagus, liver, colorectum, pancreas, and breast (ACS, 2017)
   c. Has synergistic effect with tobacco
   d. The more one drinks over the course of a lifetime, the higher the cancer risk (ACS 2017; NCI, 2013)

4. UV radiation exposure (ACS, 2017)
   a. Primarily from the sun
   b. Significant risk factor for melanoma, basal, and squamous skin cancers
    (1) Basal cell carcinoma—most common skin cancer; is rarely deadly; influenced by both long-term and intermittent sun exposure
    (2) Squamous cell carcinoma (also called *keratinocyte carcinoma* or *KC*)—often begins with small scaly lesions called *solar keratoses* or *actinic keratoses;* linked to cumulative time in the sun; both squamous and basal cell cancers typically found on the head, neck, and arms, areas most frequently exposed to sunlight
    (3) Melanoma
     (a) Accounts for 1% of all skin cancers but 75% of skin cancer deaths (Tripp, Watson, Balk, & Swetter, 2016)
     (b) Estimated 87,110 new cancers and 9730 deaths from melanoma in 2011
     (c) Risk factors include consistent UV exposure (via sun or tanning bed exposure), multiple moles, fair skin type, family and personal history, older age, and inadequate immune system
     (d) More than 410,000 cases of KC and more than 6000 cases of melanoma can be attributed to indoor tanning
     (e) As of January 1, 2017, 13 states and the District of Columbia have laws prohibiting tanning for those 18 years old and younger.
     (f) Regular UV exposure protection is lagging in the U.S. (NCI, 2017a)

5. Cancer screening (ACS, 2017)
   a. For people of average risk, recommended cancer screenings are available for breast, cervical, colorectal, lung, and prostate cancers

6. Virus exposure and vaccines
   a. Eleven bacteria, viruses, and parasites are classified as cancer-causing agents in humans (Plummer et al., 2016)
    (1) *Helicobacter pylori*
     (a) Associated with some stomach cancers
    (2) Hepatitis B virus (HBV)
     (a) HBV infection is associated with cirrhosis and liver cancer.

      i. It accounts for nearly 6 out of 10 liver cancers in undeveloped countries as opposed to 1 out of 10 liver cancers in the U.S.
    (3) Hepatitis C virus (HCV)
     (a) HCV infection is associated with cirrhosis and liver cancer.
      i. It accounts for nearly 6 out of 10 liver cancers in the U.S.
    (4) HIV type 1 (HIV-1)
     (a) HIV infection results in immunosuppression; increases the risk of Kaposi sarcoma and B-cell lymphomas.
    (5) High-risk human papillomavirus (HPV)
     (a) Endemic in human population because more than 90% of adults worldwide are seropositive
     (b) Found in virtually all cases of cervical cancers
      i. More than 150 types of HPV (Markowitz et al., 2014)
      ii. Approximately 70% of cervical cancers caused by HPV types 16 or 18
     (c) Leading cause of oral cancer
      i. HPV-16 detected in a substantial proportion of squamous cell carcinomas of the soft palate, tonsils, and base of the tongue
      ii. HPV-16 detected in 60% to 70% of all HPV-associated cancers of the oral cavity and oropharynx (Markowitz et al., 2014)
    (6) Epstein–Barr virus (EBV)
     (a) Best known for causing infectious mononucleosis, often called *"mono"* or the *"kissing disease"*
     (b) Associated with nasopharyngeal cancer, Burkitt lymphoma, Hodgkin lymphoma, and stomach cancer
    (7) Human herpesvirus type 8 (HHV-8)
     (a) Also known as Kaposi sarcoma herpesvirus
     (b) Has also been linked to some rare blood cancers
    (8) Human T-cell lymphotrophic virus type 1 (HTLV-1)
     (a) Associated with T-cell leukemias
    (9) *Opisthorichis viverrini* (the Southeast Asian river fluke parasite) and *Clonorchis sinensis* (the Chinese river fluke parasite)
     (a) Associated with cholangiocarcinoma
    (10) *Schistosoma heamatobium* (found in Africa and the Middle East; causes schistosomiasis)
     (a) Associated with bladder cancer

7. Stress and inflammation (NCI, 2015)
   a. Inflammation is the body's natural process to heal injured tissue
      (1) Acute inflammation
      (2) Chronic inflammation
   b. Causes of inflammation
      (1) Allergens
      (2) Toxins
      (3) Infectious agents
      (4) Conditions (e.g. Crohn disease and ulcerative colitis)
8. Hormonal agents and antineoplastic drugs
   a. Hormone replacement therapy (HRT)
      (1) Combined estrogen–progesterone HRT given to postmenopausal women increases risk of breast cancer (Manson et al., 2013)
      (2) Estrogens may have a protective role in preventing colorectal cancer (Barzi, Lenz, Labonte, & Lenz, 2013).
      (3) Long-term use of HRT increases risk of endometrial cancer (Trabert et al., 2013)
   b. Selective estrogen receptor modulators
      (1) Include tamoxifen and raloxifene
      (2) FDA-approved for use to reduce risk of breast cancer
      (3) Have been shown to reduce breast cancer incidence by up to 50% among high-risk women (Mocellin, Pilati, Briarava, & Nitti, 2015).
   c. Use of oral contraceptives are associated with breast cancer but may reduce the risk of cancers of ovary and uterus
   d. Daughters of women who took diethylstilbestrol (DES) during pregnancy had an increased incidence of clear cell adenocarcinoma (CCA) of the vagina, especially in their late teens and early 20s. However, after age 25, the incidence of CCA among DES-exposed daughters has decreased by over 80% (Troisi et al., 2007).
   e. Anabolic steroids may be associated with liver cancer.
   f. Certain fertility drugs (i.e., menotropins [Pergonal]) may increase the risk for ovarian cancer.
   g. Growth hormones given to children may increase the risk for leukemia.
   h. Immunosuppressive agents (for organ recipients) increase the risk of non-Hodgkin lymphoma.
   i. Prior exposure to antineoplastic agents (especially alkylating agents) and radiation therapy increases the risk of secondary cancers.
B. Nonmodifiable cancer risk factors
   1. Radiation exposure
      a. Natural radiation sources
         (1) Radon gas, x-rays, gamma rays, UV light
      b. Artificial radiation sources
         (1) Radon gas and x-rays

2. Genetics (see Chapter 10)
3. Occupational and environmental exposures
   a. Occupational cancer risks
      (1) Account for about 4% of cancers
      (2) Introduction of effective regulation of workplace exposures in the mid-twentieth century believed to have reduced these risks substantially
      (3) Asbestos: single most important known occupational carcinogen
         (a) Asbestos-related lung cancer and mesothelioma peaked during the middle to late 1980s because of extensive occupational exposure in shipyards during World War II.
         (b) Occupations exposed to asbestos include mining; shipyards; railroads; constructions; boiler plants; firefighting; oil refineries; and paper, textile, and steel mills (Dodson & Hammar, 2011).
         (c) Occupational exposures to asbestos fibers, environmental smoke, or radon have a synergistic role in elevating smoking-related lung cancer risk.
         (d) Special population concerns
            i. Blue-collar workers—tend to have higher smoking rates that increase risks associated with occupational exposures
            ii. African Americans—discriminatory work assignments have historically resulted in placement in more hazardous jobs: steel, rubber, and chemical industries
            iii. Steel workers—increased rates of lung cancer
            iv. Rubber workers—increased rates of prostate cancer
            v. Chemical workers—increased rates of bladder cancer
            vi. Miners—increased exposure to uranium and radon with a subsequent increase in gastric cancer and birth defects
III. Health promotion
   A. American Cancer Society guidelines on nutrition and physical activity for cancer prevention (Kushi et al., 2012)
      1. Nutrition: consume a healthy diet with emphasis on plant sources.
         a. Choose foods and beverages in amounts to achieve and maintain a healthy weight.
            (1) Eat smaller portions of high-calorie foods.
            (2) Choose vegetables, whole fruit, and other low-calorie foods.
            (3) Limit consumption of sugar-sweetened beverages.

(4) Avoid consuming large portion sizes.
b. Limit consumption of processed and red meats.
   (1) Minimize consumption of processed meats.
   (2) Choose fish, poultry, or beans as an alternative to red meat.
   (3) For red meat, select lean cuts and eat smaller portions.
   (4) Prepare meat, fish, or poultry by baking, broiling, or poaching rather than frying or charbroiling.
c. Eat at least 2{1/2} cups of vegetables and fruits per day.
d. Choose whole-grain instead of refined-grain products.
e. Limit alcohol intake to no more than two drinks per day for men and one drink per day for women (ACS, 2017).

2. Physical activity (Kushi et al., 2012)
   a. Intensity, duration, and frequency of physical activity to reduce cancer risk unknown
   b. ACS recommendations.
      (1) Adults—at least 150 minutes of moderate-intensity activity per week or 75 minutes of vigorous-intensity activity per week
      (2) Children—at least 60 minutes of moderate- or vigorous-intensity activity each day, with vigorous activity on at least 3 days each week
      (3) Limiting sedentary behavior (e.g. sitting, lying down, and watching television)

B. ACS guidelines on nutrition and physical activity for cancer survivors (Rock et al., 2012)
   1. Achieve and maintain a healthy weight.
      a. Limit consumption of high-calorie foods and beverages.
      b. Increase physical activity.
   2. Engage in regular physical activity.
      a. Return to normal daily activities as soon as possible after diagnosis.
      b. Exercise at least 150 minutes per week.
      c. Include strength training at least 2 days per week.
      d. Consume foods high in vegetables, fruits, and whole grains.

C. Vaccination (ACS, 2017)
   1. HPV vaccine for prevention of cervical cancer and five other cancers, in addition to genital warts
      a. Three vaccines are currently approved by the FDA for HPV chemoprevention
      b. Recommended vaccination age is 11 to 12 years (and as early as 9 years and as late as 26 years); a higher immune response is seen at this age than later adolescence.
         (1) A two-dose series is recommended for children before age 15.
         (2) After age 15, a three-dose series is recommended.
      c. HPV vaccination uptake is increasing but still lags behind other recommended vaccines potentially attributed to myths and lack of education surrounding the vaccine need

   2. Hepatitis B vaccination is the primary prevention strategy to decrease HBV rates.
      a. All unvaccinated children, adolescents, and adults at risk for hepatitis B infection should be vaccinated via a three-dose series.
         (1) The standard vaccination schedule is at 0, 3, and 6 months.
      b. Nearly 91% of adolescents 17 years and younger have had at least three HBV vaccinations.

D. Measures to prevent skin cancer (ACS, 2017)
   1. Avoid direct exposure to the sun between the hours of 10 AM and 4 PM, when UV rays are most intense.
   2. Wear hats with a brim wide enough to shade the face, ears, and neck, as well as clothing that covers as much as possible of the arms, legs, and torso.
   3. Cover exposed skin with a sunscreen lotion and sun protection factor (SPF) of ≥ 30.
   4. Avoid indoor tanning booths and sun lamps.

E. Screening and early detection of cancer (see Chapter 2)

ASSESSMENT

I. Conduct a thorough medical history and physical examination.
   A. Obtain demographic information, including age, race/ethnicity, gender, education, employment status and place of employment, insurance coverage, and area of residence.
   B. Assess for comorbidities (e.g., hepatitis infection) and previous and current medications (e.g., HRT).
   C. Assess for lifestyle risk factors such as tobacco use, alcohol consumption, exposure to UV radiation, weight, nutrition, and level of physical activity.
   D. Assess for occupational exposures (e.g., asbestos, benzene, and other chemicals).
   E. Assess for personal and family histories of cancer.
   F. Include any previous treatment with radiotherapy, chemotherapy, or both.
   G. Assess for motivation for preventive behavior (health belief model)
      1. Perceived susceptibility to cancer—evidence indicates individuals at risk often are unaware of their risks. (Ask, "How likely do you feel you are to develop cancer?")
      2. Perceived severity of cancer. (Ask, "How serious do you feel cancer is?")
      3. Perceived benefits of preventive behavior. (Ask, "Do you think you can decrease your risk for cancer by not smoking [or the habit in question]?")
      4. Perceived barriers to preventive action. (Ask, "What problems do you think you may have lowering the fat content in your diet [or the behavior in question]?")

MANAGEMENT

I. Medical management
   A. Provide cancer prevention vaccines as indicated.
II. Nursing management
   A. Provide education regarding health promotion activities.
   B. Refer to specialists (e.g., dietician, tobacco addiction treatment specialist) as needed.
   C. Encourage participation in chemoprevention trials.
      1. Tobacco cessation
         a. U.S. Public Health Service "5 A" model in treating smokers who are willing to quit (Fiore et al., 2008)
         b. For smokers unwilling to quit, the U.S. Public Health Service (USPHS) recommends brief motivational interventions that can help increase attempts.
            (1) Ask patient about smoking status.
            (2) Advise to quit.
            (3) Assess for willingness or readiness to quit.
            (4) Assist in quitting.
            (5) Arrange a follow-up visit.
               (a) Use motivational interviewing techniques such as asking, "Have you considered quitting?"
               (b) Discuss options for quitting such as use of medications (over-the-counter and prescription) to aid smoking cessation.
               (c) Assist patient with developing a quit plan.
               (d) Offer relevant and culturally appropriate cessation materials, cessation programs, and public cessation hotlines.
         c. Various pharmacologic and nonpharmacologic tools exist
      2. Encourage proper nutrition.
      3. Promote physical activity.
      4. Encourage patients to limit sun exposure.
         a. Educate persons of all ages about skin cancer prevention.
      5. Prevent viral exposures.
         a. Offer vaccinations for hepatitis B and HPV.
         b. Discuss safe sex practices.
         c. Counsel against intravenous (IV) drug use, or educate about and facilitate access to sterile needle and syringe programs.
      6. Encourage avoidance of occupational carcinogen exposures
         a. Use protective clothing and devices; follow safety procedures when exposure unavoidable

REFERENCES

American Cancer Society. (2017). *Cancer prevention & early detection: facts & figures*, 2017-2018. Retrieved from https://www.cancer.org/content/dam/cancer-org/research/cancer-facts-and-statistics/cancer-prevention-and-early-detection-facts-and-figures/cancer-prevention-and-early-detection-facts-and-figures-2017.pdf.

American Cancer Society. (2018). *Cancer facts & figures*, 2018. Retrieved from https://www.cancer.org/research/cancer-facts-statistics/all-cancer-facts-figures/cancer-facts-figures-2018.html.

Barzi, A., Lenz, A. M., Labonte, M. J., & Lenz, H. J. (2013). Molecular pathways: estrogen pathway in colorectal cancer. *Clinical Cancer Research*, 19(21), 5842–5848.

Dodson, R. F., & Hammar, S. P. (Eds.), (2011). *Asbestos: Risk assessment, epidemiology, and health effects* (2nd ed.) Boca Raton, FL: CRC Press.

Fiore, M. C., Jaén, C. R, Baker, T. B., et al. (2008). Treating tobacco use and dependence, 2008 Update. *Clinical Practice Guideline*. Rockville, MD: U.S. Department of Health and Human Services. Public Health Service.

Howlader, N., Noone, A. M., Krapcho, M., Miller, D., Bishop, K., & Kosary, C. L., et al. (2017). *SEER cancer statistics review, 1975-2014*. Bethesda, MD: National Cancer Institute.

International Agency for Research on Cancer and Cancer Research. (2018). *World cancer factsheet*. Retrieved from http://gco.iarc.fr/today/fact-sheets-cancers?cancer=29&type=0&sex=0.

Kushi, L. H., Doyle, C., McCullough, M., Rock, C. L., Demark-Wahnefried, W., Bandera, E. V., et al. (2012). American Cancer Society guidelines on nutrition and physical activity for cancer prevention. *CA: A Cancer Journal for Clinicians*, 62(1), 30–67.

Manson, J. E., Chlebowski, R. T., Stefanick, M. L., Aragaki, A. K., Rossouw, J. E., Prentice, R. L., et al. (2013). Menopausal hormone therapy and health outcomes during the intervention and extended poststopping phases of the Women's Health Initiative randomized trials update and overview of health outcomes for WHI update and overview of health outcomes for WHI. *JAMA: The Journal of the American Medical Association*, 310(13), 1353–1368.

Markowitz, L. E., Dunne, E. F., Saraiya, M., Chesson, H. W., Curtis, C. R., Gee, J., et al. (2014). *Human papillomavirus vaccination: recommendations of the Advisory Committee on Immunization Practices (ACIP)*. Retrieved from https://www.cdc.gov/mmwr/preview/mmwrhtml/rr6305a1.htm.

Mocellin, S., Pilati, P., Briarava, B., & Nitti, D. (2015). Breast cancer chemoprevention: a network meta-analysis of randomized controlled trials. *Journal of the National Cancer Institute*, 18 (108), 2.

National Cancer Institute. (2013). *Alcohol and cancer risk*. Accessed from https://www.cancer.gov/about-cancer/causes-prevention/risk/alcohol/alcohol-fact-sheet.

National Cancer Institute. (2015). *Chronic inflammation*. Retrieved from https://www.cancer.gov/about-cancer/causes-prevention/risk/chronic-inflammation.

National Cancer Institute. (2017a). *Cancer trends progress report*, 2017. Accessed from https://progressreport.cancer.gov/prevention.

National Cancer Institute. (2017b). *Cancer health disparities*. Retrieved from https://www.cancer.gov/about-cancer/understanding/disparities.

National Institutes of Health, National Health, Lung, and Blood Institute. (n.d.). Classification of overweight and obesity by body mass index. Retrieved from https://www.nhlbi.nih.gov/health/educational/lose_wt/BMI/bmi_dis.htm.

Plummer, M., de Martel, C., Vignat, J., Ferlay, J., Bray, F., & Francheschi, S. (2016). Global burden of cancers attributable to infections in 2012: a synthetic analysis. *Lancet Global Health*, 4(9), e609–e616.

Rehm, J., & Shield, K. (2014). Alcohol consumption. In B. W. Stewart & C. B. Wild (Eds.), *World Cancer Report 2014.* Lyon, France: International Agency for Research on Cancer.

Rock, C. L., Doyle, C., Demark-Wahnefried, W., Meyerhardt, J., Courneya, K. S., Schwartz, A. L., et al. (2012). Nutrition and physical activity guidelines for cancer survivors. *CA: A Cancer Journal for Clinicians, 62*(4), 242–274.

Stewart, B. W., & Wild, CP. (2014). *World Cancer Report 2014.* Retrieved from http://publications.iarc.fr/Non-Series-Publications/World-Cancer-Reports/World-Cancer-Report-2014.

Trabert, B., Wentzensen, N., Yang, H. P., Sherman, M. E., Hollenbeck, A. R., Park, Y., et al. (2013). Is estrogen plus progestin menopausal hormone therapy safe with respect to endometrial cancer risk? *International Journal of Cancer, 132*(2), 417–426.

Tripp, M. K., Watson, M., Balk, S. J., & Swetter, S. M. (2016). State of the science on prevention and screening to reduce melanoma incidence and mortality, *66*(6), 460–480.

Troisi, R., Hatch, E. E., Titus-Ernstoff, L., Hyer, M., Palmer, J. R., Robboy, S. J., et al. (2007). Cancer risk in women prenatally exposed to diethylstilbestrol. *International Journal of Cancer, 121*(2), 356–360.

U.S. Cancer Statistics Working Group. (2017). *United States cancer statistics: 1999-2014, incidence and mortality web-based report.* Retrieved from https://nccd.cdc.gov/uscs/toptencancers.aspx?printfriendly=1.

U.S. Department of Health and Human Services. (2006). *The health consequences of involuntary exposure to tobacco smoke: a report of the surgeon general.* Washington, DC: U.S. Department of Health and Human Services, Centers for Disease Control and Prevention, National Center for Chronic Disease Prevention and Health Promotion, Office on Smoking and Health.

U.S. Department of Health and Human Services. (2013). *Healthy people 2020.* Washington, D.C.: Office of Disease Prevention and Health Promotion.

U.S. Food and Drug Administration. (2018). *Vaporizers, e-cigarettes, and other electronic nicotine delivery systems (ENDS).* Retrieved from https://www.fda.gov/TobaccoProducts/Labeling/ProductsIngredientsComponents/ucm456610.htm.

World Cancer Research Fund International. (2018). *Cancer facts and figures.* Retrieved from http://www.wcrf.org/int/cancer-facts-figures/data-specific-cancers.

2

Screening and Early Detection

Jaya M. Gill

OVERVIEW

I. Levels of prevention
   A. Primary prevention – reduce risk factors or increase an individual's resistance to them; the most effective management for cancer
      1. Goal of primary prevention is to limit the incidence of cancer (e.g., vaccination)
   B. Secondary prevention – early detection and treatment of cancer through screening activities in asymptomatic individuals
      1. Goal of secondary prevention is to prevent disease progression
   C. Tertiary prevention – application of effective therapy to improve outcomes and decrease morbidity and mortality in affected individuals

II. Definitions
   A. Diagnosis – clinical problem-solving process applied to asymptomatic individuals who either screen positive or present in an already symptomatic state
   B. Epidemiology – the study of the distribution and determinants of health-related states
   C. Screening – the use of tests (e.g., physical examination and history, imaging procedures, or laboratory tests) to detect early stages of cancer aimed at reducing mortality
   D. Rates – measure of morbidity, or the rate of illness
      1. Incidence, prevalence, or mortality rates can be used to assess the value of instituting a screening test for a particular disease
         a. Involves identification of risk profiles, use of screening guidelines to enhance screening efficacy and decrease risks and costs of screening test(s)
         b. Multiple organizations publish cancer screening guidelines, including the American Cancer Society (ACS), National Comprehensive Cancer Network (NCCN), and United States Preventive Services Task Force (USPSTF)
         c. Attempts to balance risks versus benefits of screening tests
            (1) Diagnose disease early enough to favorably affect morbidity and mortality
            (2) Minimize potential harms of the screening itself, such as complications of procedure(s), cost, and false positives that may provoke anxiety (Harris, Wilt & Qaseem, 2015)
      2. Incidence – number of new cases identified in a specified population occurring in a particular time period (such as 1 year)
      3. Prevalence – percentage of all individuals affected with the disease at a given point in time

III. Attributes of effective screening tests
   A. Ease of administration (i.e., noninvasive); relatively simple, safe, and inexpensive test given to asymptomatic individuals (Glaser, 2014)
   B. Randomized clinical trials (RCTs) demonstrate effectiveness of screening tests (i.e., reduction in mortality and/or improvement in quality of life)
   C. Validity – accuracy of screening test to distinguish individuals who have the disease and those who do not
      1. Sensitivity – measure of the test's ability to correctly identify persons with the disease (true positives) among the population screened; 100% sensitivity = no false negatives
      2. Specificity – measure of the test's ability to correctly identify persons who do not have the disease in the group being screened (test will not be positive in anyone who does not have the cancer); 100% specificity = no false positives
      3. Sensitive test with a negative result rules out the disease; specific test with a positive result rules in the disease
      4. In an ideal setting, tests would be 100% sensitive and 100% specific; unfortunately, reality is more complex and there is usually overlap (Glaser, 2014)
   D. Reliability – level of agreement between measurements made at different times
   E. Predictive value – useful to assess the feasibility of screening tests; how likely disease is present or absent
      1. Negative predictive value (NPV) – the percentage of persons who screen negative who do not have the disease (true negatives)

2. Positive predictive value (PPV) – the percentage of persons who screen positive who actually have the disease (true positives)

3. Predictive values vary according to prevalence of disease; the higher the prevalence of a disease, the higher the PPV and the lower the NPV

IV. Evidence exists for screening recommendations for breast, prostate, cervical, lung, and colorectal cancer in defined populations; controversy exists for all cancers.

A. Types of screening biases
   1. Lead time bias
   2. Length time bias
   3. Selection bias
   4. Overdiagnosis

B. Confounding factors with RCTs include contamination of control group, large number of subjects required for screening diseases with low incidence rate, and ethically unacceptable to randomize subjects to nonscreened group

C. Screening allows cancer to be diagnosed earlier (before signs or symptoms), thus giving a false sense of lengthened survival; in reality, a decrease in mortality is not attributable to early diagnosis and treatment

   1. Screening most often performed on asymptomatic individuals who will generally have more indolent cancers (aggressive cancers generally cause earlier symptoms, prompting evaluation), which improves survival rates

   2. Favorable outcomes may be attributable to characteristics of "select ins" rather than to screening itself (Glaser, 2014).

   3. For very slow-growing tumors, especially in older individuals, screening may not afford a survival benefit and instead may cause unnecessary treatment, anxiety, cost, and pain (Royce, Hendrix & Stokes, 2014).

V. Characteristics of the cancers that justify the risks and costs associated with screening

A. Screening should be directed toward an important health problem

B. Effective treatment is available to reduce cause-specific mortality and is more effective if initiated during the presymptomatic stage.

C. The benefit of screening should outweigh the risks and be cost-effective

D. Potential screening participants should receive adequate information regarding risks and potential benefits of participation.

VI. Screening modalities for early detection of cancer
A. Imaging
B. Cytologic specimens
C. Chemical assays
D. Biomarkers or tumor markers
E. Proteomics
   1. Substances that may be produced by the tumor or the body's reaction to the cancer and may be detected in abnormal quantities; most often found in blood, body fluids, or tissues

   2. Although attractive for screening, most currently available biomarkers or tumor markers are neither sensitive nor specific.

VII. Screening guidelines for specific cancers
A. Breast cancer
   1. Breast cancer screening recommendations (Table 2.1)
      a. Gail model
         (1) Multivariable statistical model that has been developed to help estimate a woman's personal breast cancer risk
         (2) Model incorporates characteristics (age, age of menarche, age at first live birth, number of first-degree relatives with breast cancer, number of previous benign breast biopsies, atypical hyperplasia in a previous breast biopsy, and race) in an effort to assess 5-year and lifetime risks of developing breast cancer (Gail et al., 1989)
      b. Genetic testing for BRCA1 and BRCA2 gene mutations
         (1) Responsible for approximately 20% to 25% of hereditary breast cancers (about 5%-10% of breast cancers in women, 4%-40% in men) (ACS, 2017)
         (2) Not currently recommended for the general population
         (3) May be offered to family members of persons with features indicating an increased likelihood of a BRCA mutation (ACS, 2017; NCCN, 2017a)
   2. Impact of screening
      a. Screening reduces mortality, especially among women aged 50 to 74 years (Monticciolo et al., 2017)
      b. Smaller tumors at diagnosis associated with increased chance of survival
      c. With use of adjuvant therapy such as hormone therapy and trastuzumab (Herceptin), difficult to determine the impact of breast cancer screening on survival; two thirds of survival attributed to adjuvant therapy and one third to screening (Kalanger, Zelen, Langmark, & Adami, 2010; Park, Anderson, & Gail, 2015)
      d. Requires less invasive surgeries and less need for aggressive treatment such as chemotherapy (Esserman & Flowers, 2011)
   3. Screening modalities
      a. Screening mammography
      b. Clinical breast examination (CBE) by health care provider
      c. Breast self-awareness (formerly BSE)
      d. Breast Imaging-Reporting and Data System (BI-RADS) developed by the American

TABLE 2.1   Breast Cancer Screening Recommendations

Organization	Population	Test and Schedule
ACS, 2017a	Women ages 40–44 yr with average risk for breast cancer * Average risk – defined as those with no personal history of breast cancer, a strong family history, or a genetic mutation known to increase risk	Option to start screening with a mammogram every year
	Women age 45–54 yr with average risk	Annual mammogram
	Woman 55 yr and older with average risk for breast cancer	Option to switch to mammogram every other year or choose to continue yearly mammogram
	High-risk women (those with a >20%–25% lifetime risk, *BRCA1* or *BRCA2* gene mutation, first-degree relative)	Annual mammography at age 30 yr. MRI screening
NCCN, 2017a	Average-risk women age 25–39 yr	CBE every 1–3 yr
	Average-risk women age ≥40 yr	Annual CBE, annual mammography, consider tomosynthesis
	Increased risk: those with a prior history of breast cancer	CBE every 6–12 mo
		Annual mammography, consider risk reduction strategies (e.g., prophylactic surgery such as bilateral salpingo-oophorectomy; chemoprevention with tamoxifen, raloxifene, or exemestane)
	Increased risk: women with lifetime risk >20% largely dependent on family history	Begin CBE every 6–12 mo, annual mammography (to begin 10 yr before youngest family member but not less than age 30 yr
		Annual breast MRI recommended (to begin 10 yr before youngest family member but not less than age 25 yr), consider tomosynthesis, genetic counseling referral
	Increased risk: those who received thoracic radiation therapy (RT) between the ages of 10 and 30 yr	Age <25 yr: • CBE every 12 mo (beginning 8–10 yr after RT) Age ≥25 yr: • CBE every 6–12 mo (beginning 8–10 yr after RT • Annual screening mammogram (beginning 8–10 yr after RT but not before age 25) • Consider tomosynthesis • Annual breast MRI recommended (beginning 8–10 yr after RT but not before age 25 yr)
	Increased risk: women ≥35 yr with a 5-year risk of invasive breast cancer ≥1.7% (per Gail model)	CBE every 6–12 mo, annual screening mammogram, consider tomosynthesis, risk reduction strategies, breast awareness
	Increased risk: women with lifetime risk ≥20% based on history of LCIS or ADH/ALH	CBE every 6–12 mo, annual screening mammogram, consider tomosynthesis, risk reduction strategies, consider annual MRI (beginning at diagnosis of LCIS or ADH/ALH but not less than age 25)
	Increased risk: pedigree suggestive of or known genetic predisposition	CBE every 6–12 mo, annual mammogram, breast MRI starting at age 25 yr (or individualized by earliest age onset in family), consider risk reduction strategies
	Women with known genetic predisposition (hereditary breast and ovarian cancers)	CBE every 6–12 mo, annual mammogram, breast MRI starting at age 25 yr (or individualized by earliest age onset in family), consider risk reduction strategies
	Men with known genetic predisposition	CBE every 6–12 mo beginning at age 35, consider baseline mammography at age 40
USPSTF, 2016b	Women 40–49 yr with a first-degree relative with breast cancer	Mammography every 2 yr
	Women 50–74 yr	Mammography every 2 yr
	Women 75 yr or older	Insufficient evidence to support the benefit or harm of screening women older than 75
	Women with dense breasts	Supplemental screening of women with dense breasts is not recommended, but 24 states require women to be notified of breast density with mammography results

ACS, American Cancer Society; *BSE,* breast self-examination; *CBE,* clinical breast examination; *MRI,* magnetic resonance imaging; *NCCN,* National Comprehensive Cancer Network; *RT,* radiotherapy; *USPSTF,* U.S. Preventive Services Task Force.
Data from American Cancer Society. (2017a). *Recommendations for the early detection of cancer.* https://www.cancer.org/cancer/breastcancer/screening-tests-and-early-detection/american-cancersociety-recommendations-for-the-early-detection-of-breastcancer.html#written_by; National Comprehensive Cancer Network. (2017a). NCCN clinical practice guidelines in oncology. *Breast Cancer Screening and Diagnosis. Version, 1,* 2017. https://www.nccn.org/professionals/physician_gls/pdf/breast-screening.pdf; U.S. Preventive Services Task Force. (2016b). *Recommendations: screening for breast cancer.* https://epss.ahrq.gov/ePSS/TopicDetails.do?topicid¼198.

Society of Radiology to provide uniform reporting schema

(1) Consists of seven categories of mammographic findings, each with terminology and follow-up recommendations (D'Orsi et al., 2013)

4. Screening controversy

   a. Screening impact unclear in many subpopulations—that is, young patients—because cancer is more difficult to detect and is often associated with more aggressive tumor biology (McGuire et al., 2015)

   b. BSE was recommended routinely in the past but is no longer endorsed because of its mixed efficacy results for finding early-stage tumors and its association with high rates of false positives

   c. Digital mammography is widely available, but RCTs have not shown digital mammography to be more effective than traditional mammography.

   d. A meta-analysis of two large RCTs (nearly 400,000 women) detected no significant difference in disease-related mortality at 15 years (Kosters & Gotzsche, 2008).

B. Colorectal cancer (CRC)

   1. CRC screening recommendations (Table 2.2)

   2. Screening modalities

      a. Guaiac-based fecal occult blood test (gFOBT)—remains only CRC screening method proven consistently effective in RCTs (Bénard, Barkun, Martel, & von Renteln, 2018)

TABLE 2.2 Colorectal Cancer Screening Recommendations

Organization	Population	Test and Schedule
ACS, 2017b	Age ≥50 yr for men and women with average risk	One of the following screening tests: • Colonoscopy every 10 yr • CT colonography (virtual colonoscopy) every 5 yr* • Flexible sigmoidoscopy every 5 yr* • Double-contrast barium enema every 5 yr* • Fecal immunochemical test (FIT) every yr* • Guaiac-based fecal occult blood test (gFOBT) every yr* • Stool DNA test every 3 yr* *If any test results are positive, colonoscopy should be done
	Colorectal cancer or adenomatous polyps in any first-degree relative before age 60 yr, or in two or more first-degree relatives at any age, or in at least two second-degree relatives at any age	Starting age 40, or 10 yr before the youngest case in the immediate family, whichever is earlier; colonoscopy every 5 yr
NCCN, 2017b	Age ≥50 yr with average risk* *No history of adenoma or CRC, no history of inflammatory bowel disease, no family history for CRC	One of the following: • Colonoscopy every 10 yr • Stool-based high-sensitivity guaiac-based or immunochemical-based testing annually* • Stool-based DNA-based testing every 3 yr* • Flexible sigmoidoscopy every 5 or 10 yr* • CT colonography every 5 yr* • *If any tests are positive, must follow with colonoscopy
	>1 first-degree relative with CRC at any age	Colonoscopy beginning at age 40 or 10 yr before earliest diagnosis of CRC; repeat every 5–10 yr
	>1 second-degree relative with CRC aged <50 yr	Colonoscopy beginning at age 50; repeat every 5–10 yr
USPSTF, 2016a	Age 50–75 yr with average risk	One of the following: • gFOBT annually, FIT annually, FIT-DNA every 1 or 3 yr • Colonoscopy every 10 yr • CT colonography every 5 yr • Flexible sigmoidoscopy every 5 yr • Flexible sigmoidoscopy with FIT every 10 yr, plus FIT every yr

ACS, American Cancer Society; CRC, colorectal cancer; CT, computed tomography; FIT, fecal immunochemical test; gFOBT, guaiac-based fecal occult blood test; NCCN, National Comprehensive Cancer Network; USPSTF, U.S. Preventive Services Task Force.
Data from American Cancer Society. (2017b). *American Cancer Society recommendations for colorectal cancer early detection.* Atlanta, GA: American Cancer Society. https://www.cancer.org/cancer/colon-rectal-cancer/detection-diagnosis-staging/acsrecommendations.html; National Comprehensive Cancer Network. (2017b). NCCN clinical practice guidelines in oncology. *Colorectal cancer screening. Version V, 2,* 2017. https://www.nccn.org/professionals/physician_gls/pdf/colorectal_screening.pdf; U.S. Preventive Services Task Force. (2016a). *Screening for colorectal cancer.* https://epss.ahrq.gov/ePSS/TopicDetails.do?topicid¼205.

(1) Must evaluate any positive test with imaging, endoscopy, or both

b. Fecal immunochemical test (FIT) or immunochemical fecal occult blood test (iFOBT)

(1) Improved accuracy compared with gFOBT

c. Stool deoxyribonucleic acid (sDNA) not widely available or uniformly endorsed pending RCT results

(1) Uses antibodies specific to human globin; therefore greater specificity than FOBT while maintaining sensitivity

(2) Superior sensitivity and specificity compared with traditional FOBT (Pox, 2011)

(3) Assesses for the presence of certain DNA mutations shed in stool that are known to be associated with cancerous and precancerous lesions; does not test for presence of blood

d. Barium enema

(1) Relatively noninvasive method to visualize entire colon

(2) Does not facilitate biopsy or removal of lesions, so positive findings require flexible sigmoidoscopy or colonoscopy

e. Flexible sigmoidoscopy

f. Colonoscopy

(1) Allows more thorough examination of rectum and left colon

(2) Has ability to identify 60% to 83% of polyps and cancers and thus reduce CRC mortality by 31% (Atkin et al., 2010)

(3) Preferred screening method because it can both visualize most lesions and permit removal of polyps, thus preventing development of CRC

(4) Most invasive screening test (Haug, Knudsen, Lansdorp-Vogelaar, & Kuntz, 2015)

g. Computed tomography (CT) colonography also known as *virtual colonoscopy (VC)*

(1) Good option for older adults and frail patients

(2) Insufficient data to recommend its use as solitary screening test; multicenter RCTs currently being conducted (NCCN, 2018a)

h. Capsule endoscopy

(1) Noninvasive procedure that uses a miniature camera and light source contained in a capsule that is swallowed by the patient

(2) Used to detect sources of obscure gastrointestinal (GI) bleeding not explained by endoscopy

(3) Has the advantage of its ability to visualize the small bowel

3. Screening controversy

a. On the basis of observational studies, average timing of screening can be controversial; may take 3-5 years for polyp to develop into an invasive malignancy (Lieberman, Rex, Winawer, Giardiello, Johnson, & Levin, 2012)

b. Although colonoscopy is the preferred screening method, no direct evidence suggests that colonoscopy improves mortality.

c. Even if the noninvasive screening test (e.g., FOBT, VC, capsule endoscopy) is positive, colonoscopy is still required for cancer diagnosis.

C. Cervical cancer

1. Cervical cancer screening recommendations (Table 2.3)

TABLE 2.3	Cervical Cancer Screening Recommendations	
Organization	**Population**	**Test and Schedule**
ACS, 2013b, NCCN, 2012a	Between ages 21 and 29 yr	Cytology (Pap test) every 3 yr HPV testing is only needed after abnormal Pap results and is not recommended for routine screening in this age group.
	Ages 30–65 yr	HPV with Pap test every 5 yr (preferred) or every 3 yr with Pap alone (acceptable)
	Age >65 yr	Women >65 yr who have undergone regular cervical cancer testing with normal results should no longer be screened
	Women after hysterectomy	Cervical cancer screening not needed unless surgery was done to remove cervical cancer or precancerous lesion
USPSTF, 2012b	Ages 21–65 yr	Pap test every 3 yr or for women ages 30–65 yr, screening with a combination of Pap test and HPV testing every 5 yr
	Age <21 yr	Screening not recommended for women younger than age 21 yr, regardless of sexual history

ACS, American Cancer Society; *HPV,* human papillomavirus; *NCCN,* National Comprehensive Cancer Network; *USPSTF,* U.S. Preventive Services Task Force.
Data from American Cancer Society. (2013). *Cancer facts and figures 2013.* Atlanta, GA: American Cancer Society; National Comprehensive Cancer Network (NCCN). (2012a). NCCN clinical practice guidelines in oncology. *Cervical cancer screening. Version, 2,* 2012. http://www.nccn.org/professionals/physician_gls/pdf/cervical_screening.pdf; U.S. Preventive Services Task Force (2012b). *Screening for cervical cancer.* http://www.uspreventiveservicestaskforce.org/uspstf/uspscerv.htm.

2. Screening modalities
    a. Pap smear
        (1) Principal screening tool for cervical cancer
        (2) Low sensitivity of single Pap test because of both sampling error, in which cancerous cells do not get collected, and reading error; cumulative sensitivity of several tests is high
        (3) Incidence and mortality rates from cervical cancer decreased by use of Pap test (Meggiolaro et al., 2016).
        (4) Pap testing to begin at age 21 and performed every 3 to 5 years; yearly screening no longer recommended, because generally takes 10 to 20 years for cervical cancer to develop (ACS, 2013b)
    b. Human papillomavirus (HPV) test
        (1) HPV DNA assay is performed on liquid-based Pap specimen to identify if the oncogenic viral types are present (either as primary screening or as a "reflex test" if an abnormal Pap is reported)
        (2) Positive test only indicates viral infection (which may be transient), not its oncogenic potential. Women with persistent infection with an oncogenic HPV have a much higher risk of developing cervical cancer compared with non–HPV-infected women
    c. Colposcopy – primary method for evaluation of abnormal Pap tests
        (1) Involves viewing the cervix though a long-focal-length dissecting microscope at magnification
        (2) Acetic acid (4%) applied before viewing, which allows a directed biopsy of any grossly visible abnormalities
3. Screening controversy
    a. Controversy exists regarding frequency, ways to implement HPV testing into routine screening practices, and the lack of applicability in developing countries (because of expense and lack of equipment and clinicians).
D. Prostate cancer (PC)
    1. PC screening recommendations (Table 2.4)
    2. Screening modalities
        a. Digital rectal examination (DRE)

TABLE 2.4 Prostate Cancer Screening Recommendations

Organization	Population	Test and Schedule
ACS, 2016	Screening includes prostate-specific antigen (PSA) blood test and a digital rectal examination (DRE). Discussion about screening should take place at: • Age 50 for men with average risk • Age 45 for men with high risk (e.g., African American, first-degree relative diagnosed with prostate cancer at an early age [younger than 65]) • Age 40 for men with even higher risk (those with more than one first-degree relative who had prostate cancer at an early age) • All future screenings depend on results of the PSA blood test. Those with PSA <2.5 ng/mL may be retested every 2 yr. If PSA is ≥2.5, annual testing should be performed.	
NCCN, 2017c	Age 45–75 yr: begin risk–benefit discussions about DRE and PSA.	For men who choose to proceed with screening, offer PSA and DRE. Depending on PSA values: • If PSA <1.0 ng/mL, DRE normal (if done), repeat testing at 2–4 yr intervals • If PSA 1–3 ng/mL, DRE normal (if done), repeat testing at 1–2 yr intervals • PSA >3 ng/mL or suspicious DRE, repeat PSA, consider a percent-free PSA PHI or 4Kscore, TRUS guided biopsy, and follow-up in 6–12 mo with PSA and DRE
	Age >75 yr, testing should be done with caution and only in very healthy men with little or no comorbidity.	• If PSA <4 ng/mL, DRE normal (if done), and no other indications for biopsy, repeat testing at 1–4 yr interval • PSA ≥4 ng/mL or suspicious DRE, repeat PSA, consider a percent-free PSA PHI or 4Kscore, TRUS guided biopsy, and follow-up in 6–12 mo with PSA and DRE
USPSTF, 2012a	USPSTF recommends no screening for prostate cancer.	

ACS, American Cancer Society; *DRE,* digital rectal examination; *NCCN,* National Comprehensive Cancer Network; *ng/mL,* nanograms per milliliter; *PHI,* Prostate Health Index; *PSA,* prostate-specific antigen; *TRUS,* transrectal ultrasound; *USPSTF,* U.S. Preventive Services Task Force.
Data from American Cancer Society. (2016). *American Cancer Society recommendations for prostate cancer early detection.* Atlanta, GA: American Cancer Society. https://www.cancer.org/cancer/prostatecancer/early-detection/acs-recommendations.html. Accessed 2.11.18; National Comprehensive Cancer Network. (2017c). NCCN Clinical Practice Guidelines in Oncology. *Prostate Cancer Early Detection Version 2,* 2017. https://www.nccn.org/professionals/physician_gls/pdf/prostate_detection.pdf; U.S. Preventive Services Task Force. (2012a). *Screening for prostate cancer.* http://uspreventiveservicestaskforce.org/prostatecancerscreening.htm.

(1) DRE should not be used as a stand-alone test, but should be performed in those with an elevated serum prostate-specific antigen (PSA). DRE may be considered a baseline test in all patients, as it may identify high-grade cancers associated with "normal" serum PSA values (NCCN, 2017c)

3. Serum PSA
   a. PSA, a glycoprotein produced by prostatic epithelial cells, is the only tumor marker currently used in screening.
   b. Limited sensitivity and specificity
   c. Levels may be affected by multiple variables such as age, presence of benign prostatic hypertrophy (BPH), inflammation, urethral or prostatic trauma, and ejaculation within recent 48 hours, as well as medications

4. Ultrasound-guided prostatic biopsy is performed when PC is suspected.
   a. Multiple areas of the prostate gland are biopsied.
   b. Tumor histologic grade based on Gleason score (Gleason & Mellinger, 1974).

5. Screening controversy
   a. PSA screening has not correlated with decreases in PC mortality and has instead prompted the use of aggressive therapies, which may cause significant side effects in many men
   b. The level of PSA that should provoke biopsy is not clear, and the lower the PSA, the lower is the chance that the man has the disease (NCCN, 2017c).

(1) Results of the European Randomized Study of Screening for Prostate Cancer demonstrated 1055 men must be screened to identify 37 men who have PC; treatment only prevents one PC death over 11 years of follow-up (Schroeder et al., 2012).

E. Lung cancer
   1. Lung cancer screening guidelines (Table 2.5)
   2. Screening modalities
      a. Chest x-ray (CXR)—no RCT evidence of effect on lung cancer mortality (ACS, 2013)
      b. Sputum cytology with or without CXR—no RCT has demonstrated benefit of sputum cytology (NCCN, 2018b).
      c. Low-dose computed tomography (LDCT)
         (1) Most sensitive test available
         (2) Twenty percent reduction in lung cancer mortality demonstrated by National Lung Screening Trial using LDCT versus plain CXR in 53,454 high-risk participants (Aberle et al., 2011)
   3. Screening controversy
      a. Screening not recommended for general population; screening to be considered for those between 55 and 80 years of age with at least a 30-pack-year smoking history and either continue to smoke or have quit less than 15 years ago (Smith et al., 2017; USPSTF, 2013)
      b. Cost of screening per life saved is not known, although it is likely very high, because approximately 95% false-positive results occurred,

TABLE 2.5	Lung Cancer Screening Guidelines	
Organization	**Population**	**Test and Schedule**
ACS, 2013	Age 55–74 yr at high risk having either ≥30 pack-year smoking history, those who are currently smoking, or quit within 15 yr	Low LDCT after a process of informed and shared decision making regarding limitations, potential benefits; smoking cessation counseling remains a priority
NCCN, 2018b	High-risk population includes one of two groups: • ≥55–74 yr, have a ≥30 pack-year of smoking history, and quit smoking within 15 yr • ≥50 yr old, have a ≥20 pack-year of smoking history, and at least one additional risk factor that increases lung cancer to ≥1.3%	Screening is an option for these individuals, but LDCT is recommended
	Moderate risk population includes: • Age ≥50 yr and ≥20 pack-year history of smoking or secondhand exposure	Lung cancer screening is not recommended
	Low-risk population includes: • Age <50 yr and/or <20 pack-year history of smoking	Lung cancer screening is not recommended
USPSTF, 2013	Age 55–80 yr with a 30 or more pack-year history and currently smoke or have smoked within the past 15 yr	Annual LDCT in persons who can undergo surgical resection if tumor is discovered

ACS, American Cancer Society; *LDCT,* low-dose computed tomography; *NCCN,* National Comprehensive Cancer Network; *USPSTF,* United States Preventative Services Task Force.
Data from American Cancer Society. (2013). *Cancer facts and figures 2013.* Atlanta, GA: American Cancer Society; National Comprehensive Cancer Network. (2018b). NCCN clinical practice guidelines in oncology. *Lung cancer screening.* Version 3, 2018. https://www.nccn.org/professionals/physician_gls/pdf/lung_screening.pdf; U.S. Preventive Services Task Force (2013). *Screening for lung cancer.* http://www.uspreventiveservicestaskforce.org/uspstf13/lungcan/lungcanfinalrs.htm.

requiring additional tests, ongoing screening, and a relatively low absolute number of deaths prevented: 73 per 100,000 person-years (Haaf et al., 2017).

   c. LDCT may not be widely available.

ASSESSMENT

I. History
  A. Demographics—age, gender, race, date and place of birth, occupation
  B. Chief complaint—brief description of reason for seeking care
  C. History of present illness: onset of symptom(s), location, duration, characteristics, any aggravating and relieving factors, and timing
  D. Current medications (prescription, vitamins, herbals)
  E. Allergies (medications and environmental)
  F. Past medical history
  G. Family history—medical and cancer histories in relatives
  H. Social history (e.g., smoking, alcohol, illicit drug use, sexual habits, dietary habits, sleep patterns, and exercise)
  I. Review of systems (Table 2.6)
II. Physical examination
  A. Cancer-related physical assessment should include examination of the skin, mouth, neck, lymph nodes, breasts, cervix, pelvis, testicles, rectum, and prostate.
  B. Specific foci of physical examination are presented in Table 2.7.

III. Health counseling
  A. Teach and reinforce healthy lifestyle behaviors.
  B. Shared decision making regarding screening for cancers

MANAGEMENT

I. Interventions to improve patient participation in screening programs
  A. Assess motivation and willingness of patient to learn.
  B. Identify cultural influences regarding health and health-seeking behaviors.
  C. Provide patient with personalized risk of developing cancer by use of health history and risk profiles.
  D. Provide teaching on the risk and benefits of screening
II. Interventions for patients with positive screening test results
  A. Identify resources for cancer education and information
  B. Discuss implications of positive screening test results
  C. Ensure adherence and follow-up for persons with positive screenings for cancer
III. Interventions to promote population-based screening programs
  A. Target high-risk groups (e.g., older adults, ethnic minority, poor)
  B. Use media resources and community organizations to publicize benefits of screening
  C. Employ skilled health care educators to ensure that the target population understands the disease and the importance of screening and early detection

TABLE 2.6 Review of Cancer-Related Symptoms

System	History Components or Symptoms
Constitutional	Fatigue, malaise, recent weight gain or loss, previous and present level of activity; current performance status
Skin	Changes in warts or moles; bleeding, nonhealing lesions, change in sensation; history of skin cancer
Head and neck	Pain, tenderness; mouth lesions; difficulty swallowing or chewing; hoarseness; discharge from eyes, ears, and nose; epistaxis
Respiratory	Cough, pain, dyspnea, hemoptysis, shortness of breath; date and result of last imaging
Cardiac	Dyspnea, orthopnea, chest pain, edema, palpitations, dizziness
Gastrointestinal	Change in appetite, pain, reflux, nausea, vomiting, change in bowel pattern; dates and results of prior CRC screenings
Genitourinary	Change in urinary pattern, nocturia, dysuria, hematuria, change in force of stream, pain; testicular pain or masses; dates and results of prior PSA
Gynecologic	Vaginal discharge, nonmenstrual or intermenstrual bleeding, bloating, enlarged abdominal girth; dates and results of prior Pap screens
Breasts	Change in appearance, skin, vascular pattern, nipple direction, inversion; mass in breast or axillae; dates and results of prior mammograms
Endocrine	Flushing, sweating, orthostasis, palpitations, polyuria, polydipsia
Hematologic/ immunologic	Bruising, anemia, petechiae, purpura, bleeding disorder, anemia, fatigue, fever, infections, night sweats, chills, frequent infections, vaccines (especially HPV), enlarged lymph nodes, early satiety
Musculoskeletal	Pain and stiffness in bones and joints, limitation of movement
Neurologic	Headache, vertigo. seizures, syncope, visual disturbances; sensory, motor, memory or cognitive deficits; facial weakness, speech problems

CRC, Colorectal cancer; HPV, human papillomavirus; PSA, prostate-specific antigen.

TABLE 2.7   Physical Examination Foci

System	Components of Examination
Skin	Inspect (cutaneous and mucous membrane surfaces, sun-exposed areas). Note presence of rash, petechiae, bruising, ulcerations of color and surface.
Head, eyes	Inspect (shape, symmetry, nodules, masses, color of conjunctivae and sclerae, symmetry of pupils, reactivity, eye movements).
Ear, nose, and throat	Inspect (symmetry, presence of discharge, integrity of tissues—note polyps, exudate, friability, bleeding).
Oral cavity	Inspect (for color and integrity of mucous membranes, tongue, under tongue, lesions or plaques). Palpate (note masses and/or tenderness).
Neck	Inspect and palpate (entire neck for nodes—note, size, shape consistency, mobility, tenderness). Palpate thyroid (enlargement, consistency, nodules).
Chest	Inspect (symmetry, use of accessory muscles). Percuss for dullness. Auscultate (breath sounds—note presence of crackles, rhonchi, wheeze).
Breasts	Perform clinical breast examination. Inspect (symmetry, dimpling, skin changes, irregular venous pattern, nipple direction, and nipple discharge). Palpate (for masses, including axillae for lymph nodes).
Abdomen	Inspect (symmetry, presence of surgical scars, abnormal vascular patterns). Auscultate (bowel sounds). Percuss (liver and spleen size). Palpate (for tenderness, masses, inguinal lymph nodes).
Female genital	Inspect (masses, lesions, discharge, or bleeding). Palpate (tenderness, shape, and consistency of abdominal organs, including uterus, ovaries, and colon).
Pelvic	Inspect (mucosal integrity and color of vaginal wall and cervix; presence of lesions, polyps, or bleeding; discharge; constriction; nodules; masses).
Male genital	Inspect (for masses, cutaneous lesions, nodules.) Palpate (for tenderness, masses, consistency, contour, scrotal contents—testes, epididymis).
Rectal, prostate	Inspect (external lesions, hemorrhoids). Perform DRE (note sphincter tone, masses, tenderness, constriction, bleeding). Assess and order stool test for FOBT or FIT. In males, palpate prostate (note size, symmetry, consistency—firmness, tenderness, nodules).

EXPECTED PATIENT OUTCOMES

I. The patient will undergo systematic and regular screening and examination.

II. The patient will detect cancer early as able.

REFERENCES

Aberle, D. R., Adams, A. M., Berg, C. D., Black, W. G., Clapp, J. D., Fagerstrom, R. M., et al. (2011). Reduced lung-cancer mortality with low-dose computed tomographic screening. *New England Journal of Medicine, 365*, 395–409.

American Cancer Society. (2013). *Cancer facts and figures 2013.* Atlanta, GA: American Cancer Society.

American Cancer Society. (2016). *American Cancer Society recommendations for prostate cancer early detection.* Atlanta, GA: American Cancer Society. https://www.cancer.org/cancer/prostate-cancer/early-detection/acs-recommendations.html. Accessed 2.11.18.

American Cancer Society. (2017). *Recommendations for the early detection of cancer.* https://www.cancer.org/cancer/breast-cancer/screening-tests-and-early-detection/american-cancer-society-recommendations-for-the-early-detection-of-breast-cancer.html#written_by.

American Cancer Society. (2017). *American Cancer Society recommendations for colorectal cancer early detection.* Atlanta, GA: American Cancer Society. https://www.cancer.org/cancer/colon-rectal-cancer/detection-diagnosis-staging/acs-recommendations.html.

Atkin, W. S., Edwards, R., Kralj-Hans, I., Wooldrage, K., Hart, A. R., Northover, J. M., et al. (2010). Once-only flexible sigmoidoscopy screening in prevention of colorectal cancer: a multicenter randomized controlled trial. *The Lancet, 375*(9726), 1624–1633.

Bénard, F., Barkun, A. N., Martel, M., & von Renteln, D. (2018). Systematic review of colorectal cancer screening guidelines for average-risk adults: summarizing the current global recommendations. *World Journal of Gastroenterology, 24*(1), 124–138.

D'Orsi, C. J., Sickles, E. A., Mendelson, E. B., Morris, E. A., et al. (2013). *ACR BI-RADS Atlas, Breast Imaging Reporting and Data System.* Reston, VA: American College of Radiology.

Esserman, L. J., & Flowers, C. I. (2011). Screening for breast cancer. In V. T. Devita, T. S. Lawrence, S. A. Rosenberg, R. A. DePinho, & R. A. Wineburg (Eds.), *Cancer: Principles and practice of oncology* (9th ed., pp. 610–617). Philadelphia: Wolters Kluwer Health/Lippincott Williams & Wilkins.

Gail, M. H., Brinton, L. A., Byar, D. P., Corle, D. K., Green, S. B., Schairer, C., et al. (1989). Projecting individualized probabilities of developing breast cancer for white females who are being examined annually. *Journal of the National Cancer Institute, 81*(24), 1879–1886.

Glaser, A. (2014). *High-Yield Biostatistics, Epidemiology, and Public Health (High-Yield Series)* (4th edition, pp. 68–75). Philadelphia: Lippincott Williams & Wilkins.

Gleason, D. F., & Mellinger, G. T. (1974). Prediction of prognosis for prostatic adenocarcinoma by combined histologic grading and clinical staging. *Journal of Urology, 111*(1), 58–64.

Haaf, K., Jeon, J., Tammemägi, M. C., Han, S. S., Kong, C. Y., Plevritis, S. K., et al. (2017). Risk prediction models for selection of lung cancer screening candidates: a retrospective validation study. *PLOS Medicine, 14*(4), e1002277.

Harris, R. P., Wilt, T. J., & Qaseem, A. (2015). A value framework for cancer screening: advice for high-value care from the american college of physicians. *Annals Internal Medicine, 162*(10), 712–717.

Haug, U., Knudsen, A. B., Lansdorp-Vogelaar, I., & Kuntz, K. M. (2015 Jun 15). Development of new non-invasive tests for colorectal cancer screening: the relevance of information on adenoma detection. *Int J Cancer, 136*(12), 2864–2874.

Kalanger, M., Zelen, M., Langmark, F., & Adami, H. O. (2010). Effect of screening mammography on breast cancer mortality in Norway. *New England Journal of Medicine, 367*(13), 1203–1210.

Kosters, J. P., & Gotzsche, P. C. (2008). Regular self-breast examination or clinical examination for early detection of breast cancer. In *Cochrane Database Systematic Review.* http://onlinelibrary. wiley.com/doi/10.1002/14651858.CD003373/abstract; jsessionid=D01FBED1514E1F3A9D78B541B0B05BE7.d02t04.

Lieberman, D. A., Rex, D. K., Winawer, S. J., Giardiello, F. M., Johnson, D. A., & Levin, T. R. (2012). Guidelines for colonoscopy surveillance after screening and polypectomy: a consensus update by the US Multi-Society Task Force on Colorectal Cancer. *Gastroenterology, 143*(3), 844–857.

McGuire, A., Brown, J. A. L., Malone, C., McLaughlin, R., & Kerin, M. J. (2015). Effects of age on the detection and management of breast cancer. *Cancers, 7*(2), 908–929.

Meggiolaro, A., Unim, B., Semyonov, L., Miccoli, S., Maffongelli, E., & La Torre, G. (2016). The role of Pap test screening against cervical cancer: a systematic review and meta-analysis. *Clin Ter, 167*(4), 124–139.

Monticciolo, D. L., Newell, M. S., Hendrick, E., Helvie, M. A., Moy, L., Monsees, B., et al. (2017). Breast cancer screening for average-risk women: recommendations from the ACR commission on breast imaging. *Journal of the American College of Radiology, 14*(9), 1137–1143.

National Comprehensive Cancer Network (NCCN). (2012a). NCCN clinical practice guidelines in oncology. *Cervical cancer screening. Version, 2,* 2012. http://www.nccn.org/professionals/physician_gls/pdf/cervical_screening.pdf.

National Comprehensive Cancer Network (NCCN). (2017a). NCCN clinical practice guidelines in oncology. *Breast cancer screening and diagnosis. Version, 1,* 2017. https://www.nccn.org/professionals/physician_gls/pdf/breast-screening.pdf.

National Comprehensive Cancer Network. (2017b). NCCN clinical practice guidelines in oncology. *Colorectal cancer screening.*

Version V., 2(2017). https://www.nccn.org/professionals/physician_gls/pdf/colorectal_screening.pdf.

National Comprehensive Cancer Network. (2017c). NCCN Clinical Practice Guidelines in Oncology. *Prostate Cancer Early Detection Version 2,* 2017. https://www.nccn.org/professionals/physician_gls/pdf/prostate_detection.pdf.

National Comprehensive Cancer Network. (2018b). NCCN clinical practice guidelines in oncology. *Lung cancer screening.* Version 3.2018. https://www.nccn.org/professionals/physician_gls/pdf/lung_screening.pdf.

Park, J. H., Anderson, W. F., & Gail, M. H. (2015). Improvements in US breast cancer survival and proportion explained by tumor size and estrogen-receptor status. *Journal of clinical oncology : official journal of the American Society of Clinical Oncology, 33*(26), 2870–2876.

Pox, C. (2011). Colon cancer screening: which non-invasive filter tests? *Digestive Diseases, 29*(Suppl. 1), 56–59.

Royce, T. J., Hendrix, L. H., Stokes, W. A., et al. (2014). Cancer screening rates in individuals with different life expectancies. *JAMA Internal Medicine, 174*(10), 1558–1565.

Schroeder, F. H., Hugosson, J., Roobol, M. J., Tammela, T. L., Ciatto, S., Nelen, V., et al. (2012). Prostate-cancer mortality at 11 years of follow up. *New England Journal of Medicine, 366,* 981–990.

Smith, R. A., Andrews, K. S., Brooks, D., Fedewa, S. A., Manasssaram-Baptiste, D., Saslow, D., et al. (2017). Cancer screening in the United States, 2017: a review of current American Cancer Society guidelines and current issues in cancer screening. *CA: A Cancer Journal for Clinicians, 67*(2), 100–121.

U.S. Preventive Services Task Force. (2012a). Screening for prostate cancer. http://uspreventiveservicestaskforce.org/prostatecancerscreening.htm.

U.S. Preventive Services Task Force (2012b). Screening for cervical cancer. http://www.uspreventiveservicestaskforce.org/uspstf/uspscerv.htm.

U.S. Preventive Services Task Force. (2013). *Screening for lung cancer.* http://www.uspreventiveservicestaskforce.org/uspstf13/lungcan/lungcanfinalrs.htm.

U.S. Preventive Services Task Force. (2016a). Screening for colorectal cancer. https://epss.ahrq.gov/ePSS/TopicDetails.do?topicid=205.

U.S. Preventive Services Task Force. (2016b). Recommendations: Screening for breast cancer. https://epss.ahrq.gov/ePSS/TopicDetails.do?topicid=198.

3

Survivorship

Stacie Corcoran

OVERVIEW

I. Definition of cancer survivor (National Comprehensive Cancer Network, 2017; National Coalition for Cancer Survivorship, 2018)
   A. A patient diagnosed with cancer is considered a survivor from the time of diagnosis through the rest of his or her life.
   B. Significant others, family, and caregivers are also affected by the cancer diagnosis and are included in this definition.
II. Statistics on cancer survivors (American Cancer Society, 2017; Miller et al., 2016)
   A. In 2016, there were over 15.5 million cancer survivors in the United States (U.S.)
      1. Number of cancer survivors in the U.S. predicted to increase to 20 million by 2026
      2. Sixty percent of cancer survivors are 64 years of age or older
      3. Sixty-five percent of cancer survivors have survived 5 years or more
   B. Most common cancer sites among males
      1. Prostate, lung, and colorectal
   C. Most common cancer sites among females
      1. Breast, lung, and colorectal
III. Long-term and late effects of cancer treatment
   A. Definitions (Carver, Szalda, & Ky, 2013)
      1. Long-term side effects begin as a complication of treatment, persist throughout treatment, and may continue after treatment is completed
      2. Late effects are those that begin after treatment is completed, may be absent or subclinical at the end of treatment, and may manifest years later
   B. Cancer survivors are at risk for long-term and late effects related to their cancer and its treatment (McCabe, Faithfull, Makin, & Wengstrom, 2013; Palos & Zandstra, 2013)
   C. Long-term and late effects associated with cancer—vary according to disease, treatment, comorbid conditions, and age of patient (Carver et al., 2013; Economou, Hurria, & Grant, 2012; Stein, Syrjala, & Andrykowski, 2008)
   D. Long-term and late effects of cancer treatment (Fig. 3.1)

1. Physical consequences (Landier, Armenian, & Bhatia, 2015; Slusser, 2018)
   a. Cardiovascular—cardiomyopathy, congestive heart failure, carotid artery disease, valvular heart disease, arrhythmias, pericardial disease
   b. Pulmonary—pulmonary fibrosis, restrictive lung disease, dyspnea, pneumonitis
   c. Gastrointestinal (GI)—malabsorption, dysphagia, gastroesophageal reflux disease (GERD), hepatitis, constipation, diarrhea, weight gain, cachexia, incontinence, GI tract strictures, fistulas
   d. Bone—osteopenia, osteoporosis, avascular necrosis
   e. Endocrine—hypothyroidism, adrenal insufficiency, hypopituitarism
   f. Genitourinary—chronic kidney disease, proteinuria or albuminuria, incontinence, hypertension
   g. Oral—xerostomia, dental caries, osteonecrosis of the jaw
   h. Sensory, neurologic, or other—fatigue, hearing loss, visual changes, taste changes or loss, neuropathy, lymphedema, insomnia, skin changes after radiation
   i. Fertility—early menopause, azoospermia, alterations or injury due to surgery or radiation
   j. Sexuality
      (1) General: problems with orgasm, loss of libido, loss of intimacy, perceived or actual disfigurement
      (2) Female: vaginal dryness, stenosis, dyspareunia
      (3) Male: erectile dysfunction, retrograde ejaculation
2. Psychological concerns (National Comprehensive Cancer Network, 2017; Bevilacqua et al., 2018; Braamse et al., 2016; Yi & Syrjala, 2017)
   a. Anxiety
      (1) Higher rates in women
      (2) Shorter time since diagnosis
      (3) Living alone
      (4) Higher number of comorbidities

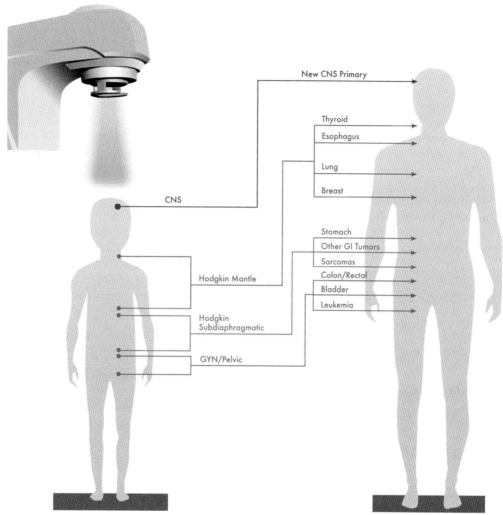

Fig. 3.1 Secondary malignancies associated with radiation therapy within the treatment field. (From Kamran, S. C., Gonzalez, A. B. d., Ng, A., Haas-Kogan, D., & Viswanathan, A. N. (2016). Therapeutic radiation and the potential risk of second malignancies. *Cancer, 122*(12), 1809–1821. https://doi.org/10.1002/cncr.29841.)

b. Depression
  (1) Underreported symptom
  (2) Impacts younger and older survivors
  (3) Associated with poor health care compliance, increased medical care use, higher mortality rates
c. Distress
  (1) Feelings ranging from vulnerability, to sadness, to trauma, to panic
  (2) Interferes with quality of life and ability to cope
  (3) May increase around transitions in care, surveillance appointments/testing, loss and other significant life events
d. Fear of recurrence (Butow et al., 2018; Simard et al., 2013)
  (1) Commonly reported problem among survivors
  (2) Strong association with younger age
  (3) Documented in all diagnostic groups
  (4) Ranges from mild to severe

  (5) Can negatively impact quality of life, adherence to follow-up recommendations
  (6) May be triggered around time of surveillance, appointments, testing, or learning of a friend's/relative's new diagnosis
  (7) Associated with depression and impaired daily functioning
3. Social concerns
  a. Changes in roles and relationships (Keesing, Rosenwax, & McNamara, 2016; Lim, Paek, & Shon, 2015)
    (1) Survivors, partners, family members, friends may experience changes in relationship, poor communication, feelings of loss related to:
      (a) Emotional withdrawal
      (b) Isolation
      (c) Guilt
      (d) Depression
      (e) Anxiety
      (f) Intimacy issues

b. Employment concerns (Lee & Yun, 2015)
   (1) Higher unemployment rate among survivors
   (2) Impacts income, health insurance and identity
   (3) Majority of survivors return to work (Heinesen, Imai, & Maruyama, 2018)
   (4) Fear of demotion, decreased wages, changing jobs, losing insurance
   (5) Potential obstacles that may impact job performance and productivity include fatigue, pain, cognitive changes and anxiety (Duijts et al., 2014)
   (6) Americans with Disabilities Act (1990) prohibits discrimination based on disability; individualized adjustments and accommodations may promote ability to continue or return to work

c. Financial concerns (Guy, et al., 2017)
   (1) Survivors have more chronic conditions than nonsurvivors; negatively impacts productivity and health care expenses

4. Cognitive impairment (Slusser, 2018)
  a. Altered attention
  b. Difficulty concentrating
  c. Mental processing speed
  d. Forgetfulness or problems with memory
  e. Difficulty finding words or expressing thoughts
  f. Visual and auditory disturbances

5. Financial issues (Konski, 2014)
  a. Change in employment status—reduced schedule, lack of employment, lost wages, or reduced earning potential
  b. Inability to obtain and retain insurance coverage
  c. Out-of-pocket expenses related to follow-up visits, radiology testing, prescription, and device costs
  d. Impact on family and lifestyle

6. Spirituality (Garssen, Uwland-Sikkema, & Visser, 2015; Jim et al., 2015)
  a. Positive correlation between greater spiritual/religious beliefs and physical health and well-being in cancer patients
   (1) Meaning of illness—its impact on individual empowerment; ability to cope
   (2) Transcendence connectedness to the unseen, comfort from believing in a higher power
   (3) Finding inner strength—connectedness to oneself
     (a) Increased psychological well-being, which impacts relationships with others; reduces stress and promotes calmness during difficult times; assists with adjustment to cancer diagnosis
     (4) Religious faith—shapes how life events are viewed
      (a) Find hope or meaning in stressful, unpredictable events
      (b) Help maintain sense of control during illness
      (c) Attending worship services and other activities—finding meaningful support through church community

E. Risk of recurrence and secondary malignancy
  1. Adult survivors of childhood cancers have a greater than nineteenfold risk of developing one or more secondary malignancies (Ater, 2015)
   a. Patients with Hodgkin lymphoma have an increased risk for recurrence and secondary malignancies related to chemotherapy and radiation
   b. Women who received chest radiation as children or adolescents have a significantly increased risk for developing breast cancer
     (1) The risk is comparable to that in women who are *BRCA1*- and *BRCA2*-positive (Swerdlow et al., 2012)
   c. Contributing factors include age, genetic predisposition, lifestyle behaviors, immunosuppression, and late effects of chemotherapy and radiotherapy (Baxi et al., 2014; Kamran, Gonzalez, Ng, Haas-Kogan, & Viswanathan, 2016)
  2. Secondary malignancies associated with radiation therapy within the treatment field (Kamran et al., 2016) (see Fig. 3.1).
   a. Surveillance recommendations for young women who have received chest radiation as a child, adolescent, or young adult (before age 30)—if received a radiation dose of 20 Gy or higher to the chest, annual breast imaging, including mammography, breast magnetic resonance imaging (MRI), or both, should be performed starting at age 25 years or at least 8 years after radiation, whichever occurs last (Mulder et al, 2013; Terenziani et al., 2015)
   b. Surveillance recommendations for survivors who have received abdominal, pelvic, or spine radiation as a child, adolescent, or young adult—survivors who received a radiation dose of 30 Gy or higher to their colon or rectum should be screened with colonoscopy every 5 years starting at age 35 years or 10 years after radiation, whichever occurs last (Daniel et al., 2015)

IV. Survivorship care
  A. Survivorship is recognized as a distinct phase of the cancer trajectory, providing multiple opportunities to promote a healthy lifestyle, monitor for recurrence, and identify and manage long-term and late effects (Fig. 3.2) (Jacobs & Vaughn, 2013).

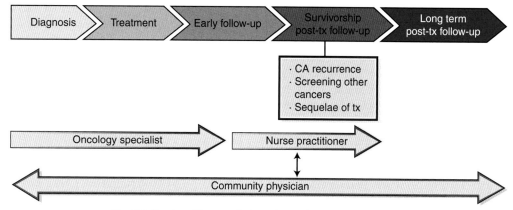

Fig. 3.2 Survivorship as a distinct phase of the cancer trajectory.

1. Many settings institute survivorship care at treatment completion or transition to maintenance therapy (e.g., androgen-blocking treatment for prostate cancer; hormone therapy for breast cancer) (McCabe, Bhatia, et al., 2013)

B. Essential components of survivorship care (Fig. 3.3)
1. Assessment to detect recurrence of cancer
2. Identification and management of long-term and late effects
3. Screening recommendations for other cancers
4. Health promotion recommendations (e.g., nutrition, exercise, smoking cessation, sun protection, dental health)
5. Treatment summary and care plan
6. Communication with primary care physician and other providers

C. Barriers to the provision of survivorship care for the future (Kirkwood, Kosty, Bajorin, Bruinooge, & Goldstein, 2013; Konski, 2014)

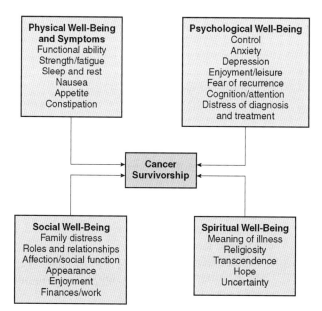

Fig. 3.3 Institute of Medicine (IOM): Components of survivorship care.

1. Demand for oncologists will outweigh supply of providers
   a. Expanding number of aging Americans
   b. Growing number of cancer survivors
   c. Significant deficits in the oncology workforce anticipated by 2020

ASSESSMENT

I. History
A. Clinical data
1. Demographic information
2. Providers' names, specialty area (e.g., primary care provider, gynecologist, cardiologist, dentist), and contact information
3. Past medical history
   a. Comorbidities
   b. Family history, including cancer diagnoses or other major illnesses
   c. Genetic history, if available
   d. Cancer diagnosis, including multiple primaries or relapses
   e. Type and duration of treatment—chemotherapy, immunotherapy, surgery, radiation therapy, hormone therapy
4. Health behaviors
   a. Tobacco/tobacco product use
   b. Alcohol intake
   c. Dietary habits
   d. Physical activity level
   e. Sun exposure
   f. Routine body mass index (BMI) assessment
5. Receipt of preventive and screening health services
   a. Cancer screening (e.g., colonoscopy, mammography)
   b. Immunizations
6. Genetic testing, as appropriate, for patients with breast, ovarian, or colon cancer (NCCN, 2017)
B. Focused review of symptoms

II. Physical examination
   A. Assessment for long-term and late effects of cancer and its treatment
   B. Focused examination to detect recurrence based on disease history and established guidelines (e.g., NCCN, American Society of Clinical Oncology [ASCO], or as developed or adapted by individual institutions or practices)
   C. Symptom management assessment
      1. Use of patient-reported outcomes (PRO) tool to assess symptoms/late effects (Kjaer et al., 2016)
      2. Oncology Nursing Society's Putting Evidence into Practice (PEP) (ONS, 2018)—symptom assessment guide; topics include fatigue, dyspnea, and anxiety
      3. National Comprehensive Cancer Network Survivorship Guidelines (NCCN), 2016)—topics include lymphedema, pain, and sexual function
III. Psychosocial assessment
   A. Social history—occupation, living situation
   B. Past coping skills
   C. Risk for anxiety, depression, fear of recurrence
      1. Contributing factors—fatigue, pain, sleep disturbances, metabolic or endocrine morbidities, medication changes
      2. Use of patient self-assessment tool (e.g., NCCN distress thermometer, Patient Health Questionnaire Hospital Anxiety and Depression Scale) per institutional practices
   D. Support systems—identification of available support from family members, friends, peers, church community
   E. Neuropsychological evaluation as appropriate
IV. Imaging and laboratory tests
   A. Assessment for recurrent disease based on established guidelines (e.g., NCCN or ASCO, or as developed or adapted by individual institutions or practices)

MANAGEMENT

I. Interventions to prevent, mitigate, and relieve adverse effects of cancer and its treatment
   A. Assess for any ongoing physiologic, psychological, emotional, social, spiritual, and financial issues
   B. Refer to appropriate specialists (e.g., physical or occupational therapist, mental health provider, chaplain, pain and palliative care specialist, speech and swallow therapist), as appropriate (Asher, 2011; Garmy & Jakobsson, 2018)
      1. Rehabilitation: identify impairments associated with cancer history and treatment exposures, develop interventions promoting health and reducing severity of actual and potential impairments; survivors have many complex needs—physical, cognitive, psychological, sexual, and vocational domains (Garmy & Jakobsson, 2018; Silver et al., 2015)
         a. Need for rehabilitation services growing as number of cancer survivors increases
         b. Significant rates of cancer-related physical impairments reported; 53% of adult-onset survivors report functional limitations
         c. Rehabilitative services go underutilized; estimated at 1% to 2%
         d. Goals are to minimize disability and improve quality of life:
            (1) Preventive—lessen effects of expected disabilities
            (2) Restorative—return survivors to previous level of functioning, maximize independence
            (3) Supportive—educate survivors regarding accommodations aimed at minimizing debilitating changes
            (4) Palliative—minimizing or removing complications, reducing symptom burden, emphasizing comfort
         e. Improve ability to work, decrease sick leave, and reduce rates of lost productivity
   C. Encourage patients to be physically active; return to daily activities as soon as possible
      1. Physical activity recommendations for cancer survivors ((NCCN), 2017)
         a. At least 150 minutes of moderate-intensity activity or 75 minutes of vigorous-intensity activity or equivalent combination per week
         b. Two to three weekly sessions of strength training that involves major muscle groups
         c. Stretch major muscle groups and tendons
         d. Avoid sedentary behaviors
         e. For physically inactive survivors, begin with one to three light- to moderate-intensity exercises, 20-minute sessions per week, with progression based on tolerance, as outlined in the previous guidelines
   D. Encourage patients to achieve and maintain healthy eating habits
      1. Plant-based diet
      2. Limit refined sugar and red meat consumption
   E. Advise patients on weight management—promote normal BMI
      1. Limit high-calorie foods, especially those with little or no nutritional benefit such as fast foods and fried foods
      2. Substitute with low-calorie, nutrient-rich foods such as fruits, vegetables, and whole grains
      3. Practice portion control
      4. Monitor food labels
      5. Routine weights
   F. Counsel patients on tobacco/tobacco product and alcohol use
      1. Avoid tobacco or tobacco products
      2. Limit alcohol to no more than one drink per day for women and two drinks per day for men

G. Refer to specialists as needed (e.g., nutritionist, smoking cessation counselor, supervised exercise program)

II. Interventions related to knowledge deficit
   A. Assess motivation and willingness of patient and caregivers to learn
   B. Determine cultural influences on health teaching
      1. Provide interpreter services as needed
      2. Provide culturally appropriate educational materials to reinforce education
   C. Provide and discuss the survivorship care plan (SCP) (McCabe, Bhatia, et al., 2013; McCabe, Faithfull, et al., 2013; Stricker, Jacobs, & Palmer, 2012)
      3. The SCP should include the following:
         a. Treatment summary—cancer site, type and stage of cancer, date of diagnosis, and any treatment(s) received
         b. Information about long-term and late effects of treatment
         c. Recommend follow-up surveillance and intervals for disease recurrence or progression (e.g., NCCN or ASCO, or as developed or adapted by individual institutions or practices)
         d. Recommend health promotion behaviors (e.g., smoking cessation, nutrition, physical activity, sun protection, safe use of complementary and alternative medicine [CAM]) and health maintenance activities (e.g., cancer screening, bone health screening, and maintaining up-to-date immunizations)
         e. Monitor and manage long-term and late effects
            (1) No established guidelines for adult survivors
            (2) Children's Oncology Group guidelines may serve as reference (www.survivorshipguidelines.org)
         f. List of health care team providers with their contact information
         g. Institutional and community resources and referral to support groups, as needed

III. Interventions to improve communication and coordination among providers
   A. Visit updates shared between providers
   B. SCP provided to the patient, primary care provider, and any specialists involved in patient's care

IV. Interventions for adolescent/young adult cancer survivors (AYA) (Lee, Khan, & Salloum, 2018; Rosenberg, Kroon, Chen, Li, & Jones, 2015)
   A. Higher-risk population requiring careful follow-up; ages 15 to 39
      1. Late physical effects (e.g., cardiomyopathy, fatigue, altered cognition, sexual dysfunction)
      2. Social concerns—relationships, education, career, finances
      3. High rates of being underinsured or uninsured
         a. Unable to afford care
         b. Limited access to treatment and surveillance
         c. Increased reports of medication nonadherence due to cost

TABLE 3.1	General Counseling Topics for Cancer Survivors

- Tests to check general health
- Dental health
- Regular measurements of weight, cholesterol levels, and blood pressure
- Immunizations ("shots") for both children and adults
- Outline special tests to be done at certain time points, such as during pregnancy and after ages 40 and 50 years
- Tobacco prevention
- Healthy diet
- Bone health
- Safe sex
- Regular exercise
- Moderate alcohol consumption
- Avoidance of illegal drugs
- Sun protection
- Use of seat belts (and car seats for children) when riding in a car or truck
- Advice about stress and accident prevention
- Regular preventive care

Adapted from American Cancer Society. (2017). American Cancer Society (ACS) facts and figures. Retrieved from. https://www.cancer.org/research/cancer-facts-statistics/all-cancer-facts-figures/cancerfacts-figures-2017.html.

EXPECTED PATIENT OUTCOMES

I. Patients will have access to information on follow-up surveillance, potential late effects of cancer and its treatment, health promotion, health maintenance activities, and available resources
   A. Patients will verbalize understanding of potential late and long-term effects of the cancer treatment
   B. Patients will adhere to recommended follow-up surveillance (Table 3.1)
   C. Patients will exhibit healthy lifestyle behaviors in their life
   D. Patients will demonstrate compliance with cancer screening recommendations
   E. Patients will use appropriate services, as directed, such as physical therapy, social work, smoking cessation specialist (Rock et al., 2012)

II. Patients will experience optimal communication and coordination of care with health care professionals
   A. Patients will identify the appropriate health care provider to consult for health prevention, promotion, and monitoring for new concerns
   B. Patients will experience collaboration and communication, particularly between oncology provider and primary care provider (PCP) (Jacobs & Vaughn, 2013)
   C. Patients will have survivorship information for PCP and nononcology providers

REFERENCES

American Cancer Society. (2017). *American Cancer Society (ACS): facts and figures.* Retrieved from https://www.cancer.org/research/cancer-facts-statistics/all-cancer-facts-figures/cancer-facts-figures-2017.html.

Asher, A. (2011). Cognitive dysfunction among cancer survivors. *Am J Phys Med Rehabil, 90*(5 Suppl 1), S16–S26. https://doi.org/10.1097/PHM.0b013e31820be463.

Ater, J. L. (2015). *Adult Survivorship of Pediatric Cancers.* Springer.

Baxi, S. S., Pinheiro, L. C., Patil, S. M., Pfister, D. G., Oeffinger, K. C., & Elkin, E. B. (2014). Causes of death in long-term survivors of head and neck cancer. *Cancer, 120*(10), 1507–1513. https://doi.org/10.1002/cncr.28588.

Bevilacqua, L. A., Dulak, D., Schofield, E., Starr, T. D., Nelson, C. J., Roth, A. J., & Alici, Y. (2018). Prevalence and predictors of depression, pain, and fatigue in older- versus younger-adult cancer survivors. *Psycho-Oncology, 27*(3), 900–907. https://doi.org/10.1002/pon.4605.

Braamse, A. M., van Turenhout, S. T., Terhaar Sive Droste, J. S., de Groot, G. H., van der Hulst, R. W., Klemt-Kropp, M., & Dekker, J. (2016). Factors associated with anxiety and depressive symptoms in colorectal cancer survivors. *Eur J Gastroenterol Hepatol, 28*(7), 831–835. https://doi.org/10.1097/meg.0000000000000615.

Butow, P., Sharpe, L., Thewes, B., Turner, J., Gilchrist, J., & Beith, J. (2018). Fear of cancer recurrence: a practical guide for clinicians. *Oncology (Williston Park), 32*(1), 32–38.

Carver, J. R., Szalda, D., & Ky, B. (2013). Asymptomatic cardiac toxicity in long-term cancer survivors: defining the population and recommendations for surveillance. *Semin Oncol, 40*(2), 229–238. https://doi.org/10.1053/j.seminoncol.2013.01.005.

Daniel, C. L., Kohler, C. L., Stratton, K. L., Oeffinger, K. C., Leisenring, W. M., Waterbor, J. W., & Nathan, P. C. (2015). Predictors of colorectal cancer surveillance among survivors of childhood cancer treated with radiation: a report from the Childhood Cancer Survivor Study. *Cancer, 121*(11), 1856–1863. https://doi.org/10.1002/cncr.29265.

Duijts, S. F. A., Egmond, M. P., Spelten, E., Muijen, P., Anema, J. R., & Beek, A. J. (2014). Physical and psychosocial problems in cancer survivors beyond return to work: a systematic review. *Psycho-Oncology, 23*(5), 481–492. https://doi.org/10.1002/pon.3467.

Economou, D., Hurria, A., & Grant, M. (2012). Integrating a cancer-specific geriatric assessment into survivorship care. *Clin J Oncol Nurs, 16*(3), E78–E85. https://doi.org/10.1188/12.cjon.e78-e83.

Garmy, P., & Jakobsson, L. (2018). Experiences of cancer rehabilitation: a cross-sectional study. *J Clin Nurs, 27*(9–10), 2014–2021. https://doi.org/10.1111/jocn.14321.

Garssen, B., Uwland-Sikkema, N. F., & Visser, A. (2015). How spirituality helps cancer patients with the adjustment to their disease. *Journal of Religion and Health, 54*(4), 1249–1265. https://doi.org/10.1007/s10943-014-9864-9.

Guy, G. P., Yabroff, K. R., Ekwueme, D. U., Rim, S. H., Li, R., & Richardson, L. C. (2017). Economic burden of chronic conditions among survivors of cancer in the United States. *Journal of Clinical Oncology, 35*(18), 2053–2061. https://doi.org/10.1200/jco.2016.71.9716.

Heinesen, E., Imai, S., & Maruyama, S. (2018). Employment, job skills and occupational mobility of cancer survivors. *J Health Econ, 58*, 151–175. https://doi.org/10.1016/j.jhealeco.2018.01.006.

Jacobs, L. A., & Vaughn, D. J. (2013). Care of the adult cancer survivor. *Annals of Internal Medicine, 158*(11), ITC6–1. https://doi.org/10.7326/0003-4819-158-11-201306040-01006.

Jim, H. S., Pustejovsky, J. E., Park, C. L., Danhauer, S. C., Sherman, A. C., Fitchett, G., & Salsman, J. M. (2015). Religion, spirituality, and physical health in cancer patients: a meta-analysis. *Cancer, 121*(21), 3760–3768. https://doi.org/10.1002/cncr.29353.

Kamran, S. C., Gonzalez, A. B. d., Ng, A., Haas-Kogan, D., & Viswanathan, A. N. (2016). Therapeutic radiation and the potential risk of second malignancies. *Cancer, 122*(12), 1809–1821. https://doi.org/10.1002/cncr.29841.

Keesing, S., Rosenwax, L., & McNamara, B. (2016). A dyadic approach to understanding the impact of breast cancer on relationships between partners during early survivorship. *BMC Women's Health. 16*, 57. https://doi.org/10.1186/s12905-016-0337-z. 57.

Kirkwood, M. K., Kosty, M. P., Bajorin, D. F., Bruinooge, S. S., & Goldstein, M. A. (2013). Tracking the workforce: the American Society of Clinical Oncology Workforce Information System. *Journal of Oncology Practice, 9*(1), 3–8. https://doi.org/10.1200/jop.2012.000827.

Kjaer, T., Dalton, S. O., Andersen, E., Karlsen, R., Nielsen, A. L., Hansen, M. K., et al. (2016). A controlled study of use of patient-reported outcomes to improve assessment of late effects after treatment for head-and-neck cancer. *Radiotherapy and Oncology, 119*(2), 221–228. https://doi.org/10.1016/j.radonc.2016.04.034.

Konski, A. (2014). Economic Consequences of Late Effects. In P. Rubin, L. S. Constine, & L. B. Marks (Eds.), *ALERT - Adverse Late Effects of Cancer Treatment* (pp. 285–291). Berlin, Heidelberg: Springer.

Landier, W., Armenian, S., & Bhatia, S. (2015). Late effects of childhood cancer and its treatment. *Pediatric Clinics of North America, 62*(1), 275–300. https://doi.org/10.1016/j.pcl.2014.09.017.

Lee, M. J., Khan, M. M., & Salloum, R. G. (2018). Recent trends in cost-related medication nonadherence among cancer survivors in the United States. *Journal of Managed Care & Specialty Pharmacy, 24*(1), 56–64. https://doi.org/10.18553/jmcp.2018.24.1.56.

Lee, M. K., & Yun, Y. H. (2015). Working situation of cancer survivors versus the general population. *Journal of Cancer Survivorship, 9*(2), 349–360. https://doi.org/10.1007/s11764-014-0418-7.

Lim, J. W., Paek, M. S., & Shon, E. J. (2015). Gender and role differences in couples' communication during cancer survivorship. *Cancer Nurs, 38*(3), E51–E60. https://doi.org/10.1097/ncc.0000000000000191.

McCabe, M. S., Bhatia, S., Oeffinger, K. C., Reaman, G. H., Tyne, C., Wollins, D. S., & Hudson, M. M. (2013). American Society of Clinical Oncology statement: achieving high-quality cancer survivorship care. *J Clin Oncol, 31*(5), 631–640. https://doi.org/10.1200/jco.2012.46.6854.

McCabe, M. S., Faithfull, S., Makin, W., & Wengstrom, Y. (2013). Survivorship programs and care planning. *Cancer, 119*(Suppl 11), 2179–2186. https://doi.org/10.1002/cncr.28068.

Miller, K. D., Siegel, R. L., Lin, C. C., Mariotto, A. B., Kramer, J. L., Rowland, J. H., & Jemal, A. (2016). Cancer treatment and survivorship statistics, 2016. *CA Cancer J Clin, 66*(4), 271–289. https://doi.org/10.3322/caac.21349.

Mulder, R. L., Kremer, L. C. M., Hudson, M. M., Bhatia, S., Landier, W., Levitt, G., & Oeffinger, K. C. (2013). Recommendations for breast cancer surveillance for female survivors of childhood, adolescent, and young adult cancer given chest radiation: a report from the International Late Effects of Childhood Cancer Guideline Harmonization Group. *The Lancet Oncology, 14*(13), e621–e629. https://doi.org/10.1016/S1470-2045(13)70303-6.

National Coalition for Cancer Survivorship. (2018). *About us: our mission.* Retrieved from https://www.canceradvocacy.org/about-us/our-mission/.

National Comprehensive Cancer Network. (2017). NCCN guidelines version 3.2017. Survivorship.

Oncology Nursing Society. (2018). *Putting evidence into practice (PEP).* Retrieved from https://www.ons.org/practice-resources/pep.

Palos, G. R., & Zandstra, F. (2013). Call for action: caring for the United States' aging cancer survivors. *Clin J Oncol Nurs, 17*(1), 88–90. https://doi.org/10.1188/13.cjon.88-90.

Rock, C. L., Doyle, C., Demark-Wahnefried, W., Meyerhardt, J., Courneya, K. S., Schwartz, A. L., & Gansler, T. (2012). Nutrition and physical activity guidelines for cancer survivors. *CA Cancer J Clin, 62*(4), 243–274. https://doi.org/10.3322/caac.21142.

Rosenberg, A. R., Kroon, L., Chen, L., Li, C. I., & Jones, B. (2015). Insurance status and risk of cancer mortality among adolescents and young adults. *Cancer, 121*(8), 1279–1286. https://doi.org/10.1002/cncr.29187.

Silver, J. K., Raj, V. S., Fu, J. B., Wisotzky, E. M., Smith, S. R., & Kirch, R. A. (2015). Cancer rehabilitation and palliative care: critical components in the delivery of high-quality oncology services. *Support Care Cancer, 23*(12), 3633–3643. https://doi.org/10.1007/s00520-015-2916-1.

Simard, S., Thewes, B., Humphris, G., Dixon, M., Hayden, C., Mireskandari, S., & Ozakinci, G. (2013). Fear of cancer recurrence in adult cancer survivors: a systematic review of quantitative studies. *J Cancer Surviv, 7*(3), 300–322. https://doi.org/10.1007/s11764-013-0272-z.

Slusser, K. M. (2018). Cancer Nursing: Principles and Practice. In *8th Ed.: Jones and Bartlett Learning.*

Stein, K. D., Syrjala, K. L., & Andrykowski, M. A. (2008). Physical and psychological long-term and late effects of cancer. *Cancer, 112*(11 Suppl), 2577–2592. https://doi.org/10.1002/cncr.23448.

Stricker, C. T., Jacobs, L. A., & Palmer, S. C. (2012). Survivorship care plans: an argument for evidence over common sense. *J Clin Oncol, 30*(12), 1392–1393. author reply 1393-1395 https://doi.org/10.1200/jco.2011.40.7940.

Swerdlow, A. J., Cooke, R., Bates, A., Cunningham, D., Falk, S. J., Gilson, D., & Williams, M. V. (2012). Breast Cancer Risk After Supradiaphragmatic Radiotherapy for Hodgkin's lymphoma in England and Wales: a national cohort study. *Journal of Clinical Oncology, 30*(22), 2745–2752. https://doi.org/10.1200/jco.2011.38.8835.

Terenziani, M., Massimino, M., Magazzu, D., Gandola, L., Capri, G., Carcangiu, M. L., & Valagussa, P. (2015). Management of breast cancer after Hodgkin's lymphoma and paediatric cancer. *Eur J Cancer, 51*(13), 1667–1674. https://doi.org/10.1016/j.ejca.2015.05.024.

Yi, J. C., & Syrjala, K. L. (2017). Anxiety and depression in cancer survivors. *Med Clin North Am, 101*(6), 1099–1113. https://doi.org/10.1016/j.mcna.2017.06.005.

4

Palliative and End-of-Life Care

Regina M. Fink and Nancy Robertson

OVERVIEW

I. Palliative care: an essential component of quality care for persons with cancer and their family caregivers
   A. Definitions
      1. "Patient/family centered care that optimizes quality of life (QOL) by anticipating, preventing, and treating suffering [and] addresses physical, intellectual, emotional, social, and spiritual needs to facilitate patient autonomy, access to information, and choice" [throughout the continuum of illness] (NCP, 2013)
      2. "An approach that improves the QOL of patients and their families facing the problem associated with life-threatening illness, through the prevention and relief of suffering by means of early identification and impeccable assessment and treatment of pain and other problems, physical, psychosocial and spiritual" (WPCA Global Atlas, WHO, 2014)
   B. Key palliative care components (Kuebler, 2017; WHO, 2014; NCP, 2013)
      1. Patient and family–centered care across the serious illness trajectory
      2. Goals of care and shared decision making (refer to Chapter 6 for detailed information) are essential elements of the palliative care approach.
         a. Elicited in an intentional and structured way
         b. Based on values and preferences of patients and caregivers
         c. Goals of care should not be confused with treatment plans or advance care planning (ACP). Palliative care goals are instead a separate conversation that can inform ACP decision and treatment preferences.
         d. May change over the course of an illness
         e. Goals of care conversations should be facilitated by the interdisciplinary team (IDT) before a health care crisis or near death, if possible

         f. Acknowledged with the primary purpose to match preferences and wishes to treatment plans
      3. IDT (physician, nurse, social worker, spiritual care provider, and other health care professionals) approach to identify and meet the needs of patients and caregivers
      4. Integration of all aspects of patient care, including physical, psychological, spiritual, emotional, social, cultural, and economic
      5. Assessment and management of distressing symptoms
      6. Support based on patient and family caregiver needs, preferences, values, and goals, regardless of prognosis
      7. Support system to help the family caregiver cope during the patient's illness and after the patient has died
      8. Enhancement of QOL for those impacted by serious illness
   C. Standards for palliative care in oncology (NCCN, 2018a)
      1. Patient and family caregiver are the focus of care
      2. Offered at the time of advanced cancer diagnosis concurrently with disease-directed, life-prolonging therapies and other health care treatments as indicated
      3. Symptom burden from disease or treatment is anticipated, prevented, and skillfully managed
      4. Psychosocial, emotional, and spiritual distress are as important as physical symptoms
      5. Patient autonomy is respected, with access to information to assist with decision making
      6. Care is provided by an IDT
      7. Life is affirmed and death is accepted as a normal process
      8. Bereavement counseling for both patient and family caregiver is included in the plan of care
      9. Palliative care may be initiated by the primary oncology team and is augmented by palliative care experts, based on the patient's and family caregiver's needs

D. Domains and competencies for quality palliative care delivery
  1. Clinical Practice Guidelines for Quality Palliative Care (NCP, 2013)
     a. Structure and processes of care
     b. Physical aspects of care
     c. Psychological and psychiatric aspects of care
     d. Social aspects of care
     e. Spiritual, religious, and existential aspects of care
     f. Cultural aspects of care
     g. Care of the patients at the end of life
     h. Ethical and legal aspects of care
  2. Hospice and Palliative Nurse Association (HPNA) competencies (Dahlin, 2014)
     a. Clinical judgment
     b. Advocacy and ethics
     c. Professionalism
     d. Collaboration
     e. Systems thinking
     f. Cultural and spiritual competence
     g. Facilitator of learning
     h. Communication
     i. Evidence-based practice and research
E. Primary, secondary, and tertiary palliative care (Kamal, Maguire, & Meier, 2015; Quill & Abernethy, 2013; von Gunten, 2002).
  1. Primary palliative care
     a. Basic palliative care skills
     b. Advance care planning
     c. Symptom assessment and management
     d. Communication among health care provider, patient, and family caregivers
     e. Support for patient and family caregiver
     f. Offered by all oncology health care providers and primary care providers to patients and family caregivers
  2. Secondary palliative care
     a. Bridge between primary and tertiary palliative care
     b. Offered by health care professionals and organizations providing specialty palliative care and consultation
     c. Accessed in community or rural settings, where needs often exceed the skill of primary care providers and access to palliative care experts is scarce
  3. Tertiary palliative care
     a. Provided at tertiary and quaternary academic centers
     b. IDT composed of physician (board-certified or fellowship-trained specialist), advanced practice registered nurse (APRN) or nurse, social worker, and spiritual care provider
     c. Complex cases (e.g., complex/refractory symptoms, existential distress, difficult goals of care discussions, conflict resolution)
     d. Formal involvement of IDT in teaching, ongoing quality improvement and safety initiatives, and research to further the palliative care field
     e. Joint Commission advanced palliative care certification of hospital inpatient programs, hospice, and home health programs (Joint Commission Advanced Palliative Care Certification, 2019)
     f. Exceptional patient and family-centered care
     g. Optimizing QOL for patients with serious illness
     h. Patient and family engagement
     i. Coordination of care and communication among providers
     j. Use of evidence-based national guidelines or expert consensus to support patient care processes
F. Palliative care is offered in multiple settings encompassing all models of delivery (Wiencek & Coyne, 2014; Higginson, 2015).
  1. Inpatient consultative teams in acute care settings, including oncology inpatient units, intensive care units, and emergency departments
  2. Palliative care inpatient units
  3. Outpatient palliative or supportive care clinics integrated within ambulatory care, oncology specialty clinics, radiation oncology, or infusion centers
  4. Home-based primary and secondary palliative care programs
  5. Hospice
  6. Telehealth connects primary rural palliative care to tertiary palliative care (Bakitas et al. 2015a)
G. Early integration of palliative care into oncology care
  1. The Oncology Nursing Society (2014) and the American Society of Clinical Oncology (Smith et al., 2012) have published palliative care position statements, suggesting that palliative care can benefit all oncology patients and should be considered early in the course of illness for any individual with metastatic cancer and/or a high symptom burden
  2. Patient-centered, symptom-focused, interprofessional palliative care improves QOL, symptom burden, depression, ACP, less aggressive care at the end of life, survival, and cost savings for patients when offered earlier in the illness trajectory (Temel et al., 2010; Zimmerman et al., 2014; Bakitas et al., 2015b; Baumann & Temel, 2014; El-Jawahri et al., 2016; Hui et al., 2015)
  3. Earlier palliative care consultation during hospital admission associated with lower cost of hospital stay for patients admitted with advanced cancer (Aldridge et al., 2016). Findings are consistent with a growing body of research suggesting that early palliative care should be more widely implemented (May et al., 2015). Limited studies, many of which have focused on rural cancer programs, have

documented cost savings of employing palliative care services in rural areas (Bakitas et al., 2015a).

II. Hospice care
   A. Definitions
      1. Both a philosophy of care and a regulated insurance benefit. The insurance benefit takes effect if the patient has been given a prognosis from two physicians of less than 6 months to live and if the patient agrees to stop all aggressive treatment.
      2. Model of high-quality, compassionate care that helps patients and family caregivers live as fully as possible when cure is not attainable (NHPCO, 2017)
      3. Hospice care is part of the palliative care continuum (Fig. 4.1)
   B. Hospice care is based on the understanding that dying is part of the life cycle and that meticulous management of physical, psychosocial, and spiritual symptoms will promote QOL for the patient–family system
   C. As an organized model of care, the hospice movement began in the early 1960s. Following is a brief history of hospice care; more detailed information is available on the NHPCO website (https://www.nhpco.org/history-hospice-care)
      1. The modern hospice movement began through the work of Dame Cicely Saunders, who began her work with the terminally ill in 1948 and eventually created the first modern hospice, St. Christopher in London, England, in 1967 (NHPCO, 2017)
      2. Dr. Florence Wald, Yale School of Nursing dean, pioneered the hospice movement in the United States (U.S.)
      3. The Connecticut Hospice, founded by Dr. Wald, two pediatricians, and a chaplain, opened in 1974 in Branford, Connecticut, and was the first U.S. hospice program
      4. The Medicare hospice benefit was approved by Congress in 1982 after demonstration projects showed that IDT care focusing on QOL and

addressing symptom burden of terminal illness improved outcomes and cost less than usual care
      5. Medicare benefit became permanent in 1986, providing a stable source of payment for hospice care; supported a steady growth of hospice programs throughout the U.S.
   D. Similar key features of palliative care apply to hospice care
   E. Focus of hospice care interventions is relief of distressing symptoms and enhancement of QOL for both patient and family caregiver
   F. Medicare hospice benefit
      1. Patient must have a prognosis of 6 months or less of remaining life to be eligible
      2. Eligibility criteria should not be confused with length of service; patients can receive hospice care for as long as they meet eligibility criteria (NHPCO, 2018a)
      3. Top five most common diagnoses of patients enrolled in the hospice benefit (NHPCO, 2018a)
         a. Alzheimer disease (13%)
         b. Congestive heart failure (8%)
         c. Lung cancer (6%)
         d. Chronic obstructive pulmonary disease (COPD) (5%)
         e. Senile degeneration of the brain (3%)
      4. Late referral to hospice is common. Median length of stay is 17 days, with 35.5% of patients dying or discharged within 7 days of admission (NHPCO, 2018a).
      5. Physicians are often overly optimistic when estimating prognosis and overestimate survival time by a factor of 4 (Soliman et al., 2018)
      6. Eligibility criteria (CMS, 2018)
         a. The patient must be eligible for Medicare Part A
         b. The referring physician and hospice medical director certify, to the best of their knowledge, that the patient has a prognosis of 6 months or less of remaining life if the disease runs its natural course
         c. Patient chooses hospice care for treatment of the terminal illness (i.e., waives right to traditional Medicare for treatment of terminal illness and its symptoms)
      7. Hospice services include (CMS, 2018)
         a. Nursing care
         b. Physician services
         c. Social services
         d. Counseling services, including but not limited to bereavement counseling, dietary counseling, and spiritual counseling
         e. Medical equipment and supplies
         f. Medications for symptom control
         g. Home health and homemaker services
         h. Physical, occupational, and speech therapy
         i. Dietary or nutrition counseling

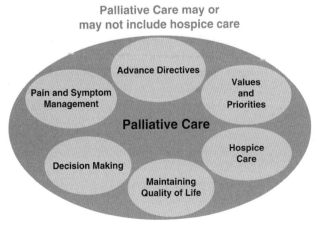

Fig. 4.1 Palliative care may or may not include hospice care.

j. Grief and loss counseling

k. Volunteer service

l. Short-term inpatient care for pain and symptom control

m. Short-term respite care

n. Routine home care—care provided in the patient's place of residence, including private home, nursing home, and residential care setting

o. Continuous home care—care provided in the patient's place of residence during a time of crisis requiring predominantly continuous nursing care

p. General inpatient care—care provided in an inpatient facility for pain or symptom control when the symptom(s) cannot be managed at home

q. Inpatient respite care—care provided in an approved facility on a short-term basis to give respite to the family caregiver

III. Grief and bereavement (refer to Chapter 50 for detailed information)

A. Definitions (Corless, 2015; Smit, 2015).

1. Loss—the absence of an object, position, ability, or attribute

2. Grief—the psychological, social, and somatic responses to loss

3. Anticipatory grief—the psychological, social, and somatic responses to an anticipated loss

4. Mourning—the outward and active expression of grief through participation in various death and bereavement rituals, which vary by culture

5. Bereavement—the state of having suffered a loss; the period during which grief and mourning occur, the first year after a loss generally being the most difficult

6. Complicated grief—a disturbance in the normal process of grief

a. Prolonged grief—persistent and severe yearning for the deceased beyond 6 to 12 months after the loss (Bryant, 2013); recognized as a mental disorder causing significant distress and disability and included in the *Diagnostic and Statistical Manual,* 5th edition (Bryant, 2013; Waldrop & Kutner, 2013a)

b. Disenfranchised grief—occurs when the loss cannot be openly acknowledged; examples include death of a person in a nonsanctioned relationship such as an extramarital affair or homosexual relationship, loss from miscarriage or abortion, loss of the essence of the individual before actual death (e.g., severe dementia)

B. Manifestations of acute grief

1. Social

a. Restlessness and inability to sit still

b. Uncomfortable around other people or social withdrawal

c. Feeling of not wanting to be alone

d. Lack of ability to initiate and maintain organized patterns of activity

2. Physical

a. Anorexia and weight loss or the opposite, overeating and weight gain

b. Heart palpitations, nervousness, tension, panic

c. Shortness of breath

d. Tightness in throat

e. Inability to sleep

f. Lack of energy and feelings of physical exhaustion

g. Headaches, muscular aches, gastrointestinal distress

3. Cognitive-emotional

a. Sadness and crying

b. Forgetfulness or difficulty concentrating

c. Feelings of anger or guilt

d. Mood swings

e. Sense of helplessness

f. Yearning for the deceased

g. Dreams of the deceased

C. Support interventions for the person experiencing grief

1. Counseling of patients and families to express feelings and heal relationships while the patient has the physical and mental capacity to participate in these conversations

2. Encouraging expression of thoughts and feelings in an accepting environment; grieving person usually benefits from the opportunity to "tell his or her story."

ASSESSMENT

I. Whole-person assessment (Chovan, Cluxton, & Rancour, 2015)

A. The traditional medical model used when assessing a health care situation is to apply a standardized, siloed technique examining parts of a person involved, rather than looking at the whole person.

B. Utilizing this approach when assessing persons with serious illness will cause the provider to overlook potential areas of suffering and miss an opportunity to enhance QOL

C. Palliative care approach incorporates the assessment of all domains of a person's being

1. Physical

2. Psychological

3. Sociocultural

4. Spiritual

5. Practical aspects

6. Economic

D. To capture the full dimension of suffering, a whole-person assessment is ideally conducted by the IDT.

1. Thorough and complete assessment may take several visits to fully address.

2. Whole-person assessments need to be repeated periodically as patient and family caregiver needs change across the illness trajectory.

E. Whole-person assessments (Table 4.1) require preparation and advanced skills. Issues approached in this type of assessment are often sensitive and filled with details not apparent to the clinician. Consider talking to the patient and family caregiver separately.

TABLE 4.1   **Approach to Whole-Person Assessment**

Action	Detail
Prepare	Read all recent history and physical or consultation reports; speak with collaborating health care team members, if possible.
Remind	Remind yourself that you are walking into a story in progress.
Introduce	Introduce yourself to the patient and family caregiver. Explain why you are there. Tell them how long you intend to spend with them. Take a seat near the patient, being alert to cultural sensitivities to closeness and eye contact.
Ask	Ask patient what name she or he would like to be called. Become familiar with close family members and friends. Find out the name of the health care agent or medical durable power of attorney.
Invite	Invite the patient to tell about how she or he learned of the diagnosis and what is understood about the situation.
Don't judge	Make the most of listening skills and be careful not to make any quick judgments.
Avoid	Avoid interrupting. Use good communication techniques.
Listen	Listen for patient and family caregiver concerns about distressing physical symptoms, emotional stress, social issues, and spiritual distress that are affecting QOL.
Take notes	Take notes quietly. You might hear something you don't completely understand. Make a note so that you can go back and ask about this once the person is done telling his or her story.
Select tools	Select appropriate clinical assessment tools to help guide the assessment.
Be alert for sensory impairments	Can the person see and hear okay? Can they understand what you are saying, or do they have a cognitive problem? Do you speak their language? Any breakdowns in this area will negatively impact the assessment.

II. Physical assessment

A. Specific disease trajectory is an important component to incorporate when helping seriously ill patients navigate their health care choices (Fig. 4.2) (Comstock Barker & Scherer, 2017; Murray, Kendall, Boyd & Sheikh, 2005)

1. Cancer illness progression can take many paths but typically follows a pattern of fairly steady functional status that drops off quickly as the end of life nears

2. Noncancer illness has more of an up–down pattern; slower decline into end of life

3. Frailty and dementia progression can follow many paths but typically exhibits a slow progressive decline

B. Impaired performance status (Table 4.2)

1. Eastern Cooperative Oncology Group (ECOG) Performance Status score of 3 or higher

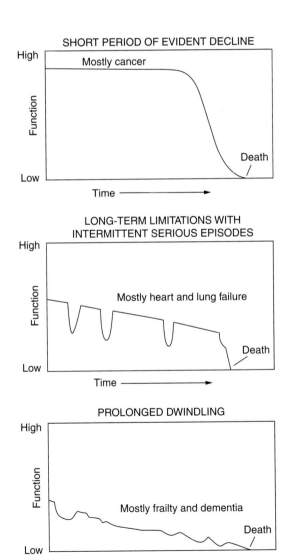

Fig. 4.2 Dying trajectories. (From Lynn, J., & Adamson, D. M. [2003]. *Living well at the end of life. Adapting health care to serious chronic illness in old age.* Washington, D.C.: Rand Health.)

TABLE 4.2 Comparison of ECOG Performance Status and Karnofsky Performance Status

ECOG Performance Status	Karnofsky Performance Status
0—Fully active, able to carry on all predisease performance without restriction	100—Normal, no complaints; no evidence of disease 90—Able to carry on normal activity; minor signs or symptoms of disease
1—Restricted in physically strenuous activity but ambulatory and able to carry out work of a light or sedentary nature (e.g., light housework, office work)	80—Normal activity with effort, some signs or symptoms of disease 70—Cares for self but unable to carry on normal activity or to do active work
2—Ambulatory and capable of all self-care but unable to carry out any work activities; up and about more than 50% of waking hours	60—Requires occasional assistance but is able to care for most of personal needs 50—Requires considerable assistance and frequent medical care
3—Capable of only limited self-care; confined to bed or chair more than 50% of waking hours	40—Disabled; requires special care and assistance 30—Severely disabled; hospitalization is indicated although death not imminent
4—Completely disabled; cannot carry on any self-care; totally confined to bed or chair	20—Very ill; hospitalization and active supportive care necessary 10—Moribund
5—Dead	0—Dead

Karnofsky, D., & Burchenal, J. (1949). The clinical evaluation of chemotherapeutic agents in cancer. In C. MacLeod (Ed.), *Evaluation of Chemotherapeutic Agents* (pp. 191–205). New York, NY: Columbia University Press; Zubrod, C. (1960). Appraisal of methods for the study of chemo-therapy in man: comparative therapeutic trial of nitrogen mustard and thiophosphoramide. *Journal of Chronic Diseases*, 11, 7–33.

    2. Karnofsky Performance Scale score of less than 50%

    3. Palliative Performance Scale (NHPCO, 2018b).

  C. Landmark SUPPORT study (Study to Understand Prognoses and Preferences for Outcomes and Risks of Treatments) focused on end-of-life suffering experienced by those nearing death and identified substantial shortcomings in caring for the seriously ill. Findings include:

    1. Forty-seven percent of physicians knew when their patients wished to avoid cardiopulmonary resuscitation (CPR)

    2. Forty-six percent of do not resuscitate (DNR) orders were written within 2 days of death

    3. Thirty-eight percent of patients who died spent at least 10 days in an intensive care unit

    4. Fifty percent of patients experienced moderate to severe pain at least half the time

  D. Systematic review/meta-analysis found pain was prevalent in 39.3% of cancer patients after curative treatment, 55% of those during anticancer treatment, and 66.4% in those with advanced, metastatic, terminal disease (van den Beuken-van et al., 2016)

  E. Fatigue in patients with cancer has been underreported, underdiagnosed, and undertreated. It is common in patients with cancer and is experienced by 80% of patients receiving chemotherapy and radiation therapy, bone marrow transplantation, or treatment with biological response modifiers (NCCN, 2018b).

  F. Incorporate a validated clinical tool to identify the beginning perception of the symptom burden and to analyze the effectiveness of interventions

III. Psychological assessment

  A. Living with a serious illness can have a major impact on the emotional and mental state of patients and their family caregivers

  B. Depression and anxiety are the most common psychological symptoms experienced by individuals with serious illness (Fulton, Newins, Porter, & Ramos, 2018)

  C. Patients can present with symptoms of anxiety, depression, grief, anticipatory grief, and thoughts of suicide (Mosher, Ott, Hanna, Jalal, & Champion, 2015)

  D. Factors that make suffering worse can be the presence of psychiatric disorders, dangerous overuse of drugs, dysfunctional and unsupportive family behaviors, poor social support, and spiritual concerns

  E. It is difficult to tell the difference between depression and normal sadness. This requires the assessment and intervention of the professional psychological team.

  F. Family caregivers are at higher risk for the development of cardiovascular disease, stroke, and mortality (Goldstein & Morrison, 2012)

  G. Listening well and using advanced communication techniques will help the suffering person feel heard and understood

IV. Sociocultural assessment

  A. The Social Work Assessment Tool (SWAT) is a validated tool that identifies problem areas (National Hospice and Palliative Care Organization, 2007)

  B. Social evaluation

    1. Safe and affordable housing

    2. Access to education

    3. Public safety

    4. Availability of healthy foods

    5. Local emergency and health services

    6. Homes and work places free of life-threatening toxins

    7. Social support network

  C. Cultural assessment

    1. Beliefs and values

    2. Language spoken

    3. Health literacy

V. Spiritual assessment
   A. Importance of religion or spirituality
   B. Individual's search for purpose and meaning to life
   C. Associated with an individual's relationship with a higher power; however, it can be associated with a structured religion or stand on its own.
   D. Goals of spiritual care within the structure of palliative care are to promote the connection between the mind, body, and spirit; to provide compassionate care; to be present; and to encourage positive and supportive thinking (Kuebler, 2017)
   E. Recent research suggests that spiritual well-being can decrease rates of depression (Unterrainer, Lewis, & Fink 2014; Abraham, 2017; Kuebler, 2017)

VI. Practical assessment
   A. Assess in the home, if possible
   B. Day-to-day challenges patients and family caregivers face such as housekeeping, shopping, care of pets, care of younger family members, dressing, bathing, and movement
   C. Katz Index of Independence of Daily Living assesses patient's function (Shelkey & Wallace, 2012)
   D. Caregiver Strain Assessment tool examines caregiver burden (Kruithof, Post, & Visser-Meily, 2015)

VII. Economic assessment
   A. Evaluate the patient's financial situation
      1. Does the patient have money for the medical care, treatments, and needed medications?
      2. Is medical insurance coverage available?
      3. Is the patient and/or family caregiver able to work, or is there a loss of income due to the health care situation?
   B. Referral to a social worker or financial counselor
   C. Community resources

VIII. Symptom assessment
   A. Common symptoms palliative care patients experience are fatigue, pain, dyspnea, nausea, and constipation. (Kelley & Morrison, 2015; Wilkie & Ezenwa, 2012)
   B. Palliative care patients may experience symptom clusters; therefore it is important not to limit a symptom assessment to a report of pain
   C. Complications or symptoms related to the disease process, such as fatigue and anxiety, may exacerbate pain
   D. Interventions to alleviate pain may cause side effects resulting in new or worsening symptoms, such as constipation or nausea
   E. Symptom assessment instruments
      1. Edmonton Symptom Assessment System-revised (ESAS-r) (Watanabe et al., 2011)
         a. Assesses nine common symptoms in palliative care (pain, tiredness, drowsiness, nausea, lack of appetite, depression, anxiety, shortness of breath, and well-being) (Fig. 4.3).
         b. Scored on a 0 to 10 scale, specifying a time frame of "now"

c. Accompanying definitions describe various symptoms
         d. If patients are unable to complete the form or are unresponsive and incapable of self-report (final days of life), observer judgments become necessary and a space is provided for the person completing the assessment
      2. Distress screening (NCCN, 2018c)
         a. Distress should be assessed in all palliative care patients and managed in all stages of the disease trajectory
         b. Distress Thermometer is the primary tool to screen for distress (NCCN, 2018c)
         c. A patient should be referred for evaluation and treatment of distress
            (1) Mild distress (<4): referral to primary oncology team with resources available
            (2) Moderate to severe distress (≥4): referral to mental health professional, social worker, spiritual care provider, counselor

MANAGEMENT

I. Medical management
   A. Employ pharmacologic supportive care interventions to ensure comfort
   B. Integrate evidence-based nonpharmacologic integrative health approaches for symptom management and psychological support

II. Nursing management
   A. Physical – primary assessment of physical symptoms, assure all physical needs are met, coordinate the plan of care, and revisit as needs change
   B. Psychological – offer psychological support and primary interventions with a follow-up referral to psychologist and counseling services
   C. Social – primary assessment of social challenges; referral to social worker and connect to community resources as needed
   D. Spiritual – primary assessment of spiritual coping, offer primary spiritual support in a culturally sensitive way; referral to spiritual care providers as needed
   E. Economic – assessment of economic challenges and coordinate referrals to social work professionals for intervention

III. Hospice and palliative care community resources
   A. Medicare-certified hospice programs
   B. Palliative care programs
      1. Inpatient palliative care consultation in U.S. hospitals (Cassel, Bowman, Rogers, Spragens, & Meier, 2018)
         a. More than 80% of U.S. patients hospitalized for serious illness have access to specialty palliative services; 1800 hospitals have palliative care programs
         b. Ninety percent of hospitals with more than 300 beds and 100% of the National Cancer

---

Edmonton Symptom Assessment System:
(revised version) (ESAS-R)

Please circle the number that best describes how you feel NOW:

| No Pain | 0 1 2 3 4 5 6 7 8 9 10 | Worst Possible Pain |

| No Tiredness *(Tiredness = lack of energy)* | 0 1 2 3 4 5 6 7 8 9 10 | Worst Possible Tiredness |

| No Drowsiness *(Drowsiness = feeling sleepy)* | 0 1 2 3 4 5 6 7 8 9 10 | Worst Possible Drowsiness |

| No Nausea | 0 1 2 3 4 5 6 7 8 9 10 | Worst Possible Nausea |

| No Lack of Appetite | 0 1 2 3 4 5 6 7 8 9 10 | Worst Possible Lack of Appetite |

| No Shortness of Breath | 0 1 2 3 4 5 6 7 8 9 10 | Worst Possible Shortness of Breath |

| No Depression *(Depression = feeling sad)* | 0 1 2 3 4 5 6 7 8 9 10 | Worst Possible Depression |

| No Anxiety *(Anxiety = feeling nervous)* | 0 1 2 3 4 5 6 7 8 9 10 | Worst Possible Anxiety |

| Best Wellbeing *(Wellbeing = how you feel overall)* | 0 1 2 3 4 5 6 7 8 9 10 | Worst Possible Wellbeing |

| No _____ Other Problem *(for example constipation)* | 0 1 2 3 4 5 6 7 8 9 10 | Worst Possible _____ |

Patient's Name _____

Date _____ Time _____

Completed by (check one):
☐ Patient
☐ Family caregiver
☐ Health care professional caregiver
☐ Caregiver-assisted

A

BODY DIAGRAM ON REVERSE SIDE

Fig. 4.3 Edmonton Symptom Assessment Scale-revised (ESAS-r). A., Rating scale.

Continued

Institute's Comprehensive Cancer Centers now have palliative care services

2. Outpatient or ambulatory palliative care services are cost-effective or offer cost savings for the health care system by avoiding inpatient care (ICER, 2016)
3. Community-based, nonhospice palliative models of care in the home and nursing home have potential to increase quality of care for persons with cancer and other chronic progressive illnesses, especially for patients who do not meet hospice eligibility criteria but who have significant symptom burden (Ornstein et al., 2013; Stephens et al., 2018)
   a. Home health aide, homemaker services, or a combination of both may or may not be covered by insurance, depending on identified needs and insurance plan
   b. Social service agencies
   c. Agencies that provide support specifically to persons with a cancer diagnosis (e.g., American Cancer Society)
   d. Agencies that provide services and support to persons with degenerative diseases and their caregivers (e.g., dementia, amyotrophic lateral sclerosis [ALS], osteoarthritis)
   e. Layperson-led and professional-led grief support programs – hospices often accept families into their grief support programs, even if the patient was not enrolled in a hospice

Please mark on these pictures where it is that you hurt:

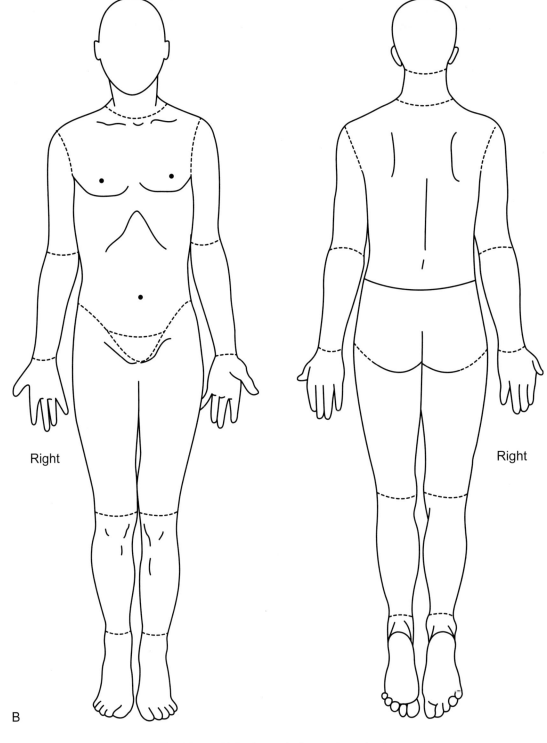

Right

Right

B

Fig. 4.3, cont'd B., Anatomic diagram to mark pain.

IV. Care of the imminently dying
- A. Patients who are in the last hours of their lives often experience unrelieved physical, emotional, spiritual, and social suffering
- B. Recognizing the signs of imminent death is critical to providing the best care possible during this phase
- C. Identifying this phase is not always easy or straightforward
- D. The place of death strongly influences the extent to which symptoms are managed
  1. Research has demonstrated that people prefer to die at home (Gomes, Calanzani, Gysels, Hall, & Higginson, 2013; Hoare, Morris, Kelly, Kuhn, & Barclay, 2015)
  2. Dying at home is associated with greater caregiver satisfaction, less aggressive care at the end of life, higher quality of death as assessed by family members, and lower overall caregiver burden (Kinoshita et al., 2014; Gomes et al., 2013)
- E. One third of patients in the United States actually die at home (Centers for Disease Control and Prevention, 2017)
- F. Hospital deaths are associated with more physical and emotional distress and more prolonged caregiver grief (Zhang, Nilsson, & Prigerson, 2012)
- G. Clinical signs of impending death may include (Sandvik, Selbaek, Bergh, Aarsland, & Husebo, 2016):
  1. Pulselessness of the radial artery
  2. Respiration with mandibular movement
  3. Decreased urine output
  4. Cheyne–Stokes breathing
  5. Terminal secretions
  6. Nonreactive pupils
  7. Decreased response to visual stimuli
  8. Palliative Performance Scale (PPS) of <10% (Fig. 4.4)
- H. Honoring preference for end-of-life care requires clear communication about the benefits and burdens of medical procedures. Ideally these goals of care conversations are held early in the disease trajectory and are revisited over time as the disease progresses.
  1. Mechanical ventilation and CPR are medical procedures of particular importance
     - a. Preferable for these discussions to take place before the dying phase, if possible
     - b. Although CPR may prolong a life in some patients, it will not reverse terminal illness
     - c. Patients imminently dying should not be subjected to CPR, as this is a nonbeneficial and potentially harmful procedure
  2. Artificial nutrition and hydration (ANH) at the end of life is a controversial topic holding emotive, physical, and ethical considerations
     - a. ANH should be considered medical interventions (AAHPM Position Statement, 2013; HPNA, 2015)
     - b. Originally developed to provide short-term support for acutely ill patients, in end-of-life situations ANH is unlikely to prolong life and can lead to complications that increase suffering
     - c. Nutrition delivered artificially does not eliminate the risk of aspiration and in some patient populations may actually increase the risk of aspiration and its complications (HPNA, 2015)
     - d. Artificial nutrition given via tube feedings is associated with increased infection, fluid overload, and skin excoriation around the tube along with the invasiveness and discomfort associated with having a tube (HPNA, 2017)
     - e. A Cochrane review of artificial hydration found no clinical difference in artificial hydration over placebo on the quality of the life; well-being; survival time; or relief of symptoms such as anxiety, pain, nausea, and sedation (Good, Richard, Syrmis, Jenkins-Marsh, & Stephens, 2014)
     - f. Many patients experience thirst or dry mouth, but this symptom is not only associated with fluid status; therefore parenteral fluids are unlikely to alleviate thirst (HPNA, 2015)
     - g. Recommendations for evidence-based care are (Good et al., 2014; HPNA Position Statement, 2017):
       (1) Acknowledge the decision made by the patient and family caregiver to initiate, withhold, or withdraw ANH
       (2) Facilitate education of patient and family caregiver about the dying process and its effects on nutrition and fluid status
       (3) Support the dying person's wishes to drink if that is their wish
       (4) Offer frequent care of the mouth and lips
       (5) Foster caregiver involvement in mouth care
       (6) Discuss risks and benefits of artificial hydration with the dying person and caregivers
       (7) Consider a therapeutic trial of artificial hydration if goals of care reflect this desire and if distressing symptoms are associated with dehydration, such as thirst or delirium
- I. Symptoms specific to end of life (EOL)
  1. Weakness, fatigue, and functional decline
     - a. Care should be taken to protect the person from injury resulting from the weakness and fatigue.
     - b. Decreased oral intake
     - c. Good oral care, offer ice chips, moistening the mouth
     - d. Diminished blood perfusion
     - e. Expect chilling of extremities as the perfusion diminishes. Offer extra blankets.

Palliative Performance Scale (PPSv2)

PPS Level	Ambulation	Activity Level & Evidence of Disease	Self-care	Intake	Conscious level
PPS 100%	Full	Normal activity & work **No evidence** of disease	Full	Normal	Full
PPS 90%	Full	Normal activity & work **Some evidence** of disease	Full	Normal	Full
PPS 80%	Full	Normal activity & work *with* effort Some evidence of disease	Full	Normal or reduced	Full
PPS 70%	Reduced	Unable normal activity & work **Significant** disease	Full	Normal or reduced	Full
PPS 60%	Reduced	Unable hobby/house work Significant disease	Occasional assistance	Normal or reduced	Full or confusion
PPS 50%	Mainly sit/lie	Unable to do any work **Extensive** disease	Considerable assistance	Normal or reduced	Full or drowsy or confusion
PPS 40%	Mainly in bed	Unable to do most activity Extensive disease	Mainly assistance	Normal or reduced	Full or drowsy +/- confusion
PPS 30%	Totally bed bound	Unable to do any activity Extensive disease	Total care	Reduced	Full or drowsy +/- confusion
PPS 20%	Totally bed bound	Unable to do any activity Extensive disease	Total care	Minimal sips	Full or drowsy +/- confusion
PPS 10%	Totally bed bound	Unable to do any activity Extensive disease	Total care	Mouth care only	Drowsy or coma
PPS 0%	Dead	-	-	-	-

Instructions: PPS level is determined by reading left to right to find a 'best horizontal fit.' Begin at left column reading downwards until current ambulation is determined, then, read across to next and downwards until each column is determined. Thus, 'leftward' columns take precedence over 'rightward' columns. Also, see 'definitions of terms' below.

Definition of Terms for PPS

As noted below, some of the terms have similar meanings with the differences being more readily apparent as one reads horizontally across each row to find an overall 'best fit' using all five columns.

1. **Ambulation** (Use item **Self-Care** to help decide the level)
   - **Full** — no restrictions or assistance
   - **Reduced ambulation** — degree to which the patient can walk and transfer with occasional assistance
   - **Mainly sit/lie vs Mainly in bed** — the amount of time that the patient is *able to* sit up or *needs* to lie down
   - **Totally bed bound** — unable to get out of bed or do self-care

2. **Activity & Evidence of Disease** (Use **Ambulation** to help decide the level.)
   - **Activity** — Refers to normal activities linked to daily routines (ADL), house work and hobbies/leisure.
   - **Job/work** — Refers to normal activities linked to both paid and unpaid work, including homemaking and volunteer activities.
   - Both include cases in which a patient continues the activity but may reduce either the time or effort involved.

Evidence of Disease
   - **No evidence of disease** — Individual is normal and healthy with no physical or investigative evidence of disease.
   - **'Some,' 'significant,' and 'extensive' disease** — Refers to physical or investigative evidence which shows disease progression, sometimes despite active treatments.

   - Example 1: Breast cancer:
     | some | = a local recurrence |
     | significant | = one or two metastases in the lung or bone |
     | extensive | = multiple metastases (lung, bone, liver or brain), hypercalcemia or other complication |

   Example 2: CHF:
     | some | = regular use of diuretic &/or ACE inhibitors to control |
     | significant | = exacerbations of CHF, effusion or edema necessitating increases or changes in drug management |
     | extensive | = 1 or more hospital admissions in past 12 months for acute CHF & general decline with effusions, edema, SOB |

3. **Self-Care**
   - **Full** — Able to do all normal activities such as transfer out of bed, walk, wash, toilet and eat without assistance.
   - **Occasional assistance** — Requires *minor* assistance from several times a week to once every day, for the activities noted above.
   - **Considerable assistance** — Requires *moderate* assistance every day, for *some* of the activities noted above (getting to the bathroom, cutting up food, etc.)
   - **Mainly assistance** — Requires *major* assistance every day, for *most* of the activities noted above (getting up, washing face and shaving, etc.). Can usually eat with minimal or no help. This may fluctuate with level of fatigue.
   - **Total care** — Always requires assistance for all care. May or may not be able to chew and swallow food.

4. **Intake**
   - **Normal** — eats normal amounts of food for the individual as when healthy
   - **Normal or reduced** — highly variable for the individual; 'reduced' means intake is less than normal amounts when healthy
   - **Minimal to sips** — very small amounts, usually pureed or liquid, and well below normal intake.
   - **Mouth care only** — no oral intake

5. **Conscious Level**
   - **Full** — fully alert and orientated, with normal (for the patient) cognitive abilities (thinking, memory, etc.)
   - **Full or confusion** — level of consciousness is full or may be reduced. If reduced, confusion denotes delirium or dementia which may be mild, moderate or severe, with multiple possible etiologies.
   - **Full or drowsy +/- confusion** — level of consciousness is full or may be markedly reduced; sometimes included in the term stupor. Implies fatigue, drug side effects, delirium or closeness to death.
   - **Drowsy or coma +/- confusion** — no response to verbal or physical stimuli; some reflexes may or may not remain. The depth of coma may fluctuate throughout a 24 hour period. Usually indicates imminent death

Fig. 4.4 Palliative Performance Scale. (The Palliative Performance Scale version 2 [PPSv2] tool is copyright to Victoria Hospice Society and replaces the first PPS published in 1996 [*J Pall Care* 9(4): 26-32]. It cannot be altered or used in any way other than as intended and described here. Programs may use PPSv2 with appropriate recognition. Available in electronic Word format by email request to judy.martell@caphealth.org. Correspondence should be sent to Medical Director, Victoria Hospice Society, 1900 Fort St, Victoria, BC, V8R 1J8, Canada.)

f. Decreased level of consciousness leading to coma and death, or terminal delirium evidenced as confusion, restlessness, and agitation

g. Monitor patient safety

2. Terminal secretions

a. Occurs when the dying patient is too weak or hypersomnolent to clear or swallow pharyngeal secretions; even small volumes of secretions will produce sounds in the resonant pharyngeal space

b. Historically, terminal secretions have been referred to as a "death rattle" and are associated with impending death. Current research supports this connection (Lokker, van Zuylen, van der Rijt & van der Heide, 2014). Reported prevalence varies widely; a range of 12% to 92% reflects a lack of large, prospective trials; differences in methodology and definitions; and the challenge of objective measurement of death rattle.

c. Though research indicates that this is not distressing to the patient, it can be distressing to the family and loved ones (Fielding & Long, 2014; Wee, Coleman, Hillier, & Holgate, 2008)

(1) Nonpharmacologic management includes raising the head of the bed to promote drainage of secretions and position the dying person on the side or semiprone

(2) Shallow oral suctioning might be of some assistance, but avoid deep suctioning, as this can be painful and not effective

(3) Although there are medications that impact terminal secretions, they are not without side effects. Multiple studies have questioned the utility of pharmacologic treatments for terminal secretions (Lokker, van Zuylen et al., 2014; Fielding & Long, 2014). Muscarinic receptor blockers (anticholinergic drugs) are the most commonly used class of medication for this symptom. Such agents include scopolamine, hyoscyamine, glycopyrrolate, and atropine.

(a) All of these agents can cause varying degrees of blurred vision, sedation, confusion, delirium, restlessness, hallucinations, palpitations, constipation, and urinary retention.

(b) Select agents based on the balance of benefits versus undesirable effects

3. Loss of sphincter control

a. Use of absorbent linens and frequent changing of soiled beddings and clothing

b. Consider good skin care

4. Inability to close eyes

a. Cool cloth over eyes

b. Normal saline lubrication

J. Care of the body after death

1. Nurses play an integral role in honoring the deceased person and family wishes for care after death.

2. Care of the body after death incorporates cultural and spiritual components

3. Kind, respectful care of the body after death impacts positively on the grief and bereavement process of loved ones.

4. Hospice utilizes policies and procedures to guide the steps of this process.

5. Nurse's role in the development of these policies and procedures is critical.

EXPECTED PATIENT OUTCOMES

I. Patient and family caregiver will be able to understand the difference between palliative care and hospice care.

II. Patient values and preferences will be recognized and supported by the health care and palliative care team.

III. Patient and/or family caregiver identifies signs and symptoms to report to the health care or palliative care team.

IV. The patient's symptoms that impact QOL will be minimized or resolved.

V. Patients will adhere to and benefit from both pharmacologic and nonpharmacologic recommendations for symptoms affecting QOL.

VI. Patients will experience fewer visits to the emergency department and admissions to the hospital in accordance to their goals of care.

VII. Patients will experience less futile end-of-life care congruent with their wishes.

VIII. Family caregivers will be supported during the patient's serious illness, thus increasing their QOL and decreasing their burden.

IX. Family caregivers' grief and bereavement will be positively impacted.

REFERENCES

Abraham, S. (2017). A correlational study of spiritual well-being and depression in the adult cancer patient. *The Health Care Manager, 36*(2), 164–172. https://doi.org/10.1097/HCM.0000000000000153.

Aldridge, M. D., Hasselaar, J., Garralda, E., van der Eerden, M., Stevenson, D., McKendrick, K., & Meier, D. E. (2016). Educations, implementation, and policy barriers to greater integration of palliative care: a literature review. *Palliative Medicine, 30*(3), 224–239. https://doi.org/10.1177/0269216315606645.

American Academy of Hospice and Palliative Medicine. (2013). *AAHPM statement on Artificial Nutrition and Hydration near the End of Life.* Retrieved from http://aahpm.org/positions/anh.

Bakitas, M. A., Elk, R., Astin, M., Ceronsky, L., Clifford, K. N., Dionne-Odom, J. N., & Ritchie, C. (2015a). Systematic review of palliative care in the rural setting. *Cancer Control, 22*(4), 450–464. https://doi.org/10.1177/107327481502200411.

Bakitas, M. A., Tosteson, T. D., Li, Z., Lyons, K. D., Hull, J. G., Li, Z., & Azuero, A. (2015b). Early versus delayed initiation of concurrent palliative oncology care: Patient outcomes in the ENABLE III randomized controlled trial. *Journal of Clinical Oncology, 33*(13), 1438–1445. https://doi.org/10.1200/JCO.2014.58.6362.

Bauman, J. R., & Temel, J. S. (2014). The integration of early palliative care with oncology care: the time has come for a new tradition. *Journal of the National Comprehensive Cancer Network, 12*(12), 1763–1771.

Bryant, R. A. (2013). Is pathological grief lasting more than 12 months grief or depression? *Current Opinion in Psychiatry, 26*, 41–46. https://doi.org/10.1097/YCO.0b013e32835b2ca2.

Cassel, J. B., Bowman, B., Rogers, M., Spragens, L. H., & Meier, D. E. (2018). Palliative care leadership centers are key to the diffusion of palliative care innovation. *Health Affairs, 37*(2), 231–239. https://doi.org/10.1377/hlthaff.2017.1122.

Center for Medicare and Medicaid Services. (2018). Hospice Medicare services. Retrieved from https://www.cms.gov/Medicare/Medicare-Fee-for-Service-Payment/Hospice/index.html.

Centers for Disease Control and Prevention. (2017). Quick Stats: percentage Distribution of deaths, by place of death—United States, 2000–2014.

Chovan, J. D., Cluxton, D., & Rancour, P. (2015). Principle of patient and family assessment. Chapter 4. In B. R. Ferrell, N. Coyle, & J. A. Paice (Eds.), *Oxford textbook of palliative nursing* (4th ed., pp. 58–80). New York, NY: Oxford University Press.

Comstock Barker, P., & Scherer, J. S. (2017). Illness trajectories: description and clinical use #326. *Journal of Palliative Medicine, 20*(4), 426–427. https://doi.org/10.1089/jpm.2016.0554.

Corless, I. B. (2015). Bereavement. In B. R. Ferrell, N. Coyle, & J. Paice (Eds.), *Oxford textbook of palliative nursing* (4th ed., pp. 487–499). New York, NY: Oxford University Press.

Dahlin, C. (2014). *Hospice and Palliative Nurses Association competencies for the hospice and palliative advanced practice nurse* (2nd ed.). Pittsburgh, PA: Hospice and Palliative Nurses Association.

El-Jawahri, A., LeBlanc, T., VanDusen, H., Traeger, L., Greer, J. A., Pirl, W. F., & McAfee, S. (2016). Effect of inpatient palliative care on quality of life 2 weeks after hematopoietic stem cell transplantation: a randomized clinical trial. *Journal of the American Medical Association, 316*(20), 2094–2103. https://doi.org/10.1001/jama.2016.16786.

Fielding, F., & Long, C. O. (2014). The death rattle dilemma. *Journal of Hospice and Palliative Nursing, 16*(8), 466–471.

Fulton, J. J., Newins, A. R., Porter, L. S., & Ramos, K. (2018). Psychotherapy targeting depression and anxiety for use in palliative care: a meta-analysis. *Journal of Palliative Medicine, 21*(7), 1024–1037. https://doi.org/10.1089/jpm.2017.0576.

Goldstein, N. E., & Morrison, R. S. (2012). *Evidence-Based Practice of Palliative Medicine E-Book*. Elsevier Health Sciences.

Gomes, B., Calanzani, N., Gysels, M., Hall, S., & Higginson, I. J. (2013). Heterogeneity and changes in preferences for dying at home: a systematic review. *BMC Palliative Care, 12*(1), 7. https://doi.org/10.1186/1472-684X-12-7.

Good, P., Richard, R., Syrmis, W., Jenkins-Marsh, S., & Stephens, J. (2014). Medically assisted hydration for adult palliative care patients. *Cochrane Database Systematic Review, 4*, 1–17. https://doi.org/10.1002/14651858.CD006274.pub3.

Higginson, I. J. (2015). Palliative care delivery models. In N. Cherny, M. Fallon, S. Kaasa, R. Portenoy, & D. C. Currow (Eds.), *Oxford textbook of palliative medicine* (pp. 112–116). Oxford, United Kingdom: Oxford University Press.

Hoare, S., Morris, Z. S., Kelly, M. P., Kuhn, I., & Barclay, S. (2015). Do patients want to die at home? A systematic review of the UK literature, focused on missing preferences for place of death. *PLoS One, 10*(11), e0142723.

Hospice and Palliative Nurses Association (HPNA). (2015). *HPNA position statement: artificial nutrition and hydration in advanced illness*. Pittsburgh, PA: HPNA.

Hui, D., Kim, Y. J., Park, J. C., Zhang, Y., Strasser, F., Cherny, N., & Bruera, E. (2015). Integration of oncology and palliative care: a systematic review. *The Oncologist, 20*(1), 77–83. https://doi.org/10.1002/14651858.CD006274.pub3.

Institute for Clinical and Economic Review (ICER). (2016). Retrieved from https://icer-review.org/wp-content/uploads/2016/03/Palliative-Care-Revised-Draft-Report-030916.pdf.

Joint Commission Advanced Palliative Care Certification. (2019). Retrieved from https://www.jointcommission.org/certification/palliative_care.aspx.

Kamal, A. H., Maguire, J. M., & Meier, D. E. (2015). Evolving the palliative workforce to provide responsive, serious illness care. *Annals of Internal Medicine, 163*(8), 637–638. https://doi.org/10.7326/M15-0071.

Karnofsky, D., & Burchenal, J. (1949). The clinical evaluation of chemotherapeutic agents in cancer. In C. MacLeod (Ed.), *Evaluation of Chemotherapeutic Agents* (pp. 191–205). New York, NY: Columbia University Press.

Kelley, A. S., & Morrison, R. S. (2015). Palliative care for the seriously ill. *New England Journal of Medicine, 373*(8), 747–755. https://doi.org/10.1056/NEJMra1404684.

Kinoshita, H., Maeda, I., Morita, T., Miyashita, M., Yamagishi, A., Shirahige, Y., & Eguchi, K. (2014). Place of death and the differences in patient quality of death and dying and caregiver burden. *Journal of Clinical Oncology, 33*(4), 357–363. https://doi.org/10.1200/JCO.2014.55.7355.

Kruithof, W. J., Post, M. W., & Visser-Meily, J. M. (2015). Measuring negative and positive caregiving experiences: a psychometric analysis of the Caregiver Strain Index expanded. *Clinical Rehabilitation, 29*(12), 1224–1233. https://doi.org/10.1177/0269215515570378.

Kuebler, K. K. (2017). *Integration of palliative care in chronic conditions: an interdisciplinary approach*. Pittsburgh, PA: Oncology Nursing Society.

Lokker, M. E., van Zuylen, L., van der Rijt, C. C., & van der Heide, A. (2014). Prevalence, impact, and treatment of death rattle: a systematic review. *Journal of Pain and Symptom Management, 47*(1), 105–122. https://doi.org/10.1016/j.jpainsymman.2013.03.011.

Lynn, J., & Adamson, D. M. (2003). *Living well at the end of life. Adapting health care to serious chronic illness in old age*. Washington, D.C.: Rand Health.

May, P., Garrido, M. M., Cassel, J. B., Kelley, A. S., Meier, D. E., Normand, C., & Morrison, R. S. (2015). Prospective cohort study of hospital palliative care teams for inpatients with advanced cancer: earlier consultation is associated with larger cost-saving effect. *Journal of Clinical Oncology, 33*(25), 2745. https://doi.org/10.1200/JCO.2014.60.2334.

Mosher, C. E., Ott, M. A., Hanna, N., Jalal, S. I., & Champion, V. L. (2015). Coping with physical and psychological symptoms: a qualitative study of advanced lung cancer patients and their family caregivers. *Supportive Care in Cancer, 23*(7), 2053–2060. https://doi.org/10.1007/s00520-014-2566-8.

Murray, S. A., Kendall, M., Boyd, K., & Sheikh, A. (2005). Illness trajectories and palliative care. *BMJ: British Medical Journal, 330*(7498), 1007. https://doi.org/10.1136/bmj.330.7498.1007.

National Comprehensive Cancer Network (NCCN). (2018a). *NCCN palliative care guidelines version 1.2018: palliative care.* Retrieved from https://www.nccn.org/professionals/physician_gls/pdf/palliative.pdf.

National Comprehensive Cancer Network (NCCN). (2018b). *NCCN guidelines cancer-related fatigue version 2.2018: cancer-related fatigue.* Retrieved from https://www.nccn.org/professionals/physician_gls/pdf/fatigue.pdf.

National Comprehensive Cancer Network (NCCN). (2018c). *NCCN guidelines for distress management version 2.2018: distress management.* Retrieved from https://www.nccn.org/professionals/physician_gls/pdf/distress.pdf.

National Consensus Project for Quality Palliative Care. (2013). *The National Consensus Project clinical practice guidelines for quality palliative care.* Retrieved from http://www.nationalcoalitionhpc.org/ncp-guidelines-2013/.

National Hospice and Palliative Care Organization. (2007). *Social Work Assessment Tool.* Retrieved from https://www.nhpco.org/social-work-assessment-tool.

National Hospice and Palliative Care Organization. (2017). *History of hospice care.* Retrieved from www.nhpco.org/history-hospice-care.

National Hospice and Palliative Care Organization (NHPCO). (2018a). *Hospice care in America.* Rev. ed. Alexandria, VA: National Hospice and Palliative Care Organization

National Hospice and Palliative Care Organization (NHPCO). (2018b). *Palliative performance scale (v2).* Retrieved from http://www.nhhpco.org/s-content/uploads/files/Palliative_Performance_Scale1.pdf.

Oncology Nursing Society. (2014). *Oncology Nursing Society position statement on palliative care for people with cancer.* Retrieved from https://www.ons.org/advocacy-policy/positions/practice/palliative-care.

Ornstein, K., Wajnberg, A., Kaye-Kauderer, H., Winkel, G., DeCherrie, L., Zhang, M., & Soriano, T. (2013). Reduction in symptoms for homebound patients receiving home-based primary and palliative care. *J Palliat Med, 16*(9), 1048–1054. https://doi.org/10.1089/jpm.2012.0546.

Quill, T. E., & Abernethy, A. P. (2013). Generalist plus specialist palliative care: creating a more sustainable model. *New England Journal of Medicine, 368*(13), 1173–1175. https://doi.org/10.1056/NEJMp1215620.

Sandvik, R. K., Selbaek, G., Bergh, S., Aarsland, D., & Husebo, B. S. (2016). Signs of imminent dying and change in symptom intensity during pharmacological treatment in dying nursing home patients: a prospective trajectory study. *Journal of the American Medical Directors Association, 17*(9), 821–827. https://doi.org/10.1016/j.jamda.2016.05.006.

Shelkey, M., & Wallace, M. (2012). Katz index of independence in activities of daily living (ADL). *The Gerontologist, 10*(1), 20–30.

Smit, C. (2015). Theories and models of grief: applications to professional practice. *Whitireia Nursing & Health Journal*, (22), 33.

Smith, T. J., Temin, S., Alesi, E. R., Abernethy, A. P., Balboni, T. A., Basch, E. M., et al. (2012). American Society of Clinical Oncology provisional clinical opinion: the integration of palliative care into standard oncology care. *Journal of Clinical Oncology, 30*(8), 880–887. https://doi.org/10.1200/JCO.2011.38.5161.

Soliman, I. W., Cremer, O. L., de Lange, D. W., Slooter, A. J., van Delden, J. H. J., van Dijk, D., & Peelen, L. M. (2018). The ability of intensive care unit physicians to estimate long-term prognosis in survivors of critical illness. *Journal of Critical Care, 43*, 148–155. https://doi.org/10.1016/j.jcrc.2017.09.007.

Stephens, C. E., Hunt, L. J., Bui, N., Halifax, E., Ritchie, C. S., & Lee, S. J. (2018). Palliative care eligibility, symptom burden, and quality-of-life ratings in nursing home residents. *JAMA Internal Medicine, 178*(1), 141–142. https://doi.org/10.1001/jamainternmed.2017.6299.

Temel, J. S., Greer, J. A., Muzikansky, A., Gallagher, E. R., Admane, S., Jackson, V. A., & Lynch, T. J. (2010). Early palliative care for patients with metastatic non-small-cell lung cancer. *New England Journal of Medicine, 363*(8), 733–742. https://doi.org/10.1056/NEJMoa1000678.

Unterrainer, H. F., Lewis, A. J., & Fink, A. (2014). Religious/spiritual well-being, personality and mental health: a review of results and conceptual issues. *Journal of Religion and Health, 53*(2), 382–392. https://doi.org/10.1007/s10943-012-9642-5.

van den Beuken-van Everdingen, M. H., Hochstenbach, L. M., Joosten, E. A., Tjan-Heijnen, V. C., & Janssen, D. J. (2016). Update on prevalence of pain in patients with cancer: systematic review and meta-analysis. *Journal of Pain and Symptom Management, 51*(6), 1070–1090. https://doi.org/10.1016/j.jpainsymman.2015.12.340.

von Gunten, C. F. (2002). Secondary and tertiary palliative care in US hospitals. *Journal of the American Medical Association, 287*(7), 875–881.

Waldrop, D., & Kutner, J. S. (2013). What is prolonged grief disorder and how can its likelihood be reduced? In N. E. Goldstein & R. S. Morrison (Eds.), *Evidence-based practice of palliative medicine* (pp. 436–442). Philadelphia: Elsevier.

Watanabe, S. M., Nekolaichuk, C., Beaumont, C., Johnson, L., Myers, J., & Strasser, F. (2011). A multicenter study comparing two numerical versions of the Edmonton Symptom Assessment System in palliative care patients. *Journal of Pain and Symptom Management, 41*(2), 456–468. https://doi.org/10.1016/j.jpainsymman.2010.04.020.

Wee, B. L., Coleman, P. G., Hillier, R., & Holgate, S. T. (2008). Death rattle: its impact on staff and volunteers in palliative care. *Palliative Medicine, 22*(2), 173–176. https://doi.org/10.1177/0269216307087146.

Wiencek, C., & Coyne, P. (2014). Palliative care delivery models. *Seminars in Oncology Nursing, 30*(4), 227–233. https://doi.org/10.1016/j.soncn.2014.08.004.

Wilkie, D. J., & Ezenwa, M. O. (2012). Pain and symptom management in palliative care and at end of life. *Nursing Outlook, 60*(6), 357–364. https://doi.org/10.1016/j.outlook.2012.08.002.

WPCA Global atlas of palliative care at the end of life. (2014). Retrieved from http://www.who.int/nmh/Global_Atlas_of_Palliative_Care.pdf.

Zhang, B., Nilsson, M. E., & Prigerson, H. G. (2012). Factors important to patients' quality of life at the end of life. *Archives of Internal Medicine, 172*(15), 1133–1142. https://doi.org/10.1001/archinternmed.2012.2364.

Zimmermann, C., Swami, N., Krzyzanowska, M., Hannon, B., Leighl, N., Oza, A., & Donner, A. (2014). Early palliative care for patients with advanced cancer: a cluster-randomised controlled trial. *The Lancet, 383*(9930), 1721–1730. https://doi.org/10.1016/S0140-6736(13)62416-2.

Zubrod, C. (1960). Appraisal of methods for the study of chemotherapy in man: comparative therapeutic trial of nitrogen mustard and thiophosphoramide. *Journal of Chronic Diseases, 11*, 7–33.

5

Nurse Navigation Across the Cancer Continuum

Shama Shrestha and Ellen Carr

OVERVIEW

I. Definitions and roles
- A. Definition: the navigator role in the oncology setting includes patient navigator, care navigator, professional nurse navigator, cancer care navigator, nurse navigator, and oncology nurse navigator (ONN) (Table 5.1).
  1. Various standards and guidelines define and recommend navigator role functions, minimum education, and operational practice settings (ONS, 2013, 2017) (Tables 5.1 and 5.2).
  2. Each navigation program differs, based on the needs and resources of the health care facility providing care (Cantril, 2014).
  3. ONS recognized that ONNs were practicing without a clear definition of the role (ONS, 2017).
  4. According to ONS, an ONN is defined as a professional registered nurse with oncology-specific knowledge, who uses the nursing process to provide quality health care to patients with timely education and resources (ONS, 2015)
- B. Role delineation (Lubejko et al., 2016)
  1. Clarification of the role was needed to support its growth and standardization
  2. In 2012, ONS conducted a role delineation study (RDS) to clearly define the role.
     - a. The RDS led to development of the ONN Core Competencies (Tables 5.3 and 5.4)
  3. A second RDS (2016) revealed differences between a clinical oncology nurse and an ONN
     - a. ONN assists with patient/family navigation of the plan of care. This includes:
       - (1) Education and coaching of colleagues about the navigation role
       - (2) Collaboration to identify and establish best practices
- C. Competencies (ONS, 2017)
  1. ONN Core Competencies outline fundamental and advanced knowledge, skills, and expertise of an ONN. Four competency areas include:
     - a. Coordination of the care of patients with a past, current, or potential diagnosis of cancer
     - b. Communication—assist patients with cancer, families, and caregivers to overcome health care system barriers
     - c. Education and resources—facilitate informed decision making and timely access to quality health and psychosocial care throughout the cancer care continuum
     - d. Establish and maintain the professional role of the ONN—to promote quality improvement of an organization's navigation program
- D. Certifications
  1. ONN demonstrates strong oncology knowledge
  2. Foundation for ONN certification, based on role delineation studies
  3. Certifications established by the Oncology Nursing Certification Corporation (ONCC) exist (but not nurse navigator–specific) (ONCC, 2018)
  4. From the Academy of Oncology Nurse & Patient Navigators (AONN+) (AONN+, 2018)
     - a. Oncology Nurse Navigator–Certified Generalist (ONN-CG)
     - b. Oncology Patient Navigator–Certified Generalist (OPN-CG)
     - c. Oncology Nurse Navigator–Certified Generalist Thoracic [ONN-CG(T)

II. History
- A. In 1990, first patient navigation program for medically underserved patients with breast cancer developed by Harold Freeman in New York City (Freeman, 2004; Freeman, 2015)
  1. Goal was to reduce cancer mortality rates by improving access to quality care
  2. High breast cancer mortality rate among poor black women
     - a. Fifty percent of the women were uninsured
     - b. Five-year survival rates improved from 39% to 70%
- B. In 2005, Cancer Patient Navigation Act was established
  1. Created to ensure patients receive high-quality care and coordination (Shockney, 2015)
- C. Patient Navigation Research Program (PNRP) data showed no difference in survival outcomes for patients with Medicaid coverage compared with

TABLE 5.1 Navigator Definitions

	Definition
Oncology Nurse Navigator (ONN)	An ONN is a professional RN with oncology-specific clinical knowledge who offers individualized assistance to patients, families, and caregivers to help overcome health care system barriers. Using the nursing process, an ONN provides education and resources to facilitate informed decision making and timely access to quality health and psychosocial care throughout all phases of the cancer continuum.
Lay Navigator	A trained nonprofessional or volunteer who provides individualized assistance to patients, families, and caregivers to help overcome health care system barriers and facilitate timely access to quality health and psychosocial care from prediagnosis through all phases of the cancer experience.
Novice ONN	A nurse who has worked 2 years or less in the ONN role and is building upon his or her academic preparation, nursing knowledge, and oncology navigation experience to develop in the ONN role.
Expert ONN	An ONN who has worked at least 3 years, is proficient in the role, and has the education and experience to use critical thinking and decision-making skills pertaining to the evolution of navigation processes and the individual ONN.

From Baileys, K., McMullen, L., Lubjeko, B., Christensen, D., Haylock, P., Rose, T., Srdranovic, D. (2018). Nurse navigator core competencies: an update to reflect the evolution of the role. Clinical Journal of Oncology Nursing, 22(3): 272–281. Retrieved from https://doi.org/10.1188/18.CJON.272-281.

TABLE 5.2 Navigator Preparation

Job Title	Recommended Preparation
Lay Patient Navigators	No professional degree, medical licensure, or credentials; education at or below a bachelor's degree
Allied health patient navigators	Professional backgrounds (i.e., medical assistants), educational degrees higher than bachelor's degree but not clinically focused
Nurse navigators	Two-year or BSN or RN, APN, NP, and other nursing backgrounds
Social worker/counselor	Education with at least a BS in social work, MS in counseling; Licensed mental health counselors
Other health navigators	Did not fit the earlier categories

From Wells, K., Valverde, P., Ustjanauskas, A., Calhoun, E., & Risendal, B. (2018). What are patient navigators doing, for whom, and where? A national survey evaluating the types of services provided by patient navigators. Patient Education and Counseling (PEC), 101(2), 285–294. Retrieved from https://doi.org/10.1016/j.pec.2017.08.017.

uninsured patients, despite the passage of the Affordable Care Act in 2010 (Freeman, 2015)
1. Data demonstrated additional nonfinancial barriers to care, including variables associated with poverty:
   a. Unemployment
   b. Lack of adequate social support
   c. Lower education levels
2. One PNRP study demonstrated delays in cancer diagnosis can be overcome by patient navigation, addressing barriers such as unemployment, housing type, and marital status.
D. Incorporated in 2009, the Academy of Oncology Nurse and Patient Navigators (AONN+) provides a network for professionals involved and interested in patient navigation and survivorship care services toward managing complex care over the cancer care treatment continuum (AONN+, 2018)
   1. ONN certification platform to demonstrate their skills, expertise, and knowledge
   2. The AONN+ created a network of nurse navigators and patient navigators interested in enhancing and promoting their roles in navigation
E. In 2010, the Oncology Nursing Society (ONS), Association of Oncology Social Work, and National Association of Social Workers published a joint position statement: *Joint Position Statement on the Role of Oncology Nursing and Oncology Social Work in Patient Navigation* (ONS/AOSW/NASW, 2010).
F. American College of Surgeons (ACOS) Commission on Cancer (CoC) added patient navigation as a requirement for CoC accreditation in 2015 (ACS, 2016; Newcomer, 2014)
   1. Although initially patient navigation included cancer prevention, it now includes the entire health continuum: prevention, detection of disease, diagnosis, treatment, and survivorship care (Freeman, 2015)
   2. In 2015, the CoC issued updated Cancer Program Standards
      a. The standards established a foundation for patient-centered care
      b. The program standards established that patient navigation was a required standard to earn and maintain CoC accreditation (ACS, 2016) (Table 5.5).
G. Oncology Nursing Society (ONS) (ONS, 2017)
   1. In 2015—then revised in 2017—ONS established a position statement: Role of the Oncology Nurse Navigator Throughout the Cancer Trajectory
   2. ONS established the Nurse Navigator Special Interest Group (SIG) in 2010
   3. ONS Nurse Navigator SIG was renamed the Navigation and Care Coordinator Community to highlight the ONN role in care coordination in 2016 (ONS, 2017)

TABLE 5.3   Oncology Nurse Navigation (ONN) Competency Categories for Novice Navigator

Competency Category 1: Coordination of Care	The Oncology Nurse Navigator (ONN) facilitates the appropriate and efficient delivery of health care services, both within and across systems, and serves as the key contact to promote optimal outcomes while delivering patient-centered care.
	Assesses patient needs upon initial encounter and periodically throughout navigation, matching unmet needs with appropriate services, referrals, and support services, such as palliative care, dietitians, medical providers, social work, pre-/rehabilitation, and legal and financial services.
	Identifies potential and realized barriers to care (e.g., transportation, child care, elder care, housing, language, culture, literacy, role disparity, psychosocial, employment, financial, insurance) and facilitates referrals as appropriate to mitigate barriers.
	Develops knowledge of available local, community, or national resources and the quality of services provided; also establishes relationships with the providers of these services.
	Develops or uses appropriate screening/assessment tools and methods (e.g., Distress Thermometer, pain scale, fatigue scale, performance status, motivational interviewing, financial) to promote a consistent, holistic plan of care.
	Facilitates timely scheduling of appointments, diagnostic testing, and procedures to expedite the plan of care and to promote continuity of care.
	Participates in coordination of the plan of care with the multidisciplinary team, promoting timely follow-up on treatment and supportive care recommendations (e.g., cancer conferences/tumor boards).
	Facilitates individualized care within the context of functional status, cultural consideration, health literacy, psychosocial, reproductive/fertility, and spiritual needs for patients, families, and caregivers.
	Applies knowledge of clinical guidelines (e.g., National Comprehensive Cancer Network, American Joint Committee on Cancer) and specialty resources (e.g., ONS Putting Evidence into Practice resources) throughout the cancer continuum.
	Assists in the identification of candidates for molecular testing and/or genetic testing and counseling, and facilitates appropriate referrals.
	Supports a smooth transition of patients from active treatment into survivorship, chronic cancer management, or end-of-life care.
	Assists patients with cancer with issues related to treatment goals, advance directives, palliative care, and end-of-life concerns using an ethical framework that is nonjudgmental and nondiscriminatory.
	Ensures documentation of patient encounters and provided services.
	Applies knowledge of insurance processes (e.g., Medicare, Medicaid, third-party payers) and their impact on staging, referrals, and patient care decisions toward establishing appropriate referrals, as needed.
Competency Category 2: Communication	The ONN demonstrates interpersonal communication skills that enable exchange of ideas and information effectively with patients, families, and colleagues at all levels. This includes writing, speaking, and listening skills.
	Builds therapeutic and trusting relationships with patients, families, and caregivers through effective communication and listening skills.
	Acts as a liaison between the patients, families, and caregivers, and the providers to optimize outcomes.
	Advocates for patients to promote patient-centered care that includes shared decision making and patients' goals of care with optimal outcomes.
	Provides psychosocial support to and facilitates appropriate referrals for patients, families, and caregivers, especially during periods of high emotional stress and anxiety.
	Empowers patients and families to self-advocate and communicate their needs.
	Adheres to established regulations concerning patient information and privacy.
	Promotes a patient- and family-centered care environment for ethical decision making and advocacy for patients with cancer.
	Ensures that communication is culturally sensitive and appropriate for identified level of health literacy.
	Facilitates communication among members of the multidisciplinary cancer care team to prevent fragmented or delayed care that could adversely affect patient outcomes.
Competency Category 3: Education	The ONN provides appropriate and timely education to patients, families, and caregivers to facilitate understanding and support informed decision making.
	Promotes lifelong learning and evidence-based practice to improve the care of patients with a past, current, or potential diagnosis of cancer.
	Demonstrates effective communication with peers, members of the multidisciplinary health care team, and community organizations and resources.
	Contributes to ONN program and role development, implementation, and evaluation within the health care system and community.
	Participates in the tracking and monitoring of metrics and outcomes, in collaboration with administration, to document and evaluate outcomes of the navigation program and report findings to the cancer committee.
	Collaborates with the cancer committee and administration to perform and evaluate data from the community needs assessment to identify areas of improvement that will affect the patient navigation process and participate in quality improvement based on identified service gaps.

TABLE 5.3	Oncology Nurse Navigation (ONN) Competency Categories for Novice Navigator—cont'd
Competency Category 4: Professional Role	In collaboration with other members of the health care team, builds partnerships with local agencies and groups that may assist with cancer patient care, support, or educational needs.
	Establishes and maintains professional role boundaries with patients, caregivers, and the multidisciplinary care team in collaboration with manager, as defined by job description.
	The ONN works to promote and advance the role of the ONN and takes responsibility to pursue personal professional growth and development. In addition, the ONN facilitates continual promotion and quality improvement of the organization's navigation program to best meet the needs of their community.
	Promotes lifelong learning and evidence-based practice to improve the care of patients with a past, current, or potential diagnosis of cancer.
	Demonstrates effective communication with peers, members of the multidisciplinary health care team, and community organizations and resources.
	Contributes to ONN program and role development, implementation, and evaluation within the health care system and community.
	Participates in the tracking and monitoring of metrics and outcomes, in collaboration with administration, to document and evaluate outcomes of the navigation program and report findings to the cancer committee.

(From Baileys, K., McMullen, L., Lubjeko, B., Christensen, D., Haylock, P., Rose, T., Srdranovic, D. (2018). Nurse Navigator core competencies: An Update to Reflect the Evolution of the Role. Clinical Journal of Oncology Nursing, 22(3): 272–281. doi: 10.1188/18.CJON.272-281.)

TABLE 5.4	Oncology Nurse Navigation (ONN): Additional Expert Competency Category (#5)
Competency Category 5: Expert Oncology Nurse Navigator	The expert ONN is proficient in the role and has the education, knowledge, and experience to use critical thinking and decision-making skills pertaining to the evolution of the ONN role and process improvement in the navigation processes.
	Contributes to development of the cancer program community needs assessment and makes suggestions to the cancer committee on navigation program changes related to community assessment outcomes and cancer program strategic plan.
	Assists in gap analysis, quality improvement, and process improvement measures, data analysis, and makes recommendations to the cancer committee for appropriate navigation program changes related to the data.
	Develops and promotes pathways for ONN patient recruitment by collaborating with internal and external stakeholders.
	Tracks use of internal and external resources of staff and patients and makes recommendations for appropriate or improved use as needed.
	Expands current or develops new processes to survey patient and/or caregiver satisfaction related to navigation services, collects results, and reports to cancer committee.
	Contributes to program growth through collaboration with cancer program administration to develop a marketing strategy to support the navigation program.
	Contributes to the knowledge base of the health care community and in support of the ONN role through activities such as involvement in professional organizations, presentations, publications, and research.
	Disseminates information about the ONN role to other health care team members through peer education, mentoring, and preceptor experiences.
	Collaborates with treating physician(s) and support staff to prevent unnecessary hospitalizations or clinic visits and improve adherence to treatment through the design and implementation of appropriate patient education and follow-up.
	Orients, mentors, and guides novice ONNs.
	Collaborates with cancer program administration and cancer committee to develop strategies to fulfill the requirements and standards of the American College of Surgeons Commission on Cancer.
	Contributes to program sustainability, improvement, and/or development through collaboration with the institutional foundation in grant writing and philanthropy.

(From Baileys, K., McMullen, L., Lubjeko, B., Christensen, D., Haylock, P., Rose, T., Srdranovic, D. (2018). Nurse Navigator core competencies: An Update to Reflect the Evolution of the Role. Clinical Journal of Oncology Nursing, 22(3): 272–281. doi: 10.1188/18.CJON.272-281.).)

TABLE 5.5   Patient Navigation Process: Comparison of Standards, 2012, 2016

	Previous Standard Description 2012	New Standard Description 2016
Standard 3.1 Patient Navigation Process	A patient navigation process, driven by a community needs assessment, is established to address health care disparities and barriers to care for patients. Resources to address identified disparities and barriers may be provided either onsite or by referral to community-based or national organizations. Each calendar year, the navigation process is evaluated, modified, or enhanced and reported to the cancer committee.	A patient navigation process, driven by a triennial community needs assessment, is established to address health care disparities and barriers to cancer care. Resources to address identified barriers may be provided either onsite or by referral.

Data from American College of Surgeons (ACS). (2016). Commission on Cancer: Cancer Program Standards. Retrieved from https://www.facs.org/quality-programs/cancer/coc/standards.

III. Measuring ONN value
 A. Components of oncology nursing navigation programs (Pratt-Chapman, 2016; Gordils-Perez et al., 2017; Harding, 2015)
  1. Relationship building: with providers, with patients and families
   a. Efficient communication
   b. Timely psychosocial support
  2. Provide expertise and education to patients and family members, based on foundation of oncology patient diagnosis, treatment, and survivorship
 B. Methods and strategies to measure ONN value, patient outcomes of care (Gordils-Perez et al., 2017; Harding, 2015. Johnson, 2015; Crane-Okada, 2013)
  1. Timeliness of care; access to care
  2. Management and monitoring of plan of care
   a. Symptom management
  3. Provider, patient, and family satisfaction scores
  4. Clinical trial accrual
  5. Health care system utilization
   a. Reduces hospital readmissions
 C. Develop template to identify essential components of care by ONNs to measure outcomes (Pratt-

Chapman, 2016; Newcomer, 2014; Hryniuk, Simpson, McGowan, & Carter, 2014). Study designs capture:
 1. Cancer patient population focus
 2. Consistent and reliable support for patients and family members
  a. Effective communication
  b. Timely and appropriate psychosocial support
   (1) Initial and ongoing administration of distress tools and evaluation of interventions to address distress, based on distress tool scoring
 3. Outcomes that eliminate barriers to treatment
  a. Expedited referrals
  b. Prompt initiation and continuation of treatment sessions
 4. ONNs provide ongoing conduit to patients and families—orientation, education, and resources
IV. Research and evidence-based practice/limitations
 A. Limitation of published research; additional published studies need to demonstrate effectiveness, improved patient outcomes due to contributions of ONN (ONS, 2017)
 B. Replicating existing navigation programs is difficult due to:
  1. Lack of standardized job descriptions
  2. Lack of standardized processes
  3. Lack of standardized ONN qualifications (credentials, competencies, education, preparation, and experience)
 C. When evaluating the benefits of navigation and ONN contributions, consider these strategies and components in study designs (Baik, Gallo, & Wells, 2016):
  1. Increasing the number of participants/patients
  2. Participants/patients representing ethnic and financial diversity
  3. After initiating navigation, conduct 5-year studies to monitor recurrence of disease and survivorship care
  4. Carefully examine processes that link navigation to improved patient outcomes
 D. To date, ONN outcome studies have limitations (Hryniuk et al., 2014):
  1. Relatively small sample sizes
  2. Poor or incomplete response rates to questionnaires
  3. Questionnaire data: lack of reliable and valid instruments to gather data
  4. Lack of data about patients who have used navigation services
   a. When ONN consulting, what services have been provided? Screening? Assessment? Providing referrals or resources?
  5. Incomplete disclosure of sensitive information, such as care costs or insufficient time to discuss costs (Spencer et al., 2018)
 E. Types of practice settings (urban vs. rural) and location in the United States and other countries—

additional need for navigation services (Spencer et al., 2017)

1. Geographic differences and the need for oncology care navigators
2. Differences in Medicaid expansion that would support navigation services
3. Oral chemotherapy parity legislation

F. Qualitative research studies are difficult to replicate: about nurse navigation and the ONN as an effective role in the delivery of patient care (Melhem & Daneault, 2017)

1. Best to compare qualitative study results to other qualitative studies with same study designs.

ASSESSMENT

I. Patient history and plan of care (Miller, 2018; Gordils-Perez et al., 2017)
   A. Assess patient's history, clinical status, barriers to care
   B. Caregiver and family support
II. Psychosocial assessment
   A. Distress assessment is focus of cancer patient clinical care (Hanes-Lewis et al., 2018; NCCN, 2018)
      1. Assessment is foundation for psychosocial support and resources
      2. Assessment includes family and caregiver support
      3. NCCN is frequent source of distress assessment tools

MANAGEMENT

I. ONN coordinates plan of care, based on health care system, options, and accessible resources

A. Goals of navigation service (Cantril, 2014; Hryniuk et al., 2014; Cantril & Haylock, 2013):
   1. Provide education about treatment plan that empowers clients to actively engage in decision making and self-care
   2. Facilitate timely access to care and treatment, based on treatment guidelines
      a. Identify and resolve barriers
   3. Provide education on symptom and side effect management to reduce early and late treatment-associated complications
      a. Access to resources
      b. Expedite referrals
   4. Reduce distress, provide psychosocial support
   5. Liaison for patient, family members, and patient's health care providers.
      a. Serve as the patient's advocate
B. Navigation models of care
C. Cancer care continuum (IOM, 2013; McMullen et al., 2016; Newcomer, 2014) (Fig. 5.1).
   1. Prevention and risk reduction
      a. Within survivorship programs—includes some community outreach, education, surveillance programs
   2. Screening—triage newly referred patients (Zibrik et al., 2016)
   3. Diagnosis
      a. In conjunction with providers and support staff, the nurse navigator ensures there are orders for stage-appropriate tests: radiology, diagnostic, and molecular tests (for example, epidermal growth factor receptor [EGFR] testing)

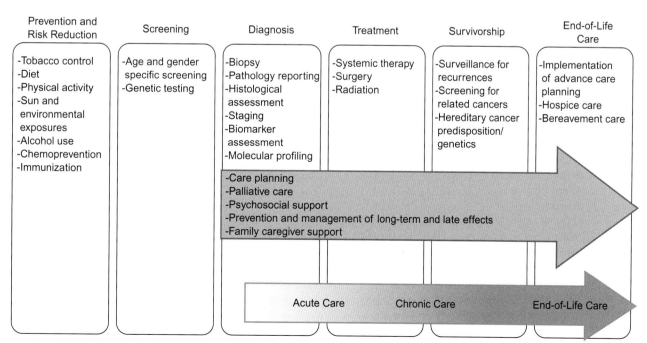

Fig. 5.1 Cancer Care Continuum Model. (From Institute of Medicine (IOM). (2013). *Delivering high-quality cancer care: charting a new course for a system in crisis.* Washington, D.C: National Academies Press.)

b. Ensure timely medical and oncology-related clinic appointments

c. Follow guidelines for workup; ensure they are complete

d. Oncology case conferences/tumor board review

e. Molecular profiling

    (1) ONN expedited genomic testing to support timely decision making (McAllister & Schmitt, 2015)

4. Treatments—consistent and available interpreter of plan of care, once established

5. Survivorship

    a. Initiate and maintain surveillance programs

    b. Screen for late and long-term side effects, recurrent disease, secondary malignancies

6. Palliative care

7. End-of-life care—coordinate and expedite referrals to hospice resources

D. Transitional care model (McMullen, 2013)

  1. Continuity of care, especially for high-risk patients

  2. Focus: hospitalized patients—goal to reduce patient complications and readmissions

E. ONN care model (ONS, 2017)

  1. Continuity of care and coordination of care, based on providers in the community

  2. Includes cultural traditions in the community, survivorship

F. Planetree model (Cantril, 2014)

  1. Holistic, patient-centered focus

  2. Supports patient autonomy and decision making

  3. Patient participation in managing illness

III. Address barriers to care

A. Access to care—patient navigation is important to reduce or eliminate barriers to access quality cancer care (Baik et al., 2016; Cantril & Haylock, 2013)

  1. Access to timely diagnosis and initiation of treatment are barriers to quality care (Baik et al., 2016; Freeman, 2015).

B. Barriers to care also include financial, transportation, language differences, cultural and ethnic diversity, and communication among the health care team and patients, as well as barriers to emotional support (Shockney, 2015)

  1. Lack of resources, lack of knowledge about resources, ability to complete complex/duplicative paperwork

    a. Child care

    b. Lodging

  2. Insufficient resources or patient ineligibility for existing resources due to living in rural areas, patients without citizenship, being underinsured, having income levels above specific program thresholds

  3. Lack of patient connection with others, reluctance to request assistance, embarrassment about situation

  4. Language and literacy as barriers

C. Psychosocial distress (NCCN, 2018)

  1. Assess, monitor, document, and intervene at all stages of disease

  2. Assess frequently (i.e., each clinic visit)

  3. Follow clinical practice guidelines for assessment and intervention

D. Managing/alleviating financial toxicity (Spencer et al., 2018; Fessele, 2017)

  1. Twenty percent to 48% of patients with cancer report significant financial burden due to their cancer treatment

  2. Patients with cancer are 2.6 times more likely to declare bankruptcy than the general population

  3. Navigators can facilitate financial assistance for patient treatment and costs associated with receiving treatment:

    a. Medication or prescription drug assistance programs

    b. Charity care

    c. Copay assistance

    d. Assistance with nonmedical expenses, such as transportation or lodging

IV. Management exemplars

A. Example #1: ONN contributions lead to thorough workups, prompt initiation of therapy (Zibrik et al., 2016)

  1. After the nurse navigator role was added as a component of care delivery, molecular testing results were more often available at the time of consultation, reducing the number of repeat visits and quicker initiation of therapy

  2. More patients received systemic therapy

  3. Rates of molecular testing increased from 62% to 91%.

  4. Thirty-seven percent of patients' molecular profiling results were available at the consultation compared with 6% before navigation implementation

  5. Patients could start systemic therapy, on average, 10 calendar days sooner than baseline (previous) start dates

B. Example #2: Patient perception of navigation services and benefits (Hryniuk et al., 2014)

  1. The CAREpath Navigation Service in Canada conducted a survey of patient perceptions about comprehensive cancer navigation services (85 of 118 patients completed). Results of CAREpath Navigation Service survey:

  2. Ninety-eight percent reported they appreciated having a designated oncology nurse

  3. Eighty-nine percent to 95% reported the navigation service was important beyond the service they received from the provincial health system

  4. Fifty-two percent to 88% reported the service was very important

  5. Sixty percent reported being grateful about the advice received about returning to work

C. Example #3: Head/neck cancer diagnosis and treatment coordination (Ohlstein et al., 2015)

  1. Study to evaluate ONN effectiveness: head/neck cancer

a. Before consult, nurse obtained and reviewed outside records

b. Records review could indicate need for additional tests

c. Patients presented at tumor board

d. Plan of care discussed with patient the next day

2. Study background: diagnostic delays can contribute to inferior treatment outcomes

a. 2011–2014 study: baseline data: >60% diagnosed at advanced stage; 5-year mean survival rate of 50%

b. This retrospective study measured the time interval between consultation and definitive treatment recommendations, with the goal being within 2 weeks

c. The clinic nurse functioned as the patient navigator to reduce costs and increase efficiency.

3. Study evaluated ONN effectiveness: head/neck cancer

a. Forty-seven out of 100 patients received treatment recommendations within 2 weeks of diagnosis

b. Two out of 100 patients had psychosocial needs/inadequate social support and could be referred to mental health care professionals by the navigator

c. Timing for patients equivalent despite different gender, races, or insurance status

D. Example #4: Palliative care coordination (Melhem & Daneault, 2017)

1. ONN coordinating palliative care was just as important to the patient as the physician in the patient's ongoing care

2. The ONN can address most relational needs and share/explain disease information

a. In addition to their medical needs, patients reported they had psychological, social, and spiritual needs addressed

3. ONN encounters increased patient satisfaction:

a. Ensured the patient understands his or her disease

b. Followed the patient from initial diagnosis, if possible

c. Provided the patient with emotional support; validated feelings; referred to other professionals, as needed

d. Listened attentively; was present without judgment; acknowledged the patient's experience and suffering

e. Ensured the patient's physical comfort; also comfort with the treatment plan and team

f. Was proactive to cooperate and communicate efficiently and effectively with other care providers

EXPECTED PATIENT OUTCOMES

I. The patient will receive timely cancer care without delays in diagnosis and treatment.

II. The patient will have access to quality cancer care throughout the cancer continuum.

REFERENCES

Academy of Oncology and Patient Navigators (AONN+). (2018). *Certification.* Retrieved from https://www.aonnonline.org/certification.

American College of Surgeons (ACS). (2016). *Commission on Cancer: Cancer Program Standards.* Retrieved from https://www.facs.org/quality-programs/cancer/coc/standards.

Baik, S., Gallo, L., & Wells, K. (2016). Patient navigation in breast cancer treatment and survivorship: a systematic review. *Journal of Clinical Oncology, 34*(30), 3686–3696. https://doi.org/10.1200/JCO.2016.67.5454.

Baileys, K., McMullen, L., Lubjeko, B., Christensen, D., Haylock, P., Rose, T., et al. (2018). Nurse Navigator core competencies: an update to reflect the evolution of the role. *Clinical Journal of Oncology Nursing, 22*(3), 272–281. https://doi.org/10.1188/18.CJON.272-281.

Cantril, C. (2014). Overview of nurse navigation. In K. Blaseg, P. Daugherty, & K. Gamblin (Eds.), *Oncology nurse navigation: delivering patient-centered care across the continuum* (pp. 1–13). Pittsburgh: Oncology Nursing Society.

Cantril, C., & Haylock, P. (2013). Patient navigation in the oncology care setting. *Seminars in Oncology Nursing, 29*(2), 76–90. https://doi.org/10.1016/j.soncn.2013.02.003.

Crane-Okada, R. (2013). Evaluation and outcome measures in patient navigation. *Seminars in Oncology Nursing, 29*(2), 128–140. https://doi.org/10.1016/j.soncn.2013.02.008.

Fessele, K. (2017). Financial toxicity: management as an adverse effect of cancer treatment. *Clinical Journal of Oncology Nursing, 21*(61), 762–764. https://doi.org/10.1188/17.CJON.762-764.

Freeman, H. (2004). A model patient navigation program. *Oncology Issues, 19,* 44–46.

Freeman, H. (2015). Patient navigation as a targeted intervention: for patients at high risk for delays in cancer care. *Cancer,* (November), 3930–3932. https://doi.org/10.1002/cncr.29610.

Gordils-Perez, J., Schneider, S., Gabel, M., & Trotter, K. (2017). Oncology nurse navigation: development and implementation of a program at a comprehensive cancer center. *Clinical Journal of Oncology Nursing, 21*(5), 581–588. https://doi.org/10.1188/17.CJON.581-588.

Hanes-Lewis, M., Clayton, M., Viswanathan, S., Moadel-Robblee, A., Clair, L., & Caserta, M. (2018). Distress and supportive care needs of ethnically diverse older adults with advanced or recurrent cancer. *Oncology Nursing Forum, 45*(4), 496–507. https://doi.org/10.1188/18.ONF.496-507.

Harding, M. (2015). Effect of nurse navigation on patient care satisfaction and distress associated with breast biopsy. *Clinical Journal of Oncology Nursing, 19*(1), E15–E20. https://doi.org/10.1188/15.CJON.E15-E20.

Hryniuk, W., Simpson, R., McGowan, A., & Carter, P. (2014). Patient perceptions of a comprehensive cancer navigation service. *Current Oncology, 21*(2), 69–76. https://doi.org/10.3747/co.21.1930.

Institute of Medicine (IOM). (2013). *Delivering high-quality cancer care: charting a new course for a system in crisis.* Washington, D.C: National Academies Press.

Johnson, F. (2015). Systematic review of oncology nurse practitioner navigation metrics. *Clinical Journal of Oncology Nursing, 19*(3), 308–313. https://doi.org/10.1188/15.CJON.308-313.

Lubejko, B., Bellfield, S., Kahn, E., Lee, C., Peterson, N., Rose, T., et al. (2016). Oncology navigation: results of the 2016 role delineation study. *Clinical Journal of Oncology Nursing, 21*(1), 43–50. https://doi.org/10.1188/17.CJON.43-50.

McAllister, K., & Schmitt, M. (2015). Impact of a nurse navigator on genomic testing and timely treatment decision making in patients with breast cancer. *Clinical Journal of Oncology Nursing, 19*(5), 510–2. https://doi.org/10.1188/15.CJON.510-512. 510-412.

McMullen, L. (2013). Oncology nurse navigators and the continuum of cancer care. *Seminars in Oncology Nursing, 29*(2), 105–117. https://doi.org/10.1016/j.soncn.2013.02.005.

McMullen, L., Banman, T., DeGroot, J., Scott, S., Srdanovic, D., & Mackey, H. (2016). Providing novice navigators with a GPS for role development: Oncology Nurse Navigator Competency Project. *Clinical Journal of Oncology Nursing, 20*(1), 33–38. Retrieved from https://doi.org/10.1188/16.CJON.20-01AP.

Melhem, D., & Daneault, S. (2017). Needs of cancer patients in palliative care during medical visits: qualitative study. *Canadian Family Physician, 63*(December), e536–e542.

Miller, E. (2018). Neuro-oncology nurse navigation: developing the role for a unique patient population. *Clinical Journal of Oncology Nursing, 22*(3), 347–349. https://doi.org/10.1188/18. CJON.347-349.

National Comprehensive Cancer Network (NCCN). (2018). *Distress Management, 2.2018.* Retrieved from www.nccn.org.

Newcomer, B. (2014). A national system approach to oncology patient population management across the continuum of care: how we standardized navigation. *Nursing Administration Quarterly, 38*(2), 138–146. https://doi.org/10.1097/ NAQ.0000000000000019.

Ohlstein, J., Brody-Camp, S., Friedman, S., Levy, J., Buell, J., & Friedlander, P. (2015). Initial experience of a patient navigation model for head and neck cancer. *JAMA Otolaryngol Head Neck Surg, 141*(9), 804–809. https://doi.org/10.1001/jamaoto. 2015.1467.

Oncology Nursing Certification Corporation (ONCC) (2018). Certifications. Retrieved from http://www.oncc.org/ certificationshttps://www.oncc.org/certifications.

Oncology Nursing Society (ONS). (2013). *Oncology nurse navigator core competencies.* Retrieved from https://www.ons.org/sites/ default/files/ONNCompetencies_rev.pdf.

Oncology Nursing Society (ONS). (2015). Oncology nurse navigation role and qualifications. *Oncology Nursing Forum, 42* (5), 447–448. https://doi.org/10.1188/15.ONF.447-448.

Oncology Nursing Society (ONS). (2017). *Oncology nurse navigator core competencies.* Retrieved from https://www.ons.org/sites/ default/files/2017ONNcompetencies.pdf.

Oncology Nursing Society (ONS) Association of Oncology Social Work (AOSW) and National Association of Social Workers (NASW). (2010). Joint position statement on the role of oncology nursing and oncology social work in patient navigation. *Oncology Nursing Forum, 37*, 251–252.

Pratt-Chapman, M. (2016). *What does a patient navigator do?* Retrieved from https://www.accc-cancer.org/docs/documents/ oncology-issues/articles/jf16/jf16-what-does-a-patient-navigator-do.pdf?sfvrsn=1d5651e3_9.

Shockney, L. (2015). Evolution of breast navigation and survivorship care. *The Breast Journal, 21*(1), 104–110. https://doi.org/10.1111/ tbj.12353. (21)1.

Spencer, J., Samuel, C., Rosenstein, D., Reeder-Hayes, K., Manning, M., Sellers, J., & Wheeler, S. (2018). Oncology navigators' perceptions of cancer-related financial burden and financial assistance resources. *Support Care Cancer, 26*(4), 1315–1321. Retrieved from https://doi.org/10.1007/s00520-017-3958-3.

Wells, K., Valverde, P., Ustjanauskas, A., Calhoun, E., & Risendal, B. (2018). What are patient navigators doing, for whom, and where? A national survey evaluating the types of services provided by patient navigators. *Patient Education and Counseling (PEC), 101*(2), 285–294. Retrieved from https://doi.org/10.1016/j.pec.2017.08.017.

Zibrik, K., Laskin, J., & Ho, C. (2016). Integration of a nurse navigator into the triage process for patients with non-small-cell-lung cancer: creating systematic improvements in patient care. *Current Oncology, 23*(3). https://doi.org/10.3747/co.23.2954. e2800-e283.

Communication and Shared Decision Making

Pamela Katz and Joseph D. Tariman

I. Shared decision making (SDM): historical background
  A. 1950s to 1970s post–World War II: model of care delivery for patient–physician relationship was predominantly patriarchal (McKinstry, 1992).
    1. Patients decline to become involved in selecting their own treatment
    2. In this case the patient is essentially saying, "It's up to you, doctor. You're the expert."
  B. Early 1970s: shared model of care is taking hold, particularly in cancer setting (Feldmann, 1973)
    1. Paternalistic model of care is becoming unpopular.
  C. Major factors for the emergence of SDM as the dominant model of care in today's health care
    1. Rising cost of health care (Ford, 1977)
    2. Increasing health care consumerism in the United States, Europe, Australia, and Canada (McDevitt, 1986; Price, 1981)
    3. Increased desire for consumer involvement, autonomy, and control over their care (Tariman et al., 2012).
    4. Emphasis of patient-centered care as an indicator of high-quality care (Institute of Medicine, 2001)
    5. Explosion of cancer treatment choices (Tariman et al., 2012)
II. Shared decision making: definition
  A. A care delivery model that facilitates treatment decision making during the patient encounter (Charles, Gafni, & Whelan, 1997, 1999)
  B. Steps in the SDM process (Agency for Healthcare Research and Quality, 2014)
    1. **Step 1: Involve your patient in the treatment decision process:** inform them of choices and invite them to be involved in the decisions.
    2. **Step 2: Assist your patient in comparing and evaluating treatment options:** discuss the risks and benefits of each option.
    3. **Step 3: Assess your patient's goals, values, and priorities:** understand and incorporate what matters most to your patient.
    4. **Step 4: Make a decision with your patient:** decide the best course of treatment as a team.
    5. **Step 5: Evaluate the treatment decision:** plan to follow up and revisit the decision, monitor progress, and revise as needed. Communication is a critical aspect of SDM (Siminoff & Step, 2005).
    6. Integrates a socially based process into the dynamics of the physician–patient relationship
    7. Examines antecedent factors that have potential to influence communication (e.g., prior medical care experiences, language and acculturation, cognitive status, education level)
    8. Emphasizes jointly constructed communication climate
    9. Outcome focuses on treatment preferences established by the patient and the treatment team (providers, nurses, interdisciplinary team)
  C. Key elements (Charles et al., 1999)
    1. At least two participants: clinician and patient; often includes other treatment team members and patient's family
    2. Both parties share information
    3. Both parties take steps to build consensus about preferred treatment, weighing risks and benefits
    4. Mutual agreement is reached between patient and clinician on treatment approach (verbal and/or written)
  D. SDM is the preferred model of care delivery by lawmakers and policymakers because it supports the patient's autonomy and empowers the patient to take responsibility of one's own health (Légaré et al., 2014)
  E. SDM has demonstrated short- and long-term benefits (Kane et al., 2014):
    1. Short-term benefits
      a. Increased confidence in treatment decisions
      b. Higher satisfaction with treatment decisions
      c. Enhanced trust with providers
      d. Improved self-efficacy
      e. Mental health—less stress and anxiety related to treatment decision making

2. Long-term benefits
   a. Patient treatment adherence
   b. Quality of life
   c. Disease remission
F. SDM care delivery model is advantageous for older adults (Ramsdale et al., 2017):
   1. Facilitates collaboration, communication, and patient-centeredness
   2. Minimizes the fragmentation that impairs the current provision of cancer care
   3. This is particularly important with older adults, given their potential for not proactively participating in their care based on a multitude of factors (generational, lessened communication abilities), as well as having multiple providers due to many comorbidities.

III. Barriers to SDM (McCarter et al., 2016)
   A. Barriers perceived by oncology nurses
      1. Practice barrier—nonnursing responsibilities (e.g., charting, administrative tasks) take away time from patients; lack of provider confidence in the ability to participate effectively.
      2. Patient barrier—lack of readiness for patient to participate in SDM; lack of knowledge to participate; age-related challenges (cognition, mindset) (Tariman et al, 2012)
      3. Institutional policy barrier—lack of institutional policy that allows specific block of nurse's time for patient education on therapy or lack of support for the process.
      4. Scope-of-practice barrier—Federal, state, and board of nursing laws and regulations that prohibit nurse practitioner from autonomous practice.
      5. Administration as a barrier—nursing administrators do not provide adequate support for nurses to actively participate in SDM process.
      6. Structural barrier—noisy environment (hospital); lack of privacy; lack of systemic alerts/triggers in the electronic medical record (to incorporate decision aids)
   B. Barriers perceived by oncologists (Charles, Gafni, & Whelan, 2004)
      1. Lack of time
      2. Patient anxiety
      3. Patient lack of information and/or misinformation
      4. Patient unwillingness or inability to participate
      5. Inability to talk in language patients can easily understand (Joseph-Williams, Elwyn, & Edwards, 2014)
      6. Lack of commonality in approaches to SDM, while maintaining flexibility for modifications (Légaré & Witteman, 2013)

IV. Patient preferences for decision making in oncology care
   A. Patients with cancer prefer to have a role in cancer care and treatment decision making (Singh et al., 2010; Tariman et al., 2010)
   B. Degner and Beaton's Pattern of Treatment Decision Making questionnaire (Fig. 6.1) (Degner & Beaton, 1987; Degner, Sloan, & Venkatesh, 1997) is the most widely used instrument to elicit patient's preferences for participation in cancer treatment decision-making process (Tariman et al., 2010)

V. Influential factors in treatment decision making in older adults; ages 60+ (Puts et al., 2015):
   A. Convenience and success rate of treatment
   B. Seeing necessity of treatment
   C. Trust in the physician
   D. Following the physician's recommendation

DEGNER and BEATON's Pattern of Decision Making

Active: Patient Controlled
Card A
   I prefer to make the final treatment decision.
Card B
   I prefer to make the final treatment decision after seriously considering my doctor's opinion.

Collaborative: Jointly Controlled
Card C
   I prefer that my doctor and I share responsibility for deciding which treatment is best.

Passive: Provider Controlled
Card D
   I prefer my doctor to make the final treatment decision, but only after my doctor has seriously considered my opinion.
Card E
   I prefer to leave all treatment decisions to my doctor.

Fig. 6.1 The most widely used instrument to elicit patient's preferences for participation in health care decision making. (From Degner, L. F., & Beaton, J. I. [1987]. *Life death decisions in health care.* New York: Hemisphere Publishing.)

VI. Patient information needs
   A. Information priorities in patients diagnosed with cancer (Tariman et al., 2014):
      1. Diagnosis
      2. Prognosis
      3. Treatment options
   B. Assertion of independence and how to maintain self-care are priority information needs in older adults diagnosed with cancer (Sattar et al., 2018; Tariman et al., 2015)
VII. Quality of communication and clinician factors
   A. Clinician characteristics that have a positive impact on quality of communication and/or patient outcomes (De Vries et al., 2014)
      1. Communication skills training
      2. An external locus of control (focus on outward aspects from their own being, such as institutional and administrative factors)
      3. Empathy
      4. Socioemotional approach
      5. Shared decision-making style
   B. Clinician characteristics that have a negative impact on patient outcomes
      1. Increased level of fatigue
      2. Burnout
      3. Expression of worry
VIII. Decision aids and SDM (Kojovic & Tariman, 2017)
   A. Decision aids for health treatment and screening decisions (Stacey et al., 2014)
      1. Explicit values clarification exercises improve informed values-based choices
      2. Positive effect on patient–practitioner communication
      3. Variable effect on length of consultation
      4. Increase patient's involvement and improve knowledge and realistic perception of outcomes
      5. Less is known about the degree of detail that decision aids need in order to have positive effects on attributes of the decision or decision-making process, but they are proven to have positive effects.
IX. Nursing roles during SDM (Tariman et al., 2016; Tariman & Szubski, 2015)
   A. Patient needs assessment
   B. Information sharing with oncology team
   C. Patient education
   D. Advocacy
   E. Psychological support
   F. Outcome evaluation
   G. Management of side effects
   H. Complex role contingent on several variables within the context of uncertainty
X. Opportunities to improve outcomes related to SDM
   A. Develop institutional policy supporting SDM model in current practice
      B. Delineate the roles of nurses during SDM, particularly advocacy and patient education on treatment options
      C. Annual education and training of nurses on SDM (as well as all treatment team members)
      D. Develop and test a conceptual model of the roles of oncology nurses during SDM
      E. Develop a measurement tool to assess the role competence of oncology nurses in SDM; nurses need more support and training to feel competent as part of the process (Katz, Tariman, Hartle, & Szubski, 2017)

REFERENCES

Agency for Healthcare Research and Quality. (2014). *The SHARE Approach Essential Steps of Shared Decision Making*. Content last reviewed April 2014. In: *Agency for Healthcare Research and Quality*. Rockville: MD. http://www.ahrq.gov/professionals/education/curriculumtools/shareddecisionmaking/tools/shareposter/index.html.

Charles, C., Gafni, A., & Whelan, T. (1997). Shared decision-making in the medical encounter: what does it mean? (or it takes at least two to tango). *Social Science & Medicine, 44*(5), 681–692. https://doi.org/S0277953696002213 [pii].

Charles, C., Gafni, A., & Whelan, T. (1999). Decision-making in the physician-patient encounter: revisiting the shared treatment decision-making model. *Social Science & Medicine, 49*(5), 651–661.

Charles, C., Gafni, A., & Whelan, T. (2004). Self-reported use of shared decision-making among breast cancer specialists and perceived barriers and facilitators to implementing this approach. *Health Expectations, 7*(4), 338–348. HEX299 [pii] https://doi.org/10.1111/j.1369-7625.2004.00299.x.

De Vries, A. M., de Roten, Y., Meystre, C., Passchier, J., Despland, J. N., & Stiefel, F. (2014). Clinician characteristics, communication, and patient outcome in oncology: a systematic review. *Psychooncology, 23*(4), 375–381. https://doi.org/10.1002/pon.3445.

Degner, L. F., & Beaton, J. I. (1987). *Life death decisions in health care.* New York: Hemisphere Publishing.

Degner, L. F., Sloan, J. A., & Venkatesh, P. (1997). The Control Preferences Scale. *Canadian Journal of Nursing Research, 29*(3), 21–43.

Feldmann, E. G. (1973). Editorial: paternalism is out. *Journal of Pharmaceutical Sciences, 62*(10), 1.

Ford, H. (1977). The rising cost of health care: the health services "crisis"—reality or fantasy? *Journal of the Tennessee Medical Association, 70*(11), 822–827.

Institute of Medicine. (2001). *Crossing the quality chasm: a new health system for the 21st century.* Washington, DC: The National Academies Press.

Joseph-Williams, N., Elwyn, G., & Edwards, A. (2014). Knowledge is not power for patients: a systematic review and thematic synthesis of patient-reported barriers and facilitators to shared decision making. *Patient Education and Counseling, 94*(3), 291–309. doi: S0738-3991(13)00472-2 [pii] https://doi.org/10.1016/j.jpec.2013.10.031.

Kane, H. L., Halpern, M. T., Squiers, L. B., Treiman, K. A., & McCormack, L. A. (2014). Implementing and evaluating shared decision making in oncology practice. *CA: A Cancer Journal for Clinicians, 64*(6), 377–388. https://doi.org/10.3322/caac.21245.

Katz, P., Tariman, J. D., Hartle, L., & Szubski, K. (2017). Development and testing of cancer treatment shared decision making scale for nurses (SDMS-N). In: *STTI 28th International Nursing Research Congress.* http://www.nursinglibrary.org/vhl/handle/10755/621570.

Kojovic, B., & Tariman, J. D. (2017). Decision aids: assisting patients with multiple myeloma and caregivers with treatment decision making. *Clinical Journal of Oncology Nursing, 21*(6), 660–664. https://doi.org/10.1188/17.CJON.660-664.

Légaré, F., & Witteman, H. O. (2013). Shared decision making: examining key elements and barriers to adoption into routine clinical practice. *Health Aff (Millwood), 32*(2), 276–284. https://doi.org/10.1377/hlthaff.2012.1078. Review. PubMed PMID: 23381520.

Légaré, F., Stacey, D., Turcotte, S., Cossi, M. J., Kryworuchko, J., Graham, I. D., & Donner-Banzhoff, N. (2014). Interventions for improving the adoption of shared decision making by healthcare professionals. *Cochrane Database of Systematic Reviews*(9), CD006732. https://doi.org/10.1002/14651858. CD006732.pub3.

McCarter, S. P., Tariman, J. D., Spawn, N., Mehmeti, E., Bishop-Royse, J., Garcia, I., & Szubski, K. (2016). Barriers and promoters to participation in the era of shared treatment decision-making. *Western Journal of Nursing Research, 38*(10), 1282–1297. https://doi.org/10.1177/0193945916650648.

McDevitt, P. K. (1986). Health care consumerism: the new force. *Journal of Hospital Marketing, 1*(1-2), 43–57.

McKinstry, B. (1992). Paternalism and the doctor-patient relationship in general practice. *British Journal of General Practice, 42*(361), 340–342.

Price, R. (1981). Consumerism in health—are we accountable and if so, how? *Australian Nurses Journal, 10*(9), 50–52.

Puts, M. T., Tapscott, B., Fitch, M., Howell, D., Monette, J., Wan-Chow-Wah, D., & Alibhai, S. M. (2015). A systematic review of factors influencing older adults' decision to accept or decline cancer treatment. *Cancer Treatment Reviews, 41*(2), 197–215. https://doi.org/10.1016/j.ctrv.2014.12.010.

Ramsdale, E. E., Csik, V., Chapman, A. E., Naeim, A., & Canin, B. (2017). *Improving quality and value of cancer care for older adults.* 37 (pp. 383–393). American Society of Clinical Oncology Education Book. https://doi.org/10.14694/EDBK_175442.

Sattar, S., Alibhai, S. M. H., Fitch, M., Krzyzanowska, M., Leighl, N., & Puts, M. T. E. (2018). Chemotherapy and radiation treatment decision-making experiences of older adults with cancer: a qualitative study. *Journal of Geriatric Oncology, 9*(1), 47–52. https://doi.org/10.1016/j.jgo.2017.07.013.

Siminoff, L. A., & Step, M. M. (2005). A communication model of shared decision making: accounting for cancer treatment decisions. *Health Psychology, 24*(4 Suppl), S99–S105. 2005-08085-015 [pii] https://doi.org/10.1037/0278-6133.24.4.S99.

Singh, J. A., Sloan, J. A., Atherton, P. J., Smith, T., Hack, T. F., Huschka, M. M., & Degner, L. F. (2010). Preferred roles in treatment decision making among patients with cancer: a pooled analysis of studies using the Control Preferences Scale. *American Journal of Managed Care, 16*(9), 688–696. doi:12718 [pii].

Stacey, D., Légaré, F., Col, N. F., Bennett, C. L., Barry, M. J., Eden, K. B., & Wu, J. H. (2014). Decision aids for people facing health treatment or screening decisions. *Cochrane Database of Systematic Reviews*(1). CD001431. https://doi.org/10.1002/14651858.CD001431.pub4.

Tariman, J. D., Berry, D. L., Cochrane, B., Doorenbos, A., & Schepp, K. (2010). Preferred and actual participation roles during health care decision making in persons with cancer: a systematic review. *Annals of Oncology, 21*(6), 1145–1151. mdp534 [pii] https://doi.org/10.1093/annonc/mdp534.

Tariman, J. D., Berry, D. L., Cochrane, B., Doorenbos, A., & Schepp, K. G. (2012). Physician, patient, and contextual factors affecting treatment decisions in older adults with cancer and models of decision making: a literature review. *Oncology Nursing Forum, 39*(1), E70–E83. doi: X90151107806H032 [pii] https://doi.org/10.1188/12.ONF.E70-E83.

Tariman, J. D., Doorenbos, A., Schepp, K. G., Singhal, S., & Berry, D. L. (2014). Information needs priorities in patients diagnosed with cancer: a systematic review. *Journal of the Advanced Practitioner in Oncology, 2014*(5), 115–122.

Tariman, J. D., Doorenbos, A., Schepp, K. G., Singhal, S., & Berry, D. L. (2015). Top information need priorities of older adults newly diagnosed with active myeloma. *Journal of the Advanced Practitioner in Oncology, 6*(1), 14–21.

Tariman, J. D., Mehmeti, E., Spawn, N., McCarter, S. P., Bishop-Royse, J., Garcia, I., & Szubski, K. (2016). Oncology nursing and shared decision making for cancer treatment. *Clinical Journal of Oncology Nursing, 20*(5), 560–563. https://doi.org/10.1188/16. CJON.560-563.

Tariman, J. D., & Szubski, K. L. (2015). The evolving role of the nurse during the cancer treatment decision-making process: a literature review. *Clinical Journal of Oncology Nursing, 19*(5), 548–556. https://doi.org/10.1188/15.CJON.548-556.

Carcinogenesis

Jennifer Alisangco Tschanz and Cathleen Sugarman

I. *Carcinogenesis:* normal cells are transformed into cancer cells through a complex and dynamic process that starts with mutations in regulatory cells and is promoted by genomic instability, inflammation, and interactions within the tumor microenvironment (Fig. 7.1).
   A. Causes of mutations
      1. Deoxyribonucleic acid (DNA) mutations can be caused by environmental factors known as *carcinogens*. Most DNA mutations are noninherited; also known as *somatic mutations.*
      2. Mutations can also be inherited or germline mutations.
         a. Currently, 853 known germline variants exist that contribute to cancer development; *BRCA1* and *BRCA2* are examples. When a person inherits one of these germline variants, he or she becomes more susceptible to certain types of cancer (Ding et al., 2018).
   B. Mutations in regulatory cells (Table 7.1):
      1. *Proto-oncogenes:* genes that code for proteins involved in normal cell growth. When mutated, they may enable a cancer cell to be self-sufficient in growth. A commonly used analogy is that the genes, when mutated, are like a car's gas pedal that is stuck.
         a. *Ras* is a commonly mutated proto-oncogene, especially in pancreatic and colorectal cancers. A point mutation (happens at a single location of DNA or a single base pair) can change *Ras* from a proto-oncogene to an oncogene.
      2. *Tumor suppressor genes:* genes that control proliferation by preventing uncontrolled growth. When mutated, these genes no longer suppress proliferation. In the car analogy, these genes, when mutated, are like the brake pedal that does not work.
         a. The *RB* gene normally inhibits cell division. This gene is mutated in childhood retinoblastoma and many lung, breast, and bone cancers (Rote & Virshup, 2017).

      3. *Caretaker genes:* DNA repair genes that correct mistakes in normal cells that might be caused by carcinogens during replication. In some individuals, these genes may not be functional, which makes it easier for a mutation to result in cancer.
      4. Chromosome translocations result when pieces of one chromosome move to another chromosome as the cell divides. This type of genetic alteration may activate an oncogene.
         a. The *MYC* proto-oncogene is normally located on chromosome 8. In the Burkitt lymphoma cells, this portion of DNA is relocated to chromosome 14.
         b. In chronic myeloid leukemia (CML), the *BCR* gene on chromosome 9 is fused to the *Abl* gene on chromosome 22. This translocation is also known as the *Philadelphia chromosome.* This fusion makes a protein called a *tyrosine kinase,* which promotes proliferation of myeloid cells. Imatinib, the original targeted tyrosine kinase inhibitor, was designed to specifically inhibit this pathway.
   C. Enabling factors: facilitate the development of cancer cells and tumor progression (Hanahan & Weinberg, 2015).
      1. Genomic instability: cancer cells have defects in mechanisms that regulate genome replication and chromosomal segregation, like the mutations previously mentioned. This defective regulation results in an increased rate of genetic alterations compared with normal cells. The genetic makeup of cancer cells is less stable than that of normal cells.
         a. Hereditary nonpolyposis colon cancer syndrome (HNPCC) is characterized by microsatellite instability (MSI). Microsatellites are a series of tandem repeated nucleotides. The variation in the number of these tandem repeated nucleotides can be identified in pathology. Normal cells have a consistent length of nucleotides (Kumar, Abbas & Aster, 2015).

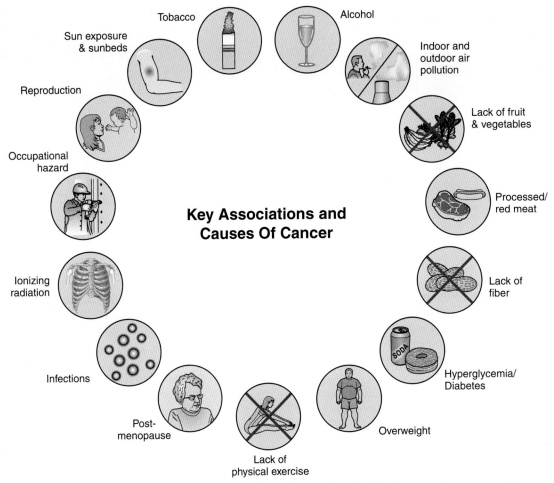

Fig. 7.1 Key associations and causes of cancer. (From McCance K. L. [2017]. Cancer epidemiology. In S. E. Huether & K. L. McCance [Eds.], *Understanding Pathophysiology* [6th ed., pp. 266–300]. St. Louis: Elsevier.)

b. *Epigenetics* describes a mechanism that may change the activity of a gene without changing the sequence of DNA.

   (1) An example of an epigenetic mechanism is DNA methylation. Adding or removing methyl groups from DNA affects the transcription of genes. The addition or subtraction of methyl groups may be affected by diet, the environment, and certain medications. One example of a medication that hypomethylates is decitabine, which is used in the treatment of myelodysplastic syndrome (MDS). If DNA is not transcribed, it is essentially silenced. Some cancers are associated with hypermethylation of the regulatory regions of genes.

   (2) Other cancers (e.g., some colon cancers) are associated with a lack of methylation, which makes it easier for genes to be overexpressed (Berman et al., 2012). Hypomethylation may contribute to cancer when it is a tumor suppressor gene not being transcribed (Kumar et al., 2015).

2. Inflammation

   a. Inflammatory cells supply signaling molecules to the tumor microenvironment, including growth factors, survival factors, proangiogenic factors, extracellular matrix-modifying enzymes, and inductive signals that lead to activation of epithelial-mesenchymal transition (EMT) and other hallmark-promoting programs. (Hanahan & Weinberg, 2015).

   b. Inflammatory cells release mutagenic agents, such as reactive oxygen species; encourages genetic evolution of cancer cells toward malignancy (Hanahan & Weinberg, 2015).

   c. One example is tumor necrosis factor (TNF), a chemical released by white blood cells in response to inflammation. This cytokine may have an antitumor effect (in immune surveillance); however, it plays a role in carcinogenesis as well.

   d. Some chronic inflammatory conditions are associated with tumor formation (Table 7.2)

3. Interactions between tumor cells and the surrounding normal tissue's stroma or the environment (Fig. 7.2)

TABLE 7.1   Comparison of Cancer Gene Types

Gene Type	Normal Function	Mutation Effect
Caretaker	DNA and chromosome stability	Chromosome instability and increased rates of mutation
Dominant oncogenes*	Encode proteins that promote growth (e.g., growth factors)	Overexpression or amplification causes gain of function
Tumor suppressors (recessive oncogenes)	Encode proteins that inhibit proliferation and prevent or repair mutations	Requires loss of function of both alleles to increase cancer risk

*Nonmutant state referred to as proto-oncogene.
From Rote N. S. & Virshup D.M. (2017). Biology of cancer. In S. E. Huether & K. L. McCance (Eds.), *Understanding Pathophysiology* (6th ed., pp. 233–265). St. Louis: Elsevier.

TABLE 7.2   Chronic Inflammatory Conditions and Infectious Agents Associated with Neoplasms

Inflammatory Condition	Associated Neoplasm(s)
Asbestosis, silicosis	Mesothelioma, lung carcinoma
Bronchitis	Lung carcinoma
Cystitis, bladder inflammation	Bladder carcinoma
Gingivitis, lichen planus	Oral squamous cell carcinoma
Inflammatory bowel disease, Crohn disease, chronic ulcerative colitis	Colorectal carcinoma
Lichen sclerosus	Vulvar squamous cell carcinoma
Chronic pancreatitis, hereditary pancreatitis	Pancreatic carcinoma
Reflux esophagitis, Barrett esophagus	Esophageal carcinoma
Sialadenitis	Salivary gland carcinoma
Sjögren syndrome, Hashimoto thyroiditis	MALT lymphoma
Skin inflammation	Melanoma

Infection Agent (Nonviral)	Associated Neoplasm(s)
Helicobacter pylori	Gastric adenocarcinoma, MALT lymphoma
Chronic bacterial cholecystitis	Gallbladder cancer
Schistosomiasis	Bladder, liver, rectal carcinoma; follicular lymphoma of spleen
Liver flukes	Cholangiocarcinoma

Infectious Agent (Viral)	Associated Neoplasm(s)
Human immunodeficiency virus type 1 (HIV-1)	Non-Hodgkin lymphoma, squamous cell carcinomas, Kaposi sarcoma
Hepatitis B and hepatitis C	Hepatocellular carcinoma
Epstein–Barr virus	B-cell non-Hodgkin lymphoma, Burkitt lymphoma, nasopharyngeal carcinoma
KSHV/HHVB and immunodeficiency	Kaposi sarcoma
HPV-16, -18, -31, others	Cervical, anogenital
HTLV-1	Adult T-cell leukemia/lymphoma

From Rote N. S. & Virshup D. M. (2017). Biology of cancer. In S. E. Huether & K. L. McCance (Eds.), *Understanding Pathophysiology* (6th ed., pp. 233–265). St. Louis: Elsevier.

a. The stroma consists of connective tissue, blood vessels, immune inflammatory cells such as macrophages and lymphocytes, and associated fibroblasts.
b. Communication and signaling between tumor cells and normal stroma cells lead to tumor growth and metastasis through a multitude of reciprocal pathways that transform both normal tissue and the tumor. For example, tumors may elicit immune and stromal responses to stimulate formation of new blood vessels (angiogenesis).
c. Example: transforming growth factor alpha (TGF-α) or the epidermal growth factor receptor (EGFR) signaling pathway plays a role in some colon cancer metastases (Langley & Fidler, 2011).
   (1) Some metastatic colon cancer cells produce five times more EGFR compared with nonmetastatic cells.
   (2) TGF-α initiates angiogenic processes in normal endothelial cells.
   (3) Signal mediated by EGFR in colon cancer and resident endothelial populations.
   (4) When combined with vascular endothelial growth factor (VEGF) production, lymphangiogenesis is stimulated; tumor cells may spread to regional lymph nodes.
   (5) Cetuximab, a monoclonal antibody, blocks ligand binding to EGFR; used in EGFR-positive patients to reduce primary tumor size and lymphatic spread.
D. Process of carcinogenesis (Fig. 7.3)
II. Hallmarks of cancer—refer to the biologic capabilities that a cancer cell acquires in a progressive multistep process that transforms a normal cell to a malignant cell (Hanahan & Weinberg, 2011; Hanahan & Weinberg, 2015; Fouad & Aanei, 2017). Tumors consist of cancer cells with various mutations and supportive tissues (the tumor microenvironment) that interact and evolve

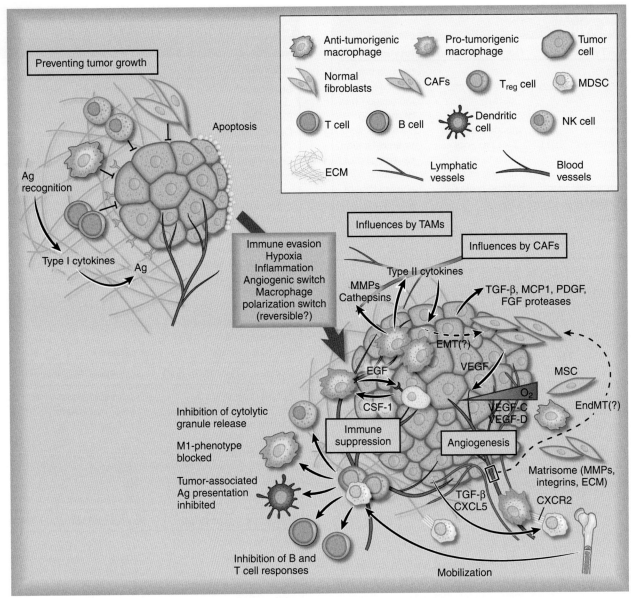

Fig. 7.2 Cancers live in a complex microenvironment. (From Rote N. S. & Virshup D. M. [2017]. Biology of cancer. In S. E. Huether & K. L. McCance [Eds.], *Understanding Pathophysiology* [6th ed., pp. 233–265]. St. Louis: Elsevier.)

together. The process is enabled by genomic instability and inflammation as described earlier. When the tumor gains a variety of clonally evolved and mutated cells that collectively have all these hallmarks of cancer, it is considered malignant (Hanahan & Weinberg, 2015).

A. Cancer cells sustain proliferative signaling.
   1. Normal cells regulate proliferation with growth-promoting signals that start and stop mitosis.
   2. Some cancer cells deregulate the signals through various means, including the following:
      a. Production of growth factors themselves.
      b. Transmission of signals to stimulate normal cells to supply cancer cells with growth factors.

   c. Presence of mutations may create proto-oncogenes, inactivate tumor suppressor genes, or disrupt negative feedback signaling.
      (1) The *Ras* oncoprotein normally signals cells to stop proliferating. Mutated *Ras* inactivates the negative feedback mechanism, and cancer cells consequently keep proliferating or producing. This is a prevalent mutation in many human cancers, such as pancreatic and colorectal cancers.
   d. May counterbalance excessive proliferative signaling by forcing some cells into senescence. This may allow high growth and avoidance of cell death pressures that ultimately allow the cancer cells to persist (Hanahan & Weinberg, 2015).

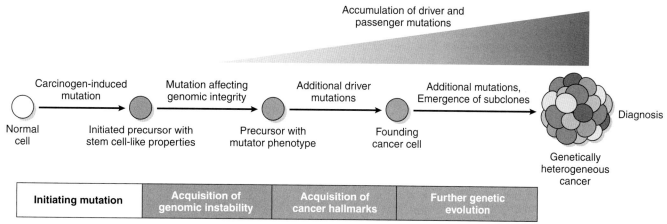

Accumulation of driver and passenger mutations

| Initiating mutation | Acquisition of genomic instability | Acquisition of cancer hallmarks | Further genetic evolution |

Fig. 7.3 Development of a cancer through stepwise acquisition of complementary mutations. A tumor is formed from a single precursor cell with genetic alterations that undergoes clonal expansion. Clonal evolution describes the process of cells within a tumor accumulating genetic changes over time that are different from one cell to the next. Thus a tumor may be heterogeneous and consist of cells that arose from the same mother cell that are genotypically different from one another. Tumors arise from the survival of the fittest collection of cancer cells. (From Kumar V., Abbas, A. K., & Aster, J. C. [2015]. Neoplasia. In V. Kumar, A. K. Abbas, & J. C. Aster [Eds.], *Robbins and Cotran Pathologic Basis of Disease* (9th ed., pp. 265–340). Philadelphia: Elsevier Saunders.)

B. Cancer cells evade growth suppressors.
  1. Normal cells regulate growth with tumor suppressor genes that lead to senescence (cellular aging) and apoptosis (programmed cell death). Cell growth is also limited by contact inhibition (cell growth and division stop on physical contact with other cells).
  2. Some cancer cells have mutations that disable gatekeeper proteins controlling mitoses, inactivating cancer inhibition.
C. Cancer cells resist cell death and enable replicative immortality.
  1. Normal cells experience apoptosis, or programmed cell death. A process called *autophagy* allows normal cells to be broken down during cellular stress so that organelles and cell contents can be reused in other cells.
  2. Necrotic cells release proinflammatory signals. Cancer cells use these proinflammatory signals to recruit inflammatory cells and enhance tumor growth through the microenvironment (Hanahan & Weinberg, 2015).
  3. Normal cells have a limited number of growth and division cycles because of senescence (a nonproliferative but viable state) and crisis (involves cell death).
    a. Cancer cells manipulate senescence and crisis mechanisms in order to survive.
  4. Normal cells have limited amounts of telomerase, an enzyme that adds telomere repeat segments. Telomeres are protective DNA at the ends of chromosomes that shorten with repeated cell duplication. An analogy for the protective effects of telomere DNA is the protective coating at the end of shoelaces

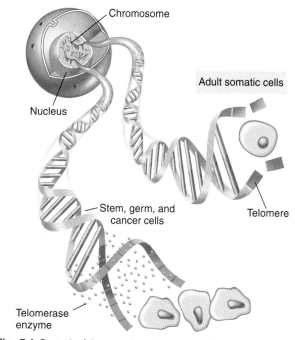

Fig. 7.4 Control of immortality: telomeres and telomerase. (From Rote N. S. & Virshup D. M. [2017]. Biology of cancer. In S. E. Huether & K. L. McCance [Eds.], *Understanding Pathophysiology* (6th ed., pp. 233–265). St. Louis: Elsevier.)

that prevent fraying. When the shortened ends reach a critical level, they signal cell death.
    a. Cancer cells contain high amounts of telomerase, which adds protective telomeres and prevents the telomere segment from shortening. This process is believed to allow continued cell replication; contributes to immortalization—cells avoid or survive crises (Fig. 7.4).

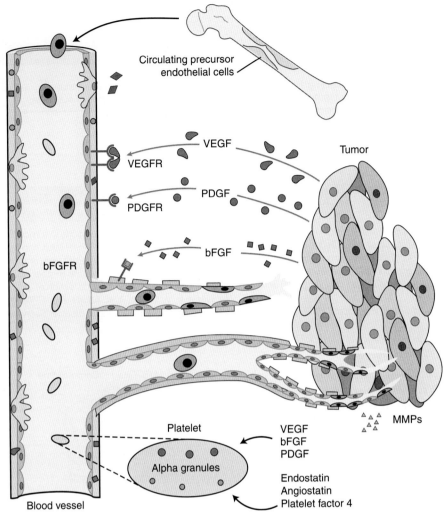

Fig. 7.5 Tumor-induced angiogenesis. (From Rote N. S. & Virshup D. M. [2017]. Biology of cancer. In S. E. Huether & K. L. McCance [Eds.], *Understanding Pathophysiology* [6th ed., pp. 233–265]. St. Louis: Elsevier.)

D. Cancer cells induce angiogenesis. Angiogenesis is the creation of new blood vessels from existing ones to provide nutrients and remove waste products.
   1. In normal tissues, angiogenesis takes place during embryogenesis with tissue and organ development. The process happens transiently in adulthood for wound healing and during female reproductive cycling. Otherwise, the process is dormant (Fig. 7.5).
   2. Cancer cells have the ability to secrete substances such as VEGFs, which stimulate angiogenesis to support continued tumor growth. The stimulation may lead to the creation of new growing vessels that supply nutrients to tumors. "Tumors cannot grow beyond 2 to 3 mm³ nor metastasize without new vasculature" (Folkman 1971, Fuoad & Aanei 2017).
   3. Tumor vasculature is less organized than normal vasculature. Consequently, blood flow is chaotic, leading to hypoxia—considered the most important trigger of angiogenesis—and acidosis that stimulates angiogenesis, decreases therapeutic

effectiveness, and contributes to resistant clonal expansion (Fuoad & Aanei, 2017).

E. Cancer cells activate invasion and metastasis
   1. Normal cells have a developmental regulatory program called *epithelial mesenchymal transition* (EMT). This process causes epithelial cells to lose cell polarity and cell–cell adhesion and have invasive properties so that they can become mesenchymal cells. This process is involved in mesoderm formation and neural tube formation during embryogenesis. It has also been found to play a role in wound healing and organ fibrosis (Kalluri & Weinberg, 2009).
   2. Cancer cells appear to use this mechanism during invasion and metastasis, which will be described further.

F. Cancer cells have altered energy metabolism
   1. Normal cells in the presence of oxygen metabolize glucose to pyruvate and then carbon dioxide. In conditions where oxygen is limited, they favor glycolysis. Embryonic cells also use the glycolysis process in the presence of oxygen.

ANTITUMOR IMMUNITY

IMMUNE EVASION BY TUMORS

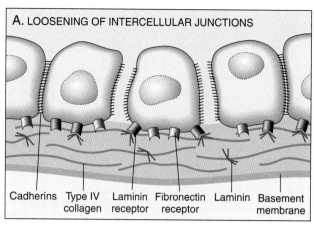

Failure to produce tumor antigen

Mutations in MHC genes or genes needed for antigen processing

Production of immunosuppressive proteins or expression of inhibitory cell surface proteins

Fig. 7.6 Mechanisms by which tumor cells evade the immune system. From Rote N. S. & Virshup D. M. [2017]. Biology of cancer. In S. E. Huether & K. L. McCance [Eds.], *Understanding Pathophysiology* [6th ed., pp. 233–265]. St. Louis: Elsevier.)

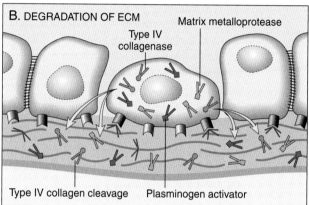

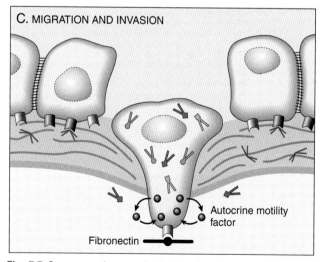

Fig. 7.7 Sequence of events in the invasion of epithelial basement membranes by tumor cells. (From Kumar V., Abbas, A. K., & Aster, J. C. [2015]. Neoplasia. In V. Kumar, A. K. Abbas, & J. C. Aster [Eds.], *Robbins and Cotran Pathologic Basis of Disease* [9th ed., pp. 265–340]. Philadelphia: Elsevier Saunders.)

2. Cancer cells use mostly glycolysis for energy production, even in the presence of oxygen, also called the *Warburg effect.*

G. Cancer cells evade immune destruction.

1. Evidence indicates that deficiencies in T lymphocytes, T helper cells, and natural killer (NK) cells increase the risk of cancer development (Mandal & Viswanathan, 2015).

2. Example: cancer cells can evade the T-cell response by expressing PDL1 to block T-cell recognition of the cancer cell that would usually initiate a cytotoxic response. There is a class of anticancer therapy called *checkpoint inhibitors* that targets PDL1 (Fig. 7.6).

III. Metastasis is the spread of cancer cells from the site of the original tumor or organ to distant tissues and organs in the body.

A. The presence of metastatic disease at diagnosis is an important prognostic factor because it indicates advanced disease. It is estimated that 30% of newly diagnosed solid tumors (excluding skin cancers other than melanomas) present with metastatic disease (Kumar et al., 2015). Ninety percent of cancer-related deaths are related to metastatic disease (Steeg, 2006).

B. Major factors of the metastatic cascade

1. Invasion of the extracellular matrix (ECM) by tumor cells (Fig. 7.7).

a. Downregulate cadherin glycoproteins that mediate cell–cell interactions.

b. Produce or stimulate stromal cells such as fibroblasts or inflammatory cells to secrete proteases that degrade the ECM.

c. Attach to ECM proteins that can assist with mobility and interact with the ECM to create an environment conducive to migration of the tumor cells.

d. Through a process called *locomotion,* which includes complex signaling involving proteases, cytokines, and motility factors, tumor cells are able to migrate through the ECM and gain access to the vascular basement membrane.

e. Process occurs in reverse when tumor cell emboli reach and invade a distant site (Fig. 7.8).

2. Survival in transport: tumor cells in circulation are susceptible to destruction by mechanical stress, immune defenses, and apoptosis because of lack of cell–cell adhesion. To survive, tumor cells tend to travel in clumps, may combine with platelets to form platelet–tumor aggregates, and may interact with coagulation factors to create emboli.

   a. Research is underway using these circulating tumor cells as a "liquid biopsy" for "cancer screening, estimation of metastatic relapse risk identification of targetable components, exploring tumor heterogeneity, and monitoring therapeutic response" (Alix-Panabières & Pantel 2016; Stegner, Dutting & Nieswandt, 2014; Zhang et al., 2016).

3. Pathways of cancer dissemination
   a. Direct invasion to an adjoining organ
   b. Seeding throughout a body cavity such as the peritoneal cavity (e.g., ovarian cancer)
   c. Dissemination through the lymphatic system
      (1) Entrapment at the first lymph node, or the "sentinel lymph node"
      (2) "Skip metastasis," where cells bypass the first node and reach more distant sites
   d. Dissemination through the blood vessels
      (1) Arterial spread
         (a) Tumor cells may be spread through the pulmonary capillary beds or pulmonary arteriovenous (AV) shunts, or when pulmonary tumors metastasize and create tumor emboli.
         (b) Because arteries have thicker walls, they are less readily penetrated than veins (Kumar et al., 2015).
      (2) Venous spread
         (a) Tumor cells often go to the first capillary bed encountered. Liver and lung are the most frequent sites of metastasis.

4. Common sites for metastasis include bones, the lungs, the liver, and the central nervous system (CNS). Predilection for certain tumors to metastasize to specific sites may be influenced by the following:

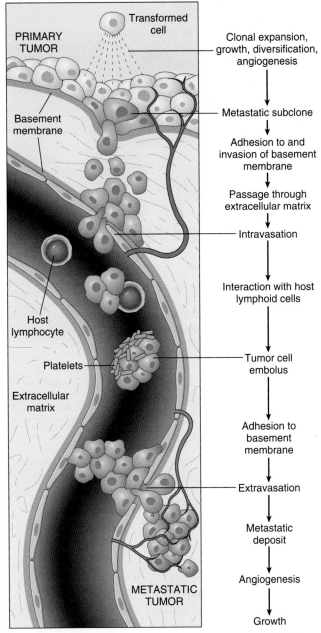

Fig. 7.8 The metastatic cascade. (From Kumar V., Abbas, A.K., & Aster, J. C. [2015]. Neoplasia. In V. Kumar, A. K. Abbas, & J. C. Aster [Eds.], *Robbins and Cotran Pathologic Basis of Disease.* [9th ed., pp. 265–340]. Philadelphia: Elsevier Saunders.)

a. Patterns of blood flow
b. Cell receptors and genes that direct the cell to travel to specific sites
c. Tumor cell production of adhesion molecules that prefer certain distant organs
d. Chemical signals and growth factors, which are found only in selected organs
e. Inhibitor substances produced by organs not typically sites for metastatic growth
f. Collectively, items b to e may be a result of "cross-talk" between cancer cells and normal host cells. That is, cancer cells may release

TABLE 7.3	Common Sites of Metastasis
Cancer Type	**Main Sites of Metastasis**
Bladder	Bone, liver, lung
Breast	Bone, brain, liver, lung
Colon	Liver, lung, peritoneum
Kidney	Adrenal gland, bone, brain, liver, lung
Lung	Adrenal gland, bone, brain, liver, other lung
Melanoma	Bone, brain, liver, lung, skin, muscle
Ovary	Liver, lung, peritoneum
Pancreas	Liver, lung, peritoneum
Prostate	Adrenal gland, bone, liver, lung
Rectal	Liver, lung, peritoneum
Stomach	Liver, lung, peritoneum
Thyroid	Bone, liver, lung
Uterus	Bone, liver, lung, peritoneum, vagina

From National Cancer Institute at the National Institute for Health. (2018). Metastatic cancer. https://www.cancer.gov/types/metastatic-cancer Accessed April 17, 2018.

cytokines that induce the host cells to produce substances that recognize receptors on the cancer cells. Hence, the cancer cells may have a "homing device" that attracts them to select host organs and may promote their growth in these distant tissues (Kumar et al., 2015) (Table 7.3).

IV. Key points

A. Metastasis contributes to the pain and suffering caused by cancer and is the major cause of death from cancer (Rote & Virshup, 2017).

B. Understanding the process of carcinogenesis and metastasis helps lead to therapies targeting the molecular changes associated with the disease.

C. Although there is a growing understanding of the genomics and the factors contributing to cancer development, cancer cells remain adaptable. This flexibility of cancer creates challenges for the development of a single cure-all therapy.

REFERENCES

Alix-Panabières, C., & Pantel, K. (2016). Clinical applications of circulating tumor cells and circulating tumor DNA as liquid biopsy. *Cancer Discovery*, 6, 479–491. https://doi.org/10.1158/2159-8290.CD-15-1483.

Berman, B. P., Weisenberger, D. J., Aman, J. F., Hinoue, T., Ramjan, Z., et al. (2012). Regions of focal DN hypermethylation and long-range hypomethylation in colorectal cancer coincide with nuclear lamina-associated domains. *Nature Genetics*, 44(1), 40–46. https://doi.org/10.1038/ng.969.

Ding, L., Bailey, M. H., Porta-Pardo, E., Thorsson, V., Colaprico, A., et al. (2018). Perspective on oncogenic processes at the end of the beginning of cancer genomics. *Cell*, 173(2), 305–320. https://doi.org/10.1016/j.cell.2018.03.033.

Folkman, J. (1971). Tumor angiogenesis: therapeutic implications. *New England Journal of Medicine*, 285, 1182–1186.

Fouad, Y. A., & Aanei, C. (2017). Revisiting the hallmarks of cancer. *American Journal of Cancer Research*, 7(5), 1016–1036.

Hanahan, D., & Weinberg, R. A. (2011). Hallmarks of cancer. The next generation. *Cell*, 144, 646–674. https://doi.org/10.1016/j.cell.2011.02.013.

Hanahan D. & Weinberg R.A. (2015) Hallmarks of cancer: an organizing principle for cancer medicine. In V.T. Devita, T.S. Lawrence & S.A. Rosenberg (Eds.), *DeVita, Hellman, and Rosenberg's Cancer: Principles and Practice of Oncology* (10th ed., pp. 24–44) Philadelphia: Wolters Kluwer Health Adis (ESP).

Kalluri, R., & Weinberg, R. A. (2009). The basics of epithelial-mesenchymal transition. *Journal of Clinical Investigation*, 119(6), 1420–1428. https://doi.org/10.1172/JCI39104.

Kumar, V., Abbas, A. K., & Aster, J. C. (2015). Neoplasia. In V. Kumar, A. K. Abbas, & J. C. Aster (Eds.), *Robbins and Cotran Pathologic Basis of Disease* (9th ed., pp. 265–340). Philadelphia: Elsevier Saunders.

Langley, R. R., & Fidler, I. J. (2011). The seed and soil hypothesis revisited—the role of tumor-stroma interactions in metastasis to different organs. *International Journal of Cancer*, 128(11), 2527–2535. https://doi.org/10.1002/ijc.26031.

Mandal, A., & Viswanathan, C. (2015). Natural killer cells: in health and disease. *Hematology/Oncology and Stem Cell Therapy*, 8(2), 47–55. https://doi.org/10.1016/j.hemonc.2014.11.006.

McCance, K. L. (2017). Cancer epidemiology. In S. E. Huether & K. L. McCance (Eds.), *Understanding Pathophysiology* (6th ed., pp. 266–300). St. Louis: Elsevier.

National Cancer Institute at the National Institute for Health. (2018). *Metastatic cancer*. https://www.cancer.gov/types/metastaticcancer. Accessed April 17, 2018.

Rote, N. S., & Virshup, D. M. (2017). Biology of cancer. In S. E. Huether & K. L. McCance (Eds.), *Understanding Pathophysiology* (6th ed., pp. 233–265). St. Louis: Elsevier.

Steeg, P. S. (2006). Tumor metastasis: mechanistic insights and clinical challenges. *Nature Medicine*, 12, 895–904.

Stegner, D., Dütting, S., & Nieswandt, B. (2014). Mechanistic explanation for platelet contribution to cancer metastasis. *Thrombosis Research*, 133, S149–S157. https://doi.org/10.1016/S0049-3848(14)50025-4.

Zhang, C., Guan, Y., Sun, Y., Ai, D., & Guo, Q. (2016). Tumor heterogeneity and circulating tumor cells. *Cancer Letters*, 374, 216–223. https://doi.org/10.1016/j.canlet.2016.02.024.

8

Immunology

Christine Boley

I. Definition of immunology
  A. Study of health maintenance and homeostasis based on identification and eradication of foreign microbes, repair of tissue damage, and defense of the host through the capacity to distinguish self from nonself, while preventing malignant proliferation (Crow, 2016)
    1. Impairment or lack of these components disrupts homeostasis by lack of immune response to allergens, antigens, infectious microbes, or tumor cells, leading to development of various disease processes
II. Basic concepts
  A. Organ and tissue components of the immune system
    1. Primary lymphoid organs—allow for the maturation of lymphocytes and includes the following organs (Vioral, 2018):
      a. Bone marrow (BM)—location of B-cell differentiation and maturation
      b. Thymus—location of T-cell differentiation and maturation
    2. Secondary lymphoid organs and tissues—sites where antigens are captured and processed (Vioral, 2018)
      a. Lymph nodes—initiate immune responses to antigens circulating in the lymph, skin, or mucosal surfaces
      b. Spleen—responds to bloodborne antigens
      c. Bone marrow—functions as both primary and secondary lymphoid organ
      d. Lymphoid tissue—gastrointestinal (GI) mucosa (Peyer patches), tonsils/adenoids (Waldeyer ring), and other body systems' mucosa-associated lymphoid tissue (MALT)
  B. Hematopoiesis—regulation, production, and development of blood cells (Vioral, 2018)
    1. Hematopoiesis begins with a single cell, a self-renewing pluripotent stem cell.
      a. Protein markers on surfaces called clusters of differentiation (CD)
        (1) CD identify cell type and function and provide molecular signaling

    2. Cells divide into undifferentiated hematopoietic stem cells that are committed to one of two cell lineages or pathways: lymphoid or myeloid progenitor cells
      a. Lymphoid—B cell, helper T cell, cytotoxic T cell, natural killer (NK) cells
      b. Myeloid—dendritic cell, macrophage, neutrophil, eosinophil, mast cell, megakaryocyte, erythrocyte (red blood cell [RBC]), basophils, monocytes
III. Cellular components of the immune system (Devine, 2013)
  A. Myeloid stem cell lineage—further divided into two lineages:
    1. Granulocyte–monocyte lineage
      a. Granulocytes—have granules in cytoplasm with enzymes that aid in digestion of foreign particles (phagocytosis) and cause inflammation.
        (1) Neutrophils or polymorphonuclear neutrophil (PMNs): rapidly produced and are first responders to bacterial and fungal microbes.
          (a) Short lived—about 6 hours, but most abundant granulocyte
          (b) Cause inflammatory response due to engulfing/destroying foreign particles/debris
        (2) Basophils: have IgE receptors that are involved in allergic responses and cause release of histamine/prostaglandins
        (3) Eosinophils: attack parasites, secrete leukotrienes/cytokines that cause inflammation during allergic responses
      b. Monocytes—migrate from BM to inflammatory site, where they divide and become macrophages (Crow, 2016)
        (1) Macrophages—rapidly recognize, ingest, and kill microbes
          (a) Present these processed antigens to T cells, called *antigen-presenting cell (APC)*.
          (b) Release proinflammatory cytokines called *M1* to initiate an immune response.

(c) Release antiinflammatory cytokines called *M2* to initiate wound healing and maintain homeostasis

(2) Mononuclear phagocytes—fixed and mobile phagocytic cells associated with blood monocytes and tissue macrophages

c. Dendritic cells (DCs)—capture foreign cells and process antigens (McCance, Huether, Brashers, & Rote, 2018)

(1) Immature DCs found in peripheral tissue possess phagocytic functions for innate immunity

(2) Function as major APC and travel from tissue to secondary lymphoid tissue to present antigen to naïve T and B cells; this process activates T cells

(3) Functions as a direct link between innate and adaptive immunity

2. Megakaryocyte–erythrocyte lineage

a. Megakaryocyte—forms into platelets before circulation

(1) Has immunologic function that releases inflammatory mediators, recruits leukocytes to tissue damage, prevents excessive bleeding

b. Erythrocytes (RBCs)—involved in tissue nourishment, oxygenation, blood viscosity

c. Mast cells—produce inflammatory response within tissues, not bloodborne, and release tumor necrosis factor/interleukin-8 (TNF/IL-8)

B. Lymphoid stem cell lineage has three types of lymphocytes that are key for immune responses:

1. B cells (B lymphocytes)—develop in the bone marrow. Two types of B cells (Devine, 2013):

a. Memory B cells: activated B cells specific to an antigen

(1) Quickly respond after a second exposure of the host.

(2) Long-term immune cells.

b. Plasma cells: produce antibodies against antigens after exposure.

(1) Secretes one of the five different specific immunoglobulins (IgA, IgG, IgE, IgD, IgM)

2. T cells (T lymphocytes)—migrate to the thymus gland for maturation; play a role in immune surveillance and response; types include (Devine, 2013):

a. T helper cells (Th): secrete cytokines that assist in activating immune responses, such as the maturation of B cells and the activation of cytotoxic T cells and macrophages.

(1) Also referred to as *CD4+ T cells* because they display CD4 cell surface molecules

(2) Recognize antigens in conjunction with class II major histocompatibility complex (MHC) molecules

(3) Th cell type I (Th1)—secretes cytokines (interferon [IFN], IL, TNF) and develops cell-mediated immunity Tc cells (Craft, 2016)

(4) Th cell type II (Th2)—secretes antiinflammatory cytokines and B-cell maturation

b. Cytotoxic T cells (Tc): destroy viral infections, cancer; play a role in autoimmunity and allogenic organ rejection

(1) Called CD8+ T cells because they display CD8 protein on their surface

(2) Recognize antigens in conjunction with class I MHC molecules

(3) Induce apoptosis of foreign cells through release of enzymes

c. T regulatory cells (Treg): previously called *suppressor T cells*

(1) Suppress T-cell–mediated immunity, as well as suppress autoreactive T cells against self.

(2) Treg and Th cells help maintain immunologic homeostasis within host.

d. Memory T cells: induce secondary cell-mediated immune response.

3. NK cells (McCance et al. 2018)

(1) Large granular cells that release cytokines, rapidly migrate to the site of inflammation, and directly kill tumor- or viral-infected cells without previous exposure to antigens

(2) Faster recognition and response without using antibodies and MHC molecules

(3) Inhibited by interaction with MHC class I molecules

(4) Activity increased with the addition of cytokines such as IL-2, IL-12, and IFN-γ

(5) Important in tumor surveillance—able to kill MHC class I–deficient tumor cells resistant to adaptive immunity (Crow, 2016)

C. Mediators of immune system function

1. Complement system—an interactive network of plasma enzymes and regulatory proteins activated in a controlled pathway; links innate and humoral immunity

a. Complement cascade (McCance et al. 2018)

(1) Classical pathway—activated by antigen–antibody complexes

(2) Lectin pathway—activated by specific bacterial carbohydrates

(3) Alternative pathway—activated on microbial surfaces

b. Functions

(1) Mast cell degranulation

(2) Leukocyte chemotaxis

(3) Opsonization—phagocytosis of antigen–antibody complexes when products of the complement cascade interact with neutrophils and macrophages

(4) Cell lysis—destruction of targeted pathogen

2. Cytokines
   a. Large variety of proteins secreted by immune cells to assist with cell signaling or communication during different immune responses, such as cellular proliferation and migration, apoptosis, and inflammation (Vioral, 2018).
      (1) Lymphokines—produced by lymphocytes to attract macrophages and other lymphocytes to site of infection for immune response, including:
         (a) IFNs—released in response to pathogens, such as viral infections, and are produced early in response to infection
         (b) ILs—help T and B lymphocytes and hematopoietic cells divide, differentiate, and activate
         (c) Colony-stimulating growth factors (CSGF)—assist with differentiation of all BM progenitor stem cells
      (2) Chemokines—induce chemotaxis, which is the activation and movement of leukocytes throughout the body in response to a chemical release
      (3) TNFs—play key roles in mediating inflammation; cause fevers, apoptosis, and acute-phase cytotoxic reactions
         (a) Produced by eosinophils, mast cells, neutrophils, NK cells, macrophages, CD4+ cells, and lymphocytes
      (4) Transforming growth factors (TGFs)—control cell division and repair
3. MHC—group of genes that controls production of glycoproteins found on the surface of all species' nucleated cells (except RBCs); help distinguish as "self antigens" (Craft, 2016)
   a. Two classes:
      (1) MHC class I molecules: displayed on almost all nucleated cells
      (2) MHC class II molecules: more specialized, or "professional" APCs, such as DCs, monocytes, macrophages, and B cells
   b. In humans, this is called human leukocyte antigen (HLA) and consists of more than 200 genes located on chromosome 6.
   c. Immune response can be mounted against foreign MHC molecules

IV. Immune system responses—body's defense against foreign substances (Vioral, 2018)
   A. Involves both innate and adaptive immunity
      1. Innate immunity—or natural immunity, is the immediate, first line of defense against invasion; does not rely on previous exposure, or "memory," to be initiated.
         a. Natural barriers—inborne to prevent damage by environmental substances and prevent infection by pathogens
            (1) Physical—epithelial cells of intact skin and mucous membranes
            (2) Chemical—bile, mucus, perspiration, tears (lysozyme), normal flora
            (3) Cellular—leukocytes, cytokines
         b. Inflammatory response—nonspecific process that results in rapid activation of several plasma protein systems; mast cell degranulation; vascular changes; and the influx of macrophages, neutrophils, NK cells, and DCs in direct response to tissue damage once natural barrier is broken (McCance et al. 2018).
            (1) Prevents infection and further damage by binding to microbes
            (2) Cascade of cells released for phagocytosis, promote inflammatory mediators, release of cytokines, and remove cellular debris
            (3) Host innate immune cells have surface receptors, called *pattern recognition receptors (PRRs),* that distinguish between self and pathogens through pathogen-associated molecular patterns (PAMPs) and cell damage/death molecules, called *damage-associated molecular patterns (DAMPs)* (Crow, 2016)
            (4) Feedback inhibition mechanisms to control damage to tissues
            (5) Unable to differentiate or memorize different types of pathogens
            (6) Macrophages and DCs produce cytokines that facilitate the development of the adaptive immune response (Crow, 2016)
      2. Adaptive immunity—occurs in later stages of immune response with specific immune cells and has memory, which allows for longer-lived immune response. Two types of adaptive immunity: humoral and cell mediated (Vioral, 2018).
         a. Humoral immunity—antibodies produced by B lymphocytes
            (1) Antigens in lymphatic fluid pass through secondary lymphatic organs, which activates B cells; antigen is processed and presented on surface with MHC-II molecule
            (2) Each B-cell lymphocyte recognizes only one type of antigen; this is called *specificity.*
            (3) Specific B cell lymphocytes quickly multiply and differentiate to become either memory or plasma cells with help from helper T cells.
            (4) Each specialized plasma cell produces one specific antibody; these committed, highly differentiated cells are not phagocytic.
               (a) These antibodies circulate, encounter antigens, and bind to them, producing cytokine reaction, which attracts macrophages/NK cells

(5) Memory B cells are capable of recognizing a particular antigen at either future exposures or at other body sites; they produce plasma cells to generate an antibody specific to the antigen

b. Cell-mediated immunity: T lymphocytes (Craft, 2016)

(1) T precursor cells migrate to thymus (primary lymphoid tissue) to mature into CD4+ helper T cells or CD8+ cytotoxic T cells, which then migrate to the secondary lymphoid organs as inactivated or naïve cells

(2) Antigens are presented to naïve T cells by APCs (macrophages or DCs)

(3) T lymphocytes specific to the presented antigen are produced: MHC class II molecules on APCs activate CD4+ T cells, and MHC class I molecules on APCs activates CD8+ T cells in the presence of costimulatory signals. This process activates T cells.

c. Activated T cells multiply, producing cytokines, and are released into lymphatic fluid from the bloodstream to navigate back and forth and perform their functions as previously mentioned.

d. T-lymphocyte memory cells are produced and respond by activating T lymphocytes when exposed to the same antigen in the future.

e. Cytotoxic T cells and NK cells are capable of directly attacking other cells and destroying them.

V. Tumor immunology (Shoushtari, Wolchok, & Hellman, 2018) (Muehlbauer, Callahan, Zlott, & Dahl, 2018)

A. Tumor recognition and rejection:

1. Cytotoxic immune response requires a complex interaction of the innate and adaptive immune systems to identify malignant cells and kill them.

(1) Cancer progression occurs due to evolution of mutated tumor cells, which evades the immune system over time, leading to immune-resistant clones, called *cancer immunoediting*

(2) Extrinsic tumor suppressor mechanism (NK cells, T cells, B cells, DCs) engages in three sequential phases:

(a) Elimination—innate and adaptive immunity destroy growing tumors before they are clinically measurable.
   i. Called immune surveillance
   ii. The host remains cancer free due to this extrinsic tumor suppression

(b) Equilibrium—a rare cancer clone acquires resistance to elimination by the immune system, where its growth is stabilized by the adaptive immune system; the innate system can no longer keep tumor in check. However, rare tumor clones persist and enter the escape phase.

(c) Escape—persistent tumor clones have acquired ability to evade the adaptive immune system, and clinical disease is apparent. Tumor cells that emerge are:

   i. No longer recognized by the adaptive immune system due to antigen loss/alteration of variants, and/or defects in tumor antigen processing or presentation.

   ii. Insensitive to immune effector mechanisms, such as upregulating immune checkpoint molecules, like PD1 and PDL-1, which promote T-cell exhaustion and dysfunction.

   iii. Able to induce an immunosuppressive state within the tumor microenvironment by manipulation of cytokines.

REFERENCES

Craft, J. (2016). The adaptive immune system. In L. Goldman, & A. I. Schafer (Eds.), *Goldman-Cecil Medicine* (25th ed). Philadelphia, PA: Elsevier Saunders.

Crow, M. K. (2016). The innate immune system. In L. Goldman, & A. I. Schafer (Eds.), *Goldman-Cecil Medicine* (25th ed). Philadelphia, PA: Elsevier Saunders.

Devine, H. (2013). Overview of Hematopoiesis and Immunology: Implications of Hematopoietic Stem Cell Transplantation. In S. A. Ezzone (Ed.), *Hematopoietic Stem Cell Transplantation: A Manual for Nursing Practice*. Pittsburgh, PA: ONS Publications Department.

McCance, K. L., Huether, S. E., Brashers, V. L., & Rote, N. S. (2018). *Pathophysiology: The Biologic Basis for Disease in Adults and Children* (8th ed.). Maryland Heights, MO: Mosby Elsevier.

Muehlbauer, P. M., Callahan, A., Zlott, D., & Dahl, B. J. (2018). Biotherapy. In C. H. Yarbro, D. Wujcik, & B. H. Gobel (Eds.), *Cancer Nursing Principles and Practice* (8th ed.). Burlington, MA: Jones & Barlett Learning.

Shoushtari, A. N., Wolchok, J., & Hellman, M. (2018). *Principles of cancer immunotherapy*. https://www.uptodate.com/contents/principles-of-cancer-immunotherapy?search=cancer%20immunotherapy&source=search_result&selectedTitle=1~150&usage_type=default&display_rank=1.

Vioral, A. (2018). Immunology. In C. H. Yarbro, D. Wujcik, & B. H. Gobel (Eds.), *Cancer Nursing Principles and Practice*. (8th ed.). Burlington, MA: Jones & Barlett Learning.

9

Precision Medicine

Marlon Garzo Saria and Santosh Kesari

I. Definition

  A. Use of specific information about a person's genes, proteins, and environment to prevent, diagnose, and treat disease (National Cancer Institute, 2017)

  B. Classifies individuals into subpopulations based on susceptibility to a particular condition, cancer biology, disease prognosis, and response to specific treatment (Lemoine, 2014)

  C. Allows for preventive or therapeutic interventions to be delivered to individuals more likely to benefit, sparing those who will not benefit from the cost and toxicities of ineffective treatment (Lemoine, 2014)

  D. Not to be confused with *personalized medicine*, defined as

    1. Receiving *personalized care* or developing patient-specific drugs (Brant & Mayer, 2017; President's Council of Advisors on Science and Technology, 2008)

    2. Ability to provide therapies specifically designed for an individual (Dodson, 2017)

    3. Tailoring of medical treatment to the individual characteristics of each patient (President's Council of Advisors on Science and Technology, 2008)

  E. Table 9.1 provides a glossary of terms to help understand precision medicine.

II. Applications of precision medicine

  A. Cancer risk assessment: tests to confirm suspected familial cancer syndromes (Blix, 2014)

    1. *BRCA1* and *BRCA2* in breast cancer syndromes

    2. *MSH2* and *MLH1* in Lynch syndrome (i.e., hereditary nonpolyposis colorectal cancer)

    3. *APC* in familial adenomatous polyposis

    4. *MEN1* and *RET* in multiple endocrine neoplasia types 1 and 2

  B. Cancer prediction tools: when specific tests are noninformative, decision aids that can be used to provide more objective information about a cancer diagnosis, treatment, or prognosis (Doyle-Lindrud, 2015)

    1. Breast Cancer Risk Assessment: estimates a woman's risk of developing invasive breast cancer (Doyle-Lindrud, 2015; National Cancer Institute, 2011).

      a. Medical, reproductive, and breast cancer history

      b. Breast cancer history of first-degree relatives, such as mother, sister, and daughter

      c. Several tools exist (e.g., Breast Cancer Risk Assessment Tool, Gail Model for Breast Cancer Risk, Tyer Cuzick)

    2. Melanoma Risk Assessment Tool: estimates a person's risk of developing invasive melanoma (Doyle-Lindrud, 2015; National Cancer Institute, 2008)

      a. Demographics (age, gender, race)

      b. Prior sunburns

      c. Complexion

      d. Current number and size of skin moles

      e. Extent of freckling

    3. Partin tables: show the probability that prostate cancer is confined to the prostate, presence of lymphatic invasion, seminal vesicle involvement, or lymph node metastases (Doyle-Lindrud, 2015; Johns Hopkins University, 2011)

      a. Serum prostate-specific antigen level

      b. Clinical stage

      c. Gleason score

    4. Colorectal cancer nomograms: predict prognosis, short-term outcome of treatments, and future development of colorectal cancer (Doyle-Lindrud, 2015; Kawai, et al., 2015)

      a. Age

      b. Preoperative carcinoembryonic antigen level

      c. Tumor location

      d. Tumor differentiation

      e. Presence of lymphovascular and perineural invasion

      f. Number of positive and negative lymph nodes

      g. Depth of tumor penetration

      h. Adjuvant chemotherapy

    5. Cancer of the Lung Evaluation and Assessment of Risk (CLEAR): determines a smoker's risk for developing lung cancer in the next 5, 10, or 15 years (Doyle-Lindrud, 2015). Many other lung cancer risk assessment tools are available, including Spitz, Liverpool Lung Project (LLP), Hoggart, and Prostate,

TABLE 9.1   Precision Medicine Definitions

Term	Definition
Actionable mutation	A genomic event that is potentially responsive to a targeted therapy (Brant & Mayer, 2017); biological molecules or processes that can be targeted by an existing or experimental drug (Lemoine, 2014)
Basket trial	Test the effect of one drug on a single mutation in a variety of tumor types (Brant & Mayer, 2017).
Biomarker	Molecule found in blood, tissues, or other body fluids that signals the presence of a condition or disease; can be used to evaluate response to treatment; also referred to as molecular marker or signature molecule (Lemoine, 2014)
Cancer genomics	Sequencing of DNA and RNA in cancer cells to identify molecular alterations that allow for cancer growth, metastasis, and drug resistance (Brant & Mayer, 2017).
Companion diagnostic test	Test carried out to specifically assist in treatment planning and decision making (Lemoine, 2014)
Drug target validation	Stage in drug development where a molecular target is evaluated for therapeutic potential; new therapies can be designed to disrupt activity of validated targets (Lemoine, 2014)
Epigenetic alteration	Heritable change that does not alter the DNA sequence but changes gene expression (Lemoine, 2014)
Gene amplification	Increase in the number of copies of a gene that may cause cancer cell growth or resistance to anticancer drugs (Lemoine, 2014)
Gene deletion	Loss of all or part of a gene found in cancer and other genetic diseases (Lemoine, 2014)
Gene overexpression	Increase in the copies of a protein made from a gene that may play a role in cancer development (Lemoine, 2014)
Genetics	The study of heredity and the variation of inherited characteristics
Genomics	Also known as *"omics"*; the study of the sequence of adenine (A), cytosine (C), guanine (G), thymine (T), or letters, within DNA (Brant & Mayer, 2017)
Multitarget inhibition	Therapeutic agents that may target more than a single biomarker (Lemoine, 2014)
Next-generation sequencing	Also known *as high-throughput sequencing*; a term used to describe modern DNA and RNA sequencing technologies (Brant & Mayer, 2017)
Omic profiling	Analysis of a tumor or other tissue to identify genomic, proteomic, or metabolomic alterations of clinical importance (Brant & Mayer, 2017)
Omics	Exploration of the roles, relationships, and actions of the molecules that comprise the organism; includes genomics, proteomics, and metabolomics (Brant & Mayer, 2017)
Pharmacodynamics	Looks at how the drug affects the individual (Dodson, 2017)
Pharmacogenomics	Study of how patient's genomes affect responses to medications (Blix, 2014)
Pharmacokinetics	Looks at how the individual affects the drug (Dodson, 2017)
Predictive biomarker	A biomarker that provides information on the effect of a therapeutic intervention (Lemoine, 2014)
Prognostic biomarker	A biomarker that provides information about the patient's overall cancer outcome, regardless of therapy (Lemoine, 2014)
Umbrella trial	Various treatment arms are available within one trial; treatment assignment is based on type of cancer and genomic makeup of the tumor (Brant & Mayer, 2017)
Wild type gene	The normal, as opposed to the mutant, gene (Lemoine, 2014)

From Brant, J. M., & Mayer, D. K. (2017). Precision medicine: accelerating the science to revolutionize cancer care. *Clin J Oncol Nurs, 21(6)*, 722–729. https://doi.org/10.1188/17.CJON.722-729. based on information from National Cancer Institute. (2017). *NCI dictionary of cancer terms—precision medicine*. Retrieved from https://www.cancer.gov/publications/dictionaries/cancer-terms/def/precision-medicine and Lemoine, C. (2014). Precision medicine for nurses: 101. *Semin Oncol Nurs, 30(2)*, 84–99. https://doi.org/10.1016/j.soncn.2014.03.002.

Lung, Colorectal, and Ovarian (PLCO) (American Association for Thoracic Surgery, 2016).
   a. Smoking history
   b. Age and gender
   c. Medical history
   d. Family history of cancer
   e. Prior exposures to asbestos
C. Diagnosing disease (Blix, 2014)
   1. Genomics is increasingly used to distinguish between cancer subtypes
   2. Whole-genome sequencing can reveal mutations that led to oncogenesis; examples:
      a. Mapping the genomic characteristics of pediatric acute myeloid leukemia
      b. Testing for gene expression subtypes of breast cancer (e.g., HER2-positive subtype)

D. Determining prognosis (Blix, 2014; Vorderstrasse, Hammer, & Dungan, 2014)
   1. Genetics and genomic testing can be used in determining disease severity and outcomes
   2. Use of clinical decision support tools to integrate patient data into treatment planning that incorporates clinical variables (extent of tumor, age, performance status, etc.)
   3. American Society of Clinical Oncology published a Clinical Practice Guideline that guides biomarker use for treatment decisions for women with early-stage invasive breast cancer (Harris et al, 2016)
E. Pharmacogenomics (Dodson, 2017)
   1. Integration of pharmacology and genomics in developing safe and effective medications

2. Dose determination based on genomics
3. Types of tests include
   a. Drug disposition testing: drug disposition genes can alter the pharmacokinetics of a drug
      - CYP2D6, a drug disposition gene, generates the metabolite endoxifen from tamoxifen
      - Endoxifen is 100 times more potent than the parent drug tamoxifen
      - High CYP2D6 activity (rapid metabolizers) has significantly higher serum concentrations of endoxifen
      - High CYP2D6 activity has been associated with higher relapse-free survival rates
   b. Drug target testing: drug target genes can change the pharmacodynamics of a drug
      - UGT1A1 is an active metabolite of irinotecan
      - Low activity of UGT1A1 enzyme associated with increased serum concentration of the active metabolite, which increases risk of adverse events, particularly neutropenia
      - Patients with two identical UGT1A1*28 alleles, which have a lower enzyme expression and activity, have a significantly higher risk of neutropenia compared with patients carrying UGT1A1*1 (normal allele)
      - Food and Drug Administration (FDA) recommended reduced irinotecan dose for patients with UGT1A1*28/*28
   c. Targeted cancer therapies: most common type of test within oncology practice; involves use of genetic and genomic information of the cancer tissue to guide selection of an appropriate targeted drug therapy
F. Identification of therapeutic targets (Lemoine, 2014)
   1. Clinically relevant biomarkers associated with specific cancers
   2. Ideal targets are present in cancer cells but not in normal cells
   3. Table 9.2 provides a list of common cancers, actionable mutations, and targeted therapies.
   4. For the most current list of FDA-approved targeted therapies and indications, refer to the Targeted Therapies Fact Sheet from the National Cancer Institute at https://www.cancer.gov/about-cancer/treatment/types/targeted-therapies/targeted-therapies-fact-sheet
G. Ethical considerations (Brant & Mayer, 2017; Lemoine, 2014)
   1. Patients provide biospecimens for biorepository and research purposes in addition to use in clinical decision making
      a. Requires informed consent and protection of patient's privacy and confidentiality
      b. Patients should be informed of purpose of biospecimen collection and associated risks and benefits
   2. The complexity of precision medicine may magnify medical mistrust, health care disparities
   3. Patients may be concerned about data security and fear government intrusion that may affect health care coverage

TABLE 9.2 Selected Common Cancers, Actionable Mutations, and Targeted Therapy

Actionable Mutations	Cancer Type	Targeted Therapy
ALK	Lung (nonsmall cell), lymphoma (large cell), neuroblastoma	Alectinib, brigatinib, crizotinib, ceritinib
BCL-2	Chronic lymphocytic leukemia	Venetoclax
BCR-ABL	Chronic myelogenous leukemia	Bafetinib, bosutinib, dasatinib, imatinib, nilotinib, ponatinib
BRAF	Colorectal, melanoma, ovarian, thyroid	Cobimetinib, dabrafenib, trametinib, vemurafenib
EGFR	Lung, colon	Afatinib, gefitinib, imatinib, osimertinib
FLT3	Acute myeloid leukemia, mastocytosis	Lestaurtinib, midostaurin, sorafenib, sunitinib
Histone deacetylase	Lymphoma (T-cell cutaneous), multiple myeloma	Panobinostat, romidepsin, vorinostat
Her2	Brain, breast, lung, ovarian, stomach	Pertuzumab, trastuzumab
KRAS	Colorectal, lung, pancreatic	Cetuximab and panitumumab
mTOR	Astrocytoma (subependymal giant cell), breast, pancreatic (neuroendocrine), renal	Everolimus, ridaforolimus, temsirolimus
MET (c-MET)	Lung (nonsmall cell), medullary thyroid	Cabozantinib, crizotinib
PARP	BRCA mutations (germline or somatic), fallopian tube, ovarian (epithelial), peritoneal	Niraparib, olaparib, rucaparib
PDL-1	Head and neck squamous cell, Hodgkin lymphoma, Merkel cell carcinoma, urothelial carcinoma	Atezolizumab, avelumab, durvalumab, nivolumab, pemrolizuma

Source: Modified from Brant, J. M., & Mayer, D. K. (2017). Precision Medicine: Accelerating the Science to Revolutionize Cancer Care. *Clin J Oncol Nurs, 21(6)*, 722–729. https://doi.org/10.1188/17.CJON.722-729.

4. Genetic Information Nondiscrimination Act of 2008 mandates fairness in the use of genetic information

H. Patient care considerations

1. Genetic testing results may take up to 8 weeks and cause waiting-related patient anxiety when treatment is dependent on results (Wujcik, 2016)

2. Discussion of costs/insurance coverage should occur before testing (Brant & Mayer, 2017)

3. Genetic testing results may have implications for reproduction (Brant & Mayer, 2017) or include non-medical information such as a discovery of nonpaternity (Holt, Hussain, Wachbroit, & Scott, 2017)

4. Effective communication is needed, especially for patients with limited resources, education, or health literacy (Holt et al., 2017)

5. Unclear or ineffective communication about genetic testing and results can widen health disparities (Holt et al., 2017)

REFERENCES

American Association for Thoracic Surgery. (2016). *Lung cancer risk assessment tool.* Retrieved from http://aats.org/aatsimis/AATS/Applications/Lung_Screening_Calculator.aspx?WebsiteKey=81f79f5f-4a27-4146-913d-cffea0ac81f7.

Blix, A. (2014). Personalized medicine, genomics, and pharmacogenomics: a primer for nurses. *Clin J Oncol Nurs, 18*(4), 437–441. https://doi.org/10.1188/14.CJON.437-441.

Brant, J. M., & Mayer, D. K. (2017). Precision medicine: accelerating the science to revolutionize cancer care. *Clin J Oncol Nurs, 21*(6), 722–729. https://doi.org/10.1188/17.CJON.722-729.

Dodson, C. H. (2017). Pharmacogenomics: principles and relevance to oncology nursing. *Clin J Oncol Nurs, 21*(6), 739–745. https://doi.org/10.1188/17.CJON.739-745.

Doyle-Lindrud, S. (2015). Risk prediction tools in oncology. *Clin J Oncol Nurs, 19*(6), 665–666. https://doi.org/10.1188/15.CJON.665-666.

Harris, L. N., Ismaila, N., McShane, L. M., Andre, F., Collyar, D. E., Gonzalez-Angulo, A. M., et al. (2016). American Society of Clinical Oncology. Use of biomarkers to guide decisions on Adjuvant systemic therapy for women with early-stage invasive breast cancer: American Society of Clinical Oncology Clinical Practice Guideline. *J Clin Oncol, 34*(10), 1134–1150. https://doi.org/10.1200/JCO.2015.65.2289.

Holt, C. L., Hussain, A., Wachbroit, R., & Scott, J. (2017). Precision medicine across the cancer continuum: implementation and implications for cancer disparities. *JCO Precision Medicine.* Retrieved February 12, 2018 from http://ascopubs.org/doi/full/10.1200/PO.17.00102.

Johns Hopkins University. (2011). *New Partin nomogram.* Retrieved from http://urology.jhu.edu/support/partinTables.php.

Kawai, K., Sunami, E., Yamaguchi, H., Ishihara, S., Kazama, S., Nozawa, H., et al. (2015). Nomograms for colorectal cancer: a systematic review. *World J Gastroenterol, 21*(41), 11877–11886. https://doi.org/10.3748/wjg.v21.i41.11877. Central PMCID: PMC4631985.

Lemoine, C. (2014). Precision medicine for nurses: 101. *Semin Oncol Nurs, 30*(2), 84–99. https://doi.org/10.1016/j.soncn.2014.03.002.

National Cancer Institute. (2008). *Melanoma risk assessment tool.* Retrieved from https://www.cancer.gov/melanomarisktool/.

National Cancer Institute. (2011). *Breast cancer risk assessment tool.* Retrieved from https://www.cancer.gov/bcrisktool/.

National Cancer Institute. (2017). *NCI dictionary of cancer terms—precision medicine.* Retrieved from https://www.cancer.gov/publications/dictionaries/cancer-terms/def/precision-medicine.

President's Council of Advisors on Science and Technology. (2008). *Priorities for personalized medicine : report of the President's Council of Advisors on Science and Technology.* Retrieved from http://cdm266901.cdmhost.com/cdm/ref/collection/p266901coll4/id/1735.

Vorderstrasse, A. A., Hammer, M. J., & Dungan, J. R. (2014). Nursing implications of personalized and precision medicine. *Semin Oncol Nurs, 30*(2), 130–136. https://doi.org/10.1016/j.soncn.2014.03.007.

Wujcik, D. (2016). Scientific advances shaping the future roles of oncology nurses. *Semin Oncol Nurs, 32*(2), 87–98. https://doi.org/10.1016/j.soncn.2016.02.003.

10

Genetic Risk Factors

Julie Eggert

OVERVIEW

I. The "central dogma" of molecular biology, that is, "DNA makes RNA and RNA makes protein," guides the production of protein for all body functions.

II. Cancer is a common disease associated with changes in the DNA (genetic information) due to inheritance or environmental damage.

A. Chromosomes: threadlike structures of DNA containing genetic information.

B. Forty-six chromosomes in the body include 23 chromosome pairs, one copy from each parent.

1. Small arm of the chromosome identified as the "petite," or "p,'" arm.

2. The long arm is labeled the "q" arm, because "q" follows "p" in the alphabet.

C. Two types of nucleic acid exist.

1. Deoxyribonucleic acid (DNA) comprises two nucleotide chains; held together by oxygen bonds, coiled around one another to form a double helix. Two bases:

   a. Purines: adenine (A) and guanine (G)

   b. Pyridines: thymine (T) and cytosine (C)

   c. DNA base pairs are complementary; A attaches to T, and G attaches to C.

2. Ribonucleic acid (RNA) consists of a single nucleotide chain and represents a complementary copy of a strand of DNA.

   a. DNA sequence order determines RNA code for amino acids and the protein.

   b. In RNA, the base uracil (U) replaces thymine (T).

   c. Transcription refers to the process of making RNA from DNA (Fig. 10.1).

   (1) Loosening DNA wound around the histone allows transcription.

   (2) Tightening the DNA around the histone prevents transcription.

   d. Primary types of RNA

   (1) Messenger RNA (mRNA) directs the order of the amino acids in a protein.

   (2) A codon is a sequence of three mRNA nucleotides (e.g., ACG) yielding one (threonine) of the 20 amino acids.

(3) Multiple codons can code for a specific amino acid (e.g., ACC and ACG code for threonine).

(4) A change in the first position of the codon usually will cause a different amino acid to be produced, allowing an error in building the protein.

(5) An mRNA nucleotide change in the third position of the codon rarely causes an amino acid change.

(6) mRNA changes are the direct cause of polymorphisms and mutations.

   (a) A single nucleotide polymorphism (SNP) change in a nucleotide of a gene causing variation in the DNA sequence affects 1% of population.

   (b) A mutation is a permanent alteration of nucleotide sequence of a gene causing a rare and abnormal variant; more likely responsible for a disease.

   e. Translation refers to the process of creating protein from the chains of amino acids translated from mRNA.

   (1) A variety of RNA types are involved in the protein development process, including transfer RNA (tRNA), ribosomal RNA (rRNA), small silencing RNAs (smRNA), piwi interacting RNAs (piRNA), and small interfering RNA (siRNA) (Siomi et al., 2011; Gorski et al., 2017).

   (2) Sequences of the amino acids determine the structure of the protein.

   (3) Any alteration in characteristics of the 20 amino acids can allow cancer, causing structural changes of the protein.

D. Genes—individual units of hereditary information located at a specific position on the chromosome.

1. Consist of sequence of amino acids that code for a specific protein (see Fig. 10.1).

2. Genes consist primarily of exons and introns.

   a. Exons: protein-coding segments of a gene.

   b. Introns: non–protein-coding segments, the sequence-interrupting piece of a gene.

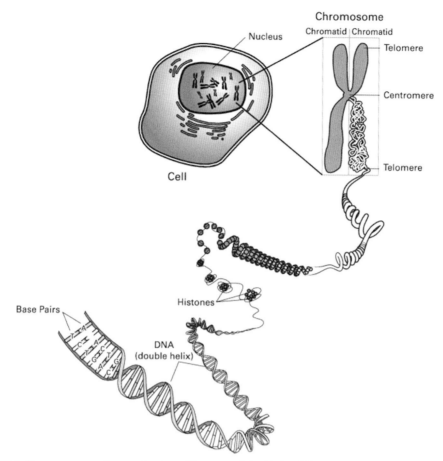

Fig. 10.1 Chromosome and gene structure. (Courtesy of the National Human Genome Research Institute, Bethesda, MD.)

E. Epigenetics: switching genes on and off with a variety of "chemical tails" attached to the DNA structure, without changing the DNA sequence.
  1. DNA transcription controlled by opening or closing the tightly wound histone structure
  2. This occurs by opening (allowing transcription) and closing the histone structure to alter the "DNA to RNA to protein" outcome.
  3. Diet, exercise, aging, drugs and addiction, parenting, and environment can affect epigenetics positively or negatively.
  4. Epigenetic changes can cause or prevent cancer.

III. Basic mechanisms of mutations and heredity
  A. Cancer has a multifactorial etiology with genetic, environmental, and personal factors interacting to produce a malignant transformation.
  B. Genetic mutations and genetic instability are the core of cancer development.
    1. Most cancers are the result of environmentally caused mutations in single cells over the lifetime of an individual.

  2. A malignant tumor arises after a series of genetic mutations have accumulated.
  C. Variations in the sequence of DNA.
    1. Mutations
      a. Germline mutations occur in the reproductive cells of a person with an inherited predisposition to cancer.
      b. Somatic mutations occur in body cells (except gametes) after conception and are acquired over a lifetime.
      c. A variety of mutation types result in an altered form or different protein than required for correct function of a gene; mutations include frameshift, missense, nonsense, silent point, RNA-negative, and splicing changes (Griffith et al., 2000).
    2. SNPs are changes in one of the DNA sequences of the nucleotides of a gene that often are not disease related, occur at variable frequency, and are associated with changes in the general population; create individual differences (NCI Dictionary of Terms, n.d.).

3. Chromosomal abnormalities
   a. Translocations refer to segments of one chromosome that break off and attach themselves to other chromosomes, resulting in altered protein production.
   b. Aneuploidy is an abnormal number of chromosomes.
   c. Loss of heterozygosity refers to the loss of the second segment of both copies (alleles) of a chromosome.
   d. Microsatellite instability (MSI) is a change in the DNA in some cells, like tumor cells, where short, repeated sequences of nucleotide repeats (microsatellites) are different from the inherited DNA. MSI identifies germline abnormality in mismatch repair genes in colorectal cancer, also known as *Lynch syndrome* (NCI Dictionary of Terms, N.D.).
D. A malignant tumor is derived from genetic instability and genetic mutations in genes that control cell growth and proliferation.
   1. Types of regulatory genes
      a. Proto-oncogenes: normal genes essential for usual cell growth and regulation (e.g., *HER2*). Mutations occurring in proto-oncogenes convert to oncogene activation to cause uncontrolled cell division.
      b. Tumor suppressor genes: function as regulators of cell growth (e.g., *p53*). Some tumor suppressor genes appear to play a role in cell cycle regulation or DNA repair. Mutation of a tumor suppressor gene may cause uncontrolled cell growth.
      c. DNA repair genes
         (1) Mismatch repair (MMR) genes: a type of DNA repair gene responsible for keeping the DNA free of "changes" during DNA synthesis; associated with MSI in Lynch syndrome.
         (2) Mutations in DNA repair genes may be inherited from a parent or acquired over time due to aging or impact of carcinogens from the environment.
   2. Mutator gene phenotype
      a. Allows increased mutation of genes due to poor proofreading or insertion of incorrect nucleotides left unrepaired.
      b. Efficient at acquiring mutations with both clonal and random mutations, allowing thousands of mutations versus lower rates seen with normal cells (Loeb, 2016).
   3. Driver and passenger mutations
      a. Driver mutations—overlooked DNA damage with increased chance of oncogene mutations. These mutations offer a selective growth advantage.
      b. Passenger mutations—nucleotide changes that *do not* provide a growth advantage.

IV. Common hereditary cancer syndromes and cancer susceptibility genes
   A. Approximately 10% of all cancers are passed from generation to generation
   B. More than 45 cancer syndromes are suggestive of hereditary cancer (NCI PDQ, 2018a).
   C. Features suggestive of risk for hereditary cancer include:
      1. Family member with a known germline-deleterious mutation in a cancer susceptibility gene
      2. Predisposition of a family to common types of cancer such as breast, ovarian, colon, and/or endometrial
      3. Multiple primary cancers found in one individual
      4. Bilateral cancer in paired organs and/or multifocal disease
      5. Close relatives with three generations of family history who have same type of cancer
         a. First-degree relatives are siblings, children, and parents.
         b. Second-degree relatives include aunts/uncles and grandparents.
         c. Cousins and great-aunts/great-uncles are third-degree relatives.
      6. Autosomal-dominant inheritance; multiple generations having same type of cancers.
         a. Trait is passed to future generations on both alleles of the chromosome.
         b. Most cancer syndromes are autosomal dominant.
      7. Cancers diagnosed at an early age or earlier than normal (e.g., familial adenomatous polyposis [FAP])
      8. Rare cancers
         a. Types such as retinoblastoma, adrenocortical carcinoma, or duodenal cancer.
         b. Uncommon histology such as medullary thyroid cancer.
         c. Unusual presentation such as male breast cancer.
         d. Birth defects associated with rare cancers (e.g., Wilms tumor)
         e. Cancers associated with strong founder effect such as Ashkenazi heritage and the *BRCA1/ BRCA2* pathogenic variants.
         f. Examples of common hereditary cancer syndromes, clinical manifestations, genes, and inheritance patterns are listed in Table 10.1.
   D. Pedigree documentation (NCI PDQ, 2018a).
      1. A recorded disease history for at least three generations of family.
      2. Utilize common pedigree nomenclature (Fig. 10.2).
      3. Paternal lineage on the left side and maternal lineage on the right side of the pedigree.

TABLE 10.1   Common Hereditary Cancer Syndromes and Cancer Susceptibility Genes

Syndrome	Clinical Manifestations	Common Gene(s)	Mode of Inheritance
Birt–Hogg–Dube syndrome (OMIM 135150)	Classic noncancerous skin lesions (30–40 yr), bilateral and multifocal renal tumors and multiple bilateral lung cysts associated with spontaneous pneumothorax.	FLCN	Autosomal dominant
Cowden syndrome, also known as PTEN hamartoma tumor syndrome (OMIM 158350)	Characterized by benign skin findings, increased lifetime risks for breast, follicular thyroid, renal cell, endometrial, and colorectal cancers, and possibly melanoma. Macrocephaly >97th percentile; 58 cm for women and 60 cm for men. Multiple mucocutaneous lesions Multiple hamartomas	PTEN	Autosomal dominant
Familial adenomatous polyposis and attenuated familial adenomatous polyposis (OMIM 175100)	Colon polyposis (adenomas), desmoid tumors, osteomas, thyroid cancer, and hepatoblastoma Increased lifetime risk of colorectal cancer (nearly 100% for FAP [>100 adenomatous polyps in colon] and 70% for attenuated FAP [30–100 adenomatous polyps]). Elevated lifetime risk for duodenal, pancreatic, and papillary thyroid cancers, plus hepatoblastoma by age 5 and medulloblastoma.	APC MUTYH	Autosomal dominant Autosomal recessive
Familial gastrointestinal stromal tumor (OMIM 606764) [GIST]	Mutations in: KIT = hyperpigmentation, mast cell tumors, or dysphagia PDGFRA = large hands Diagnosis of neurofibromatosis type 1 can also develop GISTs. Wild-type GISTs are defined as GISTs that **do not have detectable mutations** in KIT, PDGFRA, or BRAF.	KIT PDGFRA	Most GIST is sporadic. Autosomal dominant if familial in these two genes.
	Sporadic wild-type GIST, small number are SDHB or SDHC mutations.	SDHB, and SDHC	Autosomal recessive if mutations in these or other genes.
	Small number of wild-type GISTs with SDHA mutation (all of which exhibited loss of the SDHA protein by immunohistochemistry).	SDHA	
Familial pancreatic cancer (OMIM 260350)	Common in Lynch syndrome, Peutz–Jeghers syndrome, FAP, hereditary melanoma, and hereditary breast–ovarian cancer syndrome.	BRCA2, most common CDKN2A, PALB2, ATM	Autosomal dominant
Hereditary breast–ovarian cancer syndrome (OMIM 604370 and 612555)	Early-onset breast, multiple breast primaries, male breast, and epithelial ovarian, fallopian tube, or primary peritoneal cancers. In addition, cancers of the pancreas, prostate, and melanoma seem to be more common. Negative markers for estrogen receptor, progesterone receptor, and HER2 receptors (triple-negative phenotype). Founder mutations in Ashkenazi Jewish, Icelandic, and Mexican Hispanic populations.	BRCA1 BRCA2	Autosomal dominant

Continued

TABLE 10.1 **Common Hereditary Cancer Syndromes and Cancer Susceptibility Genes—cont'd**

Syndrome	Clinical Manifestations	Common Gene(s)	Mode of Inheritance
Hereditary diffuse gastric cancer (OMIM 137215)	Diffuse gastric cancer, lobular breast cancer, adenocarcinoma and epithelial ovarian cancer, prostate, signet ring colon cancer	*CDH1*	Autosomal dominant
Hereditary papillary RCC (OMIM 605074)	Papillary type 1 renal cell cancer with bilateral disease and history of *MET* mutation.	*MET*	Autosomal dominant
Hereditary retinoblastoma (OMIM 180200)	Malignant tumor of the retina, usually before age 5. Family history of retinoblastoma, bilateral tumors, and multifocal tumors have the highest chance to have hereditary retinoblastoma. Individuals with hereditary retinoblastoma. Also increased risk for pinealoblastoma, osteosarcomas, sarcoma (especially radiogenic), and melanoma.	*RBl*	Autosomal dominant
Li–Fraumeni syndrome (OMIM 151623)	Cancers of brain, breast, adrenocortex, and non-Ewing sarcoma with onset before age 50.	*TP53*	Autosomal dominant
Lynch syndrome (OMIM 120435 and 120436) (previously known as *hereditary nonpolyposis colorectal cancer* [HNPCC])	Cancers of the colon, rectum, stomach, small intestine, esophagus, biliary tract, brain, endometrium, and ovary. Other cancers at elevated risk are transitional cell carcinoma of the ureters and renal pelvis plus pancreatic.	*MLH1* *MSH2* (including methylation due to *EPCAM* deletion) *MSH6* *PMS2* Characterized by microsatellite instability (MSI) due to defective mismatch repair	Autosomal dominant
Muir–Torre syndrome (variant of Lynch syndrome)	Gastrointestinal and genitourinary cancers, skin, breast cancer, and benign breast tumors Glioblastoma Endometrial cancer and other Lynch syndrome–associated cancers such as sebaceous adenomas and carcinomas. Keratoacanthomas	*MSH2* *MLH1* *MSH6*	Autosomal dominant
Multiple endocrine neoplasia type I (OMIM 131100)	Endocrine and nonendocrine tumors, including parathyroid glands, pituitary gland, and the pancreas.	*MEN1*	Autosomal dominant
Multiple endocrine neoplasia type II (OMIM 171400, 155240, and 162300)	Medullary thyroid cancer and pheochromocytoma. Subtypes 2A = hyperparathyroidism 2B = Familial medullary thyroid carcinoma (FMTC) 4 = symptoms similar to MEN type 1, especially hyperparathyroidism, pituitary gland, and other endocrine glands and organs.	*RET*	Autosomal dominant
MUTYH-associated polyposis (MAP) (OMIM 608456)	Colon cancer and duodenal cancer, as well as colon, duodenal, and gastric fundic gland polyps, osteomas, sebaceous gland adenomas, and pilomatricomas (Polyps range from few to >1000 with biallelic *MUTYH* mutations	*MYH*, biallelic mutations	Autosomal recessive

TABLE 10.1 Common Hereditary Cancer Syndromes and Cancer Susceptibility Genes—cont'd

Syndrome	Clinical Manifestations	Common Gene(s)	Mode of Inheritance
Neurofibromatosis type 1 (OMIM 162200)	Malignant peripheral neural sheath tumors, neurofibromas, benign pheochromocytomas, meningiomas, hamartomatous intestinal polyps, gastrointestinal stromal tumors, optic gliomas, café-au-lait macules, axillary or inguinal freckles, iris hamartomas, and sphenoid wing dysplasia or congenital bowing or thinning of long bones, as well as other malignancies	NF1	Autosomal dominant
Neurofibromatosis type 2 (OMIM 101000)	Neurofibromas, gliomas, vestibular schwannoma, schwannomas of other cranial and peripheral nerves, meningioma, ependymomas, and astrocytoma	NF2	Autosomal dominant
Nevoid basal cell carcinoma syndrome (Gorlin syndrome) (OMIM 109400)	Multiple jaw keratocysts beginning in the teens and multiple basal-cell carcinomas beginning in the twenties. Common features include macrocephaly, bossing of the forehead (unusually pronounced), coarse facial features, facial milia, and skeletal anomalies	PTCH	Autosomal dominant
Von Hippel–Lindau (OMIM 193300)	Renal cell cancer; hemangioblastoma of brain, spinal cord, and retina; renal cysts; pheochromocytomas; endolymphatic sac tumors; and pancreatic islet cell tumors	VHL	Autosomal dominant, but two copies of VHL gene must be altered to trigger tumor and cyst formation of von Hippel–Lindau syndrome.
Xeroderma pigmentosum OMIM 278700	Basal and squamous cell skin cancer, melanoma, and sarcoma, as well as brain, lung, breast, uterus, kidney, and testicle cancers, leukemia, conjunctival papillomas, actinic keratosis, lid epithiomas, keratoacanthomas, angiomas, fibromas	XPA ERCC3 XPC ERCC2 DDB2 ERCC4 ERCC5 POLH	Autosomal recessive

From Genetics Home Reference (2018). Retrieved from https://ghr.nlm.nih.gov/; Guarinos, C., Sanchez-Fortun, C., Rodriguez-Soler, M., Alenda, C., Paya, A., & Joyer, R. (2012). Serrated polyposis syndrome: molecular, pathological and clinical aspects. *World Journal of Gastroenterology, 18(20)*, 2452–2461; and Online Mendelian Inheritance in Man (OMIM) (2018), Retrieved from https://www.omim.org/.

4. Include three generations, minimum, for both lineages with at least first- and second-degree relatives.
5. Add distant relatives (greater than third-degree relatives) in one lineage when information available. "Singleton" children can affect gender-related disease probabilities (e.g., male children when there is ovarian cancer history in females of the earliest generation or prostate cancer with primarily female generations).
6. Include race, ancestry, and ethnicity of all grandparents.
7. Relatives with cancer diagnosis should also be designated with:
   a. Primary site of cancer(s) with treatment type.
   b. Age at diagnosis for primary cancers.
   c. History of surgery or treatments that may have reduced risk of cancer:
      (1) Bilateral salpingo-oophorectomy in premenopausal woman to decrease risk of ovarian and breast cancers or colectomy for hereditary nonpolyposis colorectal cancer (HNPCC).
      (2) Chemoprevention (e.g., tamoxifen for breast or aspirin for colon cancers).
   d. Current age or age at and cause of death (if deceased).

Standard Pedigree Nomenclature

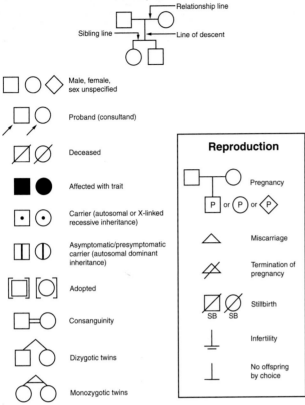

Fig. 10.2 Pedigree nomenclature symbols. Symbols used in drawing pedigrees of persons with family history of cancer. (Retrieved March 10, 2018, from https://visualsonline.cancer.gov/details.cfm?imageid = 10346.)

e. Carcinogenic exposures (e.g., tobacco use or World War II veterans stationed in the South Pacific and exposure to uncovered asbestos in submarines)

f. Physical characteristics indicative of hereditary cancer (e.g., macrocephaly, café-au-lait spots)

g. Other significant health problems (e.g., history of blood clots in the patient/family could be related to factor V Leiden; need for genetic testing before colectomy).

8. Relatives without cancer
   a. Current age or age at death with cause (if deceased).
   b. History of surgeries or treatment that may have reduced risk of cancer.
   c. Cancer screening practices.
   d. Nonmalignant features associated with the syndrome in question (e.g., benign tumors of the parathyroid gland are associated with multiple endocrine neoplasia type II [MEN II] syndrome).
   e. Carcinogenic exposures.
   f. Other significant health problems (e.g., chronic obstructive pulmonary disease [COPD], history of multiple adenomatous colon polyps).

V. Genetic testing
   A. Results sharing of inherited cancer predisposition testing
      1. The predictive value of a negative test result varies, depending on whether a known genetic mutation exists in the family.
         a. A negative test result with a known familial genetic mutation indicates
            (1) The patient is within the "general population risk of cancer" associated with that branch of the family. No additional high-risk screening required.
            (2) Family history from the other parent influences the risk of developing cancer.
         b. A negative result with "no known family genetic mutation" may occur because:
            (1) Identification of a mutation in a cancer susceptibility gene may not be possible because of the limited sensitivity of the techniques used.
            (2) Function of the gene may be affected by a mutation in a different gene.
            (3) The cancer in the family may be associated with a cancer susceptibility gene other than the one tested.
            (4) The cancer in the family is not the result of a germline genetic mutation.
      2. A "variant of uncertain clinical significance" (VUS) is identified (Strom, 2016; Maxwell et al., 2016).
         a. Mutations in which the association with cancer risk cannot be established.
         b. Labs report VUS differently; some always, some never, and some only when specific conditions are met.
         c. VUS is not a pathogenic mutation; did not identify a genetic diagnosis of disease.
         d. Explain how VUS classification works and if it is a "good fit" based on the gene, inheritance pattern, patient's phenotype, and family history.
         e. A VUS diagnosis is common and may be familial or benign for traits like freckles, blue eyes, or red hair.
         f. Caution about going to websites to learn about the gene. Many phenotypes exist; may or may not be applicable to their personal or family situation.
         g. VUS may be reclassified as benign or pathogenic in the future. Explain how the patient/family will be notified (e.g., phone call from the clinic or office).
         h. Offer genetic testing to the family (parents or siblings especially), if appropriate, to determine whether the VUS is associated with a disease in other members of the family. Depending on laboratory policy, may be free to certain members of the family.

3. Predictive value of a positive test result varies, depending on the type of genetic mutation identified and degree of certainty that the gene function has been affected.
   a. Penetrance refers to the proportion of all individuals with a specific genotype that express the specific trait such as cancer.
   b. Expression refers to the degree to which a single individual with a specific genotype will exhibit a specific trait (e.g., cancer).
      (1) Expression may be different for different genetic mutations in the same cancer susceptibility gene.
      (2) Expression may also be affected by other genetic variations, as well as by the environment and other personal factors.
   c. Direct to consumer testing
      (1) Food and Drug Administration (FDA) approved breast cancer predisposition testing from 23andMe.
      (2) Includes only the three *BRCA1/2* (selected variants) mutations most common in persons of Ashkenazi descent. The most common out of thousands of mutations are *not* included (FDA, 2018).
      (3) Direct to consumer testing is not meant to be used for diagnosis of disease and/or clinical decision making (FDA, 2018).

B. Predisposition genetic testing and tumor profiling
   1. Techniques for identifying mutations in patients
      a. Cytogenetic reports include modal number of chromosomes, sex chromosome designation (XX or XY or aberrations of these chromosomes); abnormality abbreviation—first chromosome separated with a semicolon from the second chromosome t(14;16), then the arm and band number (q32; q23) (Palumbo & Russo, 2016) (Table 10.2).
      b. Direct sequencing (Sanger sequencing)
         (1) Determines the sequence of a gene being tested and detects sequence changes in regions being analyzed
         (2) May miss mutations outside the coding region or mutations that are large genomic rearrangements or large deletions
      c. Genome-wide association studies (GWAS) (NCI Dictionary of Terms, n.d.)
         (1) Survey the entire genome for small nucleotide alterations
         (2) Purpose is to:
            (a) Detect SNPs or small mutations to determine association with disease
            (b) Review for changes with specific disease (cancer type) versus people without the disease
            (c) Design high-throughput genome sequencing techniques for faster and

TABLE 10.2	Common Cytogenetic Nomenclature
Nomenclature	**Meaning**
'	Separate different elements of a cytogenetic report
( )	Surround structurally altered chromosomes
+	Gain of chromosome
-	Loss of chromosome
;	Separate rearranged chromosomes when >1 involved
/	Separates cell lines or clones
//	Separates recipient and donor cell lines in bone marrow transplants
cd	Cell or cluster of differentiation on surface of cell membrane
del	Deletion of chromosomal material
der	Derivative chromosome (used when only one chromosome from a translocation is present or when one chromosome has two or more structural abnormalities)
dic	Dicentric chromosome
dn	New chromosomal abnormality; not inherited from parents
dup	Duplication of chromosomal material
h	Heterochromatic region of chromosome
i	Isochromosome (both arms of chromosome are the same)
ins	Insertion
inv	Inversion
.ish	Precedes karyotype results from fluorescence in situ hybridization (FISH) analysis
mar	Unidentifiable piece of chromosome (marker)
p	Petite (short) arm of the chromosome
q	Long arm of the chromosome
r	Ring chromosome
t	Translocation or move of genetic material
ter	Terminal end of arm
tri	Trisomy
trp	Triplication of a chromosome piece
Example	46, XY, t(14;16)(q32;q23) = normal number of chromosomes, male, translocation of chromosome 14 and 16; specifically, with position 32 on the long arm of chromosome 14 rearranging with position 23 on the long arm of chromosome 16

Data from *Basic nomenclature for cytogenetics*. <http://www.slh.wisc.edu/clinical/cytogenetics/basics/> Accessed March 5, 2018.

cheaper ways to obtain genetic data, with potential impact on personalized profiling for diagnosis, pharmacogenomics, and disease monitoring (Soon, Hariharan & Snyder, 2013).
   d. Large genomic rearrangements (LGRs) detect large rearrangements, deletions, and duplications (like pages or paragraphs missing or rearranged in a mystery novel) (Park et al., 2017).

(1) Found in *BRCA1* family mutations with following characteristics:
  (a) At least two persons <50 years diagnosed with breast cancer
  (b) Family history of breast and ovarian cancers
  (c) Only ovarian cancer, with at least two members diagnosed with ovarian cancer
  (d) A single breast cancer case before the age of 36 years
  (e) None identified in only one breast cancer case before age 51 (Engert et al., 2008).
  e. Microarray
  (1) Microarray is used for mutation detection and gene expression.
  (2) Large numbers (hundreds to thousands) of DNA, RNA, protein, or tissue segments attached to slides at specific locations, followed by application of a fluorescent label.
  (3) Slide is scanned to measure the brightness of each fluorescent dot. The brighter the dot, the greater the fluorescent activity.
  f. Next-generation DNA sequencing (second-generation sequencing)
  (1) New, lower-cost, higher-efficiency techniques to target the whole genome, whole exome, and whole transcriptome
  (2) Detects somatic cancer genome alterations of the nucleotide (substitutions, small insertions, deletions, variations in copy number)
  (3) Enables results of more mutations. Many more "variants of unknown significance" are identified. These can be confusing for determining how to determine prevention, early detection
  g. Whole-exome sequencing (WES) or targeted exome capture
  (1) Low-cost alternative technique to sequence exon (gene to protein-coding regions) pieces of the genome
  (2) Identifies area of protein function change in mendelian and common diseases.
  h. Other genetic testing is available, including transcriptome, protein truncation assays, histone modifications, and chromosome conformation.
C. Tumor profiling
  1. Somatic mutations occur in all cells (except the gametes) due to damage by variety of environmental carcinogens
  a. Colon cancer (somatic cells)—profiling examples include OncotypeDX and ColoPrint.
  b. Breast cancer (somatic cells)—gene profiling examples include Mammaprint, Symphony, and OncotypeDX.

  2. Germline mutations occur in the gametes; eggs and sperm
  a. Passed from generation to generation.
  b. De novo mutation—change in a gene, present for the first time in one family member due to mutation in a germ cell (egg or sperm) of one of the parents or in the fertilized egg.
  c. Determines whether mutation is inherited and can be passed from generation to generation.
VI. Ethical, legal, and social issues associated with genetic information (NCI PDQ, 2018a; NCI PDQ, 2018b)
  A. Implications of predisposition genetic testing
  1. Psychological consequences, some of which could impact subsequent health behaviors and family communication.
  a. Survivor guilt is often observed in persons who have not inherited the genetic mutation that is present in other close family members.
  b. Transmitter guilt is often observed when family members pass on the genetic mutation to one of their offspring.
  c. Heightened anxiety may result when patients learn that they are at a substantially increased risk for developing cancer or another primary lesion.
  d. Depression and anger may occur, regardless of genetic status.
  e. Personal identity issues result because genetic information involves the very essence of an individual.
  f. Regret for previous decisions may be present in patients who have made decisions based on their perceived cancer risk and testing results are inconsistent with what they had previously thought.
  g. Uncertainty occurs because predisposition genetic testing does not provide information about if or when cancer develops. In many instances, no proven risk-reducing strategy exists.
  h. Intrafamilial issues arise because predisposition genetic testing affects all family members. These issues include but are not limited to the following:
  (1) Coercion regarding testing, disclosure of testing results to family members, and cancer risk management approaches
  (2) Effect of the genetic information on the partner, who is not at risk physically but whose children may be impacted
  2. Stigmatization both within the family and the individual's social network
  B. Social implications
  1. Financial considerations
  a. Predisposition genetic testing may be expensive; not all insurers cover testing and counseling.
  b. Insurers may be reluctant to cover enhanced surveillance programs unless efficacy has been proven.

c. Insurers may not be willing to cover the expense of prophylactic surgery unless it has proven benefit.

2. Quality assurance of laboratory testing uncertain because no regulation exists beyond approval for molecular laboratories that perform testing based on the Clinical Laboratory Improvement Amendments (CLIA).

3. Availability and quality assurance of genetic counseling are of concern, given the small number of trained providers in cancer genetics.

C. Legal issues may involve the following:

1. Discrimination may occur for those harboring an altered cancer susceptibility gene because they may be considered as having a preexisting condition or may be too high a risk to insure or employ (NCI PDQ, 2018a; NCI PDQ, 2018b).
   a. Health insurance
   b. Life insurance
   c. Disability insurance
   d. Long-term care insurance
   e. Education
   f. Employment

2. State and federal legislative approaches have been proposed or enacted, depending on the issue and state (NCI PDQ, 2018a; NCI PDQ, 2018b).
   a. The Health Insurance Portability and Accountability Act (HIPAA), a federal law enacted in 1996, states that genetic information cannot be used as a preexisting condition or to determine eligibility for insurance.
      (1) Applies only to group and self-funded plans.
      (2) Law does not protect against rate hikes, access of insurers to individual's genetic information, or insurer requiring genetic testing as condition of insurance coverage.
   b. The Genetic Information Nondiscrimination Act (GINA), federal legislation enacted in 2008, applies to health insurance and employment discrimination based on genetic information (NCI PDQ, 2018a; NCI PDQ, 2018b).
      (1) Health insurance protections include protections against accessing an individual's genomic information, requirements for an individual to undergo a genetic or genomic test, and using genomic information against a person during medical underwriting.
      (2) Employment protections include prohibiting employers from accessing an individual's genetic information, use of genomic information to deny employment, or collecting genomic information without consent.
      (3) GINA does not supersede state legislation that provides for more extensive protections.
      (4) GINA does not apply to active-duty military personnel, Veterans Administration, or Indian Health Service because the laws amended for GINA do not apply to these groups.
   c. The U.S. Equal Employment Opportunity Commission released guidelines in March 1995 on the definition of "disability" under the Americans with Disabilities Act (ADA), which is now extended to include discrimination based on genetic information. This set of guidelines is not law but is an interpretation of the language of the ADA and may be overturned in a court of law.

3. Self-insured employers may also be exempt from state laws and regulations on health insurance because of the Employee Retirement Income Security Act of 1974 (ERISA), which governs employer pension plans as well as other benefits.

D. Genetic technology raises legal liability issues for the health care provider.

1. Privacy and confidentiality
   a. Genetic information of all types should be handled in a confidential manner to prevent unauthorized access.

2. Genetic testing should be preceded by genetic counseling by a genetic health care professional to include education, counseling, and informed consent.

ASSESSMENT

I. Models/tools used to assess high risk to develop cancer in disease-free populations

A. BRisk app—based on age-adjusted calculations for women with family history of breast or ovarian cancer (previously known as Claus tables) (COH, 2014).

B. Gail (Breast Cancer Risk Assessment Tool)—assesses risk to develop invasive breast cancer based on number of first-degree relatives with breast cancer diagnosis, current age, age at menarche, age at menopause, age at first live birth, number of breast biopsies plus history of atypical hyperplasia, race/ethnicity (NCI Breast Cancer Risk Assessment Tool, n.d.).

C. BRCAPRO—a computer program that calculates the possibility of an individual having an inherited mutation in the *BRCA1* or *BRCA2* gene (NCI, n.d.).

D. Pedigree Assessment Tool (PAT)—assigns 3 to 8 points to each family member with an ovarian or breast cancer diagnosis (Hoskins, Zwaagstra, & Ranz, 2006).

E. Tyrer-Cuzick/IBIS—assesses genes predisposing to breast cancer in addition to the *BRCA1/2* genes. The woman's family history (maternal and paternal) for first- and second-degree relatives is used to calculate the likelihood of carrying an adverse gene. Questions on age at menarche and menopause, breast biopsy, LCIS, and affected cousins and half-siblings are included. Height and body mass index (BMI) plus use of estrogen are also included. The lifetime risk and the risk of having a *BRCA1/2* gene mutation is calculated (Cuzik, 2017).

F. Melanoma Risk Assessment Tool (MRAT)—estimates a person's risk of developing invasive melanoma. The variables of demographics (age, gender, race), tanning ability, complexion, and current number and size of skin moles, plus extent of freckling are used to calculate risk (MRAT, n.d.).

G. Lung Cancer Screening—Assesses low-, moderate-, and high-risk status of previously undiagnosed individuals with 10-year life expectancy for development of lung cancer. Assesses symptoms, diagnostic results, and pack-year history of smoking to calculate risk (Lung Cancer Screening, 2017).

H. NCI Colorectal Cancer Risk Assessment Tool—estimates risk of colorectal cancer for men and women between ages of 50 and 85, or from African American, Asian American/Pacific Islander, Hispanic/Latino, or white ethnic groups. Unable to accurately estimate risk of colorectal cancer in those with a diagnosis of ulcerative colitis, Crohn disease, Lynch syndrome, HNPCC, or FAP (NCI CRAT, 2014).

I. Other risk assessment tools are in development for use in early detection and prevention clinics for patients at high risk to develop cancer. Websites for the American Cancer Society, National Cancer Institute, and Centers for Disease Control monitor literature for new tools being researched for specificity, validity, and reliability.

II. Assess indications for cancer predisposition testing (NCI PDQ, 2018a).

A. Designation of high-risk status on models/tools.

B. Universal criteria for predisposition genetic testing vary, depending on the suspected inherited cancer syndrome and mutations in the gene or genes associated with that syndrome. Criteria include:

1. Individual's medical history is suspicious for genetic predisposition to cancer.

2. The confirmed family history is consistent with the hereditary cancer syndrome.

3. Tests that are ordered should have results information that:

   a. Can be interpreted with sufficient sensitivity and specificity

   b. Is "actionable" to assist in medical decision making

   c. Will assist in diagnosis and management of cancer

   d. Can assist with clarification of cancer risk in family members

MANAGEMENT

I. Chemoprevention (ASCO Cancer.net, 2016)

A. Tamoxifen (for *BRCA2* mutations) prevention

B. Aspirin and nonsteroidal anti-inflammatory drugs (NSAIDs) for colorectal cancer prevention

C. Calcium and vitamins or other substances; the role is unclear.

II. Provide ongoing surveillance that detects cancer as early as possible, when chances for cure are greatest

III. Risk-reducing surgery (also called *prophylactic surgery*) as indicated, which is the removal of as much of the tissue at risk as possible to reduce the risk of developing a cancer. Follow guidelines based on evidence-based literature and specialists working with the cancer subtype (e.g., 23-year-old female with *BRCA2* mutation can have children and breastfeed without having a risk-reducing bilateral mastectomy or salpingo-oophorectomy until she is 40 years of age [NCCN Guidelines, 2018)])

IV. Provide informed consent—precedes genetic testing for the patient to be tested and should include the following: (Riley et al., 2012; Weitzel, Blazer, Macdonald, Culver, & Offit, 2011; NCI PDQ, 2018a; NCI PDQ, 2018b):

A. Purpose of the genetic test

B. Motivation for testing

C. Risks and benefits of genetic testing

D. Limitations of genetic testing

E. Inheritance pattern of the gene(s) being tested

F. Risk of misidentified paternity, if applicable

G. Accuracy and sensitivity of genetic testing method

H. Outcomes of genetic testing

I. Confidentiality of genetic testing results

J. Possibility of discrimination

K. Alternatives to genetic testing

L. How testing will impact health care decision making

M. Cost of testing

N. Right to refuse

O. Testing in children (<18 years of age)—performed only when clinical utility has been established

V. Offer genetic testing and services as indicated

A. Provide genetic counseling—physicians, nurses, or genetic counselors with specialized training in genetics.

1. Inform patients regarding their potential for increased cancer risk from an inherited susceptibility and the availability of predisposition genetic testing (NCI PDQ, 2018a; NCI PDQ, 2018b).

2. Provide genetic counseling before testing (NCI PDQ, 2018a; NCI PDQ, 2018b).

   a. Individuals with personal and family history.

   b. Discuss results from collected information:

      (1) Genetic and other laboratory tests

      (2) Procedures and imaging studies

      (3) Physical examination findings

VI. Discuss clinical and genetic aspects of a suspected diagnosis to include:

A. Mode of inheritance

B. Identification of family members at risk, including:

1. Effect on cancer susceptibility.

2. Clarification of increased risk status.

C. Benefits, risks, limitations of genetic testing plus alternative to *not* testing

1. Costs

2. Logistics of follow-up

D. Assistance to help patients make informed decisions (without coercion or personal opinions) about genetic testing with consideration for their health care needs, preferences, and values

E. Encourage avoidance of exposures that may increase the risk of certain cancers (e.g., smoking and lung or bladder cancer) and healthy behaviors that include diet and exercise

EXPECTED PATIENT OUTCOMES

I. Patients and families will understand their genetic risks of developing cancer.

II. Patients and families will make an informed decision regarding genetic testing and management.

REFERENCES

American Society of Clinical Oncology (ASCO) Cancer.Net. (2016). *Chemoprevention.* Retrieved from https://www.cancer.net/navigating-cancer-care/prevention-and-healthy-living/chemoprevention.

City of Hope (COH). (2014). *Have breast cancer in family? Need to know risk? There's an app for that.* Retrieved from https://www.cityofhope.org/blog/breast-cancer-app-risk.

Cuzik, J. (2017). *IBIS Breast cancer risk evaluation tool.* Retrieved at http://www.ems-trials.org/riskevaluator/.

Engert, S., Wappenschmidt, B., Betz, B., Kast, K., Kutsche, M., Hellebrand, H., et al. (2008). MLPA screening in the BRCA1 gene from 1,506 German hereditary breast cancer cases: novel deletions, frequent involvement of exon 17, and occurrence in single early-onset cases. *Human Mutation, 7*(7), 948–958.

Genetics Home Reference (2018), Retrieved from https://ghr.nlm.nih.gov/.

Gorski, S. A., Vogel, J., & Doudna, J. A. (2017). RNA-based recognition and targeting: sowing the seeds of specificity. *Nature Review: Molecular Cell Biology, 18,* 215–228. https://doi.org/10.1038/nrm.2016.174.

Griffiths, A. J. F., Miller, J. H., Suzuki, D. T., et al. (2000). An introduction to genetic analysis. In *How DNA changes affect phenotype* (7th ed.). New York: W. H. Freeman. Available from: https://www.ncbi.nlm.nih.gov/books/NBK21955/.

Guarinos, C., Sanchez-Fortun, C., Rodriguez-Soler, M., Alenda, C., Paya, A., & Joyer, R. (2012). Serrated polyposis syndrome: molecular, pathological and clinical aspects. *World Journal of Gastroenterology, 18*(20), 2452–2461.

Hoskins, K. F., Zwaagstra, A., & Hoskins, K. F. (2006). Validation of a tool for identifying women at high risk for hereditary breast cancer in population-based screening. *Cancer, 107*(8), 1769–1776.

Loeb, L. A. (2016). Human cancers express a mutator phenotypes: hypothesis, origin, and consequence. *Cancer Research, 76*(8), 2057–2059. https://doi.org/10.1158/0008-5472.CAN-16-079.

Lung Cancer Risk Screening Tool. (2017). Available at https://www.mdanderson.org/content/dam/mdanderson/documents/for-physicians/algorithms/screening/screening-lung-web-algorithm.pdf.

Maxwell, K. N., Hart, S. N., Vijai, J., Kasmintan, A., Schrader, T. P., Slavin, T. T., et al. (2016). Evaluation of ACMG-Guideline-Based variant classification of cancer susceptibility and non-can-associated genes in families affected by breast cancer. *The American Journal of Human Genetics, 98*(5), 801–817. https://doi.org/10.1016/j.ajhg.2016.02.024.

Melanoma Risk Assessment Tool. (n.d.) Available from: https://www.cancer.gov/melanomarisktool/.

National Cancer Institute (NCI) PDQ Cancer Genetics Editorial Board. (2018a) PDQ Cancer Genetics Risk Assessment and Counseling. Bethesda, MD: National Cancer Institute. Updated 03/02/2018. Available at: https://www.cancer.gov/about-cancer/causes-prevention/genetics/risk-assessment-pdq. Accessed 03/10/2018.

National Cancer Institute (NCI) PDQ Genetics Editorial Board. (2018b, 2/15/2018). Risk assessment and counseling: employment and insurance discrimination. Available from, https://www.cancer.gov/about-cancer/causes-prevention/genetics/risk-assessment-pdq#section/all.

National Cancer Institute (NCI) (n.d.). Breast Cancer Assessment Tool. Retrieved from https://www.cancer.gov/bcrisktool/about-tool.aspx#gail.

National Cancer Institute (NCI) (n.d.). The Colorectal Cancer Risk Assessment Tool. (2014) Retrieved from https://ccrisktool.cancer.gov/.

National Cancer Institute (NCI) Dictionary of Genetic Terms. (n.d.). BRCAPRO. Retrieved from https://www.cancer.gov/publications/dictionaries/cancer-terms/def/brcapro.

National Cancer Institute (NCI) Dictionary of Genetic Terms. (n.d.). Genome wide association study (GWAS). Retrieved from http://www.cancer.gov/geneticsdictionary?cdrid=636780.

National Cancer Institute (NCI) Dictionary of Genetic Terms. (n.d.). Microsatellite instability (MSI). Retrieved from https://www.cancer.gov/publications/dictionaries/cancer-terms/search?contains=false&q=microsatellite+instability.

National Cancer Institute (NCI) Dictionary of Genetic Terms. (n.d.). Single Nucleotide Polymorphism Retrieved from https://www.cancer.gov/publications/dictionaries/genetics-dictionary/def/single-nucleotide-polymorphism.

National Comprehensive Cancer Network. (2018). *NCCN guidelines for detection, prevention and risk reduction.* Available at https://www.mdanderson.org/content/dam/mdanderson/documents/for-physicians/algorithms/screening/screening-lung-web-algorithm.pdf.

Online Mendelian Inheritance in Man (OMIM) (2018), Retrieved from https://www.omim.org/.

Palumbo, E., & Russo, A. (2016). Chromosome imbalances in cancer: molecular cytogenetics meets genomics. *Cytogenetic and Genome Research. 150*(pp. 176–184). Retrieved from https://doi.org/10.1159/000455804.

Park, B., Sohn, J. Y., Yoon, K.-A., Lee, K. S., Cho, E. H., Lim, M. C., et al. (2017). Characteristics of BRCA1/2 mutations carriers including large genomic rearrangements in high risk breast cancer patients. *Breast Cancer Research and Treatment, 163*(1), 139–150. https://doi.org/10.1007/s10549-017-4142-7.

Riley, B. D., Culver, J. O., Skrzynia, C., Senter, L. A., Peters, J. A., Costalas, J. W., et al. (2012). Essential elements of genetic cancer risk assessment, counseling, and testing: updated recommendations of the National Society of Genetic Counselors. *Journal of Genetic Counseling, 21*(2), 151–161. https://doi.org/10.1007/s10897-011-9462-x.

Siomi, M. C., Sato, K., Pezic, D., & Aravin, A. A. (2011). PIWI-interacting small RNAs: the vanguard of genome defence. *Nature Reviews: Molecular Cell Biology, 12,* 246–258. https://doi.org/10.1038/nrm3089.

Soon, W. W., Hariharan, M., & Snyder, M. P. (2013). High-throughput sequencing for biology and medicine.

Molecular Systems Biology, 9, 640. https://doi.org/10.1038/msb.2012.61.

Strom, S. P. (2016).Current practices and guidelines for clinical next-generation sequencing oncology testing. *Cancer Biology & Medicine, 13*(1), 3–11.

U.S. Food & Drug Administration (FDA). (2018). FDA authorizes, with special controls, direct-to-consumer test that reports three mutations in the BRCA breast cancer genes.

Retrieved from https://www.fda.gov/NewsEvents/Newsroom/PressAnnouncements/ucm599560.htm.

Weitzel, J. N., Blazer, K. R., Macdonald, D. J., Culver, J. O., & Offit, K. (2011). Genetics, genomics, and cancer risk assessment: State of the art and future directions in the era of personalized medicine. CA: A Cancer Journal for Clinicians, 61, 327–351. https://doi.org/10.3322/caac.20128.

11

Clinical Trials and Research Protocols

Marlon Garzo Saria and Santosh Kesari

I. Definitions (ClinicalTrials.gov, 2018; National Cancer Institute, 2016)
   A. Research protocol: detailed written plan of a clinical trial
   B. Clinical research: studies that involve human volunteer participants
   C. Clinical trials: studies that test new treatments or new ways of using existing treatments, also referred as *experimental* or *interventional studies*

II. Types of clinical research (ClinicalTrials.gov, 2018; National Cancer Institute, 2016; Saria, 2017; Schmotzer, 2015)
   A. Observational studies: participants are not assigned to specific interventions; assesses health outcomes
      1. Case report/case studies series: explore a single individual (case report) or small group (case series) to determine the likelihood of an association between an observed effect and a specific event
      2. Cross-sectional studies: describe the association between a condition and other characteristics that may exist in a specific group
      3. Case control studies: compare cases (subjects with outcome of interest) to controls (similar subjects who do not have the disease or condition) with respect to exposure
      4. Cohort studies: subjects who do not have the outcome or condition are followed and compared based on the exposure
      5. Outcomes research: explores the results of health care practices and interventions; includes patient-based outcomes as well as the study of populations, databases, and the delivery of health care
   B. Experimental or interventional studies (clinical trials): participants receive specific interventions; each type is designed to answer different research questions
      1. Prevention trials: evaluate the safety and efficacy of various risk reduction strategies
         a. Action studies (e.g., being more active, quitting smoking, eating more fruits and vegetables)
         b. Agent or chemoprevention studies (e.g., taking certain medications, vitamins, and supplements)
      2. Screening trials: evaluate the effectiveness of new techniques for early detection of cancer in the general population
      3. Diagnostic trials: evaluate tests or procedures that may better identify cancer in symptomatic individuals
      4. Quality-of-life or supportive care trials: explore pharmacologic or nonpharmacologic therapies to minimize cancer- and cancer treatment–related toxicities on persons with cancer and their families
      5. Treatment or therapeutic trials: evaluate the safety and efficacy of new drugs, vaccines, biological agents, approaches to surgery or radiation therapy, treatment combinations, or other interventions
   C. Expanded access or compassionate use (Standafer, 2015)
      1. Expanded access protocols: provide a means for patients and their physicians to use an investigational drug outside of a designated clinical trial; restricted to patients with a serious condition or disease who no longer have satisfactory medical options available and who may benefit from the investigational therapy
      2. Compassionate use or special exemption: individual patient accesses investigational therapy; risk from the investigational drug is not greater than the risk from the disease; approval from Food and Drug Administration (FDA) may be obtained within 24 hours in emergency situations

III. Clinical trials
   A. Clinical trial designs (Ness & Cusack, 2015)
      1. Parallel design: participant is randomized to one of several treatment groups (Fig. 11.1)
      2. Crossover design: allows participants to receive more than one treatment (Fig. 11.2)
      3. Factorial design: allows for multiple factors (i.e., multiple treatments) to be studied simultaneously (Fig. 11.3)

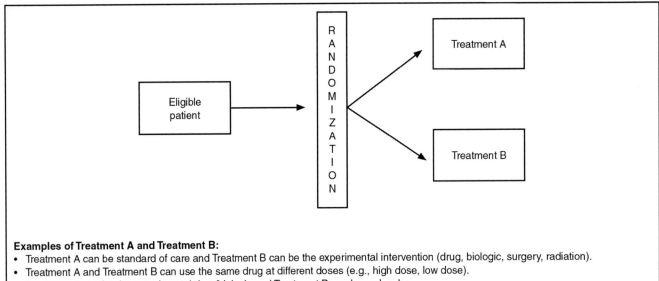

Examples of Treatment A and Treatment B:
- Treatment A can be standard of care and Treatment B can be the experimental intervention (drug, biologic, surgery, radiation).
- Treatment A and Treatment B can use the same drug at different doses (e.g., high dose, low dose).
- Treatment A can be the experimental drug/biologic and Treatment B can be a placebo.
- Treatment A can be the experimental drug/biologic + standard of care and Treatment B can be the experimental drug/biologic alone.

Note. Based on information from Stoney & Johnson, 2012a.

Fig. 11.1 Parallel design: two study groups. From Stoney, C.M., & Johnson, L.L. (2012a). Design of clinical studies and trials. In J.I. Gallin & F.P. Ognibene (Eds.), Principles and practice of clinical research (3rd ed., pp. 225–242). https://doi.org/10.1016/B978-0-12-382167-6.00019-9.)

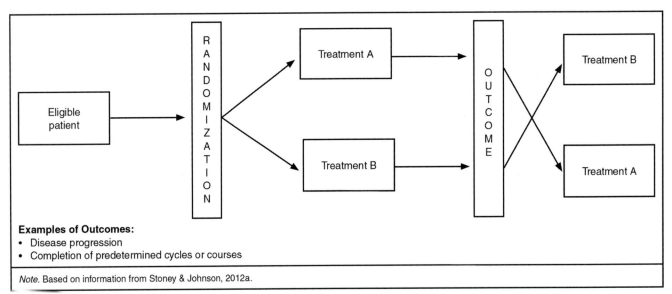

Examples of Outcomes:
- Disease progression
- Completion of predetermined cycles or courses

Note. Based on information from Stoney & Johnson, 2012a.

Fig. 11.2 Crossover design. From Stoney, C.M., & Johnson, L.L. (2012a). Design of clinical studies and trials. In J.I. Gallin & F.P. Ognibene (Eds.), Principles and practice of clinical research (3rd ed., pp. 225–242). https://doi.org/10.1016/B978-0-12-382167-6.00019-9.)

4. Randomized discontinuation design: all participants receive experimental treatment and randomized to continue or discontinue after significant response or stable disease is achieved

5. Adaptive design: allows investigators to change trial design without compromising the integrity and validity of the trial (Mahajan & Gupta, 2010)
   a. Allows for identifying the best clinical benefit of the treatment as the trial progresses
   b. An example is the "3 + 3" phase I trial design to determine maximum tolerated dose. Three

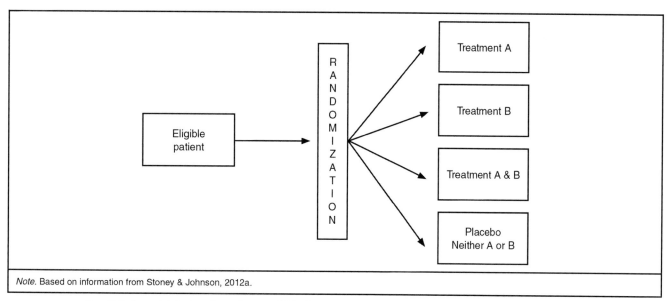

Note. Based on information from Stoney & Johnson, 2012a.

Fig. 11.3 Factorial design. From Stoney, C.M., & Johnson, L.L. (2012a). Design of clinical studies and trials. In J.I. Gallin & F.P. Ognibene (Eds.), Principles and practice of clinical research (3rd ed., pp. 225–242). https://doi.org/10.1016/B978-0-12-382167-6.00019-9.)

patients start the trial at a given dose, and if no dose-limiting toxicities are observed, three more patients are added at a higher dose until the first instance of limiting toxicity is observed, then three more patients will be added at the same dose. Dose-limiting toxicity in two or all three patients will identify the next lower dose as the maximum tolerated dose.

6. Basket trials: enroll patients with any cancer type sharing specific target; patients receive the same novel treatment that targets the specific target (West, 2017)

7. Umbrella trials: enroll patients with the same cancer but different potential targets; patients assigned to a study arm based on the presence of a mutation that is matched with a potentially effective treatment (West, 2017)

B. Phases of clinical trials (Table 11.1)

C. Considerations in clinical trials

1. Research team: led by a principal investigator and consists of professionals who study the safety and efficacy of drugs, devices, and interventions before approval for use with confidence on the public (Schmotzer & Ness, 2015)

   a. Principal investigator ensures the ethical conduct of the research study

   b. The only research team roles defined in regulations and guidance documents are those of the investigator and subinvestigator

   c. Other members of the research team include nurses, study coordinators, and clinical data managers; roles and job descriptions of each member vary greatly per study site

   d. Additional members may include statisticians; pharmacists, radiology department staff, and infusion center staff; and those who work in administrative roles such as contracting and billing

2. Ethics of clinical research: clinical research is dependent on the voluntary consent of human participants (Ulrich & Wallen, 2015)

   a. Research studies must demonstrate social and scientific value, address relevant problems or significant health-related questions

   b. Research studies must be methodologically rigorous

   c. Codes of ethics and codes of conduct

      (1) Nuremberg Code: voluntary consent

      (2) Declaration of Helsinki: informed consent, therapeutic versus nontherapeutic research, surrogate decision making

      (3) Belmont Report: beneficence, respect for persons, justice

      (4) Common Rule [Protection of Human Research Subjects (2009) 45 C.F.R. pt. 46, subpt. A, §§ 46.101–46.124]: informed consent; institutional review boards (IRBs); protections for pregnant women, fetuses, neonates, children, and prisoners

      (5) Council for International Organizations of Medical Sciences (CIOMS): conduct of research for developing countries

   d. Issues with ethical conduct of research

      (1) Therapeutic misconception: patient-participants believe that they will

TABLE 11.1   Phases of Clinical Trials

Phase	Description	Goals	Approximate Subjects
0	• Exploratory study using small doses of investigational agent • Very limited drug exposure with limited duration of dosing (approx. ≤7 days) • No therapeutic (or diagnostic) intent • Conducted before traditional phase I study • Conducted under an exploratory investigational new drug (IND) application	• Provide human pharmacokinetic (PK) or pharmacodynamic (PD) data • Determine whether mechanism of action defined in preclinical models could be observed in humans • Refine biomarker assay using human tumor tissue, surrogate tissue, or both • Enhance efficiency and increase chance of success of subsequent development of the agent	• 10–12
I	• Traditional first-in-human (FIH) dose-finding study for single agent • Dose-finding study when using multiple agents or multiple interventions (e.g., drug + radiation)	• Evaluate the safety and tolerability • Determine the maximum tolerated dose (MTD): • Single agent • Combination of agents • Combination interventions • Determine dose-limiting toxicity (DLT) • Define optimal biologically active dose (BAD) • Evaluate PK or PD data • Observe preliminary response (e.g., antitumor activity)	• 20–100 • Healthy volunteer • Patient volunteer • Usually many cancer types (e.g., solid tumors) • Refractory to standard therapy or no remaining standard therapy • Adequate organ function, specifically bone marrow, liver, kidney • Pediatric studies conducted after safety and toxicity evaluation in adults
II	Phase IIA • Proof-of-concept study to provide initial information on activity of intervention to justify conducting a larger study Phase IIB • Optimal dosing study to target population	Phase IIA • Demonstrate activity of the intervention in the intended patient condition or targeted population • Establish proof of concept Phase IIB • Establish optimal dosing for the intended patient condition or targeted population to be used in phase III study • Evaluate for safety	• 80–300 • More homogenous population deemed likely to respond based on phase I data, preclinical models, and/or mechanisms of action • Subject needs to have disease that can be accurately and reproducibility measured • May limit number of prior treatments
III	Randomized controlled trial (RCT)	• Compare efficacy of intervention being studied to a control group • Evaluate for safety	• Hundreds to thousands • Homogenous population
IV	Postmarketing study	• Evaluate safety during postmarketing period • May or may not be required by the U.S. Food and Drug Administration (FDA) • Compare the drug to another similar product that is already being marketed • Monitor for long-term and additional safety, efficacy, and quality of life • Assess drug–food interactions • Assess effect in specific populations (e.g., pregnant women, children) or determine cost-effectiveness	• Hundreds to thousands • With the labeled indication of the newly marketed drug or biologic

Adapted from Ness, E., & Cusack, G. (2015). Types of clinical research: experimental. In A. D. Klimaszewski, M. Bacon, J. A. Eggert, E. Ness, J. G. Westendorp, & K. Willenberg (Eds.), *Manual for Clinical Trials Nursing* (3rd Ed.). Pittsburgh, PA: Oncology Nursing Society.

personally benefit or receive therapeutic gain from all aspects of research participation

(2) Scientific integrity: authenticity, transparency, and honesty in all aspects of the research process, from study design to dissemination of results; fairness in peer review, collegiality, and adherence to standards of practice

(3) Research misconduct: fabrication, falsification, or plagiarism in proposing, performing, or reviewing research, or in reporting research results (Steneck, 2007)

(4) Conflict of interest: personal, financial, professional, or political interests that are likely to undermine the ability to meet or fulfill primary professional, ethical, or legal obligations (Shamoo & Resnik, 2009)

IV. Research protocol

A. Clear, detailed, and transparent action plan that guides the conduct of a clinical trial (Saria, 2017)

1. For investigators: written plan to carry out the clinical trial

2. For trial participants: precise description of the methodology

3. For ethics committees and IRBs: information on a safety plan and assurances to protect participants' welfare and rights

4. For funding agencies: mechanism to evaluate proposed methodologies

5. For reviewers: description of a priori methods to address potential biases

B. Essential elements of a protocol (Table 11.2) (Mitchell & Smith, 2015)

1. Schema: brief description of the treatment plan provided in a diagram format (see Figs. 11.1 and 11.2).

2. Eligibility criteria: characteristics that potential participants must meet to be enrolled into the trial; includes demographic, disease-specific, and treatment-related variables (Saria, 2017)

a. Common inclusion criteria: must be satisfied before a patient can enter a trial

(1) Cancer status or stage of disease, for example, remission, progressive disease, failed previous treatment

(2) Health and performance status, for example, laboratory values, Eastern Cooperative Oncology Group (ECOG) or Karnofsky Performance status

(3) Measurable disease, for example, tumor size measured using computed tomography (CT) or positron emission tomography/computed tomography (PET/CT) scans

(4) Presence or absence of tumor biomarkers

b. Common exclusion criterion: history of certain prior treatment and comorbidities

TABLE 11.2 **Elements of a Protocol**
Title page
Schema
Objectives
Background and rationale
Patient eligibility criteria
Pharmaceutical information
Treatment plan
Procedures for patient entry on study
Adverse events list and reporting requirements
Dose modifications for adverse events
Criteria for response assessment
Monitoring of patients
Off-study criteria
Statistical considerations
Records to be kept
Participation
Multicenter trials

From A Handbook for Clinical Investigators Conducting Therapeutic Clinical Trials Supported by CTEP, DCTD, NCI [v.1.2], by National Cancer Institute Cancer Therapy Evaluation Program, 2014. Retrieved from http:// ctep.cancer.gov/investigatorResources/docs/InvestigatorHandbook.pdf.

3. Pharmaceutical information: details on experimental agents (i.e., investigational or commercial agent)

4. Treatment plan: includes aspects of experimental treatment, including dose, route, and schedule

5. Adverse events list and reporting requirements: identify previously reported side effects associated with the experimental treatment; include procedures for reporting (i.e., method, time frame, regulatory and administrative agencies)

a. Common Terminology Criteria for Adverse Events (CTCAE v5.0): provides standardization and consistency in the definition of treatment-related toxicity

6. Criteria for response assessment: objective study endpoints, including definitions of complete and partial response, stable disease, and progressive disease

a. Clinical trial endpoints (Table 11.3)

b. Response Evaluation Criteria in Solid Tumors (RECIST): solid tumor response assessment

(1) Complete response: disappearance of all target lesions, and any pathologic lymph nodes (whether target or nontarget) must have reduction in short axis to less than 10 mm

(2) Partial response: at least a 30% decrease in the sum of the diameters of target lesions

(3) Progressive disease: at least a 20% increase in the sum of the diameters of target lesions

(4) Stable disease: neither partial response nor progressive disease

TABLE 11.3 Clinical Trial Endpoints

Endpoint	Definition
Overall survival	Time from randomization until death
	Intent-to-treat population
Disease-free survival	Randomization until recurrence of tumor or death from any cause
	Adjuvant setting after definitive surgery or radiotherapy
	Large percentage of patients achieve complete response after chemotherapy
Objective response rate	Proportion of patients with reduction of tumor size of a predefined amount and for a minimum period
	Measure from time of initial response until progression
	Sum of partial-response patients and complete-response patients
	Uses standardized criteria when possible
Progression-free survival	Randomization until objective tumor progression or death
	Preferred regulatory endpoint
	Assumes deaths are related to progression
Time to progression	Randomization until objective tumor progression, excluding deaths
Time to treatment failure	Randomization to discontinuation of treatment for any reason (e.g., progressive disease, toxicity, death)
	Not recommended for regulatory drug approval

From Madsen, L. & Ness, E. (2016). Protocol development and response assessment. In Klimaszewski, A. D., Bacon, M., Eggert, J., Ness, E., Westendorp, J. & Willenberg, K. (Eds.), *Manual for clinical trials nursing*. Pittsburgh: Oncology Nursing Society.

    c. Internationally agreed-upon response standards exist for hematologic malignancies (refer to Chapters 18, 20, and 21)

    7. Off-study criteria: circumstances that prevent the participant from continuing the trial (e.g., progressive disease, adverse events, or delay in study treatment)

V. Nursing implications

  A. Provide information related to clinical trials participation

    1. Reinforce information received from principal investigator (PI), clinical trial nurse, or members of the research team regarding the research study in which they are considering participation

    2. Discuss the risks and benefits of the research study

    3. Explain that participating is voluntary and that refusal to participate or withdrawal later will not result in penalty or loss of benefits to which the research participant is otherwise entitled

    4. Review alternatives for treatment

  B. Assist patient and family in decision making

    1. Encourage patient to discuss the research study with family, friends, and a trusted non–family member advisor (i.e., pastor, attorney)

    2. Instruct patient and family to write down pros and cons of, and alternatives to, participation in the research study

    3. Read and discuss with significant others the informed consent form and educational information provided by the principal investigator or clinical trial nurse (CTN)

    4. Instruct patient and family to write down questions for principal investigator or research nurse. Provide patient with sample questions.

    5. Encourage patient and family to approach PI or CTN to ask questions

    6. Allow patient and family time to make a decision

    7. Provide resources, including websites that have patient information about clinical trials

REFERENCES

ClinicalTrials.gov. (2018). Glossary of common site terms Retrieved from https://clinicaltrials.gov/ct2/about-studies/glossary.

Madsen, L., & Ness, E. (2016). Protocol development and response ssessment. In A. D. Klimaszewski, M. Bacon, J. Eggert, E. Ness, J. Westendorp, & K. Willenberg (Eds.), *Manual for clinical trials nursing*. Pittsburgh: Oncology Nursing Society.

Mahajan, R., & Gupta, K. (2010). Adaptive design clinical trials: methodology, challenges and prospect. *Indian Jorunal of Pharmacology*, 42(4), 201–207.

Mitchell, W., & Smith, Z. (2015). Elements of a protocol. In A. D. Klimaszewski, M. Bacon, J. A. Eggert, E. Ness, J. G. Westendorp, & K. Willenberg (Eds.), *Manual for Clinical Trials Nursing* (3rd ed.). Pittsburgh, PA: Oncology Nursing Society.

National Cancer Institute. (2016). Types of clinical trials. Retrieved from https://www.cancer.gov/about-cancer/treatment/clinical-trials/what-are-trials/types.

Ness, E., & Cusack, G. (2015). Types of clinical research: experimental. In A. D. Klimaszewski, M. Bacon, J. A. Eggert, E. Ness, J. G. Westendorp, & K. Willenberg (Eds.), *Manual for Clinical Trials Nursing* (3rd ed.). Pittsburgh, PA: Oncology Nursing Society.

Saria, M. G. (2017). Clinical trials. In S. Newton, M. Hickey, & J. M. Brant (Eds.), *Mosby's Oncology Nursing Advisor* (2nd ed.). St. Louis, MO: Elsevier.

Schmotzer, G. (2015). Types of clinical research. In A. D. Klimaszewski, M. Bacon, J. A. Eggert, E. Ness, J. G. Westendorp, & K. Willenberg (Eds.), *Manual for Clinical Trials Nursing* (3rd ed.). Pittsburgh, PA: Oncology Nursing Society.

Schmotzer, G., & Ness, E. (2015). The research team. In A. D. Klimaszewski, M. Bacon, J. A. Eggert, E. Ness, J. G. Westendorp, & K. Willenberg (Eds.), *Manual for Clinical Trials Nursing* (3rd ed.). Pittsburgh, PA: Oncology Nursing Society.

Shamoo, A. E., & Resnik, D. B. (2009). *Responsible conduct of research*. New York, NY: Oxford University.

Standafer, D. (2015). Expanded access to investigational drugs. In A. D. Klimaszewski, M. Bacon, J. A. Eggert, E. Ness, J. G. Westendorp, & K. Willenberg (Eds.), *Manual for Clinical Trials Nursing* (3rd ed.). Pittsburgh, PA: Oncology Nursing Society.

Steneck, N. H. (2007). *Office of Research Integrity: introduction to the responsible conduct of research.* Retrieved from https://ori.hhs.gov/sites/default/files/rcrintro.pdf.

Ulrich, C., & Wallen, G. (2015). Ethics of clinical research. In A. D. Klimaszewski, M. Bacon, J. A. Eggert, E. Ness, J. G. Westendorp, & K. Willenberg (Eds.), *Manual for Clinical Trials Nursing* (3rd ed.). Pittsburgh, PA: Oncology Nursing Society.

West, H. (2017). Novel precision medicine trial designs: umbrellas and baskets. *JAMA Oncology, 3*(3), 423.

12

Bone and Soft Tissue Cancers

Ellen Carr

I. Physiology and pathophysiology (Broadowicz et al., 2017; Handforth et al., 2017; NCI, 2018b)
   A. Primary bone and soft tissue cancers
      1. From mesoderm and ectoderm
      2. Pseudocapsule contains tumor then breaks through to surrounding tissue (called *skip metastasis*)
      3. Patterns of growth (Samuel, 2018)
         a. Compression of normal tissue
         b. Resorption of bone by reactive osteoclasts
         c. Destruction of normal tissue (when malignant)
      4. Soft tissue sarcomas (ACS, 2018b; Frezza et al., 2017; Hatcher et al., 2017)
         a. May appear anywhere because of the body's widespread connective tissue; most found in the lower extremities or trunk
         b. More than 50 different types of soft tissue sarcoma (ACS, 2018b)
         c. Table 12.1 lists common types.
   B. Metastatic spread to bone from primary solid tumors, including lung, breast, kidney, thyroid, and prostate (Samuel, 2018)
II. Epidemiology: low incidence of primary malignant bone and soft tissue tumors (ACS, 2018a)
   A. 2018 estimates (bone and joints)—3450 new cases; deaths, 1590 (ACS, 2018a)
      1. Approximately 68% survival at 5 years (NCI, 2018b)
      2. Bone cancers in pediatrics/adolescents: (ACS, 2018a)
         a. Osteosarcoma (2% of all childhood cancers)
         b. Ewing sarcoma (1% of all childhood cancers)
   B. Soft tissue sarcoma 2018 estimates—13,040 new cases; incidence slightly higher for men (ACS, 2018b)
III. Risk factors
   A. Soft tissue (ACS, 2018b; NCI, 2018a)
      1. Risk factors include radiation, certain family cancer syndromes, a damaged lymph system, and exposure to certain chemicals
   B. Osteosarcoma (osteogenic sarcoma, osseous tissue) (NCI, 2018e)

1. Males affected more frequently than females (Samuel, 2018)
   C. Ewing family tumors (EFT, reticuloendothelial tissue) (NCI, 2018c)
      1. 50% of patients diagnosed are adolescents (NCI, 2018c; Samuel, 2018)
      2. Associated with retinoblastoma and skeletal anomalies
   D. Chondrosarcoma (cartilaginous tissue) (Samuel, 2018)
      1. Occurs most often in adults aged 30 to 60 years and more often in men
   E. Fibrosarcoma (fibrous tissue) (Samuel, 2018)
      1. Most often seen in adolescents and young adults
   F. Kaposi sarcoma (NCI, 2018d)
      1. Caused by infectious virus: Kaposi sarcoma–associated herpesvirus (KSHV)
         a. Virus also known as *human herpesvirus 8* (HHV8)
         b. KSHV is in the same family as Epstein–Barr virus (EBV)
IV. Histopathology
   A. Classified or staged by cell type, origin—connective tissue (fat, muscle, tendons, fibrous tissue) (American Joint Committee on Cancer [AJCC], 2015)
   B. Sarcomas classified by histology, not location (ACS, 2018b)
   C. Pathology evaluation can include (NCI, 2018a, 2018b)
      1. Cell type or tissue of origin
      2. Genetic factors: alterations and variants
      3. Immunohistochemistry testing results
V. Diagnosis and staging
   A. Clinical symptoms
      1. Bone (NCI, 2018b)
         a. Can present as painless or painful swollen mass (>5 cm)
            (1) Variety of presenting symptoms—peripheral neuralgias, vascular ischemia, paralysis, bowel obstruction, but often no symptoms reported
         b. Pain (worsening) in time, dull, aching; increasing at night (Milgrom et al., 2017)

TABLE 12.1	Major Types of Soft Tissue Sarcomas in Adults	
Tissue of Origin	**Type of Cancer**	**Usual Location in the Body**
Fibrous tissue	Fibrosarcoma	Arms, legs, trunk
	Malignant fibrous histiocytoma	Legs
	Dermatofibrosarcoma	Trunk
Fat	Liposarcoma	Arms, legs, trunk
Muscle	Rhabdomyosarcoma	Arms, legs
Striated muscle	Leiomyosarcoma	Uterus, digestive tract
Smooth muscle		
Blood vessels	Hemangiosarcoma	Arms, legs, trunk
	Kaposi sarcoma	Legs, trunk
Lymph vessels	Lymphangiosarcoma	Arms
Synovial tissue (linings of joint cavities, tendon sheaths)	Synovial sarcoma	Legs
Peripheral nerves	Neurofibrosarcoma	Arms, legs, trunk
Cartilage and bone-forming tissue	Extraskeletal chondrosarcoma	Legs
	Extraskeletal osteosarcoma	Legs, trunk (not involving the bone)

Data from National Cancer Institute. (2018a). *Adult soft tissue sarcoma treatment (PDQ®). Health professional version.* Retrieved from https://www.cancer.gov/types/soft-tissue-sarcoma/hp/adultsoft-tissue-treatment-pdq.

(1) Note onset, location, duration, quality; may be radicular; gradual onset; increases with tumor burden; swelling in affected area

c. Bone—injury has to be ruled out
(1) If pathologic fracture, acute, sudden pain may be present

d. Recurrence of lesions after resection, reappearing deeper and larger, more aggressive with metastasis

2. Soft tissue sarcoma (ACS, 2018b)
a. New lump anywhere in body
(1) Half appear on leg or arm
b. Worsening abdominal pain (location retroperitoneum)
(1) Blood in stool or vomit

B. Physical examination
1. Characteristics:
a. Mass may or may not be visible, palpable; may be firm, nontender, warm
b. Size noted, bilateral comparison
c. Many soft tissue lesions can be benign (ACS, 2018b)
d. Limited range of motion

2. Specifics, related to physical examination:
a. Osteosarcoma (NCI, 2018b)
(1) In children and adolescents, >50% of these tumors originate from long bones around the knee
b. Soft tissue sarcoma (ACS, 2018a)
(1) Workup of unexplained lumps and symptoms
(a) Biopsy and imaging
c. Chondrosarcoma (cartilaginous tissue) (Samuel, 2018)

(1) Commonly affects pelvis, femur, and shoulder
d. Fibrosarcoma (fibrous tissue)
(1) Commonly affects the femur and tibia
e. EFT (NCI, 2018c)
(1) Clinical symptoms can be vague; pain progressing, lump progressing; sometimes feel heat over lump; flulike symptoms (fever, fatigue, anemia)
(2) Swelling, progressing in affected area

C. Diagnostic imaging
1. Radiography (cannot see changes until tumor is advanced)
a. Bone scan—shows additional skeletal lesions
b. Other imaging: computed tomography (CT), magnetic resonance imaging (MRI), positron emission tomography (PET)
2. For example related to imaging, EFT (reticuloendothelial tissue) (NCI, 2018c)
a. Appear onionlike on radiographs from multiple layers of subperiosteal new bone reacting to tumor invading the bone cortex
b. Similar diagnostic studies as for osteosarcoma

D. Laboratory values
1. Elevated serum alkaline phosphatase level because of increased osteoblastic activity (Samuel, 2018)

E. Staging based on biologic behavior and tumor aggressiveness (AJCC, 2015)
1. Staging identified subcategories, size, or depth of tumors (Samuel, 2018)
2. Common malignant bone and soft tissue cancers (with cell or tissue of origin) (Samuel, 2018) (see Fig. 12.1 and Table 12.2)
3. Staging not standard; grading system based on mitotic activity (ACS, 2018b; AJCC, 2015)

TABLE 12.2	Cancers of the Bone		
Type of Cancer	**Tissue of Origin**	**Common Locations**	**Common Ages (yr)**
Osteosarcoma	Osteoid	Knees, upper legs, upper arms	10–25
Chondrosarcoma	Cartilage	Pelvis, upper legs, shoulders	50–60
Ewing sarcoma	Immature nerve tissue, usually in bone marrow	Pelvis, upper legs, ribs, arms	10–20

Data from National Cancer Institute. (2018b). *Bone cancer.* Retrieved from https://www.cancer.gov/types/bone/hp; National Cancer Institute. (2018c). *Ewing sarcoma treatment (PDQ®).* Health professional version. Retrieved from https://www.cancer.gov/types/bone/hp/ewing-treatment-pdq.

a. Staging (TNM: tumor, nodes, metastasis)

b. Grade (French system = three stages: differentiation, mitotic count, tumor necrosis)

VI. Prognosis and survival

A. Sarcomas

1. Prognosis depends on tumor size, grade, resection margin (NCI, 2018a)

a. Prognosis poor with metastasis

b. Spread from primary lesions to lung, breast, colon, pancreas, kidney, thyroid, prostate, stomach, and testes (ACS, 2018b; NCI, 2018e)

c. Other early metastatic sites—spine, ribs, pelvis (90% in axial skeleton) (ACS, 2018b) (Fig. 12.1)

d. Tumor infiltrates may be distant from the site of origin

B. Osteosarcoma (osteogenic sarcoma, osseous tissue) (NCI, 2018e)

1. Between 1975 and 2010, childhood osteosarcoma mortality decreased by more than 50%

2. In adolescents (15–19 years), 5-year survival rate increased 56% to approximately 66%

C. EFT (reticuloendothelial tissue) (NCI, 2018c)

1. Highly malignant (approximately 25% with metastases at time of diagnosis to lungs, lymph nodes, other bones) (NCI, 2018c)

2. 5-year disease-free survivors—73% (because of multimodality therapies, precision in surgery [wide resections]) (ACS, 2018a; Samuel, 2018)

D. Soft tissue sarcoma (ACS, 2018b)

1. In 2018 in U.S., about 13,040 adults newly diagnosed; 5150 will die

VII. Management

A. Treatment (ACS 2018b; Samuel, 2018)

1. Goals: survival, removal of tumor, preserve functioning

B. Treatment: surgery

1. Treatment of choice with osteosarcoma, fibrosarcoma, chondrosarcoma

2. Types of surgery:

a. Amputation

b. Limb salvage

c. Rotationplasty

3. Amputation versus limb salvage issues—increased effort to salvage rather than amputate; issues that affect the decision include:

a. Acceptable surgical margins

b. Blood vessels and nerves involved with the tumor

c. Age (in children younger than 10 years, surgery affects limb growth)

d. Typical treatment strategy: if limb salvage, radiation therapy follows

4. Amputation issues

a. When tumor extends to incisional surface

b. When location necessitates (e.g., tumor extends to vertebral body and pelvis)

c. Infection, skeletal immaturity

d. Major neurovascular involvement

5. Reconstruction (Samuel, 2018)

a. Bone autografts, allografts

b. After soft tissue resection, three common methods:

(1) Arthrodesis or fusion (with implants or grafts)

(2) Arthroplasty for joints

(3) Allografts (since the 1960s)—bone, tendon, ligament, connective tissue

6. Issues—nonunion, infections, healing, functional concerns (especially with limb salvage) ⚠️

C. Treatment: adjuvant radiotherapy (RT) (Samuel, 2018)

1. Soft tissue tumors can be radiosensitive and radioresponsive

2. Usually, external-beam RT, before or after surgery

a. Used when tumor is localized or after surgical debulking or tumor removal

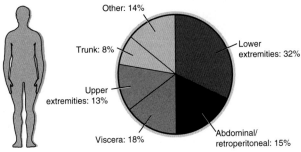

Other: 14%
Trunk: 8%
Upper extremities: 13%
Viscera: 18%
Lower extremities: 32%
Abdominal/retroperitoneal: 15%

Fig. 12.1 Sites of soft tissue sarcomas.

3. For palliative care, pain relief (Pina et al., 2018)

D. Treatment: chemotherapy or immunotherapy (NCCN, 2018a, 2018b)

1. Adjuvant or neoadjuvant with surgery/RT (Samuel, 2018)

   a. Outcomes show better local control, increased time to treatment failure, especially in EFT, rhabdomyosarcoma, and osteosarcomas (NCI, 2013c, 2013d; Samuel, 2018)

   b. Treats occult micrometastases (Samuel, 2018)

   c. In advanced tumors, treatments can include sequential and/or multiagent protocols (Frezza et al., 2017; Samuel, 2018; Zer et al., 2018)

      (1) Exception—highly active antiretroviral therapy (HAART) for Kaposi sarcoma (NCI, 2018d)

   d. Targeted molecular therapies are promising (oncogene activation triggered by viruses or antibodies) (Samuel, 2018; Zustrovich & Barsanti, 2018)

2. Food and Drug Administration (FDA)–approved chemotherapeutic agents—doxorubicin (Adriamycin), cisplatin (Platinol), cyclophosphamide (Cytoxan), dacarbazine (DTIC-Dome), ifosfamide (Ifex), methotrexate (Mexate), vincristine (Oncovin), cosmegen (Dactinomycin), and denosumab (Xgeva) (NCI, 2018b)

   a. Combination regimens: soft tissue sarcoma subtypes, nonspecific histologies. Selected therapies (NCCN, 2018b):

      (1) AD: doxorubicin, dacarbazine
      (2) AIM: doxorubicin, ifosfamide, Mesna
      (3) MAID: Mesna, doxorubicin, ifosfamide, dacarbazine

3. Systemic treatment using molecular and cell biology (antiangiogenesis, monoclonal antibodies, vaccines, T cells) (Zustovich & Barsanti, 2018):

   a. As an example for gastrointestinal stromal tumor (GIST) with disease progression after standard therapies, some selected molecular/cell biology therapies (NCCN, 2018b):

      (1) Sorafenib
      (2) Nilotinib
      (3) Pazopanib

VIII. Nursing implications ⚠

A. Care related to phantom limb pain or sensation (Samuel, 2018)

1. 1 to 4 weeks postoperatively; usually resolves in a few months; can be chronic

2. Client aware of itching, pressure, tingling, severe cramping, throbbing, burning pain

3. Usually triggered by fatigue, stress, excitement, other stimuli

B. Care related to preoperative care when client will lose limb (Samuel, 2018)

1. For anticipated amputation, many psychological needs exist (especially with adolescents); issues to address include anxiety, depression; grief about lost limb—physical as well as emotional and social losses; altered body image; fear of disability; coping with deformity; short-term loss of independence and self-sufficiency

2. Rehabilitation plan after surgery—awareness of possible symptoms after surgery, including phantom limb sensation, pain (throbbing, burning), itching pressure, tingling, and severe cramping

3. Postoperative care when client has lost limb (Gerrand & Furtado, 2017)

   a. Observation of drainage from site; also for redness, hemorrhage, increased pain, tenderness and swelling, blisters, abrasion

   b. If need for stump care

      (1) Elevation of stump (usually at least 24 hours) to prevent edema and promote venous return

      (2) Frequent wrapping of stump with elastic bandages or stump shrinkers

      (3) Dangling and transfer to chair after day of surgery

         (a) Assisting client into prone position three or four times per day for 15 minutes minimum to prevent hip contractures

         (b) Coordination of collaborative services (e.g., physical therapy, social services, occupational therapy)

4. Postoperative management of limb salvage (Gerrand & Furtado, 2017)

   a. Neurovascular checks distal to surgical site

   b. Monitor for blood loss and anemia from extensive tumor resection and reconstruction

   c. Monitor wound site for signs of infection

   d. Pain management

5. Many other areas for nurses to address in plan of care (Samuel, 2018)

   a. Pathologic fractures/weight-bearing
   b. Radiation effects
   c. Chemotherapy effects
   d. Body image
   e. Impaired sexuality and fertility
   f. Psychosocial support and coping
   g. Survivorship and follow-up

REFERENCES

American Cancer Society. (2018a). *Cancer facts & figures*, 2018. Retrieved from https://www.cancer.org/research/cancer-facts-statistics.html.

American Cancer Society. (2018b). *Soft tissue sarcoma.* Retrieved from https://www.cancer.org/cancer/soft-tissue-sarcoma.html

American Joint Committee on Cancer. (2015). Musculoskeletal sites (bone; soft tissue sarcoma). In *AJCC cancer staging manual* (7th ed., pp. 279–298). New York: Springer.

Broadowicz, T., Hadji, P., Niepel, D., & Diel, I. (2017). Early identification and intervention matter: a comprehensive review of current evidence and the monitoring of bone health in patients with cancer. *Cancer Treatment Review, 61,* 23–34. https://doi.org/10.1016/j.ctrv.2017.09.008.

Frezza, A., Stacchiotti, S., & Gronchi, A. (2017). Systemic treatment in advanced soft tissue sarcoma: what is standard, what is new. *BMC Medicine, 15,* 109. https://doi.org/10.1186/s12916-017-0872-y.

Gerrand, C., & Furtado, S. (2017). Issues of survivorship and rehabilitation in soft tissue sarcoma. *Clinical Oncology, 29,* 538–545. https://doi.org/10.1016/j.clon.2017.04.001.

Handforth, C., D'Oronzo, S., Coleman, R., & Brown, J. (2017). Cancer treatment and bone health. *Calcified Tissue International, 102,* 251–264. https://doi.org/10.1007/s00223-017-0369-x.

Hatcher, H., Benson, C., & Ajithkumar, T. (2017). Systemic treatments in soft tissue sarcomas. *Clinical Oncology, 29,* 507–515. https://doi.org/10.1016/j.clon.2017.05.002.

Milgrom, D., Lad, N., Koniaris, L., & Zimmers, T. (2017). Bone pain and muscle weakness in cancer patients. *Curr Osteoporos Rep, 15,* 76–87. https://doi.org/10.1007/s11914-017-0354-3.

National Comprehensive Cancer Network (NCCN). (2018a). *NCCN clinical practice guidelines in oncology: bone cancer.* Retrieved from https://www.nccn.org/professionals/physician_gls/pdf/bone.pdf.

National Comprehensive Cancer Network (NCCN). (2018b). *NCCN clinical practice guidelines in oncology: soft tissue sarcoma.* Retrieved from https://www.nccn.org/professionals/physician_gls/pdf/sarcoma.pdf *formerly Deimetri.*

National Cancer Institute. (2018a). *Adult soft tissue sarcoma treatment (PDQ®). Health professional version.* Retrieved from https://www.cancer.gov/types/soft-tissue-sarcoma/hp/adult-soft-tissue-treatment-pdq.

National Cancer Institute. (2018b). *Bone cancer.* Retrieved from https://www.cancer.gov/types/bone/hp.

National Cancer Institute. (2018c). *Ewing sarcoma treatment (PDQ®). Health professional version.* Retrieved from https://www.cancer.gov/types/bone/hp/ewing-treatment-pdq.

National Cancer Institute. (2018d). *Kaposi sarcoma.* Retrieved from https://www.cancer.org/cancer/kaposi-sarcoma.html

National Cancer Institute. (2018e). *Osteosarcoma and malignant fibrous histiocytoma of bone treatment (PDQ®). Health Professional Version.* Retrieved from https://www.cancer.gov/types/bone/hp/osteosarcoma-treatment-pdq.

Pina, Y., Paix, A., Fevre, C., Antoni, D., Blondet, C., & Noel, G. (2018). A systematic review of palliative bone radiotherapy based on pain relief and retreatment rates. *Critical Reviews in Oncology/ Hematology, 123,* 132–137. https://doi.org/10.1016/j.critrevonc.2018.01.006.

Samuel, L. C. (2018). Bone and soft tissue sarcomas. In C. H. Yarbro, D. Wujcik, & B. H. Gobel (Eds.), *Cancer nursing: principles and practice* (8th ed., pp. 1243–1277). Sudbury, MA: Jones & Bartlett.

Zer, A., Prince, R., Amir, E., & Razak, A. (2018). Multi-agent chemotherapy in advanced soft tissue sarcoma (STS)—a systemic review and meta-analysis. *Cancer Treatment Reviews, 63,* 71–78. https://doi.org/10.1016/j.ctrv.2017.12.003.

Zustovich, F., & Barsanti, R. (2018). Targeted α therapies for the treatment of bone metastases. *Int. J. Mol. Sci., 19,* 74. https://doi.org/10.3390/ijms19010074.

13

Breast Cancer

Jan Petree

I. Anatomy and physiology
   A. Anatomy of the breast—both men and women develop breasts from the same embryologic tissues. At puberty, female sex hormones, mainly, estrogen, promote (Knauer et al., 2010) development of tissue; this does not occur in men because of higher amounts of testosterone. Women's breasts become more prominent than those of men (NIH, 2018a). Female adult breast tissue overlies the chest (pectoral) muscles; it lies between the sternum and the midaxillary line (axilla) from the second to the sixth ribs and below the clavicle (NIH, 2018a; Osborne & Boolbol, 2010).
      1. Breast consists of connective tissues (collagen and elastin), nerves (peripheral nerves, with front and side branches of the fourth, fifth, and sixth intercostal nerves, and T4 [thoracic spinal nerve, innervates the skin and dermatome of the nipple and areola complex]), blood vessels, lymphatic vessels, fat, lobules, ducts, suspensory Cooper ligaments, and nipple and areola (NIH, 2018a).
      2. Two main aspects of the breast—functional breast and anatomic breast
         a. Functional breast—composed of glandular and adipose tissues (NIH, 2018a).
            (1) Glandular tissue—14 to 18 lactiferous lobes with lobules and milk ducts that are 2.0 to 4.55 mm in diameter, heading toward the nipple and surrounded by dense connective tissue, are called *terminal duct lobular units* (TDLUs), which produce fatty breast milk (NIH, 2018a).
            (2) Adipose tissue—becomes more prominent after menopause; 2:1 ratio of milk glands to fat in lactating breast; 1:1 ratio of milk glands to fat in nonlactating breast (NIH, 2018a).
         b. Anatomic breast
            (1) Size and shape of breasts vary from woman to woman and will change over the course of her life.
            (2) Men may develop increased breast tissue; this condition is called *gynecomastia* (NIH, 2018b).
      3. Lymphatic tissues—consist of lymph nodes and lymph channels; 75% of lymph fluid flows toward the axilla (pectoral, subscapular, humeral); 25% flows toward the parasternal lymph nodes, other breast, or abdomen (NIH, 2018a).

II. Epidemiology (Maisonneuve, 2017)
   A. Most common cancer in women worldwide, with 1.7 million new cases in 2012 (International Agency for Research on Cancer and Cancer Research UK, 2012).
   B. In the U.S. approximately 268,670 new cases diagnosed (266,120 women and 2550 men); about 41,400 deaths (40,920 women and 480 men) reported from breast cancer in 2018. Breast cancer accounts for 30% of new cases in women (ACS, 2018a; Siegel, 2017).
   C. Second leading cause of cancer-related deaths in U. S. women (ACS, 2018a; Siegel, 2017).
   D. Mortality trends
      1. Death rate peaked at 33.2/100,000 in 1989, declined to 39% in 2015, attributed to improvements in screening and treatment, with 322,600 fewer breast cancer deaths (ACS, 2018a; NIH, 2018c).
      2. Male breast cancer (estimated): incidence: in 2018 2550 men in U.S. diagnosed, with black men having a higher incidence (2.7 per 100,000) compared with white men (1.9 per 100,000).
      3. An estimated 480 men will die of breast cancer. Five-year survival rate is 84% in men with all stages: stage 0 and 1 (100% survival rate), stage II (91%), stage III (72%), metastatic or stage IV (20%) (ACS, 2018a).
   E. Trends in incidence rates
      1. Between 2002 and 2003, breast cancer incidence rate dropped by 7%, largely because of reduction in the use of hormone replacement therapy.
      2. Slight increase in breast cancer risk from 2005 to 2014 due to an increased rate (0.3% to 0.4%) in Hispanic and black women. A 1.7% increase in women from Asia/Pacific Islands (Siegel, 2017).

3. An estimated 63,960 U.S. women were newly diagnosed with in situ breast cancer in 2018 (Seigel, 2017).
    a. Two types of in situ breast cancer (NIH, 2018b)
        (1) Ductal carcinoma in situ (DCIS) (NIH, 2018b)
            (a) Noninvasive breast cancer involving the duct cells
            (b) Accounts for 85% of diagnosed in situ cases
        (2) Lobular carcinoma in situ (LCIS) (NIH, 2018b)
            (a) Involves milk-producing lobule cells
            (b) Pleomorphic LCIS, an aggressive variant, is more likely to develop into invasive lobular carcinoma (National Comprehensive Cancer Network [NCCN], 2018; NIH, 2018b).

III. Risk factors (ACS, 2018e, 2018g)
    A. Gender—100 times more common in women than men
    B. Age—incidence higher with aging; only 5% women before age 40 develop breast cancer, but 60% age 60 years or older; rates decline after 75 (ACS, 2018g).
    C. Race and ethnicity
        1. 1 in 8 (12.4%) white women will develop breast cancer from birth until death.
        2. 1 in 10 African American women will develop breast cancer.
            a. More African American women are diagnosed with breast cancer at a younger age (<45 years old).
            b. Lower rates in Hispanic, Asian, and Pacific Islanders (ACS, 2018g)
    D. Reproductive and hormonal factors: late age of first full-term pregnancy (first child after age 30), less risk if first pregnancy before age 20 (ACS, 2018g)
    E. Number of births—lower risk seen in higher number of births (ACS, 2018g)
    F. Lactation or breastfeeding—decreased risk of breast cancer in women who breastfed their babies, especially for long duration (Andersen, 2014; Loibl et al., 2017).
    G. Age at menopause/menarche—delay in menarche decreases risk, 2.9% increased risk for older when becoming menopausal.
    H. Nulliparity—never pregnant (ACS, 2018f)
    I. Use of hormone replacement therapy, oral contraceptives, or both
    J. Postthoracic radiation therapy to chest (e.g., radiation therapy to the chest for Hodgkin lymphoma and non-Hodgkin lymphoma) (ACS, 2018g)
    K. Family history—increased risk in women who have first-degree relative(s) (mother, father, sister, daughter) with breast cancer (ACS, 2018g)

L. Genetic factors—hereditary breast cancer syndromes or mutations: account for 5% to 10% of all female breast cancers; 4% to 40% chance of genetic abnormality of all male breast cancers (additional information in Chapter 10) (NCCN, 2018).
    1. *BRCA1*: 50% to 85% lifetime risk of developing breast cancer (NCCN, 2018).
    2. *BRCA2* gene mutation, risk 50% to 85% (Chaves de Gouvea & Garber, 2017; NCCN, 2018).
    3. *TP53*–Li-Fraumeni syndrome risk 65% to 90% (NCCN 2018).
    4. *ATM* (ataxia telangiectasia mutated) gene—causes ataxia-telangiectasia disease, which is associated with higher rate of breast cancer (Chaves de Gouvea & Garber, 2017).
    5. *PTEN*: causes Cowden disease; lifetime risk of developing breast cancer, 85% (NCCN, 2017; Chaves de Gouvea & Garber, 2017)
    6. *STK11/LKB*—can cause Peutz–Jeghers syndrome; risk 32% (Chaves de Gouvea & Garber, 2017; NCCN, 2018).
    7. *CHEK2*: cell cycle checkpoint kinase gene (NCCN, 2018).
    8. Lynch syndrome: hereditary nonpolyposis colorectal cancer (HNPCC) (NCCN, 2018).
    9. *PALB2*: making a protein called *partner and localizer of BRCA2* (NCCN, 2018).
    10. *BRIP1*: *BRCA1* interacting protein gene (NCCN, 2018).
    11. *RAD51C* and *RAD51D* (NCCN, 2018), *RAD50* (Chaves de Gouvea & Garber, 2017).
    12. *NBN* and *NF1, BARD1* (NCCN, 2018), *MRE11A* (NCCN, 2018).
    13. *CDH1*: increase risk 45% for lobular cancer (NCCN, 2018).
    14. Male breast cancers (Ottini & Capalbo, 2017): incidence: generally very low, 1/1000.
        a. Genetics: family history of inherited breast cancer, less common 5% to 10% of all breast cancers. One out of five men who develop breast cancer has a family history of the disease. All men should undergo genetic testing after diagnosis of breast cancer. Multigene testing should be done (NCCN, 2018; Pruneri & Boggio, 2017).
            (1) *BRCA1* and *BRCA2*
                (a) *BRCA1* (1/100) chance of developing breast cancer
                (b) *BRCA2* (6/100) chance of developing breast cancer
            (2) Klinefelter syndrome: extra X chromosome has increased risk of breast cancer due to higher levels of estrogen and lower levels of male hormones, androgens.
            (3) Other genetic syndromes seen in men (*P53*, Cowden *PTEN, ATM, PALB2, CDH1, CHEK2, NF1*, Li-Fraumeni) (NCCN, 2018; Pruneri & Boggio, 2017).

15. Age: average age of men diagnosed with breast cancer is 65.
16. Lifestyle factors:
    a. Obesity
    b. Lack of exercise: exercise lowers hormone levels, alters metabolism (ACS, 2018b).
M. Diets high in fat, especially polyunsaturated fats (Maisonneuve, 2017).
N. Monounsaturated fats such as olive oil may be protective (Maisonneuve, 2017).
O. Obesity/weight gain (increased postmenopausal breast cancer), premenopausal decreased risk associated (Maisonneuve, 2017).
P. Alcohol intake—risk increases with amount of alcohol consumed, three to four drinks daily 30% increased risk (Maisonneuve, 2017).
Q. Smoking—starting at a young age and continuing for more than 20 years, increased risk (ACS, 2018g).
R. Lack of physical activity, risk reduction 20% to 80% with exercise (Maisonneuve, 2017).

IV. Primary prevention of breast cancer in high-risk individuals (NCCN, 2018; Pagani, 2017).
A. Tamoxifen (Nolvadex)—first-generation selective estrogen receptor modulator (SERM) used in men and women (NCCN, 2018).
B. Raloxifene (STAR trial) tamoxifen versus raloxifene (SERM) (not used in men in trial) (NCCN, 2018).
C. Aromatase inhibitors (exemestane) used in women but not commonly used in men.
    1. Exemestane—showed benefit in reducing invasive breast cancers in postmenopausal women who were at moderate risk for breast cancer
    2. Anastrozole (Cuzick et al., 2014)
    3. Fulvestrant (not commonly used in men) (NCCN, 2018)
D. Adjuvant investigational treatments (NCCN, 2018; Pagani, 2017)
    1. Poly (ADP-ribose) polymerase inhibitors (PARP) triple negative breast cancer *BRCA* mutations
    2. Epidermal growth factor receptor (EGFR) tyrosine kinase inhibitors (TKI) inhibit HER1 and HER2 pathways
    3. Metformin reduced Ki67 proliferation
    4. Retinoids: regulate cell growth, differentiation, apoptosis ER+ and ER- tumors
    5. COX-2 inhibitors
    6. Bisphosphonates: prevent skeletal events

V. Screening and early detection (see Chapter 2) (Lauby-Secretan et al., 2015)
A. Early detection—increases chance of survival if breast cancer is diagnosed at an early stage

VI. Diagnostic measures
A. Biopsy—considerations based on location in breast or axilla; microscopic evaluation to make the diagnosis (NIH, 2018a).
    1. Gives the patient the opportunity to decide on type of surgery to receive
    2. Enough cells are needed for estrogen-receptor (ER), progesterone-receptor (PR), and HER-2-Neu testing, Ki67 (NIH, 2018b).
    3. Types of biopsies (NIH, 2018b)
        a. Core needle biopsy
        b. Stereotactic vacuum-assisted breast biopsy
        c. Fine-needle aspiration (FNA)
        d. Incisional biopsy
        e. Excisional biopsy
    4. Magnetic resonance imaging (MRI), mammography, or ultrasonography may be used to localize the site to be biopsied (Frigerio, Sardanelli, & Podo, 2017).

VII. Classic histopathologic classifications of breast cancer (NCCN, 2018; Pegram, Takita, & Casciato, 2011).
A. Ductal adenocarcinoma—70% to 80% of breast cancer cases (NCCN, 2018).
    1. Invasive ductal carcinoma (IDC)—most common type
    2. Clinical prognosis highly variable; depends on cellular morphologic characteristics: ER, PR, Ki67 (marker of cell proliferation), and HER-2Neu.
B. Lobular carcinoma—10% to 15% of breast cancer cases (NCCN, 2018)
    1. Invasive lobular carcinoma (ILC)—capable of metastasis; has a range of prognosis similar to IDC.
    2. Difficult to diagnose because of radial pattern of spread, not easily detected on mammography, usually nonpalpable, and more likely to affect bilateral breasts compared with IDC.
    3. Metastasizes to unusual surfaces, such as the pericardium, abdomen, ovary, uterus, stomach, and eye.
C. Special subtypes with a favorable prognosis—less than 10% of cases (NCCN, 2018).
    1. Includes papillary, tubular, mucinous, pure medullary carcinomas, and metaplastic carcinoma
D. Inflammatory breast cancer—1% of cases (NCCN, 2018)
    1. Aggressive subtype
    2. Based on presence of dermolymphatic invasion with erythema, which mimics mastitis
    3. Exhibits edema in skin (peau d'orange) with palpable border
E. Paget disease of the breast—characterized by unilateral eczematous changes in the nipple; frequently seen with DCIS (NCCN, 2018).
F. Cystosarcoma phyllodes—less than 1% of breast neoplasms (NCCN, 2018).
    1. 90% benign and 10% malignant
    2. Rarely metastasizes but may recur locally
G. Rare tumors—include squamous cell carcinoma, lymphoma, and angiosarcoma

H. Nonmalignant tumors
  1. DCIS—also referred to as *intraductal carcinoma*
     a. Proliferation of cells inside the ducts
     b. Staged as stage 0
     c. May become invasive if not removed, so surgical excision recommended
     d. Usually not palpable, often detected by mammography and pleomorphic (broken glass dispersal pattern of calcifications) calcifications; highly suspicious of malignancy and need further evaluation; biopsy recommended—FNA or core biopsy
     e. Architectural patterns—micropapillary, solid, comedo, papillary, cribiform
        (1) Comedonecrosis often more aggressive and at higher risk of recurrence or becoming invasive
  2. LCIS—also called *lobular neoplasia*
     a. Often multicentric (more than one tumor) and multifocal (involves more than one quadrant of the breast).
     b. Usually not detected on mammography or in physical examination but may be an incidental finding on pathology report or may be seen on breast MRI.
     c. Staged as stage 0
     d. Surgical excision recommended
  3. Atypical ductal hyperplasia and atypical lobular hyperplasia
     a. Surgical excision recommended (Pegram et al., 2011)

VIII. Molecular classification of breast cancer
  A. Molecular classification of breast tumors may be based on
     1. Single-gene arrays: ER, PR, HER-2/neu, Ki67, and proliferation index
     2. Multigene expression
        a. Multigene transcript profiles use gene chip expression microarray (e.g., Oncotype DX Assay) or real-time polymerase chain reaction (RT-PCR) (e.g., Mammaprint, Prosigna, EndoPredict, Breast Cancer Index, other tests) (Sparano et al., 2015).
     3. Recent reports indicate distinct gene expression profiles for inflammatory breast cancer, HER2-positive breast cancer, lobular breast cancer, and *BRCA*-mutant breast cancer.
  B. Breast cancer has been divided into at least five subgroups with distinct clinical outcomes and biologic features (Veronesi, 2017)
     1. Luminal A tumors (Pruneri & Boggio, 2017)
        a. Have the highest levels of ER expression: ER-positive and/or PR-positive, HER2Neu positive or HER2-negative
        b. Tend to be low grade
        c. Most likely to respond to endocrine therapy and have a favorable prognosis

d. Tend to be less responsive to chemotherapy (Veronesi, 2017)
  2. Luminal B tumors (Pruneri & Boggio, 2017)
     a. Tumor cells' gene patterns—ER-positive, PR-negative, HER2-positive an unfavorable subset with aggressive behavior can be tamoxifen resistant; this subset of patients may benefit from chemotherapy and aromatase inhibitor (AI) or fulvestrant (Thakkar & Mehta, 2011).
     b. Prognosis worse than luminal A tumors
     c. Tend to be high grade
     d. May benefit from chemotherapy and targeted HER2 therapy (Veronesi, 2017)
  3. Normal-like breast tumors (Pruneri & Boggio, 2017).
     a. Gene expression profile similar to the nonmalignant normal breast epithelium
     b. Prognosis similar to the luminal B tumors (Veronesi, 2017)
  4. HER2-amplified (Hart, Biganzoli, & Di Leo, 2017)
     a. Tumors have amplification of HER2 gene on chromosome 17q and may have overexpression of other genes adjacent to HER2.
     b. HER2-positive cancers have decreased expression of ER and PR and upregulation of vascular endothelium growth factor (VEGF).
     c. Clinical prognosis of these tumors was poor, but with the advent of trastuzumab (Herceptin) therapy, clinical outcome has improved.
  5. Basal tumors
     a. Tumors negative for ER, PR, and HER2, or "triple-negative" (Hart et al., 2017).
     b. Tend to be high grade and express cytokeratins (5/6 and 17), vimentin, p63, CD10, smooth muscle actin, and EGFR.
     c. *BRCA1* breast cancers may fall into this group and often have a poor prognosis; therefore will likely benefit from chemotherapy (Veronesi, 2017).

IX. Histologic grade (NCCN, 2018).
  A. Bloom–Richardson or Nottingham grading system most often used
     1. Grade 1: low grade or well differentiated
     2. Grade 2: intermediate grade or moderately differentiated
     3. Grade 3: high grade or poorly differentiated

X. Staging
  A. Staging workup includes the following:
     1. Computed tomography (CT) of chest (if pulmonary symptoms present). Abdominal pelvic ± CT or MRI (if there is elevated alkaline phosphatase, abnormal liver function test, abdominal symptoms, or clinical stage IIA or higher).
     2. Bone scan (if indicated for bone pain or elevated alkaline phosphatase).
     3. Positron emission tomography (PET) or CT (optional)—not recommended for all women

4. Bilateral breast MRI (stages I–III optional)—not recommended for all women
5. Blood work, including complete blood cell count (CBC), platelets (plts), liver, and alkaline phosphatase (NCCN, 2018).

B. Stages of breast cancer give anatomic, pathologic, or prognostic staging; will determine risk of recurrence (Schnitt, 2010).

C. Metastatic pattern
   1. Most common organs involved in metastases in the local area are regional lymph nodes (axillary, internal mammary, inferior, supraclavicular lymph nodes) or in the skin
      a. Internal mammary nodes—involved in about 25% of patients with tumors in the upper inner quadrant and 15% with outer quadrant lesions
   2. Contralateral breast—most common in invasive lobular carcinomas
   3. Distant metastatic sites—include bone, skin, lung, liver, abdomen, eyes, bladder, brain, and spinal cord
      a. Hematogenous spread—to liver, lung, bone, brain, and abdomen

D. Lymphatic spread—to intramammary lymph nodes, axillary nodes, mediastinal nodes, other lymphatics
   1. Unusual sites of distant metastasis—eye, bladder, ovary, peritoneum
      a. More common with invasive lobular cancers (NCCN, 2018).

XI. Prognosis and survival rates
   A. 5-year survival rate by stage: stage 0 (100%), I (100%), II (93%), III (72%), and IV (22%) (ACS, 2018a). New AJCC staging, eighth edition, takes in other prognostic features to either upgrade or downgrade the staging system based on ER, PR, Her2Neu, and grade of tumor and looks at assay, such as Oncotype DX or Mammaprint, to help clinicians decide what patient's risk of recurrence is (AJCC, 2018).
   B. Factors affecting prognosis and treatment (NCCN, 2018).
      1. Lymph node status—poorer prognosis with more lymph node involvement
      2. Tumor size—better prognosis with smaller tumors
      3. Histologic grade—more aggressive disease with higher-grade tumors
      4. Hormone receptor status—better prognosis with ER- and/or PR-positive tumors
      5. Histologic tumor type—invasive tumors have ability to metastasize
      6. Ki-67 (MIB1) proliferation rate—Ki67 ratio in percentage of cells that are actively proliferating
      7. Oncogene HER2/Neu and EGFR overexpression
      8. Breast cancer assay—Oncotype DX, MammaPrint (new profiles: Prosigna, Breast Cancer Index, EndoPredict, IHC4) (Dowsett et al., 2010, Gluz et al., 2016; Sparano et al., 2015).

a. Oncotype DX—a 21-gene assay used to predict chemotherapy benefit and estimate the 10-year risk of distant recurrence in women with early-stage, node-negative, estrogen receptor–positive (ER+) invasive breast cancer (Genomic Health, 2014; Peethambaram et al., 2017).
   (1) Ribonucleic acid (RNA) extracted from the breast cancer specimen is analyzed by RT-PCR assay.
   (2) Recurrence score result is calculated from the gene expression results (Peethambaram et al., 2017).
      (a) Low risk: recurrence score of 0 to 17
      (b) Intermediate risk: recurrence score of 18 to 31
      (c) High risk: recurrence score ≥ 32
b. MammaPrint—70-gene array used to identify women with early-stage breast cancer (either hormone receptor–positive or hormone receptor–negative) who are at risk of distant recurrence after surgery (Drukker, Bueno-de-Mesquita, & Retel, 2013).
   (1) Seventy genes affect all the steps known to be important for metastasis, including cell cycle regulation, angiogenesis, invasion, cell migration, and signal transduction (Knauer et al., 2010).
   (2) Recurrence score is assigned as low risk or high risk.
   (3) No intermediate-risk group.

XII. Treatment
   A. Locoregional treatment of clinical stage I, IIA, or IIB disease or T3 N1 M0 (NCCN, 2018; Vila, Ripoll, & Gentilini, 2017)
      1. Lumpectomy with surgical axillary staging followed by radiation therapy and possible chemotherapy, antihormonal therapy, and antibody therapy (Andre, Volovat, & Cardosa, 2017; Mahmood et al., 2012; Murphy & Sacchini, 2013; NCCN, 2018; Veronesi, 2017) followed by radiation therapy (Murphy & Sacchini, 2013).
      2. Total mastectomy with surgical axillary staging, with or without reconstruction (Intra, 2017; Luini, 2017).
         a. Consider chemotherapy followed by radiation therapy for those with close margins (<1 mm), positive margins, and/or positive lymph nodes.
         b. Breast reconstruction for mastectomy can be performed at the same time as mastectomy or at some time after completion of cancer treatment (Mahmood et al., 2012; NCCN, 2018; Veronesi, 2017).
            (1) Options for breast reconstruction include the following (De Lorenzi, 2017):
               (a) Implants alone
               (b) Tissue expanders with implants later

(c) Latissimus dorsi alone

(d) TRAM (transverse rectus abdominus myocutaneous) or DIEP (deep inferior epigastric perforator) tissue flap

(e) Pedicle or gluteal flap

3. Sentinel lymph node biopsy—preferred method of axillary lymph node staging (NCCN, 2018).

a. Sentinel node—most likely the first lymph nodes to which cancer may spread from a primary tumor.

4. Axillary lymph node dissection—done if sentinel nodes positive or if palpable or biopsy-proven positive lymph nodes in axilla.

B. Adjuvant endocrine therapy—ER+ and/or PR+ (NCCN, 2017; Pagani, 2017).

1. Premenopausal: SERMS

a. Tamoxifen for 5 to 10 years, with or without ovarian suppression or ablation; if ovarian suppression or ablation, may use an aromatase inhibitor (anastrozole, letrozole, exemestane) (Vogel et al., 2006).

2. Postmenopausal at diagnosis (Cuzick et al., 2010; NCCN, 2017; Pagani, 2017).

a. AI for 5 years, nonsteroidal: anastrozole, letrozole, or addition of tamoxifen for total 10 years, or tamoxifen for 5 years, AI for 5 years; do not know currently if AI optimal length is 5 to 10 years (NCCN, 2018). Unclear of sequence of tamoxifen or AI first for 2 to 3 years, then switching over to other drug to complete 5 to 10 years. Benefit in adding AI to treatment (NCCN, 2018). Do not take AI and tamoxifen at same time.

(1) Potential side effects include hot flashes, joint aches, loss of bone density, dry skin, vaginal dryness, and decreased libido.

b. Aromatase inhibitors, steroidal inactivator: exemestane 5 years, unknown if 10 years is beneficial (Goss et al., 2011; NCCN, 2018).

C. Tamoxifen for 5 to 10 years for women with contraindications or who are intolerant of aromatase inhibitors (Hackshaw et al., 2011; Thakkar & Mehta, 2011) or have HER2-positive disease (Hart et al., 2017; NCCN, 2018).

1. Trastuzumab (Herceptin)—a monoclonal antibody (Baselga et al., 2012; Gianni et al., 2012; LoRusso et al., 2011)

a. Given intravenously (IV)

b. Potential side effects include allergic reaction, decreased left ejection fraction, pulmonary toxicity with interstitial pneumonitis, and pulmonary fibrosis, interval prolongation, palmar and plantar erythrodysesthesia, rash, and fatigue.

2. Pertuzumab (Perjeta)—a monoclonal antibody (Gianni, Nicoletti, & Arcangeli, 2017)

a. Given IV

b. Given IV in combination with trastuzumab and/or chemotherapy neoadjuvantly (Baselga et al., 2012; NCCN, 2018)

c. Given IV in combination with chemotherapy in the adjuvant setting with node-positive disease (NCCN, 2018)

D. Chemotherapy for locally advanced and/or metastatic disease

1. Antihormonal therapy:

a. SERMS tamoxifen (Hackshaw et al., 2011) and toremifine (Cuzik et al., 2010; Dowsett et al., 2010; NCCN, 2018)

b. AIs (anastrozole, letrozole) (NCCN, 2018)

c. Steroidal aromatase inactivator: exemestane (Goss et al., 2011)

2. Antihormonal therapy with other agents

a. Cyclin-dependent kinase (CDK 4/6 inhibitors) for metastatic disease (Malorni et al., 2017; NCCN, 2018)

(1) Palbociclib with letrozole, anastrozole, or fulvestrant

(2) Abemaciclib plus fulvestrant (Sledge et al., 2017)

(3) Ribociclib and AI

b. mTor inhibitors; everolimus with aromatase inhibitor or SERM, or steroid aromatase (AI) for metastatic disease (NCCN, 2018).

c. Megestrol acetate

d. Ethinyl estradiol

3. Chemotherapy agents: preferred regimens (Hart et al., 2017; NCCN, 2018).

a. TAC (docetaxel, doxorubicin, and cyclophosphamide)

b. Dose-dense AC (doxorubicin and cyclophosphamide) for four cycles followed by paclitaxel for four cycles every 2 weeks

c. AC (doxorubicin and cyclophosphamide) followed by weekly paclitaxel

d. TC (docetaxel and cyclophosphamide)

e. EC (epirubicin, cyclophosphamide) then ± docetaxel

f. CMF (cyclophosphamide, methotrexate, 5-fluorouracil)

g. Taxanes: paclitaxel and docetaxel, abraxane

h. Taxotere, carboplatin, Herceptin

i. Capecitabine (CREATE -X trial) (Zujewski & Rubenstein, 2017)

4. Trastuzumab/Her2Neu positive-containing regimens (Munzone, 2017)

a. Preferred regimens (NCCN, 2018)

(1) AC followed by T plus concurrent trastuzumab (doxorubicin and cyclophosphamide followed by paclitaxel plus trastuzumab) or AC followed by trastuzumab and Taxotere

(2) TCH (docetaxel, carboplatin, trastuzumab) (Andre et al., 2017; Baselga et al., 2012)

(3) Traztuzumab, pertuzumab, carboplatin, and docetaxel—approved in metastatic disease and in neoadjuvant setting (Andre et al., 2017; Baselga et al., 2012; Gianni et al., 2012; Hart et al., 2017; NCCN, 2018).

(4) Lapatinib (Tykerb)—a kinase inhibitor for use in metastatic HER2-positive disease in combination with chemotherapy agents (recurrent or metastatic disease). Must be taken at least 1 hour before or 1 hour after a meal (Blackwell et al., 2010; Frenel et al., 2009).

(5) Trastuzumab emtansine (Krop et al., 2012; LoRusso et al., 2011; Verma et al., 2012)

XIII. Nursing implications (ACS, 2018a, 2018b, 2018c)

A. Nurses play a vital role in educating patients regarding disease process, treatment options, side effects, self-care, body image, fertility, and pregnancy after treatment.

1. Interventions to increase patient knowledge regarding disease process, treatment, and side effects (ACS, 2018a, 2018b).

a. Explaining disease process and treatment options in a nonjudgmental way and at the patient's level of understanding (ACS, 2018a, 2018b).

b. Encouraging discussion regarding potential physical and emotional changes resulting from treatment and exploration of personal values and beliefs as they relate to treatment options (ACS, 2018a, 2018d).

c. Facilitating patient's involvement in treatment decision making to the extent desired.

d. Providing education regarding the risk for lymphedema; teaching the patient how to measure the circumference of the affected arm and to notify the provider if increases.

(1) Teaching the patient about precautions to take with regard to the affected arm to prevent trauma and infection, which could lead to lymphedema (ACS, 2018a, 2018b).

e. Informing the patient about altered arm and breast sensations (numbness and tingling of arm, lack of sensation on chest wall, phantom breast sensation after mastectomy) that may persist indefinitely after surgery (ACS, 2018a, 2018b).

f. Assessing for menopausal symptoms (hot flashes, vaginal dryness) that may be associated with adjuvant endocrine therapy or chemotherapy-induced ovarian failure.

g. Monitoring for and managing side effects of surgery, radiation, biotherapy, and chemotherapy (ACS, 2018a).

2. Interventions to promote self-care and enhance adaptation and rehabilitation

a. Facilitating communication between patient and health care providers; alerting the health care team to the patient's concerns about breast cancer and its treatment.

b. Assessing coping skills, support system, feelings about body image, sexually identity, role relationships (ACS, 2018b).

c. Providing the patient with information regarding community resources available for support, rehabilitation, and breast prostheses (ACS, 2018a).

d. Survivorship visit (see Chapter 3) with provider for transition visit and discussing long-term follow-up, surveillance, exercise, diet, and symptoms to be aware of, as well as future office visits (ACS, 2018b, 2018c).

e. Teaching the patient about the importance of practicing breast self-examination (BSE) and examining the axillary for any lymphadenopathy (ACS, 2018a, 2018b).

REFERENCES

AJCC Cancer Staging Manual. (8th ed.) (2018). *The American College of Surgeons (ACS)*. Chicago, Illinois.

American Cancer Society. (2018a). *Cancer facts & figures, 2018*. Atlanta, Georgia.

American Cancer Society. (2018b). *Breast cancer risk and prevention, (2018)*. www.cancer.org.

American Cancer Society. (2018c). *Special issues women with breast cancer face*. https://www.cancer.org/cancer/breast-cancer/living-as-a-breast-cancer-survivor/body-image.

American Cancer Society. (2018d). *Special issues women with breast cancer face*. https://www.cancer.org/cancer/breast-cancer/living-as-a-breast-cancer-survivor/emotions.

American Cancer Society. (2018e). *Special issues women with breast cancer face*. https://www.cancer.org/cancer/breast-cancer/risk-and-prevention/factors.

American Cancer Society. (2018f). *Special issues women with breast cancer face*. https://www.cancer.org/cancer/breast-cancer/screening-tests-and-early-detection/experiment.

American Cancer Society. (2018g). *What are the risk factors for breast cancer?* http://www.cancer.org/cancer/breastcancer/detailedguide/breast-cancer-risk-factors.

Anderson, K. N., Schwab, R. B., & Martinez, M. E. (2014). Reproductive factors and breast cancer subtypes: A review of the literature. *Breast Cancer Research and Treatment*, *144*(1), 1–10.

Andre, R., Volovat, S. R., & Cardosa, F. (2017). Treatment of advanced disease: Guidelines. In U. Veronesi, & P. Veronesi (Eds.), *Breast Cancer: Innovations in Research and Management*. Milan, Italy: Springer International Publishing.

Baselga, J., Cortes, J., Kim, S.-B., Im, S., Hegg, R., Im, Y., et al. (2012). Pertuzumab plus trastuzumab plus docetaxel for metastatic breast cancer. *New England Journal of Medicine*, *366*(2), 109–119.

Blackwell, K. L., Burstein, H. J., Storniolo, A. M., Rugo, H., Sledge, G., Koehler, M., et al. (2010). Randomized study of lapatinib alone or in combination with trastuzumab in women with ErbB2-positive, trastuzumab-refractory metastatic breast cancer. *Journal of Clinical Oncology, 28*(7), 1124–1130.

Chaves de Gouvea, A. C., & Garber, J. E. (2017). Breast cancer genetics. In U. Veronesi, & P. Veronesi (Eds.), *Breast Cancer: Innovations in Research and Management*. Milan, Italy: Springer International Publishing.

Cuzick, J., Sestak, I., Baum, M., Buzdar, A., Howell, A., Dowsett, M., et al. (2010). Effect of anastrozole and tamoxifen as adjuvant treatment for early-stage breast cancer: 10-year analysis of the ATAC trial. *Lancet Oncology, 11*(12), 1135–1141.

Cuzick, J., Sestak, I., Forbes, J. F., Dowsett, M., & Knox, J. (2014). Anastrozole for prevention of breast cancer in high-risk postmenopausal women (IBIS-ll): an international, double-blind, randomised, placebo-controlled trial. *Lancet, 383*(9922), 1041–1048.

De Lorenzi, F. (2017). How to manage complication in breast reconstruction. In U. Veronesi, & P. Veronesi (Eds.), *Breast Cancer: Innovations in Research and Management*. Milan, Italy: Springer International Publishing.

Dowsett, M., Cuzick, J., Wale, C., Forbes, J., Mallon, E., Salter, J., et al. (2010). Prediction of risk of distant recurrence using the 21-gene recurrence score in node-negative and node-positive postmenopausal breast cancer patients treated with anastrozole or tamoxifen: a trans ATAC study. *Journal of Clinical Oncology, 28*(11), 1829–1834.

Drukker, C. A., Bueno-de-Mesquita, J. M., & Retel, V. P. (2013). A prospective evaluation of a breast cancer prognosis signature in the observational RASTER study. *International Journal of Cancer, 133*(4), 929–936.

Frenel, J. S., Bourbouloux, E., Berton-Rigaud, D., Sadot-Lebouvier, S., Zanetti, A., & Campone, M. (2009). Lapatinib in metastatic breast cancer. *Women's Health, 5*(6), 603–612.

Frigerio, A., Sardanelli, F., & Podo, F. (2017). Radiological screening of breast cancer: evolution. In U. Veronesi, & P. Veronesi (Eds.), *Breast Cancer: Innovations in Research and Management*. Milan, Italy: Springer International Publishing.

Genomic Health, (2014). *Oncotype DX. (2014)*. http://www.genomichealth.com/OncotypeDX.

Gianni, L., Nicoletti, M. V. S., & Arcangeli, V. (2017). Emergencies in breast cancer. In U. Veronesi, & P. Veronesi (Eds.), *Breast Cancer: Innovations in Research and Management*. Milan, Italy: Springer International Publishing.

Gianni, L., Pienkowski, T., Im, Y. H., Roman, L., Tseng, L. M., Liu, M. C., et al. (2012). Efficacy and safety of neoadjuvant pertuzumab and trastuzumab in women with locally advanced, inflammatory, or early HER2-positive breast cancer (NeoSphere): a randomised multicentre, open-label, phase 2 trial. *The Lancet Oncology, 13*(1), 25–32.

Gluz, O., Nitz, U. A., Christgen, M., et al. (2016). West German study group phase III plan B trial: first prospective outcome data for the 21-gene recurrence score assay and concordance of prognostic marker by central and local pathology assessment. *Journal of Clinical Oncology, 34*(20), 2341–2349.

Goss, P. E., Ingle, J. N., Alés-Martínez, J. E., Cheung, A. M., Chlebowski, R. T., Wactawski-Wende, J., et al. (2011). Exemestane for breast-cancer prevention in postmenopausal women. *New England Journal of Medicine, 364*(25), 2381–2391.

Hackshaw, A., Roughton, M., Forsyth, S., Monson, K., Reczko, K., Sainsbury, R., & Baum, M. (2011). Long-term benefits of 5 years of tamoxifen: 10-year follow-up of a large randomized trial in women at least 50 years of age with early breast cancer. *Journal of Clinical Oncology, 29*(13), 1657–1663.

Hart, C. D., Biganzoli, L., & Di Leo, A. (2017). Chemotherapy regimens in the adjuvant and advanced disease settings. In U. Veronesi, & P. Veronesi (Eds.), *Breast Cancer: Innovations in Research and Management*. Milan, Italy: Springer International Publishing.

International Agency for Research on Cancer and Cancer Research UK. (2012). *Cancer worldwide*. http://gicr.iarc.fr/public/docs/20120906-WorldCancerFactSheet.pdf.

Intra, M. (2017). Surgical treatment of the primary tumor in patients with metastatic breast cancer (stage IV disease). In U. Veronesi & P. Veronesi (Eds.), *Breast Cancer: Innovations in Research and Management*. Milan, Italy: Springer International Publishing.

Knauer, M., Mook, S., Rutgers, E. J., Bender, R. A., Hauptmann, M., Van de Vijver, M. J., et al. (2010). The predictive value of the 70-gene signature for adjuvant chemotherapy in early breast cancer. *Breast Cancer Research and Treatment, 120*(3), 655–661.

Krop, I. E., LoRusso, P., Miller, K. D., Modi, S., Yardley, D., Rodriguez, G., et al. (2012). A phase II study of trastuzumab emtansine in patients with human epidermal growth factor receptor 2-positive metastatic breast cancer who were previously treated with trastuzumab, lapatinib, an anthracycline, a taxane, and capecitabine. *Journal of Clinical Oncology, 30*(26), 3234–3241.

Lauby-Secretan, B., Scoccianti, C., Loomis, D., Benbrahim-Tallaa, L., Bouvard, V., Bianchini, F., et al. (2015). Breast-cancer screening-viewpoint of IARC working group. *New England Journal of Medicine, 372*(24), 2353–2357.

Loibl, S., Schmidt, A., Gentilini, O. D., Kaufman, B., et al. (2017). Breast cancer (diagnosed) during pregnancy: adapting recent advances in breast cancer care for pregnant patients. In U. Veronesi, & P. Veronesi (Eds.), *Breast Cancer: Innovations in Research and Management*. Milan, Italy: Springer International Publishing.

LoRusso, P. M., Weiss, D., Guardino, E., Girish, S., & Sliwkowski, M. X. (2011). Trastuzumab emtansine: a unique antibody-drug conjugate in development for human epidermal growth factor receptor 2–positive cancer. *Clinical Cancer Research, 17*(20), 6437–6447.

Luini, A. (2017). The conservative mastectomy. In U. Veronesi & P. Veronesi (Eds.), *Breast Cancer: Innovations in Research and Management*. Milan, Italy: Springer International Publishing.

Mahmood, U., Morris, C., Neuner, G., Koshy, M., Kesmodel, S., Buras, R., et al. (2012). Similar survival with breast conservation therapy or mastectomy in the management of young women with early-stage breast cancer. *International Journal of Radiation Oncology, Biology, Physics, 83*(5), 1387–1393.

Maisonneuve, P. (2017). Epidemiology, lifestyle, and environmental factors. In U. Veronesi & P. Veronesi (Eds.), *Breast Cancer: Innovations in Research and Management*. Milan, Italy: Springer International Publishing.

Malorni, L., Migliaccio, I., Guarducci, C., Benelli, M., & Di Leo, A. (2017). Targeting the CD K 4/6 pathway in breast cancer. In U. Veronesi, & P. Veronesi (Eds.), *Breast Cancer: Innovations in Research and Management*. Milan, Italy: Springer International Publishing.

Munzone, E. (2017). Anti-HER2 therapies in the adjuvant and advanced disease settings. In U. Veronesi & P. Veronesi (Eds.), *Breast Cancer: Innovations in Research and Management*. Milan, Italy: Springer International Publishing.

Murphy, J. O., & Sacchini, V. S. (2013). New innovative techniques in radiotherapy for breast cancer. *Minerva Chirurgica, 68*(2), 139–154.

National Comprehensive Cancer Network. (2017). *NCCN practice guidelines in oncology: Breast cancer, invasive breast cancer [v.4.2017].* http://www.nccn.org/professionals/physician_gls/pdf/breast.pdf.

National Comprehensive Cancer Network. (2018). *NCCN clinical practice guidelines in oncology: genetic/familial high risk assessment: breast and ovarian. [v1.2018]* http://www.nccn.org/professionals/physician_gls/pdf/genetics.screening.pdf.

National Institutes of Health. (2018a). www.cancer.gov/types/breast/patient/breast-treatment-pdq.

National Institutes of Health. (2018b). www.cancer.gov/types/common-cancers/breast.

National Institutes of Health. (2018c). https://seer.cancer.gov/statfacts/html/breast.html.

Osborne, M. P., & Boolbol, S. K. (2010). Breast anatomy and development. In J. R. Harris, M. E. Lippman, M. Morrow, & C. K. Osborne (Eds.), *Diseases of the breast.* (4th Ed.). Philadelphia: Lippincott Williams & Wilkins.

Ottini, L., & Capalbo, C. (2017). Male breast cancer. In U. Veronesi & P. Veronesi (Eds.), *Breast Cancer: Innovations in Research and Management.* Milan, Italy: Springer International Publishing.

Pagani, O. (2017). Endocrine therapies in the adjuvant and advanced disease settings. In U. Veronesi, & P. Veronesi (Eds.), *Breast Cancer: Innovations in Research and Management.* Milan, Italy: Springer International Publishing.

Peethambaram, P., Hoskin, T., Day, C., Goetz, M., Habermann, E., & Boughey, J. (2017). Uses of 21-gene recurrence score assay to individualize adjuvant chemotherapy recommendations in ER+/HER 2- node positive breast cancer—a National Cancer Database study. *Nature Partner Journals, 47,* 1–8.

Pegram, M. D., Takita, C., & Casciato, D. A. (2011). Breast diseases. Breast cancer. In D. A. Casciato & M. C. Territo (Eds.), *Manual of clinical oncology* (7th ed.). Philadelphia: Lippincott Williams & Wilkins.

Pruneri, G., & Boggio, F. (2017). Prognostic and predictive role of genetic signatures. In U. Veronesi & P. Veronesi (Eds.), *Breast Cancer: Innovations in Research and Management.* Milan, Italy: Springer International Publishing.

Schnitt, S. J. (2010). Classification and prognosis of invasive breast cancer: from morphology to molecular taxonomy. *Modern Pathology, 23,* S60–S64.

Siegel, R. L. (2017). Cancer statistics. *CA: A Cancer Journal for Clinicians, 67*(1), 7–30.

Sledge, G. W., Toi, M., Neven, P., Sohn, J., Inoue, K., Pivot, X., et al. (2017). Monarch 2: abemaciclib in combination with fulvestrant in women with HR+/Her2− advanced breast cancer who had progressed while receiving endocrine therapy. *Journal of Clinical Oncology, 35*(25), 2875–2886.

Sparano, J. A., Gray, R. J., Makower, D. F., Pritchard, K. I., Albain, K. S., Hayes, D. F., et al. (2015). Prospective validation of a 21-gene expression assay in breast cancer. *New England Journal of Medicine, 373,* 2005–2014.

Thakkar, J. P., & Mehta, D. G. (2011). A review of an unfavorable subset of breast cancer: estrogen positive progesterone receptor negative. *Oncologist, 16*(3), 276.

Verma, S., Miles, D., Gianni, L., Krop, I. E., Welslau, M., Baselga, J., et al. (2012). Trastuzumab emtansine for HER2-positive advanced breast cancer. *New England Journal of Medicine, 367*(19), 1783–1791.

Veronesi, U. (2017). Conservative surgery. In U. Veronesi & P. Veronesi (Eds.), *Breast Cancer: Innovations in Research and Management.* Milan, Italy: Springer International Publishing.

Vila, J., Ripoll, F., & Gentilini, O. D. (2017). Surgical treatment of local recurrence in breast cancer patients. In U. Veronesi, & P. Veronesi (Eds.), *Breast Cancer: Innovations in Research and Management.* Milan, Italy: Springer International Publishing.

Vogel, V. G., Costantino, J. P., Wickerham, D. L., Cronin, W. M., Cecchini, R. S., Atkins, J. N., et al. (2006). Effects of tamoxifen vs raloxifene on the risk of developing invasive breast cancer and other disease outcomes. *Journal of the American Medical Association, 295*(23), 2727–2741.

Zujewski, J., & Rubinstein, L. (2017). CREATE-X: a role for capecitabine in early-stage breast cancer: an analysis of available data. *Nature Partner Journal, Breast Cancer, 3*(27), 1–5.

14

Gastrointestinal Cancers

Christa Braun-Inglis

ESOPHAGEAL CANCER

Overview

I. Arise from either the glandular or squamous epithelium and have different risk factors for each. At present, there is a shifting in the location of upper gastrointestinal (GI) tract tumors in the Western world due to a decrease in tobacco use but increase in obesity.

II. Epidemiology
   A. Estimated 17,290 new esophageal cancer cases diagnosed; 15,850 deaths from esophageal cancer in 2018
   B. Esophageal cancer—1% of all cancers diagnosed in the U.S.; much more common in some other parts of the world (American Cancer Society [ACS], 2018)

III. Risk factors
   A. Modifiable
      1. Smoking (squamous cell); alcohol (squamous cell)
      2. Occupational exposure (dry cleaners, asbestos)
      3. Obesity (adenocarcinoma)
      4. Diet—low consumption of fruits and vegetables
      5. Gastroesophageal reflux disease (GERD) (adenocarcinoma)
      6. Barrett esophagus (BE) (adenocarcinoma) (ACS, 2018a)
   B. Nonmodifiable
      1. Gender—more prevalent in men
      2. Genetic syndromes (e.g., tylosis, Howel–Evan syndrome, Bloom syndrome, Fanconi anemia)
      3. Achalasia—cancers are found about 15 to 20 years after the achalasia began
      4. Esophageal webs
      5. History of other cancers
      6. Hiatal hernia (NCCN, 2018a)

IV. Prevention
   A. Avoid alcohol and tobacco
   B. Control diet and body weight
   C. Treat Barrett's esophagitis and/or GERD
   D. Aspirin and nonsteroidal anti-inflammatory drugs (NSAIDS), but have increased bleeding, risk more evidence needed
   E. No evidence for vitamin D as preventive agent (ACS, 2018a; Rouphael, Kamal, Sanaka, & Thota, 2018)

V. Histopathology
   A. Squamous cell carcinoma
      1. Arises from squamous cell epithelium
      2. More common in developing countries
   B. Adenocarcinoma
      1. Arises from glandular epithelium
      2. Affects mostly distal esophagus
      3. Appears to be related to GERD and BE (ACS, 2018a; NCCN, 2018)

VI. Molecular classification
   A. MSI-H/dMMR testing if metastatic disease is suspected
   B. HER2 and PD-L1 testing if metastatic adenocarcinoma suspected (NCCN, 2018)

VII. Diagnosis and staging
   A. Diagnosis
      1. Endoscopy and biopsy
      2. Computed tomography (CT) scan of chest and abdomen with oral and intravenous (IV) contrast, positron emission tomography (PET) scan
      3. Endoscopic ultrasound (EUS)
      4. Bronchoscopy (NCCN, 2018)
   B. Staging
      1. American Joint Committee on Cancer (AJCC) (AJCC, 2018)
      2. Separate staging for adenocarcinoma versus squamous cell carcinoma (NCCN, 2018)

VIII. Prognosis and survival
   A. The 5-year survival rate is 18%
   B. 5-year survival rates depend on several factors, including the stage at diagnosis: stages I and II are 41%, stage III is 23%, stage IV is 5% (ACS, 2018a)
   C. HER2-positive tumors associated with poor overall survival and higher 5-year mortality rate (Nagaraja & Eslick, 2015)
   D. Prognostic significance of epidermal growth factor receptor (EGFR) overexpression remains controversial (Guo, Yu, Zhu, Guo, 2015)

Management

I. Surgery
   A. Endoscopic resection/ablation for carcinoma in situ or tumor in situ (CIS/TIS) in selected stage I patients
   B. Esophagectomy for patients with stages I to III
II. Radiation
   A. Concurrent with chemotherapy—usually in neoadjuvant setting
   B. May be used with concurrent chemotherapy as definitive therapy if patient declines surgery or is not a surgical candidate
   C. In palliative setting for pain control, alleviate obstruction/restore swallowing
III. Systemic therapy
   A. Chemotherapy is used with radiation therapy as neoadjuvant or definitive therapy
   B. Chemotherapy is primary treatment for stage IV disease
   C. Trastuzumab added to chemotherapy for HER2+ metastatic adenocarcinoma
   D. Ramucirumab alone or in combination with paclitaxel
   E. Pembrolizumab for patients with MSI-H/dMMR for second-line therapy and third-line therapy for patients PD-L1 positive (NCCN, 2018)
   F. Common chemotherapy regimens for esophageal cancer (Table 14.1) (NCCN, 2018)

TABLE 14.1 Common Chemotherapy Regimens Used in Esophageal and Gastric Cancers

Type of Chemotherapy	Preferred Regimen per NCCN
Preoperative chemoradiation	Paclitaxel and carboplatin; cisplatin and 5-fluorouacil (5-FU); oxaliplatin and 5-FU
Perioperative chemotherapy (three cycles preoperative and three cycles postoperative)	cisplatin and 5-FU; epirubicin, cisplatin, 5FU (ECF), oxaliplatin, and 5-FU
Definitive chemoradiation	Cisplatin and 5-FU; oxaliplatin and 5-FU*, cisplatin and paclitaxel and carboplatin *May use capecitabine instead of 5FU
Postoperative chemoradiation	Infusional 5-FU or capecitabine
Metastatic	Docetaxel, cisplatin, 5-FU (DCF); ECF, cisplatin and 5-FU or capecitabine; oxaliplatin and 5-FU or capecitabine; irinotecan and 5-FU

Data from National Comprehensive Cancer Network. (2018). *NCCN practice guidelines in oncology: esophageal and esophagastric junction cancer [v.2.2018]*. https://www.nccn.org/professionals/physician_gls/pdf/esophageal.pdf; National Comprehensive Cancer Network. (2018a). *NCCN practice guidelines in oncology: gastric cancer [v.2.2018]*. https://www.nccn.org/professionals/physician_gls/gastric.pdf.

STOMACH CANCER

Overview

I. In Western countries, the proximal lesser curvature, cardia, and esophagogastric junction (EGJ) are the most common sites. Gastric cancer is not very common in North America; however, it is rampant in other parts of the world.
II. Epidemiology
   A. Estimated 26,240 cases of stomach cancer diagnosed, and about 10,800 people will die of this type of cancer in 2018
   B. Fourth most common cause of cancer-related death in the world
   C. Higher incidence in Asians and males (ACS, 2017; WHO, 2018)
III. Risk factors (ACS, 2017)
   A. Modifiable
      1. Diet high in salted and smoked foods, low in fruits and vegetables
      2. Alcohol use greater than four drinks per day, smoking
      3. Obesity—high body mass index (BMI) associated with gastric cardia cancer
      4. *H. pylori*; gastric ulcers (ACS, 2017; Chen et al., 2013)
   B. Nonmodifiable
      1. Age, male sex, family history
      2. Epstein–Barr virus
      3. Previous gastric surgery
      4. Gastric polyps
      5. Inherited cancer syndromes
         a. Hereditary diffuse gastric cancer (rare)
         b. Familial adenomatous polyposis (FAP)
         c. Peutz–Jeghers syndrome (PJS)
         d. Juvenile polyposis syndrome
         e. Lynch syndrome (NCCN, 2018a)
IV. Prevention
   A. Avoid diet high in smoked/pickled foods and salted meats/fish
   B. Diet high in fresh fruits and vegetables can lower stomach cancer risk
   C. Regular exercise
   D. Healthy body weight
   E. Treat *H. pylori*, gastric ulcers (ACS, 2017)
V. Histopathology—95% are adenocarcinomas
VI. Molecular classification
   A. MSI-H/dMMR testing if metastatic disease is suspected
   B. HER2 and PD-L1 testing if metastatic adenocarcinoma suspected (NCCN, 2018a)
VII. Diagnosis and staging
   A. Endoscopy and biopsy
   B. CT chest, abdomen, and pelvis; PET scan
   C. EUS
   D. Staging (AJCC, 2018)

1. Prognostic staging for gastric cancer is complex; based on multiple principles—clinical, pathologic, and response to neoadjuvant therapy

VIII. Prognosis and survival
   A. Poor prognosis, as it is typically diagnosed in later stages
   B. 5-year relative survival rate in the U.S. is about 31% (ACS, 2017)

Management

I. Surgery
   A. TIS or T1 may be eligible for ER
   B. Stage T1B to T3: gastric resection
   C. Stage T4: en-bloc resection

II. Radiation
   A. Used in adjuvant setting with concurrent chemotherapy
   B. May be used in neoadjuvant setting with concurrent chemotherapy
   C. Given concurrently with chemotherapy in nonsurgical candidates (definitively)
   D. Palliative

III. Systemic therapy—same principles as discussed for esophageal cancer
   A. See Table 14.1 for common chemotherapy regimens used for gastric cancer
   B. Trastuzumab added for HER2-overexpressing metastatic adenocarcinoma
   C. Ramucirumab alone or in combination with paclitaxel
   D. Pembrolizumab for patients with MSI-H/dMMR for second-line therapy and third-line therapy for patients PD-L1 positive (NCCN, 2018b)

COLORECTAL CANCER (CRC)

Overview

I. CRC usually begins as a noncancerous growth called a *polyp;* develops on the inner lining of the colon or rectum and grows slowly over a period of 10 to 20 years. Typical slow growth pattern is why screening is so important to prevent cancers.

II. Epidemiology
   A. Estimated 97,220 new cases of colon cancer, 43,030 of rectal cancer in the U.S. in 2018
   B. Third most common cancer diagnosed in both men and women in the U.S.
   C. Third leading cause of cancer-related deaths in men and women in the U.S. and world
   D. Expected to cause about 50,630 deaths in 2018 (ACS, 2018b; WHO, 2018)

III. Risk factors
   A. Modifiable
      1. Smoking, alcohol
      2. High-fat diet or high intake of red meats
      3. Obesity
         a. Relative risk higher in men compared with women
         b. Relative risk higher in colon than colorectal cancer
      4. Inadequate intake of fruits and vegetables
      5. Physical inactivity
   B. Nonmodifiable
      1. Age >50
      2. Familial clustering—20% of cases associated
         a. Personal or family history of colon cancer or inflammatory bowel disease
         b. Hereditary cancer syndromes—5% of cases have germline mutations
            (1) FAP—attenuated familial polyposis (AFAP), MUTYH-associated polyposis (MAP-1)
            (2) Lynch syndrome (hereditary nonpolyposis colorectal cancer, or HNPCC)
      3. Other syndromes can also increase CRC risk, including PJS-1, serrated polyposis syndrome (SPS-1), colonic adenomatous polyposis of unknown etiology (CPUE-1)
      4. Presence of edematous polyps (Jochem & Leitzman, 2016; NCCN, 2018b)

IV. Screening and prevention
   A. Screening (see Chapter 2)
   B. Prevention
      1. Keep a healthy weight
      2. Limit red and processed meats and eat more vegetables and fruits—may lower risk
      3. Limit alcohol intake—fewer than two drinks/day for males, one drink/day for females
      4. Avoid tobacco
      5. Acetylsalicylic acid (ASA), NSAIDS (however, not always recommended due to risk of adverse events) (ACS, 2018b; Jochem & Leitzman, 2016)

V. Histopathology
   A. Adenocarcinoma accounts for 95% of all cases, originates from the glandular epithelium

VI. Molecular classification
   A. KRAS/NRAS (in patients with metastatic disease)
   B. BRAF (in patients with metastatic disease)
   C. MMR or MSI in appropriate patients (NCCN, 2018c, 2018d)

VII. Diagnosis and staging (AJCC, 2018)
   A. Colonoscopy; CT chest, abdomen, and pelvis
   B. Colectomy with minimum 12 lymph nodes (LN) for correct staging (NCCN 2018b, 2018c)

VIII. Prognosis and survival
   A. Prognosis depends on the stage at which the colorectal cancer is diagnosed
   B. The 5-year survival rate for colorectal cancer is 65%; localized disease is as high as 90%, but only 39% of patients are diagnosed at an early stage
   C. Stage IV 12%; average overall survival is 23 months (ACS, 2018b)

Management

I. Surgery
   A. Coloncolectomy (Fig. 14.1)
   B. Rectal
      1. Transanal resection
      2. Transabdominal resection
   C. Metastectomy—liver and/or lung
II. Radiation
   A. Used in adjuvant setting for rectal cancer due to high risk for local recurrence—neoadjuvant setting preferred
   B. Palliative setting for both colon and rectal for pain control, obstruction
III. Systemic
   A. Used concurrently in neoadjuvant setting—typically capecitabine
   B. Adjuvant setting FOLFOX, CAPEOX, capecitabine/5-FU/leucovorin
   C. Metastatic setting
      1. FOLFOX, FOLFIRI ± bevacizumab or cetuximab/panitumumab depending on KRA/NRAS status
      2. Regorafenib
      3. Trifluridine + tipiracil
      4. Pembrolizumab or nivolumab—dMMR/MSI-H (NCCN, 2018c, 2018d)

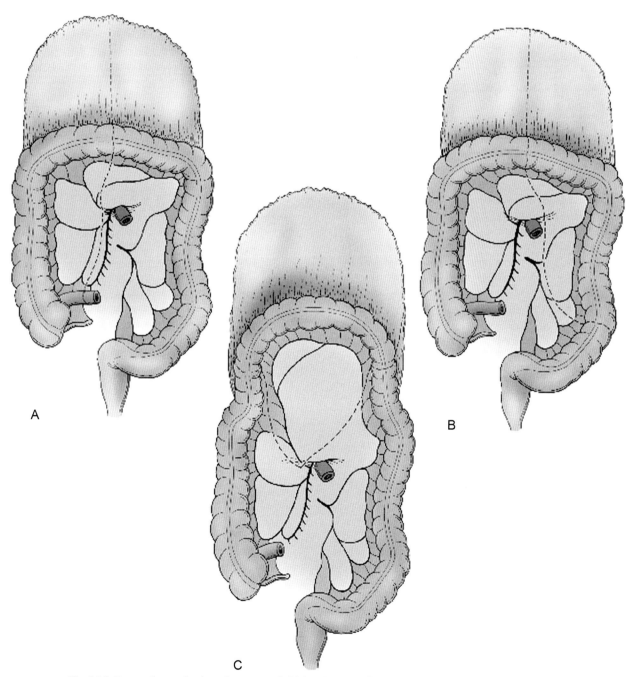

Fig. 14.1 Extent of resection for colon cancer. **A,** Right colectomy. **B,** Left colectomy. **C,** Transverse colectomy. (From Rothrock, J. (2011). *Alexander's care of the patient in surgery* (14th ed.). Philadelphia: Mosby.)

ANAL CANCER

Overview

I. Rare cancer arising from the squamocolumnar epithelium; directly linked to human papillomavirus infection (HPV) (particularly serotypes 16 and 18) (ACS, 2017a)

II. Epidemiology
   A. Estimated 8580 new cases and 1160 deaths related to anal cancer in 2018
   B. More common in women than men
   C. Incidence is rising (ACS, 2017a)

III. Risk factors
   A. HPV-16—nearly universal in men who have sex with other men (MSM)
   B. Other cancers associated with HPV
   C. HIV infection
   D. Smoking
   E. Anal sex
   F. Lowered immunity (ACS, 2017a)

IV. Prevention
   A. HPV vaccination—recommended in boys and girls 11 to 12 years, females 13 to 26, males 13 to 21, and for MSM up to age 26
   B. Condom use
   C. Treat HIV
   D. Not smoking (NCCN, 2018e)

V. Histopathology—squamous cell cancer, HIV associated or non-HIV associated

VI. Diagnosis and staging
   A. Biopsy—needs to confirm squamous cell origin
   B. CT chest, abdomen, and pelvis; anoscopy
   C. Gynecologic examination for women
   D. Staging (AJCC, 2018)
   E. Prognosis and survival—5-year survival for stage I about 75%; stage IV is estimated at 15% (ACS, 2017a)

Management

I. Surgery—local incision for stage I well-differentiated

II. Radiation
   A. Definitive therapy with stages I to III with concurrent chemotherapy
   B. Palliative for stage IV disease if indicated

III. Systemic therapy
   A. Definitive chemotherapy with stages I to III 5FU/mitomycin
   B. Palliative chemotherapy stage IV disease—cisplatin/5FU, FOLFOX, carboplatin/paclitaxel
   C. Palliative immunotherapy—nivolumab, pembrolizumab (NCCN, 2018e)

HEPATOCELLULAR CANCER (HCC)

Overview

I. Occurs predominantly in patients with underlying chronic liver disease and cirrhosis. Cell(s) of origin believed to be the hepatic stem cells. Some begin as a single tumor that grows larger; spreads late in the disease to other parts of the liver. Second type seems to start as small cancer nodules throughout the liver, not just a single tumor—seen most often in people with cirrhosis (chronic liver damage), most common in the U.S. (ACS, 2016)

II. Epidemiology
   A. HCC is second leading cause of cancer death worldwide
   B. Estimated 42,220 new cases diagnosed, 30,200 deaths in the U.S. in 2018
   C. Liver cancer incidence has more than tripled since 1980; peak of the epidemic may have passed due to improved treatments for hepatitis C and hepatitis B immunization
   D. Largest increases occurring in African Americans and Latinos (Altekruse, Henley, Cucinelli, & McGlynn, 2014)

III. Risk factors
   A. Trends: increased obesity, type 2 diabetes, and non-alcoholic fatty liver disease (NAFLD) replacing viral and alcohol-related liver disease
   B. Modifiable
      1. High-fat diet, obesity, including childhood obesity
      2. NAFLD
      3. Diabetes
      4. Alcohol, smoking
      5. Exposure to chemical carcinogens
      6. Anabolic steroids
   C. Nonmodifiable
      1. Primary biliary cirrhosis
      2. Nonalcoholic steatohepatitis (NASH)
      3. Hepatitis B or C
      4. Genetic disorders such as hemochromatosis and Wilson's disease can cause chronic inflammation leading to liver damage and increased HCC risk
      5. Parasitic infection (ACS, 2016; NCCN, 2018f)

IV. Screening and prevention
   A. Screening
      1. Ultrasound every 6 months is recommended for high-risk individuals, which include patients with all types of cirrhosis and hepatitis B virus (HBV) carriers without cirrhosis
   B. Prevention
      1. Avoiding/treating hepatitis infection
      2. Limiting alcohol and tobacco use
      3. Maintaining healthy weight
      4. Limiting exposure to cancer-causing chemicals
      5. Treating diseases that increase hepatocellular cancer risk (ACS, 2016a; NCCN, 2018f)

V. Pathology
   A. Gross morphology
      1. Nodular—associated with cirrhosis
      2. Massive—noncirrhosis type
      3. Diffuse—small distinct areas throughout the liver (NCCN, 2018f)

VI. Diagnosis and staging
   A. Ultrasound
   B. Abdominal multiphasic CT

C. MRI

D. Alpha fetoprotein is a predictor of advanced disease and poor prognosis

E. Biopsy if indicated only—not routinely done

F. For staging, refer to https://www.cancer.org/cancer/liver-cancer/detection-diagnosis-staging/staging.html

VII. Prognosis and survival

A. Prognosis based on tumor burden, liver function, and general health status

B. Generally poor—majority of patients are diagnosed with advanced disease

C. Localized tumors have approximately 30% survival at 5 years

D. Advanced tumors have an estimated 7% 5-year survival (ACS, 2016)

Management

I. May be limited because of underlying liver function

II. Surgery

A. Partial hepatectomy—potentially curative in patients with early-stage HCC, only in setting of preserved liver function, Child–Pugh score A (assess prognosis of chronic liver disease)

III. Transplantation

A. Additional potentially curative option for early-stage HCC

B. Removes both detectable and undetectable tumor lesions and treats underlying cirrhosis

C. Treatment before transplantation may include bridge therapy or downstaging therapy with transarterial chemoembolization (TACE) or thermal/radiofrequency ablation (RFA)

IV. Local-regional therapies

A. Ablation—RFA, microwave ablation (MWA), cryoablation

B. Arterially directed therapies—transarterial bland embolization (TABE), TACE, yttrium-90 transarterial radioembolization (TARE), TACE with drug-eluting beads (DEB)

V. Radiation—external beam radiation allows high-dose radiation to focal liver tumors while sparing surrounding tissue

A. Intensity modulated radiation therapy (IMRT)

B. Stereotactic body radiation therapy (SBRT)

VI. Systemic

A. First line—sorafenib

B. Second line—regorafenib, nivolumab

1. Child–Pugh score A to B7 only

C. Systemic chemotherapy recommended in context of clinical trial only (NCCN, 2018f)

PANCREATIC CANCER

Overview

I. Pancreatic adenocarcinoma is the most common form of pancreatic cancer. It accounts for almost 95% of cases and arises from the exocrine pancreas. Pancreatic neuroendocrine tumors are less common but tend to have a better prognosis. For the purpose of this chapter, pancreatic adenocarcinoma will be discussed, which is a tumor of the exocrine pancreas. Pancreatic adenocarcinoma is most commonly found in the head of the pancreas but may also be found in the body and the tail. It is often found at advanced stages, when it is found in the tail as it does not typically produce symptoms until it has spread. It typically first metastasizes to regional lymph nodes, then to the liver and, less commonly, to the lungs. It may also directly invade surrounding visceral organs such as the duodenum, stomach, and colon. It may also spread via the peritoneal cavity causing peritoneal carcinomatosis (NCCN, 2018g).

II. Epidemiology

A. In 2018, an estimated 55,440 people will be diagnosed with pancreatic cancer and 44,330 people will die of the disease in the U.S.

B. Fourth most common cause of cancer death in the U.S. (ACS, 2016, 2018)

III. Risk factors

A. Modifiable

1. Tobacco use

2. Obesity

3. Lack of exercise

4. Chemical exposure (heavy metals, benzidine, pesticides, asbestos, benzene)

5. Alcohol consumption

6. Periodontal disease

B. Nonmodifiable

1. Age

2. Higher incidence in African Americans (50%–90%)

3. Family history

4. Inherited genetic syndromes such as hereditary breast and ovarian cancer syndrome (HBOC), Lynch syndrome, FAP, PJS, familial atypical multiple mole melanoma, hereditary pancreatitis, cystic fibrosis, and ataxia-telangiectasia (AT)

5. Diabetes, both type 1 and 2

6. Chronic pancreatitis, which is usually related to alcohol abuse

7. Liver cirrhosis (NCCN, 2018g)

IV. Screening and prevention

A. Screening—routine screening for pancreatic cancer is generally not recommended for asymptomatic persons. However, EUS or MRI/magnetic resonance cholangiopancreatography (MRCP) may be used for persons with genetic mutations such as HBOC, Lynch syndrome, or PJS.

B. Prevention

1. Avoid tobacco

2. Keep healthy weight

3. Exercise regularly

4. Avoid heavy alcohol use

5. Limit exposure to certain chemicals in the workplace (ACS, 2016; NCCN, 2018g)
V. Histopathology
   A. Adenocarcinoma—accounts for 95% of all cases
   B. Neuroendocrine tumors—rare (carry better prognosis) (NCCN, 2018g)
VI. Diagnosis and staging
   A. Clinical presentation
   B. Pancreatic protocol CT—helps to see tumor in relation to blood vessels, which is critical for surgical planning
   C. Multidisciplinary review
   D. Consider EUS if no mass seen on CT
   E. Chest CT
   F. Biopsy if surgery not planned
   G. Biomarkers—CA 19-9 (NCCN, 2018g)
   H. For staging, refer to https://www.cancer.org/cancer/pancreatic-cancer/detection-diagnosis-staging/staging.html
VII. Prognosis and survival
   A. Typically caries poor prognosis, as less than 20% of patients are surgical candidates at the time of diagnosis and the median overall survival (OS) for nonresected patients is 3.5 months
   B. 5-year survival rate for stage 1 disease is approximately 13%, and for stage 4 disease is 1% (ACS, 2018c)

Management

I. Disease is typically classified as resectable, borderline resectable, locally advanced unresectable, or disseminated
II. Surgery
   A. Pancreatoduodenectomy (Whipple procedure) is the most common procedure done. It removes the head of the pancreas, duodenum, a portion of the common bile duct, gallbladder, and sometimes part of the stomach.
   B. Distal pancreatectomy. A procedure in which the tail of the pancreas and/or portion of the body of the pancreas is removed but not the head.
   C. Total pancreatectomy. A procedure in which the entire pancreas and spleen are surgically removed. Rarely performed.
   D. Goals of surgery are for negative margins, as a positive margin is associated with poor OS
III. Radiation
   A. Neoadjuvant setting with concurrent chemotherapy or SBRT
   B. Adjuvant setting
   C. Palliative therapy
IV. Systemic therapy
   A. Adjuvant chemotherapy
      1. Gemcitabine, 5FU, gemcitabine/capecitabine
   B. Unresectable and/or metastatic setting

1. FOLFIRINOX (5FU, leucovorin, irinotecan, oxaliplatin), gemcitabine/nab-paclitaxel, gemcitabine/cisplatin
2. Immunotherapy—second line for MSI-H, dMMR type tumors (NCCN, 2018g)

CHOLANGIOCARCINOMA

Overview

I. Cholangiocarcinomas encompass all tumors originating from the epithelium of the bile duct. Cholangiocarcinomas are diagnosed throughout the biliary tree and are typically classified as intrahepatic or extrahepatic. Intrahepatic cholangiocarcinomas are located within the hepatic parenchyma. Extrahepatic occur anywhere within the extrahepatic bile duct, from the junction of the right and left hepatic ducts to the common bile duct (NCCN, 2018f).
II. Epidemiology
   A. Rare—only about 8000 cases diagnosed in the U.S. annually.
   B. The incidence is increasing but may be due to the ability to accurately diagnose intrahepatic cholangiocarcinoma.
   C. More common in Southeast Asia due to parasitic infections (ACS, 2018c).
III. Risk factors
   A. No predisposing risk factors can be identified in most patients. However, associations have been found to include hepatitis C virus (HCV), HBV, cirrhosis, diabetes, obesity, alcohol, NAFLD, tobacco
IV. Screening and prevention: no screening methods identified. Preventive measures—see potential risk factors as noted earlier (NCCN, 2018f).
V. Histopathology—more than 90% are adenocarcinomas
   A. Extrahepatic more common than intrahepatic
   B. Broadly divided into three histologic types based on growth patterns: mass forming, periductal infiltrating, intraductal growing (NCCN, 2018f)
VI. Diagnosis and staging (AJCC, 2018)
   A. Clinical presentation
   B. Multiphasic abdominal/pelvic CT/MRI
   C. CT chest, liver function tests (LFTs), possible EUS
   D. Surgical consultation (NCCN, 2018f)
VII. Prognosis and survival
   A. Prognosis typically better for extrahepatic compared with intrahepatic
   B. Intrahepatic: for early stage, the 5-year survival rate is 15%; lymphatic spread, 5-year survival rate is 6%; distant spread, 5-year survival rate is 2%
   C. Extrahepatic: early stage, 5-year survival rate is 30%; lymphatic spread, 5-year survival rate is 24%; distant spread, 5-year survival rate is 2% (ACS, 2018c)

Management

I. Surgery
   A. Complete resection only potentially curative treatment for intrahepatic and extrahepatic cholangiocarcinoma; if possible, carries a much better prognosis.
   B. Liver transplantation sometimes a curative option with lymph node negative, nondisseminated, locally advanced hilar cholangiocarcinomas
II. Local-regional therapies for intrahepatic cholangiocarcinoma similar to HCC; include RFA, TACE, DEB-TACE, and TARE; hepatic arterial infusion (HAI) also used in certain settings
III. Radiation
   A. Employed as local regional therapy in intrahepatic
   B. Sometimes used in adjuvant setting combined with chemotherapy
IV. Systemic therapies—used in adjuvant and advanced settings: fluoropyridine based or gemcitabine based (NCCN, 2018f)
V. Nursing implications
   A. Assist with primary and secondary prevention strategies such as tobacco cessation, minimize alcohol use, promote appropriate vaccinations: HPV, hepatitis B; encourage healthy diet and regular exercise; educate the public about screening when appropriate
   B. Educate patients with GI malignancy about the disease process, diagnostic and treatment plans, and potential side effects of treatment
      1. Educate patient about treatment (rationale, type, and duration of treatment)
      2. Provide teaching on potential side effects and how to manage them based on patient's learning style (written, verbal, audiovisual presentation, or combination of these)
      3. Discuss nonpharmacologic and pharmacologic interventions to manage side effects
   C. Assist with palliative and/or hospice referral as appropriate
   D. Continuously monitor for alterations in GI function, fluid volume, nutrition
   E. See Chapter 37 for management of GI symptoms; see Chapter 43 for management of patients with nutritional issues

REFERENCES

Altekruse, S. F., Henley, S. J., Cucinelli, J. E., & McGlynn, K. A. (2014). Changing hepatocellular carcinoma incidence and liver cancer mortality rates in the United States. *Am J Gastroenterol*, *109*(4), 542–553. https://doi.org/10.1038/ajg.2014.11.

American Cancer Society. (2018). *Cancer facts & figures, 2018*. Atlanta: American Cancer Society.

American Cancer Society. (2018a). *Esophagus cancer detailed guide*. http://www.cancer.org/cancer/esophagus-cancer.html

American Cancer Society. (2018b). *Colorectal cancer detailed guide*. http://www.cancer.org/cancer/colon-rectal-cancer.html

American Cancer Society. (2018c). *Bile Duct Cancer detailed guide*. https://www.cancer.org/cancer/bile-duct-cancer.html.

American Cancer Society. (2017). *Stomach cancer detailed guide*. http://www.cancer.org/cancer/stomach-cancer.html.

American Cancer Society. (2017a). *Anal cancer detailed guide*. http://www.cancer.org/cancer/anal-cancer.html

American Cancer Society. (2016). *Liver cancer detailed guide*. http://www.cancer.org/cancer/liver-cancer.html.

American Cancer Society. (2016a). *Pancreatic cancer detailed guide*. http://www.cancer.org/cancer/pancreatic-cancer.html

American Joint Committee on Cancer. (2018). *Implementation of AJCC 8th Edition Cancer Staging System*. https://cancerstaging.org/About/news/Pages/Implementation-of-AJCC-8th-Edition-Cancer-Staging-System.aspx.

Chen, Y., Liu, L., Wang, X., Wang, J., Yan, Z., Cheng, J., & Li, G. (2013). Body mass index and risk of gastric cancer: a meta-analysis of a population with more than ten million from 24 prospective studies. *Cancer Epidemiol Biomarkers Prev*, *22*(8), 1395–1408. https://doi.org/10.1158/1055-9965.EPI-13-0042.

Guo, Y. M., Yu, W. W., Zhu, M., & Guo, C. Y. (2015). Clinicopathological and prognostic significance of epidermal growth factor receptor overexpression in patients with esophageal adenocarcinoma: a meta-analysis. *Dis Esophagus*, *28*(8), 750–756. https://doi.org/10.1111/dote.12248.

Jochem, C., & Leitzmann, M. (2016). Obesity and colorectal cancer. In T. Pshon, & K. Nimptsch (Eds.), *Obesity and Cancer*. SUI: Springer. Recent Results in cancer Research. Cham.

Nagaraja, V., & Eslick, G. D. (2015). HER2 expression in gastric and oesophageal cancer: a meta-analytic review. *J Gastrointest Oncol*, *6*(2), 143–154. https://doi.org/10.3978/j.issn.2078-6891.2014.107.

National Comprehensive Cancer Network. (2018). *NCCN practice guidelines in oncology: esophageal and esophagastric junction cancer [v.2.2018]*. https://www.nccn.org/professionals/physician_gls/pdf/esophageal.pdf.

National Comprehensive Cancer Network. (2018a). *NCCN practice guidelines in oncology: gastric cancer [v.2.2018]*. https://www.nccn.org/professionals/physician_gls/gastric.pdf.

National Comprehensive Cancer Network. (2018b). *Colorectal cancer screening [v.1.2018]*. https://www.nccn.org/professionals/physician_gls/pdf/colorectalscreening.pdf.

National Comprehensive Cancer Network. (2018c). *NCCN practice guidelines in oncology: colon cancer [v.2.2018]*. https://www.nccn.org/professionals/physician_gls/pdf/colon.pdf.

National Comprehensive Cancer Network. (2018d). *NCCN practice guidelines in oncology: rectal cancer [v.2.2018]* https://www.nccn.org/professionals/physician_gls/rectal.pdf

National Comprehensive Cancer Network. (2018e). *NCCN practice guidelines in oncology: anal cancer [v.2.2018]*. https://www.nccn.org/professionals/physician_gls/anal.pdf.

National Comprehensive Cancer Network. (2018f). *NCCN practice guidelines in oncology: hepatobiliary cancer [v.2.2018]*. https://www.nccn.org/professionals/physician_gls/hepatobiliary.pdf.

National Comprehensive Cancer Network. (2018g). *NCCN practice guidelines in oncology: pancreatic adenocarcinoma cancer [v.2.2018]*. https://www.nccn.org/professionals/physician_gls/pancreatic.pdf.

Rouphael, C., Kamal, A., Sanaka, M. R., & Thota, P. N. (2018). Vitamin D in esophageal cancer: is there a role for chemoprevention? *World J Gastrointest Oncol*, *10*(1), 23–30. https://doi.org/10.4251/wjgo.v10.i1.23.

World Health Orgnization. (2018). *Cancer Key Facts. (2018)*. http://www.who.int/en/news-room/fact-sheets/detail/cancer.

15

Genitourinary Cancers

Sally Maliski

KIDNEY CANCER

I. Physiology and pathophysiology (OpenStax, 2018)
  A. Anatomy
    1. The kidneys are on either side of the spine in the retroperitoneal space between the parietal peritoneum and posterior abdominal wall
    2. Protected by muscle, fat, and ribs
    3. The adrenal gland is located on the superior aspect of each kidney, with the adrenal cortex influencing renal function through aldosterone production
    4. The inner structure consists of the renal cortex, medulla, renal columns separating the renal pyramids, and renal papillae
    5. Receive about 25% of cardiac output at rest
  B. Physiology
    1. The nephron is the basic structural and functional unit of the kidney
      a. Cleanses blood and balances constituents in circulation through filtration, reabsorption, and secretion
      b. Regulates blood pressure
      c. Controls red blood cell (RBC) production and calcium absorption
      d. Comprises glomerulus, a tuft of high-pressure capillaries formed from the afferent arterioles, surrounded by the proximal end of a continuous, sophisticated tubule creating Bowman capsule
  C. Kidney cancer classifications (Jonasch, 2014; Motzer, 2017)
    1. Clear cell carcinoma, also known as *conventional* or *nonpapillary*
      a. Comprises 70% to 80% of cases
      b. Thought to arise from proximal renal tubule
      c. Hereditary and sporadic forms
    2. Papillary renal cell carcinoma (RCC)
      a. Comprises 10% of cases
      b. Thought to arise from proximal renal tubular epithelium
      c. Hereditary and sporadic forms
    3. Chromophobe renal cell carcinoma
      a. Comprises 5% of cases
      b. Arises from renal tubular epithelium; proposed to originate in collecting ducts
      c. Excellent prognosis—better than papillary or clear cell carcinoma
    D. Collecting duct carcinoma or Bellini duct carcinoma of the kidney
      1. Comprises fewer than 1% of all cases
      2. Arises in medullary collecting ducts
      3. Aggressive with rapid metastasis
      4. Subtype of collecting duct carcinoma
        a. Renal medullary carcinoma (RMC)
        b. Occurs almost exclusively in African American men with sickle cell disease (Jonasch, 2014)
    E. Unclassified RCC
      1. Remains as diagnostic category for tumors that do not fit into other categories
      2. Sarcomatoid is no longer considered a distinct category but is viewed as a manifestation of high-grade carcinoma
      3. Includes rare tumors—may be misclassified subtypes of RCC (Jonasch, 2014)
    F. Tumors of the renal pelvis (Board, 2018)
      1. Very rare
      2. 5% or less of all cases (Liu, 2013)
    G. Urothelial or transitional cell carcinomas
      1. May occur at any site within the upper urinary collecting system
      2. Generally multifocal
      3. Decreased incidence over past decades (Board, 2018)
    H. Renal cell cancers—tend to grow toward the medullary portion of the kidney and spread via direct extrusion to the renal vein or the vena cava
      1. Metastasis at diagnosis in 30% of patients; recurrence in 40%, even among those with early-stage disease (Motzer, 2017)

II. Epidemiology
  A. Kidney cancers rare in the U.S., accounting for only 3% of all cancers (Motzer, 2017; Siegel, Naishadham, & Jemal, 2013)
    1. Incidence and death rates have been rising since 1998
    2. Rising incidence may be related to common use of high-resolution imaging and incidental

finding of tumors among asymptomatic persons

3. Two thirds of renal carcinomas are now discovered incidentally during pelvic and abdominal scanning (Jonasch, 2014)

4. Renal cell cancer incidence rates vary by race/ethnicity (Chow, 2010)

B. Male predominance, 1.5:1 (Jonasch, 2014)

III. Risk factors (Chow, Dong, & Devesa, 2010; Steele, 2017)

A. Tobacco use, obesity, hypertension, unopposed estrogen use, diuretic treatment, prior radiation therapy (RT), occupational exposure to petroleum products or heavy metals, asbestos exposure, and dialysis-acquired cystic kidney disease

B. Dietary factors: high-fat diets, high-protein diets, diets low in antioxidants

C. Genetic predisposition, von Hippel–Lindau (VHL) disease, non-Hodgkin lymphoma, and sickle cell disease linked to an increased risk of kidney cancer

D. Clear cell carcinomas associated with loss/inactivation of short arm of chromosome 3p (Liu, 2013)

1. Alterations found in 80% of patients (Liu, 2013; Morrissey et al., 2001)

2. Association also found with von Hippel-Lindau disease

a. Papillary renal cell carcinoma

(1) Normal 3p but often trisomies 3q, 8, 12, 17, and 20 noted

(2) Trisomies 7 and 17 and the loss of the Y chromosome also reported (Jonasch, 2014)

b. Chromophobe RCC associated with loss of chromosomes 1, 2, 6, 10, 13, and 21 and alterations of chromosome 17

c. Common metastatic sites: lungs, abdominal and mediastinal lymph nodes, liver, and bone (Fig. 15.1) (Motzer, 2017)

IV. Screening and diagnostic measures (Motzer, 2017)

A. Screening—no screening tests available for kidney cancer; patients with multiple affected relatives should be referred for genetic counseling, possible surveillance

B. Diagnostic measures (Table 15.1)

1. Kidney, ureter, and bladder (KUB) radiography

2. Intravenous pyelography (IVP; also referred to as *excretory urography*): commonly used to evaluate patients presenting with hematuria

3. Renal ultrasonography

4. Pelvic or abdominal computed tomography (CT)—diagnostic test of choice

5. Renal angiography—less commonly performed; may be necessary because of large vascular mass if renal artery embolization is planned

6. Magnetic resonance imaging (MRI)—especially important if vena cava involvement

7. Retrograde urography

V. Grading and staging

A. Grading (Jonasch, 2014)

1. Fuhrman grading system on a scale of 1 (least aggressive) to 4 (most aggressive)

2. Higher nuclear grade associated with worse 5-year overall survival

B. Staging

1. No known tumor or molecular marker to confirm diagnosis, remission, progression, or relapse

2. Research for potential urinary and serum biomarkers promising (Pastore, 2015)

3. Staging—based on tumor size, lymph node involvement, and distant metastasis

4. American Joint Committee on Cancer (AJCC) staging system used for grading (AJCC, 2017; Motzer, 2017)

VI. Prognosis

A. Prognostic factors: patient age, histologic grade and type, disease stage, performance status, low hemoglobin level, elevated serum calcium and lactate dehydrogenase (LDH or LD) levels, number and location of metastatic sites, time to appearance of metastasis, and prior nephrectomy (Jonasch, 2014)

B. Antithyroid antibodies stimulated by interleukin-2 (IL-2) immunotherapy may be associated with improved survival (Motzer, 2017)

C. The 5-year survival rate is determined by the stage of kidney cancer: stage I (81%), stage II (74%), stage III (53%), and stage IV (8%) (ACS, 2018c)

VII. Management

A. Active surveillance (stage 1A RCC)—option should be considered for patients with decreased life expectancy or extensive comorbidities that would place them at risk for more invasive treatment (Motzer, 2017)

B. Surgery

1. Radical nephrectomy—primary treatment since 1960 (Motzer, 2017)

2. Partial nephrectomy—preferred whenever feasible, especially in patients with limited renal function, bilateral tumors, or a solitary kidney (Motzer, 2017)

3. Open, laparoscopic, robotic surgical techniques used to perform radical and partial nephrectomies

4. Cryosurgery and radiofrequency ablation (RFA)—option for patients with clinical stage T1 lesions who are not surgical candidates (Motzer, 2017)

5. Cytoreductive nephrectomy before systemic therapy for patients with surgically resectable primary tumor and multiple metastatic sites (Motzer, 2017)

a. Patients most likely to benefit are those with lung-only metastases, good prognostic features, and good performance status

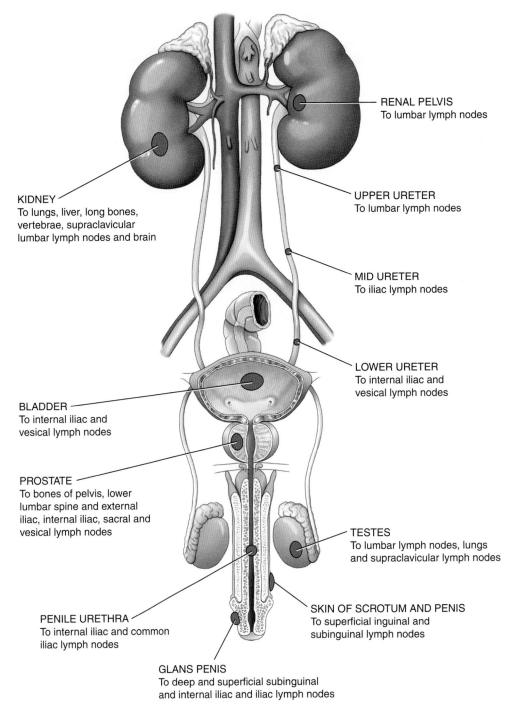

Fig. 15.1 Sites of tumor origin and metastases in the male.

KIDNEY
To lungs, liver, long bones,
vertebrae, supraclavicular
lumbar lymph nodes and brain

RENAL PELVIS
To lumbar lymph nodes

UPPER URETER
To lumbar lymph nodes

MID URETER
To iliac lymph nodes

LOWER URETER
To internal iliac and
vesical lymph nodes

BLADDER
To internal iliac and
vesical lymph nodes

PROSTATE
To bones of pelvis, lower
lumbar spine and external
iliac, internal iliac, sacral and
vesical lymph nodes

TESTES
To lumbar lymph nodes, lungs
and supraclavicular lymph nodes

SKIN OF SCROTUM AND PENIS
To superficial inguinal and
subinguinal lymph nodes

PENILE URETHRA
To internal iliac and common
iliac lymph nodes

GLANS PENIS
To deep and superficial subinguinal
and internal iliac and iliac lymph nodes

C. Radiation therapy (ACS, 2018c; Motzer, 2017)
   1. Renal cell cancers unresponsive to radiotherapy
   2. May be used for palliation (e.g., skeletal metastasis, brain metastasis)
D. Chemotherapy—has not been shown to improve survival (ACS, 2018c)
E. Immunotherapy
   1. IL-2
      a. Overall response rate of 14%, with 5% complete responses

      (1) Majority who had complete response had durable complete remissions (ACS, 2018c; Motzer, 2017)
      (2) Patients should have good performance status, normal organ function
   2. Interferon-alpha (IFN-α) (ACS, 2018c)
      a. Produced response rates of 10% to 15% given as a single agent
      b. Can be given in combination with IL-2 or bevacizumab

TABLE 15.1	Urologic Diagnostic Tests and Nursing Interventions	
Test	**Preparation**	**Nursing Interventions**
Radiographic examination of kidneys, ureter, bladder (KUB)	None—plain film of abdomen	Explain to the patient the need to lie flat on examination table. Do not schedule after barium studies (will obscure kidneys).
Excretory urography	Dye excreted unchanged by kidneys; notify radiologist if kidney function is impaired; limit fluid intake to assist the kidneys in concentrating the substance in the urine. Dye injected intravenously; anaphylactic or allergic reaction to dye may occur; may need to premedicate with antihistamines.	Assess history of allergy to iodine dyes or contrast media before test; pretesting may be indicated. Use of iodine dyes may be contraindicated in patients with severe renal or hepatic disease or clinical hypersensitivity (severe allergies, asthma). Have emergency equipment and personnel available before injection (anaphylaxis and cardiovascular reactions may occur) and 30–60 min after test (delayed reactions). Observe for adverse reactions to dye—angina, chest pain, arrhythmias, hypotension, dizziness, blurred vision, headache, fever, convulsions, dyspnea, rhinitis, laryngitis, and nausea.
Retrograde urography	General anesthesia or opioid analgesia may be used; cystoscope is inserted; iodinated dye is injected via the urethral catheter. Laxatives at bedtime before test may be used to cleanse bowel.	Observe for reaction to anesthetic or analgesic. Monitor for bleeding, symptoms of urinary tract infections, dysuria, or difficulty voiding after test.

3. Immune checkpoint inhibitors (ACS, 2018c; Motzer, 2017)
   a. Checkpoints turn on or off to start an immune process
   b. Prevents immune system from attacking normal cells
   c. Cancer cell may use checkpoints to avoid being attacked
   d. Drugs being developed to target checkpoints
  F. Targeted therapies
   1. Everolimus (RAD001), axitinib (Inlyta), sorafenib (Nexavar), sunitinib (Sutent), temsirolimus (Torisel), bevacizumab (Avastin), pazopanib (Votrient)
   2. Common side effects—fatigue, skin rash, diarrhea, hand–foot syndrome, increased glucose and cholesterol levels, and delayed wound healing
VIII. Nursing implications
  A. Maximize safety postoperatively
   1. Pulmonary hygiene—teach patients to perform cough and deep-breathing exercises
   2. Observe for signs of hemorrhage
   3. Monitor vital signs, hemoglobin, hematocrit, kidney function tests, and urine output
   4. Provide pharmacologic and nonpharmacologic pain relief measures
  B. Provide patient education regarding follow-up care and surveillance
   1. Teach patient to identify and manage symptoms, including when to report symptoms

2. Refer to mental health specialist, community resources, support groups as needed
3. Provide education and cancer survivorship care plan, which includes treatment summary and follow-up plan

BLADDER CANCER

I. Physiology and pathophysiology
  A. Primary function
   1. The bladder is a hollow muscular organ that serves as a temporary reservoir for urine, which is then discharged through the urethra.
   2. In men, critical adjacent structures include the prostate, seminal vesicles, urethra, nerves at the base of the penis, and local lymph nodes (see Fig. 15.1).
   3. In women, critical adjacent structures include the uterus, ovaries, fallopian tubes, urethra, and local lymph nodes (Fig. 15.2).
  B. Changes associated with cancer
   1. Proliferation of abnormal tissue in one or more places within the bladder
   2. Clinical manifestations—hematuria (especially with bladder wall invasion), dysuria, burning, frequency, pelvic pain (ACS, 2018a)
  C. Major classifications of bladder cancer (ACS, 2018a)
   1. Urothelial carcinoma (formerly known as *transitional cell carcinoma*)
    a. Arises from epithelial layer of the bladder, which rests on basement membrane

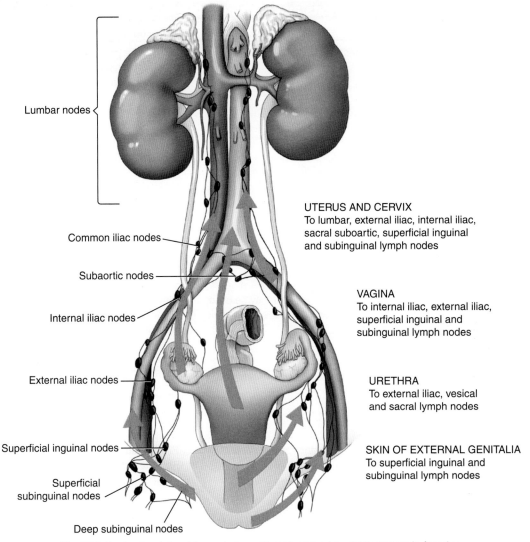

Lumbar nodes

Common iliac nodes

Subaortic nodes

Internal iliac nodes

External iliac nodes

Superficial inguinal nodes

Superficial subinguinal nodes

Deep subinguinal nodes

UTERUS AND CERVIX
To lumbar, external iliac, internal iliac, sacral suboartic, superficial inguinal and subinguinal lymph nodes

VAGINA
To internal iliac, external iliac, superficial inguinal and subinguinal lymph nodes

URETHRA
To external iliac, vesical and sacral lymph nodes

SKIN OF EXTERNAL GENITALIA
To superficial inguinal and subinguinal lymph nodes

Fig. 15.2 Anatomic relationships and sites of lymph nodes for urinary tumors in females.

b. Comprises about 95% of bladder tumors (ACS, 2018a)

c. Can be further subdivided—carcinoma in situ (CIS), noninvasive papillary carcinoma, invasive papillary carcinoma, and solid tumors
  (1) 70% to 80% considered "superficial" disease—World Health Organization has recommended the term be abandoned; referred to as *nonmuscle invasive bladder cancer* (NMIBC) (NCI, 2018a)
  (2) Papillary tumors confined to the first two layers of the bladder but project toward the lumen (ACS, 2018a)
    (a) These tumors demonstrate changes to chromosome 9 and an overexpression of vascular endothelial growth factor, leading to angiogenesis (NCI, 2018a)

2. Squamous cell carcinomas—make up approximately 1% to 2% of cases

3. Adenocarcinomas—make up approximately 1% of cases

4. Small cell tumors—make up less than 1% of cases (ACS, 2018a)

II. Epidemiology
  A. Incidence rates high in the U.S. and Africa, especially Egypt, where schistosomiasis is endemic (ACS, 2018a)
  B. Estimated new cases in the U.S. in 2013—72,570 (ACS, 2018a)
  C. Estimated deaths in U.S.—17,240; male-to-female ratio nearly 3:1 (ACS, 2018b)
  D. Median age at diagnosis 65 years; rarely diagnosed before age 40 years (ACS, 2018b)
  E. African Americans lag behind whites in 5-year survival rates (ACS, 2018b)

III. Risk factors
  A. Tobacco use
    1. Most significant risk factor, accounting for 50% to 66% of all bladder tumors in men, 25% in women (ACS, 2018b)
  B. High body mass index (BMI) may increase risk and risk of recurrence, but results are inconsistent (Westhoff, et al., 2017; Westhoff, et al., 2018)
  C. Dietary supplements containing aristocholic acid (ACS, 2018a)
  D. Arsenic in drinking water (ACS, 2018a)
  E. Not drinking enough fluids (ACS, 2018a)
  F. Chronic bladder irritations and infections have unclear link (ACS, 2018a)
  G. History of bladder or other urothelial cancer (ACS, 2018a)
  H. Genetics and family history (ACS, 2018a)
  I. No strong evidence suggesting that supplementation with any micronutrient reduces bladder cancer risk (Piyathilake, 2016)
  J. Diets rich in fruits and vegetables, low in processed meats, in addition to smoking cessation may be somewhat protective for bladder cancer (Piyathilake, 2016)
  K. Common metastatic sites—lymph nodes, bones, lung, liver, and peritoneum (NCI, 2018b)
IV. Screening and diagnostic measures
  A. Screening—not currently recommended by any major preventive group in the U.S.
    1. No specific serologic tumor markers
    2. Urinary assays for bladder cancer
      a. Food and Drug Administration (FDA)–approved nuclear matrix protein 22 (NMP-22) assay: a noninvasive test used for the surveillance and monitoring of patients with bladder cancer. Studies have demonstrated a sensitivity ranging anywhere from 47% to 100% with a specificity of 60% to 90% (Xylinas, Kluth, Rieken, Karakiewicz, Lotan, & Shariat, 2014).
      b. Other FDA-approved urinary assays for bladder cancer detection and monitoring—bladder tumor–associated antigen (BTA) assays, ImmunoCyt test, and UroVysion fluorescence in situ hybridization (FISH) assay. Sensitivity and specificity of the BTA stat test are 57% to 83% and 60% to 92%, respectively.
      c. Elevated urine levels of COL4A1 and COL13A1 show promise for diagnosis and prognosis (Miyake, 2017)
  B. Diagnostic measures
    1. IVP, also referred to as *excretory urography*—allows visualization of upper tracts to determine whether the source is within the bladder (intravesicular) or located elsewhere (see Table 15.1)
    2. Cystoscopy with bladder washings and biopsies

    3. Urinary cytology—specimens obtained from late-morning or early-afternoon urine
    4. CT—aids to define extent of local tumor, identifying pelvic lymph node metastasis
    5. MRI—distinguishes the tumor from the normal bladder wall and identifies the presence of pelvic lymph node involvement
V. Grading and staging
  A. Grading
    1. Tumor grade (grades X, 1, 2, 3, 4)—refers to the degree of tumor cell differentiation and aggressive nature of the tumor cells
      a. This grading system has changed to a low- and high-grade designation to match current World Health Organization/International Society of Urologic Pathology (WHO/ISUP)–recommended grading system
      b. High-grade tumors tend to grow more quickly and are more likely to metastasize
  B. Staging
    1. AJCC staging system (www.cancerstaging.org)
VI. Prognosis
  A. Prognostic indicators—tumor grade, size, location, biomarkers such as the p21 gene and ki67 antigen, cellular adhesion models, and response to therapy
  B. 5-year survival rate by stage of bladder cancer—stage 0 (98%), stage I (88%), stage II (63%), stage III (46%), and stage IV (15%) (ACS, 2018a)
VII. Management
  A. NMIBC
    1. Goal—prevent disease progression/invasion, avoid bladder loss, increase survival
      a. Primary mode of treatment—cystoscopy to confirm tumor presence, then transurethral resection of bladder tumor (TURBT); tumor removal achieved by fulguration (burning with electrical current) or laser therapy
        (1) Most common side effects—bleeding and infection
        (2) Perforation of surrounding tissues also risk of treatment
    2. Intravesical therapy—includes intravesical chemotherapy and immunotherapy
      a. Indications based on probability of recurrence and progression to muscle-invasive disease such as size, number, and grade (Clark, 2016)
      b. Intravesicular chemotherapy has been found to be more effective than TUR alone in preventing tumor recurrence
      c. Most common agents: mitomycin C (MMC), Bacillus Calmette–Guerin (BCG), thiotepa (Thioplex), valrubicin, doxorubicin (Adriamycin)
        (1) Combination of these drugs has also been used

(2) Thiotepa is infrequently used in clinical practice due to higher systemic side effects, such as myelosuppression

B. Treatment of muscle invasive disease

1. Radical cystectomy with urinary diversion

a. Removal of the bladder and prostate in men

b. Hysterectomy in women

c. Bilateral pelvic lymphadenectomy, including at a minimum common internal iliac, external iliac, and obturator nodes in both men and women

d. Potential complications—infection, bleeding, and sexual dysfunction

e. Presurgical chemotherapy using MVAC (methotrexate [Mexate], vinblastine [Velban], doxorubicin [Adriamycin], cisplatin [Platinol]) demonstrated to double survival rates in patients with advanced bladder cancer compared with surgery alone (NCI, 2018a)

f. Cisplatin-based combination chemotherapy strongly recommended by NCCN guidelines (Clark, 2016)

g. Types of urinary diversions (see Chapter 38)

(1) Ileal conduit (Fig. 15.3)—urinary diversion performed with cystectomy

(a) A portion of the terminal end of the ileum is isolated, the proximal end is closed, and the distal end is brought out through an opening in the abdominal wall and sutured to the skin, creating a stoma.

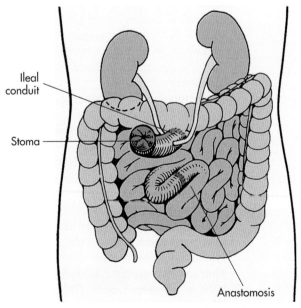

Fig. 15.3 Urinary diversion using a segment of ileum. As short a segment as possible is used and positioned in the right lower quadrant of the abdomen in an isoperistaltic direction. (From Christensen, B. L., & Kockrow, E. O. (2010). *Adult health nursing care* (6th ed.). St. Louis: Mosby.)

(b) Ureters are implanted into the ileal segment, urine flows into the conduit, and peristalsis propels urine out through the stoma.

(2) Continent ileal reservoir (Fig. 15.4)—technique that provides an intraabdominal pouch for storage of urine

(a) Typically, the stoma has a nipple valve to prevent ureteral reflux. The stoma is generally placed below the undergarment line.

(b) No external collecting device needed; urine remains in reservoir until patient self-catheterizes through stoma, approximately every 6 hours.

(3) Orthotopic neobladder—a technique that provides a creation of a new bladder that is made from the intestine; better quality of life reported compared with ileal conduit.

2. Bladder preservation therapy

a. Although radical cystectomy is the current primary treatment modality, some patients cannot tolerate cystectomy or are unwilling to undergo the procedure

b. Bladder preservation strategies include the following:

(1) External beam radiation therapy (XRT)

(2) Trimodality therapy—transurethral resection (TUR), radiation therapy, and systemic chemotherapy

3. Chemotherapy

a. Advanced bladder cancer is often treated with systemic chemotherapy.

(1) NCCN guidelines indicate first-line combination chemotherapy for metastatic disease includes the following (Clark, 2016:

(a) Dose-dense MVAC with growth factor support

(b) Gemcitabine and cisplatin

(2) For second-line therapy, single-agent taxane or gemcitabine preferred

(3) For concurrent treatment with radiation therapy, radiosensitizing chemotherapy regimens include the following:

b. Cisplatin alone or in combination with 5-fluorouracil (5-FU)

c. Mitomycin C in combination with 5-FU

d. Clinical trial

4. Radiation therapy

a. Useful in the management of invasive disease

b. Linear accelerator with multiple fields, daily or twice daily

c. An empty bladder required for both simulation and treatment

d. Radiation usually preceded by TUR

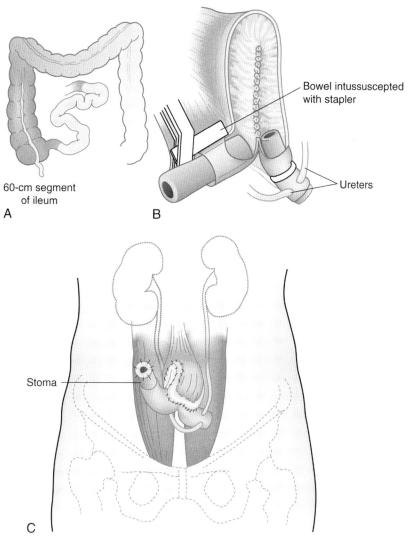

Fig. 15.4 Kock pouch urinary reservoir. **A,** Shaded area indicates section of small intestine selected for reservoir construction. **B,** Afferent (nonrefluxing) limb for ureteral implantation and efferent limb (with nippled valve) for stoma are created by using stapling devices. **C,** Completed reservoir with the efferent limb drawn through the abdominal wall and stoma created. (From Tanagho, E.A., & McAninch, J.W. (Eds.) (1992). *Smith's general urology* (13th ed.). San Mateo, CA: Appleton & Lange.)

e. Often used as combined modality therapy with chemotherapy
f. Dose range to whole bladder—40 to 55 gray (Gy), with an additional boost of 9 to 11 Gy, for a total of 49 to 66 Gy (Clark, 2016)

VIII. Nursing implications
  A. Maximize safety postoperatively
    1. Pulmonary hygiene—teach patient to perform cough and deep-breathing exercises; use of incentive spirometry
    2. Observe for signs of hemorrhage
    3. Monitor vital signs, hemoglobin, hematocrit, kidney function tests, and urine output
    4. Provide pharmacologic and nonpharmacologic pain relief measures

  B. Interventions related to the management of radiation therapy (see Chapter 27); targeted therapies and biotherapies (see Chapter 29)
  C. Interventions for patients receiving intravesical chemotherapy
    1. BCG—contraindicated in patients with immune system compromise because of HIV or steroid use, urinary tract infection, or past reactions to tuberculosis strains; systemic tuberculosis may develop.
    2. Thiotepa—low molecular weight leads to high rates of systemic absorption and severe myelosuppression.
    3. Mitomycin C—may cause dysuria, frequency, and, less commonly, allergic reactions and myelosuppression
  D. Management of common ileal conduit problems (Table 15.2).

TABLE 15.2 Management of Common Ileal Conduit Problems

Problem	Interventions
Urinary odor	Avoid use of rubber pouch.
	Soak appliance in vinegar and water, 1:4.
Rash around stoma or under pouch	Dry and powder skin except under adhesive.
	Use a skin barrier (e.g., Stomahesive).
Macerated skin around stoma	Dry skin, and apply a hydroponic skin barrier.
	Decrease size of pouch opening.
Crystals on or around stoma	Apply vinegar compresses on stoma and inside pouch.
Ulcerated stoma	Enlarge pouch opening.
	Consult enterostomal therapist if not partially healed in 1 week.
Monilial infection after antibiotic therapy	Dry skin, and apply nystatin (Mycostatin) powder.
	Encourage oral fluids.
Hyperplasia of skin around stoma	Decrease pouch-opening size.
Fistula	Revise stoma at new site.

PROSTATE CANCER

I. Physiology and pathophysiology
   A. Primary function
      1. Located posterior to the symphysis pubis, inferior to the bladder, in front of the rectum (see Fig. 15.1)
      2. Prostate gland—encircles the urethra as it leaves the bladder
      3. Comprises three zones—transitional zone, central zone, and peripheral zone
      4. Functions as a secondary sex organ that secretes a component of seminal fluid
   B. Changes associated with cancer
      1. Most cancers develop in the peripheral zone.
      2. Malignant cell growth spreads locally to the seminal vesicles, bladder, and peritoneum (see Fig. 15.1).
         a. Lymphatic, hematogenous spread is also common, pelvic lymph node invasion
   C. Major classifications
      1. Adenocarcinomas—95%
      2. Remaining 5% are sarcomas, mucinous or signet ring tumors, adenoid cystic carcinomas, and small cell undifferentiated cancers (ACS, 2018b)

II. Epidemiology
   A. National trend in prostate cancer incidence—increased rates 1988 to 1992 coinciding with the advent of widespread prostate-specific antigen (PSA) testing; sharp declines 1992 to 1995, followed by a leveling off 1995 to 2013; decrease of 8% 2009 to 2013 likely due to the United States Preventive Services Task Force (USPSTF) recommendation against routine testing (ACS, 2018b).
   B. Approximately 161,360 men newly diagnosed and 26,730 are estimated to die of the disease yearly; third leading cause of cancer death among men (ACS, 2018b).
   C. Accounts for one third of all male cancers; most commonly diagnosed noncutaneous cancer among men.
   D. 5-year survival rates—steady improvement since 1974 for both whites and African Americans; however, continuing lower 5-year survival rates for all stages of prostate cancer among African Americans (ACS, 2018b).
   E. Risk for prostate cancer is 74% higher in African American men than Caucasian men.

III. Risk factors
   A. Increasing age—only well-established risk factor (ACS, 2018b).
      1. More than 75% of prostate cancers are diagnosed in men 65 years or older.
      2. Autopsy studies reveal 30% of men aged 50 have evidence of adenocarcinoma of the prostate; by age 90 that percentage rises to 57%.
   B. Ethnicity
      1. Higher mortality rates in Western countries compared with non-Western countries (e.g., developing countries such as in Asia and the Middle East) (Kumst, 2017)
      2. Highest incidence and mortality rates in the world among African Americans (ACS, 2018b; Kumst, 2017)
   C. Dietary factors
      1. Possible role of high-fat or high-dairy diets in promotion of prostate cancer
      2. Diets high in vitamins E, D, and selenium possibly inhibit or prevent prostate cancer (Chhabra, Chandra, Ndiaye, Fedorowicz, Molot, & Ahmad, 2018)
      3. Studies are inconsistent on the role of obesity (ACS, 2018b)
      4. Diets high in lycopene linked to a low incidence of prostate cancer (ACS, 2018b)
   D. Occupational exposures
      1. Farming and cadmium exposure through welding and battery manufacturing associated with increased risk, as is Agent Orange among veterans who served in Vietnam (ACS, 2018b; Chamie, 2008)
   E. Genetic factors
      1. Prostate cancer susceptibility locus, called HPC1, located on chromosome 1—thought to be

responsible for 33% of all hereditary prostate cancer and 3% of cases overall

2. Mutations of *BRCA1* and *BRCA2* genes—implicated in breast cancer, as well as in prostate cancer

3. Having a single first-degree relative with prostate cancer—increases risk twofold to threefold; having a first- and second-degree relative affected increases risk sixfold

F. Common metastatic sites—lung, liver, adrenal glands, kidneys, and bones

IV. Screening and diagnostic measures

A. Screening

1. High level of controversy continues at the national level with regard to routine screening for prostate cancer with PSA testing.

a. Central issue—PSA testing may reveal clinically insignificant tumors; ensuing treatment causes significant side effects, resulting in diminished quality of life.

2. Following USPSTF recommendations, the American Urologic Association (AUA) published new guidelines for prostate cancer screening in 2013 (Smith, 2017)

a. PSA screening in men younger than 40 years not recommended

b. Routine screening in men 40 to 54 years at average risk not recommended; at-risk men may benefit from shared decision making at this earlier age

c. Shared decision making about PSA screening for men ages 55 to 69 years; greatest screening benefit in this age group

d. Screening interval of 2 or more years for those deciding on screening

e. PSA screening not recommended for men 70 years or older or for those with less than a 10- to 15-year life expectancy

3. Normal range for PSA varies by age, race, and prostate size—0 to 4 ng/mL considered standard norm. Other markers: PSA density, PSA velocity.

B. Diagnostic tests

1. Digital rectal examination (DRE)—assess for size, lesions, symmetry, texture

a. Simple and inexpensive, but only the posterior and lateral areas can be palpated

2. Transrectal ultrasound (TRUS)—evaluation of the prostate volume

3. Biopsy

a. Performed with TRUS for guidance

b. Transrectal route preferred; six specimens obtained from both sides of the prostate

4. Pelvic MRI to evaluate capsular penetration, seminal vesicle involvement, lymph node metastasis

5. Bone scans—to evaluate possible bone metastasis; generally not performed unless PSA level is above 10 ng/mL or patient complains of skeletal symptoms (Mohler, 2016b)

6. Laboratory studies

a. PSA—increased levels may be significant as an adjunct in differential diagnosis or as a marker for disease progression

(1) Men should avoid ejaculation for 48 hours before test

(2) Finasteride (Propecia), androgen receptor blockers, PC-SPES may also affect PSA levels (Mohler, 2016b)

V. Grading and staging

A. Grading—based on the Gleason score (Mohler, 2016a)

1. Primary grade—based on evaluation of architecture of malignant glands in the largest portion of the specimen; most common cell grade seen

2. Secondary grade—assigned to the next largest area of malignant growth; second most common cell grade seen

3. Score computed by adding the primary and secondary grades together; order reveals most common cell grade (i.e., 3 + 4 = 7 versus 4 + 3 = 7); scores 2 to 10 possible

4. Higher scores (8–10) indicate aggressive disease, with a poor prognosis

B. Staging

1. AJCC staging system (www.cancerstaging.org)

VI. Prognosis

A. 5-year survival rate by stage of prostate cancer—local (near 100%), regional (near 100%), and distant disease (29%)

B. 5-year survival for all stages combined—89.9% for whites, 65.5% for African Americans (Kumst, 2017)

VII. Management

A. Early-stage disease

1. Treatment options—active surveillance, observation or expectant management, radical prostatectomy with lymph node dissection, three-dimensional conformal radiotherapy (3D-CRT), or brachytherapy

a. Radical prostatectomy—complete removal of prostate; lymph node sampling

(1) Alternative approaches—laparoscopic prostatectomy and robotic laparoscopic prostatectomy (Mohler, 2016b)

b. 3D-CRT—radiation doses to prostate greater than 81 Gy (Mohler, 2016a) intensity-modulated radiation therapy (IMRT) replacing 3D

c. Androgen deprivation therapy (ADT) increasingly being used adjuvantly with radiation (Mohler, 2016a)

d. Brachytherapy—guided by TRUS, radioactive seed placement into the prostate gland via the perineum through a grid template (Mohler, 2016a)

(1) Isotopes used—iodine-125 or palladium-103

e. Active surveillance, expectant management for lower Gleason score (<6)—follow-up with PSA testing, needle biopsy, DRE, followed by active treatment if disease progression noted (Mohler, 2016a)

f. Cryosurgery—direct application of freezing temperatures to the prostate via percutaneously inserted cryogenic probes (Mohler, 2016a)

2. Complications of treatment

a. Incontinence—conflicting data because of imprecise measurement; estimated range from 3% to 87% after radical prostatectomy, 3% to 7% for external beam radiotherapy, 6% for brachytherapy; other complications: urethral stricture, urethral sloughing, and bladder outlet obstruction.

b. Erectile dysfunction—nerve-sparing prostatectomy techniques lessen incidence; comparisons difficult because of imprecise definitions and measurement; high rates reported after surgery, and some form of impotence seen in 6% to 61% of cases after brachytherapy

c. Gastrointestinal dysfunction—diarrhea, proctitis, and rectal bleeding associated with both radiation therapy and brachytherapy

3. Treatment for advanced prostate cancer

a. Hormonal manipulation—accepted standard for metastatic prostate cancer and in patients at high risk for relapse; also used in neoadjuvant setting

(1) Orchiectomy—surgical removal of testicles; produces rapid response; for patients unreliable in taking medication or when estrogen is contraindicated

(a) Not acceptable as an option for many men

(b) Psychological trauma as a result of surgical castration

(2) Luteinizing hormone–releasing hormones (LHRH analogs; such as leuprolide [Lupron], goserelin [Zoladex])—decrease production of testosterone; may produce fewer side effects compared with estrogens; used with flutamide (Eulexin) to reduce "flare," which is the sudden exacerbation of symptoms (Mohler, 2016a)

(a) Flare can be life threatening, with spinal cord compression and ureteral obstruction (Mohler, 2016a)

(b) Other side effects: hot flashes, loss of libido, erectile dysfunction, gynecomastia

(3) Antiandrogens (flutamide [Eulexin], enzalutamide [Xtandi], megestrol acetate [Megace])—interfere with intracellular androgen activity; effects may be delayed 1 to 2 months

(4) Estrogen therapy—generally, diethylstilbestrol (DES)

(a) Used in castration-resistant prostate cancer

(b) Results in decreased pain, decreased tumor size, decreased urinary symptoms (Mohler, 2016a)

(c) Complications—gynecomastia, sodium retention, weight gain, and severe cardiovascular and thrombotic complications

(d) Associated with relapse within 2 to 3 years; at the time of relapse, disease often becomes resistant to further hormone treatment

(5) Ketoconazole (Nizoral)—suppresses adrenal testosterone production

(a) Used in castration-resistant prostate cancer

(b) Administered with hydrocortisone to reduce risk of adrenal insufficiency (Mohler, 2016a)

(c) Abiraterone (Zytiga)—used in combination with prednisone for castration-resistant prostate cancer (Mohler, 2016a)

4. Radiation therapy—for local extension and distant metastases

a. Primary treatment option for stage D lesions if hormone manipulation ineffective or contraindicated; may be used as a component of combined-modality therapy

b. Used for palliation of pain from bone metastasis or spinal cord compression

c. Radium-223 for symptomatic bone metastases

5. Chemotherapy

a. Optimal timing of initiation of chemotherapy in men with castration-resistant prostate cancer undetermined (Mohler, 2016a)

b. Docetaxel (Taxotere) preferred (Mohler, 2016a)

c. Other options—sipuleucel-T, mitoxantrone, cyclophosphamide, estramustine, vinblastine, and vinorelbine; cabazitaxel preferred after docetaxel

VIII. Nursing implications

A. Manage physical, psychological, social, and spiritual distress during and after treatment

1. Encourage patient to verbalize feelings about disease and treatment

2. Refer to mental health specialist, community resources, support groups (e.g., ACS, UsToo), as needed

3. Teach patient to identify and manage symptoms and when to report

4. Manage pain and other side effects

B. Promote optimal sexual functioning

1. Facilitate discussion among the physician, nurse, patient, and caregiver about the potential impact of treatment on sexual functioning, interventions to minimize effects

a. Obtain permission, before and after treatment, to discuss functional and anatomic changes with treatment and resultant sexual concerns

b. Respect the patient's reticence in discussing sexual concerns

2. Use terminology appropriate to social and cultural level

3. Provide written information and anatomic drawings, as indicated, for clarifications and to reinforce teaching

4. Provide specific suggestions related to treatment used and alternatives

a. Teach patient and caregiver about options for the treatment of impotence—pharmacologic, mechanical, surgical. See Chapter 38 for management of genitourinary symptoms.

b. Refer to physical therapy, sexual counseling, if indicated.

REFERENCES

ACS. (2018a). *Bladder Cancer*. ACS Facts and Statistics.

ACS. (2018b). *Cancer Facts & Figures 2018*.

ACS. (2018c). *Kidney Cancer*.

AJCC (2017). *Cancer Staging System*. 8 (8th ed.).

Board, P. A. T. E. (2018). *PDQ Transitional cell cancer of the renal pelvis and uretery. Clinical Guidelines*.

Chamie, K., DeVere White, R. W., Lee, D., Ok, J. H., & Ellison, L. M. (2008). Agent Orange exposure, Vietnam War veterans, and the risk of prostate cancer. *Cancer, 113*(9), 2404–2470. https://doi.org/10.1002/cncr.23695.

Chhabra, G., Singh, C. K., Ndiaye, M. A., Fedorowicz, S., Molot, A., & Ahmad, N. (2018). Prostate cancer chemoprevention by natural agents: clinical evidence and potential implications. *Cancer Lett, 422*, 9–18. https://doi.org/10.1016/j.canlet.2018.02.025.

Chow, W. H., Dong, L. M., & Devesa, S. S. (2010). Epidemiology and risk factors for kidney cancer. *National Reviews in Urology, 7*(5), 245–257. https://doi.org/10.1038/nrurol.2010.46.

Clark PE, S. P., Agarwal, N., Bangs, R., Boorjian, S. A., Buyyounouski, M. K., Efstathiou, J. A., Flaig, T. W., Friedlander, T., Greenberg, R. E., Guru, K. A., Hahn, N., Herr, H. W. , Hoimes, C., Inman, B. A., Kader, A. K., Kibel, A. S., Kuzel, T. M., Lele, S. M., Meeks, J. J., Michalski, J., Montgomery, J. S., Pagliaro, L. C., Pal, S. K., Patterson, A., Petrylak, D., Plimack, E. R., Pohar, K. S., Porter, M. P., Sexton, W. J., Siefker-Radtke, A. O., Sonpavde, G., Tward, J.,

Wile, G., Dwyer, M. A., & Smith, C. (2016). NCCN guidelines insights: bladder cancer, version 2. *2016 Journal of the National Comprehensive Cancer Network, 14*(10), 1213–1224.

Jonasch, E., Gao, J., & Rathmell, W. K. (2014). Renal cell carcinoma. *BMJ, 349.* https://doi.org/10.1136/bmj.g4787.

Kumst, D., Singh, R., Malik, S., Manne, U., & Mishra, M. (2017). Prostate cancer health disparities: an immuno-biological perspective. *Cancer Letters, 414*, 153–165.

Liu, K. W., Lin, V. C., & Chang, I. W. (2013). Clear cell adenocarcinoma of the renal pelvis: an extremely rare neoplasm of the upper urinary tract. *Pol Journal of Pathology, 64*(4), 308–311.

Miyake M, M. Y., Hori, S., Tatsumi, Y., Onishi, S., Owari, T., Iida, K., Onishi, K., Gotoh, D., Nakai, Y., Anai, S., Chihara, Y., Torimoto, K., Aoki, K., Tanaka, N., Shimada, K., Konishi, N., & Fujimoto, K. (2017). Diagnostic and prognostic role of urinary collagens in primary human bladder cancer. *Cancer Science, 108*(11), 2221-1118. https://doi.org/10.1111/cas.13384.

Mohler, J. L., Armstrong, A. J., Bhnson, R. R., D'Amico, A. V., Davis, B. J., Eastham, J. A., … Freedman-Cass, D. A. (2016a). Prostate cancer, version 1.2016: Featured updates to the NCCN Guidelines. *Journal of the National Comprehensive Cancer Network, 14*(1), 19–30.

Mohler, J. L., Armstrong, A. J., Bhnson, R. R., D'Amico, A. V., Davis, B. J., Eastham, J. A., … Freedman-Cass, D. A. (2016b). Prostate cancer, version 1.2016: Featurered updates to the NCCN guidelines. *Journal of the National Comprehensive Cancer Network, 14*(1), 19–30.

Motzer, R. J., Jonasch, E., Agarwal, N., Bhayani, S., Bro, W. P., Chang, S. S., … Plimack, E. R. (2017). Kidney cancer, version 2.2017: clinical practice guidelines in oncology. *Journal of the National Comprehensive Cancer Network, 15*(6), 804–834. https://doi.org/10.6004/jnccn.2017.0100.

National Cancer Institute (NCI). (2018a). *Bladder Cancer*.

National Cancer Institute (NCI). (2018b). *Bladder Cancer*.

NCI. (2018). *Genetics of prostate cancer (PDQ)*.

OpenStax. (2018). *Anatomy & Physiology*. OpenStax CNX. Retrieved from https://cnx.org/contents/FPtK1zmh@8.119:7l9EIHui@4/Gross-Anatomy-of-the-Kidney.

Pastore, A. L., Palleschi, G., Silvestri, L., Moschese, D., Ricci, V., Petrozza, A., Carbone, A., & Di Carlo, A. (2015). Serum and urine biomarkers for human renal cell carcinoma. *Disease Markers, 2015*, 9 pages https://doi.org/10.1155/2015/251403.

Piyathilake, C. (2016). Dietary factors associated with bladder cancer. *Investigative Clinical Urology, 57*(Suppl 1), S14–S25. https://doi.org/10.4111/icu.2016.57.S1.S14.

Smith, R. A., Andrews, K. S., Brooks, D., Fedewa, S. A., Manassaram-Batiste, D., Saslow, D., Brawley, O. W., & Wender, R. C. (2017). Cancer screening in the United States, 2017: a review of current American Cancer Society guidelines and current issues in cancer screening. *CA Cancer J Clin, 67*(2), 100–121. https://doi.org/10.3322/caac.21392.

Steele, C. B., Thomas, C. C., Henley, S. J., Massetti, G. M., Galuska, D. A., Agurs-Collins, T., Puckett, M., & Richardson, L. C. (2017). Vital signs: trends in incidence of cancers assoiacted with overweight and obesity - United States, 2005-2014. *MMWR, 66*(39), 1052–1058. https://doi.org/10.15585/mmwr.mm6639e1.

Westhoff, E., Witjes, J. A., Fleshner, N. E., Lerner, S. P., Shariat, S. R., Kampman, E., Kliemeney, L. A., Vrieling, A., & Tu, H. (2018). Body mass index, diet-related factors, and bladder cancer prognosis: a systematic review and meta-analysis. *Bladder Cancer, 4*(1), 91–112. https://doi.org/10.3233/BLC-170147.

Westhoff, E. W. X., Kliemeney, L. A., Lerner, S. P., Huang, M., Dinney, C. P., Vrieling, A., & Tu, H. (2017). Dietary patterns amd riski of recurrence and progression in non-muscle-invasive bladder cancer. *International Journal of Cancer.* https://doi.org/10.1002/ijc.312`14.

Xylinas, E., Kluth, L. A., Rieken, M., Karakiewicz, P. I., Lotan, Y., & Shariat, S. F. (2014). Urine markers for detection and surveillance of bladder cancer. *Urol Oncol, 32*(3), 222–229. https://doi.org/10.1016/j.urolonc.2013.06.001. Epub 2013 Sep 17. Review.

16

Head and Neck Cancers

Beverly Hudson and Ellen Carr

I. Physiology and pathophysiology (Carr, 2018)
   A. Includes cancers of the oral cavity, oropharynx, nasal cavity, paranasal sinuses, nasopharynx, larynx, hypopharynx, and salivary glands; cancers of the thyroid and parathyroid
   B. Anatomy of the head and neck (H-N) (Fig. 16.1)
      1. Oral cavity—extends from the lips to the hard palate above and the circumvallate papillae below; structures include lips, buccal mucosa, floor of the mouth, upper and lower alveoli, retromolar trigone, hard palate, and anterior two thirds of the tongue
      2. Oropharynx—extends from the circumvallate papillae below and hard palate above to the level of the hyoid bone; structures include the base of the tongue (posterior one third), soft palate, tonsils, and posterior pharyngeal wall
      3. Nasal cavity and paranasal sinuses—include nasal vestibule; paired maxillary, ethmoid, and frontal sinuses; and a single sphenoid sinus
      4. Nasopharynx—located below the base of the skull and behind the nasal cavity; continuous with the posterior pharyngeal wall
      5. Larynx—extends from the epiglottis to the cricoid cartilage; protected by the thyroid cartilage, which encases it; subdivided into three areas
         a. Supraglottis—below the base of the tongue, extending to but not including the true vocal cord; includes epiglottis, aryepiglottic folds, arytenoid cartilages, and false vocal cords
         b. Glottis—area of the true vocal cord
         c. Subglottis—below the true vocal cord, extending to the cricoid cartilage
      6. Hypopharynx—extends from the hyoid bone to the lower border of the cricoid cartilage; structures include pyriform sinuses, postcricoid region, and the lower posterior pharyngeal wall
   C. Critical adjacent structures
      1. Regional lymph nodes of the neck drain the anatomic structures of the H-N; the area includes the submental submaxillary, upper and lower jugular, posterior triangle (spinal accessory), and preauricular nodes (Fig. 16.2)
      2. H-N structures are contiguous with the lower aerodigestive tract—trachea, lungs, and esophagus
      3. The nasopharynx and paranasal sinuses are close to the brain

II. Epidemiology (ACS, 2018a)
   A. 2018 estimated incidence and death rates:
      1. Larynx cancer: 13,150 (incidence); 3710 (death rate)
      2. Oral cavity and pharynx cancers: 51,540 (incidence); 10,030 (death rate)
      3. Thyroid cancer: 53,990 (incidence); 2060 (death rate)
   B. Most H-N tumors occur in the oral cavity, oropharynx, larynx, nasal cavity, paranasal, nasopharynx, laryngeal, and hypopharyngeal
   C. Higher incidence rates (NCI, 2018):
      a. >50 years of age
      b. Men 2× higher incidence than women

III. Risk factors (ACS, 2018b, 2018e; Lechelt et al., 2018)
   A. Tobacco use, excessive alcohol intake increases risk of developing oral or pharyngeal cancer. Smokeless tobacco types; chewing, oral, or spit tobacco; snuff or dipping tobacco; dissolvable tobacco.
   B. Tobacco and alcohol do not contribute to salivary tumors.
   C. Estimated from 2011 to 2015 in men, 81% of all human papillomavirus (HPV)–associated cancers are oropharynx cancers. In women, 15% of all HPV-associated cancers are oropharynx cancers (CDC, 2018).
   D. Additional risk factors (Tamaki et al., 2018)
      1. Gastroesophageal reflux
      2. Diet
      3. History of neck radiation
      4. Familial history of cancer
      5. Environmental exposure (wood, dust, asbestos)
      6. Polycyclic hydrocarbons

IV. Prevention
   A. Smoking cessation; limiting alcohol intake; preventing exposure to tobacco, nicotine, and environmental carcinogenic agents; early detection of infection by HPV (ACS, 2018a)

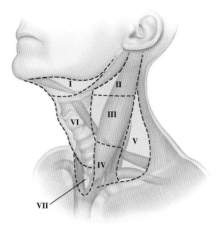

Fig. 16.1 Regional lymphatic pattern in the head and neck. (From Friedman, M., Kelley, K., & Maley, A. [2011]. Central neck dissection. *Operative Techniques in Otolaryngology—Head and Neck Surgery*, 22(2): 169–172.)

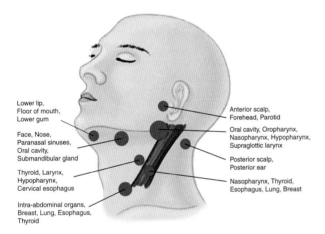

Lower lip, Floor of mouth, Lower gum

Face, Nose, Paranasal sinuses, Oral cavity, Submandibular gland

Thyroid, Larynx, Hypopharynx, Cervical esophagus

Intra-abdominal organs, Breast, Lung, Esophagus, Thyroid

Anterior scalp, Forehead, Parotid

Oral cavity, Oropharynx, Nasopharynx, Hypopharynx, Supraglottic larynx

Posterior scalp, Posterior ear

Nasopharynx, Thyroid, Esophagus, Lung, Breast

Fig. 16.2 Likely sites of metastasis from various areas of the head and neck.

B. Smoking cessation programs are encouraged to successfully help at-risk H-N cancer patients to quit smoking (ACS, 2018b, 2018f; Smokefree.gov, 2018).

V. Histology classification of H-N tumors
   A. Squamous cell carcinomas (SCCs), verrucous SCC, adenocarcinoma, minor salivary gland tumors, spindle cell carcinoma, fibrosarcomas, chondrosarcomas, neuroendocrine tumors, and metastatic disease (Tamaki et al., 2018)

VI. Molecular classification
   A. Pathology/histologic diagnosis from molecular pathway expression, targeted markers (NCCN, 2018a)
      1. Identification of p16 and p53 protein expression and high-risk HPV (HPV-HR) types have been associated with poorer survival in H-N malignancies.
      2. Multiple molecular pathways better predict the outcomes and potentially the type of treatment targeted to those markers.
         a. Based on pathology results and clinical staging, treatment based on algorithms.

b. Example: SCC base of tongue with HPV+
   (1) Depending on the clinical stage (i.e., T1), treatment would be surgery or chemotherapy-radiation (NCCN, 2018a).

VII. Diagnosis and staging
   A. Screening
      1. Detection
         a. Many laryngeal and some hypopharyngeal cancers can be found early. They usually cause symptoms, such as hoarseness or voice changes (ACS, 2018c, 2018d)
         b. Screening strategies: inspection of the oral cavity is often part of the physical examination by a primary care physician and/or dentist.
            (1) For 20- to 40-year-olds, every 3 years; for >40, every year (ACS, 2018d)
   B. Diagnosis of H-N tumors (NCCN 2018a; NIDCR, 2018):
      1. History (risk factors)
      2. Signs and symptoms of disease (Box 16.1)
      3. Physical examination: visualization, mirror examination of the pharynx and larynx, palpation via a bimanual examination to assess the oral cavity and upper neck
      4. Radiologic studies, among them:
         a. Computed tomography (CT)—to assist in determining the extent of the primary tumor and to identify metastasis to the cervical lymph nodes
         b. Magnetic resonance imaging (MRI)—superior to CT in staging nasopharyngeal primaries
         c. Positron emission tomography (PET) with CT (PET-CT)—useful in determining specific areas for biopsy, lymph node involvement, and extent of disease to aid in treatment planning
      5. Laboratory studies—complete blood cell count, chemistry studies, liver function tests
      6. For histologic diagnosis, procedures to obtain specimen:
         a. Fine-needle aspiration—preferred over open biopsy for treatment planning and management
         b. Excisional biopsy of the lesion
            (1) On small oral cavity, lip, or skin lesions
            (2) An open or excisional biopsy of suspicious neck nodes can be contraindicated because it may alter or interfere with subsequent treatment
               (a) Exception—when all other examinations fail to identify a primary site or when lymphoma is suspected
         c. Incisional biopsy—tumor sample along with adjoining normal tissue
         d. Panendoscopy (passing an endoscope along the entire mucosa of the upper aerodigestive

---

BOX 16.1 Signs and Symptoms of Head and Neck Cancers*

- A lump or sore that does not heal in mouth, lip, or throat
- A sore throat that does not go away
- A change or hoarseness in the voice
- A white or red patch in the mouth
- A feeling that something is caught in the throat
- Difficulty chewing or swallowing
- Difficulty moving the jaw or tongue
- Swelling in the jaw
- Numbness in the tongue or other areas of the mouth
- Pain in one ear without hearing loss

- Loose teeth or dentures that no longer fit well
- Blocked sinuses that do not clear, or sinus pressure or pain
- Double vision or the eyes pointing in different directions
- Pain in the upper teeth
- Pain, pressure, or drainage in the ear
- A lump (usually painless) in the area of the ear, cheek, jaw, lip, or inside the mouth
- Fluid draining from the ear
- Weight loss for no known reason
- Ear pain or hearing loss

Check with a provider about any of these symptoms.

Other Possible Symptoms

- White or red patch on the gums, tongue, or lining of the mouth
- Bleeding, pain, or numbness in the lip, mouth, or nose

---

* These symptoms may be caused by a malignancy or other, less serious causes.
Data from National Cancer Institute. (NCI) (2018). *Head and neck cancers*. Retrieved from https://www.cancer.gov/types/head-and-neck/head-neck-fact-sheet; National Institute of Dental and Craniofacial Research. (NIDCR) (2018). *Oral cancer*. Retrieved from https://www.nidcr.nih.gov/health-info/oral-cancer/more-info.

---

tract)—to examine and perform a biopsy on suspicious areas, determine the full extent of disease, and identify synchronous primary tumors

   (1) Lymph node biopsies/eval to determine spread of tumor regionally or distant (Talmi et al., 2018)

  e. From biopsies and specimens, molecular and genetics studies (Eskander, Ghanem, & Agrawal, 2018; Fulcher, Haigentz, & Ow, 2018; Gill, Vasan, Givi, & Joshi, 2018; MLCWG, 2018; NCCN, 2018a)

C. Staging—TNM (tumor–node–metastasis) classification system for specific diagnoses developed by the American Joint Committee on Cancer (AJCC, 2017)

  1. Metastatic patterns

    a. H-N cancer is a locally aggressive disease that can spread regionally to the lymphatics of the neck.

    b. Most patients present with stage III or IV disease (tumor is very large, has invaded adjacent tissue, or is a primary tumor that has spread to the lymphatics).

    c. At the time of initial diagnosis, distant metastases are uncommon at presentation (NCCN, 2018a).

      (1) H-N cancers tend to recur locally; can also develop second primary H-N cancers; usually of the upper aerodigestive tract or lung; depend on original cancer site and if patients continue to use tobacco and drink alcohol

    d. Most common sites of distal metastasis for laryngeal cancer are the lungs followed by the liver (Tamaki et al., 2018)

VIII. Prognosis and trends in survival

  A. Survival rates

    1. The 5-year relative survival rate for all stages of oral cavity and pharynx cancers combined is 65%,

but is much lower in blacks (48%) than in whites (66%). Studies indicate survival is better for patients with cancer who test positive for HPV (ACS, 2018a; Boggs, 2015; Zenga et al., 2018).

    2. For laryngeal cancer (all stages), 5-year survival rate is 60.7% (NCI, 2018).

    3. For thyroid cancer, 5-year relative survival rate is 98% (ACS, 2018a).

  B. The rate of new cases of laryngeal cancer is decreasing by about 2% to 3% a year, most likely because fewer people are smoking (ACS, 2018c).

IX. Management

  A. Developments in care and treatment—reduced deformities and improved cosmetic effect because of prosthetic devices and surgical flaps (myocutaneous and free flaps) (McEwen et al., 2018; Tamaki et al., 2018)

    1. Since the early 1970s, more conservative surgical technique and reconstruction has improved quality of life—decreasing dysfunctional airway, communication, swallowing (NCCN, 2018a)

  B. Management strategies

    1. Based on TNM classification tumor volume and grade, as well as patient age, performance status, and goals of care (Eskander et al., 2018; Fulcher et al., 2018; Gill et al., 2018; MLCWG, 2018; NCCN, 2018a)

    2. Surgery and radiation—the primary treatment modalities for managing malignant H-N tumors; adjuvant chemotherapy for recurrent and metastatic disease (NCCN, 2018a)

      a. Best to implement interdisciplinary (interprofessional) approach to managing the patient and family with H-N cancers on admission (e.g., nurses, various physicians, dental, social worker, nutritionists, physical therapist [PT], occupational therapist [OT]) (Brunner et al., 2015)

b. In general, for early-stage H-N cancers (i.e., T1 and T2 lesions of the oral cavity, larynx, nose, and paranasal sinuses), treatment is surgery or radiation (Fulcher et al., 2018; Gill et al., 2018; NCCN, 2018a)

(1) T2 can involve metastasis (NCCN, 2018a)

3. For later-stage H-N cancers (i.e., T3 and T4 tumors), treatment is combination therapy (NCCN, 2018a)

4. For N1, N2, and N3

5. For clinically negative neck nodes and a large primary lesion (T2, N0) of the oral cavity, oropharynx, hypopharynx, or larynx, treatment is either lymphadenectomy or radiation (because tumor cells can spread) (NCCN, 2018a)

C. Management: surgery
  1. Common surgical procedures (Table 16.1)
D. Management: radiation therapy (see Chapter 27)
  1. Primary treatment to control the primary tumor and adjacent lymph nodes while maintaining structure and function—external beam (over 5–7 weeks) in dose fractions; dose range 62 to 72 gray (Gy) for gross disease, 44 to 63 Gy for subclinical disease (NCCN, 2018a)

TABLE 16.1 Surgical Procedures for Head and Neck Cancers

Procedure	Physical Alteration	Nursing Implications
Laser	Little to none	Minimal bleeding
Composite resection	Resection of oral cavity, oropharyngeal lesion in continuity with neck dissection Portion of mandible is resected Reconstruction with myocutaneous flaps is usually required, with resections of large amounts of tissue	May experience problems with speech (decreased articulation with tongue involvement), swallowing (impaired mastication, salivary drooling, aspiration), altered facial contour
Cordectomy	Removal of all or part of the vocal cords	All: normal speech no longer possible Part: may cause hoarse voice
Supraglottic laryngectomy	Resection of structures above the false vocal cords, including the epiglottis (preserves the true vocal cords)	Aspiration until swallowing techniques are learned Maintains a relatively normal voice
Hemilaryngectomy	Vertical excision of one true and one false cord and underlying cartilage	Hoarse voice Minimal or no swallowing problems
Total laryngectomy	Excision of the entire larynx from the hyoid bone to the second tracheal ring	Permanent tracheostomy Aphonia Decreased sense of smell Unable to perform Valsalva maneuver
Maxillectomy	Partial or total en-bloc resection of the cavity May include the ethmoid sinus, lateral nasal wall, palate, and floor of orbit	Preoperatively, maxillofacial prosthodontist makes dental obturator to fill the large surgical defect and to facilitate swallowing Requires daily care to cavity and placement of obturator
Orbital exoneration	Resection of orbit secondary to extension of maxillary sinus tumor or recurrent disease	Facial defect Unilateral vision loss Requires daily care and cleansing of cavity
Craniofacial, skull base resection	Surgical approach to inaccessible midfacial and extensive paranasal sinus and nasopharyngeal lesions	May have facial defect and cranial nerve (III, IV, V) deficits
Radical neck dissection	Resection of sternocleidomastoid muscle, jugular vein, spinal accessory nerve, and cervical lymph nodes	Shoulder droop Concave contour of neck
Modified neck dissection	Radical neck dissection with preservation of the sternocleidomastoid muscle, jugular vein, or spinal accessory nerve	Shoulder droop if spinal accessory nerve resected Concave contour of neck
Lymphadenectomy	Resection of lymph nodes in neck	Surgical scars
Thyroidectomy	Removal of all or part of the thyroid gland	Surgical scars Possibly radioactive iodine ([radioiodine] therapy) daily thyroid hormone (levothyroxine) pill

Data from American Cancer Society (ACS) (2018d). *Laryngeal and hypopharyngeal cancers.* Retrieved from https://www.cancer.org/cancer/laryngeal-and-hypopharyngeal-cancer.html; National Cancer Institute (NCI) (2018). *Head and neck cancers.* Retrieved from https://www.cancer.gov/types/head-and-neck/head-neck-fact-sheet; National Comprehensive Cancer Network (NCCN) (2018a). *Head and neck cancers 2.2018.* Retrieved from https://www.nccn.org/professionals/physician_gls/pdf/head-and-neck.pdf; National Comprehensive Cancer Network (NCCN) (2018b). *Thyroid cancers 1.2018.* Retrieved from https://www.nccn.org/professionals/physician_gls/pdf/thyroid.pdf.

2. Adjuvant treatment for stage III and IV disease and tumors that can spread toward the midline (e.g., oropharyngeal lesions)
   a. On average 50 to 66 Gy (in 2.0-Gy dose fractions) over 5 to 6 weeks is adjuvant treatment for locally advanced H-N cancers (NCCN, 2018a)
3. External beam radiation therapy (RT) performed approximately 4 to 6 weeks after surgery
4. Preoperative radiation or permanently placed iodine-125 seeds used to debulk large or unresectable lesions
5. Treatment for nasopharyngeal cancer primarily radiation
   a. Surgery avoided because area is close to vital structures of the brain
   b. Carefully selected clients who experience treatment failure with RT treated with base-of-skull resection of tumor
6. Brachytherapy—treatment for lesions of the anterior and posterior tongue, floor of mouth, and nasal vestibule (implanted iridium-192 or cesium-137)
7. A low dose of radioactive iodine given after surgery for thyroid cancer destroyed (ablated) residual thyroid tissue as effectively as a higher dose, but with fewer side effects and less exposure to radiation (NCCN, 2018b)

E. Management: chemotherapy (see Chapter 28)
   1. Chemotherapy alone is not curative
      a. Reduces tumor volume or rids clinically detectable SCCs
      b. Treatment for recurrent or metastatic disease
   2. As adjuvant and neoadjuvant therapy, single-agent or combination chemotherapy regimens—cisplatin (Platinol), bleomycin (Blenoxane), fluorouracil (5-fluorouracil, 5-FU), paclitaxel (Taxol), and methotrexate (Mexate); also used for palliative therapy for recurrent or unresectable lesions (NCCN, 2018a)
      a. First-line single agents: cisplatin, carboplatin, 5-FU, docetaxel (Taxotere), paclitaxel (Taxol), epirubicin (NCCN, 2018a)
      b. Combination protocols of chemotherapy with RT used because of sensitizing effect of chemotherapy
         (1) Example—RADPLAT (protocol for mouth cancers; strategy is concurrent RT and cisplatin-based infusion to the tumor)

F. Management: targeted therapies (see Chapter 29)
   1. Treatment for those diagnosed with HPV-positive oropharyngeal cancer may be different from that for those with oropharyngeal cancers that are HPV-negative. Patients with HPV-positive oropharyngeal tumors may have a better prognosis and may do just as well on less intense treatment (Boggs, 2015; Haddad & Glass, 2017)

2. Food and Drug Administration (FDA) has approved targeted therapies for H-N cancer: cetuximab (Erbitux), pembrolizumab (Keytruda), nivolumab (Opdivo) (NCCN, 2018a)
   3. Targeted therapies may be combined with radiation therapy (NCCN, 2018a)

G. Management: combined chemotherapy and radiation therapy (NCCN, 2018a)
   1. Concomitant treatment provides synergy to treatment strategy

H. Management: palliative therapy (Hendriks-Ferguson & Ott, 2016)
   1. Surgery, radiation, chemotherapy, or combination therapy for unresectable lesions or recurrent tumors or when surgery is considered high risk
   2. To relieve pain, bleeding, or obstruction, short courses of radiation (30 Gy over 2 to 3 weeks) (NCCN, 2018a)

X. Nursing implications
A. Assessment: head and neck function (McEwen et al., 2018; NCCN 2018a)
   1. Respiration
      a. H-N cancers affect the structures of the upper airway, which transports warmed, filtered, and humidified air into the lungs.
      b. When disease and treatment affect this area, the natural air-conditioning function of the upper air passageways is bypassed. The effect—cooling and dryness of the trachea and lungs—may lead to infection.
      c. When the upper airway is altered, the sense of smell changes (e.g., inability to sniff).
   2. Speech
      a. When the larynx is removed (all or part), it results in loss of vibrating component for speech; thus sound waves cannot be produced (total laryngectomy) or are diminished (partial).
      b. Surgery to the mouth, tongue, or palate causes changes in the person's ability to articulate clear, understandable speech.
      c. Cancer or treatment of the nose or paranasal sinuses influences the tone and quality of the speech.
      d. Altered speech: phonation (from larynx), articulation (from the lips, tongue, and soft palate), resonation (tone and quality of speech from resonators—pharynx, mouth, nose, paranasal sinuses)
   3. Swallowing (Balusik, 2014; NCCN, 2018a)
      a. Components—26 muscles and six cranial nerves orchestrate the transport of food from the mouth to the stomach in four phases of swallowing
         (1) Oral preparatory—in the oral cavity, bolus of food is chewed and combined with saliva; the tongue, using front and

back movement, propels bolus into the pharynx

(2) Taste receptors are on the tongue, soft palate, glossopalatine arch, and posterior wall of the pharynx

(3) Pharyngeal—the bolus moves through the pharynx and is propelled toward the esophagus; the vocal cords close, and the larynx moves upward and forward, preventing aspiration

(4) Esophageal—the bolus moves through the esophagus and enters the stomach

b. Supraglottic laryngectomy affects the pharyngeal phase of swallowing, undermining the protection of the glottis. Until swallowing techniques are mastered, aspiration is a risk.

c. When the structures in the oral cavity and oropharynx undergo extensive resections (requiring flap reconstruction), swallowing phases (oral preparatory and oral) change and may result in drooling of saliva, decreased mastication, aspiration, and pooling of food and fluids.

d. RT to this area causes decreased saliva production (xerostomia), with loss of lubrication of food bolus and taste changes

(1) Thorough dental care is necessary before RT treatment begins

(2) With RT, the risk for dental caries or osteoradionecrosis is increased

(3) With RT, it is important to adhere to fluoride treatment protocol

4. Trismus (restriction in opening the mouth)—may be a side effect of RT

a. Affects ability to eat a regular diet. It also may affect speech, swallowing, mastication, and adequate oral hygiene.

b. Jaw exercises to increase opening of the mouth may help reduce the stiffness of trismus

5. Hormone regulation

a. Thyroid—the thyroid makes hormones that help control heart rate, blood pressure, body temperature, and weight

b. Parathyroid—the parathyroid glands make parathyroid hormone (PTH), which helps the body use calcium and keeps the amount of calcium in the blood at normal levels

B. Preoperative care (Bressler, 1999) ⚠️

1. Preoperative teaching; discuss disease, treatment, side effects, and anticipated postoperative changes

2. Provide instruction about equipment (tracheostomy tube, drains, nasogastric tube, tonsil-tip suction catheter)

3. Provide counseling, support, economic, and rehabilitation resources

4. Determine the reading ability and planning for postoperative communication preoperatively.

a. Options: paper and pencil, magic slate, picture board, nonverbal cues, electronic communication board or device

C. Postoperative care: maximize safety (Baehring & McCorkle, 2012; Bressler, 1999; NCCN 2018a) ⚠️

1. Patient in proximity to nurses' station to monitor client with altered airway

2. For tracheotomy patients, tracheotomy is securely held in place

a. Keep an extra tracheostomy tube of the same size (inner and outer cannulas and obturator), scissors, cotton-free gauze, and a tracheal dilator at the bedside

3. Call bell within reach at all times

4. If patient has a tracheostomy, identify a method of communication

5. Observe for signs and symptoms of delirium tremens in patients with recent history of alcohol abuse

6. Observe for aspiration in patients who have had a supraglottic laryngectomy (includes resection of structures in the oropharynx, or cranial nerve [IX, X, XII] deficits)

7. For patients at risk for carotid rupture (i.e., after neck dissection), implement carotid precautions

8. Manage the airway (Bressler, 1999; Loerzel, Woodfin, Reising, & Sole, 2014) ⚠️

a. Tracheostomy (i.e., total laryngectomy):

(1) Airway

(a) Use of a cuffed tracheostomy tube when client needs mechanical ventilation; may be removed by postoperative day 2 or 3

(b) Laryngectomy tube used if stoma begins to narrow

(2) Humidity

(a) Humidified air or oxygen via a tracheostomy collar to prevent mucosa drying and crusting of secretions

(b) Apply moistened 4 × 4 gauze pads over stoma

(c) A stoma bib worn over the stoma helps lessen drying of mucosa

(d) Teach about symptoms of inadequate humidity—thick, tenacious secretions that are difficult to expectorate

(3) Stoma care

(a) Cleanse stoma with 50% peroxide/50% normal saline solution

(b) Remove all mucus crusting twice each day and as needed

(c) Remove visible mucus plugs with a Kelly clamp

(d) Apply thin layer of prescribed ointment around the stoma twice each day

(4) Suction to clear airway

(a) To prevent hypoxemia and arrhythmia, the lungs are hyperoxygenated, hyperinflated, or both before and after suctioning.

(b) To precipitate coughing and mobilize secretions if needed, 2 to 5 mL of normal saline solution is instilled into the tracheostomy for lavage. Then the trachea and bronchi are stimulated.

(c) To mobilize secretions and prevent atelectasis, an incentive spirometer is attached via a female adapter to a plastic tracheostomy tube, chest physical therapy is provided (as indicated), or both.

(d) Record the color, amount, and odor of sputum produced, frequency of suctioning.

(5) Tracheostomy care

(a) Initially remove and cleanse inner cannula of all mucus and crusts with a solution of 50% peroxide/50% normal saline every 4 to 8 hours, then twice daily and as needed.

(b) Replace soiled tracheostomy ties, as needed. To determine tightness, one fingerbreadth should be allowed underneath the ties.

9. Wound care (Baehring & McCorkle, 2012; Bressler, 1999)

a. Every 3 to 4 hours, assess the surgical wounds, noting color (pink versus cyanotic), temperature, and capillary refill (immediately after blanching) of skin and muscle flaps

b. Avoid excessive pressure that interferes with flap perfusion and viability (e.g., tight tracheostomy ties, oxygen collars, hyperextension of the neck, and the client lying on the flap)

c. Assess the integrity of suture lines, both external and intraoral (if applicable); breakdown may be the first sign of wound infection or fistula formation

d. Clean the external suture lines with a solution of 50% peroxide/50% normal saline; then the prescribed ointment is applied every 4 to 8 hours

e. If the patient has had nasal surgery, a maxillectomy, an orbital exoneration, or a combination of all these, as ordered by the physician, clean the cavities to remove accumulated crusts

(1) Use a solution of 50% normal saline/50% sodium bicarbonate or normal saline solution

f. Assess wound drains for color, amount, and odor of drainage, and drain patency

(1) If not prevented or treated early, clotting and air leaks may lead to wound infections.

D. Posttreatment nursing care ⚠

1. Oral care (NCCN, 2018a; NCI, 2016)

a. Prevention—thorough and frequent mouth care

(1) As ordered by physician, perform systematic oral care at least every 4 hours with soft toothbrush and a rinse of normal saline or a solution of 50% normal saline/50% baking soda. Use nonabrasive (waxed) dental floss.

b. Use a fluoridated toothpaste or a fluoride treatment recommended by the dentist

c. To gently cleanse the cavity, use a gravity gavage or jet-spray dental cleansing system

2. Nutrition (NCCN, 2018a; van den Berg et al., 2014)

a. Assessment and management (NCCN, 2018a)

(1) Evaluate patients for nutritional risks

(2) Assess the patient's nutritional status before surgery; 60% of head and neck patients initially present with malnutrition

(a) Nutrition should be protein-rich, easy to swallow (e.g., protein shakes, soups, pudding), given in small and frequent meals (if needed) to meet daily caloric requirements and promote adequate, continuous hydration

(3) Nutritional counseling from a registered dietician and/or indicated treatment with various nutritional interventions such as feeding tubes, for example, nasogastric (NG) tubes, percutaneous endoscopic gastrostomy (PEG), or intravenous (IV) nutrition support (but only if enteral feeding is not feasible) (Mays et al., 2018; NCCN, 2018a)

b. Identify patients who have nutritional deficiencies and require oral, enteral, or parenteral nutritional supplements

(1) Greater than 10% body weight loss during any treatment phase

(2) More than 20% below ideal body weight

c. With the physician, coordinate methods of nutritional support—enteral tube feedings, other methods

d. Assess after surgery for swallowing dysfunction

3. Mobility (NCCN, 2018a)
   a. Neck dissection—the spinal accessory nerve and the sternocleidomastoid muscles may be resected; physical therapy referral needed to evaluate and treat
      (1) Could result in shoulder droop, atrophy of the trapezius muscle, forward curvature of the spine, and limited range of motion (approximately 90 degrees) of the shoulder
      (2) Treatment—after wound drains removed and patient has progressed to resistive exercises, initiate passive and active range of motion shoulder exercises; optimal goal is functional range of 150 degrees

4. Symptom management
   a. Review strategies to manage side effects: chemoradiation or radiation alone (NCI, 2016)
   b. On discharge, nursing should provide patient education and support to avoid emergency room visits and readmissions due to post-treatment complications (Baskin et al., 2018)
   c. Focus on issues of survivorship (Berkowitz et al., 2018)
      (1) Disease and treatment side effect management
      (2) Ways to address hearing loss, sleep, tiredness, and anxiety
      (3) Strategies to reduce alcohol and tobacco intake (ACS, 2018f; Penfold, Thomas, Waylen, & Ness, 2018)

5. Body image changes (Baehring & McCorkle, 2012; McEwen et al., 2018)
   a. Promote control of secretion and odor; teach wound, oral, and tracheostomy care
   b. Encourage self-care activities (e.g., tracheostomy care, tube feeding, suctioning) and activities of daily living (e.g., grooming, hair combing, shaving, applying makeup)
   c. Encourage resocialization: progressive ambulation, social interactions, support group participation (e.g., Voice Masters, Lost Chord Club, I Can Cope, CanSurmount)
   d. Inform the patient of resources to purchase tracheostomy covers, scarves, makeup, or other cosmetic assistance; consulting with the ACS Look Good, Feel Better programs (e.g., hair care, scarves)
   e. Support patients and their families to grieve; allowing them to voice concerns, fears, and anxieties

6. Communication (van den Berg et al., 2014; Balusik, 2014)
   a. Cancers in the oral cavity affect the function of articulation; therapy includes:
      (1) Exercises to increase strength, range of motion, coordination, and accuracy of tongue movement
      (2) Use of oral prostheses to compensate for tissue loss and allow for greater contact of the tongue with the palate, creating more intelligible speech
   b. Cancers in the larynx affect phonation.
      (1) After a partial laryngectomy, exercises to improve voice quality, pitch, and loudness
      (2) After a total laryngectomy (Loerzel, et al., 2014)
         (a) Use of artificial larynx that transmits sound into the vocal tract
      (3) Use of esophageal speech—air is swallowed and trapped in the esophagus, then released, allowing air to vibrate against the walls of the esophagus
      (4) Use of tracheoesophageal prosthesis—placement of a prosthesis in a surgically created tracheoesophageal fistula; sound is formed by air from the lungs, creating a better quality of esophageal speech

7. Swallowing (Balusik, 2014)
   a. Surgeries and RT as treatment for H-N cancer may affect swallowing
   b. To assess the oral and pharyngeal stages of the swallow, a barium swallow and radiography or cine-esophagography are performed
   c. Swallowing plan for the patient (Balusik, 2014)
      (1) Compensatory strategies—postural changes that facilitate passage of food into the oral cavity and pharynx (head elevated, upper body upright positioning); changes in food consistency (i.e., thin versus thick fluids, semisolid versus pureed foods)
      (2) Indirect swallowing therapy—jaw and tongue range of motion exercises; adduction of tongue exercises to improve laryngeal closure
         (a) Direct swallowing therapy using supraglottic swallow, with the following instructions to the patient:
            i. Prepare the bolus of food in the oral preparatory phase
            ii. Before initiating the swallow, hold breath to close vocal cords
            iii. Swallow while still holding breath
            iv. Cough while exhaling after the swallow to expectorate remaining food or fluids on top of vocal cords

     v. Repeat steps (iii) and (iv) (swallow and cough)

(b) To avoid aspiration, inflate the cuff on the tracheostomy tube partially or totally during meals and 30 minutes afterward

(c) With some patients, remove the tracheostomy tube to improve swallowing, allowing the larynx to elevate

(d) Until the patient can take adequate amounts by mouth, enteral tube feedings maintain nutritional requirements

(e) Speech and swallowing: assessment and management (NCCN, 2018a)

     i. Evaluation at baseline with follow-up recommendations for speech and/or swallowing dysfunction from the tumor or treatment

     ii. Regular evaluation/assessment by speech pathologists

     iii. Videofluoroscopic and/or swallowing studies

8. Psychosocial issues (Berkowitz et al., 2018; Henricks-Ferguson & Ott, 2016; McEwen et al., 2018; Peeters et al., 2018)

a. Priority focus on emotional support of patients and families as they cope with treatment and posttreatment sequalae (see earlier) (Lechelt et al., 2018)

b. Psychological impact is significant, affects physical functioning, mental health status, and quality of life

    (1) Depression (Fan et al., 2018; Rhoten, Murphy, Dietrich, & Ridner, 2018)

      (a) For H-N cancer patients, $3\times$ incidence of depressive disorder compared with those not diagnosed with H-N cancer

      (b) H-N patients score higher on social anxiety

    (2) Quality of life (Lechelt et al., 2018)

      (a) Constant adjustment to balance treatment side effects, posttreatment new normal status, and quality of life

REFERENCES

American Cancer Society (ACS). (2018a). *Cancer facts & figures 2018*. Retrieved from https://www.cancer.org/content/dam/cancer-org/research/cancer-facts-and-statistics/annual-cancer-facts-and-figures/2018/cancer-facts-and-figures-2018.pdf.

American Cancer Society (ACS). (2018b). *Health risks of smokeless tobacco*. Retrieved from https://www.cancer.org/cancer/cancer-causes/tobacco-and-cancer/smokeless-tobacco.html.

American Cancer Society (ACS). (2018c). *Key statistics for laryngeal and hypopharyngeal cancers*. Retrieved from https://www.cancer.org/cancer/laryngeal-and-hypopharyngeal-cancer/about/key-statistics.html.

American Cancer Society (ACS). (2018d). *Laryngeal and hypopharyngeal cancers*. Retrieved from https://www.cancer.org/cancer/laryngeal-and-hypopharyngeal-cancer/detection-diagnosis-staging/detection.html.

American Cancer Society (ACS). (2018e). *Oral cavity and oropharyngeal cancers*. Retrieved from https://www.cancer.org/cancer/oral-cavity-and-oropharyngeal-cancer/about/what-is-oral- cavity-cancer.html

American Cancer Society (ACS). (2018f). *Tobacco and cancer fact sheet*. Retrieved from https://www.cancer.org/content/dam/cancer-org/cancer-control/en/booklets- flyers/tobacco-and-cancer-fact-sheet.pdf

American Joint Committee on Cancer (AJCC). (2017). *Head and neck cancers. AJCC cancer staging manual* (8th ed.). Retrieved from https://cancerstaging.org/references-tools/deskreferences/Pages/default.aspx.

Baehring, E., & McCorkle, R. (2012). Postoperative complications in head and neck cancer. *Clin J Oncol Nurs, 16*(6), E203–E209. https://doi.org/10.1188/12.CJON.E203-E209.

Balusik, B. (2014). Management of dysphagia in patients with head and neck cancer. *Clin J Oncol Nurs, 18*(2), 149–150. https://doi.org/10.1188/14.CJON.149-15.

Baskin, R., Zhang, J., Dirain, C., Lipori, P., Fonseca, G., Sawhney, R., et al. (2018). Predictors of returns to the emergency department after head and neck surgery. *Head Neck, 40*(3), 498–511. https://doi.org/10.1002/hed.25019.

Berkowitz, C., Allen, D., Tenhover, J., Zullig, L., Fischer, J. Pollak, K., et al. (2018). Head and neck cancer survivors: specific needs and their implications for survivorship care planning. *Clin J Oncol Nurs, 22*(5), 523-528 DOI: https://doi.org/10.1188/18.CJON.523-528

Boggs, K. (2015). Significance of human papillomavirus in head and neck cancers. *J Adv Pract Oncol, 6*(3), 256–262.

Bressler, C. (1999). Post operative care of the laryngectomy patient. *Perspectives, 2*(1), 1. 5-7. Retrieved from www.perspectivesinnursing.org/assets/perspectives5.pdf.

Brunner, M., Gore, S. M., Read, R., Alexander, A., Mehta, A., Elliot, M., et al. (2015). Head and neck multidisciplinary team meetings: effect on patient management. *Head Neck, 37*(7), 1046–1050. https://doi.org/10.1002/hed.23709. Epub 2014 Jul 11.

Carr, E. (2018). Head and neck malignancies. In C. H. Yarbro, D. Wujcik, & B. H. Gobel (Eds.), *Cancer nursing: principles and practice* (8th ed., pp. 1573–1598). Sudbury, MA: Jones and Bartlett.

Centers for Disease Control and Prevention (CDC). (2018). *United States cancer statistics data brief, #4*. Retrieved from https://www.cdc.gov/cancer/hpv/pdf/USCS-DataBrief-No4-August2018-508.pdf.

Eskander, A., Ghanem, T., & Agrawal, A. (2018). AHNS Series: do you know your guidelines? Guideline recommendations for head and neck cancer of unknown primary site. *Head & Neck, 40*, 614–621. https://doi.org/10.1002/hed.25026. Epub 2017 Nov 21.

Fan, C.-Y., Chao, H.-L., Lin, C.-S., et al. (2018). Risk of depressive disorder among patients with head and neck cancer: a nationwide population-based study. *Head & Neck, 40*, 312–323. https://doi.org/https://doi.org/10.1002/hed.24961.

Fulcher, C., Haigentz, M., & Ow, T. (2018). AHNS Series: do you know your guidelines? Principles of treatment for locally advanced or unresectable head and neck squamous cell carcinoma. *Head & Neck, 40*, 676–686. https://doi.org/10.1002/hed.25025. Epub 2017 Nov 24.

Gill, A., Vasan, N., Givi, B., & Joshi, A. (2018). AHNS Series: do you know your guidelines? Evidence-based management of oral cavity cancers. *Head & Neck, 40,* 406–416. https://doi.org/10.1002/hed.25024. Epub 2017 Dec 5.

Haddad, R., & Glass, J. (2017). Advances in collaborative practice for patients with head and neck cancers. *J Adv Pract Oncol, 8*(3), 261–265.

Henricks-Ferguson, V., & Ott, R. (2016). Palliative care considerations for patients with head and neck cancer with children at home. *Clin J Oncol Nurs, 20*(6), 585–587. https://doi.org/10.1188/16.CJON.585-587.

Lechelt, L., Rieger, J., Cowan, K., et al. (2018). Top 10 research priorities in head and neck cancer: results of an Alberta priority setting partnership of patients, caregivers, family members, and clinicians. *Head & Neck, 40,* 544–554. https://doi.org/10.1002/hed.24998.

Loerzel, V., Woodfin, W., Reising, E., & Sole, M. (2014). Developing the Tracheostomy Care Anxiety Relief through Education and Support (T-CARES) Program. *Clin J Onco Nurs, 18*(5), 522–527. https://doi.org/10.1188/14.CJON.522-527.

Mays, A., Bartels, H., Wistermayer, P., et al. (2018). Potential for health care cost savings with preoperative gastrostomy tube placement in the head and neck cancer population. *Head & Neck, 40,* 111–119. https://doi.org/10.1002/hed.24992. Epub 2017 Nov 13.

McEwen, S., Dunphy, C., Rios, J., et al. (2018). Evaluation of a rehabilitation planning consult for survivors of head and neck cancer. *Head & Neck, 40,* 1415–1424. https://doi.org/10.1002/hed.25113. Epub 2018 Mar 22.

Multidisciplinary Larynx Cancer Working Group (MLCWG), Mulcahy, C., Mohamed, A., et al. (2018). Age-adjusted comorbidity and survival in locally advanced laryngeal cancer. *Head & Neck, 40,* 2060–2069.

National Cancer Institute (NCI). (2016). *Oral complications of chemotherapy and head/neck radiation (PDQ®)–health professional version.* Retrieved from https://www.cancer.gov/about-cancer/treatment/side-effects/mouth-throat/oral-complications-hp-pdq.

National Cancer Institute (NCI). (2018). *Head and neck cancers.* Retrieved from https://www.cancer.gov/types/head-and-neck/head-neck-fact-sheet.

National Comprehensive Cancer Network (NCCN). (2018a). *Head and neck cancers 2.2018.* Retrieved from https://www.nccn.org/professionals/physician_gls/pdf/head-and-neck.pdf.

National Comprehensive Cancer Network (NCCN). (2018b). *Thyroid cancers 1.2018.* Retrieved from https://www.nccn.org/professionals/physician_gls/pdf/thyroid.pdf.

National Institute of Dental and Craniofacial Research (NIDCR). (2018). *Oral cancer.* Retrieved from https://www.nidcr.nih.gov/health-info/oral-cancer/more-info.

Peeters, M., Braat, C., Been-Dahmen, J., Verduijn, G., Oldenmenger, W., & van Staa, A. (2018). Support needs of people with head and neck cancer regarding the disease and its treatment. *Oncology Nursing Forum, 45*(5), 587–596. https://doi.org/10.1188/18.ONF.587-596.

Penfold, C., Thomas, S., Waylen, A., & Ness, A. (2018). Change in alcohol and tobacco consumption after a diagnosis of head and neck cancer: findings from Head and Neck 5000. *Head & Neck, 40,* 1389–1399. https://doi.org/10.1002/hed.25116. Epub 2018 Feb 27.

Rhoten, B., Murphy, B., Dietrich, M., & Ridner, S. (2018). Depressive symptoms, social anxiety, and perceived neck function in patients with head and neck cancer. *Head & Neck, 40,* 1443–1452. https://doi.org/10.1002/hed.25129. Epub 2018 Mar 23.

Smokefree.gov. (2018). *Smoking Cessation.* Retrieved from https://smokefree.gov/sites/default/files/pdf/clearing-the-air-accessible.pdf.

Talmi, Y., Takes, R., Alon, E., et al. (2018). Prognostic value of lymph node ratio in head and neck squamous cell carcinoma. *Head & Neck, 40,* 1082–1090. https://doi.org/10.1002/hed.25080. Epub 2018 Feb 2. Review.

Tamaki, A., Miles, B., Lango, M., Kowalski, L., & Zender, C. (2018). AHNS Series: Do you know your guidelines? Review of current knowledge on laryngeal cancer. *Head & Neck, 40,* 170–181. https://doi.org/10.1002/hed.24862. Epub 2017 Oct 27.

van den Berg, M., Rütten, H., Rasmussen-Conrad, E., Knuijt, S., Takes, R., van Herpen, C., et al. (2014). Nutritional status, food intake, and dysphagia in long-term survivors with head and neck cancer treated with chemoradiotherapy: a cross-sectional study. *Head & Neck, 36*(1), 60–65. https://doi.org/10.1002/hed.23265. Epub 2013 Apr 4.

Zenga, J., Pipkorn, P., Graboyes, E., et al. (2018). Oncologic outcomes of extended neck dissections in human papillomavirus-related oropharyngeal squamous cell carcinoma. *Head & Neck, 40,* 955–962. https://doi.org/10.1002/hed.25060. Epub 2018 Jan 29.

17

HIV-Related Cancers

Brenda K. Shelton

HUMAN IMMUNODEFICIENCY VIRUS

I. Pathophysiology
   A. HIV—viral illness that produces widespread immune dysfunction due to viral DNA replacement of the normal immune cells
   B. Normal immunologic structures (see Chapter 8)
   C. Physiologic basis of HIV infection (U.S. Department of Health and Human Services, 2018f)
      1. Infects vital cells of the immune system (CD4 T cells, macrophages, dendritic cells)
      2. Direct viral destruction of affected cells and CD8 cytotoxic lymphocyte recognition and destruction of infected cells
      3. Results in reduced immune cells and immune surveillance competence
   D. Pathophysiology of malignancy with HIV (Carr, 2013; U.S. Department of Health and Human Services, 2018f)
      1. Cytopathic retrovirus member of retroviridae, genus *Lentivirus* (Moss, 2013; Relf, Shelton, & Jones, 2017)
      2. Transmission (Moss, 2013; Relf, Shelton, & Jones, 2017)
         a. Two species of HIV—HIV-1 (more virulent and infective) and HIV-2 (Selik, Mokotoff, Branson, Whitmore, & Hall, 2014)
            (1) Most HIV-2 found only in West Africa
            (2) Viral combinations—assume HIV-1 unless confirmatory diagnostic criteria met through use of Food and Drug Administration (FDA)–approved HIV-1/2 differentiating antibody test interpreted as HIV-2 by expert pathologist (Selik et al., 2014)
               (a) HIV-1 positive, HIV-2 negative
               (b) HIV-1 negative, HIV-2 positive
               (c) HIV-1 positive and HIV-2 positive
               (d) Undifferentiated
            (3) Major subtypes: M-trophic, N-trophic, O-trophic, and other subtypes labeled by letters A, B, C, D, E, F, G, H, I, J, and K that are associated primarily by geographic region of prevalence (Selik et al., 2014)
               (a) M-trophic replicates in macrophages and CD4+ T lymphocytes and is active in almost 90% HIV-1 viral strains; early infection manifests as high amounts of disease in tonsils and adenoids
               (b) Other subtypes correlate only to viral infecting mechanisms and origin of transmission
         b. Long incubation and gradual progression typical (Shiels et al., 2018; Thrift & Chiao, 2018; U.S. Department of Health and Human Services, 2018f)
            (1) Average time from HIV infection to symptomatic disease depends on inoculation method, exposure, preexisting health, and prompt initiation of treatment for antiretroviral disease.
            (2) Average time from infection to active AIDS is approximately 10 years, but shorter with children and older adults.
            (3) Average life expectancy is near normal if viral illness is well controlled and associated cancers or adverse effects of antiretroviral therapy do not occur.
         c. Transmission through body fluids (blood, semen, vaginal secretions, breast milk)
         d. Virus entry via the bloodstream; infection occurs with transmission across mucosal barriers, attaching to dendritic or Langerhans cells
         e. Surface antigen gp120—attracted to host CD4 surface marker
         f. Human cells with most abundant CD4—T lymphocytes; CD4 cell surface marker also found on macrophages, monocytes, microglial cells, Langerhans, and dendritic cells
         g. Initial occurrence in partially activated CD4 cells, followed by spread via the CD4 cells in gut-associated lymphoid tissue
         h. For replication—HIV uses reverse transcriptase, an enzyme that mediates transcription of viral RNA to DNA in infected CD4 cell.
         i. Viral protein integrated into the cells by integrase
         j. After incorporation into cells' DNA, cellular components broken down into functional infectious virions by the enzyme protease

k. Components for more virions made by host cells

l. Process called *coating* undergone by the new virions, which are then expelled from the host cell by budding

m. Daughter cells disseminate in the bloodstream, infecting new cells

n. Approximately 30% of the viral burden in HIV-positive patients regenerated daily, weakening cellular stability of normal CD4 and progenitor cells, causing apoptosis and reduced circulating CD4 cells (Relf, Shelton & Jones, 2017)

3. HIV effect on CD4 lymphocytes—apoptosis and reduced quantity

4. May remain dormant for variable period, or immediate viral production by infected cell may occur

5. Clinical staging and classification of HIV infection

a. Three stages

(1) Acute infection

(2) Chronic/progressive infection—leads to qualitative and quantitative T4-lymphocyte dysfunction, with resultant defect in both cellular and humoral immunity as immunoregulatory function of T4 cells is gradually impaired (Relf, Shelton, & Jones, 2017)

(3) AIDS—disorder of severe immune deficiency

b. Cofactors in disease progression (Relf, Shelton, & Jones, 2017)

(1) Lifestyle factors—for example, inadequate nutrition, general poor health, smoking, activities that may result in infection with other strains of HIV, may also influence course of infection

(2) Definitive role of specific cofactors in disease progression controversial; may be difficult to distinguish between comorbid infection and true causal relationship

(3) Infectious cofactors including presence of cytomegalovirus (CMV), Epstein–Barr virus (EBV), hepatitis C virus, human papillomavirus (HPV), herpes simplex 6 (HSV-6), herpes simplex 8 (HSV-8), and other viruses (D'Aleo, Ceccerelli, Venanzi Rullo, Facciola, Di Rosa, Pinzone, ⋯ Nunnari, 2017; De Paoli, & Carbone, 2015).

(4) Approximately 67% of cases in gay, bisexual, and other men who have sex with men; comprises half of newly infected HIV infections and half of people living with the disease (U.S. Department Health and Human Services, 2018c)

(5) Increased risk of infection in uncircumcised males related to dendritic cells on foreskin (Heyns, Smit, van der Merwe, & Zarrabi, 2013)

c. Clinical status—may change rapidly and improve or decline

(1) Centers for Disease Control (CDC) classification system for disease staging—guides therapeutic intervention and support (Selik et al., 2014).

(2) Impaired immune surveillance function and chronically stimulated B cells may result in growth of malignantly transformed cells.

(3) Patients may experience abnormal sites of presentation and poor duration of response to therapy (Carr, 2013; Reid et al., 2018).

II. Incidence and risk

A. HIV (Shiels et al., 2018; Thrift & Chiao, 2018)

1. Estimated 1.1 million people in the U.S. living with HIV, and one in seven did not know they were infected (U.S. Department Health and Human Service, 2018f).

2. In 2016, 39,782 Americans newly infected with HIV, decreasing yearly since 2011 (U.S. Department Health and Human Services, 2018f).

3. Incidence among African Americans and white gay individuals is stable, but diagnoses increased among young Hispanic/Latino gay and bisexual men (Moss, 2013; U.S. Department Health and Human Services, 2018c).

4. Heterosexual contact with HIV-infected individual accounts for about 24% of new HIV diagnoses in 2016 (U.S. Department of Health and Human Services, 2018e).

5. Those older than 50 years are the fastest-growing HIV-positive population and are at increased risk for diseases and cancers not included among the defining AIDS malignancies. Increases attributable to prolonged survival with disease, age-related physiologic changes enhancing risk of transmission, and propensity to engage in unprotected sex (U.S. Department of Health and Human Services, 2018d).

6. Approximately one third of individuals with HIV infection will die of cancer during their disease trajectory (Jensen et al., 2017).

7. Cancer, liver disease, and concomitant cardiovascular disease are the most common causes of death among HIV-infected individuals whose viral load is effectively managed (Goehringer, Bonnet, Salmon, Cacoub, Paye, Chene, ⋯ May, 2017; Jensen, Oette, Haes, & Haussinger, 2017).

B. Malignancy risks—presence of typical malignancy risks enhances likelihood of developing cancer with HIV infection (Reid, et al., 2018; Shiels et al., 2018; Suneja, et al., 2018; Thrift & Chiao, 2018; Yarchoan & Uldrick, 2018).

1. AIDS-defining malignancies—malignancies related specifically to HIV infection and the subsequently altered immune system

a. AIDS-defining cancers include non-Hodgkin lymphoma (NHL), Burkitt lymphoma, Kaposi sarcoma, and cervical cancer.

b. B-cell lymphoma is the most frequently diagnosed AIDS-defining malignancy.

c. HIV-infected women are at increased risk for cervical dysplasia that rapidly progresses to cervical cancer; histology is often characterized by more aggressive disease progression (Chen, Li, Liu, Lee, Ko, & Ko, 2014).

d. Proportional decreases in HIV-related cervical cancers may have not matched other AIDS-related cancers because of the link to HPV (Chen et al., 2014).

e. AIDS-defining malignancies are more common shortly after initiation of active retroviral therapy, particularly among patients with low CD4 counts.

2. Non–AIDS-defining malignancies (D'Aleo et al., 2017; Jensen et al., 2017; Palefsky, 2017; Reid et al., 2018; Shiels et al., 2018; Sigel, Makinson, & Thaler, 2017; Thrift & Chaio, 2018)

a. Cancers classified as non–AIDS defining—cancers of the anus, head and neck, kidney, liver, and lung and Hodgkin lymphoma

b. Others with possible association—acute myelogenous leukemia colon, esophageal, and gastric cancers; melanoma; oral cancer, prostate cancer, and squamous cell skin cancer

c. Increased incidence of non–AIDS-defining malignancies with extended time living with the disease

d. Malignancies associated with viral infection (e.g., hepatitis B and C and hepatocellular cancer, EBV, Hodgkin disease)—more accelerated conversion to malignancy in HIV-infected individuals (Reid et al., 2018)

(1) Longer life expectancy with antiretroviral therapy; chronic immune suppression leads to late lymphoproliferative cancers

(2) May be related to lifestyle commonalities—higher incidence with sexually transmitted diseases, hepatitis; smoking has led to emergence of other cancers

(3) Increased incidence of non–AIDS-defining malignancies—disproportionate compared with incidence in the normal population (Yarchoan & Uldrick, 2018)

(4) Comprise 58% of all cancers in HIV (in 1990 was 31%)

(5) Less likely related to viral load or CD4 count compared with AIDS-defining malignancies

(6) More likely to present with aggressive disease and higher risk of metastasis compared with other non–HIV-infected patients

(7) More common in whites, males

(8) Occur at younger age compared with same cancers in non-HIV malignancies

C. General principles of HIV-related malignancies (Goncalves, Uldrick, & Yarchoan, 2017; Jensen et al., 2017; Reid, 2018; Shiels et al., 2018)

1. HIV-infected patients are also at risk for other age- and behavior-associated malignancies related to smoking and alcohol intake.

2. Average onset of malignancies has increased by 9 years because of combined antiretroviral therapy (cART), also known as *highly active antiretroviral therapy* (HAART) (Yanik et al., 2013).

3. Decreased overall incidence of HIV-related malignancies attributed to antiretroviral therapy (Cobucci, Lima, de Souza, Costa, Cornetta Mda, Fernandes, ⋯ Goncalves 2015; Yarchoan & Uldrick, 2018).

4. Since the advent of highly active cART and recognized connection to HSV-8, the incidence of Kaposi sarcoma has declined dramatically (Goncalves, Uldrick, & Yarchoan, 2017).

a. Found equally in all subpopulations of HIV-infected persons; reflects same epidemiology as non–HIV-related lymphoma

b. Still prevalent disease in Africa

5. The coexistence of cancer and HIV may be related to the presence of HIV or other cofactors or lifestyle factors.

6. Staging and diagnosis of HIV-associated cancers are the same as with non–HIV-related cancers of the same pathology (Reid et al., 2018).

a. Imaging is more complex to interpret due to concomitant HIV-related lymphadenopathy

b. Brain and bone lesions often nonmalignant in this population

c. Concurrent diagnosis of HIV infection may affect treatment planning

7. The treatment of cancer usually follows near the same therapy plan as would be used even in the absence of HIV (Reid et al., 2018).

a. Steroids often avoided in usual cancer treatment regimens due to high risk of immune reconstitution syndrome

b. Vaccines during or after cancer treatment may be modified due to continued immune defect

c. Ideally should be comanaged with an HIV specialist

8. Every attempt should be made to continue cART through antineoplastic therapy because a temporary reduction in CD4+ lymphocyte counts is likely to occur during antineoplastic therapy and CD4+ levels correlate to long-term outcomes (Achhra, Petoumenos, & Law, 2014; Carr, 2013; Reid et al., 2018; US Department Health and Human Services, 2018a).

a. Interactions between antiretroviral and antineoplastic agents may be caused by disruption of the CYP pathways.

b. Even when the metabolism is not disrupted by concomitant antiretroviral and antineoplastic medications, overlapping toxicities may be problematic with combination therapy (Table 17.1).

c. Nononcologic medications may also be affected by cART (Greene, Steinman, McNicholl, & Valcour, 2014; Kumar, Rao, Earlia, & Kumar, 2015; Patel, Borg, Haubrich, & McNicholl, 2018).

(1) Frequent and thorough assessment of concomitant medications that result in inadequate absorption or altered effectiveness is recommended.

(2) Nononcologic medications have adverse interactions with antiretroviral agents such as alcohol, amiodarone, anticonvulsants, antihyperlipidemics, antimicrobials (metronidazole, rifabutin, rifampin), azole antifungals (posaconazole, voriconazole), benzodiazepines, cocaine, contraceptives, dexamethasone, digitalis derivatives, histamine-2 receptor agonists, methamphetamine opioids, proton pump inhibitors, and warfarin.

HIV-RELATED LYMPHOMA (CARBONE, VOLPI, GUALENI, & GLOGHINI, 2017; CARR, 2013; REID ET AL., 2018; YARCHOAN & ULDRICK, 2018)

I. Pathophysiology

A. Traditionally considered a late manifestation of HIV infection, occurring in the setting of significant immune suppression with CD4 counts less than $200/mm^3$

B. Characteristics specific to HIV include lower CD4 counts (below $200/mm^3$), older age, lack of CD20+ marker, and lack of cART-related lymphoma (Reid et al., 2018).

C. Systemic lymphomas seem to have more complex pathophysiology (Reid et al., 2018).

D. EBV is present in 33% to 67% of HIV lymphomas (Carbone et al., 2017).

E. Genetic analyses of patient cohorts have begun to reveal host-related factors relevant to the risk of lymphoma.

F. Tat protein is an HIV gene product implicated in the pathogenesis of Burkitt and Burkitt-like lymphomas

II. Common presentation and metastatic sites

A. In systemic disease, extranodal involvement is common; the most commonly affected sites are the

TABLE 17.1 Overlapping Toxicities Between Antiretroviral and Antineoplastic Agents That May Require Changing the Antiretroviral

Toxicity Concern	Antiretrovirals	Antineoplastic Interactions
Diarrhea	Darunavir, fosamprenavir, lopinavir, saquinavir, tipranavir	When given with antineoplastic agents such as fluoropyrimidines, irinotecan, may produce intolerable diarrhea
Hepatotoxicity	Didanosine, maraviroc, raltegravir, stavudine, tipranavir, zidovudine	Do not administer concomitantly with antineoplastic agents that have hepatic metabolism at standard doses
Hyperbilirubinemia	Didanosine, stavudine, zidovudine	Overlapping toxicities with chemotherapy may produce confusion about source of elevated bilirubin and premature discontinuation of antineoplastic therapies
Hyperglycemia	Atazanavir, darunavir, fosamprenavir, indinavir, ritonavir, saquinavir, tipranavir	Exacerbated hyperglycemia with mTOR inhibitors
Myelosuppression, neutropenia	Zidovudine	Approximately 8% of patients will develop severe neutropenia, so may be discontinued if antineoplastic therapy is also myelosuppressive Antineoplastics that have been associated with exacerbated neutropenia when given with zidovudine include bevacizumab, etoposide, gemcitabine, irinotecan, pemetrexed, platinols, taxanes, topotecan
Pancreatitis	Didanosine, stavudine	Avoid concomitant administration with antineoplastics such as L-asparaginase
Peripheral neuropathy	Didanosine, stavudine	May want to discontinue if preferred antineoplastic therapy includes platinum, taxanes, vinca agents
Prolonged QT segment	Atazanavir, ritonavir, lopinavir, saquinavir	May be altered if given concomitantly with antineoplastics causing prolonged QT segment—anthracyclines, arsenic trioxide, dasatinib, lapatinib, nilotinib, sunitinib, tamoxifen
Renal toxicity	Tenofovir, zidovudine	Platinols
Vasculitis	Atazanavir, darunavir, fosamprenavir, indinavir, ritonavir, saquinavir, tipranavir	May enhance radiosensitivity, but may also enhance hypertension and idiosyncratic bleeding tendency of vascular endothelial growth factor (VEGF) inhibitors such as bevacizumab, lenalidomide, and thalidomide

gastrointestinal (GI) tract, central nervous system (CNS), and bone marrow.

B. The presentation of primary effusion lymphoma (body cavity lymphoma) is associated with human herpesvirus type 8 (HHV-8) (Goncalves, Uldrick, & Yarchoan, 2017; Goncalves, Ziegelbauer, Uldrick, & Yarchoan, 2017).

C. Metastasis—CNS, GI tract, and bone marrow involvement more frequent in HIV-infected persons; every organ system may be involved.

D. Primary CNS involvement—only the CNS involved; no other organs or tissues involved (Gupta, Nolan, Omuro, Reid, Wang, Jaglal, ⋯ Rubenstein, 2017).

   1. Multifocal lesions are common; ocular involvement occurs in 20%

   2. BCL6 mutation is common

   3. Primary CNS lymphoma (PCNSL) highly associated with HIV and EBV; linked to lower CD4+ counts

III. Diagnostic measures—usual diagnostic testing with inclusion of serum and tumor HIV testing

IV. Prognosis based on control of HIV disease, specific disease-related variables (Carbone et al., 2017; Goncalves, Uldrick, & Yarchoan, 2017; Reid et al., 2018; Yarchoan & Uldrick, 2018)

V. Classification of HIV-related lymphomas is not altered from usual malignancy classification (Reid et al., 2018) (see Chapter 20)

VI. Staging and grading are not altered from usual malignancy staging and grading

VII. Principles of management

A. Treatment based on approaches used for uninfected persons; underlying immune deficiency, presence of opportunistic infections, polypharmacy, and generalized poor health status may require dose reduction, scheduling modifications, and selection of alternative approaches (Reid et al., 2018).

   1. Need to confirm HIV positivity—diagnosis of HIV infection usually made on basis of positive antibody test, although tumor biopsy is helpful when other lymphoma risk factors are present or the causal link is unclear

   2. Diagnosis of HIV-related lymphoma—similar to testing for non–HIV-related infection; because of the wide variance in presenting symptoms, workup in HIV-infected person may have more aggressive disease

      a. Because HIV-related malignancies may occur at abnormal sites, diagnostic imaging, endoscopic examinations, or both may be more extensive than in HIV-negative persons

      b. Histology same as immunocompetent hosts—Burkitt, Burkitt-like, diffuse large cell, peripheral T-cell, extranodal marginal zone

c. Staging for HIV-related lymphoma typically follows the same schema as that for non–HIV-related lymphoma (see Chapter 20)

d. Majority intermediate or high-grade B-cell tumors

3. Presentation factors to consider with diagnosis

   a. Brain biopsy may be performed to establish a diagnosis of PCNSL versus opportunistic infection; night sweats may be related to infection with *Mycobacterium avium*-intracellulare, and CNS symptoms are related to cerebral toxoplasmosis (Gupta et al., 2017).

   b. In the absence of brain biopsy, diagnosis of PCNSL is by exclusion. Response to treatment for toxoplasmosis may indicate infection. Lack of response presumes PCNSL (Gupta et al., 2017).

   c. CNS lesions may cause changes in cognitive function, memory loss, decreased attention span, headaches, personality change, focal neurologic deficits, or generalized seizure activity.

   d. GI tract lesions may cause malabsorption, diarrhea, constipation, or focal or diffuse abdominal discomfort; may present as an asymptomatic abdominal mass.

   e. Patients with primary effusion lymphomas present with effusions (pericardial, pleural, or ascites) and no discrete mass.

   f. Involvement of the oral cavity is linked to HIV disease, low CD4+ counts (<100 µL), associated with EBV (Gennaro, Naidoo, & Berthold, 2008).

   g. Blood counts are usually normal despite bone marrow involvement.

4. Survival depends on multiple factors, including cART, degree of immunosuppression, presence of opportunistic infection(s), nutritional status, presenting lesion location, lifestyle, and accessibility of adequate care.

   a. Factors associated with shorter survival include CD4 cell count below 100 cells/mm³, stage III or IV disease, age older than 35 years, history of intravenous drug use, and elevated lactate dehydrogenase (LDH). The International Prognostic Index (IPI) for aggressive lymphoma has also been validated in patients with AIDS-related lymphoma.

   b. Median survival time ranges from 4 to 10 months. Shortest survival time is with CNS primary tumor (median, 1–2 months); longest survival time is with low-grade lymphomas (1–4 years). Lymphomas specific to HIV—primary effusion lymphoma, plasmablastic lymphoma of the oral cavity or other variants.

5. Lymphomas occurring in other patients with immune suppression; for example, polymorphic B-cell lymphoma (posttransplant lymphoproliferative disorder)

6. Hodgkin disease, multiple myeloma, and B-cell acute lymphocytic leukemia are examples of other lymphoid malignancies diagnosed in HIV-infected persons

7. Large-cell lymphomas mostly found in the GI tract; small-cell lymphomas more likely to involve the bone marrow and meninges

8. Aggressive disease, poor prognosis; better outcomes with early clinical stage and complete response to therapy
   a. Lesions painful and rapidly proliferative; occasionally mistaken for Kaposi sarcoma
   b. May be preceded by Castleman disease or plasmacytoma (Goncalves, Uldrick, & Yarchoan, 2017).

9. PCNSL (Gupta et al., 2017)

10. Systemic NHL
    a. Typically, a CD4 count less than 100 cells/mm^3, often less than 50 cells/mm^3; less common since the advent of cART
    b. Uniformly associated with EBV
    c. Less dramatically reduced by cART; overall estimated twofold to sevenfold decline in incidence
    d. Declines in specific subsets of NHL, specifically immunoblastic lymphoma and PCNSL; incidence of Burkitt lymphoma and Hodgkin disease unchanged, suggests possible variable involvement of immune function in tumor development

11. Antiretroviral therapy should be continued during antineoplastic therapy

12. Surgery—rarely used; exceptions include excisional or incisional biopsy in patients with HIV-related NHL

13. Chemotherapy—regimens are unchanged from usual therapies used to treat NHL, although choices may vary based upon the prescribed antiretroviral agents and their potential interactions with antineoplastic agents, and steroids are avoided

14. Radiotherapy
    a. For palliation or consolidation (e.g., involved-field radiotherapy after chemotherapy)
    b. May be used to attempt to control otherwise unresponsive disease

15. Biologic response modifiers—the addition of rituximab a standard therapy for HIV-related non-Hodgkin lymphoma; no dose adjustments appear to be necessary, but increased incidence of hemophagocytic syndrome has been noted (Reid et al., 2018)

16. Combined-modality treatment not well documented; synergistic therapeutic effects and side effects must be weighed carefully
    a. Continuation of cART therapy during anticancer treatment desirable, if tolerated by patient; ability to treat cancer while continuing cART therapy associated with reduced incidence of opportunistic infections and higher complete response rates
    b. Increased risk if resistance with inconsistent administration or absorption of cART; sometimes influences response to entire categories of cART medications
    c. Immune recovery inflammatory response syndrome/immune reconstitution syndrome (IRIS) (Goncalves, Uldrick, & Yarchoan, 2017; Reid et al., 2018)
       (1) A brisk inflammatory response when the white blood cell (WBC) count rapidly increases
       (2) Manifestations—fever, edema and effusions, weight loss, myalgias, fatigue, hepatomegaly, lymphadenopathy, splenomegaly, respiratory symptoms, mental status changes, diarrhea and gastrointestinal distress, anemia, hypoalbuminemia, thrombocytopenia, and hyponatremia
       (3) More often occurs with initial cART therapy or with severe inflammatory or infectious reactions; has occurred with toxoplasmosis, pneumocystis, other opportunistic infections in HIV disease, and EBV reactivation
       (4) More often reported with lymphoma compared with other cancer; has been linked to administration of rituximab, although also commonly reported with Kaposi sarcoma
       (5) cART delayed in patients with simultaneously diagnosed HIV and malignancy because of risk of severe immune reconstitution syndrome (Reid et al., 2018)
    d. Dose adjustment indicated on the basis of CD4 count, treatment-related side effects, response, and concomitant infections
    e. HIV-related lymphoma treated with combination chemotherapy using agents such as cyclophosphamide (Cytoxan), vincristine (Oncovin), methotrexate (Mexate), etoposide (VP-16, VePesid), cytosine arabinoside (Ara-C, Cytosar), bleomycin (Blenoxane), and steroids; methotrexate, bleomycin, doxorubicin (Adriamycin), cyclophosphamide, vincristine (Oncovin), and dexamethasone (M-BACOD) regimen common (Reid et al., 2018)

f. Burkitt lymphoma common in HIV disease; outcomes equivalent to other patients

g. PCNSL usually resistant to systemic chemotherapy because few agents cross the blood–brain barrier; exceptions are high-dose methotrexate ($>3 \text{ g/m}^2$) and high-dose cytarabine (Ara-C) ($>2 \text{ g/m}^2$); rituximab recommended and usually well tolerated (Reid et al., 2018)

h. Intrathecal administration of chemotherapy considered to treat lymphomatous meningitis; not useful in bulky disease

i. Concomitant cART plus chemotherapy to be used cautiously when giving chemotherapy with zidovudine (AZT) because of significant bone marrow compromise; increased febrile neutropenia risk with older age, lower CD4 counts

j. Hematopoietic stem cell transplantation may be a treatment option for lymphoma with well-controlled viral load (Reid et al., 2018)

k. Response short lived in high-grade tumors; in low-grade tumors, good control of symptoms, often with longer duration of response

HIV-RELATED KAPOSI SARCOMA (KS)

I. Pathophysiology—soft tissue malignancy characterized by malignant growth of reticuloendothelial cell origin in HIV-infected persons

A. Before HIV, KS endemic in geographic regions such as the Mediterranean basin and sub-Saharan Africa

B. Persons receiving immunosuppressive agents after organ transplantation

C. Malignantly transformed cells reproducing as a result of underlying immune defect in patients with HIV-related KS (epidemic KS)

   1. Disproportionate risk for KS among select immunodeficient populations raised suspicion of secondary infectious factor

   2. KSHV genome—encodes several gene products; host response to the virus critical in determining outcome of infection and tumor development

   3. HIV-associated tat gene product—may enhance KSHV replication, increase expression of various chemokines, potentiate KSHV effects, and indirectly contribute to oncogenesis

      a. Confirmed by identification of HHV-8, also known as *KS herpesvirus* (KSHV)

      b. Causative association of KSHV with KS

      c. KSHV infection necessary but not sufficient for KS; malignant potential appears to be quite low outside the setting of immune compromise

II. Clinical manifestations and metastatic sites (Robey & Bower, 2015; Suneja et al., 2018)

A. Types of KS

   1. Endemic KS—locoregional and related to viral cause

   2. Classic KS—rare angiogenic malignancy

   3. Pediatric (lymphadenopathic) KS—occurs in children in developing countries

   4. Epidemic KS (AIDS-related)

B. Presentation—includes skin lesions ranging from pink to purple to brownish, flat or raised, usually painless (unless in a sensitive area), and do not blanch with pressure; body organ lesions usually nodular and hemorrhagic (Goncalves, Uldrick, & Yarchoan, 2017)

C. Common locations—lower extremities or face, oral cavity and palate, GI tract, respiratory tract (especially endobronchial)

III. Diagnostic measures (Goncalves, Uldrick, & Yarchoan, 2017)

A. Similar to testing done when not related to HIV infection

B. Once tissue diagnosis of KS lesions confirmed, biopsy of new skin lesions not always performed; biopsy of visceral lesions may be performed

IV. Prognosis (Goncalves, Uldrick, & Yarchoan, 2017)

A. Dramatic increase in survival in the era of cART

B. Survival for several years possible; shorter in patients with GI tract lesions or B symptoms (fever, night sweats, unintentional weight loss); worse with prior or comorbid major opportunistic infection, with median survival time of less than 1 year

C. Survival—depends on cART, degree of immunosuppression, presence of opportunistic infection(s), nutritional status, presenting lesion location, lifestyle, care accessibility

V. Classification, staging, and histology (Goncalves, Zieglebauer, Uldrick, & Yarchoan, 2017)

A. All schemas include parameters of cutaneous, lymph node, and visceral involvement and the occurrence of B symptoms.

B. Classic KS is typically indolent; HIV-related KS may be aggressive and progress rapidly.

C. Spectrum of tumors varies by risk group; dramatically influenced by HAART.

D. The incidence of KS was already on the decline in the U.S. even before introduction of cART; since then, KS has become a relative rarity in the U.S.

E. Estimates of reduction of KS in HIV-infected persons are as much as eightyfold; in areas where cART is not available (sub-Saharan Africa), KS remains a major problem, and in some areas, it is the major cancer diagnosis.

VI. Principles of management

A. Risk stratification into good risk and poor risk is helpful (Suneja et al., 2018).

   1. Good risk—confined to skin or lymph nodes or minimal oral disease, CD4 greater than 200/μL,

no oral thrush or B symptoms; Karnofsky performance greater than 70

2. Poor risk—edema or ulceration of tumor; extensive oral, GI, nonnode visceral tumors; CD4 less than 200/μL, history of oral thrush or B symptoms, poor performance status, other HIV-related illness

3. Treatment based on approaches used for uninfected persons; treatment adjustment required for underlying immune deficiency, presence of other opportunistic infections, polypharmacy, and poor health status

B. Surgery—rarely used in the treatment of KS; exceptions include removal of lesions that interfere with function or cause significant pain

C. Chemotherapy (Sharma, Sharma, & Pathak, 2015; Suneja et al., 2018)
1. Most contain an anthracycline; often liposomal formulation or doses adjusted for overlapping myelosuppression
2. Taxanes, etoposide, biological response modifiers (e.g., pomalidomide, thalidomide) also commonly used in conjunction with anthracyclines
3. mTOR inhibitors show promise but interact with antiretroviral therapy

D. Radiotherapy—may be given as photon radiotherapy or superficial electron beam ((Sharma, Sharma, & Pathak, 2015; Suneja et al., 2018)
1. Doses from 10 to 30 Gy by 45 to 70 kV x-ray or 4-MV photon
2. Better response rates with multiple fractions
3. Effective short to moderate local control may be achieved, especially for cosmetic effects or relief of lymphedema caused by lymphatic lesions; response rates 92% for cutaneous lesions; 100% for oral lesions; 89% for eyelids, conjunctiva, and genitals
4. Permanent alteration in the radiated skin and lymphatics, with subsequent persistent edema and tissue breakdown
5. Interferon-alpha (IFN-α), with or without concomitant zidovudine, approved as treatment for HIV-related KS

E. Biologic response modifiers
1. Dose adjustment possibly indicated on the basis of CD4 count, treatment-related side effects, response, concomitant infections
2. HIV-related KS treated with cART (up to 86% response rate, durable responses); if recurrent or persistent, may be treated with single-agent therapy (liposomal doxorubicin, paclitaxel) or combination chemotherapy (vincristine, doxorubicin, and bleomycin)
3. mTOR inhibition (e.g., sorafenib, sunitinib)—reduces tumor angiogenesis and leads to tumor regression (Roy, Sin, & Lucas, 2013; Suneja et al., 2018)

4. Because of the vascular nature of KS lesions, antiangiogenic compounds are a natural strategy for treatment; ongoing trials include thalidomide (Thalomid), fumagillin, and metastat (a matrix metalloproteinase inhibitor) (Suneja et al., 2018)

OTHER MALIGNANCIES

I. Cervical cancer (Chen et al., 2014; Palefsky, 2017; Reid et al., 2018) (see also Chapter 23)
A. Squamous cell carcinoma (SCC) of the cervix added to HIV-related malignancies in 1993 because of incidence of HPV and cervical dysplasia found in women infected with HIV
B. Risk four times higher than general U.S. population, higher in developing countries (Chen et al., 2014)
C. Cervical cancer screening in HIV-infected individuals low—influenced by age, ethnicity/race, tobacco use, weight, education, economic issues, risky behaviors (Chapman Lambert, 2013)
D. HPV increases risk of development of, or rapid progression to, cervical cancer
E. HIV infection increases risk for cervical cancer recurrence after treatment
F. Management
1. Lesions may regress or be controlled with antiretroviral therapy alone
2. Colposcopy—primary therapy if lesions persist on cART
3. Cryotherapy—for persistent lesions
4. Radiation therapy—in form of brachytherapy; may be administered for locally advanced disease; radiation toxicity increased in the population receiving antiretroviral agents

II. Anal cancer (D'Souza et al., 2016; Jensen et al., 2017; Palefsky, 2017; Reid et al., 2018; Wells, Holstad, Thomas, & Bruner, 2014) (see also Chapter 14)
A. Incidence normally 1.5% of GI malignancies, increased in HIV-infected persons.
B. More common among men practicing anal-receptive intercourse.
C. Like cervical cancer, has been highly associated with HIV infection with HPV.
D. Minimal regression with cART.
E. Prophylactic screening of high-risk individuals recommended but not validated as helpful to reduce incidence or associated mortality. Poor compliance with screening recommendations (<40% among highest risk) (D'Souza et al., 2016; Wells et al., 2014).
F. Management—combined chemotherapy and radiation

III. Hepatocellular carcinoma (HCC) (D'Aleo, Ceccarelli, Venanzi Rullo, Facciola, Di Rosa, Pinzone, ⋯ Nunnari, 2017; Jensen et al., 2017; Reid et al., 2018) (see also Chapter 14)
   A. Three to six times increased incidence of HCC in HIV-infected patients; if HCC is related to HIV disease, longevity of survival is better
   B. More common in hepatitis C and HIV dual infection than hepatitis B and HIV infection
   C. More likely in HIV-1 disease
   D. Increased risk with advanced age and hepatic cirrhosis, suggesting contribution of progressive liver dysfunction
   E. HCC with HIV more aggressive and refractory to treatment, with shorter life expectancy compared with HCC from other causes
   F. Highly responsive to sorafenib
IV. Lung cancer (Reid et al., 2018; Sigel, Makinson, & Thaler, 2017) (see also Chapter 19)
   A. Third most common malignancy in patients with HIV
   B. Presentation usually at younger age compared with lung cancer; mean age 46 years
   C. Highest incidence of mortality among HIV-related cancers
   D. Average life expectancy 6 to 7 months after diagnosis; usually diagnosed at late stage with significant symptoms (cough, chest pain, dyspnea, hemoptysis)
   E. Lung infection, which often precedes diagnosis, delays diagnosis because of overlapping symptoms; up to 30% of one cohort had radiographic changes more typical of lung infection
   F. Possible link to chronic pulmonary inflammation and infection unclear
   G. Increased survival with concomitant cART
   H. Significant hematologic toxicity in most patients receiving concomitant cART
V. Hodgkin disease (Reid et al., 2018; Yarchoan & Uldrick, 2018) (see also Chapter 20)
   A. Most common non–AIDS-defining malignancy; relative risk 11 to 31.7 times that for normal population
   B. Often occurs within 1 year of diagnosis and cART initiation
   C. Common pathology—mixed cellularity and lymphocyte depleted subtypes; most express herpesvirus
   D. More aggressive and less responsive than non-HIV Hodgkin disease
   E. Late-stage presentation
   F. Common for multiple node groups
   G. Less sensitive to chemotherapy or radiotherapy compared with de novo Hodgkin disease

NURSING IMPLICATIONS

I. Maximize patient safety ⚠
   A. Ensure environmental safety for patients experiencing sensorimotor changes (e.g., adequate lighting, especially at night) (Theroux, Phipps, Zimmerman, & Relf, 2013)
   B. Instruct patient about avoidance of potential environmental sources of opportunistic infection—for example, animal waste from pets; or uncooked, undercooked, or improperly stored food (Relf et al., 2017).
II. Decrease incidence and severity of symptoms
   A. Assess for peripheral neuropathies that may occur from HIV, antiretroviral, or antineoplastic therapy
   B. Baseline and ongoing assessment for neurocognitive disorders may be related to HIV disease, neurologic malignancies, opportunistic infections, and adverse effects of therapy (Rumbaugh & Tyor, 2015)
   C. Assess for balance and strength; cachexia and muscle wasting common in combined HIV and cancer cluster; referral to physical and occupational therapy with functional deficits
   D. Teach (or referral for teaching) about ways to enhance appearance—for example, use of covering cosmetics to hide KS lesions in cosmetically sensitive areas; use of scarves or other clothing to cover swollen lymph nodes; use of clothing appropriate to changing body mass with weight loss
   E. Instruct the patient to avoid aspirin because it may interfere with platelet function and recommend use of acetaminophen instead to control fevers and pains
   F. Monitor for jaw pain in patients receiving vinca alkaloids; this neuropathy seems to occur more frequently in the HIV population
   G. Overlapping toxicities between antiretroviral therapy and chemotherapy must be considered in determining the best treatment plan and supportive measures (see Table 17.1)
      1. Diarrhea—lopinavir, tenofovir
      2. Hepatotoxicity—nonnucleoside reverse transcriptase inhibitors, nucleoside reverse transcriptase inhibitors, protease inhibitors
      3. Myelosuppression—zidovudine
      4. Neuropathy—didanosine, stavudine
      5. Nephrotoxicity—indinavir, tenofovir
      6. Nausea and vomiting—didanosine, protease inhibitors, zidovudine
   H. Many antiretroviral medications affect the CYP pathway enzymes and may interfere with chemotherapy-related therapeutic or toxic effects
      1. CYP inhibitors may require dose reductions.
      2. CYP inducers may require lead to reduced benefit of specific chemotherapy agents, but insufficient research is available with most malignancies to make recommendations. Changes in antiretroviral therapy may be preferable in these situations.
   I. Palliative care referral—particularly helpful for patients experiencing significant physical symptoms or distress (Relf et al., 2017)

1. Helps patients with multiple or overlapping symptoms
2. Assists with management of complexities of polypharmacy
3. Pain complex in this population because of multiple causes
4. May help patients explore and rally support systems and informal care resources
5. Sensitive assessment and interventions for spiritual distress
6. Supportive and consistent caregivers helpful in recognizing psychosocial distress or mental incapacity related to disease

III. Prevent infection due to immune suppression from disease and treatment
   A. Assess for opportunistic infections that occur from HIV but are compounded in patients undergoing cancer treatment.
   B. Oral lesions may be due to HIV-related malignancies, opportunistic infections, nutrition deficits (Gennaro, Naidoo, & Berthold, 2008).
   C. Immunosuppressive effects of chemotherapy are associated with up to 50% temporary reduction in CD4 counts, even if lymphopenia is not a normal adverse effect of that chemotherapy agent. CD4 counts should be monitored during chemotherapy and more frequently in high-risk groups (e.g., older age).
   D. Appropriate antimicrobial prophylaxis based on CD4 counts, if indicated.
   E. Concomitant administration of hematopoietic growth factors is based on increased risk of HIV-related cancer.

IV. Interventions to enhance nutritional status
   A. Teaching techniques to enhance nutritional intake (e.g., use of supplements, keeping ready-to-eat foods available, smaller and more frequent meals)
   B. Providing or encouraging frequent oral hygiene

V. Interventions to monitor for sequelae of disease and treatment that may be different from those for non–HIV-related malignancies
   A. Assess and document location, appearance, size of KS lesions, lymphadenopathy, organomegaly, or other tumor effects (e.g., abdominal masses, oral lesions, ascites)
   B. Monitor for changes in size or appearance of the abnormalities
   C. Monitor for tumor lysis syndrome in patients with HIV-related NHL as presentation, with bulky disease common and highly responsive to treatment.
   D. Assess neurologic status frequently, as neurologic symptoms may signal advanced HIV disease, chemotherapy toxicity, or opportunistic infections (Theroux et al., 2013)

VI. Monitor response to medical management
   A. Assess usual tolerance to antineoplastic therapies
   B. Consider overlapping toxicities between antiretroviral agents and antineoplastic agents (see Table 17.1)
   C. Assess absorption and metabolic drug interactions between antiretroviral and antineoplastic agents (many antiretroviral agents are metabolized through CYP pathways)
   D. Careful consideration of initiation of antiretroviral therapy with concomitant newly diagnosed cancer and HIV disease given risk for immune reconstitution syndrome or with significant opportunistic infections

VII. Provide cancer screening and disease prevention (Reid et al., 2018; U.S. Department Health and Human Services, 2018b, 2018c, 2018d, 2018e; Wells et al., 2014)
   A. Organizational recommendations for cancer screening—not delineated for HIV-infected patients despite clear risks for specific cancers. Evidence-based literature suggests the following enhanced screening activities in HIV-infected individuals:
      1. Papanicolaou (Pap) testing—every 6 to 12 months for early detection of cervical cancer (Chen et al., 2014)
      2. Anal screening with cytology or high-resolution anoscopy for early detection of SCC—has not been adopted by professional organizations, but a growing body of literature suggests that at-risk individuals can benefit from screening: digital anal examination also a proven cost-effective method to screen for this cancer in high-risk individuals (D'Souza et al., 2016)
      3. Computed tomography (CT) of the chest—as indicated to assess high-risk individuals for lung cancer
      4. Sigmoidoscopy—controversy about value in patients with HIV disease because most cancers are right-sided; full colonoscopy required to assess for colon cancer
      5. Periodic oral or dental examination—to detect early oropharyngeal masses that can signal HPV-related squamous cell head and neck cancers
      6. Vaccines (Moss, 2013)
         a. Hepatitis vaccines are recommended to prevent hepatitis and associated cancers.
         b. HPV vaccines have been proven safe in HIV-infected men.

VIII. Address the psychosocial issues of HIV and its malignancies
   A. Thorough psychosocial assessment of all patients (Carr, 2013)
   B. Assess self-image in patients with KS who have visible lesions that may contribute to distress and social isolation
   C. Determine past experience with HIV disease; in areas of high incidence, multiple losses may occur without adequate time for effective grieving

D. Recognize that a significant other not infected with HIV may experience feelings of guilt, uncertainty about own health, concern for the future

E. Monitor for maladaptive coping strategies, especially if history of substance use disorder is present; assisting with learning alternative behaviors to manage stress and cope

IX. Incorporate patient and significant other in care (Relf et al., 2017)

A. Recognize that the patient's family of choice may not be the biologic family of origin

B. Include persons identified by the patient as significant others in teaching and care decisions when appropriate.

X. Teach to reduce possibility of HIV transmission (Moss, 2013; Relf et al., 2017)

A. Provide education about the use of latex condom with a water-based lubricant to reduce risk (petroleum-based lubricants or cosmetic creams weaken the condom, increasing the chance of breakage during use) during every episode of vaginal, rectal, or oral intercourse

B. Provide information about avoidance of sharing toothbrushes, razors, personal care items

C. Wearing gloves and using a solution of 1 part household bleach to 10 parts water during cleanup of emesis or other body fluid spills

D. Use universal precautions as recommended by the CDC to reduce the risk of occupational exposure to HIV

E. Assess health literacy and ability to comply with complex therapies, multiple appointments with medical specialists

1. Low literacy associated with only 17% to 40% maintaining regular medical care

2. Low literacy associated with lack of understanding of CD4 counts, viral load, medications

3. Studies of antiretroviral adherence reflect low rates of medication adherence among individuals with low health literacy

4. Low health literacy associated with English not being the first language, mental health disorder, lack of understanding of how to access care and support

REFERENCES

Achhra, A. C., Petoumenos, K., & Law, M. G. (2014). Relationship between CD4 cell count and serious long-term complications among HIV-positive individuals. *Current Opinions HIV/ AIDS, 9*(1), 63–71. https://doi.org/10.1097/COH.0000000000000017.

Carbone, A., Volpi, C. C., Gualeni, A. V., & Gloghini, A. (2017). Epstein-barr virus associated lymphomas in people with HIV. *Current Opinion in HIV/ AIDS, 12*(1), 39–46.

Carr, E. R. (2013). HIV-and AIDS-associated cancers. *Clinical Journal of Oncology Nursing, 17*(2), 201–204. https://doi.org/10.1188/13.CJON.201-204.

Chapman Lambert, C. L. (2013). Factors influencing cervical cancer screening in women infected with HIV: a review of the literature. *Journal Association AIDS Care, 24*(3), 189–197. https://doi.org/10.1016/j.jana.2012.06.010.

Chen, Y. C., Li, C. Y., Liu, H. Y., Lee, N. Y., Ko, W. C., & Ko, N. Y. (2014). Effect of antiretroviral therapy on the incidence of cervical neoplasia among HIV-infected women: a population-based cohort study in Taiwan. *AIDS, 28*(5), 709–715. https://doi.org/10.1097/QAD.0000000000000132.

Cobucci, R. N., Lima, P. H., de Souza, P. C., Costa, V. V., Cornetta Mda, C., Fernandes, J. V., … Goncalves, A. K. (2015). Assessing the impact of HAART on the incidence of defining and non-defining AIDS cancers among patients with HIV/AIDS: a systematic review. *Journal Infections in Public Health. 8*, https://doi.org/10.1016/j.jiph.2014.08.003.

D'Aleo, F., Ceccarelli, M., Venanzi Rullo, E., Facciola, A., Di Rosa, M., Pinzone, M. R., … Nunnari, G. (2017). "Hepatitis C-related hepatocellular carcinoma" diagnostic and therapeutic management in HIV-patients. *European Review for Medical and Pharmacological Sciences. 21*, https://doi.org/10.26355/eurrev_201712_14035. 5859-4867.

De Paoli, P., & Carbone, A. (2015). Microenvironmental abnormalities induced by viral cooperation: impact on lymphomagenesis. *Seminars In Cancer Biology, 34*, 70–80. https://doi.org/10.1016/j.semcancer.2015.03.009.

D'Souza, G., Wentz, A., Wiley, D., Shah, N., Barrington, F., Darragh, T. M., & Cranston, R. D. (2016). Anal cancer screening in men who have sex with men in the Multicenter AIDS Cohort Study. *Journal Acquired Immunodeficiency Syndrome, 71*(5), 570–576. https://doi.org/10.1097/QAI.0000000000000910.

Gennaro, S., Naidoo, S., & Berthold, P. (2008). Oral health & HIV/ AIDS. *MCN. American Journal Maternal Child Nursing, 33*(1), 50–57.

Goehringer, F., Bonnet, F., Salmon, D., Cacoub, P., Paye, A., Chene, G., & May, T. (2017). Causes of death in HIV-infected individuals with immunologic success in a National Prospective survey. *AIDS Research and Human retroviruses, 33*(2). Accessed at https://www.liebertpub.com/doi/full/10.1089/aid.2016.0222.

Goncalves, P. H., Uldrick, T. S., & Yarchoan, R. (2017). HIV-associated Kaposi sarcoma and related diseases. *AIDS, 31*(14), 1903–1916. https://doi.org/10.1097/QAD.0000000000001567.

Goncalves, P. H., Ziegelbauer, J., Uldrick, T. S., & Yarchoan, R. (2017). Kaposi sarcoma herpesvirus-associated cancers and related diseases. *Current Opinions in HIV/ AIDS, 12*(1), 47–56.

Greene, M., Steinman, M. A., McNicholl, I. R., & Valcour, V. (2014). Polypharmacy, drug-drug interactions, and potentially inappropriate medications in older adults with human immunodeficiency virus infection. *Journal American Geriatric Society, 62*(3), 447–453. https://doi.org/10.111/jgs.12695.

Gupta, N. K., Nolan, A., Omuro, A., Reid, E. G., Wang, C. C., Jaglal, M., … Rubenstein, J. L. (2017). Long-term survival in AIDS-related primary central nervous system lymphoma. *Neurologic Oncology, 19*(1), 99–108. https://doi.org/10.1093/neuonc/now155.

Heyns, C. F., Smit, S. G., van der Merwe, A., & Zarrabi, A. D. (2013). Urological aspects of HIV and AIDS. *National Review Urology, 10*(12), 713–722. https://doi.org/10.1038/nrurol.2013.230.

Jensen, B. E. O., Oette, M., Haes, J., & Haussinger, D. (2017). HIV-associated gastrointestinal cancer. *Oncology Research and Treatment, 40*, 115–118. https://doi.org/10.1159/000456714.

Kumar, S., Rao, P. S., Earlia, R., & Kumar, A. (2015). Drug-drug interactions between anti-retroviral therapies and drugs of abuse in HIV systems. *Expert Opinions Drug Metabolism Toxicology, 11*(3), 343–355. https://doi.org/10.1517/17425255.2015.996546.

Moss, J. A. (2013). HIV/AIDS review. *Radiology Technology, 84*(3), 247–267.

Palefsky, J. M. (2017). Human papillomavirus-associated anal and cervical cancers in HIV-infected individuals: incidence and prevention in the antiretroviral era. *Current Opinions HIV / AIDS, 12*(1), 26–30.

Patel, N., Borg, P., Haubrich, R., & McNicholl, I. (2018). Analysis of drug-drug interactions among patients receiving antiretroviral regimens using data from a large open-source prescription database. *American Journal Health System Pharmacy. 14*, https://doi.org/10.2146/ajhp170613. *Jun.*

Reid, E., Suneja, G., Ambinder, R., Ard, K., Baiocchi, R., Barta, S., & Wang, C. J. (2018). *NCCN guidelines: cancer in people living with cancer. Version 1.2018.* Accessed at on July 1, 2018, (2018). www.nccn.org.

Relf, M. V., Shelton, B. K., & Jones, K. M. (2017). Common immunological disorders (oncologic emergencies). In P. G. Morton, & D. K. Fontaine (Eds.), *Critical Care Nursing.* (ed 11). Philadelphia: Elsevier Publishing (pp.949-981).

Robey, R. C., & Bower, M. (2015). Facing up to the ongoing challenge of Kaposi's sarcoma. *Current Opinion Infectious Disease, 28*(1), 31–40. https://doi.org/10.1097/QCO.0000000000000122.

Roy, D., Sin, S. H., Lucas, A., Venkataramanan, R., Wang, L., Eason, A., … Tamburro, K. M. (2013). mTOR inhibitors block Kaposi sarcoma growth by inhibiting essential autocrine growth factors and tumor angiogenesis. *Cancer Research, 73*(7), 2235–2246. https://doi.org/10.1158/0008-5472.CAN-12-1851.

Rumbaugh, J. A., & Tyor, W. (2015). HIV-associated neurocognitive disorders: five new things. *Neurology Clinical Practice, 5*(3), 224–231.

Selik, R. M., Mokotoff, E. D., Branson, B., Owen, S. M., Whitmore, S., & Hall, H. I. (2014). Revised surveillance case definition for HIV infection- United States, 2014. *MMWR, Mortality and Morbidity Weekly Report, 63*(3), 1–10.

Sharma, M., Sharma, V., & Pathak, K. (2015). Therapy stratifications and novel approach in pursuit of AIDS related Kaposi sarcoma management- a paradigm for noninvasiveness. *Current Drug Delivery, 12*(6), 770–781.

Shiels, M. S., Islam, J. Y., Rosenberg, P. S., Hall, I., Jacobson, E., & Engels, E. A. (2018). Projected cancer incidence rates and burden of incident cancer cases in HIV-infected adults in the United States through 2030. *Annals Internal Medicine, 168*(12), 866–873. https://doi.org/10.7326/Mi7-2499.

Sigel, K., Makinson, A., & Thaler, J. (2017). Lung cancer in persons with HIV. *Current Opinion in HIV/AIDS, 12*(1), 31–38.

Suneja, G., Reid, E., Ambinder, R. F., Ard, K., Baiocchi, R., Barta, S. K., & Wang, C. J. (2018). *NCCN guidelines: AIDS-related Kaposi sarcoma, Version 1.2018.* Accessed at www.nccn.org on July 1, 2018.

Theroux, N., Phipps, M., Zimmerman, L., & Relf, M. V. (2013). Neurological complications associated with HIV and AIDS: clinical implications for nursing. *J Neurosci Nurs, 45*(1), 5–13. https://doi.org/10.1097/JNN.0b013e318275b1b2.

Thrift, A. P., & Chiao, E. Y. (2018). Are non-HIV malignancies increased in the HIV-infected population? *Current Infectious Disease Reports, 20*, 22–28. https://doi.org/10.1007/s11908-018-0626-9.

U.S. Department Health and Human Services. (2018a). *AIDSinfo: FDA-approved HIV medications, 2018.* Accessed at: https://aidsinfo.nih.gov/understanding-hiv-aids/fact-sheets/19/58/fda-approved-hiv-medicines.

U.S. Department Health and Human Services. (2018b). *AIDSinfo: HIV and specific populations: HIV and children and adolescents, 2018.* Accessed at: https://aidsinfo.nih.gov/understanding-hiv-aids/fact-sheets/25/82/hiv-and-children-and-adolescents.

U.S. Department Health and Human Services. (2018c). *AIDSinfo: HIV and specific populations: HIV and gay and bisexual men, 2018.* Accessed at: https://aidsinfo.nih.gov/understanding-hiv-aids/fact-sheets/25/81/hiv-and-gay-and-bisexual-men.

U.S. Department Health and Human Services. (2018d). *AIDSinfo: HIV and specific populations: HIV and older adults, 2018.* Accessed at: https://aidsinfo.nih.gov/understanding-hiv-aids/fact-sheets/25/80/hiv-and-older-adults.

U.S. Department Health and Human Services. (2018e). *AIDSinfo: HIV and specific populations: HIV and women, 2018.* Accessed at: https://aidsinfo.nih.gov/understanding-hiv-aids/fact-sheets/25/69/hiv-and-women.

U.S. Dept Health and Human Services, (2018f). *AIDSinfo: HIV overview,* Accessed at: https://aidsinfo.nih.gov/understanding-hiv-aids/fact-sheets/19/45/hiv-aids—the-basics

Wells, J. S., Holstad, M. M., Thomas, T., & Bruner, D. W. (2014). An integrative review of guidelines for anal cancer screening in HIV-infected persons. *AIDS Patient Care STDS, 28*(7), 350–357. https://doi.org/10.1089/apc.2013.0358.

Yanik, E. L., Napravnik, S., Cole, S. R., Achenbach, C. J., Gopal, S., Olshan, A., … Eron, J. J. (2013). Incidence and timing of cancer in HIV-infected individuals following initiation of combination antiretroviral therapy. *Clinical Infectious Disease, 57*(5), 756–764. https://doi.org/10.1093/cid/cit369.

Yarchoan, R., & Uldrick, T. S. (2018). HIV-associated cancers and related diseases. *New England Journal Medicine, 378*(11), 1029–1041. https://doi.org/10.1056/NEJMra15896.

18

Leukemia

Stephanie Jackson and Jeannine M. Brant

LEUKEMIA OVERVIEW

I. Physiology and pathophysiology
   A. Leukemia (Leukemia & Lymphoma Society, 2017a)
      1. Blood cancer that is caused by an accumulation of neoplasms in the bone marrow, blood cells, and lymph nodes
      2. Mutations in the DNA stimulate abnormal cells to replicate without recognition by the adaptive immune system
      3. This cascade results in multiplication of abnormal cells and interferes with the production and function of the white blood cells, red blood cells, and platelets
      4. Acute leukemia grows rapidly, whereas the chronic form progresses slowly, which influences their treatment modalities ranging from several months to years

ACUTE LYMPHOBLASTIC LEUKEMIA (ALL)

I. Physiology and pathophysiology
   A. Originates from the immature lymphocytes and inhibits the body's ability to fight bacterial and viral infections. Lymphocytes do not develop into mature cells and therefore impair human immunity.
   B. Three subtypes include the B cells, T cells, and natural killer cells.
II. Epidemiology (Leukemia & Lymphoma Society, 2017a)
   A. Accounts for 5970 cases among all ages each year in the United States.
   B. It is the most common form of leukemia among children and adolescents representing 20% of all cancers among persons <20 years, or >3000 new cases annually (Siegel, Henley, Li, Pollack, Van Dyne, & White, 2017). The risk declines after 5 years of age until the middle twenties and then rises again after the age of 50. Adults have a prevalence of 4 out of 10 cases of acute lymphoblastic leukemia (American Cancer Society, 2018).
   C. Advancements in treatment have resulted in an increased 5-year survival to 34% of cases diagnosed between 2006 and 2012 (Leukemia & Lymphoma Society, 2017a). Children under the age of 15 have a 5-year survival of 92%, with an increased risk for long-term complications associated with secondary cancers, cardiac disease, and pulmonary diseases related to treatments (Leukemia & Lymphoma Society, 2017a).
III. Risk factors (Leukemia & Lymphoma Society, 2017a; Shah & Wayne, 2013)
   A. Genetic conditions
      1. Down syndrome, ataxia telangiectasia, Li–Fraumeni syndrome, Klinefelter syndrome, and Fanconi anemia
      2. Age—children, adolescents, and young adults less than 20 and adults greater than 50
   B. Race
      1. Caucasians have a twofold increased risk compared with African Americans
      2. Hispanic children have the highest incidence of developing ALL
   C. High-dose radiation
      1. Exposure to atomic bombs, electromagnetic fields, or high-voltage electronic lines
   D. Viruses
      1. Epstein–Barr virus
      2. Human T-cell leukemia virus-1
IV. Histopathology
   A. The bone marrow is usually hypercellular with auer rods in 70% of blasts
   B. Erythroid and megakaryocyte precursors may have dysplastic abnormalities
   C. Eosinophil precursors and basophils are increased with rare mast cell hyperplasia
V. Molecular classification
   A. ALL is classified histologically as follows:
      1. B-cell lymphoblastic leukemia/lymphoma not otherwise specified
      2. B-cell lymphoblastic leukemia/lymphoma, with recurrent genetic abnormalities
      3. B-cell lymphoblastic leukemia/lymphoma with hypodiploidy
      4. B-cell lymphoblastic leukemia/lymphoma with hyperdiploidy
      5. B-cell lymphoblastic leukemia/lymphoma with t(9;22) (q34;q11.2) (BCR-ABL1)

6. B-cell lymphoblastic leukemia/lymphoma with t (v;11q23) (MLL rearranged)
7. B-cell lymphoblastic leukemia/lymphoma with (12;21) (p13;q22) (ETV6-RUNX1)
8. B-cell lymphoblastic leukemia/lymphoma with t(1;19) (q23;p13.3) (TCF3-PBX1)
9. B-cell lymphoblastic leukemia/lymphoma with intrachromosomal amplification of chromosome (iAMP21)
10. B-cell lymphoblastic leukemia/lymphoma with translocations involving tyrosine kinases or cytokine receptors (BCR-ABL1-like ALL)
11. T-cell lymphoblastic leukemia/lymphomas
12. Early T-cell precursor lymphoblastic leukemia

VI. Histologic-grade French-American-British classification (Seiter, 2018) (Table 18.1)
   A. L1—small cells with a homogeneous chromatin and a regular nuclear shape and a scanty cytoplasm. Occurs in 25% to 30% of adults with leukemia.
   B. L2—large and heterogeneous cells with irregularly shaped nucleus; seen in 25% to 30% of patients and is the most common.
   C. L3—large, homogenous cells with multiple nucleoli; accounts for 1% to 2% of adults with leukemia.

VII. Diagnosis and staging
   A. Complete blood count and leukocyte differential
   B. Bone marrow aspiration and biopsy
   C. Flow cytometry immunophenotyping
   D. Cytogenetic analysis
   E. Molecular genetic studies
   F. Lumbar puncture (for those suspected of cerebrospinal leukemia involvement)
   G. Imaging tests: computed tomography (CT) scan, magnetic resonance imaging, and positron emission tomography (PET) scan as indicated for specific concerns

VIII. Assessment (Leukemia & Lymphoma Society, 2017a)
   A. Fever, night sweats, lethargy, weight loss
   B. Infections
   C. Bleeding or petechiae
   D. Palpable lymphadenopathy
   E. Disseminated intravascular coagulation (DIC)
   F. Splenomegaly
   G. Pain related to invasion of leukemia cells in the bone marrow
   H. Leukostasis
   I. Hyperuricemia
   J. Renal failure

IX. Prognosis and survival
   A. The survival rate in children is 94%, while adults is 40%.
   B. Unfavorable prognosis is seen in patients with an elevated white blood cell count greater than 50,000 at diagnosis, central nervous system involvement, early relapse, and lack of response to chemotherapy measured by the minimal residual disease on bone marrow biopsy.
   C. Predictors for survival include age and genetic abnormalities (Tsang, 2018). Patients younger than 50 years of age have a more favorable prognosis due to fewer chromosomal abnormalities.

X. Management
   A. Systemic therapy (National Comprehensive Cancer Network, 2018a)
      1. Induction Philadelphia-positive: to induce complete remission
         a. Adolescents and young adults (AYAs) and patients <65 years of age
            (1) Tyrosine kinase inhibitor (TKI)—targeted therapy that blocks the action of BCR-ABL fusion gene (imatinib, dasatinib, ponatinib, or nilotinib); given with corticosteroids
            (2) Multiagent chemotherapy may be given with a TKI—vincristine, pegasparagase, steroid (prednisone or dexamethasone), and an anthracycline (doxorubicin or daunorubicin). This regimen may also include cyclophosphamide.
            (3) Central nervous system prevention or treatment—methotrexate or cytarabine is given during a lumbar puncture (IT chemotherapy).
            (4) Clinical trials are also an option for patients who meet the inclusion criteria.
         b. Patients >65 years of age or those with significant comorbidities
            (1) These patients are not eligible for intensive therapy.
            (2) General health, organ function, and comorbidities must be considered by the provider to determine the best regimen for this population.
      2. Induction Philadelphia-negative:
         a. AYA and patients <65 years of age—clinical trial, pediatric chemotherapy regimen, or multiagent chemotherapy

TABLE 18.1	French-American-British Classification	
French-American-British Morphology	Bone Marrow Involvement	Cerebrospinal Fluid
L1 homogeneous blasts, minimal cytoplasm	M1 <5% blasts	CNS 1 no blasts
L2 heterogeneity, prominent nucleoli	M2 5%–25% blasts	CNS 2 WBC <5 UL with blasts
L3 basophilic cytoplasm with prominent vascuolization	M3 >25% blasts	CNS 3 WBC ≥ 5 UL with blasts

Seiter, K. (2018). What is the French-American-British (FAB) classification of acute lymphoblastic leukemia (ALL)? Retrieved from https://www.medscape.com/answers/207631-105131what-is-the-french-american-british-fab-classification-of-acutelymphoblastic-leukemia-all on March 11, 2019.

b. >65 years of age
   (1) Clinical trial or multiagent chemotherapy
   (2) Multiagent chemotherapy or palliative corticosteroids with signficant comorbidities

3. Postremission consolidation and maintenance therapy—treatment given to maintain remission
   a. AYA and patients <65 years of age
     (1) Philadelphia-positive: consolidation should be considered with an allogeneic hematopoietic cell transplantation (HCT) if a donor is available; if a donor is unavailable, multiagent chemotherapy and a TKI will be given.
     (2) Philadelphia-negative: blinatumomab for B-ALL, HCT, or multiagent chemotherapy depending on minimal residual disease (MRD).
   b. Patients >65 years of age
     (1) Philadelphia-positive: allogeneic HCT or continue the TKI with or without corticosteroids, or TKI plus or minus chemotherapy for consolidation chemotherapy.
     (2) Maintenance chemotherapy includes a TKI for 1 year for Philadelphia-positive.

B. Radiation therapy (NCCN, 2018a; Shah & Wayne, 2013)
   1. Treatment may be needed to destroy cancer cells that have invaded the brain and spine. Central nervous system involvement is seen in 90% of children (Cousins et al., 2017) and 5% of adults (Del Principe et al., 2014).

C. Allogeneic HCT (NCCN, 2018a; Shah & Wayne, 2013)
   1. Stem cell transplant is a curative treatment for patients with complex cytogenetics with likelihood for relapsing disease that provides patients with human leukocyte–matched hematopoietic stem cells from a relative or unrelated donor after administration of high-dose chemotherapy and/or radiation.

D. Chimeric antigen receptor therapy (CAR T cells)
   1. Tisagenlecleucel (Kymriah) is a CD 19–directed, genetically modified, T-cell immunotherapy used to treat patients with pre–B-cell ALL between ages 18 and 25. This therapy was approved in 2017 for patients who have refractory disease, failed two prior lines of chemotherapy, or relapsed. Associated side effects include cytokine release syndrome (CRS), neurologic toxicity (CRES), hypersensitivity reactions, prolonged cytopenias, and hypogammaglobulinemia (McLaughlin, Cruz, & Bollard, 2015; Novartis Pharmaceuticals Corporation, 2018).

XI. Nursing implications
A. Conduct ongoing assessments to monitor for pancytopenia.
B. Safely administer systemic therapy based on the Oncology Nursing Society (ONS) chemotherapy/biotherapy guidelines for administration.

C. Monitor for adverse events related to stem cell transplantation.
D. Explain schedule for taking medications.
E. Discuss the impact of decreased drug adherence in taking oral medications.

ACUTE MYELOID LEUKEMIA (AML)

I. Physiology and pathophysiology
A. Heterogenous disease with a rapid onset characterized by abnormal hematopoietic stem cells of the myeloid layer of the bone marrow.

II. Epidemiology (American Cancer Society, 2018)
A. The American Cancer Society estimated 19,520 new cases of AML in 2018.
B. Most common among male adults over 45 years of age, with average age being 68.
C. The lifetime risk of developing AML among males and females is 1%.

III. Risk factors (Leukemia & Lymphoma Society, 2017b; Yin & Malkovska, 2013)
A. Genetic disorders—Fanconi anemia, Bloom syndrome, ataxia-telangiectasia, Down syndrome, Li–Fraumeni syndrome, Diamond–Blackfan anemia, neurofibromatosis type 1
B. Familial history of AML
C. History of myelodysplastic syndrome (MDS)
D. Long-term exposure to benzene
   1. Benzene is a chemical used in oil refineries, chemical plants, gasoline industries, cigarette smoke, vehicle exhaust, glue, detergent, art supplies, and paint
E. Smoking
F. Chemotherapy
   1. Alkylating agents—cyclophosphamide, mechlorethamine, procarbazine, chlorambucil, melphalan, busulfan, carmustine
   2. Platinum agents—cisplatin and carboplatin
G. Radiation exposure
   1. Atomic bomb and nuclear accident survivors have an increased risk 6 to 8 years after exposure

IV. Histopathology (Arber, 2016)
A. AML with characteristic genetic abnormalities—World Health Organization classification
   1. AML with t (8;21) (q22;q22); RUNX-1-RUNX1T1
   2. AML with inv (16) (p13q22) or t (16;16) (p13; q22) (CBFB-MYH11)
   3. APL with PML-RARA
   4. AML with t(9;11)(p21.3q26.2) or t(3;3) (q21.3; q26.2); GATA2, MECOM
   5. AML (megakaryoblastic) with t(1;22)(p 13.3; q13.3);RBM15-MKL1
   6. AML with mutated NPM1
   7. AML with biallelic mutations of CEBPA
   8. AML with MDS-related changes
   9. Therapy-related myeloid neoplasms
   10. AML, NOS (not otherwise specified)

a. AML with minimal differentiation
b. AML without maturation
c. AML with maturation
d. Acute myelomonocytic leukemia
e. Acute monoblastic/monocytic leukemia
f. Pure erythroid leukemia
g. Acute megakaryoblastic leukemia
h. Acute basophilic leukemia
i. Acute panmyelosis with myelofibrosis
11. Myeloid sarcoma
12. Myeloid proliferations related to Down syndrome
   a. Transient abnormal myelopoiesis (TAM)
   b. Myeloid leukemia associated with Down syndrome
  B. French-American-British classification.
V. Diagnosis and staging (Leukemia & Lymphoma Society, 2017b)
  A. Complete blood count with peripheral smear
  B. Bone marrow aspiration and biopsy
  C. Skin biopsy when there is suspected myeloid sarcoma
  D. Lumbar puncture (central nervous system involvement)
  E. Cytogenetic analysis
  F. Assessment (Leukemia & Lymphoma Society, 2017b; Yin & Malkovska, 2013)
    1. Pancytopenia
     a. Fatigue
     b. Shortness of breath
     c. Fever
     d. Bacterial infections
     e. Petechiae, bruising
     f. Bleeding, cerebral bleeding, pulmonary hemorrhage
     g. Splenomegaly, hepatomegaly
     h. Gingival hyperplasia
     i. Loss of appetite
     j. Blurry vision, blindness
     k. Headaches
    2. Laboratory studies (Yin & Malkovska, 2013)
     a. Complete blood count
     b. Hyperuricemia
     c. Elevated blood urea nitrogen
     d. High lactic dehydrogenase
     e. Hypokalemia or hyperkalemia
     f. Lactic acidosis
     g. Hypercalcemia
     h. Hypoglycemia
     i. Hypoxemia
VI. Prognosis and survival
  A. To achieve a complete remission (CR), the treatment for AML should be aggressive.
  B. Approximately 60% to 70% of adults can achieve a CR after induction therapy.
  C. 25% of adults survive 3 or more years and can be cured.

D. Shorter duration of remission and advanced age may decrease survival.
E. Prognostic factors associated with survival include systemic infections, white blood cell count greater than 100,000/mm^3, history of MDS, neurologic involvement with leukemia, and treatment-related leukemia development.
F. Patients who have an FLT3 gene mutation have higher rates of relapse.
G. Survival (American Cancer Society, 2018)
    1. The 5-year survival of adults with AML is approximately 24%. Statistics vary based on biologic features of the disease, advanced age, and comorbidities of the patient.
VII. Management (NCCN, 2018b; Yin & Malkovska, 2013)
  A. Systemic therapy
    1. Induction chemotherapy
     a. Cytarabine and an anthracycline antibiotic (most often daunorubicin; can use doxorubicin or idarubicin)—traditional 7 + 3 regimen
     b. Additional agents: clofarabine, azacytidine, decitabine, and lenalidomide
     c. Gemtuzumab ozogamicin
      (1) Food and Drug Administration (FDA) approved for newly diagnosed AML with tumors that express CD33-positive antigens
     d. Midostaurin
      (1) FDA approved for FLT3 mutation positive in combination with standard cytarabine and daunorubicin induction and consolidation chemotherapy
     e. Daunorubicin and cytarabine (Vyxeos)
      (1) FDA approved for the treatment of therapy-related AML or MDS. Patients who are newly diagnosed with this form of leukemia will receive the standard 7 + 3 regimen.
  B. Day 14 evaluation
    1. A bone marrow biopsy is performed on day 14 postinduction chemotherapy to assess for response to induction chemotherapy. Reinduction chemotherapy is recommended for patients with a residual leukemia of >5% blasts.
    2. Postremission chemotherapy—dependent on risk and age
     a. Consolidation chemotherapy
      (1) High-dose cytarabine (HDAC)
  C. HCT
    1. Patients with a poor prognosis and complex cytogenetics receive allogeneic stem cells from a human leukocyte antigen (HLA)–matched donor, which includes siblings, parents, unrelated donors, and cord blood.
    2. This form of transplant provides graft vs. leukemia with a goal of complete eradication of leukemia.

VIII. Nursing implications
  A. Assess for modifiable and nonmodifiable risk factors of AML.
  B. Assess for pancytopenia and additional new-onset symptoms of leukemia.
  C. Assess for oral chemotherapy adherence to minimize risk for medication resistance.
  D. Educate patient on the proper schedule with oral chemotherapy.
  E. Appropriate pharmacologic and nonpharmacologic management through chemotherapy administration and safe infusion of stem cell transfusion.

ACUTE PROMYELOCYTIC LEUKEMIA (APL)

  I. All-transretinoic acid (ATRA) plus arsenic trioxide is the initial treatment for APL. It may be given with an anthracycline in low-risk disease and is recommended in high-risk disease in the absence of cardiac disease. This therapy restores the normal growth of cells and promotes differentiation of hematopoietic cells.
  II. Other options: cytarabine for high risk; cytarabine/anthracycline combination for relapsed APL; gemtuzumab ozogamicin for high risk, relapse, or inability to tolerate arsenic trioxide due to QT prolongation or other reason
  III. Intrathecal chemotherapy is given during consolidation for patients with high-risk APL.
  A. This regimen is used to treat acute promyelocytic leukemia and is the most curable subtype of acute myeloid leukemia.
  B. The curative rate is >90%.

CHRONIC LYMPHOCYTIC LEUKEMIA

  I. Physiology and pathophysiology
  A. Chronic lymphocytic leukemia (CLL) is the most frequent form of leukemia and originates from mature B lymphocytes. The median age at diagnosis is 60, and less than 15% are diagnosed under the age of 50.
  II. Epidemiology (American Cancer Society, 2018)
  A. 20,940 new cases of CLL estimated to occur in 2018 with 4510 deaths in 2018.
  B. The lifetime risk of CLL is 1 in 175 and is most commonly diagnosed at 70 years of age.
  C. CLL accounts for 25% of all leukemias and is more frequently seen in Caucasians compared with Asians, as well as Hispanics.
  III. Risk factors (Farooqui, Wiestner, & Aue, 2013; Leukemia & Lymphoma Society, 2017c, 2017e)
  A. Familial history
  B. Exposure to Agent Orange
  IV. Histopathology (Inamdar & Bueso-Ramos, 2007)
  A. Clusters of round lymphoid cells protrude beneath endothelial veins and enlargement of mantle zone.

  B. The nuclear contours of lymphocytes are irregular, and there is a presence of extensive granulomas. Lymphoma may be masked by the presence of abnormal granulomas (Mansouri, 2018).
  V. Molecular classification (Lamanna, Weiss, & Dunleavy, 2015)
  A. There is rearrangement of immunoglobulin (Ig) genes, somatic hypermutation, or unmutated subtype.
  B. Unmutated immunoglobulin heavy-chain variable (IgVH) subtype accounts for 80% of patients with a ZAP 70 expression (Mansouri, 2018).
  VI. Histologic grade (None)
  VII. Diagnosis and staging (Mansouri, 2018)
  A. Peripheral blood—presence of at least 5000 peripheral clonal B cells/mcL (5×10^9/L); confirmed by flow cytometry
  B. Lymph node and bone marrow biopsy
  C. Immunohistochemistry
  D. Flow cytometry
  E. Cytogenetics
  F. Assessment (Farooqui et al., 2013; Leukemia & Lymphoma Society, 2017c, 2017e)
    1. Symptoms—fever, night sweats, weight loss, and fatigue
    2. Lymphadenopathy—abdominal discomfort, fullness, and malaise
    3. Splenomegaly
    4. Hepatomegaly
    5. Gastrointestinal bleeding
    6. Extranodal involvement—pulmonary nodules or skin lesions
    7. Recurrent infections
    8. Autoimmune disorders—hemolytic anemia, immune thrombocytopenia purpura
    9. Rai staging system for CLL (Table 18.2) (Rai et al., 1975)
    10. Binet staging system (Binet et al., 1981)
  VIII. Prognosis and survival (Mansouri, 2018)
  A. The 5-year survival is 83%; 10-year survival, 59.5% (American Cancer Society, 2018; Pulte et al., 2016)

| TABLE 18.2 | Rai Staging System | |
Rai Staging System	Risk Group	Clinical Presentation
0	Low	Lymphocytosis
I	Intermediate	Adenopathy and lymphocytosis
II	Intermediate	Splenomegaly, lymphocytosis, or hepatomegaly
III	High	Anemia Hgb <11g/dL and lymphocytosis
IV	High	Thrombocytopenia <100,000 μl and lymphocytosis

Rai, K. R., Sawitsky, A., Cronkite, E. P., Chanana, A. D., Levy, R. N., & Pasternack, B. S. (1975). Clinical staging of chronic lymphocytic leukemia. *Blood*, 46(2), 219–234.

B. Favorable factors: wild type TP53, isolated del 13q; low clinical staging based per Rai and Binet (Amin & Malek, 2016)

C. Unfavorable factors: TP53 mutated, del 11q, del 17p; increased CD38, ZAP70 and, CD49d expression; elevated B-2 microglobulin; high clinical stage based on Rai and Binet (Amin & Malek, 2016)

IX. Management (Farooqui et al., 2013; NCCN, 2018c)

A. Systemic therapy—dependent on 17p deletion and TP53 mutation

1. Standard chemotherapy
   a. Fludarabine, cyclophosphamide, bendamustine, chlorambucil, doxorubicin, prednisone, vincristine, cladribine, pentostatin

2. Targeted therapies
   a. Ibrutinib: used for patients with 17p deletion (NCCN, 2018c)
   b. Idelalisib: for younger patients and those with significant comorbidities

3. Monoclonal antibodies
   a. Rituximab: humanized antibody that targets CD20 (ofatumumab and obinutuzumab): Antigen target site is CD 20—used in patients with relapsed or refractory disease (NCCN, 2018c).
   b. Alemtuzumab—targets CD 52

B. Allogeneic HCT

1. This is a potentially curable treatment that provides patients with graft-versus-tumor effect. The risk vs. benefit must be evaluated, given that the patient population is older.

X. Nursing implications

A. Assess for signs and symptoms of CLL.

B. Safe administration of systemic therapy according to the ONS chemotherapy/biotherapy administration guidelines.

C. Prompt management of any adverse events related to chemotherapy, targeted therapies, and monoclonal antibodies.

D. Medication education that includes administration, side effect recognition, and safe handling in the home setting to maximize adherence

CHRONIC MYELOGENOUS LEUKEMIA

I. Physiology and pathophysiology

A. Chronic myelogenous leukemia (CML) is a clonal disorder that originates from the Philadelphia chromosome translocation BCR-ABL oncogene. The translocation between chromosome 9 and 22 fuse together, causing tyrosine kinase activity, which results in initiation of leukemia (Philadelphia chromosome). There are three phases of this disorder, which include chronic, accelerated, and blast crisis phase (Leukemia & Lymphoma Society, 2018d).

II. Epidemiology (American Cancer Society, 2018)

A. 8430 new cases of CML estimated to be diagnosed in 2018 with a death rate of 1090.

B. Average age at diagnosis >60 with half of the total cases being over the age of 65.

C. Imatinib mesylate (Gleevec) became widely known for causing arrest of the tyrosine kinase activity and producing favorable outcomes.

III. Risk factors (Leukemia & Lymphoma Society, 2017d; Yong & Barrett, 2013)

A. Gender—males have a 1.5:1 risk greater than women of developing CML

B. Age—patients over the age of 60 have a higher risk of developing this form of leukemia

C. Radiation exposure

1. Patients who have been treated with radiation in the past for other cancers have a risk of developing chronic leukemia.

IV. Prevention

A. Avoiding high-dose radiation exposure is the only avoidable risk factor for CML (American Cancer Society, 2018)

V. Histopathology

A. Greater than 100,000 white blood cells with neutrophilia, significant involvement of the metamyelocytes, basophilia, eosinophilia, monocytosis. Thrombocytosis will be present in 50% of patients.

B. Up to 100% increased precursors of granulocytes, basophils, and eosinophils in the bone marrow; no visible nodules present; infarcts present in the spleen (Sangle, 2017).

VI. Molecular classification

A. (q34;q11) t(9;22) Philadelphia chromosome or ABL gene (#9q34) and BCR gene (#22q11) fusion is necessary for a diagnosis to be made (Sangle, 2017)

VII. Histologic grade (none)

VIII. Diagnosis and staging (Leukemia & Lymphoma Society, 2017d)

A. Complete blood count with differential

B. Bone marrow aspiration and biopsy

C. Cytogenetic analysis (including BCR-ABL)

D. Fluorescence in situ hybridization

E. Quantitative polymerase chain reaction for BCR-ABL gene

F. Assessment (Leukemia & Lymphoma Society, 2017d; Yong & Barrett, 2013)

1. Weakness, fatigue
2. Bone pain
3. Unexplained weight loss
4. Fevers
5. Fullness below the ribs
6. Night sweats
7. Petechiae, bruising
8. Chloroma

G. Laboratory studies (Leukemia & Lymphoma Society, 2017d; Yong & Barrett, 2013)

TABLE 18.3 Stages of Chronic Myelogenous Leukemia

Chronic Phase	Accelerated Phase	Blast Phase
Increased leukocyte count	≥15% to <30% myeloblasts in the blood >30% myeloblasts and promyelocytes combined ≥20% basophils ≤100,000 platelets	≥30% blasts in the blood, bone marrow, or both
Symptoms may or may not be present	B symptoms: fever, night sweats, weight loss Fatigue Splenomegaly	B symptoms Fatigue Shortness of breath Bone and abdominal pain Splenomegaly Bleeding Infection

From Leukemia & Lymphoma Society. (2017). Chronic Myeloid Leukemia. Retrieved from https://www.lls.org/leukemia/chroniclymphocytic-leukemia and National Comprehensive Cancer Network. (2018d). *Chronic myeloid leukemia, v. 1.2019.* Retrieved October 4, 2018 from https://www.nccn.org/professionals/physician_gls/pdf/cml.pdf.

1. Complete blood count with differential
   a. Patients may have a slightly elevated white blood cell count over $200 \times 10^{9/}$ L
   b. Anemia
   c. Normal platelets or thrombocytopenia
2. Peripheral blood smear
   a. Abnormal size of the white blood cells
   b. Larger amount of blast counts
   c. Normal or giant platelets
   H. Stages of CML (Table 18.3)
IX. Prognosis and survival
   A. The 5-year survival for CML depends on the phase of disease, response to treatment, and biological features.
   B. Given the evolution of imatinib, survival has doubled from 31% in the 1990s to 90% in those who take their medications consistently (American Cancer Society, 2018).
X. Management
   A. Systemic therapy (NCCN, 2018d; Yong & Barrett, 2013)
      1. TKI
         a. First generation: imatinib
         b. Second generation: bosutinib, dasatinib, nilotinib
      2. Low-risk disease—TKI or clinical trial
      3. High-risk disease—second-generation TKI or clinical trial
      4. Second-line therapy depending on mutation
         a. Dasatinib, nilotinib, bosutinib, ponatinib, omacetaxine
      5. Remission induction
         a. Daunorubicin, cytosine arabinoside
   B. Allogeneic transplantation—survival 70%
XI. Nursing implications
   A. Assess patient adherence to oral chemotherapy and knowledge of medication regimen.
   B. Discuss the importance of follow-up and the significance of the treatment plan.
   C. Discuss the importance of continuing therapy and risk of nonadherence to therapy.
   D. Educate the patient and family on environmental risk factors and exposure to hazardous drugs in the home setting.

REFERENCES

American Cancer Society. (2018). *Facts and figures 2018.* Retrieved from https://www.cancer.org/research/cancer-facts-statistics/all-cancer-facts-figures/cancer-facts-figures-2018.htm.

Amin, N. A., & Malek, S. N. (2016). Gene mutations in chronic lymphocytic leukemia. *Semin Oncol, 43*(2), 215–221. https://doi.org/10.1053/j.seminoncol.2016.02.002.

Binet, J. L., Auquier, A., Dighiero, G., Chastang, C., Piguet, H., Goasguen, J., & Gremy, F. (1981). A new prognostic classification of chronic lymphocytic leukemia derived from a multivariate survival analysis. *Cancer, 48*(1), 198–206.

Cousins, A. F., Olivares, O., Michie, A. M., Gottlieb, E., & Halsey, C. (2017). Association of CNS involvement in childhood acute lymphoblastic leukaemia with cholesterol biosynthesis upregulation. *The Lancet, 389*, S35. https://doi.org/10.1016/S0140-6736(17)30431-2.

Del Principe, M.I., Maurillo,L., Buccisano, F., Sconocchia, G., Cefalo, M., De Santis, G., et al. (2014). Central nervous system involvement in adult acute lymphoblastic leukemia: diagnostic tools, prophylaxis, and therapy. *Mediterranean Journal of Hematology and Infectious Diseases, 6* (1), e2014075. https://doi.org/10.4084/MJHID.2014.075.

Farooqui, M., Wiestner, A., & Aue, G. (2013). Chronic lymphocytic leukemia. In G. Rodgers & N. Young (Eds.), *The Bethesda Handbook of Clinical Hematology* (pp. 186–196). Philadelphia, PA: Lippincott Williams & Wilkins.

Inamdar, K. V., & Bueso-Ramos, C. E. (2007). Pathology of chronic lymphocytic leukemia: an update. *Ann Diagn Pathol, 11*(5), 363–389. https://doi.org/10.1016/j.anndiagpath.2007.08.002.

Lamanna, N., Weiss, M. A., & Dunleavy, K. (2015). *Chronic lymphoblastic leukemia and hairy-cell leukemia.* Retrieved from http://www.cancernetwork.com/cancer-management/chronic-lymphocytic-leukemia-and-hairy-cell-leukemia.

Leukemia & Lymphoma Society. (2017a). *Acute lymphoblastic leukemia.* Retrieved from https://www.lls.org/leukemia/acute-lymphoblastic-leukemia

Leukemia & Lymphoma Society. (2017b). *Acute myeloid leukemia.* Retrieved from https://www.lls.org/leukemia/acute-myeloid-leukemia.

Leukemia & Lymphoma Society. (2017c). *Chronic lymphocytic Leukemia.* Retrieved from https://www.lls.org/leukemia/chronic-lymphocytic-leukemia.

Leukemia & Lymphoma Society. (2017d). *Chronic myeloid leukemia*. Retrieved from https://www.lls.org/leukemia/chronic-lymphocytic-leukemia.

Leukemia & Lymphoma Society. (2017e). *Facts and statistics*. Retrieved from https://www.lls.org/leukemia/chronic-lymphocytic-leukemia.

Mansouri, J. (2018). Hematogenous neoplasms: small lymphocytic lymphoma/chronic lymphocytic leukemia. *Pathology Outlines*. http://www.pathologyoutlines.com/topic/spleensllcll.html.

McLaughlin, L., Cruz, C. R., & Bollard, C. M. (2015). Adoptive T-cell therapies for refractory/relapsed leukemia and lymphoma: current strategies and recent advances. *Ther Adv Hematol, 6*(6), 295–307. https://doi.org/10.1177/2040620715594736.

National Comprehensive Cancer Network (NCCN). (2018a). *Acute lymphoblastic leukemia, v. 1.2018*. Retrieved October 4, 2018 from https://www.nccn.org/professionals/physician_gls/pdf/all.pdf.

National Comprehensive Cancer Network (NCCN). (2018b). *Acute myeloid leukemia, v. 2.2018*. Retrieved October 4, 2018 from https://www.nccn.org/professionals/physician_gls/pdf/aml.pdf.

National Comprehensive Cancer Network (NCCN). (2018c). *Chronic myeloid leukemia, v. 1.2019*. Retrieved October 4, 2018 from https://www.nccn.org/professionals/physician_gls/pdf/cll.pdf.

National Comprehensive Cancer Network (NCCN). (2018d). *Chronic myeloid leukemia, v. 1.2019*. Retrieved October 4, 2018 from https://www.nccn.org/professionals/physician_gls/pdf/cml.pdf.

Novartis Pharmaceuticals Corporation. (2018). *KYMRIAH™ (tisagenlecleucel) [package insert]*. NJ: East Hanover.

Pulte, D., Castro, F. A., Jansen, L., Luttmann, S., Holleczek, B., Nennecke, A., & GEKID Cancer Survival Working Group. (2016). Trends in survival of chronic lymphocytic leukemia patients in Germany and the USA in the first decade of the twenty-first century. *Journal of Hematology & Oncology, 9*, 28. https://doi.org/10.1186/s13045-016-0257-2.

Rai, K. R., Sawitsky, A., Cronkite, E. P., Chanana, A. D., Levy, R. N., & Pasternack, B. S. (1975). Clinical staging of chronic lymphocytic leukemia. *Blood, 46*(2), 219–234.

Sangle, N. (2017). Chronic myelogenous leukemia (CML). In *PathologyOutlines.com website*. http://www.pathologyoutlines.com/topic/myeloproliferativecml.html.

Siegel, D.A., Henley, S.J., Li, J., Pollack, L.A., Van Dyne, E.A., & White, A. (2016). Rates and trends of pediatric acute lymphoblastic leukemia - United States, 2001–2014. *MMWR Morb Mortal Wkly Rep, 15*:66(36):950–954. https://doi.org/10.15585/mmwr.mm6636a3.

Seiter, K. (2015). *Acute Myeloid Leukemia Staging*. Retrieved from https://emedicine.medscape.com/article/2006750-overview on January 23, 2019.

Seiter, K. (2018). What is the French-American-British (FAB) classification of acute lymphoblastic leukemia (ALL)? Retrieved from https://www.medscape.com/answers/207631-105131/what-is-the-french-american-british-fab-classification-of-acute-lymphoblastic-leukemia-all on March 11, 2019

Shah, N., & Wayne, A. (2013). Acute lymphoblastic leukemia. In G. Rodgers & N. Young (Eds.), *The Bethesda Handbook of Clinical Hematology* (pp. 158–169). Philadelphia, PA: Lippincott Williams & Wilkins.

Tsang, P. (2018). *Acute lymphocytic leukemia (ALL)*. http://www.pathologyoutlines.com/topic/lymphnodesALL.html.

Walter, R. B., Othus, M., Burnett, A. K., Lowenberg, B., Kantarjian, H. M., Ossenkoppele, G. J., & Estey, E. H. (2013). Significance of FAB subclassification of "acute myeloid leukemia, NOS" in the 2008 WHO classification: analysis of 5848 newly diagnosed patients. *Blood, 121*(13), 2424–2431. https://doi.org/10.1182/blood-2012-10-462440.

Yin, F., & Malkovska, V. (2013). Acute myeloid leukemia. In G. Rodgers & N. Young (Eds.), *The Bethesda Handbook of Clinical Oncology* (pp. 137–157). Philadelphia, PA: Lippincott Williams & Wilkins.

Yong, A., & Barrett, A. (2013). Chronic myelogenous leukemia. In G. Rodgers & N. Young (Eds.), *Chronic myelogenous leukemia* (pp. 170–185). Philadelphia, PA: Lippincott Williams & Wilkins.

19

Lung Cancer

Geline J. Tamayo

I. Anatomy and physiology (Knoop, 2018)
   A. Lung
      1. The right and the left lung are contained within the thorax and separated by the mediastinum
      2. The right lung has three lobes (upper, middle, and lower) and 10 segments
      3. The left lung has two lobes (upper and lower) and eight segments
   B. Pleura:
      1. The pleura is a thin membrane lining the surface of the lungs and the inside of the chest wall.
      2. The pleural space is bounded by the parietal (lining of the lung surface) and visceral (lining the chest wall) membranes.
      3. The volume of fluid in the pleural space results from a balance of fluid production thought to be made by the visceral pleura and absorption by the lymphatics of the parietal pleura.
      4. Pleural effusion occurs when the production of fluid in the pleural space exceeds the absorption.
   C. Lung cancer, or bronchogenic carcinoma, refers to malignancies that originate in the airways or pulmonary parenchyma
      1. Cancer may be incidentally diagnosed with a chest radiography or other radiographic views that may capture an image of the lungs
      2. Early signs and symptoms may be absent in part because of the large lung surface area.
      3. The most common metastatic sites are the liver, adrenal glands, bones, and brain.
      4. Individuals with small cell lung cancer (SCLC) are at risk for paraneoplastic syndromes, more commonly in the late stages. This group of patients can also experience oncologic emergencies such as hypercalcemia, syndrome of inappropriate antidiuretic hormone (SIADH), spinal cord compression (SCC), superior vena cava syndrome (SVC), and cardiac tamponade.
   D. Clinical manifestations (Knoop, 2018)
      1. Patients may not exhibit symptoms until they have locally advanced or metastatic disease.
      2. Symptoms can result from local effects of the tumor, from regional or distant spread, or from distant effects not related to metastasis (paraneoplastic syndromes).
      3. There are intrathoracic and extrathoracic effects of lung cancer.
         a. Intrathoracic effects: it is common for individuals to have both respiratory and constitutional symptoms, including cough, hemoptysis, chest pain, and dyspnea.
            (1) Pleural effusions can cause dyspnea and cough.
            (2) SVC syndrome is more common in SCLC. Symptoms include facial swelling, upper extremity edema, headache, and venous distension.
            (3) Pancoast syndrome is characteristic of lung cancer arising in the superior sulcus and is manifested by shoulder pain.
         b. Extrathoracic sites include the liver, bone, adrenal gland, and brain, and can cause the following:
            (1) Liver: enzyme abnormalities
            (2) Bone: pain to the back, chest, or extremities, as well as elevated serum alkaline phosphatase and elevated serum calcium
            (3) Adrenal: rarely symptomatic. Sometimes detected on staging computed tomography (CT) scans.
            (4) Brain: headache, vomiting, visual field loss, hemiparesis, and seizures.
II. Epidemiology (de Groot, Wu., Carter, & Munden, 2018; Knoop, 2018; Mountzios, 2018; Siegel, Miller, & Jemal, 2018)
   A. The major types of lung cancer are non–small cell lung cancer (NSCLC), SCLC, and neuroendocrine tumors. NSCLC and SCLC account for 95% of all lung cancers.
      1. Neuroendocrine tumors include SCC, large cell neuroendocrine carcinoma, typical carcinoid, and atypical carcinoid.
         a. SCCs and large cell neuroendocrine carcinomas typically have a more aggressive course compared with the carcinoid types.

B. As of 2018, lung cancer is the second most common cancer in both men and women in the United States.
   1. A combined total of 234,030 estimated new cases annually: 14% in men and 13% in women
   2. The leading cause of cancer mortality in the United States, 26% for men and 25% for women, with 154,050 combined estimated deaths for 2018
   3. Both incidence and mortality rates are slowly declining in the United States for both genders, with changes correlating with decreased smoking

C. The median age of diagnosis is 70 years old for both men and women
   1. 53% occur in individuals 55 to 74 years old.
   2. 37% occur over 75 years old.
   3. 10% of cases occur in individuals less than 55 years.

D. Non-Hispanic black men have the highest incidence, as well as poor outcomes, and are diagnosed at a more advanced stage of disease.

E. In nonsmokers, lung cancer is the seventh leading cause of cancer deaths, approximately 10% to 15% of lung cancer cases in the U.S.

III. Risk factors (Alberg et al., 2013; de Groot et al., 2018; NCCN 2018a; NCCN, 2018b)

A. Smoking
   1. Cigarette smoking remains the predominant risk factor for developing lung cancer; accounts for approximately 85% to 90% of lung cancers and is closely associated with all histologic types.
   2. Accounts for cancers caused by voluntary or involuntary (secondhand) cigarette smoking.
   3. Evidence shows a 20% to 30% increase in the risk for lung cancer from exposure to secondhand smoke associated with living with a smoker.
   4. Risk increases with number of years smoked and number of cigarettes per day. To quantify tobacco exposure, the number of packs of cigarettes per day is multiplied by the number of years smoked to obtain pack history.
      a. For example, one pack per day for 30 years = 30 pack/year smoking history.
   5. Tobacco smoke also promotes the carcinogenic effect of other carcinogens, such as radon, asbestos, and air pollution.
   6. Electronic cigarettes have been sold in the U.S. since 2007, and the risk factor for developing lung cancer from this is not well established.

B. Environmental and occupational factors that increase the risk of developing lung cancer
   1. Asbestos exposure (especially for mesothelioma)
   2. Radon gas
   3. Air pollution

C. DNA changes
   1. Potent carcinogens in tobacco smoke can cause genetic and epigenetic changes. Carcinogens can bind to DNA and cause cancer-causing mutations.
   2. Genetic testing is not standard of care.
   3. Some genetic mutations associated with SCLC: p53, RB1, PARP.
   4. Some genetic mutations associated with NSCLC: EGFR, KRAS, ALK, PARP, p16.

D. Genetic risk factors have also been identified
   1. Patients who smoke and have TP53 germline sequence variations are three times more likely to develop lung cancer than nonsmokers; three genes within chromosome 15 risk for lung cancer—30% increased risk with one marker, 70% to 80% increased risk with all three markers (Zappa and Mousa, 2016).
   2. Lung cancer risk increased two to four times in first-degree relatives of lung cancer patients, controlled for personal smoking history.

E. Preexisting pulmonary disease (chronic obstructive pulmonary disease [COPD], pulmonary fibrosis, tuberculosis) is associated with an increased incidence.

IV. Prevention (Fintelmann et al., 2015; Knoop, 2018; NCCN, 2018a; Wiener et al., 2015)

A. Lung cancer screening guidelines based on the National Lung Screening Trial (NLST)
   1. The NLST completed in 2011 found fewer lung cancer deaths with spiral low-dose computed tomography (LDCT).
   2. Lung cancer screening is recommended by National Comprehensive Cancer Network (NCCN), Centers for Medicare and Medicaid Services (CMMS), American Cancer Society (ACS), U.S. Preventive Services Task Force (USPSTF), American College of Chest Physicians (ACCP), and European Society for Medical Oncology (ESMO).
   3. Current screening guidelines are for current or former smokers (≥30 pack-years or quit <15 years), asymptomatic, age 55 to 74, to have annual screening with LDCT (Weiner, et al., 2015).
   4. LDCT must be performed in settings that have expertise in lung cancer screening, diagnosis, and treatment (NCCN, 2018a).
   5. Screening guidelines do not recommend routine use of chest radiography or sputum cytology because these have not been shown to reduce the risk of mortality.
   6. Screening results in increased detection of early-stage lung cancer, which is more treatable; however, screening also results in the identification of many nodules that may be benign and may result in unnecessary procedures and psychological distress (Bach et al., 2012).

7. Early-stage lung cancer may be curable; effective population-based screening could decrease mortality rates.

8. Results of ongoing trials may prompt further changes in the screening recommendations. Specifically, the U.S. Preventive Services Task Force has issued draft guidelines that expand the age range to 55 to 79 years (U.S. Preventive Services Task Force [USPSTF], 2013).

  B. Smoking cessation (Knoop, 2018)

1. Smoking cessation can decrease the risk of developing comorbidities such as cardiovascular disease and other malignancies such as head and neck cancers, colorectal cancer, and liver cancer.

2. Five or more years must lapse before an appreciable decrease in risk occurs.

3. Supportive therapy
   a. Assessing a patient's desire to stop smoking
   b. Teaching stress management and relaxation techniques
   c. Referring patients to tobacco cessation resources such as the national quitline network (1-800-QUIT-NOW).

4. Pharmacologic treatments: nicotine replacement therapy (NRT), for example, varenicline and bupropion

5. Behavioral counseling and cognitive behavioral therapy

V. Histopathology (NCCN, 2018a; NCCN 2018b; NCI, 2018c)

  A. Cancer classification systems commonly in use include identification of the primary site or anatomic location in the body (lung) and the tissue of origin (histologic type).

1. Establishment of lung cancer as the primary diagnosis may be challenging, as the lung is a common metastatic site and lung cancer may first appear elsewhere in the body (e.g., brain).

2. Determining the lungs as the primary site has been aided by the development of immunohistochemical staining (e.g., thyroid transcription factor 1 [TTF-1], multiple creatinine kinase [CK] stains), which may assist in differentiating the histology and primary versus metastatic adenocarcinoma.

VI. Molecular classification (NCCN, 2018a; NCCN, 2018b)

  A. Since the early 2000s, there has there has been increased understanding of molecular pathways that have contributed to the development of targeted therapy.

  B. Adequate tissue availability is necessary to complete multiple molecular testing.

  C. Molecular testing is available for both epidermal growth factor receptor (EGFR) and anaplastic lymphoma kinase (ALK) gene rearrangements to determine appropriate treatment recommendations:

1. EGRF mutations are critical, as these mutations are associated with a sensitivity to tyrosine kinase inhibitor (TKI) responses.

2. EGRF mutations occur in up to 50% of patients with adenocarcinoma, being more common in Asians, women, and never-smokers.

3. ALK gene rearrangements in NSCLC associated with response to crizotinib.

  D. KRAS mutations: associated with TKI resistance. Presence of KRAS is associated with poor survival compared with patients without KRAS mutation.

VII. Histologic grade See Table 19.1.

VIII. Diagnosis and staging (ACCP 2013; NCCN, 2018a; NCCN, 2018b; NCI, 2018c)

  A. Complete history and physical examination to include:

1. Identification of findings related to local or systemic spread

2. Evaluation of pulmonary status

3. Identification of any comorbidities, all of which influence treatment options

  B. To date, no specific tumor markers for disease status have been identified.

  C. Imaging begins with a chest x-ray and CT of the chest, liver, and adrenal glands.

1. If spread is suspected, additional imaging may include positron emission tomography (PET) (particularly helpful for nodal evaluation and to identify metastatic sites) and additional imaging of suspicious sites (bone scan, abdominal imaging).

2. Magnetic resonance imaging (MRI) is recommended for stage II to IIIA lung cancer to evaluate for brain metastasis.

  D. Tissue sample to be obtained for diagnosis

1. The least invasive and safest method that is likely to provide the highest yield of tissue for histopathology is recommended.

2. Bronchoscopy is recommended for a centrally located lung lesion to confirm diagnosis. If negative, further tests are recommended
   a. Transbronchial needle aspiration (TBNA)
   b. Navigation bronchoscopy (NB)
   c. Endobronchial ultrasound-guided needle aspiration (EBUS-NA)

3. Endoscopic ultrasound-guided needle aspiration (EUS-NA)

4. Transthoracic needle aspiration (TTNA)

5. Mediastinoscopy: a minor procedure used to obtain samples of all accessible lymph nodes

  E. In the presence of pleural effusion, a thoracentesis is performed to determine malignancy. Malignant cells present in the pleural fluid alter the stage of lung cancer.

  F. Lung cancer is staged clinically on the basis of clinical examination and imaging findings, and pathologically on surgical and pathologic findings.

TABLE 19.1 Lung Cancer: Proposed IASLC Histology Classification

Small Biopsy and Cytology: IASLC/ATS/ERS

Morphologic adenocarcinoma patterns clearly present:
Adenocarcinoma—describe identifiable patterns present (including micropapillary pattern not included in 2004 WHO classification).
Comment: If pure lepidic growth, mention that an invasive component cannot be excluded in this small specimen.

Adenocarcinoma with lepidic pattern (if pure, add note: an invasive component cannot be excluded)

Mucinous adenocarcinoma (describe patterns present)

Adenocarcinoma with fetal pattern

Adenocarcinoma with colloid pattern

Adenocarcinoma with (describe patterns present) and signet ring features

Adenocarcinoma with (describe patterns present) and clear cell features

Morphologic adenocarcinoma patterns not present (supported by special stains):
Non–small cell carcinoma, favor adenocarcinoma

Morphologic squamous cell patterns clearly present:
Squamous cell carcinoma

Morphologic squamous cell patterns not present (supported by stains):
Non–small cell carcinoma, favor squamous cell carcinoma

Small cell carcinoma

Non–small cell carcinoma, not otherwise specified (NOS)

Non–small cell carcinoma with neuroendocrine (NE) morphology (positive NE markers), possible LCNEC

Non–small cell carcinoma with NE morphology (negative NE markers); see comment.
Comment: This is a non–small cell carcinoma where LCNEC is suspected but stains failed to demonstrate NE differentiation.

Morphologic squamous cell and adenocarcinoma patterns present:
Non–small cell carcinoma, with squamous cell and adenocarcinoma patterns
Comment: This could represent adenosquamous carcinoma.

Morphologic squamous cell or adenocarcinoma patterns not present but immunostains favor separate glandular and adenocarcinoma components
Non–small cell carcinoma, NOS (specify the results of the immunohistochemical stains and the interpretation)
Comment: This could represent adenosquamous carcinoma.

Poorly differentiated NSCLC with spindle and/or giant cell carcinoma (mention if adenocarcinoma or squamous carcinoma are present)

ATS, American Thoracic Society; *ERS,* European Respiratory Society; *IASLC,* International Association for the Study of Lung Cancer; *LCNEC,* large cell neuroendocrine carcinoma; *NSCLC,* non–small cell lung carcinoma; *WHO,* World Health Organization.
Reprinted courtesy of the International Association for the Study of Lung Cancer. Copyright © 2011.

1. A biopsy is not required before surgery if a strong clinical suspicion of stage I or II lung cancer exists.
2. Mediastinoscopy (invasive mediastinal staging) is recommended before surgical resection for most patients with clinical stage I or II lung cancer. Performed as the initial step before planned resection (during the same anesthetic procedure).
3. For strong clinical suspicion of N2 or N3 nodal disease, a preoperative invasive mediastinal staging is appropriate.
4. Bronchoscopy is recommended to be performed during the planned surgical resection in order to limit procedural risks, limit costs, and avoid multiple procedures (NCCN, 2018a).

G. Staging system (refer to American Joint Committee on Cancer [AJCC] Lung Cancer Staging, 8th edition www.cancerstaging.org)

1. Stage of disease at time of diagnosis is a critical element in determining appropriate treatment, as well as a key factor in defining prognosis.
2. SCLC uses a simplified staging system of clinical limited or clinical extensive disease.
3. TNM (T = tumor size, N = nodal status, M = metastasis) staging was revised for lung cancer in the AJCC Cancer Staging, 8th edition.
   a. Changes were based on analysis of a large multinational data set of lung cancer cases
   b. More accurately differentiate staging and prognosis
   c. Primary changes made in cutoff for tumor size and subdivisions in T staging
   d. Changes in M category made to include contralateral lung nodules and pleural effusions, with subdivisions added

IX. Prognosis and survival (American Cancer Society [ACS], 2018)
   A. Leading cause of cancer-related deaths worldwide, in part because the disease is diagnosed at advanced stages and survival is poor
      1. Worldwide, lung cancer remains an epidemic, and deaths from lung cancer are four times more common than from any other cancer.
      2. Overall survival rate for lung cancer at 5 years is only 18.6% in all patients.
      3. One-year survival rates increased in the U.S. to 44%.
      4. Five-year relative survival rates for all types of cancer of the lung depend on stage of disease:
         a. 56.3% for localized disease
         b. 29.7% for regional disease
         c. 4.7% for distant disease
         d. 7.3% for unknown
      5. SCLC is difficult to cure because at the time of diagnosis, it is already widely disseminated.
         a. Limited disease: 5-year survival is 14%
         b. Extensive disease: long-term survival is rare
      6. Positive prognostic factors include early stage of disease, good performance status, less than 5% weight loss, and female gender.
X. Management (Detterbeck, et al., 2013; NCCN, 2018a; NCCN, 2018b)
   A. Principles for medical management
      1. Delivery of care should be timely and efficient
      2. A multidisciplinary team approach is recommended for lung cancer patients who require multimodality therapy
      3. Treatment decisions are influenced by the stage of disease, histologic subtype, performance status (PS), pulmonary status, comorbidities, age, and patient-informed decisions
      4. Evidence-based treatment algorithms are readily available electronically from multiple national organizations:
         a. American Society of Clinical Oncology (ASCO, 2018)
         b. National Comprehensive Cancer Network (NCCN)
         c. National Cancer Institute (NCI, 2018a, b, d)
         d. American College of Chest Physicians (ACCP, 2013)
         e. Clinical trials: NCCN recommends the participation of anyone with cancer in a clinical trial; clinical trials can be found at http://clinicaltrials.gov.
   B. Surgery (ACCP, 2013; NCCN, 2018a; Knoop, 2018)
      1. Surgery is the primary treatment for the management of early-stage NSCLC (stages I and II).
         a. Surgery is the best option for curative therapy.
         b. Role of surgery in stage III disease is controversial; reserved for select cases (NCCN, 2018a).

(1) Stage IIIA: lymph nodes involved, no distant metastatic disease
(2) Stage IIIB: tumor size is larger, more lymph nodes involved, no distant metastatic disease
         c. Only 25% to 35% of cases are candidates for surgical resection.
         d. Surgery also plays a major role in the establishment of the diagnosis by obtaining tissue and has a role in the palliation of symptoms.
         e. Individuals considered for lung surgery should undergo pulmonary function tests to measure forced expiratory volume in the first second (FEV1) and diffusing capacity of the lungs for carbon monoxide (DLCO).
         f. As primary treatment, the surgical procedure selected depends on both the extent of the disease and the patient's cardiopulmonary status.
            (1) In general, lung-sparing resection is preferred; lobectomy remains the standard approach.
            (2) Minimally invasive techniques such as video-assisted thoracic surgery (VATS) are recommended; this surgery may be done in conjunction with wedge resection and has been associated with decreased morbidity.
            (3) Systematic lymphadenectomy is recommended (rather than complete lymph node dissection).
            (4) Not all patients with lung cancer are candidates for surgery, and in those who are undergoing surgery, resection may be halted if evidence of metastasis is found.
            (5) Surgery may also be indicated for metastatic sites of disease that are symptomatic (i.e., resection of a solitary brain metastasis).
         g. Patients who are considered for surgery after neoadjuvant therapy should undergo pulmonary function tests to measure diffusion capacity
   C. Radiation therapy (RT) (NCCN, 2018a)
      1. In all stages of NSCLC, RT has a potential role for either definitive or palliative therapy.
      2. For early-stage NSCLC (stage I or node-negative stage IIa disease), stereotactic body radiation therapy (SBRT) or stereotactic ablative radiotherapy (SABR) is recommended for the individual who is not a surgical candidate or refuses surgery.
      3. Postoperative radiation administered to those with positive surgical margins.
      4. May be administered for stage III and stage IV disease.
      5. May be effective for palliation of symptoms and management of brain metastasis.

6. Advanced techniques—conformal simulation and intensity-modulated radiotherapy, which reduce toxicity and increase survival.
   a. Commonly prescribed dosing is 60 to 70 gray (Gy) in 2-Gy fractions.
   b. Treatment planning standard is a minimum of three-dimensional conformal RT.
   c. Radiofrequency ablation (RFA) involves whole-brain RT and stereotactic radiosurgery for the management of brain metastasis and improves quality of life.
D. Chemotherapy—NSCLC (NCCN, 2018a)
   1. Chemotherapy may be administered as neoadjuvant therapy, concurrently with RT, or as single modality (see NCCN guidelines for treatment recommendations).
   2. Rapid advancements in targeted therapy specific to the tumor histology have been developed to treat lung cancer; multiple changes have been made to therapy options and first-line recommendations. It is important to seek out the latest information and nationally recommended guidelines.
   3. Chemotherapy can be indicated for individuals with a performed status measured by Eastern Cooperation Oncology Group (ECOG) of 0 to 2 and may be contraindicated in individual scenarios.
   4. Chemotherapy is considered in as many as 80% of NSCLC cases.
E. Molecular targeted therapy for NSCLC involves the following considerations:
   1. Effective in individuals with certain genetic mutations
   2. Holds promise for further development of targeted therapies for specific pathways of mutations
   3. EGRF-targeted therapies—include oral TKIs now indicated for treatment in selected cases
   4. Bevacizumab—in addition to chemotherapy, recommended in select patients with advanced NSCLC
   5. Erlotinib—first-line therapy for individuals with advanced, recurrent, or metastatic non–squamous NSCLC (NCCN, 2018b)
   6. Crizotinib—first-line therapy for individuals with advanced disease and who are ALK-positive
F. Immunotherapy, an upcoming treatment strategy in cancer therapeutics, involves modulation of regulatory mechanisms to boost the immune response against cancer cells.
   1. Immune-checkpoint inhibitors are drugs that block specific proteins involved in downregulation of immune response in cancer cells.
   2. Anti–PD-1 human monoclonal antibody, nivolumab and pembrolizumab, atezolimab, and durvalumab are approved immune-checkpoint inhibitors for NSCLC.

3. Pembrolizumab was approved to replace chemotherapy as first-line treatment for NSCLC with high PD-L1 expression.
4. The optimal duration of therapy is an area of active study; current options include close surveillance, maintenance, and switch therapy.
E. Palliative care (NCCN, 2018a)
   1. Early palliative care combined with standard therapy is recommended because it improves quality of life, mood, and, in one study, survival (Ferrell, et al., 2016).
F. Recurrent disease
   1. The management of recurrent or progressive NSCLC is an area of active investigation, but few guidelines are available for the use of second- and third-line agents.
   2. With systemic therapy, different agents are often tried, with disease response monitored after two cycles of therapy. Careful attention paid to toxicities and tolerance (NCCN, 2018a).
   3. Treatment decisions need to be individualized to the specific context with chemotherapy, RT, and surgery. Goals are symptom relief, treatment of emergencies, and disease stabilization.
   4. Maximization of palliative care, consideration of hospice care, or a combination of both is recommended.
G. SCLC (NCI, 2018d; NCCN, 2018b)
   1. Accounts for approximately 15% of cases and is responsive to chemotherapy and RT
   2. Prognosis poor with overall 5-year survival at 5% to 10%
   3. Untreated median survival 2 to 4 months
   4. Standard of care for individuals with limited disease—concurrent combined modality with chemotherapy or RT
   5. Prophylactic cranial RT indicated for individuals with complete response to chemotherapy or RT to reduce the risk of developing brain metastasis
   6. Maintenance chemotherapy outside of a clinical trial not supported by current evidence
   7. Standard therapy for individuals with extensive disease—a doublet chemotherapy regimen (i.e., cisplatin, etoposide).
      a. Carboplatin used if contraindications present; duration of treatment generally four to six cycles
XI. Nursing implications
A. Patient or family understanding of diagnosis and treatment options
   1. Establish goals of care
   2. Assess coping with diagnosis and prognosis
   3. Allow the patient to maintain roles and activities most important to him or her
   4. Emphasize short-term goals in daily care and priority setting
   5. Refer to community resources as appropriate and available

6. Teach supportive care skills
7. Maintain realistic hope and yet prepare for changes in lifestyle if prognosis is poor
8. Recognize needs related to anticipatory grieving
9. Assist to resume previous roles and responsibilities if prognostic factors are favorable

B. Treatment
1. Communication is essential in the coordination of care within the multidisciplinary team.
2. Includes teaching, side effect prevention, and monitoring
3. Pain management with metastatic disease, pleural catheter management, and reinforcement of deep-breathing exercises helpful to increase physical activity.
4. Individuals who receive radiation therapy may experience localized skin reactions, esophagitis, fatigue, and symptoms specific to the treatment field.
5. Individuals who receive chemotherapy or targeted agents will have side effect profiles specific to the regimen.
   a. In addition to risk for neutropenia, cisplatin-based regimens may cause nausea and vomiting and peripheral neuropathies, which require monitoring of kidney functioning.
   b. Some of the targeted therapies may cause rash, diarrhea, or both.

C. Decrease severity of symptoms associated with the disease, treatment, or both
1. Individuals diagnosed with lung cancer are known to be at high risk for pain and multiple other symptoms such as shortness of breath, fatigue, and weakness.
2. Maximal palliative care interventions for all symptoms are essential.
3. Refer to Oncology Nursing Society PEP resources (www.ons.org/Research/PEP/)(ONS, 2017) for evidence-based guidelines for symptom management

REFERENCES

Alberg, A., Brock, M., Ford, J., Samet, J., & Spivack, S. (2013). Diagnosis and management of lung cancer, 3rd ed: American College of Chest Physicians evidenced-based practice guidelines. *Chest, 143*(5 Suppl), e1S–e29S.

American Cancer Society [ACS]. (2018). *Cancer facts & figures 2018.* Atlanta: American Cancer Society.

American College of Chest Physicians [ACCP]. (2013). Lung cancer. www.chestnet.org/Publications/CHEST-Publications/Guidelines-Consensus-Statements.

American Joint Commission on Cancer [AJCC]. (2018). *Lung cancer staging. (8th ed.) (2018).* www.cancerstaging.org.

American Society Clinical Oncology [ASCO]. (2018). *Lung cancer treatment guidelines.* www.asco.org/guidelines/lung-cancer.

Bach, P., Mirkin, J., Oliver, T., Azzoli, C., Berry, D., Brawley, O., et al. (2012). Benefits and harms of CT screening for lung cancer: a systematic review. *JAMA, 307,* 2418–2429. (2012). https://doi.org/10.1001/jama.2012.5521.

de Groot, P. M., Wu, C. C., Carter, B. W., & Munden, R. F. (2018). The epidemiology of lung cancer. *Translational Lung Cancer Research, 7*(3), 220–233. https://doi.org/10.21037/tlcr.2018.05.06.

Detterbeck, F. C., Lewis, S. Z., Diekemper, R., Addrizzo-Harris, D., & Alberts, W. M. (2013). Executive summary: diagnosis and management of lung cancer, 3rd ed: American College of Chest Physicians evidence-based clinical practice guidelines. *Chest, 143* (5 Suppl), 7S–37S. https://doi.org/10.1378/chest.12-2377.

Ferrell, B. R., Temel, J. S., Temin, S., Alesi, E. R., Balboni, T. A., Basch, E. M., et al. (2016). Integration of palliative care into standard oncology care: American Society of Clinical Oncology Clinical Practice Guideline Update. *Journal of Clinical Oncology, 35,* 96–112. https://doi.org/10.1200/JCO.2016.70.1474.

Fintelmann, F. J., Bernheim, A. B., Digumarthy, S. R., Lennes, I. T., Kalra, M. K., Gilman, M. D., et al. (2015). The 10 pillars of lung cancer screening: rationale and logistics of a lung cancer screening program. *Chest Imaging, 35,* 1893–1908. https://doi.org/10.1148/rg.2015150079.

Knoop, T. (2018). Lung cancer. In C. H. Yarbro, D. Wujcik, & B. H. Gobel (Eds.), *Cancer Nursing: Principles and Practice* (8th ed., pp. 1679–1720). Boston: Jones and Bartlett.

Mountzios, G. (2018). Lung cancer: biology and technology foster therapeutic innovation. *Annals Translational Medicine, 6*(8), 137. https://doi.org/10.21037/atm.2018.04.19.

National Cancer Institute [NCI]. (2018a). Clinical trials for lung cancer. www.cancer.gov/cancertopics/types/lung.

National Cancer Institute [NCI]. (2018b). Non-small cell lung cancer treatment PDQ. Retrieved from, www.cancer.gov/cancertopics/pdq/treatment/non-small-cell-lung/healthprofessional/page1/AllPages.

National Cancer Institute [NCI]. (2018c). SEER training modules; cancer classification. Retrieved from, https://training.seer.cancer.gov/disease/categories/classification.html.

National Cancer Institute [NCI]. (2018d). Small cell lung cancer treatment PDQ. www.cancer.gov/cancertopics/pdq/treatment/small-cell-lung/healthprofessional/page4/AllPages.

National Comprehensive Cancer Network [NCCN]. (2018a). Non-small cell lung cancer. *In NCCN clinical practice guidelines in oncology.* Version 6.2018. Retrieved from. www.nccn.org/professionals/physician_gls/f_guidelines.asp#site.

National Comprehensive Cancer Network. (2018b). Small cell lung cancer. *In Version 2.2018.* Retrieved from. https://www.nccn.org/professionals/physician_gls/pdf/sclc.pdf.

Oncology Nursing Society. (2017). *PEP resources.* www.ons.org/Research/PEP.

Siegel, R. L., Miller, K. D., & Jemal, A. (2018). Cancer statistics, 2018. *CA Cancer J Clin, 68*(1), 7–30. https://doi.org/10.3322/caac.21442.

U.S. Preventive Service Task Force. (USPSTF). (2013). Screening for lung cancer. http://www.uspreventiveservicestaskforce.org/uspstf/uspslung.htm.

Wiener, R. S., Gould, M. K., Arenberg, D. A., Au, D. H., Fennig, K., Lamb, C. R., et al. (2015). An official American Thoracic Society/American College of Chest Physicians statement: implementation of low-dose computed tomography lung cancer screening programs in clinical practice. *American Journal of Respiratory and Critical Care Medicine, 192*(7), 881–891. https://doi.org/10.1164/rccm.201508-1671ST.

Zappa, C., & Mousa, S. A. (2016). Non-small cell lung cancer: current treatment and future advances. *Translational Lung Cancer Research, 5*(3), 288–300. http://doi.org/10.21037/tlcr.2016.06.07.

20

Lymphoma

Judy Petersen

I. Pathophysiology of the lymphoid system
   A. Malignancies of the lymphoid system—heterogenous group of malignancies of B cells, T cells, and, rarely, natural killer (NK) cells; usually originate in the lymph nodes; can affect any organ of the body.
II. Hodgkin lymphoma (HL)
   A. Pathophysiology (Press & Lichtman, 2015; Ansell, 2016; Portlock, Kumar, & Armitage, 2017)
      1. The two distinct types are classic HL (cHL) and nodular lymphocyte-predominant HL (NLPHL).
      2. cHL—multinucleated giant Reed–Sternberg cell within characteristic reactive cellular background
      3. NLPHL lacks typical Reed–Sternberg cells; characterized by a malignant population of large cells with folded lobulated nuclei—lymphocytic and histiocytic cells.
   B. Epidemiology (American Cancer Society [ACS], 2018; SEER, 2018a; Ansell, 2016)
      1. Estimated 8500 new cases diagnosed and 1050 deaths from HL in 2018. Overall, incidence rates stable from 2005 to 2014. HL represents 0.5% of all new cancer cases in the U.S.
      2. Age-related bimodal incidence—most common among teens and adults aged 15 to 35 years and adults aged 55 years and older.
      3. Mortality—death rates declining since 1975; decreased by about 3% per year from 2006 to 2015.
   C. Risk factors and prevention (NCI, 2018a; Press & Lichtman; 2015, Ansell, 2016)
      1. The exact cause of HL is unknown
      2. Factors that increase the risk of HL
         a. Age—most often between ages 15 and 35 years and in those 55 years or older
         b. Infection with the Epstein–Barr virus (EBV) and human immunodeficiency virus (HIV)
         c. More common in males
         d. Family history of lymphoma
         e. Primary immunodeficiencies, prior solid organ and allogeneic bone marrow transplantation
         f. Prior treatment with cytotoxic chemotherapy drugs for other diseases
      3. No known preventive measures
   D. Classification (Swerdlow et al., 2016; Portlock, et al., 2017) (Box 20.1)
      1. 95% HL are cHL, which includes four subtypes: nodular sclerosis HL, mixed cellularity HL, lymphocyte depletion HL, and lymphocyte-rich cHL.
      2. Typical immunophenotype for cHL is CD15+, CD40+, and CD30+.
      3. NLPHL clinicopathologic entity of B-cell origin is distinct from cHL.
      4. Common immunophenotype for NLPHL is CD15-, CD20+, CD30-, and CD45+.
   E. Diagnosis and staging (Younes et al., 2014; NCCN, 2018a; Ansell, 2016)
      1. Clinical presentation—enlarged lymph nodes, spleen, other immune tissue, with/without systemic symptoms; each histologic subtype has its own clinical features.
         a. cHL—most common presentation (half of patients) is localized disease (stage I or II) in painless cervical and supraclavicular nodes and mediastinal lymph node
         b. NLPHL—more than 80% present with localized disease in cervical, axillary, or inguinal nodes; extranodal disease rare; earlier-stage disease has more indolent course than those with cHL.
         c. Tends to spread first to adjacent lymph nodes
         d. Systemic symptoms (B symptoms)—fever, weight loss, fatigue, and night sweats; present in approximately 40% of patients, less common with NLPHL. Another characteristic symptom can be generalized pruritus, and some patients report pain at the nodal site when drinking, but the significance of these symptoms is unknown.
      2. Diagnostic measures
         a. Excisional lymph node biopsy required
         b. Presence of Reed–Sternberg cells on pathologic examination with cHL
         c. Fluordeoxyglucose positive emission tomography (FDG-PET) ± radiographic studies (contrast computed tomography [CT] of the chest, abdomen, and pelvis); FDG-PET shown to be important tool in staging to support treatment selection and monitoring treatment response

BOX 20.1 2016 WHO Classification of Mature B-Cell, T-Cell, and NK-Cell Neoplasms*

Mature B-Cell Neoplasms
Chronic lymphocytic leukemia/small lymphocytic lymphoma
Monoclonal B-cell lymphocytosis
B-cell prolymphocytic leukemia
Splenic marginal zone lymphoma
Hairy cell leukemia
Extranodal marginal zone lymphoma of mucosa-associated lymphoid tissue (MALT lymphoma)
Nodal marginal zone lymphoma (MZL)
Follicular lymphoma
   In situ follicular neoplasia
   Duodenal-type follicular lymphoma
Pediatric-type follicular lymphoma
Primary cutaneous follicle center lymphoma
Mantle cell lymphoma
   In situ mantle cell neoplasia
Diffuse large B-cell lymphoma (DLBCL), not otherwise specified (NOS)
   Germinal center B-cell type
   Activated B-cell type
T-cell/histiocyte-rich large B-cell lymphoma
Primary DLBCL of the central nervous system (CNS)
Primary cutaneous DLBCL, leg type
Epstein–Barr virus (EBV)–positive DLBCL, NOS
DLBCL associated with chronic inflammation
Lymphamatoid granulomatosis
Primary mediastinal (thymic) large B-cell lymphoma
Intravascular large B-cell lymphoma
ALK-positive large B-cell lymphoma
Plasmablastic lymphoma
Primary effusion lymphoma
HHV8-positive DLBCL, NOS
Burkitt lymphoma
High-grade B-cell lymphoma with MYC and BCL2 and/or BCL6 rearrangements

High-grade B-cell lymphoma, NOS
B-cell lymphoma, unclassifiable, with features intermediate between DLBCL and classical Hodgkin lymphoma

Mature T-Cell and NK-Cell Neoplasms
T-cell prolymphocytic leukemia
T-cell large granular lymphocytic leukemia
Aggressive NK-cell leukemia
Systemic EBV-positive T-cell lymphoma of childhood
Hydroa vacciniforme–like lymphoproliferative disorder
Adult T-cell leukemia/lymphoma
Extranodal NK-/T-cell lymphoma, nasal type
Enteropathy-associated T-cell lymphoma
Monomorphic epitheliotropic intestinal T-cell lymphoma
Hepatosplenic T-cell lymphoma
Subcutaneous panniculitis–like T-cell lymphoma
Mycosis fungoides
Sézary syndrome
Primary cutaneous CD30-positive T-cell lymphoproliferative disorders
   Lymphomatoid papulosis
   Primary cutaneous anaplastic large cell lymphoma
Primary cutaneous gamma-delta T-cell lymphoma
Peripheral T-cell lymphoma, NOS
Angioimmunoblastic T-cell lymphoma
Anaplastic large cell lymphoma, ALK-positive
Anaplastic large cell lymphoma, ALK-negative

Hodgkin Lymphoma
Nodular lymphocyte predominate Hodgkin lymphoma (NLPHL)
Classical Hodgkin lymphoma
   Nodular sclerosis classical Hodgkin lymphoma
   Lymphocyte-rich classical Hodgkin lymphoma
   Mixed-cellularity classical Hodgkin lymphoma
   Lymphocyte-depleted classical Hodgkin lymphoma

* Several histologic types were identified as provisional in the 2016 WHO classification system. They have been left out of this box. Plasma cell neoplasms are not included here; see Chapter 21. Two additional categories *not* included are the rare posttransplant lymphoproliferative disorders (PTLD) and histiocytic and dendritic cell neoplasms.
Excerpted from Swerdlow, S. H., Campo, E., Pileri, S. A., Harris, N. L., Stein, H., Siebert, R., et al. (2016). The 2016 revision of the World Health Organization classification of lymphoid neoplasms. *Blood, (127)*, 2375–2390.

   d. Bone marrow biopsy may be required for accurate staging
   e. Immunohistochemistry and cytogenetic evaluation
   f. HIV testing and additional testing based on recommended treatment plan (e.g., evaluation of ejection fraction, pulmonary function tests)
   g. Fertility counseling
  3. Staging
   a. The Lugano Classification modification of the Ann Arbor Staging System. Staging based on the extent of disease and the presence of systemic symptoms (B symptoms) (American Joint Committee on Cancer [AJCC], 2017; Barrington, et al., 2014).

   b. Patients divided into three major prognostic groups that support treatment decisions (Box 20.2) (NCCN, 2018a; NCI, 2018a; Hasenclever & Diehl, 1998; AJCC, 2017).
  F. Prognosis and survival (SEER, 2018a; Ansell, 2016)
   1. Combination chemotherapy and/or radiation therapy (RT) cures >80% of newly diagnosed HL patients.
   2. Adverse prognostic factors for advanced HL (see Box 20.2). An International Prognostic Score (IPS) has been defined by the number of adverse prognostic factors identified at diagnosis. The IPS helps support treatment decisions and predict prognosis for patients with stage III to IV disease.

BOX 20.2 **Hodgkin Lymphoma Prognostic Categories by Stage and Clinical Features**

- **Early favorable:** Clinical stage I or II without any risk factors
- **Early unfavorable:** Clinical stage I or II with one or more of the following risk factors:
  - Large mediastinal mass (>33% of the thoracic width on the chest radiography; ≥10 cm on CT scan)
  - Extranodal involvement
  - Involvement of three or more lymph node areas
  - Elevated erythrocyte sedimentation rate (≥50 mm/hr)
  - B symptoms

- **Advanced:** Clinical stage III or IV with zero to seven adverse risk factors:*
  - Male gender
  - Age ≥45 years
  - Albumin level <4.0 g/dL
  - Hemoglobin level <10.5 g/dL
  - Stage IV disease
  - White blood cell (WBC) count ≥15,000/mm^3
  - Absolute lymphocytic count <600/mm^3 or lymphocyte count that was <8% of the total WBC count

* An International Prognostic Score (IPS) has been defined by the number of these adverse prognostic factors identified at diagnosis. The IPS helps support treatment decisions and predict prognosis for patients with stage III to IV disease.
Data from National Cancer Institute. (2018a). *PDQ Adult Hodgkin lymphoma treatment.* Bethesda, MD: National Cancer Institute. https://www.cancer.gov/types/lymphoma/hp/adult-hodgkintreatment-pdq; National Comprehensive Cancer Network (NCCN). (2018a). *NCCN guidelines v.1.2018 Hodgkin lymphoma* http://www.nccn.org/professionals/physician_gls/f_guidelines.asp; Hasenclever, D., & Diehl, V. (1998). A prognostic score for advanced Hodgkin's disease. International Prognostic Factors Project on Advanced Hodgkin's Disease. *N Engl J Med, 339(21),* 1506–1514.

G. Treatment—standard treatment approaches defined by prognostic groups (Younes, et al., 2014; Ansell, 2016; NCCN, 2018a; Barrington, et al., 2014; Meyer, et al., 2012)

1. Initial therapy based on the histology, anatomic stage, presence of poor prognostic features, "B" symptoms, and bulky disease.
2. Because this disease often affects young people, the goal of treatment is to avoid preventable long-term side effects while achieving maximum tumor control.
3. During treatment, FDG-PET scanning supports treatment decisions to complete therapy as planned or add or omit treatment.
4. Early favorable stages (see Box 20.2)—limited amount of chemotherapy (typically two or three cycles) plus involved field radiation
5. Unfavorable stages (see Box 20.2)—moderate amount of chemotherapy (typically four cycles) plus involved field radiation
6. Advanced stages (see Box 20.2)—extensive chemotherapy (typically eight cycles), with or without consolidation RT (usually to residual tumors)
7. Management of relapsed/refractory disease
   a. High-dose chemotherapy (HDCT) followed by an autologous stem cell (ASC) transplant
   b. Other options include the drugs everolimus, brentuximab vedotin, bendamustine, or lenalidomide.
8. For patients who fail HDCT with ASCT options include nivolumab, pembrolizumab, or clinical trials.
9. Survivorship issues and monitoring for long-term effects (see Chapter 3)

III. Non-Hodgkin lymphoma (NHL)
A. Pathophysiology (Pasqualucci, & Dalla-Favera, 2014)
   1. Heterogeneous group of lymphoproliferative cancers with wide range of histologic appearances, clinical features, behavior, and response to treatment. Diffuse large B-cell lymphoma (DLBCL) is the most common.

2. 85% to 90% arise from B lymphocytes, the rest from T lymphocytes or NK lymphocytes
B. Epidemiology
   1. Estimated 74,680 new cases diagnosed and 19,910 deaths from NHL in 2018 (ACS, 2018); incidence rates falling on average 0.6% each year over the last 10 years; however, NHL encompasses a wide variety of disease subtypes for which incidence patterns may vary (ACS, 2018). Twenty-five percent of NHL cases in U.S. are follicular lymphoma (Press & Lichtman, 2015).
   2. Mortality rates—began decreasing in the late 1990s; decrease on average 2.3% per year from 2005 to 2014. Seventy-one percent survive 5 years (SEER, 2018b).
   3. Most frequently diagnosed among people aged 65 to 74; median age at diagnosis is 67 years (SEER, 2018b).
C. Risk factors and prevention
   1. Cause of most cases of NHL unknown
   2. Risk factors for NHL (Press & Lichtman, 2015; Portlock, et al., 2017)
      a. Immunodeficiency—inherited, acquired, solid organ transplantation
      b. Infectious agents
         (1) Infection with EBV—associated with Burkitt lymphoma
         (2) Infection with the HTLV-1—increases risk for T-cell lymphoma
         (3) Hepatitis viruses B and C—seropositivity higher in DLBCL and follicular lymphoma
         (4) HIV
         (5) *Helicobacter pylori* bacterial infection linked to mucosa-associated lymphoid tissue (MALT) lymphoma in the stomach
      c. Environmental and occupational exposure to radiation, chemicals, pesticides, and solvents
   3. No known preventive measures

D. Classification (Swerdlow et al., 2016)
1. New diseases and subtypes added in the updated 2016 World Health Organization (WHO) classification system (see Box 20.2)
2. Cell of origin (B, T, or NK) considered, then further subdivided into precursor lymphocyte vs. mature lymphocyte; further refinement based on immunophenotype and genetic and clinical features

E. Diagnosis and staging
1. Clinical presentation
   a. Dependent on site of involvement and natural history of the subtype
   b. Painless lymphadenopathy more generalized, less predictable than HL; more commonly spreads to extranodal sites
   c. Other possible symptoms—pruritus, fatigue, abdominal pain (enlarged spleen or liver; bulky adenopathy), bone pain
   d. Involvement of bone marrow, liver, or other extranodal site common; most often presents as disseminated disease
2. Diagnostic measures (NCI, 2018b; Sorenson, Johnson, & Gilliam, 2016: NCCN, 2018b)
   a. Excisional lymph node core biopsy required.
   b. Radiographic studies (contrast CT of the chest, abdomen, and pelvis) to assess disease burden. PET used for initial staging and for follow-up after therapy as a supplement to CT scanning.
   c. Bone marrow biopsy may be required for accurate staging.
   d. Immunohistochemistry and cytogenetic evaluation.
   e. HIV testing and additional testing based on recommended treatment plan (i.e., evaluation of ejection fraction, pulmonary function tests).
   f. Laboratory monitoring (complete blood count [CBC], comprehensive metabolic panel [CMP], lactate dehydrogenase [LDH], uric acid) to monitor for tumor lysis syndrome as therapy initiated.
3. Staging
   a. Lugano Classification modification of Ann Arbor Staging System—based on the extent of disease (AJCC, 2017). Recent analyses show that the presence of systemic symptoms (B symptoms) do not have prognostic significance for NHL (Press & Lichtman, 2015).
   b. Most patients with advanced (stage III or stage IV) disease at presentation.
   c. Additional factors not included in the staging system important to consider for prognosis and treatment; age, performance status, tumor size, LDH values, and number of extranodal sites (AJCC, 2017).

F. Prognosis and survival (NCI, 2018b; SEER, 2018b; Sorenson, et al., 2016)
1. NHL can be divided into two prognostic groups: the indolent lymphomas and the aggressive lymphomas.
   a. Low-grade lymphomas have an indolent course with median survival as long as 20 years without aggressive therapy; not considered curable and characterized by recurrences, especially in advanced stages; occasionally can transform into high-grade NHL
   b. Aggressive or high-grade lymphomas—prognosis depends on tumor bulk, responsiveness to therapy, and patient's ability to tolerate treatment; majority of patients with localized disease curable with radiation plus chemotherapy or combination chemotherapy alone; overall survival at 5 years is over 60%. Of patients with aggressive NHL, more than 50% can be cured. Most relapses occur in the first 2 years after therapy.
2. Pretreatment prognostic models based on identification of risk factors from large groups of patients have been developed that assign patients to risk groups and predict outcomes (Ziepert, et al., 2010; Solai-Celigny, et al., 2004).
3. Relapse—may occur; requires biopsy and restaging

G. Treatment (Freedman & LaCasce, 2017; Sorenson, et al., 2016: NCI, 2018b; NCCN, 2018b)
1. Therapeutic choices are increasingly tailored to the immunologically classified lymphoma.
2. The most common NHL types are indolent (follicular lymphoma [FL] 20%) and aggressive (DLBCL 30%) NHL; treatment plans are representative for NHL.
3. Standard treatment options for indolent FL include the following:
   a. For stage I or II disease:
      (1) RT to involved site
      (2) Monoclonal antibodies (rituximab [Rituxan]) alone or in combination with chemotherapy (single-agent or combination therapy)
      (3) Observation until symptomatic
   b. For stage III or IV disease—optimal treatment is controversial, not curative
      (1) Observation recommended if no symptoms, cytopenias, or end-organ dysfunction
      (2) Numerous drug therapy options available, including rituximab, idelalisib, alkylating agents, bendamustine, combination therapy
      (3) RT for palliation of symptomatic disease

4. Intermediate- and high-grade DLBCL are considered systemic disease. Standard treatment options include the following:
   a. For stage I or contiguous II disease
      (1) Chemotherapy with or without involved-field radiation therapy (IF-XRT)
      (2) R-CHOP (rituximab [Rituxan], cyclophosphamide, doxorubicin [Adriamycin], vincristine, prednisone)
   b. Treatment for aggressive, noncontiguous stage II, III, or IV disease:
      (1) R-CHOP or other combination chemotherapy
      (2) Clinical trials including new therapies such as CAR T cells
5. Recurrent NHL
   a. Other chemotherapy regimens (single agent or combination)
   b. Autologous peripheral blood stem cell (PBSC) or allogeneic PBSC for aggressive NHL
   c. Palliative radiation therapy
6. Supportive care

IV. Nursing implications
   A. An individualized and holistic plan of care is needed when caring for the patient with a lymphoid malignancy.
   B. The plan of care is developed and implemented in cooperation with the patient, family, and multidisciplinary team.
   C. Interventions related to physical, emotional, psychological, social, and spiritual distress during extensive diagnostic testing and treatment regimen.
      1. Encourage patient to verbalize feelings about disease and treatment.
      2. Explore coping options with the patient and family, and validate effective mechanisms.
      3. Refer to mental health specialist, community support groups (Leukemia and Lymphoma Society, American Cancer Society, adolescent and young adult [AYA] cancer programs) as needed.
      4. Teach patient to identify and manage symptoms and to report symptoms to health care providers.
      5. Provide pharmacologic and nonpharmacologic interventions to managing side effects.
   D. Interventions related to the prevention of complications
      1. Ongoing assessment for potential disease and treatment-related complications is important: tumor lysis syndrome, superior vena cava syndrome, anemia, and infection. The type of complications depend on the subtype of lymphoma, treatment, and patient variables.
      2. Long-term survival, especially for young HL patients, results in increased risk for long-term complications, that is, second malignancies, various organ toxicities (pulmonary, cardiac, renal), fatigue, sexuality/fertility issues. Teach patients about the importance of monitoring for late effects and yearly evaluations (NCCN, 2018a).

REFERENCES

American Cancer Society. (2018) *Cancer facts and figures 2018.* Atlanta, Ga: American Cancer Society.https://www.cancer.org/research/cancer-facts-statistics/all-cancer-facts-figures/cancer-facts-figures-2018.html.

American Joint Committee on Cancer. (2017). Hodgkin and non-Hodgkin lymphomas. In M. B. Amin, S. Edge, F. Greene, D. R. Byrd, R. K. Brookland, M. K. Washington, et al. (Eds.), *AJCC Cancer Staging Manual.* (8th ed.). New York: Springer.

Ansell, S. M. (2016). Hodgkin lymphoma: 2016 update on diagnosis, risk-stratification, and management. *Am J Hematol, 91*(4), 434–442.

Barrington, S. F., Mikhaeel, N. G., Kostakoglu, L., Meignan, M., Hutchings, M., Müeller, S. P., et al. (2014). Role of imaging in the staging and response assessment in lymphoma: consensus of the International Conference on Malignant Lymphomas Imaging Work Group. *J Clin Oncol, 32,* 3048–3058.

Cheson, B. D., Fisher, R. I., Barrington, S. F., Cavalli, F., Schwartz, L. H., Zucca, E., & Lister, T. A. (2014). Recommendations for initial evaluation, staging, and response assessment of Hodgkin lymphoma and non-Hodgkin lymphoma: the Lugano classification. *J Clin Oncol, 32*(27), 3059–3068.

Freedman, A. S., & LaCasce, A. S. (2017). Non-Hodgkin's Lymphoma. In R. C. Bast, C. M. Croce, W. N. Hait, W. K. Hong, D. W. Kufe, M. Pocart-Gebhart, et al. (Eds.), *Holland-Frei Cancer Medicine* (9th ed., pp. 1605–1614). Hoboken, New Jersey: John Wiley & Sons, Inc.

Hasenclever, D., & Diehl, V. (1998). A prognostic score for advanced Hodgkin's disease. International Prognostic Factors Project on Advanced Hodgkin's Disease. *N Engl J Med, 339*(21), 1506–1514.

Meyer, R. M., Gospodarowicz, M. K., Connors, J. M., Pearcey, R. G., Wells, W. A., Winter, J. N., et al. (2012). ABVD alone versus radiation-based therapy in limited-stage Hodgkin's lymphoma. *N Engl J Med, 366,* 399–408.

National Cancer Institute. (2018a). *PDQ Adult Hodgkin lymphoma treatment.* Bethesda, MD: National Cancer Institute. https://www.cancer.gov/types/lymphoma/hp/adult-hodgkin-treatment-pdq.

National Cancer Institute. (2018b). *PDQ Adult Non-Hodgkin lymphoma treatment.* Bethesda, MD: National Cancer Institute. https://www.cancer.gov/types/lymphoma/hp/adult-nhl-treatment-pdq.

National Comprehensive Cancer Network (NCCN). (2018a). *NCCN guidelines v.1.2018 Hodgkin lymphoma* http://www.nccn.org/professionals/physician_gls/f_guidelines.asp.

National Comprehensive Cancer Network (NCCN). (2018b). *NCCN guidelines v.7.2017 B-cell lymphomas* https://www.nccn.org/professionals/physician_gls/pdf/b-cell.pdf.

Pasqualucci, L., & Dalla-Favera, R. (2014). Molecular biology of lymphomas. In V. DeVita, Jr., Hellman, & S. Rosenberg (Eds.), *Cancer: Principles & Practice in Oncology.* (12 ed.). Philadelphia: Lippincott Williams & Wilkins.

Portlock, C. S., Kumar, A., & Armitage, J. (2017). Hodgkin lymphoma. In R. C. Bast, C. M. Croce, W. N. Hait, W. K. Hong, D. W. Kufe, M. Pocart-Gebhart, et al. (Eds.), *Holland-Frei Cancer Medicine* (9th ed., pp. 1605–1614). Hoboken, New Jersey: John Wiley & Sons, Inc.

Press, O. W., & Lichtman, M. A. (2015). General considerations for lymphomas: epidemiology, etiology, heterogeneity, and primary extranodal disease. In K. Kaushansky, M. A. Lichtman,

J. T. Prchal, M. M. Marcel, O. W. Press, L. J. Burns, & M. Caligiuri (Eds.), *Williams Hematology.* (9th ed.). New York: McGraw Hill.

Solai-Celigny, P., Roy, P., Colombat, P.,White, J., Armitage, J. O., Arranz-Saez, R., et al. (2004). Follicular lymphoma international prognostic index. *Blood, 104*, 1258–1265.

Sorenson, E., Johnson, J., & Gilliam, M. (2016). Lymphomas. In C. H. Yarbro, D. Wujcik, & B. H. Gobel (Eds.), *Cancer Nursing: Principles and Practice.* (8th Ed.). Sudbury, MA: Jones and Bartlett.

Surveillance, Epidemiology, and End Results (SEER) Program (www.seer.cancer.gov) (2018a) *Cancer stat facts: Hodgkin lymphoma* http://seer.cancer.gov/statfacts/html/hodg.html Bethesda, MD: National Cancer Institute.

Surveillance, Epidemiology, and End Results (SEER) Program (www.seer.cancer.gov) (2018b) *Cancer stat facts: Non-Hodgkin lymphoma.* https://seer.cancer.gov/statfacts/html/nhl.html Bethesda, MD: National Cancer Institute.

Swerdlow, S. H., Campo, E., Pileri, S. A., Harris, N. L., Stein, H., Siebert, R., et al. (2016). The 2016 revision of the World Health Organization classification of lymphoid neoplasms. *Blood,* (127), 2375–2390.

Younes, A., Carbone, A., Johnson, P., Dabaja, B., Ansell, S., & Kuruvilla, J. (2014). Hodgkin lymphoma. In V. DeVita, Jr., Hellman, & S. Rosenberg (Eds.), *Cancer: Principles & Practice in Oncology.* (12 ed.). Philadelphia: Lippincott Williams & Wilkins.

Ziepert, M., Hasenclever, D., Kuhn, E., Glass, B., Schmitz, N., Pfreundschuh, M., & Loeffler, M. (2010). Standard international prognostic index remains a predictor of outcome for patients with aggressive CD20 + B-cell lymphoma in the rituximab era. *J Clin Oncol, 28*, 2373–2380.

21

Multiple Myeloma

Joseph D. Tariman and Jazel Dolores Sugay

I. Epidemiology
   A. Estimated 30,770 new cases diagnosed and 12,770 deaths from multiple myeloma (MM) in 2018
      1. Incidence in men slightly higher
      2. Men have a slightly higher number of deaths than women (Siegel, Miller, & Jemal, 2018)
   B. Second most common hematologic malignancy in the U.S.; constitutes approximately 1% of all cancers (Siegel et al., 2018)

II. Risk factors (Gleason, 2015)
   A. Veterans exposed to Agent Orange during deployment in Vietnam in the 1960s and early 1970s
   B. Environmental exposure to ionizing radiation
   C. Exposure to low-level radiation (e.g., radiologists, those employed in the nuclear industry)
   D. Exposure to metals (especially nickel), agricultural chemicals, benzene, petroleum products, aromatic hydrocarbons, and silicone
   E. Family history
   F. Immunologic factors—several studies have linked AIDS with an increased risk for myeloma
   G. Obesity (Lichtman, 2010)
   H. History of monoclonal gammopathy of undetermined significance (MGUS)
   I. Ethnicity—two times higher incidence of MM among African Americans compared with their white counterparts
   J. Older age—most diagnosed with this disease in their sixties (Faiman, Richards, & Tariman, 2018)

III. Pathophysiology
   A. Multiple myeloma is a B-cell clonal malignancy of the plasma cells that is characterized by monoclonal plasmacytosis in the bone marrow, excessive production of M protein (myeloma-produced immunoglobulin), osteolytic bone lesions, renal disease, anemia, hypercalcemia, and immunodeficiency (Noonan, 2015).
   B. The pathophysiology of MM is complicated but includes a well-orchestrated and organized sequence of interactions between various tumor cells and the bone marrow microenvironment. Specific interactions occur with cytokines and growth factors (particularly IL-6, SDF-1, VEGF, IGF-1, TNF-α, and TGF-β), osteoclasts and osteoblasts in the bone marrow microenvironment, and bone marrow stromal cells. Myeloma cells also produce osteoclast-activating factor (OAF).
      1. The various interactions produce lytic bone lesions, resulting in a "punched-out" appearance on radiographs and often in pathologic fractures
      2. OAF specifically increases bone resorption, which may cause hypercalcemia (Noonan, 2015)
   C. MM affects many genes such as KRAS, NRAS, TP53 [aka deletion of the short arm of chromosome 17 or del(17p)], FAM46C, BRAF, DIS3, ATM, and CCND1. KRAS and NRAS are "mutational drivers" for both translocations in chromosomes 4 and 14 or t(4;14) and chromosomes 11 and 14 or t(11;14). TP53 and ATM play a role in drug resistance. CCND1 is involved in early myeloma pathogenesis (Weaver & Tariman, 2017).
   D. Although a solitary plasmacytoma (defined as a localized plasma cell tumor) could occur, multiple myeloma is a systemic disease.

IV. Clinical presentation (Noonan, 2015)
   A. Commonly presents with bone pain from lytic lesions affecting thoracic and lumbar spine
   B. Multiple lytic bone lesions, high serum M protein, and extensive bone marrow plasmacytosis (>30%) common presentation
   C. Multiple systemic symptoms—anemia, uremia, recurrent infections, hypercalcemia, hyperviscosity, polyneuropathy, and spinal cord compression
   D. Patients who present with hypercalcemia, renal dysfunction, and bone fractures were associated with inferior overall survival

V. Diagnostic measures (Kehrer, Koob, Strauss, Wirtz, & Schmolders, 2017; National Comprehensive Cancer Network [NCCN], 2018). Smoldering or asymptomatic MM:
   A. Bone marrow biopsy—demonstrates presence of more than 10% clonal plasma cells
   B. Serum protein immunoelectrophoresis—demonstrates increased levels of heavy-chain M proteins.

Serum immunofixation confirms presence of monoclonal heavy chain immunoglobulin (IgG, IgA, IgM or IgD). IgM and IgD subtypes are rare; account for less than 2% of all MM cases.

C. Urine protein immunoelectrophoresis demonstrates increased levels of light-chain proteins. Urine immunofixation confirms presence of a monoclonal kappa or lambda light chain protein. The initials of Greek terms kappa and lambda honor the two scientists, Korngold and Lipari, who identified these proteins in relation to MM (Korngold & Lipari, 1956)

D. Serum-free light chains—directly measure light chain proteins (kappa or lambda) from a peripheral blood source. The normal kappa-to-lambda ratio is 0.26 to 1.65.

E. Serum lactate dehydrogenase (LDH) levels higher than upper-normal limit—a prognostic indicator

F. Urinary light chain M proteins (Bence–Jones proteins)

G. Myeloma-related organ dysfunction (SLiM CRAB criteria) (NCCN, 2018). Diagnostic criteria for active or symptomatic MM requiring therapy:
   1. **S**ixty percent clonal bone marrow plasma cells
   2. Serum-free **L**ight chain ratio kappa:lambda >100
   3. **M**agnetic resonance imaging (MRI) studies with >1 focal lesion (>5 mm in size)
   4. **C**alcium elevation in blood—calcium level greater than 10.5 ng/L or upper limit of normal
   5. **R**enal insufficiency—serum creatinine level greater than 2 mg/dL
   6. **A**nemia—hemoglobin less than 10 g/dL
   7. **B**one lytic lesions—metastatic bone survey, MRI or positron emission tomography/computed tomography (PET/CT) imaging
   8. Bone marrow biopsy—demonstrates presence of more than 10% plasma cells

H. Serum albumin and beta-2-microglobulin levels; level of beta-2-microglobulin reflects tumor mass, standard measure for tumor burden; beta-2-microglobulin used as a marker for multiple myeloma but not specific to myeloma

I. Additional blood studies, biologic assessment differentiates symptomatic and asymptomatic myeloma (i.e., decreased kidney function)

J. Pathologic fractures in the spine—MRI or CT scan

K. Nonsecretory-type myeloma (no detectable M protein in blood or urine)—PET/CT is indicated

L. Differential diagnosis: MGUS. Bone marrow biopsy shows less than 10% monoclonal plasma cells. Absence of CRAB symptoms.

VI. Classification
   A. MM is a blood cancer of the bone marrow, and the World Health Organization (WHO) classified it as a plasma cell neoplasm (Kehrer et al., 2017)

VII. Staging
   A. Historical Durie–Salmon staging system (stages I to III)—quantifies tumor volume on the basis of the amount of M proteins in urine and blood, along with clinical parameters, hemoglobin, serum calcium level, and presence of bone lesions (Durie & Salmon, 1975).
   B. More recently the International Myeloma Working Group developed the Revised International Staging System (R-ISS) stages I to III based on the serum levels of beta-2-microglobulin, LDH, albumin, and genetic factors on bone marrow biopsy, as these factors are better predictors of patient survival (Greipp et al., 2005; Palumbo et al., 2015).
   C. Genetic factors and risk groups—support individualized treatment strategies
      1. Genetic abnormalities identified by fluorescence in situ hybridization (FISH) have defined prognostic groups in retrospective and prospective analyses.
         a. Mayo myeloma risk stratification based on genetic translocations (Dispenzieri et al., 2007; Mikhael et al., 2013)
            (1) Standard risk—trisomies t(11;14) and t (6;14) translocations
            (2) Intermediate risk—t(4;14) translocation and 1q gain by FISH
            (3) High risk—del17p, t(14;16), and t (14;20) translocations by FISH gene expression profile (GEP)—high-risk signature
   D. EMC92 gene expression profiler plus the ISS (aka EMC92-ISS) is a novel prognostic tool that classifies MM into four group-risk classifications (Kuiper et al., 2015)
   E. Resultant risk group stratification; standard versus high risk

VIII. Prognosis
   A. No cure exists for MM. Improvements in survival continue with newer therapies. Among patients 65 to 74 years of age, 10-year relative survival rates improved for non-Hispanic whites (11.3% vs. 20.5%; $p < .001$) and Hispanics (10.6% vs. 20.2%; $p = .02$), but not for non-Hispanic blacks (12.6% vs. 19.5%; $p = .06$). Older and minority patients lag behind improvement in survival (Costa et al., 2017)

IX. Principles of medical management (NCCN, 2018)
   A. Diagnostic challenge—identification of stable, asymptomatic patients who do not require treatment versus those with symptomatic myeloma, which requires immediate treatment
   B. Treatment choices for symptomatic myeloma based on therapy for transplantation candidate versus nontransplantation candidate (NCCN, 2018) (Table 21.1)

TABLE 21.1   Chemotherapy Agents for Multiple Myeloma

Population/Treatment Phase	Preferred	Options
Nontransplant Primary Therapy	Bortezomib, lenalidomide, dexamethasone (category 1 NCCN Guidelines) Lenalidomide, low-dose dexamethasone (category 1) Bortezomib, cyclophosphamide, dexamethasone Daratumumab, melphalan, bortezomib, and prednisone (category 1)	Carfilzomib, lenalidomide, dexamethasone Carfilzomib, cyclophosphamide, dexamethasone Ixazomib, lenalidomide, dexamethasone Bortezomib, dexamethasone
Nontransplant Maintenance Therapy	Lenalidomide (category 1)	Bortezomib
Transplantation Candidates (avoid alkylating agents, which compromise stem cell collection)	Bortezomib, lenalidomide, and dexamethasone (category 1) Bortezomib, cyclophosphamide, and dexamethasone (category 1)	Other recommended options Bortezomib, doxorubicin, and dexamethasone (category 1) Carfilzomib, lenalidomide, and dexamethasone Ixazomib, lenalidomide, and dexamethasone (category 2b) Others Bortezomib and dexamethasone (category 1) Bortezomib, thalidomide, and dexamethasone (category 1) Lenalidomide and dexamethasone (category 1) Bortezomib, thalidomide, dexamethasone–cisplatin, doxorubicin, cyclophosphamide, etoposide (VTD-PACE)
Transplant Induction	No clear choice of induction therapy currently exists	Steroids (e.g., dexamethasone and prednisone) Antiangiogenesis agents and immunomodulating agents (e.g., lenalidomide) Proteasome inhibitors (e.g., bortezomib, carfilzomib, or ixazomib) Alkylating agents (e.g., melphalan and cyclophosphamide) Other cytotoxic drugs (e.g., vincristine, doxorubicin, liposomal doxorubicin)
Previously treated MM	Carfilzomib (twice weekly), dexamethasone (category 1) Carfilzomib, lenalidomide, and dexamethasone (category 1) Daratumumab, lenalidomide, and dexamethasone (category 1) Daratumumab, bortezomib, and dexamethasone (category 1) Elotuzumab, lenalidomide, and dexamethasone (category 1) Ixazomib, lenalidomide, and dexamethasone (category 1)	Bortezomib, lenalidomide, and dexamethasone

C. Transplant induction considerations
   1. Steroids usually given in high doses
      a. Given the median age of patients with MM, it is important to monitor for potential toxicities: hyperglycemia, hypokalemia, sodium and water retention, weight gain, cushingoid changes, mood changes, euphoria, psychosis, and insomnia (Faiman, Bilotti, Mangan, & Rogers, 2008).
      b. It may be necessary to adjust the warfarin (Coumadin) and insulin doses.

D. Stem cell transplantation (SCT)— for eligible, newly diagnosed patients (Miceli et al., 2013)
   1. Types of SCT
      a. Autologous SCT—standard of care after primary therapy for eligible patients
      b. Tandem SCT—planned second course of high-dose therapy and SCT within 6 months of the first course
         (1) May be an option as salvage therapy for relapse or progressive disease (Koniarczyk, Ferraro, & Miceli, 2017)

c. Allogeneic SCT—an option as part of a clinical trial or salvage therapy in patients with progressive disease

E. Different maintenance therapies studied for lenalidomide (Pulte et al., 2018) or bortezomib to sustain remission; maintenance therapy is beneficial for improving progression-free survival (PFS) and overall survival (OS) (Chakraborty et al., 2018)

F. For relapse—treatment with alternative chemotherapy; choice dependent on prior treatment used for induction and toxicities (e.g., neuropathy, cytopenias, deep vein thrombosis [DVT])

1. Assess response after each cycle
2. Repeat primary induction therapy if relapse occurs after 6 months
3. There are many other recommended regimens for relapsed/refractory myeloma. Refer to NCCN guidelines for myeloma for more details.

G. Supportive care

1. Bisphosphonates—for all patients receiving myeloma therapy
2. Radiation therapy (RT)—for painful lytic lesions, spinal cord compression
3. Ongoing treatment for disease complications—hypercalcemia, hyperviscosity, renal impairment, anemia, infection, coagulation disorders

X. Nursing implications (Brigle et al., 2017; Faiman et al., 2017; Rome, Noonan, Bertolotti, Tariman, & Miceli, 2017)

A. Individualized, holistic, and evidence-based plan of care for patients with lymphoid malignancy

B. Develop and implement plan of care with the patient, family, and multidisciplinary team

C. Interventions related to physical, emotional, psychological, social, and spiritual distress during extensive diagnostic testing and treatment regimen

1. Encourage patient to verbalize feelings about disease and treatment
2. Explore coping options with the patient and family and validate effective mechanisms
3. Refer to mental health specialist, community resources, support groups (Leukemia and Lymphoma Society, American Cancer Society, International Myeloma Foundation), as needed
4. Teach patient and family to identify, manage, and report symptoms
5. Provide pharmacologic and nonpharmacologic interventions to manage side effects

D. Interventions related to the prevention of complications

1. Ongoing assessment for potential disease and treatment-related complications: tumor lysis syndrome, superior vena cava syndrome, hypercalcemia, hyperviscosity, renal impairment, skeleton-related events, anemia, infection, cardiac toxicity, and coagulation disorders

E. Use evidence-based nursing interventions for steroid-related side effects (Faiman et al., 2008), diarrhea (Faiman, 2016), distress, fatigue, sexuality issues (Catamero et al., 2017), renal and peripheral nerve complications (Faiman et al., 2017), DVT (Rome, Doss, Miller, & Westphal, 2008), and myelosuppression and bone complications (Brigle et al., 2017) to maintain quality of life while living with myeloma.

F. Critical nursing considerations for patients receiving therapy for MM (Bertolotti, Pierre, Rome, & Faiman, 2017; Tariman et al., 2016)

1. DVT prevention during immunomodulatory-based (i.e., thalidomide, lenalidomide, or pomalidomide) therapy—daily aspirin or therapeutic anticoagulation with warfarin (Coumadin) for patients with a known history of DVT or pulmonary embolism
2. Shingle prophylaxis during proteasome inhibitor-based (i.e., bortezomib, carfilzomib, ixazomib)—daily acyclovir or valacyclovir
3. Peripheral neuropathy assessment for patients receiving proteasome inhibitor therapy
4. Close monitoring of complete blood counts for any cytopenia
5. Cardiopulmonary assessment for patients receiving carfilzomib or doxorubicin therapy
6. Advocate shared decision-making when two or more treatment options exist

REFERENCES

Bertolotti, P., Pierre, A., Rome, S., & Faiman, B. (2017). Evidence-based guidelines for preventing and managing side effects of multiple myeloma. *Seminars in Oncology Nursing, 33*(3), 332–347. https://doi.org/10.1016/j.soncn.2017.05.008.

Brigle, K., Pierre, A., Finley-Oliver, E., Faiman, B., Tariman, J. D., & Miceli, T. (2017). Myelosuppression, bone disease, and acute renal failure: evidence-based recommendations for oncologic emergencies. *Clinical Journal of Oncology Nursing, 21*(5), 60–76. https://doi.org/10.1188/17.CJON.S5.60-76.

Catamero, D., Noonan, K., Richards, T., Faiman, B., Manchulenko, C., Devine, H., & Gleason, C. (2017). Distress, fatigue, and sexuality: understanding and treating concerns and symptoms in patients with multiple myeloma. *Clinical Journal of Oncology Nursing, 21*(5 Suppl), 7–18. https://doi.org/10.1188/17.CJON.S5.7-18.

Chakraborty, R., Muchtar, E., Kumar, S. K., Buadi, F. K., Dingli, D., Dispenzieri, A., & Gertz, M. A. (2018). Outcomes of maintenance therapy with lenalidomide or bortezomib in multiple myeloma in the setting of early autologous stem cell transplantation. *Leukemia, 32*(3), 712–718. https://doi.org/10.1038/leu.2017.256.

Costa, L. J., Brill, I. K., Omel, J., Godby, K., Kumar, S. K., & Brown, E. E. (2017). Recent trends in multiple myeloma incidence and survival by age, race, and ethnicity in the United States. *Blood Advances, 1*(4), 282–287. https://doi.org/10.1182/bloodadvances.2016002493.

Dispenzieri, A., Rajkumar, S. V., Gertz, M. A., Fonseca, R., Lacy, M. Q., Bergsagel, P. L., & Stewart, A. K. (2007). Treatment of newly diagnosed multiple myeloma based on Mayo Stratification of Myeloma and Risk-adapted Therapy (mSMART): consensus statement. *Mayo Clinic Proceedings, 82*(3), 323–341.

Durie, B. G., & Salmon, S. E. (1975). A clinical staging system for multiple myeloma. Correlation of measured myeloma cell mass with presenting clinical features, response to treatment, and survival. *Cancer, 36*(3), 842–854.

Faiman, B. (2016). Diarrhea in multiple myeloma: a review of the literature. *Clinical Journal of Oncology Nursing, 20*(4), E100–E105. https://doi.org/10.1188/16.CJON.E100-E105.

Faiman, B., Bilotti, E., Mangan, P. A., & Rogers, K. (2008). Steroid-associated side effects in patients with multiple myeloma: consensus statement of the IMF Nurse Leadership Board. *Clinical Journal of Oncology Nursing, 12*(3 Suppl), 53–63. doi:PV352137P5058783 [pii]. https://doi.org/10.1188/08.CJON.S1.53-62.

Faiman, B., Doss, D., Colson, K., Mangan, P., King, T., & Tariman, J. D. (2017). Renal, GI, and peripheral nerves: evidence-based recommendations for the management of symptoms and care for patients with multiple myeloma. *Clinical Journa of Oncology Nursing, 21*(5), 19–36. https://doi.org/10.1188/17.CJON.S5.3-6.

Faiman, B., Richards, T., & Tariman, J. D. (2018). Multiple myeloma. In C. H. Yarbro, D. Wujcik, & B. H. Gobel (Eds.), *Cancer Nursing: Principles and Practice* (pp. 6167–6324). Burlington, MA: Jones and Bartlett Learning.

Gleason, C. (2015). Epidemiology. In J. D. Tariman, & B. Faiman (Eds.), *Multiple myeloma: A textbook for nurses* (2nd ed., pp. 53.69). Pittsburgh, PA: Oncology Nursing Society.

Greipp, P. R., San Miguel, J., Durie, B. G., Crowley, J. J., Barlogie, B., Blade, J., & Westin, J. (2005). International staging system for multiple myeloma. *Journal of Clinical Oncology, 23*(15), 3412–3420. doi:JCO.2005.04.242 [pii]. https://doi.org/10.1200/JCO.2005.04.242.

Kehrer, M., Koob, S., Strauss, A., Wirtz, D. C., & Schmolders, J. (2017). Multiple myeloma - current status in diagnostic testing and therapy. *Z Orthop Unfall, 155*(5), 575–586. https://doi.org/10.1055/s-0043-110224.

Koniarczyk, H. L., Ferraro, C., & Miceli, T. (2017). Hematopoietic stem cell transplantation for multiple myeloma. *Seminars in Oncology Nursing, 33*(3), 265–278. https://doi.org/10.1016/j.soncn.2017.05.004.

Korngold, L., & Lipari, R. (1956). *Multiple-myeloma proteins.* III. The antigenic relationship of Bence Jones proteins to normal gammaglobulin and multiple-myeloma serum proteins. *Cancer, 9*(2), 262–272.

Kuiper, R., van Duin, M., van Vliet, M. H., Broijl, A., van der Holt, B., El Jarari, L., & Sonneveld, P. (2015). Prediction of high- and low-risk multiple myeloma based on gene expression and the International Staging System. *Blood, 126*(17), 1996–2004. https://doi.org/10.1182/blood-2015-05-644039.

Lichtman, M. A. (2010). Obesity and the risk for a hematological malignancy: leukemia, lymphoma, or myeloma. *Oncologist, 15*(10), 1083–1101. https://doi.org/10.1634/theoncologist.2010-0206.

Miceli, T., Lilleby, K., Noonan, K., Kurtin, S., Faiman, B., & Mangan, P. A. (2013). Autologous hematopoietic stem cell transplantation for patients with multiple myeloma: an overview for nurses in community practice. *Clinical Journal of Oncology Nursing, 17*, 13–24. https://doi.org/10.1188/13.CJON.S2.13-24 Suppl.

Mikhael, J. R., Dingli, D., Roy, V., Reeder, C. B., Buadi, F. K., Hayman, S. R., & Mayo, C. (2013). Management of newly diagnosed symptomatic multiple myeloma: updated Mayo Stratification of Myeloma and Risk-Adapted Therapy (mSMART) consensus guidelines 2013. *Mayo Clinic Proceedings, 88*(4), 360–376. https://doi.org/10.1016/j.mayocp.2013.01.019.

National Comprehensive Cancer Network (NCCN) (2018). *NCCN clinical practice guidelines in oncology: multiple myeloma version 4.2018 February 12, 2018.* Retrieved from https://www.nccn.org/professionals/physician_gls/pdf/myeloma.pdf.

Noonan, K. (2015). Pathophysiology. In J. D. Tariman & B. Faiman (Eds.), *Multiple myeloma: A textbook for nurses* (pp. 35–52). Pittsburgh, PA: Oncology Nursing Society.

Palumbo, A., Avet-Loiseau, H., Oliva, S., Lokhorst, H. M., Goldschmidt, H., Rosinol, L., & Moreau, P. (2015). Revised International Staging System for Multiple Myeloma: a report from International Myeloma Working Group. *Journal of Clinical Oncology, 33*(26), 2863–2869. https://doi.org/10.1200/JCO.2015.61.2267. 10.

Pulte, E. D., Dmytrijuk, A., Nie, L., Goldberg, K. B., McKee, A. E., Farrell, A. T., & Pazdur, R. (2018). FDA approval summary: lenalidomide as maintenance therapy after autologous stem cell transplant in newly diagnosed multiple myeloma. *Oncologist.* https://doi.org/10.1634/theoncologist.2017-0440.

Rome, S., Doss, D., Miller, K., & Westphal, J. (2008). Thromboembolic events associated with novel therapies in patients with multiple myeloma: consensus statement of the IMF Nurse Leadership Board. *Clinical Journal of Oncology Nursing, 12*(3 Suppl), 21–28. doi:0JV17R8057786240 [pii]. https://doi.org/10.1188/08.CJON.S1.21-27.

Rome, S., Noonan, K., Bertolotti, P., Tariman, J. D., & Miceli, T. (2017). Bone health, pain, and mobility: evidence-based recommendations for patients with multiple myeloma. *Clinical Journal of Oncology Nursing, 21*(5), 47–59. https://doi.org/10.1188/17.CJON.S5.47-59.

Siegel, R. L., Miller, K. D., & Jemal, A. (2018). Cancer statistics, 2018. *CA: A Cancer Journal for Clinicians, 68*(1), 7–30. https://doi.org/10.3322/caac.21442.

Tariman, J. D., Mehmeti, E., Spawn, N., McCarter, S. P., Bishop-Royse, J., Garcia, I., & Szubski, K. (2016). Oncology nursing and shared decision making for cancer treatment. *Clinical Journal of Oncology Nursing, 20*(5), 560–563. https://doi.org/10.1188/16.CJON.560-563.

Weaver, C. J., & Tariman, J. D. (2017). Multiple myeloma genomics: a systematic review. *Seminars in Oncology Nursing, 33*(3), 237–253. https://doi.org/10.1016/j.soncn.2017.05.001.

Neurologic System Cancers

Mady C. Stovall

I. Physiology and pathophysiology
  A. Brain anatomy and physiology (National Brain Tumor Society, 2018) (Fig. 22.1)
  B. Pathophysiology of central nervous system (CNS) cancers
    1. Primary CNS tumors
      a. Benign—"benign" may suggest a nonmalignant process but has the potential to cause significant morbidity/mortality depending on location, size, and affected structures
        (1) Benign primary brain tumors (PBTs)
        (2) Benign primary spinal tumors—more likely to occur inside the dura but outside the spinal cord (extramedullary); examples include meningiomas, neurofibromas, and schwannomas
      b. Malignant
        (1) Malignant PBT—arise from any cell in the CNS
          (a) Rare for PBT to metastasize outside of CNS
          (b) PBT may invade dura and adjacent structures
          (c) PBT may have drop metastases to spine
        (2) Malignant primary spine tumors
          (a) Frequently arise from intramedullary (within the spinal cord) support cells
          (b) Symptoms determined by tumor location, size, compression of nearby structures (including cerebrospinal fluid [CSF] flow, spinal nerves, or blood vessels)
    2. Metastatic CNS tumors
      a. Spread through hematogenous seeding, direct extension, or invasion to the CNS
II. Epidemiology
  A. CNS tumors—pediatric
    1. Brain and spinal cord tumors are the second most common cancers in children (after leukemia) (American Cancer Society [ACS], 2018)
      a. Prevalence of CNS tumors (Ostrom et al., 2017)
        (1) Pilocytic astrocytoma
          (a) World Health Organization (WHO) grade I glioma
          (b) The most common glioma in children; accounts for 37% of all glioma diagnoses among those under age 20 (Walsh, Ohgaki, & Wrensch, 2016)
        (2) Malignant glioma
        (3) Medulloblastoma
        (4) Neuronal and mixed neuronal-glial tumors
        (5) Ependymoma
      b. Pediatric brain tumors are the leading cause of cancer-related death among children and adolescents ages 0 to 19, surpassing leukemia.
    2. More than 4000 primary CNS tumors are diagnosed in children and teens each year
    3. 75% of children/teens survive more than 5 years after their CNS tumor diagnosis
    4. Tumors most frequently associated with CNS metastases are germ cell tumors and sarcomas (Ostrom, Wright, & Barnholtz-Sloan, 2018)
  B. CNS tumors—adult (ACS, 2018)
    1. Primary CNS tumors
      a. About 23,880 (13,720 males; 10,160 females) primary brain or spinal cord tumors diagnosed in adults each year
        (1) Incidence higher if benign (noncancer) tumors were also included
        (2) About 16,830 people (9490 males; 7340 females) die annually
      b. PBTs (PDQ Adult Treatment Editorial Board, 2018)
        (1) Incidence in decreasing order of frequency
          (a) Glioblastoma and anaplastic astrocytomas (38% of PBT)
          (b) Meningiomas and other mesenchymal tumors (27% of PBT)
          (c) Pituitary tumors
          (d) Schwannomas
          (e) Primary CNS lymphoma
          (f) Oligodendroglioma
          (g) Ependymoma
          (h) Low-grade astrocytoma
          (i) Medulloblastoma

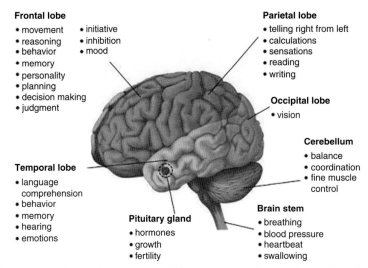

Frontal lobe
- movement
- reasoning
- behavior
- memory
- personality
- planning
- decision making
- judgment
- initiative
- inhibition
- mood

Parietal lobe
- telling right from left
- calculations
- sensations
- reading
- writing

Occipital lobe
- vision

Cerebellum
- balance
- coordination
- fine muscle control

Temporal lobe
- language comprehension
- behavior
- memory
- hearing
- emotions

Pituitary gland
- hormones
- growth
- fertility

Brain stem
- breathing
- blood pressure
- heartbeat
- swallowing

Fig. 22.1 Brain anatomy and physiology. (Courtesy of Schering Corporation, Kenilworth, NJ. In Vassall, E. (2004). *The essential guide to brain tumors*. National Brain Tumor Foundation.)

c. Prevalence (Ostrom et al., 2017)
  (1) Meningiomas make up 36.6% of all PBT
  (2) Gliomas (such as glioblastoma, ependymomas, astrocytomas, and oligodendrogliomas) make-up 74.6% of malignant brain tumors
  (3) An estimated 700,000 Americans are living with a brain tumor
    (a) 80% are benign
    (b) 20% are malignant
d. Primary spine tumors (PDQ Adult Treatment Editorial Board, 2018)
  (1) Incidence in decreasing order of frequency
    (a) Schwannomas, meningiomas, and ependymomas (comprise 79%)
    (b) Sarcomas
    (c) Astrocytomas
    (d) Vascular tumors
    (e) Chordomas
2. CNS metastatic disease
  a. Site of CNS metastatic presentation (Nolan & DeAngelis, 2018)
    (1) Brain 10% to 35%
    (2) Skull 15% to 20%
    (3) Spine 20%
    (4) Leptomeningeal 4% to 15%
    (5) Dura 9% to 10%
  b. Brain metastases (BM) (Ostrom, Wright, & Barnholtz-Sloan, 2018)
    (1) Incidence (PDQ Adult Treatment Editorial Board, 2018)
      (a) 72.2% of individuals across all histologies have solitary BM
      (b) Nearly 37% of individuals across all histologies have at least three BM
    (2) Most common metastatic histologies to brain
      (a) Lung (18%–64%), breast (2%–21%), cancer of unknown primary (1%–18%), colorectal (2%–12%), kidney (1%–8%)
      (b) Lung
        i. Non–small cell lung cancer (NSCLC) accounts for 85% of lung cancer diagnoses; most common primary tumor metastasizing to brain; about 9% of patients with NSCLC develop BM
        ii. About 50% to 60% of those newly diagnosed with small cell lung cancer (SCLC) will develop BM within 2 years
        iii. More likely to present with multiple BMs
        iv. Younger age, larger tumor size, hilar node involvement, lymphovascular space invasion associated with increased risk of BM
        v. 5-year risk of developing BM ≈10% in those who received surgical treatment for stage I to II NSCLC, 24% to 55% in those with stage III
      (c) Breast
        i. Most common type of BM in women
        ii. Likely to present with a single metastasis
        iii. Risks for BM: age <35 years old at time of primary breast cancer

diagnosis, high histologic grade, tumor size >2 cm, node positive

    iv. Higher odds of developing BM in HER2-positive breast cancers compared with other subtypes

(d) Melanoma

    i. Of all tumors, melanoma has strongest affinity to metastasize to CNS

    ii. Likely to present with multiple BMs

    iii. High incidence of hemorrhagic BM

(e) Renal—Likely to present with a single metastasis

(f) Colorectal

    i. Likely to present with a single metastasis

    ii. Survival after diagnosis with BM from gastrointestinal tumors is significantly decreased compared with breast, lung, and renal cancers

(g) Leukemia and lymphoma (American Society of Clinical Oncology Cancer. Net, 2017) also commonly metastasize to the CNS

(h) Biomarker predictors of BM

    i. HER2 in breast cancer

    ii. Anaplastic lymphoma kinase (ALK) gene rearrangement in NSCLC

    iii. BRAF mutations in melanoma

c. Spinal metastases

(1) Leptomeningeal carcinomatosis (PDQ Adult Treatment Editorial Board, 2018)

    (a) Occurs in 5% of all cancer patients

    (b) Median overall survival is ≈ 12 weeks

    (c) Breast tumors (35%), lung tumors (24%), hematologic malignancies (16%)

(2) Site of spinal metastatic presentation

    (a) Epidural 95%

    (b) Intradural extramedullary 4%

    (c) Intramedullary 1%

(3) Vertebral body metastases (Barzilai et al., 2017; Nolan & DeAngelis, 2018)

    (a) Breast, prostate, lung most common

    (b) 40% of tumors that originate outside CNS will metastasize to spine: thoracic 70%, lumbar 20%, cervical 10%

III. Risk factors (Table 22.1)

IV. Diagnostics

A. Neurologic examination (Armitage, 2015)

1. A detailed and accurate history

2. Mental status testing

3. Cranial nerve testing

4. Motor strength testing

5. Sensation testing: light touch, pain, temperature, vibration, proprioception, dermatomal sensory patterns

6. Reflexes

7. Balance and gait

8. Coordination testing

B. Diagnostic imaging examinations (Larsson & Wikström, 2018; Stupp et al., 2014)

1. Computed tomography (CT) of brain and spine

a. Without contrast—helpful at initial presentation to evaluate stroke versus intracranial lesions in persons with new-onset neurologic symptoms

b. With intravenous radiocontrast—surgical and radiation planning or for surveillance of patients not able to get magnetic resonance imaging (MRI)

c. Malignant tumors best visualized with contrast-enhanced scans

(1) CT is test of choice for evaluating spinal bony metastases

    (a) Superior for detecting hemorrhage and calcification

    (b) Less expensive than MRI

(2) MRI of brain and spine

    (a) Without gadolinium—helpful in evaluating edema, nonenhancing tumors, radiation-induced leukoencephalopathy, or acute blood products

    (b) With intravenous gadolinium—test of choice for visualizing brain and spine lesions and for ongoing disease surveillance

    (c) Diagnostic choice in persons with symptoms of brain tumor, soft tissue tumors involving the spine

    (d) High-grade tumors best visualized with contrast

    (e) Superior contrast resolution and multiplanar capability

    (f) MRI CSF flow study for evaluating the flow of CSF around the brain, brainstem, and spinal cord when concern about obstruction exists

    (g) Functional MRI—for identifying areas of eloquent brain preoperatively

    (h) MR spectroscopy—to differentiate normal versus abnormal tissues

(3) Nuclear medicine studies—provide physiologic as opposed to structural picture

    (a) Positron emission tomography (PET)—high sensitivity to high-grade malignancies and radiation necrosis but low specificity

TABLE 22.1 Central Nervous System Tumor Risk Factors

Type of Risk Factor	Risk Factors	References
Known intrinsic risk factors	• Age—children and older adults • Gender—men, glioma; women, meningioma • Race/ethnicity—Caucasian northern European; meningioma more common in African American populations	• American Cancer Society (ACS), 2017 • American Society of Clinical Oncology (ASCO) Cancer.net, 2017
Known situational risk factors	• Epstein–Barr virus increases risk of CNS lymphoma • Exposure to vinyl chloride • Immunocompromised—HIV/AIDS, immunosuppressive medical therapies, congenital immunodeficiency • Injury—history of head trauma associated with meningiomas • Personal history of cancer	• ACS, 2017 • ASCO Cancer.net, 2017 • PDQ Adult Treatment Editorial Board, 2018
Known extrinsic risk factors	• Ionizing radiation (IR)—causal relationship between therapeutic irradiation of doses >2500 cGy and development of brain tumors; risk higher for nerve sheath tumors and meningiomas than gliomas • Children with leukemia—risk highest if treated before age 5 years • Panorex radiography before age 10 associated with increased risk of meningioma • Prior radiation for treatment of *Tinea capitus*—common in the 1950s	• ACS, 2017 • ASCO Cancer.net, 2017
Genetic/inherited risk factors (5%–17% of primary brain tumors associated with genetic disorders)	• Neurofibromatosis 1 (*NF1* gene, 17q11) • Neurofibromatosis 2 (*NF2* gene, 22q12) • Turcot syndrome type 1 (*APC* gene, 3p21, 7p22) • Turcot syndrome type 2 (APC gene, 5q21) • Gorlin syndrome (*PTCH* gene) • Tuberous sclerosis (*TSC1,* 9q34, and *TSC2,* 16p13, genes) • Li–Fraumeni syndrome (*TP53* gene, 17p13) • von-Hippel–Lindau disease (*VHL* gene, 3p25–26) • *BRCA1, BRCA2,* and *PALB2* germline mutations • *P14 (ARF)* germline mutations • Nevoid basal cell carcinoma syndrome (9q22.3) • Brain cancer "clusters" in families without known genetic cause	• ACS, 2017 • ASCO Cancer.net, 2017 • Jackson, LaDuca, & Bergner, 2017 • Kyritsis, Bondy, Rao, & Sioka, 2010 • Zhang et al., 2015 • PDQ Adult Treatment Editorial Board, 2018
Unproven risk factors currently under investigation	• Late menarche in females • Obesity • Exposures—pesticides, vinyl chloride, petrochemicals, electromagnetic fields, inks and solvents, dietary N-nitroso compounds, long-term use of black or brown hair dyes, cell phones, aspartame, and certain viral exposures	• ACS, 2017 • ASCO Cancer.net, 2017

(b) Octreotide scan—may be useful in evaluating malignant meningioma or primitive neuroectodermal tumors

(c) Bone scan—indicated for staging medulloblastoma

(4) Radiography (spine)

(5) Myelography—aids in finding source of spinal compression

(6) Electromyography—detects muscular innervation dysfunctions peripherally

(7) Points of care where neuroimaging is indicated (Stupp et al., 2014)

(a) Preoperatively—identify patterns of cerebral edema or location of lesions

(b) Postoperative imaging with CT or MRI recommended within 24 hours of surgical resection to assess residual tumor volume and establish new baseline to measure treatment effect

(c) Follow-up examinations—every 3 to 4 months is typical standard practice outside of clinical trials unless clinically indicated

C. Diagnostic lumbar puncture

1. Laboratory and pathology evaluations

a. Cell count and differential, glucose level, protein concentration
b. Gram stain, culture, and sensitivity
c. Tumor markers, cytopathology

D. Diagnostic blood tests
1. Serum tests—vary according to primary disease diagnosis; no serum evaluation for diagnosis of gliomas
2. Tumor markers—may include beta-human chorionic gonadotropin (beta-hCG), alpha-fetoprotein (AFP), and placental isoenzyme of alkaline phosphatase (PLAP) for germinoma tumors or teratomas

E. Bone marrow biopsy—workup with CNS lymphoma

F. Neuro-ophthalmology examination—evaluate for intraocular CNS lymphoma

V. Staging, histopathology, genetic, and molecular classification of CNS tumors
A. Brain and spine tumor staging
1. Metastatic CNS malignancies
a. A non-CNS primary tumor metastasizing to brain or spine is a stage IV according to classic tumor–node–metastasis (TNM) staging
2. Primary CNS malignancy staging (PDQ Adult Treatment Editorial Board, 2018)
a. TNM classification not used because two of three indicators are not applicable (no nodes and extracranial metastases extraordinarily rare)
b. WHO classification of CNS that is universally applicable and prognostically valid

(1) WHO grade I—lesions with low proliferative potential, frequently discrete nature, possibility of cure after surgical resection alone.
(2) WHO grade II—lesions generally infiltrating, low in mitotic activity, recur more frequently than grade I, some progress to higher grades
(3) WHO grade III—lesions with histologic evidence of malignancy, for example, nuclear atypia and increased mitotic activity, anaplastic histology and infiltrative capacity. They are usually treated with aggressive adjuvant therapy.
(4) WHO grade IV—lesions mitotically active, necrosis prone, generally associated with a rapid preoperative/postoperative progression and fatal outcomes. Lesions are usually treated with aggressive adjuvant therapy.
c. See Table 22.2 for biomarkers with diagnostic/prognostic value in PBT

VI. Prognosis and survival
A. Primary brain and spine tumors
1. Gliomas
a. Extent of tumor resection, patient age, tumor histology, performance status, molecular markers (1p19q codeletion, isocitrate dehydrogenase (IDH) status, O6-methylguanine-DNA methyltransferase (MGMT) promoter methylation status, Alpha thalassemia/mental retardation syndrome X-linked (ATRX)

TABLE 22.2 Biomarkers in Primary Brain Tumors

Biomarker/Description	Clinical Significance	Source
1p19q codeletion • 1p and 19q chromosome arms	• 1p/19q codeletion has predictive value for response to chemotherapy in surgically diagnosed anaplastic oligodendrogliomas with nearly a doubling of survival in those treated with procarbazine–lomustine–vincristine plus radiotherapy compared with those being treated with radiotherapy alone • 1p/19q codeletion is a strong independent prognostic biomarker associated with improved survival in both diffuse low-grade and anaplastic brain tumors • With very few exceptions, 1p/19q codeletion is mutually exclusive with *TP53* and *ATRX* mutation	Cairncross et al., 2013 van den Bent et al., 2013
ATRX • Alpha thalassemia/mental retardation syndrome X-linked (ATRX) gene • A telomere maintenance–related gene	• 90% of IDH-mutant diffuse gliomas have mutations in ATRX and/or TERT • IDH wild-type glioblastomas, ATRX alterations are associated with favorable outcomes	Pekmezci et al., 2017
BRAF • Human gene that encodes a protein belonging to the RAF family of serine/threonine protein kinases	• Tandem duplication at 7q34 leading to a fusion between KIAA1549 and BRAF is found in approximately 70% of pilocytic astrocytomas	PDQ Adult Treatment

Continued

TABLE 22.2   Biomarkers in Primary Brain Tumors—cont'd

Biomarker/Description	Clinical Significance	Source
• Plays a role in regulating the MAP kinase/ERK signaling pathway, which affects cell division, differentiation, and secretion • Mutation of valine 600 to glutamic acid (V600E) is the most prevalent BRAF mutation	• An activating point mutation in BRAF (V600E) is found in an additional 5%–9% of these tumors, and in general, RAF alterations occur in approximately 80% of pilocytic astrocytomas • BRAF V600E mutations are observed (in about 60%) of other benign glioma variants, including pleomorphic xanthoastrocytoma and ganglioglioma, whereas BRAF tandem duplications are not found in these variant glioma tumors.	Editorial Board, 2018

EGFR
• Epidermal growth factor receptor
• Tyrosine kinase ligand
• Exists on cell surface
• Activated by various growth factors, which leads to cell proliferation
	• EGFR expression
	  • Amplified ≈50% of primary glioblastoma
	  • Associated with poor prognosis
	• Coexpression of *EGFR* deletion mutant variant III (*EGFRvIII*) with PTEN poor prognostic indicator
	• *EGFRvIII* expression associated with worse prognosis than wild-type EGFR expression (amplification) alone
		Abdullah, Adamson, & Brem, 2016

IDH • Isocitrate dehydrogenase 1 (IDH1) • Isocitrate dehydrogenase 2 (IDH2) • Enzyme mutations found in multiple human cancers	• *IDH1* and *IDH2* mutations occur in a mutually exclusive manner in nearly 80% of grades II and III oligodendrogliomas and astrocytomas and secondary glioblastomas • IDH-mutant tumors frequently have other molecular alterations, including 1p/19q codeletion, *CIC*, *FUBP* and *TERT* promoter mutations • Presence of IDH2 mutation predicts improved sensitivity of glioma to radiation	Pekmezci et al., 2017
INI$_1$ • A member of the SWI/SNF chromatin remodeling complex located on chromosome 22q11.2, hSNF5/SMARCB1 • *INI$_1$* gene deletion or mutation	• Deletion or mutation in atypical teratoid/rhabdoid tumors	Abdullah et al., 2016
PTEN • Phosphatase and tensin homolog • Protein encoded by PTEN gene • Plays roll in cancer suppression	• PTEN loss (mutation) associated with proliferation of glioblastoma	Abdullah et al., 2016
TERT • Telomerase reverse transcriptase gene promoter mutation • A telomere maintenance-related gene	• In IDH-mutant 1p/19q-codeleted oligodendrogliomas, those tumors with TERT wild type have significantly worse overall survival than those with TERT mutation • In IDH wild-type astrocytomas, TERT wild type has significantly better overall survival than the TERT mutation group	Pekmezci et al., 2017
MGMT • Methyl-guanine methyl transferase (MGMT) gene • The protein encoded by MGMT is a DNA repair protein that is involved in cellular defense against mutagenesis and toxicity from alkylating agents. The protein catalyzes transfer of methyl groups from O(6)-alkylguanine and other methylated moieties of the DNA to its own molecule, which repairs the toxic lesions.	• Methylation of the MGMT promoter has been associated with several cancer types, including colorectal cancer, lung cancer, lymphoma, and glioblastoma • MGMT promoter methylation is associated with more favorable response to alkylating agents	Stupp et al., 2014

mutation) predictive of outcome (Hervey-Jumper & Berger, 2016).

  b. Expected median survival with glioma (Stupp et al., 2014)

    (1) Grade II

      (a) Astrocytoma—7 to 10 years

      (b) Oligodendroglioma with 1p/19q codeletion—>10 to 15 years

    (2) Grade III

      (a) Anaplastic astrocytoma—3.5 years

      (b) Anaplastic oligodendroglioma with 1p/19q codeletion—> 10 years

    (3) Grade IV – Glioblastoma—15 months, 2-year survival 27%

      (a) MGMT methylated—23 months, 2-year survival 49%

      (b) MGMT unmethylated—13 months, 2-year survival 12%

  c. Malignant transformation of low-grade gliomas ranges from 4 to 29 months; roughly 45% of patients with diffuse low-grade WHO grade II glioma undergo transformation to anaplastic (WHO grade III) glioma within 5 years (Hervey-Jumper & Berger, 2016).

B. Metastatic brain and spine tumors

  1. BMs (Nolan & DeAngelis, 2018)

    a. Prognostic factors vary according to the cancer type and include number of BM, age, Karnofsky Performance Score, and extent of systemic disease.

    b. Survival for patients with BM is poor, typically in the range of 3 to 6 months.

    c. Age <65 years, Karnofsky Performance Score >70, and controlled systemic disease are predictors of better overall survival (OS), with median OS of 7.1 months versus an OS of 2.3 months if all factors were poor

  2. Spine metastases (SM)

    a. Only 10% to 20% of patients with SM will be alive 2 years after initial diagnosis

    b. Poor performance status at diagnosis strongest predictor of poor OS; low systemic disease load and favorable tumor histology are associated with increased OS

  3. Leptomeningeal carcinomatosis

    a. Median overall survival 10 to 12 weeks

VII. Management—surgery, radiation, chemo/biotherapy, clinical trials, active surveillance

A. Surgery

  1. Brain tumor surgical management (Hervey-Jumper & Berger, 2016)

    a. Goals of brain surgery

      (1) Symptom relief (i.e., reduction in mass effect)

      (2) Obtaining a diagnosis (initial or restaging)

      (3) Cytoreduction

    b. Brain surgical intervention—provides tissue diagnosis and may improve outcomes (survival and global functioning)

      (1) Gross total—removal of all measurable tumor tissue; may improve response to therapy due to smaller residual tumor volume

      (2) Subtotal resection—removal of measurable tumor volume; preferred resection type if tumor near eloquent areas and aggressive surgical approach could result in worse neurologic deficits

      (3) Stereotactic brain biopsy—goal is to obtain a tissue diagnosis

        (a) Preferred method if tumor near eloquent areas, location difficult to access, or very poor surgical candidate

        (b) Risk for sampling error due to small volume obtained with needle sample; may result in underdiagnosis

  2. Spine tumor surgical management (Barzilai et al., 2017)

    a. Goals for spinal surgery

      (1) Obtain tissue diagnosis: biopsy, surgical resection

      (2) Symptom relief

        (a) Preservation or restoration of neurologic function and ambulation

        (b) Maintain spinal stability

        (c) Durable local tumor control

        (d) Improved quality of life (e.g. pain control, neurologic preservation)

    b. Indications for spinal surgery

      (1) Neurologic status is deteriorating

      (2) Unknown tumor type

      (3) Tumor is not radiosensitive

B. Radiation (see Chapter 27)

  1. Primary brain tumor radiation (PDQ Adult Treatment Editorial Board, 2018)

    a. High-grade gliomas (WHO grade III or IV) or other high-grade PBT

      (1) External beam radiation therapy (EBRT)

        (a) Conformal or intensity-modulated radiation therapy (RT)

        (b) Thirty fractions over 6 weeks totaling 60 Gy

        (c) Treat tumor plus 2- to 3-cm margins on the MRI-based volumes

        (d) EBRT is standard first-line adjuvant therapy with or without concurrent adjuvant chemotherapy after surgical diagnosis

        (e) Provides a significant survival advantage compared with no EBRT

      (2) No survival or quality-of-life benefit has been demonstrated with alternative RT

strategies (i.e., radiosurgery with or without EBRT, hypofractionated RT, brachytherapy)
  b. Low-grade gliomas (WHO I or II) or other low-grade PBT
     (1) Although there is a delayed time to progression in low-grade tumors treated with EBRT up-front, there is no difference in overall survival compared with waiting until progression of disease to treat with EBRT
     (2) Treatment plan would be the same as with high-grade gliomas
  c. Maximum tolerable dose to normal brain is considered 60 Gy
2. Primary spine tumor radiation (NCCN, 2017)
  a. Intradural intramedullary tumor well defined/well circumscribed
     (1) EBRT only if symptomatic
  b. Intradural intramedullary tumor poorly defined/infiltrative
     (1) EBRT depends on tumor histology, presentation, and symptoms
  c. Intradural extramedullary
     (1) Single versus multiple lesions
     (2) RT decision depends on surgical candidacy, symptoms, and goals of therapy
  d. Multidisciplinary input for treatment planning
3. Metastatic CNS malignancy radiation
  a. BMs (Nolan & DeAngelis, 2018)
     (1) Single BM—radiosurgery ± surgical resection
     (2) Multiple BMs
        (a) Whole brain radiation therapy (WBRT) is the mainstay of treatment
        (b) Radiation is palliative
        (c) If one to three BM, consider stereotactic radiosurgery (SRS) alone (16–24 Gy); more than four BM, consider WBRT
        (d) Hypofractionated radiosurgery (21–25 Gy over three to five fractions) recommended for BM >3 cm due to high risk of radiation necrosis
  b. SMs (Barzilai et al., 2017)
     (1) Neurologic, oncologic, mechanical instability, and systemic disease (NOMS) framework for principled assessments in treatment decision making for SM
     (2) Location of disease in the spine, mechanical instability, neurology, oncology, and patient fitness; prognosis; and response to prior therapy (LMNOP) framework is intended to provide general guidance

based on key principles to radiation oncologists and spine surgeons (Spratt et al., 2017)
     (3) Surgery and radiation are the mainstay of treatment for SM
     (4) Conventional EBRT (cEBRT)
        (a) Typically 30 Gy over 10 fractions
        (b) Tumor histology is most important predictor for response to cEBRT
     (5) SRS—single (16–24 Gy) or hypofractionated (24–30 Gy over two to three fractions)
C. Chemotherapy/biotherapy (NCCN, 2017; PDQ Adult Treatment Editorial Board, 2018; Stupp et al., 2014)
  1. PBT
     a. Gliomas
        (1) Low-grade gliomas
           (a) Temozolomide depending on disease burden or progression status
           (b) Consider lomustine or carmustine, procarbazine with lomustine and vincristine (PCV), or platinum-based therapy after temozolomide failure
        (2) High-grade gliomas
           (a) Anaplastic gliomas and glioblastoma
              i. Temozolomide is the standard of care for adjuvant treatment of anaplastic astrocytoma after surgery and radiation and in glioblastoma concurrently with radiation therapy, then adjuvant
              ii. Other cytotoxic treatments after temozolomide has failed to provide benefit include lomustine or carmustine, PCV, or platinum-based therapy
              iii. Implanted carmustine-impregnated wafers—Food and Drug Administration (FDA)–approved therapy; used more at second or third craniotomy resecting recurrent or progressive high-grade gliomas in heavily treated individuals
              iv. Bevacizumab—for progressive glioblastoma
                 ◆ Generally, well tolerated; risks include hypertension, proteinuria, vascular events such as stroke and intracranial bleed, gastrointestinal perforation
                 ◆ To manage radiation necrosis–related cerebral edema (Levin et al., 2011)

(b) Anaplastic oligodendrogliomas
   i. Patients with 1p/19q codeleted tumors should be treated with PCV after RT, depending on ability to tolerate therapy
   ii. At progression, temozolomide and nitrosoureas should be considered
   iii. Other regimens include cyclophosphamide, platinum-based regimens, irinotecan, or etoposide
b. Medulloblastoma and supratentorial primitive neuroectodermal tumors (PNET)
   (1) Optimal use of adjuvant chemotherapy for adults is unclear
   (2) At recurrence, drugs used include etoposide, temozolomide, and high-dose chemotherapy with autologous stem cell transplant
c. CNS lymphoma
   (1) High-dose methotrexate (MTX)–based regimens (3.5 g/m^2 or higher)
   (2) If CSF or spinal MRI positive, intra-CNS chemotherapy considered
   (3) If eye examination positive, intraocular chemotherapy considered
   (4) Other agents used in combination with MTX include dexamethasone, vincristine, procarbazine, cytarabine, rituximab, and ifosfamide
2. Ependymoma
   a. The role of chemotherapy is poorly defined
   b. Sometimes considered palliative after RT has failed to control the disease with drugs such as carboplatin or cisplatin, etoposide, lomustine or carmustine, bevacizumab, and temozolomide
3. Meningiomas
   a. Cytotoxic therapies generally not efficacious
   b. Refractory meningiomas may benefit from somatostatin analogs or α interferon
4. Metastatic brain and spine tumors
   a. Systemic chemo/biotherapy not routine treatment for brain/spine metastasis due to
      (1) Poor penetration through blood–brain barrier (BBB)
      (2) Heavily pretreated tumors are less chemosensitive
   b. Breast cancer
      (1) MTX may be an option
      (2) Platinum plus etoposide
      (3) Capecitabine with or without lapatinib
   c. Melanoma
      (1) Ipilimumab and BRAF inhibitors (dabrafenib and vemurafenib)
      (2) Temozolomide may be useful in some patients

d. Leptomeningeal metastases (LM)
   (1) Intrathecal chemotherapy
      (a) MTX for breast cancer, lymphoma, and leukemia
      (b) Cytarabine and liposomal cytarabine for lymphoma and leukemia
      (c) Thiotepa
      (d) Rituximab for lymphoma
      (e) Topotecan
      (f) Etoposide
      (g) Trastuzumab for breast cancer
      (h) Interferon alpha
   (2) High-dose MTX for breast LM
   (3) Weekly pulse erlotinib for NSCLC with epidermal growth factor receptor (EGFR) exon 19 or exon 21 deletions
e. Corticosteroids to manage spinal cord compression range from 10 to 96 mg per day
D. Tumor-treating fields (TTFields) (Mehta et al., 2017)
   1. Optune is a portable, battery-operated device that generates TTFields and is designed to be worn continuously for the treatment of supratentorial glioblastoma
   2. TTFields produce antimitotic effects by physically interacting with highly charged macromolecules and organelles in rapidly dividing cancer cells to disrupt their proper alignment during different stages of mitosis
   3. TTFields plus temozolomide (TMZ) compared with TMZ alone after concomitant TMZ and radiotherapy in newly diagnosed glioblastoma patients demonstrated statistically significant improvement in survival (Mehta et al, 2017; Stupp et al., 2015)
   4. TTFields approved as monotherapy in patients with recurrent glioblastoma; approved treatment option without systemic side effects for patients with recurrent glioblastoma who did not have TTFields plus TMZ as first-line therapy
E. Blood and marrow transplantation—used for treatment of recurrent medulloblastoma
F. Clinical trials—experimental treatment regimens should be considered at all stages of disease as appropriate based upon availability, functional status, and desire
G. Medical interventions for symptom management
   1. Glucocorticoids
      a. High dose to manage acute cerebral edema
      b. High dose to manage extradural spinal lesions causing compression of spinal cord
      c. Dosed 16 mg or more per day; use the lowest possible dose for the shortest time possible to reduce serious steroid-related complications such as myopathy, diabetes, infections, and other comorbid conditions

2. Mannitol
   a. Generally used only in emergency situations to capitalize on the osmotic properties of mannitol effects on brain edema resulting from leakage of plasma into the brain parenchyma through dysfunctional cerebral capillaries
   b. Only administered in intensive care unit (ICU) setting
   c. Often last effort for cerebral edema management if bevacizumab is not an option
3. Ventricular interventions
   a. Ventriculoperitoneal (VP) shunt—placed for management of hydrocephalus
      (1) Programmable VP shunt—may be affected by magnetic fields during MRI; patient will require plain film within 4 hours of MRI to assess valve settings.
      (2) Nonprogrammable VP shunt
   b. Ommaya reservoir—placed for delivery of intrathecal chemotherapy
   c. Ventriculostomy—performed to relieve pressure within the CNS

VIII. Nursing implications
   A. Assessment and management of symptoms—symptoms are related to the tumor or related to the treatment, as there is frequent overlap
      1. Fatigue (Cahill et al., 2012; Stupp et al., 2014)- most frequent and severe symptom reported by persons with PBT
      2. Headache
         a. Head pain or headache in PBT is the strongest independent predictor of BM
         b. Less prevalent in survivors of PBT
      3. Nausea and vomiting (N/V)—common at diagnosis in 30% to 40% PBT
      4. Neurologic/mental status symptoms
         a. Sensory changes with vision, hearing, or smelling are common at presentation for all BT types; numbness and tingling may be present in 15% of PBT
         b. Dizziness, weakness, gait instability, coordination, and balance symptoms are broadly associated with BM from all tumor types
      5. Seizures
         a. Presenting symptom in 15% of PBT, in 20% of BM
         b. Risk highest with cortical tumors; temporal tumors tend to be most epileptogenic
         c. Antiepileptic drug (AED) therapy indicated in those with seizures and during the perioperative craniotomy setting; prophylactic use of anticonvulsants not indicated otherwise
            (1) First-line agents: lamotrigine, levetiracetam, pregabalin, or valproic acid
            (2) First-generation AEDs are strong inducers of hepatic metabolism and are not preferred (i.e., phenytoin, carbamazepine,

phenobarbital, and their derivatives) due to numerous drug interactions
6. Venous thrombotic events, for example, deep vein thrombosis (DVT), pulmonary embolism (PE)
   a. Glioma patients at increased risk due to tumor-induced hypercoagulable state, neurologic deficits, immobility, steroid use, and chemotherapy treatments
   b. 20% to 30% of glioma patients will have a DVT or PE
   c. Standard anticoagulant treatment not contraindicated in patients with brain tumor
7. Corticosteroid use and associated complications
   a. Dexamethasone (8–16 mg/day) to manage tumor-associated cerebral edema and improve clinical symptoms
   b. Monitor blood glucose
   c. Long-term therapy complications: hyperglycemia, myopathy, weakness, lymphopenia, increased risk of infection, osteoporosis, insomnia, agitation, Cushing syndrome
8. Toxicities of treatment
   a. Radiation complications
      (1) Acute effects (during and immediately after radiation therapy)
         (a) Global—headaches, neurocognitive changes, seizures, and somnolence
         (b) Focal—specific neurologic deficits based on tumor location
      (2) Subacute effects (within weeks to 4–6 months after radiation)
         (a) Somnolence, exacerbation of tumor-related symptoms
      (3) Late radiation effects (occurring >6 months to several years after RT)
         (a) Radiation necrosis
         (b) Diffuse white matter changes
         (c) Neurocognitive effects
         (d) Cerebrovascular events
         (e) Optic nerve toxicities
         (f) Endocrine toxicities
         (g) Secondary malignancies
            i. Most common—meningiomas, gliomas, and nerve sheath tumors
            ii. Risk greatest with cranial radiation given to young children
   B. Oncologic emergencies (see Chapters 52 and 53)
   C. Caregiver burden (Saria et al., 2017) (see Chapter 48)

REFERENCES

Abdullah, K. G., Adamson, C., & Brem, S. (2016). The molecular pathogenesis of glioblastoma. In S. Brem, & K. G. Abdullah (Eds.), *Glioblastoma* (pp. 21–31). https://doi.org/10.1016/B978-0-323-47660-7.0003-3.

American Cancer Society. (2017). *Risk factors for brain and spinal cord tumors*. Retrieved 3/11/2018 from: https://www.cancer.org/cancer/brain-spinal-cord-tumors-adults/causes-risks-prevention/risk-factors.html.

American Cancer Society. (2018). *Key statistics for brain and spinal cord tumors in children*. Retrieved 3/11/2018 from: https://www.cancer.org/cancer/brain-spinal-cord-tumors-children/about/key-statistics.html.

American Society of Clinical Oncology (ASCO) Cancer.net. (2017). *Brain tumor: risk factors*. Retrieved 3/11/2018 from: https://www.cancer.net/cancer-types/brain-tumor/risk-factors.

Armitage, A. (2015). *Advanced Practice Nursing Guide to the Neurological Exam*. New York: Springer Publishing Company.

Barzilai, O., Laufer, I., Yamada, Y., Higginson, D. S., Schmitt, A. M., Lis, E., et al. (2017). Integrating evidence-based medicine for treatment of spinal metastases into a decision framework: neurologic, oncologic, mechanical stability, and systemic disease. *Journal of Clinical Oncology, 35*(21), 2419–2427. https://doi.org/10.1200/JCO.2017.72.7362.

Cahill, J., LoBiondo-Wood, G., Bergstrom, N., & Armstrong, T. (2012). Brain tumor symptoms as antecedents to uncertainty: an integrative review. *Journal of Nursing Scholarship, 44*(2), 145–155. https://doi.org/10.1111/j.1547-5069.2012.01445.x.

Cairncross, G., Wang, M., Shaw, E., et al. (2013). Phase III trial of chemoradiotherapy for anaplastic oligodendroglioma: long-term results of RTOG 9402. *Journal of Clinical Oncology, 31*, 337–343.

Hervey-Jumper, S. L., & Berger, M. S. (2016). Maximizing safe resection of low- and high-grade glioma. *Journal of Neuro-Oncology, 130*(2), 269–282. https://doi.org/10.1007/s11060-016-2110-4.

Kyritsis, A. P., Bondy, M. L., Rao, J. S., & Sioka, C. (2010). Inherited predisposition to glioma. *Neuro-Oncology, 12*(1), 104–113. https://doi.org/10.1093/neuonc/nop011.

Larsson, E.M. & Wikström, J. (2018). Overview of neuroradiology. In G.G. Kovacs and I. Alafuzoff (Eds.), *Handbook of Clinical Neurology: Neuropathology 145*, 579-599. doi: https://doi.org/10.1016/B978-0-12-802395-2.00037-7

Levin, V. A., Bidaut, L., Hou, P., Kumar, A. J., Wefel, J. S., Bekele, B. N., et al. (2011). Randomized double-blind placebo-controlled trial of bevacizumab therapy for radiation necrosis of the central nervous system. *International Journal of Radiation Oncology, Biology, and Physics, 79*(5), 1487–1495. https://doi.org/10.1016/j.ijrobp.2009.12.061.

Mehta, M., Wen, P., Nishikawa, R., Reardon, D., & Peters, K. (2017). Critical review of the addition of tumor treating fields (TTFields) to the existing standard of care for newly diagnosed glioblastoma patients. *Critical Reviews in Oncology/Hematology, 11*, 60–65. https://doi.org/10.1016/j.critrevonc.2017.01.005.

National Brain Tumor Society. (2018). *Brain structures and their functions*. Available online http://braintumor.org/brain-tumor-information/signs-and-symptoms/.

National Comprehensive Cancer Center Network. (2017). NCCN guidelines version 1.2017. In *Central nervous system cancers*.

Nolan, C., & Deangelis, L. M. (2018). Overview of metastatic disease of the central nervous system. *Handb Clin Neurol, 149*, 3–23. https://doi.org/10.1016/B978-0-12-811161-1.00001-3.

Ostrom, Q. T., Gittleman, H., Liao, P., Vecchione-Koval, T., Wolinsky, Y., Kruchko, C., et al. (2017). CBTRUS Statistical report: primary brain and other central nervous system tumors diagnosed in the United States in 2010–2014. *Neuro-Oncology, 19*(S5), v1–v88. https://doi.org/10.1093/neuonc/nox158.

Ostrom, Q. T., Wright, C. H., & Barnholtz-Sloan, J. S. (2018). Brain metastases: epidemiology. In: D.Schiff and M.J. van den Bent (Ed.), 149. *Handbook of Clinical Neurology, Metastatic Disease of the Nervous System* (pp. 2–287). https://doi.org/10.1016/B978-0-12-811161-1.00002-5.

PDQ Adult Treatment Editorial Board. (2018) Adult Central Nervous System Tumors Treatment (PDQ®). Health Professional Version. *PDQ Cancer Information Summaries* [Internet]. Bethesda (MD): National Cancer Institute (US); 2002. Available online https://www.ncbi.nlm.nih.gov/pubmedhealth/PMH0032627

Pekmezci, M., Rice, T., Molinaro, A. M., Walsh, K. M., Decker, P. A., Hansen, H., et al. (2017). Adult infiltrating gliomas with WHO 2016 integrated diagnosis: additional prognostic roles of ATRX and TERT. *Acta Neuropathologica, 133*(6), 1001–1016. https://doi.org/10.1007/s00401-017-1690-1.

Saria, M. G., Nyamathi, A., Philips, L. R., Stanton, A. L., Evangelista, L., Kesari, S., et al. (2017). The hidden morbidity of cancer: burden in caregivers of patients with brain metastases. *Nursing Clinics of North America, 52*(1), 159–178. https://doi.org/10.1016/j.cnur.2016.10.002.

Spratt, D.E., Beeler, W.H., de Moraes, F.Y., Rhines, L.D., Gemmete, J.J., Chaudhary, N., ... and Szerlip, N.J. (2017). An integrated multidisciplinary algorithm for the management of spinal metastases: an International Spine Oncology Consortium report. *Lancet Oncology, 18*(12), e720-e730. doi: https://doi.org/10.1016/S1470-2045(17)30612-5

Stupp, R., Brada, M., van den Bent, M. J., Tonn, T.-C., & Pentheroudakis, G. (2014). High-grade glioma: ESMO clinical practice guidelines for diagnosis, treatment and follow-up. *Annals of Oncology, 25*(S3), iii93–iii101. https://doi.org/10.1093/annonc/mdu050.

Stupp, R., Taillibert, S., Kanner, A. A., Kesari, S., Steinberg, D. M., Toms, S. A., et al. (2015). Maintenance therapy with tumor-treating fields plus temozolomide vs temozolomide alone for glioblastoma: a randomized clinical trial. *JAMA, 314*(23), 2535–2543. https://doi.org/10.1001/jama.2015.16669.

van den Bent, M., Brandes, A., Taphoorn, M., et al.(2013). Adjuvant procarbazine, lomustine, and vincristine chemotherapy in newly diagnosed anaplastic oligodendroglioma: long-term follow-up of EORTC brain tumor group study 26951. *Journal of Clinical Oncology, 31*, 344–350.

Walsh, K. M., Ohgaki, H., & Wrensch, M. R. (2016). Epidemiology. In: M. S. Berger, & M. Weller (Eds.), 134. *Handbook of Clinical Neurology, Gliomas*, (pp. 3–18). https://doi.org/10.1016/B978-0-12-802997-8.00001-3.

Zhang, J., Walsh, M., Wu, G., Edmonson, M. N., Gruber, T. A., Easton, J., Hedges, M. N., & Downing, J. (2015). Germline mutations in predisposition genes in pediatric cancer. *New England Journal of Medicine, 373*, 2336–2346. https://doi.org/10.1056/NEJMoa1508054.

23

Reproductive System Cancers

Denise Falardeau

OVERVIEW

Cervical Cancer

I. Physiology and pathophysiology of the cervix uteri
  A. The cervix is the narrow lower end of the uterus that forms a canal between the uterine cavity and vaginal canal.
  B. The exocervix (squamous epithelial cells) and endocervix (columnar glandular epithelial cells) meet at the squamocolumnar junction (transition zone), which is the site of most pathologic changes.

II. Epidemiology
  A. Fourth most common cancer in women worldwide, with 90% of associated deaths in low- to middle-income countries (WHO, 2017) due to lack of prevention, screening, and early treatment resources.
  B. Deaths in the U.S. have decreased since implementation of Papanicolaou (Pap) test screening for preinvasive disease (Siegel, Miller, & Jemal., 2017).

III. Risk factors
  A. Infection with oncogenic HPV type 16, 18, 31, 33, 35, 39, 45, 51, 52, 56, 58, or 59
  B. Multiple partners, early age at intercourse, history of dysplasia, family history, smoking, born to a mother using DES during pregnancy (ACOG, 2015), chronic immunosuppression, and oral contraceptive (OCP) use (NCCN, 2018a)

IV. Prevention
  A. Vaccination for HPV type 16, 18, 31, 33, 45, 52, and 58 (Bailey et al., 2016)
  B. Screening per guidelines (see Chapter 2) with cervical cytology/Pap test, human papillomavirus (HPV) DNA testing, and visual inspection (Jeronimo et al., 2017)

V. Histopathology: two main histology types include squamous cell carcinomas (80% of cases) and adenocarcinoma (20% of cases) (NCCN, 2018a)

VI. Histologic grade
  A. Precancerous changes include cervical intraepithelial neoplasia (CIN grades 1, 2, 3), atypical squamous cells (ASC), and adenocarcinoma in situ (AIS) (Jeronimo et al., 2017).
  B. Grading by degree of differentiation: unable to assess (GX), well (G1), moderately (G2), or poorly/undifferentiated (G3) (Amin, et al., 2017).

VII. Diagnosis and staging (NCCN, 2018a)
  A. Carcinoma in situ is stage 0 noninvasive disease
  B. Clinical diagnosis: watery vaginal discharge, postcoital bleeding, intermittent spotting, and abnormal pelvic examination.
  C. Tissue diagnosis by Pap smear, colposcopy, cone, or LEEP (loop electrosurgical excision procedure) biopsy, endocervical curettage, and indicated imaging with chest radiograph, computed tomography (CT), positron emission tomography/computed tomography (PET/CT), magnetic resonance imaging (MRI), cystoscopy, proctoscopy, barium enema

VIII. Prognosis and survival
  A. Prognosis is related to stage at diagnosis.
  B. U.S. 5-year relative survival by stage at diagnosis: localized (91.5%), regional (57.1%), distant (17.3%), unstaged (52.2%) (NCI, 2017a)

IX. Treatment (NCCN, 2018a)
  A. Preinvasive disease (CIN1–3) may be treated by diagnostic modality (LEEP, cone biopsy), local cauterization or cryotherapy, or hysterectomy if fertility sparing is not desired.
  B. Treatments for early-stage disease (IA1–IB1)
    1. Fertility sparing: conization with cold knife or LEEP procedure, lymph node evaluation if lymphovascular space invasion (LVSI) is present, radical trachelectomy.
    2. Non–fertility sparing: simple or modified radical hysterectomy with or without lymph node evaluation.
  C. Treatments for more advanced stages
    1. Select IIA1 disease: radical hysterectomy, lymph node evaluation
    2. IB2, IIA2, or greater nonsurgical candidates: definitive chemoradiation (with or without ovarian transposition if premenopausal), possibly neoadjuvant chemotherapy followed by resection
    3. Primary treatment followed by observation, external beam radiation therapy (EBRT), and/or adjuvant chemotherapy

D. Recurrent disease: radiation therapy (RT), systemic therapy, local ablation, surgical resection

E. Metastatic disease: RT with or without chemotherapy, palliative systemic agents, best supportive care

X. Nursing implications

A. Client safety and risk reduction: identify high-risk populations, limit sexual partners, HPV vaccination, regular screening examinations, smoking/tobacco cessation.

B. Manage treatment- and cancer-related symptoms

1. Cancer-related symptoms can include significant bleeding, pain, urinary or bowel obstruction/invasion, and complications of metastatic sites of local structures, lymph nodes, and distant sites.

2. Abdominal/pelvic surgery: alterations in urinary, bowel, and vaginal function. Management of catheterization, urinary tract infection, constipation, bowel obstruction, and shortening of the vagina. Preoperative and postoperative care, including risks for bleeding, infection, deep vein thrombosis (DVT), lymphedema after lymph node dissection (LND). See Chapter 25.

3. Abdominal/pelvic RT: changes in bowel and urinary function may include loose stools, obstructions, fistula formation, ulceration, pain, radiation cystitis, and urinary frequency or retention. Changes in vaginal function may involve stenosis, dryness, and atrophy. See Chapter 27.

4. Systemic agents and toxicities: cisplatin, fluorouracil, carboplatin, paclitaxel, topotecan, and bevacizumab. Particular attention to renal and hepatic function, CINV, hypersensitivity reactions, myelosuppression, and neuropathy. See Chapter 28 for more information on chemotherapies.

C. Assess for signs of recurrent disease: pain, changes in bowel/bladder, vaginal bleeding, leg swelling, groin mass/changes, abnormal follow-up examination.

D. Sexual and reproductive function

1. Even with fertility-sparing treatment, changes in vaginal function may still affect sexual function. Encourage open communication with the patient, provider, and sexual partner. Contraception should be used during and for a period after active treatment, depending on treatment type.

2. Non–fertility sparing: discuss infertility with patient, partner, and provider before treatment starts.

3. Use vaginal dilators, different sexual positions, and vaginal lubricants.

Uterine Cancer

I. Physiology and pathophysiology

A. The uterus is the female reproductive organ consisting of the endometrium (most common site of uterine cancers), myometrium, and perimetrium.

B. The endometrium is the innermost layer of the uterus, hormonally driven (estrogen, progesterone) for vascular proliferation to support the fetus.

II. Epidemiology

A. Sixth most common cancer in women worldwide (WCRF, 2017a)

B. U.S. and trends (NCCN, 2018b; NCI, 2017d)

1. Most common cancer of the female genital tract in the U.S. with stable incidence but increasing mortality annually 2005 to 2014.

2. Incidence is highest in women age 55 to 64, mortality highest age 65 to 74, and disproportionately represented in African American women.

III. Risk factors (NCCN, 2018b).

A. Modifiable: increased estrogen caused by obesity, diabetes, high-fat diet.

B. Early age at menarche, late menopause, hereditary nonpolyposis colorectal cancer (HNPCC)/Lynch syndrome (60% lifetime risk of endometrial cancer), age ≥55 years, tamoxifen use, nulliparity.

IV. Prevention

A. Weight and dietary management should be encouraged, along with urgent evaluation of any postmenopausal bleeding.

B. HNPCC is indicated for personal/family history of endometrial or colon cancer before age 50. For individuals with HNPCC: annual endometrial biopsy (fertility sparing) or prophylactic hysterectomy if desired (NCCN, 2018b).

V. Histopathology (NCCN, 2018b)

A. Atypical hyperplasia is not malignant, but should be further evaluated and treated.

B. Epithelial tumors: pure endometrioid cancer (most common), uterine serous carcinoma, clear cell carcinoma, carcinosarcoma (malignant mixed mullerian tumor), and undifferentiated carcinoma.

C. Stroma tumors: uterine leiomyosarcoma, endometrial stromal sarcoma, undifferentiated sarcoma, adenosarcoma, and perivascular epithelioid cell neoplasm

VI. Molecular classification

A. Estrogen receptor/progesterone receptor testing (NCCN, 2018b)

B. Testing for microsatellite instability (DNA mismatch repair system)

VII. Histologic grade: reported as degree of differentiation (Gx, G1, G2, G3)

VIII. Diagnosis and staging (NCCN, 2018b)

A. Clinical presentation of irregular or postmenopausal bleeding, thickened endometrium, or abnormal pelvic examination. Clinical staging with imaging studies (CT, MRI, PET/CT).

B. Pathologic diagnosis by endometrial biopsy, fractional dilation and curettage (D&C), and/or endocervical curettage to rule out cervical cancer. Hysteroscopy to evaluate polyps or persistent undiagnosed bleeding.

C. Surgical staging with total hysterectomy with bilateral salpingo-oophorectomy (TH/BSO), peritoneal washings, evaluation of lymph nodes, and detailed pathologic review.

IX. Prognosis and survival (NCI, 2017d)
  A. U.S. overall 5-year survival 81.3% and by stage at diagnosis: localized (95%), regional (68.5%), distant (16.2%), unstaged (50.3%)
  B. Prognosis favorable in younger patients with early-stage, low-grade disease
  C. Prognosis less favorable with increased age, positive lymph nodes (LNs), larger tumor, LVSI, or involvement of the lower uterine segment (NCCN, 2018b)

X. Treatment (NCCN, 2018b)
  A. Fertility-sparing treatment is not the standard of care but may be considered for limited, well-differentiated, early-stage (IA) endometrial adenocarcinoma along with genetic counseling, continuous progestin-based suppression, and hysterectomy after childbearing, or on progression of disease.
  B. Generally up-front TH/BSO is the standard of care with or without neoadjuvant chemotherapy, RT and possible adjuvant systemic therapy, EBRT, and/or brachytherapy. Highly dependent on extent of disease and histopathologic type.
  C. Premenopausal patients with stage I: ovarian preservation if desired.
  D. If not a surgical candidate: EBRT and/or brachytherapy, systemic therapy, or hormonal therapy for ER/PR-positive endometrioid histology.
  E. Recurrent disease
    1. Local/confined recurrence or isolated metastasis: second-line systemic therapy, RT, and/or secondary surgery
    2. Low-grade, disseminated disease: hormonal or systemic chemotherapy
    3. High-grade, disseminated disease: systemic therapy with or without palliative RT

XI. Nursing implications
  A. Client safety and risk reduction: weight and dietary management, identify high-risk populations due to genetic, socioeconomic, and reproductive risk factors and screen for abnormal bleeding and report to provider.
  B. Manage treatment- and cancer-related symptoms
    1. Cancer-related symptoms may include abnormal bleeding, vaginal discharge, changes in urinary function, and discomfort.
    2. Surgery and radiation therapy of the abdomen/pelvis and associated pretreatment and post-treatment care, including hypoestrogenism after BSO, which may induce hot flashes, mood changes, vaginal dryness, pelvic tissue atrophy, osteoporosis, and increased cardiovascular disease (CVD) risk (NCCN, 2018b).
    3. Management of systemic therapies and toxicities: common agents include cisplatin, carboplatin, doxorubicin, docetaxel, gemcitabine, paclitaxel, ifosfamide, everolimus, and aromatase inhibitors (Chapter 28).

C. Assess for recurrent disease: typically, within 3 years of initial diagnosis, presenting with vaginal bleeding, poor appetite, weight loss, pain, cough, abdominal or leg swelling (NCCN, 2018b).
  D. Sexual and reproductive functioning
    1. Appropriate use of lubricants, changes in sexual position, and teaching.
    2. Encourage communication with patient and sexual partner regarding fertility concerns and sexual function before, during, and after treatment.
  E. Genetic risk factors may have implications for extended family members.

Ovarian Cancer

I. Pathology and pathophysiology of ovaries
  A. Female reproductive glands located bilaterally at the termination of the fallopian tubes, providing ova and reproductive hormone regulation and production.
  B. Ovarian cancer originates from tissue of the ovary or fallopian tube and may seed the peritoneal cavity and adjacent pelvic and lymphatic structures.

II. Epidemiology
  A. Seventh most common cancer in women worldwide (WCRF, 2017b).
  B. In the U.S. ovarian cancer is relatively rare with decreased incidences and deaths, and increased survival over the past 10 years. Most new cases diagnosed in women age 55 to 64 and deaths age 65 to 74 (NCCN, 2018c; NCI, 2017b).

III. Risk factors (NCCN, 2018c)
  A. Smoking, nulliparity, older age at first birth, hormone replacement therapy (HRT), pelvic inflammation disease (PID), ovarian stimulation for in vitro fertilization (IVF) (in some cases), family/genetics: *BRCA* mutation, HNPCC, hereditary breast and ovarian cancer (HBOC) (see Chapter 10).
  B. Protective factors: younger age at first pregnancy, use of OCPs, breastfeeding.

IV. Prevention (NCCN, 2018c)
  A. Tobacco/smoking prevention, prevention/treatment for PID
  B. There is currently no screening recommendation for ovarian cancer. CA125 serum levels and/or ovarian ultrasound may be investigated (ACOG, 2017).
  C. Prophylactic BSO in high-risk patients with *BRCA1* or *BRCA2* mutations.

V. Histopathology (NCCN, 2018c)
  A. Epithelial ovarian cancer (90%). Most common subtype is serous (70%).
  B. Less common ovarian histology (LCOH) tumors include carcinosarcoma, clear cell, mucinous, low-grade serous, borderline epithelial, and malignant sex cord-stromal/germ cell tumors.

VI. Histologic grade (NCCN, 2018c)
  A. Serous ovarian cancer is low grade (grade 1) or high grade (grade 2, 3).
  B. Endometrioid/mucinous carcinomas and stable 1C tumors are graded G1 to G3.
VII. Diagnosis and staging (NCCN, 2018c)
  A. Clinical presentation of bloating, pain, early satiety, urinary urgency/frequency, pelvic mass, and tumor marker evaluation (CA125, inhibin, alpha-fetoprotein (AFP), beta-human chorionic gonadotropin [hCG]). Image with CT/MRI, PET/CT.
  B. Pathologic diagnosis of biopsy or operative specimen with surgical staging.
VIII. Prognosis and survival (NCI, 2017b)
  A. Many ovarian cancers are diagnosed in later stages, which carries poor prognosis.
  B. Overall 5-year survival has increased, and survival by stage is localized (92.5%), regional (73.0%), distant (28.9%), and unstaged (25.1%).
IX. Treatment (NCCN, 2018c)
  A. Fertility sparing: USO may be adequate for unilateral stage I tumors. For stage IB tumors a BSO with preservation of the uterus may be an option.
  B. Surgical staging with TAH/BSO and LND as indicated, debulking, and adjuvant chemotherapy (platinum/taxane).
    1. Consider neoadjuvant chemotherapy for bulky disease/poor surgical candidates
    2. Intraperitoneal chemotherapy if stage II/III disease is optimally debulked
  C. Relapsed ovarian cancer
    1. For those with poor response to chemotherapy or short interval from completion of chemotherapy to relapse (<6 m): clinical trials, supportive care, second-line systemic therapy
    2. If complete remission and relapse >6 months after primary chemotherapy
      a. Biochemical relapse (elevated CA125): clinical trial, observe until clinical relapse, platinum-based therapy, supportive care
      b. Clinical relapse: surgery, clinical trials, best supportive care, platinum-based recurrence therapy, PARP inhibitor
  D. Indications for hormonal therapy or treatment of LCOH according to diagnosis.
X. Nursing implications
  A. Risk mitigation depends on early identification of risk factors, referral for genetic risk evaluation, and addressing of modifiable risk factors such as tobacco cessation and prevention of PID/sexually transmitted disease (STD) infection (NCCN, 2018c).
  B. Manage treatment- and cancer-related symptoms
    1. Cancer-related symptoms commonly include gastrointestinal dysfunction, ascites, and abdominal pain.
    2. Surgery and RT of the abdomen/pelvis and associated pretreatment and posttreatment care as described previously.

    3. Management of systemic toxicities for common agents such as carboplatin, cisplatin, paclitaxel, docetaxel, bevacizumab, gemcitabine, pegylated liposomal doxorubicin, PARP inhibitors, and many others. Many patients will require more than one line of therapy.
    4. Address fertility and surgically/chemotherapy induced menopause for patients who were previously premenopausal.
  C. Recurrent disease is frequent due to later stages of diagnosis.
    1. Assess for abdominal bloating, bowel/bladder changes, weight loss, early satiety, nausea, vomiting, ascites.
    2. CA125/tumor markers, imaging surveillance per guidelines.

Gestational Trophoblastic Neoplasia (GTN)

I. Physiology and pathophysiology (Seckl et al., 2013)
  A. Arise from components of the placenta.
  B. Malignant GTN: malignant invasive mole, choriocarcinoma, placental site trophoblastic tumor/epithelioid trophoblastic tumor (PSTT/ETT).
  C. Result of abnormal conception leading to molar pregnancy: hydatidiform mole.
II. Epidemiology: relatively uncommon overall and is more common in Asia than Europe or North America (Seckl et al., 2013)
III. Risk factors (Seckl et al., 2013)
  A. Very young or geriatric pregnancy (under 16 or over 45)
  B. Autosomal-recessive familial recurrent hydatidiform mole (HM)
  C. Some evidence for menarche after age 12, history of light menses, OCP use
IV. Prevention (Seckl et al., 2013)
  A. Early detection with hCG level monitoring after molar pregnancies facilitates earlier treatment and better outcomes
V. Histopathology (Seckl et al., 2013)
  A. Villous trophoblast: complete or partial hydatidiform mole (CHM/PHM)
  B. Epithelial tumor: choriocarcinoma (CC)
  C. PSTT: lower hemorrhage risk, lower hCG levels. ETT behaves similarly.
VI. Diagnosis and staging (Seckl et al., 2013)
  A. HM presents with vaginal bleeding in the first trimester. Diagnosed and staged by suction D&C and histologic examination, hCG monitoring, pelvic ultrasound, chest x-ray with or without CT and brain MRI.
  B. CC, PSTT/ETT: may also include lumbar puncture to determine occult central nervous system disease
  C. PSTT/ETT: occurs after any pregnancy; diagnosis commonly delayed. hCG monitoring indicated for metastatic disease in women of childbearing potential

D. Staging
   1. For CHM/PHM, CC: patient age, pregnancy history, hCG, metastases, largest tumor, and history of prior chemotherapy to determine overall prognostic score as low (0–6) or high (≥7) risk.
   2. PSTT/ETT is staged I, II, III, or IV depending on spread of disease.

VII. Prognosis and survival
  A. Prognostic factors: interval from pregnancy to diagnosis, stage at presentation, and high mitotic index (poor prognosis for PSTT) (Seckl et al., 2013).
  B. Five-year survival: approximately 100% for low-risk and 90% for high-risk groups.

VIII. Treatment (Seckl et al., 2013)
  A. GTN after HM, CC: single-agent chemotherapy for low risk and multiagent therapy for high risk. Treatment continues until hCG normalized 6 to 8 weeks.
  B. PSTT/ETT: stage I recommended for hysterectomy with lymph node sampling, chemotherapy, and secondary surgical resection of residual masses. Advanced stages recommended for combination/high-dose chemotherapy.
  C. Recurrent disease: 3% overall relapse rate, most common within 1 year of treatment. For GTN after HM, second-line and salvage chemotherapy with or without resection has excellent cure rates.

IX. Nursing implications
  A. Risk factors and prevention: review family/personal history of molar pregnancies, encourage regular prenatal and OB/GYN care.
  B. Cancer- and treatment-related symptoms (Seckl et al., 2013)
   1. Due to rise in hCG many cancer-related symptoms are similar, but more severe, than those in pregnancy, bleeding.
   2. Chemotherapy regimens for more advanced or recurrent disease have many significant side effects, and toxicities should be managed closely. Common agents for GTN include methotrexate, etoposide, cyclophosphamide, vincristine, actinomycin-D.
   3. Postsurgical care after hysterectomy and/or surgical resections.
  C. Assess for recurrent disease; will include timely follow-up even beyond the first year of hCG surveillance (Seckl et al., 2013).
  D. Sexual and reproductive function (Seckl et al., 2013)
   1. No obvious increase in risk of congenital malformations or decrease in fertility after treatment, but avoid pregnancy for at least 1 year after completion of therapy.
   2. Infertility in case of hysterectomy (with or without surgical menopause).
   3. Involve sexual partners and patient in discussion surrounding fertility issues, contraception recommendations before, during, and after treatment.

Vulvar Cancer

I. Physiology and pathophysiology
  A. External female genitalia from mons pubis to perineum, including labia majora and minora, with smooth internal mucosal membranes that are continuous with the female urogenital tract.
  B. Premalignant and malignant changes may involve only the vulva; malignant changes may extend to lymph nodes, local structures, distant sites (Saito et al., 2018)

II. Epidemiology (NCI, 2017e)
  A. Relatively rare worldwide and in the U.S.; most commonly diagnosed in women aged 55 to 75 years, with most associated deaths occurring over 84 years.
  B. The trend for associated deaths has increased over the past 10 years.

III. Risk factors (NCCN, 2018f): oncogenic HPV infection, cigarette smoking, inflammatory conditions of the vulva, immunodeficiency.

IV. Prevention
  A. Vaccination for HPV subtype 16, 18 (NCCN, 2018f)
  B. Identification and early treatment of preinvasive disease

V. Histopathology (NCCN, 2018f; Saito et al., 2018)
  A. The most common histology is squamous (90%)
   1. Noninvasive vulvar intraepithelial neoplasia (VINs) and VINs related to HPV infection are classified as squamous intraepithelial lesions (SILs).
   2. Squamous cell carcinoma (SCC)
  B. Less common histology: melanoma, extramammary Paget disease, Bartholin gland adenocarcinoma, verrucous carcinoma, basal cell carcinoma, sarcoma

VI. Histologic grade (Saito et al., 2018)
  A. VIN1/low-grade SIL (LSIL): considered nonneoplastic
  B. VIN2/VIN3/high-grade SIL (HSIL): neoplastic with chance of carcinogenesis

VII. Diagnosis and staging (NCCN, 2018f)
  A. Visual inspection with or without acetic acid staining and diagnostic biopsy.
  B. Staging involves biopsy, lymph node evaluation, imaging and/or cystoscopy, proctoscopy.

VIII. Prognosis and survival
  A. Prognosis is most influenced by involvement of lymph nodes.
  B. Poorer prognosis with larger primary tumor, greater depth of invasion, and LVSI.
  C. Postsurgically influenced by status of the tumor margin after primary resection.
  D. Overall 5-year survival in the U.S. is 72.1% (NCI, 2017e) and by stage is localized (86.4%), regional (56.9%), distant (17.4%), unstaged (56.2%)

IX. Treatment (NCCN, 2018f)
  A. Early stage (I/II): conservative tumor excision and lymph node evaluation
  B. Locally advanced (stage III/IVA): concurrent chemoradiation, surgical resection (modified or radical vulvectomy), and lymph node evaluation

C. Distant metastatic (IVB —→ extrapelvic disease): EBRT for local control and /or chemotherapy, treatments extrapolated from cervical cancer

D. RT may be used if not a surgical candidate and for nodal involvement

E. Local recurrence: reexcision, EBRT with or without concurrent chemotherapy, brachytherapy.

F. Distant/nodal recurrence or metastatic disease: dependent on prior treatments and recurrence site(s). RT, chemotherapy, rarely resection, and may involve best supportive care.

X. Nursing implications

A. Client safety and risk reduction: early detection of history of vulvar chronic inflammation, lesions, or HPV infection; encourage HPV vaccination, tobacco cessation, regular pelvic examinations, and posttreatment surveillance.

B. Cancer- and treatment-related symptoms

1. Cancer-related symptoms may involve local site irritation, mass, pain, or complications of LN involvement or metastases.

2. Local care of excision and/or biopsy sites and nursing care after abdominal/pelvic surgery or RT.

3. Management of chemotherapy and systemic toxicities.

Vaginal Cancer

I. Physiology and pathophysiology

A. The vaginal canal consists of connective, muscular, and erectile tissue covered with mucosal membrane with many rugae, extending from the vulvar opening to the uterine cervix, in proximity with lymphatics and blood vessels.

B. Preinvasive and invasive changes of the vagina may be similar to those found in cervical cancers or an extension of a cervical cancer.

II. Epidemiology

A. Occurrence is rare in the U.S.: less than 1 of every 1000 women (ACS, 2018b).

B. Elderly women are more commonly affected (Saito et al., 2018)

III. Risk factors (Saito et al., 2018)

A. Oncogenic HPV infection (in 80% of vaginal cancer SCCs)

B. Diethylstilbestrol (DES) exposure in utero increases risk of clear cell adenocarcinoma

IV. Prevention: HPV vaccination and early detection of preinvasive lesions

V. Histopathology (ACS, 2016; Saito et al., 2018)

A. Most commonly SCC or VIN, which involves squamous epithelial cells but not underlying tissue

B. Less common: adenocarcinoma, clear cell carcinoma, vaginal melanoma

VI. Histologic grade (Saito et al., 2018)

A. VIN associated with HPV infection stratified by low- or high-grade squamous intraepithelial lesions (LSIL/HSIL)

B. VIN1 is considered LSIL; VIN2/VIN3 are considered HSIL

VII. Diagnosis and staging: visual inspection, biopsy with pathologic examination, FIGO staging.

VIII. Prognosis and survival (ACS, 2016)

A. Prognostic factors influenced by histologic type and extent of disease

1. SCC and adenocarcinoma (highest 5-year survival rates—about 50%)

2. Vaginal melanoma (poor survival, about 13% at 5 years)

B. Five-year relative survival by stage at diagnosis in the U.S.: stage 1 (84%), stage II (75%), stage III/IV (57%)

IX. Treatment (Saito et al., 2018)

A. Treatments are dependent on the degree of invasion and LN status.

B. Preinvasive disease may be treated with local agents, excision, or brachytherapy.

C. The mainstay of invasive disease involves surgical excision, RT, brachytherapy, chemotherapy, or a combination of modalities.

D. Surgical: partial or total vaginectomy (high morbidity) or pelvic exenteration.

E. Recurrent disease is retreated dependent on site and extent of recurrence.

X. Nursing implications

A. Client safety and risk reduction involves early detection for the development of lesions, HPV vaccination, screen patients for congenital abnormalities and/or DES exposure in utero.

B. Cancer- and treatment-related symptoms

1. Beyond abdominal/pelvic surgery/RT, reproductive and sexual function affected by significant surgical loss of vaginal length and changes secondary to chemotherapy or radiotherapy modalities (may include stenosis, dryness). Use of dilators and/or lubricants as indicated.

2. Management of chemotherapy-induced toxicities.

3. Management of complications from distant metastatic sites

Testicular Cancer

I. Physiology and pathophysiology

A. Male ovoid reproductive glands descending from the inguinal canal during gestation into the scrotal sac, producing testosterone and spermatogenesis.

B. Testicular cancer is usually unilateral, arising from the germinal epithelium.

II. Epidemiology in the U.S. (NCI, 2017c)

A. Rare in the U.S. overall with most cases of diagnosis or death in males aged 20 to 43 and less common in African American or Asian/Pacific Islander males.

B. Over 10 years the incidence has risen; death rates are stable (NCCN, 2018e).

III. Risk factors include personal or family history of germ cell tumor (GCT), cryptorchidism, testicular dysgenesis, and Klinefelter syndrome. (NCCN, 2018e).

IV. Prevention
   A. Early screening, detection, and treatment for excellent options of cure.

V. Histopathology (NCCN, 2018e)
   A. Most tumors in testes are GCTs (95%)
   B. Nonseminomatous germ cell tumors (NSGCT), mixed seminoma/nonseminomas, seminomas with elevated AFP: more clinically aggressive.
   C. Pure seminomas are less aggressive and spread more slowly.

VI. Diagnosis and staging (NCCN, 2018e)
   A. Usually a painless unilateral mass, confirmed on ultrasound. May initially be suspected as epididymitis or orchitis if pain or swelling is present. Extragonadal disease confirmed on biopsy, and possible diagnostic orchiectomy for gonadal tumors may also be therapeutic.
   B. Tumor markers: seminoma will have elevated beta-hCG and lactate dehydrogenase (LDH). Nonseminomas indicated with elevated AFP levels
   C. Staging
      1. CT, MRI as indicated and TNM staging based on postorchiectomy values of beta-hCG, LDH, and AFP
      2. Prognostic groupings combine TNM (clinical and pathologic) with serum tumor markers (AFP, LDH, beta-hCG) and report as SX, S0, S1, S2, and S3 per AJCC guidelines (NCCN, 2018e).
   D. Risk classifications are based on primary tumor location, presence/absence of nonpulmonary visceral metastases, and tumor marker status.
      1. Nonseminoma: good, intermediate, or poor risk status.
      2. Seminoma: good or intermediate risk status (none are poor risk status).

VII. Prognosis and survival
   A. Initial prognosis by tumor marker status and disease bulk (NCCN, 2018e)
   B. Prognostic factors at relapse (NCCN, 2018e)
      1. Favorable: complete response to first-line therapy, low postorchiectomy tumor markers, low volume disease
      2. Unfavorable: incomplete first-line response, high tumor markers, high-volume disease, extratesticular primary
   C. Five-year relative survival by stage at diagnosis in the U.S.: localized (99.2%), regional (96.1%), distant (73.2%), unstaged (76.7%), with overall 50year survival of 95.1% (NCI, 2017c)

VIII. Treatment (NCCN, 2018e).
   A. Treatments
      1. Radical inguinal orchiectomy with or without open inguinal biopsy of contralateral testis.
      2. Fertility preservation: consider sperm banking before surgery, RT, or chemotherapy.
      3. Seminoma: orchiectomy is followed by surveillance, RT, and/or chemotherapy
      4. Nonseminoma: orchiectomy is followed by surveillance, chemotherapy, and retroperitoneal LND (RLND)
   B. Recurrent disease
      1. Favorable: standard second-line chemotherapy. Possible surgical salvage if solitary resectable relapse site
      2. Unfavorable: clinical trial chemotherapy, second-line or high-dose chemotherapy, palliative chemotherapy, salvage surgery

IX. Nursing implications
   A. Client safety and risk reduction centers around early detection (testicular self-examination and clinical examination), detection of recurrent cancer, patient education, and family history or presence of other risk factors.
   B. Cancer- and treatment-related symptoms
      1. Surgical issues may involve local pain and discomfort or more extensive postoperative care for RLND.
      2. Chemotherapy toxicity management should be aggressive due to intensive GCT regimens (BEP, VIP, TIP).
      3. Radiation therapy may cause local irritation and affect fertility.
      4. Metastatic symptoms of advanced disease/palliation
   C. Sexual and reproductive function should be discussed with client and sexual partner at the time of diagnosis (NCCN, 2018e)
      1. Esthetic changes may be mitigated by a testicular implant, which may be placed at the time of initial surgery (NCCN, 2018e)
      2. Sperm banking may be done before or after surgery, but ideally before any RT or chemotherapy
      3. Retrograde ejaculation after bilateral retroperitoneal LND, infertility

Penile Cancer

I. Physiology and pathophysiology (Diorio, Leone, & Speiss, 2016)
   A. Penile root and shaft terminates at the glans and urinary meatus. In uncircumcised males the glans is covered with the prepuce (foreskin).
   B. Composed of fascia, nerves, lymphatics, sebaceous glands, and vascular erectile tissue. The glans is the most common site of penile cancers.
   C. Functions: excretion of urinary waste, internal fertilization, and reproduction.

II. Epidemiology
   A. More common in parts of Asia, Africa, and South America than in North America or Europe; rare in the U.S. with usual presentation at 50 to 70 years (ACS, 2018a; Diorio, Leone, & Speiss, 2016; NCCN, 2018d; NCCN, 2018e).

III. Risk factors (Diorio, Leone, & Speiss, 2016; NCCN, 2018d)
   A. HIV/HPV infection (positive in 60%–80% of penile cancers, type 16, 18).
   B. Phimosis, balanitis, chronic inflammation, penile trauma, lack of circumcision, lichen sclerosis, tobacco use, poor hygiene, and low socioeconomic status.
IV. Prevention: control of modifiable risk factors such as vaccination for HPV, prevention of HIV infection, avoiding tobacco use, and early detection of lesions.
V. Histopathology (Diorio, Leone, Speiss, 2016; NCCN, 2018d)
   A. Premalignant penile intraepithelial neoplasia (PIN)
   B. SCC (95% of penile cancers) subtypes: verrucous (low malignant potential), papillary squamous, warty, basaloid
VI. Histologic grade: degree of differentiation Gx, G1, G2, G3 (NCCN, 2018e)
VII. Diagnosis and staging
   A. Clinical presentation of palpable/visible lesion with or without pain, discharge, or bleeding, or constitutional symptoms of cancer and diagnosed on biopsy.
   B. Staging: TNM staging criteria and can involve MRI and/or ultrasound evaluation of primary lesion, depth of invasion and of lymph nodes that are otherwise difficult to assess.
VIII. Prognosis and survival
   A. Prognostic factors (Diorio, Leone, & Speiss, 2016; NCCN, 2018d)
      1. Inguinal LN metastasis is most prognostic factor.
      2. Earlier stage at diagnosis and treatment is favorable, up to 80% cure rate.
   B. Overall 5-year survival is 50%, with 5-year relative survival affected by LN status: negative nodes: (>85%), positive nodes (29%–40%), pelvic lymph node involvement (0%).
IX. Treatment (Diorio, Leone & Speiss, 2016; NCCN, 2018d)
   A. Treatments
      1. Penile organ–sparing approaches are available for Tis, ta, some T1 lesions, which include topical treatments, laser therapy, wide or local excision, glansectomy, and Mohs surgery, and are often followed by surveillance.
      2. To preserve functional anatomy and control primary tumor, radiation/brachytherapy or concurrent chemoradiation may be recommended.
      3. Treating penile cancer with higher grades or deeper invasion may involve partial or total penectomy, with inguinal LN dissection/lymphadenectomy for high-risk penile cancers.
      4. Neoadjuvant chemotherapy, chemoradiation, or adjuvant chemotherapy may be recommended based on LN status.
   B. Treatment for recurrent disease varies based on prior surgery, radiation, systemic treatment/chemotherapy, and LN status at recurrence. May involve retreatment or best supportive care.
X. Nursing implications (Diorio, Leone & Speiss, 2016)
   A. Encourage modification of risk factors: HPV vaccination, prevent HIV infection, circumcision before puberty, maintain good hygiene (retraction of foreskin and cleansing of the glans regularly), smoking cessation
   B. Cancer- and treatment-related symptoms
      1. Care related to treatment involves teaching and safety of topical treatments (imiquimod, 5-FU) and site care/wound care after minor and major surgical resection (including risks for sexual dysfunction and lymphedema) and during RT.
      2. Manage toxicities such as myelosuppression, renal or liver dysfunction, and neuropathy of agents such as cisplatin, ifosfamide, and paclitaxel.
      3. Advanced disease requires supportive care.
   C. Assess for recurrent disease after topical treatment for early stages; may involve teaching for weekly self-checks in reliable patients.
   D. Sexual and reproductive function should be discussed at diagnosis with client and sexual partner.
      1. Sexual function is best preserved with topical, less invasive, or RT treatments, and is significantly affected by partial or full penectomy.
      2. Prosthetics and alternative ways to express sexual intimacy may be explored.

REFERENCES

American Cancer Society. (2016). *Survival rates for vaginal cancer.* Retrieved September 10, 2018, from https://www.cancer.org/cancer/vaginal-cancer/detection-diagnosis-staging/survival-rates.html.

American Cancer Society. (2018a). *Key statistics for penile cancer.* Retrieved September 10, 2018, from https://www.cancer.org/cancer/penile-cancer/about/key-statistics.html.

American Cancer Society. (2018b). *Key statistics for vaginal cancer.* Retrieved September 10, 2018, from https://www.cancer.org/cancer/vaginal-cancer/about/key-statistics.html.

American College of Obstetricians and Gynecologists. (2015). *FAQ: frequently asked questions gynecologic problems (FAQ163) - cervical cancer.* Retrieved September 10, 2018, from https://www.acog.org/Patients/FAQs/Cervical-Cancer.

American College of Obstetricians and Gynecologists. (2017). *Patient Education Fact Sheet: BRCA1 and BRCA2 mutations (PFS007).* Retrieved September 10, 2018, from https://www.acog.org/Patients/FAQs/BRCA1-and-BRCA2-Mutations.

Amin, M. B., Edge, S. B., & American Joint Committee on Cancer, & Springer Science Business Media. (2017). *AJCC Cancer Staging Manual* (8th ed.). In *Chicago; [S.l.]: American Joint Committee on Cancer: Springer International Publishing AG Switzerland.*

Bailey, H. H., Chuang, L. T., duPont, N. C., Eng, C., Foxhall, L. E., Merrill, J. K., ... Blanke, C. D. (2016). American Society of Clinical Oncology statement: human papillomavirus vaccination for cancer prevention. *Journal of Clinical Oncology, 34*(15), 1803–1812. https://doi.org/10.1200/JCO.2016.67.2014.

Diorio, G. J., Leone, A. R., & Spiess, P. E. (2016). Management of penile cancer. [Urology]. *Urology, 96,* 15–21. https://doi.org/10.1016/j.urology.2015.12.041.

Jeronimo, J., Castle, P. E., Temin, S., Denny, L., Gupta, V., Kim, J. J., … Shastri, S. S. (2017). Secondary prevention of cervical cancer: ASCO resource-stratified clinical practice guideline. *Journal of Global Oncology, 3*(5), 635–657. https://doi.org/10.1200/JGO.2016.006577.

National Cancer Institute (NCI). (2017a). *Cancer Stat Facts: cervical cancer.* Retrieved September 10, 2018, from http://seer.cancer.gov/statfacts/html/cervix.html.

National Cancer Institute. (2017b). *Cancer Stat Facts: ovarian cancer.* Retrieved September 10, 2018, from https://seer.cancer.gov/statfacts/html/ovary.html.

National Cancer Institute. (2017c). *Cancer Stat Facts: testicular cancer.* Retrieved September 10, 2018 from https://seer.cancer.gov/statfacts/html/testis.html.

National Cancer Institute. (2017d). *Cancer Stat Facts: uterine Cancer.* Retrieved September 10, 2018, from https://seer.cancer.gov/statfacts/html/corp.html.

National Cancer Institute. (2017e). *Cancer Stat Facts: vulvar cancer.* Retrieved September 10, 2018, from https://seer.cancer.gov/statfacts/html/vulva.html.

National Comprehensive Cancer Network. (NCCN). (2018a). *Clinical practice guidelines in oncology-cervical cancer. Version, 1,* 2018.

National Comprehensive Cancer Network. (2018b). *Clinical practice guidelines in oncology-endometrial/uterine cancer. Version* 1.2018.

National Comprehensive Cancer Network. (2018c). *Clinical practice guidelines in oncology-ovarian cancer. Version 1.2018.*

National Comprehensive Cancer Network. (2018d). *Clinical practice guidelines in oncology-penile cancer.* Version 1.2018.

National Comprehensive Cancer Network. (2018e). *Clinical practice guidelines in oncology-testicular cancer.* Version 1.2018.

National Comprehensive Cancer Network. (2018f). *Clinical practice guidelines in oncology-vulvar cancer.* Version 1.2018.

Saito, T., Tabata, T., Ikushima, H., Yanai, H., Tashiro, H., Niikura, H., … Katabuchi, H. (2018). Japan Society of Gynecologic Oncology guidelines 2015 for the treatment of vulvar cancer and vaginal cancer. *International Journal of Clinical Oncology, 23*(2), 201–234. https://doi.org/10.1007/s10147-017-1193-z.

Seckl, M. J., Sebire, N. J., Fisher, R. A., Golfier, F., Massuger, L., Sessa, C., & Group, E. G. W. (2013). Gestational trophoblastic disease: ESMO clinical practice guidelines for diagnosis, treatment and follow-up. *Annals of Oncology.* 24(Suppl 6). https://doi.org/10.1093/annonc/mdt345 vi39-50.

Siegel, R. L., Miller, K. D., & Jemal, A. (2017). Cancer statistics, 2017. *CA: A Cancer Journal for Clinicians, 67*(1), 7–30. https://doi.org/10.3322/caac.21387.

World Cancer Research Fund International. (2017a). *Cancer facts & figures: endometrial cancer (cancer of the lining of the womb) statistics.* Retrieved September 10, 2018, from http://www.wcrf.org/int/cancer-facts-figures/data-specific-cancers/endometrial-cancer-cancer-lining-womb-statistics.

World Cancer Research Fund International. (2017b). *Cancer facts & figures: ovarian cancer statistics.* Retrieved September 10, 2018, from www.wcrf.org/int/cancer-facts-figures/data-specific-cancers/ovarian-cancer-statistics.

World Health Organization. Cervical cancer. (2017). Retrieved September 10, 2018, from http://www.who.int/cancer/prevention/diagnosis-screening/cervical-cancer/en/.

24

Skin Cancer

Krista M. Rubin and Christine Boley

I. Physiology and pathophysiology
  A. Pathogenesis of skin cancer (Coelho et al., 2016)
    1. Ultraviolet radiation (UVR) includes solar and artificial (from tanning beds)
    2. UVR causes multiple types of DNA damage resulting in mutations in key cancer genes controlling cell survival, proliferation, and differentiation
    3. Two main types of UVR:
      a. Ultraviolet A (UVA)—passes deeper into skin: DNA damage is indirect, mediated by free radical formation and damage to cellular membranes
      b. Ultraviolet B (UVB)—1000 to 10,000 times more carcinogenic than UVA; most is absorbed in the epidermis; causes erythema or sunburn; directly damages DNA
    4. Genetics—inherited predisposition for skin cancer
      a. Xeroderma pigmentosum (XP): inability to repair UV-induced DNA damage, resulting in multiple skin cancers at an early age (Vandergriff, 2018; Coehlo et al., 2016)
      b. Oculocutaneous albinism: a group of autosomal-recessive disorders in which there is partial or total absence of melanin pigment within melanocytes of the skin, hair follicles, and eyes (Vandergriff, 2018)
      c. Basal cell nevus syndrome (Gorlin syndrome): an inherited disorder characterized by abnormal facial features and development of numerous basal cell carcinomas (BCCs) at an early age (Didona et al., 2018; Coehlo et al., 2016)
      d. Familial atypical multiple mole and melanoma syndrome (dysplastic nevus syndrome): an autosomal-dominant group of disorders characterized by hundreds of dysplastic nevi on individuals with an increased risk of melanoma (Shi & Leventhal, 2017; Soura et al., 2016)
II. Epidemiology
  A. Nonmelanoma skin cancer (NMSC)
    1. BCC (also known as *keratinocyte carcinoma*) (Bichakjian et al., 2018)
      a. Most common cancer: ≈3.3 million cases/year in U.S. with increasing incidence
      b. Prevalence has increased by 35% over the past 20 years
    2. Squamous cell carcinoma (SCC) (Alam et al., 2018; Didona et al., 2018)
      a. Second most common skin cancer: 200,000 to 400,000 new cases/year; increasing incidence
      b. Prevalence has increased by 133% over the past 20 years
    3. Merkel cell carcinoma (MCC) (Paulson et al., 2018; Coggshall et al., 2018)
      a. Approximately 1600 cases/year; new MCC cases increased 95% 2000 to 2013
      b. Incidence rates are expected to climb to 2835 cases/year in 2020 and 3284 cases/year in 2025 due to aging Baby Boomers
    4. Cutaneous melanoma (ACS, 2018)
      a. Approximately 91,270 new cases in U.S. with 9320 deaths
      b. Fifth most common cancer in men; sixth in women
III. Risk factors (Tables 24.1 to 24.3; Box 24.1)
  A. Fitzpatrick skin types (Table 24.4) (High et al., 2018)
    1. A scale representing the effect and response to UV irradiation. It also refers to other shared characteristics, such as hair and eye color and a tendency toward certain reaction patterns in the skin as a response to an insult (UV exposure).
    2. Variations in skin color are due to differences in the amount and distribution of melanin and not the number of melanocytes
IV. Prevention (Box 24.2)
 V. Histology and histopathology (see Tables 24.1 to 24.3)
  A. NMSC
    1. BCC: A neoplasm arising from basal cell layer of the epidermis (Christensen & Leffell, 2016; Didona et al., 2018)
      a. Subtypes (Table 24.5)
    2. SCC: arises from squamous cell layer of the epidermis (Christensen & Leffell, 2016)
      a. Precursors and premalignant states
        (1) Actinic keratoses (AK): approximately 60% to 65% of SCCs arise from prior AKs
        (2) SCC in situ (SCCis): confined to the epidermis

TABLE 24.1 Risk Factors and Characteristics of BCC

Risk Factors	Characteristics
• Major risk is UVR; specifically, intermittent exposure early in life • Family history of skin cancer • Male gender • Age >65 • Immunosuppression • Prior PUVS therapy for psoriasis • Fitzpatrick skin types I and II • Exposure to carcinogenic chemicals, especially arsenic • Genetics: Gorlin syndrome (basal cell nevus syndrome)	• Develops primarily on sun-exposed skin; rarely found on palmoplantar surfaces and never appears on the mucosa • 80% arise on the head and neck • Slow growing • Arise without precursor lesions • Locally invasive tumor • Can develop at sites of chemical exposure or chronic trauma

Approximately 40% of patients who have had a primary BCC will develop a new BCC within 5 years of their first occurrence.

Adapted from Didona, D., Paolino, G., Bottoni, U., & Cantisani, C. (2018). Non-melanoma skin cancer pathogenesis overview. *Biomedicines, 6*(1), 6. https://doi.org/10.3390/biomedicines6010006; Coelho, M. M. V., Matos, T. R., & Apetato, M. (2016). The dark side of the light: mechanisms of photocarcinogenesis. *Clinics in Dermatology, 34*(5), 563–570. https://doi.org/10.1016/j.clindermatol.2016.05.022.

TABLE 24.2 Risk Factors and Characteristics of cuSCC

Risk Factors	Characteristics

• Chronic UV exposure, especially in childhood and youth
• Fitzpatrick skin types I and II
• Increasing age
• Male gender
• Presence of precursor lesions
• Immunosuppression, particularly solid-organ transplant recipients
• Chronic skin ulcers, nonhealing wounds, or burn scars
• Chronic use of photosensitizing medications such as voriconazole (an antifungal)
• Exposure to carcinogenic chemicals, specifically arsenic
• Outdoor occupation
• Genetics
	• Typically arise in sun-exposed areas.
	  • 55% head and neck locations
	  • 18% on extensor surfaces of the hands and forearms
	  • Up to 13% on the legs
	• Often presents as a new or enlarging lesion that may bleed, weep, be tender, or be painful
	• Slightly raised papule, plaque, or nodule; may be flesh-colored, pink, or red
	• Surface of the tumor may be smooth, crusted, or ulcerated
	• Typically slow growing; however, those arising in in non–sun-exposed sites (i.e., lips, genitalia, perianal areas) are more aggressive with a higher risk of metastases
	• The most common type of skin cancer that occurs in African Americans and Asian Indians

Adapted from Didona, D., Paolino, G., Bottoni, U., & Cantisani, C. (2018). Non-melanoma skin cancer pathogenesis overview. *Biomedicines, 6*(1), 6. https://doi.org/10.3390/biomedicines6010006; Farberg, A. S., & Goldenberg, G. (2018). New guidelines of care for the management of nonmelanoma skin cancer. *Cutis, 101*(5), 319; Christensen, S. R., & Leffell, D. J. (2016). Cancer of the Skin. In V. T. DeVita, T. S. Lawrence, & S. A. Rosenberg (Eds.), *Cancer: Principles and Practice of Oncology* (pp. 838–886 Chapter 6). Philadelphia: Wolters Kluwer Health; Coelho, M. M. V., Matos, T. R., & Apetato, M. (2016). The dark side of the light: mechanisms of photocarcinogenesis. *Clinics in Dermatology, 34*(5), 563–570. https://doi.org/10.1016/j.clindermatol.2016.05.022.

    3. MCC: a neoplasm of neuroendocrine cell origin located in the epidermis (Christensen & Leffell, 2016; Paulson et al., 2018)

       a. 80% of MCCs are caused by a common virus (Merkel cell polyomavirus), and the remaining 20% are attributed to UV exposure

  B. Melanoma: arises from melanocytes; pigment-producing cells originate from the neural crest and migrate to the skin, meninges, mucous membranes, upper esophagus, and eyes

    1. Precursors and premalignant states

       a. Atypical nevi/dysplastic nevi

       b. Malignant melanoma in situ (MMIS)—confined to the epidermis

    2. Subtypes (Table 24.6)

VI. Molecular classification

  A. NMSC

    1. BCC (Didona et al., 2018)

       a. Most BCCs result from somatic mutations in key receptors in the Hedgehog (Hh) signaling pathway

       b. Inhibitors of the Hh pathway are available for advanced or recurrent BCC not amenable to local therapies

    2. SCC and MCC not clinically relevant currently

  B. Melanoma (Sullivan & Fisher, 2018)

    1. Genomic mutations are present in the majority of cutaneous melanoma

       a. *BRAF* mutation the most common; occurring in 40% to 50% of cutaneous melanoma

       b. *NRAS* mutations are the second most common; occurring in 15% to 20%

       c. *cKIT* mutations are rare; seen with acral and mucosal melanomas or those arising in chronically sun-damaged skin

VII. Diagnosis and staging

  A. Diagnosis

    1. NMSC (Farberg & Goldenberg 2018; Bichakjian et al., 2018; Alam et al., 2018)

       a. Presumptive diagnosis and biopsy type based on the clinician's interpretation of clinical information, including appearance and morphology, anatomic location, genetic risk factors,

TABLE 24.3 Risk Factors and Characteristics of MCC

Risk Factors	Characteristics

• Age ≥65; the average age at diagnosis is 70 years
• Male gender
• Fair skin or a history of extensive sun exposure
• Whites of European ancestry
• Prior PUVA* treatment for psoriasis
• Chronic immunosuppression, especially solid-organ transplant recipients
	• Most commonly presents as an erythematous or violaceous, tender, dome-shaped nodule on sun-exposed areas on the head or neck of an elderly white male
	• Can also present as papules, plaques, and cystlike structures or pruritic tumors on the lower extremities
	• Perianal and vulvar sites have the worst prognosis of all primary sites
	• Rapid growth is common
	• Most lesions are <2 cm in diameter at the time of diagnosis; rapid growth is common
	• 4% of cases present with no known primary
	• The mnemonic "AEIOU" is used to describe common clinical features:
	  • **A**symptomatic
	  • **E**xpanding rapidly
	  • **I**mmunosuppression
	  • **O**lder than 50 years
	  • **U**ltraviolet exposed/fair skin

*PUVA, Psoralen and ultraviolet A radiation.
Adapted from Paulson, K. G., Park, S. Y., Vandeven, N. A., Lachance, K., Thomas, H., Chapuis, A. G., & Nghiem, P. (2018). Merkel cell carcinoma: Current US incidence and projected increases based on changing demographics. *Journal of the American Academy of Dermatology, 78*(3), 457–463. https://doi.org/10.1016/j.jaad.2017.10.028; Harms, P. W. (2017). Update on Merkel Cell Carcinoma. *Clinics in Laboratory Medicine, 37*(3), 485–501. Available at https://doi.org/10.1016/j.cll.2017.05.004; Christensen, S. R., & Leffell, D. J. (2016). Cancer of the Skin. In V. T. DeVita, T. S. Lawrence, & S. A. Rosenberg (Eds.), *Cancer: Principles and Practice of Oncology* (pp. 838–886 Chapter 6). Philadelphia: Wolters Kluwer Health.

BOX 24.1 Risk Factors for Melanoma

- Personal history of melanoma
- Family history of melanoma or NMSC
- Number of moles (typical and atypical)
- UV exposure, especially burns and/or blistering
- Fair skin, red or blonde hair, blue or green eyes, freckling
- Immunosuppression
- Age: risk increases with age >60 years
- Gender: males > females
- Genetics

Adapted from American Cancer Society (ACS). (2018). *Melanoma Skin Cancer.* Atlanta: American Cancer Society. Available at https://www.cancer.org/cancer/melanoma-skin-cancer.html; Garbe, C., & Bauer, J. (2018). Melanoma. In J. L. Bologna, J. V. Schaffer, & L. Cerooni (Eds.): *Dermatology (4th ed) (pp. 1989–2019 Section 18 Melanoma).* Elsevier. Retrieved August 19, 2018 from https://phstwlp2.partners.org:2093/#!/content/book/3-s2.0-B9780702062759001070?scrollTo¼%23s0050; Shi, V. J., & Leventhal, J. S. (2017). Epidemiology and screening of pigmented lesions. In H. Kluger, & S. Aryan (Eds.), *The Melanoma Handbook.* New York: Demos Medical. Springer.

TABLE 24.4 Fitzpatrick Skin Types

Skin Type	Skin Color	Features	Ability to Tan
I	White	Very light complexion, blue or green eye color, blonde or red hair	Always burns, never tans
II	White	Fair complexion, light eye color	Burns easily, rarely tans
III	Beige	Darker light complexion, light brown or dark hair	Sometimes burns, sometimes tans
IV	Brown	Olive or light brown skin, dark hair	Rarely burns, tans easily
V	Dark brown	Olive or dark complexion	Very rarely burns, tans very easily
VI	Black	Black skin, dark hair	Never burns, tans very easily

Adapted from High, W.A., Tomasini, C.F., Argenziano, G., & Zalaudek, I. (2018). Basic principles of dermatology. In J.L. Bologna, J.V. Schaffer, & L. Cerooni (Eds.) Dermatology (4th ed) (pp. 1–43, Section 0). Elsevier. Retrieved August 19, 2018 from: https://phstwlp2.partners.org:2093/#!/content/book/3-s2.0. Skin Cancer Foundation (SCF). (2018). *Skin types and at-risk groups.* Available at: https://www.skincancer.org/prevention/are-you-atrisk/skin-types-and-at-risk-groups.

and patient reported history. Clinical diagnosis is routinely confirmed by biopsy findings before treatment.

    b. Biopsy types—shave (saucerization or scoop technique to penetrate to deep dermis), punch, excisional; shave most commonly used for nonpigmented lesions

2. Melanoma (Buzaid & Gershenwald, 2018)

    a. Signs and symptoms

      (1) ABCDEs of mole/melanoma recognition (Table 24.7)

      (2) Choice of biopsy technique depends on level of size, location, and shape and should include the full epidermal/dermal thickness down to subcutaneous fat

B. Staging

1. BCC and SCC (Farberg & Goldenberg 2018; Bichakjian et al., 2018)

    a. No formal staging system due to exceedingly low incidence of metastases

    b. National Comprehensive Cancer Network (NCCN) guideline framework is favored for clinical practice, as it stratifies localized tumors into low- or high-risk BCC; provides practical guidelines to treat SCC (NCCN, 2018)

BOX 24.2 Skin Cancer Prevention Measures

- Avoid excessive exposure to UVR, particularly prolonged midday sunlight exposure
- UVR penetrates even on cloudy or hazy days; UVR reflects off surfaces like water, sand, cement, and snow
- Do not burn
- Seek shade
- Avoid tanning and UV tanning booths
- Use clothing: whenever possible, long-sleeved shirts, long pants, and skirts offer protection from UVR. Tightly woven fabric offers the most protection. SPF clothing: Wear protective clothing and wide-brim hat
- Use a broad-spectrum (UVA/UVB), water-resistant sunscreen with an SPF of 30+ and reapply every 2 hours and/or after swimming or sweating
- Wear sunglasses that protect against UVA/UVB; use eye and lip protection
- Keep infants under 6 months old out of the sun

Adapted from Didona, D., Paolino, G., Bottoni, U., & Cantisani, C. (2018). Non-melanoma skin cancer pathogenesis overview. *Biomedicines*, 6(1), 6. https://doi.org/10.3390/biomedicines6010006; American Cancer Society (ACS). (2018). *Melanoma Skin Cancer*. Atlanta: American Cancer Society. Available at https://www.cancer.org/cancer/melanoma-skin-cancer.html; Christensen, S. R., & Leffell, D. J. (2016). Cancer of the Skin. In V. T. DeVita, T. S. Lawrence, & S. A. Rosenberg (Eds.), *Cancer: Principles and Practice of Oncology* (pp. 838–886 Chapter 6). Philadelphia: Wolters Kluwer Health.

2. MCC (American Joint Committee on Cancer [AJCC], 2017)
   a. AJCC tumor–node–metastasis (TNM) staging system commonly used; separates clinical and pathologic groups; reclassifies staging for unknown primary tumors
   b. Sentinel lymph node biopsy (SLNBx) should be considered for all patients, as one third of patients with clinically localized disease at the time of presentation have occult lymph node involvement
3. Melanoma (Buzaid & Gershenwald, 2018)
   a. AJCC staging most commonly used (AJCC, 2017)
   b. SLNBx used to evaluate regional nodal status and prognosis

VIII. Prognosis and survival
   A. NMSC: when detected and managed early, most have excellent prognosis
      1. BCC (Bichakjian et al., 2018; Coehlo et al., 2016)
         a. Rarely metastasize; if untreated, can become ulcerated and locally invasive
      2. SCC (Didona et al., 2018; Alam et al., 2018)
         a. Favorable prognosis, 4% of the patients develop metastases; 1.5% eventually die
      3. MCC (Harms, 2017)
         a. Five-year overall survival rates of 51% for local disease, 35% for nodal disease, and 14% for distant disease
         b. The strongest indicator of metastatic risk is primary tumor size

TABLE 24.5 Most Common Subtypes of BCC

Type	Characteristics	Risk
Nodular	- Most common; approximately 50%–80% - Most likely to occur on the head and neck - Typically presents as a round, pink, pearly, flesh-colored papule with a central depression - Often see telangiectasias within the lesion - May or may not be crusted, ulcerated, or bleeding - Pigmented BCCs are a variant of the subtype	Low
Superficial	- 15% - Most commonly found on the trunk - Typically presents as a bright red-to-pink, often scaly patch - Lesions are slowly progressive	Low
Micronodular	- Aggressive subtype - May appear yellow to white when stretched - Firm to touch	High
Infiltrative	- 5%; develops primarily in the head and neck region of older individuals - Mean age at presentation is 66 years	High
Morpheaform Variant	- 3%–6% - A high-risk subtype - May appear yellow to white when stretched - Firm to touch	High

Adapted from Colegio, O. R., O'Toole, E. A., Ponten, F., Lundeberg, J., & Asplund, A. (2018). Principles of tumor biology and pathogenesis of basal cell carcinoma and squamous cell carcinomas. In J. L. Bolognia, J. V. Schaffer, & L. Cerooni (Eds.), *Dermatology* (4th ed) (pp. 1858–1871, Section 18 Neoplasms of the Skin): Elsevier. Retrieved July 8, 2018 from https://phstwlp2.partners.org:2093/#!/content/book/3-s2.0-B9780702062759001070?scrollTo¼%23s0050; Christensen, S. R., & Leffell, D. J. (2016). Cancer of the Skin. In V. T. DeVita, T. S. Lawrence, & S. A. Rosenberg (Eds.), *Cancer: Principles and Practice of Oncology* (pp. 838–886 Chapter 6). Philadelphia: Wolters Kluwer Health.

B. Melanoma (Buzaid & Gershenwald, 2018)
   1. Prognostic stage group based on TNM staging (AJCC, 2017)
      a. Prognostic stage, age, performance status, tumor burden, pathologic features, and mutation status influence prognosis.
         (1) Most important prognostic features in localized melanoma include:
            (a) Depth of invasion measured in millimeters (Breslow depth)
            (b) Ulceration and mitosis of the primary lesion
         (2) Metastasis to regional lymph nodes, distant skin, subcutaneous, lung, liver, and brain. Risk of metastases is dependent on stage at time of diagnosis.

TABLE 24.6 Subtypes and Features of Melanoma

Type	Frequency	Features
Superficial spreading (SSM)	60%–75%	- Most common subtype - Type seen most often in young persons - About 30% arise from a preexisting mole, and the remainder de novo - Can be found anywhere on the body, but more likely to occur on the trunk in men and legs in women - Begins as an asymptomatic brown-to-black macule with color variations
Nodular (NM)	15%–30%	- Most aggressive type - Appears as a darkly pigmented, pedunculated, or polypoid nodule but may also be red or flesh-colored (amelanotic) - Most often found on the trunk, legs, and arms, or the scalp in men - Tend to be diagnosed at a thicker and more advanced stage
Lentigo maligna (LMM)	5%–10%	- Typically arises from the precursor lentigo maligna; in chronically sun-exposed skin on the face, ears, arms, and upper trunk of older individuals - Often begins as a frecklelike, tan-brown macule that gradually enlarges and develops darker, asymmetric foci - About 5% of LMs will progress to LMM
Acral lentiginous (ALM)	<5%	- Usually appears as a black or brown discoloration under the nails or on the soles of the feet or palms of the hands and occasionally on mucosal surfaces - Most common type among Asians and dark-skinned individuals, with a particular predilection for the soles of the feet - Least common type among Caucasians

Adapted from American Cancer Society (ACS). (2018). *Melanoma Skin Cancer*. Atlanta: American Cancer Society. Available at https://www.cancer.org/cancer/melanoma-skin-cancer.html; Galan, A. (2017). Pathologic and molecular features of melanocytic nevi and melanoma. In H. Kluger & S. Aryan (Eds.), *The Melanoma Handbook*. New York: Demos Medical. Springer; Garbe, C., & Bauer, J. (2018). Melanoma. In J. L. Bolognia, J. V. Schaffer, & L. Cerooni (Eds.): *Dermatology* (4th ed) (pp. 1989–2019 Section 18 Melanoma). Elsevier. Retrieved August 19, 2018 from https://phstwlp2.partners.org:2093/#!/content/book/3-s2.0-B9780702062759001070?scrollTo¼%23s0050.

TABLE 24.7 ABCDEs of Mole/Melanoma Recognition

A	Asymmetry	Normal moles are symmetrical in appearance (half of the lesion is a mirror image of the other half), whereas melanomas tend to be asymmetrical
B	Border	Normal moles tend to have even, regular, borders, whereas melanomas tend to have irregular, jagged borders
C	Color	Normal moles are uniformly one color, whereas melanomas tend to have color variegation
D	Diameter	Normal moles tend to be ≤6 mm in size, whereas melanomas tend to be larger than 6 mm
E	Evolving	Normal moles should not change (evolve) in size, shape, or color, whereas melanomas may possess features such as evolving size, shape, color, or concerning symptoms such as itching or bleeding

Adapted from American Cancer Society (ACS). (2018). *Melanoma Skin Cancer*. Atlanta: American Cancer Society. Available at https://www.cancer.org/cancer/melanoma-skin-cancer.html; Shi, V. J., & Leventhal, J. S. (2017). Epidemiology and screening of pigmented lesions. In H. Kluger, & S. Aryan (Eds.), *The Melanoma Handbook*. New York: Demos Medical. Springer.

2. General estimate of 5-year survival rate (ACS, 2018)
   a. Local early-stage disease—99%
   b. Regional stage—63%
   c. Metastatic disease—20%

IX. Treatment (Alam et al., 2018; Bichijkian et al., 2018; Didona et al., 2018; Farberg & Goldenberg 2018; Christensen & Leffell, 2016)

A. NMSC
   1. Surgical—treatment of choice for majority of lesions
      a. Electrodessication and curettage (ED&C)—uses curette to scrape tumor cells with a margin, then cautery or electrodessication destroys the remainder of the tissue
         (1) Reserved for small (<1 cm), low-risk BCC, AKs, SSCis
      b. Excision—removal of the tumor and a margin of clinically uninvolved tissue; used for low-risk, small (<1 cm) lesions
      c. Mohs micrographic surgery (MMS)—removes tissue in multiple progressive thin layers; preserves maximum amount of tissue
   2. Topical—primarily for low-risk lesions
      a. Cryotherapy—destroys tissue by exposing to subzero temperatures, causing tissue damage and subsequent cell death

(1) Used for low-risk lesions or for those when more effective therapies are contra-indicated or not practical

b. Imiquimod (an immunomodulator) used to treat AKs and superficial BCCs on the trunk, neck, or extremities.

c. 5 fluorouracil (5-FU) (chemotherapy)
   (1) Used to treat AKs and superficial BCCs

d. Photodynamic therapy (PDT)—combines photosensitizing medications with light or lasers to induce cell death
   (1) Used primarily to treat large numbers of AKs
   (2) May be combined with ED&C as adjuvant modality for invasive SCC in high-risk patients (i.e., solid organ transplant recipients) (Alam et al., 2018)

e. Radiation
   (1) Used as adjuvant therapy for positive margins after surgical removal
   (2) Lesions with perineural invasion (PNI)
   (3) Local regional nodal metastasis

f. Systemic therapy
   (1) Hh inhibitors for unresectable/recurrent BCC: vismodegib, sonidegib
   (2) Platinum-based chemotherapy for unresectable or distant metastatic SCC or for recurrence after surgery or radiation
   (3) Anti–PD-L1 antibody, avelumab recently approved for metastatic or unresectable MCC

B. Melanoma (NCCN, 2018)
   1. Surgery for primary melanomas
      a. Wide local excision is the preferred treatment for primary melanoma lesions
      b. Tumor thickness determines appropriate surgical margins (see Table 24.2)
      c. SLNBx is recommended for lesions >1.0 mm or <1 mm if there are adverse pathologic factors such as ulceration, mitoses, or lymphovascular invasion
         (1) Tumor thickness most reliable predictor of positive SLNBx, which also predicts overall survival
         (2) Highly sensitive for the detection of microscopic nodal metastases, with a high negative predictive value
         (3) Complete lymph node dissection no longer advised when positive sentinel node identified due to lack of increase in overall survival (Faries, et al., 2017)
   2. Surgery for advanced melanoma
      a. Elective nodal dissection clinically palpable metastasis
      b. Other treatments in certain clinical situations (NCCN, 2018)
         (1) Isolated limb perfusion

(2) Metastasectomy for patients with oligometastases
(3) Those with a solitary metastasis involving skin, lungs, distant lymph nodes, or gastrointestinal tract
(4) Those with a long disease-free interval between disease recurrence and metastatic focus can be completely resected.

3. Palliative surgery—resection of troublesome tumors causing pain or wounds

4. Radiotherapy
   a. Adjuvant radiotherapy may be used to increase regional control
   b. Palliative for patients with bone or brain metastases

5. Adjuvant therapy for high-risk, resected stage II B/C, III, IVA melanoma (NCCN, 2018)
   a. Immunotherapy (Weber et al., 2017)
      (1) Nivolumab every 2 weeks for 1 year
      (2) Pembrolizumab every 3 weeks for 1 year (*not yet Food and Drug Administration [FDA] approved; approval expected by end of 2018)
      (3) Ipilimumab—every 3 weeks × four doses (less favored due to increased risk of associated toxicity)
   b. Targeted therapy
      (1) *BRAF* + *MEK* inhibitor therapy with dabrafenib + trametinib for 1 year

6. Metastatic disease and systemic treatments (NCCN, 2018)
   a. Immunotherapy: considered standard treatment regardless of mutation status
      (1) Anti–PD-1 monotherapy with pembrolizumab or nivolumab
      (2) Combination anti-CTLA-4 + anti–PD-1 with ipilimumab and nivolumab
   b. Targeted therapy: considered standard treatment for melanoma tumors with an identified *BRAF* V600 mutation
      (1) Combination therapy with oral *BRAF/ MEK* inhibitors:
         (a) Vemurafenib + cobimetinib
         (b) Dabrafenib + trametinib
         (c) Encorafenib + binimetinib
   c. Chemotherapy
      (1) Dacarbazine or temozolomide (an oral analog of dacarbazine, or paclitaxel with/without carboplatin, used primarily as salvage therapy)
   d. Clinical trial
   e. Best supportive care for poor performance status

X. Nursing implications
   A. Provide patient education
      1. Skin cancer prevention strategies (see Box 24.2), especially parents with young children

2. Self-skin examination with ABCDEs
3. Importance of ongoing follow-up to assess for potential recurrence
4. Critical for managing immune checkpoint inhibitors and targeted therapy toxicity

B. Coping (see Chapter 50)

REFERENCES

Alam, M., Armstrong, A., Baum, C., Bordeaux, J. S., Brown, M., Busam, K. J., & Messina, J. (2018). Guidelines of care for the management of cutaneous squamous cell carcinoma. *Journal of the American Academy of Dermatology, 78*(3), 560–578. https://doi.org/10.1016/j.jaad.2017.10.007.

American Cancer Society (ACS). (2018). *Melanoma skin cancer.* Atlanta: American Cancer Society. Available at https://www.cancer.org/cancer/melanoma-skin-cancer.html.

American Joint Committee on Cancer. (2017). In AJCC Cancer Staging Manual. (8th ed.). New York, NY: Springer; 563.

Bichakjian, C., Armstrong, A., Baum, C., Bordeaux, J. S., Brown, M., Busam, K. J., & Messina, J. (2018). Guidelines of care for the management of basal cell carcinoma. *Journal of the American Academy of Dermatology, 78*(3), 540–559. https://doi.org/10.1016/j.jaad.2017.10.006.

Buzaid, A. C., & Gershenwald, J. E. (2018). *Tumor node metastasis (TNM) staging system and other prognostic factors in cutaneous melanoma.* Retrieved May 5, 2018 from https://www.uptodate.com/contents/tumor-node-metastasis-tnm-staging-system-and-other-prognostic-factors-in-cutaneous-melanoma?search=melanoma&source=search_result&selectedTitle=5~150&usage_type=default&display_rank=5.

Christensen, S. R., & Leffell, D. J. (2016). Cancer of the skin. In V. T. DeVita, T. S. Lawrence, & S. A. Rosenberg (Eds.), *Cancer: Principles and Practice of Oncology* (pp. 838–886 Chapter 6). Philadelphia: Wolters Kluwer Health.

Coelho, M. M. V., Matos, T. R., & Apetato, M. (2016). The dark side of the light: mechanisms of photocarcinogenesis. *Clinics in Dermatology, 34*(5), 563–570. https://doi.org/10.1016/j.clindermatol.2016.05.022.

Coggshall, K., Tello, T. L., North, J. P., & Yu, S. S. (2018). Merkel cell carcinoma: an update and review: pathogenesis, diagnosis, and staging. *Journal of the American Academy of Dermatology, 78*(3), 433–442. https://doi.org/10.1016/j.jaad.2017.12.001.

Colegio, O. R., O'Toole, E. A., Pontén, F., Lundeberg, J., & Asplund, A. (2018). Principles of tumor biology and pathogenesis of basal cell carcinoma and squamous cell carcinomas. In J. L. Bolognia, J. V. Schaffer, & L. Cerooni (Eds.), *Dermatology* (4th ed) (pp. 1858-1871, Section 18 Neoplasms of the Skin). Elsevier. Retrieved July 8, 2018 from https://phstwlp2.partners.org:2093/#!/content/book/3-s2.0-B9780702062759001070?scrollTo=%23s0050.

Didona, D., Paolino, G., Bottoni, U., & Cantisani, C. (2018). Non-melanoma skin cancer pathogenesis overview. *Biomedicines, 6*(1), 6. https://doi.org/10.3390/biomedicines6010006.

Farberg, A. S., & Goldenberg, G. (2018). New guidelines of care for the management of nonmelanoma skin cancer. *Cutis, 101*(5), 319.

Faries, M. B., Thompson, J. F., Cochran, A. J., Andtbacka, R. H., Mozzillo, N., Zager, J. S., & Hoekstra, H. J. (2017). Completion dissection or observation for sentinel-node metastasis in melanoma. *New England Journal of Medicine, 376*(23), 2211–2222. https://doi.org/10.1056/NEJMoa1613210.

Galan, A. (2017). Pathologic and molecular features of melanocytic nevi and melanoma. In H. Kluger & S. Aryan (Eds.), *The Melanoma Handbook.* New York: Demos Medical. Springer.

Garbe, C., & Bauer, J. (2018). Melanoma. In J. L. Bolognia, J. V. Schaffer, & L. Cerooni (Eds.): *Dermatology* (4th ed) (pp. 1989-2019 Section 18 Melanoma). Elsevier. Retrieved August 19, 2018 from https://phstwlp2.partners.org:2093/#!/content/book/3-s2.0-B9780702062759001070?scrollTo=%23s0050.

Harms, P. W. (2017). Update on Merkel cell carcinoma. *Clinics in Laboratory Medicine, 37*(3), 485–501. Available at https://doi.org/10.1016/j.cll.2017.05.004.

High, W.A., Tomasini, C.F., Argenziano, G., & Zalaudek, I. (2018). Basic principles of dermatology. In J.L. Bolognia, J.V. Schaffer, & L. Cerooni (Eds.) Dermatology (4th ed) (pp. 1-43, Section 0). Elsevier. Retrieved August 19, 2018 from: https://phstwlp2.partners.org:2093/#!/content/book/3-s2.0 B9780702062759001616?scrollTo=%23top

National Comprehensive Cancer Network. (2018). *Melanoma.* Retrieved January 28, 2018, from www.nccn.org/professionals/physician_gls/default.aspx#melanoma.

Paulson, K. G., Park, S. Y., Vandeven, N. A., Lachance, K., Thomas, H., Chapuis, A. G., & Nghiem, P. (2018). Merkel cell carcinoma: current US incidence and projected increases based on changing demographics. *Journal of the American Academy of Dermatology, 78*(3), 457–463. https://doi.org/10.1016/j.jaad.2017.10.028.

Shi, V. J., & Leventhal, J. S. (2017). Epidemiology and screening of pigmented lesions. In H. Kluger, & S. Aryan (Eds.), *The Melanoma Handbook.* New York: Demos Medical. Springer.

Skin Cancer Foundation (SCF). (2018). *Skin types and at-risk groups.* Available at: https://www.skincancer.org/prevention/are-you-at-risk/skin-types-and-at-risk-groups.

Soura, E., Eliades, P. J., Shannon, K., Stratigos, A. J., & Tsao, H. (2016). Hereditary melanoma: update on syndromes and management. Genetics of familial atypical multiple mole melanoma syndrome. *Journal of the American Academy of Dermatology, 74*(3), 395–407. https://doi.org/10.1016/j.jaad.2015.08.037.

Sullivan, R. J., & Fisher, D. E. (2018). *The molecular biology of melanoma.* Retrieved July 8, 2018 from: https://www.uptodate.com/contents/the-molecular-biology-of-melanoma?search=melanoma%20braf&source=search_result&selectedTitle=4~150&usage_type=default&display_rank.

Vandergriff, T. W. (2018). Anatomy and physiology. In J. L. Bolognia, J. V. Schaffer, & L. Cerooni (Eds.), *Dermatology* (4th ed) (pp. 44-55. Section 1, Overview of Basic Science). Elsevier Retrieved July 8, 2018 from https://phstwlp2.partners.org:2093/#!/content/book/3-s2.0-B9780702062759000015.

Weber, J., Mandala, M., Del Vecchio, M., Gogas, H. J., Arance, A. M., Cowey, C. L., & Grob, J. J. (2017). Adjuvant nivolumab versus ipilimumab in resected stage III or IV melanoma. *New England Journal of Medicine, 377*(19), 1824–1835. https://doi.org/10.1056/NEJMoa1709030.

25

Surgery

Gail W. Davidson

OVERVIEW

I. Principles of cancer surgery
   A. Surgery is the mainstay treatment for most solid tumors (Hoekstra et al., 2016)
   B. Surgical oncologists often lead the multidisciplinary cancer care team (Balch, 2018)
   C. Before surgery, it is important to define:
      1. Goal of surgery (e.g., prevention, cure, palliation)
      2. Functional importance of the involved organ or structure
      3. Ability to reconstruct or restore function if needed
      4. Patient's condition to undergo procedure
         a. "Operable" describes the patient's physiologic condition
         b. "Resectable" describes ability to safely remove cancer with appropriate outcomes (Davidson, 2014)
II. Role of surgery in the oncology patient (Table 25.1 lists surgical approaches)
   A. Diagnosis and staging—histologic examination of tissue is necessary to determine the diagnosis and treatment of most cancers (Guillem, Berchuk, Moley, Norton, & Gabram-Mendola, 2015). Tissue sampling methods are included in Table 25.2.
   B. Curative surgery—achieve "R0" microscopic complete resection (Avital, Stojadinovik, Pisters, Kelsen, & Willett, 2015): remove primary tumor, lymph nodes, adjacent affected organs with negative margins attained via the least invasive means
      1. Local excision—removal of cancer and a small margin of surrounding tissue
      2. Wide excision—removal of cancer and adjacent tissue ± regional lymph nodes
      3. En bloc resection—removal of bulky cancer with contiguous tissues, lymph nodes, and vascular structures required to attain safe margins
   C. Surgery for cancer prevention—prophylactic risk-reducing surgery (e.g., mastectomy, oophorectomy, total colectomy) when found to have a genetic link/mutation such as *BRCA1, BRCA2, TP53, PTEN, STK11, CDH1,* Lynch syndrome (Guillem, Berchuk, Moley, Norton, & Gabram-Mendola, 2015)
   D. Palliative cancer surgery—to improve comfort when curative resection is not possible; includes surgical debulking, decompression, or diversion via stent or ostomy (e.g., gastrojejunostomy, colostomy) (Avital, Stojadinovik, Pisters, Kelsen, & Willett, 2015).
   E. Restorative "oncoplastic" surgery—to improve function or appearance of a surgical defect improving the quality of life (e.g., restoration of a limb posthemipelvectomy, breast reconstruction after mastectomy) (Stubblefield, 2015)
   F. Surgery for oncologic emergencies such as hemorrhage, organ ischemia or perforation, drainage/washout for abscess or infection, cord compression

ASSESSMENT

I. Principles of patient selection (Are et al., 2016)
   A. Select patient based on appropriate indication and benefit outweighs risk
      1. Use objective tools for risk stratification, for example, American College of Surgeons National Surgical Quality Improvement Program (NSQIP) risk calculator (ACS, 2018)
      2. Evaluate functional assessment with standardized tools (e.g., Karnofsky scale)
      3. Cardiopulmonary clearance and American Society of Anesthesiologists (ASA) class for anesthesia preparation
      4. Patient preoperative assessment and education
   B. History
      1. Preexisting conditions, allergies
      2. Previous surgery, reaction to anesthesia and blood products

TABLE 25.1 Surgical Approaches

Approach/ Procedure	Description	Example
Open resection	Requires extended, full-thickness incision to allow thorough exploration and manipulation of tissues	Exploratory laparotomy
Laparoscopic	Multiple small incisions ("ports") are made for surgical camera insertion and application of operative tools allowing less tissue manipulation	Laparoscopic cholecystectomy
Robotic	Remotely controlled instruments allowing less invasion, improved optics, finer control, and ergonomics to lessen tissue manipulation (Owen, 2014)	Robotic prostatectomy
Endoscopic or "natural orifice transluminal endoscopic surgery" (NOTES)	Surgical tools passed through an existing orifice (mouth, nares, anus, urethra) without external incision/scar	Transvaginal cholecystectomy
Laser	Used alone or in combination with photosensitive agents to apply precise beams to damage tumors at the cellular level	Photodynamic therapy
Ablative techniques	Thermal (heat- or cold-based) radiofrequency or microwave ablation may be applied during open, laparoscopic, or percutaneous procedures	Percutaneous ablation of primary liver cancer

Data from Owen, D. (2014). Robotic minimally invasive surgery. In G.W. Davidson, J. L. Lester, & M. Routt (Eds.), *Surgical Oncology Nursing* (pp. 199–204). Pittsburgh: Oncology Nursing Society; Thompson, K. R., Kavnoudias, H., & Neal, R. E. (2015). Introduction to irreversible electroporation—principles and techniques. *Techniques in vascular and interventional radiology, 18.* 1280134. https://doi.org/10.1053/j.tvir.2015.06.002.

TABLE 25.2 Tissue Sampling Methods

Tissue Sampling Procedure	Description
Fine needle aspiration	Percutaneous fine needle guided to mass to remove tissue fragments
Core or needle biopsy	Larger needle used to sample tissue via percutaneous stick
Incisional biopsy	Small incision over mass to remove tissue sample
Excisional biopsy	Removal of entire mass through an incision
Sentinel lymph node biopsy	Intradermal injection of isosulfan blue (dye) for lymphatic mapping to identify primary (sentinel) node(s) for histopathic examination for metastatic disease; spares regional node dissection and associated morbidity (Ribas, Slingluff, & Rosenberg, 2017)
Endoscopic/ laparoscopic biopsy	Direct visualization of mass, adjacent lymph nodes through scopes, cameras for tissue samples or washings for cytology

3. Previous chemotherapy or radiation and effects that could influence surgical selection and outcomes (Lorusso et al., 2018)
4. Current medications (beta blockers, anticoagulants), herbal and vitamin supplements
5. Social history (smoking, alcohol, illicit drug use), social support for after-care

C. Physical examination
   1. Cardiovascular changes—increased risk of cardiac event if previous injury (e.g., myocardial infarction/ischemia, stroke), anemia, venous thromboembolism (VTE)
   2. Pulmonary function alterations related to anemia, obstructive sleep apnea, aerodigestive cancers with increased aspiration risk, pleural effusions, or pneumonia
   3. Hematologic—assess for anemia, coagulopathy, bone marrow suppression related to chemotherapy, immunotherapy, radiation
   4. Gastrointestinal, hepatic—assess for malnutrition, malabsorption, cachexia, coagulopathy, fluid balance, vomiting, diarrhea, constipation, which can affect surgery readiness and recovery
   5. Renal—evaluate function and fluid and electrolyte balance, renal dose medications and dialysis the day before surgical procedures if end-stage renal disease exists
   6. Endocrine—glycemic control before surgery is optimal; hyperglycemia can lead to volume depletion, electrolyte imbalance, osmotic diuresis, diabetic ketoacidosis, increased surgical site infections, and poor wound healing (Morgan, 2014)

D. Psychosocial evaluation, patient and caregiver education
   1. Assess for psychosocial support, stressors, coping mechanisms
   2. Plan for postdischarge care and recovery site
   3. Caregiver readiness, access to services/supplies
   4. Advance directive discussion and access
   5. Preoperative directions—report in time/place, home medication instructions, expectations related to surgery and discharge
   6. Enhanced recovery after surgery (ERAS) instruction as prescribed—approach to care allows clear carbohydrate-enriched fluid intake up to 2 hours before surgery (decreases nausea, fatigue, dehydration, hunger), VTE prevention, antimicrobial prophylaxis, patient/caregiver education to decrease cost and length of stay (LOS) related to surgery (Segelman & Nygrem, 2017)

MANAGEMENT

I. Surgery as part of the multimodal cancer treatment plan
   A. Chemotherapy or radiation may be delivered before surgery (neoadjuvant) to downsize disease or improve margins—can affect wound healing
   B. Intraoperative chemotherapy delivered directly to tissue or vasculature (e.g., hyperthermic intraperitoneal chemotherapy [HIPEC], isolated limb perfusion)
   C. Intraoperative radiation (IORT)—a single dose of radiation delivered directly to tissue via open incision typically to deep margins that cannot be resected without significant morbidity; or via brachytherapy—surgically implanted device is sourced with a radioactive agent (Williams & Burke, 2014)
   D. Postoperative chemotherapy (adjuvant) may be given if cancer was incompletely resected or if cytoreduction/debulking surgery was planned to improve chemotherapy delivery to active tumors (Cannistra, Gershenson, & Recht, 2015), or via an implanted chemotherapy pump (hepatic arterial infusion pump)
   E. Postoperative radiation (adjuvant) to treat potential microscopic disease when conservative surgery performed (e.g., radiation after lumpectomy)
II. Interventional radiology as part of the interdisciplinary team
   A. Before surgery, may perform biopsy, tissue sampling, central line placement
   B. Instead of surgery may perform minimally invasive procedures such as percutaneous ablation, vascular embolization
   C. Postoperative and supportive care—drain or stent placement
III. Safety and management of the perioperative/procedural patient
   A. Safety, teamwork, and collaboration are critical competencies within the perioperative environment.

(QSEN, 2018) (Burke, 2014). Multiple agencies have collaborated to develop safety goals, procedures, and tools to improve safe caregiving, including:
   1. Association of periOperative Registered Nurses (AORN) (AORN, 2016) comprehensive tool includes aspects from each of the following agencies:
      a. World Health Organization checklist (WHO, 2009)—ensures patient confirmation, consent, site marking, safe environment, team collaboration through all perioperative phases
      b. The Joint Commission National Patient Safety Goals (TJC, 2018) ensures patient, team, and equipment preparation, site marking, "universal protocol" and "time out" safety goals
      c. The Surgical Care Improvement Project (SCIP) embellished by The Joint Commission—developed from the Centers for Medicare and Medicaid, the Centers for Disease Control, and the Institute of Healthcare Improvement to decrease complications, cost, LOS (Williams & Burke, 2014), (Chou, et al. 2016).
   B. Postanesthesia recovery
      1. Close monitoring until discharge/transition criteria met
      2. Postoperative report handoff communication includes patient name, diagnosis, history, reason for surgery, type of surgery and anesthesia, patient condition, vital signs, oxygenation, level of consciousness, counts correct, length of time in operating room (OR), deep vein thrombosis (DVT) prophylaxis, specimens sent, pain level, last medication and time due, location of incision, bandage, drains, urinary catheter/urine output, intravenous (IV) fluid, amount, location, medications given and due, specific care, any complications, estimated blood loss and replacement if planned (Flexner, 2017)
      3. Employ pulmonary toilet to prevent atelectasis, pneumonia, aspiration with cough and deep breathing, incentive spirometry, early ambulation, oral hygiene, elevate head of bed (Kazaure, Martin, Yoon, & Wren, 2014)
      4. VTE prophylaxis (sequential compression, early ambulation/return to preoperative activity level, antithrombotic therapy) to avoid DVT, pulmonary embolism (NCCN, 2018 to review guidelines)

EXPECTED PATIENT OUTCOMES

I. The patient will be kept safe during surgery: correct procedure, correct site, correct person; perioperative positioning without harm to skin, nerves, joints; correct instrument and sponge count; preoperative antibiotic, skin prep, antisepsis maintained; incision/wound intact for healing without surgical site infection (Torres-Berrios et al., 2017).

II. Hemodynamic and cardiopulmonary stability will occur.

III. Postoperative pain will be controlled with pharmacologic and nonpharmacologic measures.

IV. Patient and caregiver will demonstrate readiness to manage care or resources arranged and understand when to follow up.

REFERENCES

American College of Surgeons. (2018) ACS NSQIP Surgical Risk Calculator. Retrieved from https://riskcalculator.facs.org/RiskCalculaotr/PatientInfo.jsp.

Are, C., Berman, R. S., Wuld, L., Cummings, C., Lecoq, C., & Audisio, R. A. (2016). Global curriculum in surgical oncology. *Annals of Surgical Oncology, 23*, 1782–1795. https://doi.org/10.1245/s10434-016-5239-7.

Association of periOperative Registered Nurses. (2016). *AORN Comprehensive Surgical Checklist.* Retrieved from https://www.aorn.org.443/-media/aorn/guidelines/tool-kits/correct-site-surgery/aorn_comprehensive_surgical_checklist_2016.pdf.

Avital, I., Stojadinovik, A., Pisters, P. W. T., Kelsen, D. P., & Willett, C. G. (2015). Cancer of the stomach. In V. T. Devita, T. S. Lawrence, & S. Rosenberg (Eds.), *DeVita, Hellman, and Rosenberg's Cancer: Principles & Practice of Oncology* (10th ed., pp. 613–641). Philadelphia: Lippincott Williams and Wilkins.

Balch, C. (2018). What is a surgical oncologist. *Annals of Surgical Oncology, 25*, 7–9. https://doi.org/10.1245/s10434-017-6287-3.

Burke, S. A. (2014). Perioperative care of the patient with cancer. In G. W. Davidson, J. L. Lester, & M. Routt (Eds.), *Surgical Oncology Nursing* (pp. 39–52). Pittsburgh: Oncology Nursing Society.

Cannistra, S. A., Gershenson, D. M., & Recht, A. (2015). Ovarian cancer, fallopian tube carcinoma, and peritoneal carcinoma. In V. T. Devita, T. S. Lawrence, & S. Rosenberg (Eds.), *DeVita, Hellman, and Rosenberg's Cancer: Principles & Practice of Oncology* (10th ed., pp. 1075–1097). Philadelphia: Lippincott Williams and Wilkins.

Chou, R., Gordon, D. B., de Leon-Casasola, O. A., Rosenberg, J. M., Bickler, S., Brennan, T., & Wu, C. L. (2016). Guidelines on the management of postoperative pain. *The Journal of Pain, 17*(2), 131–157. https://doi.org/10.1016/j.jpain.2015.12.008.

Davidson, G. (2014). Overview. In G. W. Davidson, J. L. Lester, & M. Routt (Eds.), *Surgical Oncology Nursing* (pp. 1–11). Pittsburgh: Oncology Nursing Society.

Flexner, R. (2017). *Operative report post-op rubric.* Retrieved from http://qsen.org/wp-content/uploads/formidable/OPERATIVE-REPORT-Post-op-rubric.docx.

Guillem, J. G., Berchuk, A., Moley, J. F., Norton, Z. J. A., & Gabram-Mendola, S. G. A. (2015). Role of surgery in cancer prevention. In V. T. Devita, T. S. Lawrence, & S. Rosenberg (Eds.), *DeVita, Hellman, and Rosenberg's Cancer: Principles & Practice of Oncology* (10th ed., pp. 335–348). Philadelphia: Lippincott Williams and Wilkins.

Hoekstra, H. J., Wobbes, T., Heineman, E., Haryomo, S., Aryanduno, T., & Balch, C. K. (2016). Fighting global disparities in cancer care: a surgical oncology view. *Annals of Surgical Oncology, 23*, 2131–2136. https://doi.org/10.1245/s10434-016-5194-3.

Kazaure, H. S., Martin, M., Yoon, J. K., & Wren, S. M. (2014). Long-term results of a postoperative pneumonia prevention program for the inpatient surgical ward. *JAMA Surgery, 149*(9), 914–918. https://doi.org/10.1001/jamasurg.2014.1216.

Lorusso, R., Vizzardi, E., Johnson, D., Mariscalco, G., Sciatti, E., Maessen, J., … Gelsomino, S. (2018). Cardiac surgery in adult patients with remitted or active malignancies: a review of preoperative screening, surgical management and short- and long-term postoperative results. *European Journal of Cardio-Thoracic Surgery, 2018*, 1–9. https://doi.org/10.1093/ejcts/ezy019. 0.

Morgan, S. W. (2014). Preoperative care of the patient with cancer. In G. W. Davidson, J. L. Lester, & M. Routt (Eds.), *Surgical Oncology Nursing* (pp. 25–38). Pittsburgh: Oncology Nursing Society.

National Comprehensive Cancer Network. (NCCN) (2018). *NCCN clinical practice guidelines in oncology: cancer-associated venous thromboembolic disease [v.1.2018].* Retrieved from https://www.nccn.org/professionals/physician_gls/pdf/vte.pdf.

Owen, D. (2014). Robotic minimally invasive surgery. In G. W. Davidson, J. L. Lester, & M. Routt (Eds.), *Surgical Oncology Nursing* (pp. 199–204). Pittsburgh: Oncology Nursing Society.

Quality and Safety Education for Nurses (QSEN, 2018) Competencies. Retrieved from http://qsen.org/competencies/pre-licensure-ksas/#teamwork_collaboration.

Ribas, A., Slingluff, C. L., & Rosenberg, S. A. (2017). Cutaneous melanoma. In V. T. Devita, T. S. Lawrence, & S. Rosenberg (Eds.), *DeVita, Hellman, and Rosenberg's Cancer: Principles & Practice of Oncology* (10th ed., chapter 94). Retrieved from http://ovidsp.ovid.com.proxy.lib.ohio-state.edu/ovidweb.cgi?T=JS&CSC=Y&NEWS=N&PAGE=booktext&D=books1&AN=01833060/10th_Edition/12&XPATH=/OVIDBOOK%5b1%5d/TXTBKBD%5b1%5d/DIVISIONA%5b5%5d/DIVISIONB%5b9%5d/CHAPTER%5b3%5d.

Segelman, J., & Nygren, J. (2017). Best practice in major elective rectal/pelvis surgery: enhanced recovery after surgery (ERAS). *Updates in Surgery, 69*, 435–439. https://doi.org/10.1007/s13304-017-0492-2.

Stubblefield, M. D. (2015). Rehabilitation of the cancer patient. In V. T. Devita, T. S. Lawrence, & S. Rosenberg (Eds.), *DeVita, Hellman, and Rosenberg's Cancer: Principles & Practice of Oncology* (10th ed., pp. 2141–2161). Philadelphia: Lippincott Williams and Wilkins.

The Joint Commission National Patient Safety Goals effective. (January 2018). Retrieved from https://www.jointcommission.org/assets/1/6/NPSG_Chapter_HAP_Jan2018.pdf.

Thompson, K. R., Kavnoudias, H., & Neal, R. E. (2015). Introduction to irreversible electroporation- principles and techniques. *Techniques in vascular and interventional radiology, 18*. 1280134. https://doi.org/10.1053/j.tvir.2015.06.002.

Torres-Berrios, S., Umscheid, C., Bratzler, D. W., Leas, B., Stone, E. C., Kelz, R. R., & Schecter, W. P. (2017). Centers of disease control and preventions guideline for the prevention of surgical site infection. *JAMA Surgery, 152*(8), 784–791. https://doi.org/10.1001/jamasurg.2017.0904.

Williams, L., & Burke, S. A. (2014). Intraoperative radiation therapy. In G. W. Davidson, J. L. Lester, & M. Routt (Eds.), *Surgical Oncology Nursing* (pp. 225–236). Pittsburgh: Oncology Nursing Society.

World Health Organization. (WHO) (2009). *Surgical Safety Checklist.* Retrieved from http://www.who.int/patientsafety/safesurgery/ss_checklist/en/.

26

Nursing Implications of Hematopoietic Stem Transplantation

Terry Wikle Shapiro

OVERVIEW

I. Principles of hematopoietic stem cell transplantation (HSCT) (Forman, Negrin, Antin, & Appelbaum, 2016; Brown, 2018; Wikle Shapiro, 2017)

A. A dose-related response to chemotherapy or radiation therapy (RT) exhibited by many malignancies

1. Increasing the dose raises the number of cells destroyed.

2. Chemotherapy or RT dose delivered is limited by the degree of marrow toxicity.

3. High-dose chemotherapy or RT may be administered to treat more aggressive, higher-risk diseases.

4. A potent antitumor effect can be immunologically derived from donor T lymphocytes known as the *graft-versus-tumor effect* (GVT) in allogeneic HSCT.

B. Process of bone marrow transplantation (Forman, Negrin, Antin & Appelbaum, 2016 et al., 2016; Brown, 2018; Wikle Shapiro, 2017) (Fig. 26.1)

1. Marrow source is identified. Bone marrow or stem cells from either the patient (autograft) or a donor (allograft) are infused and engraft to "rescue" the patient's hematopoietic function from the toxic effects of antineoplastic therapy or RT. Box 26.1 outlines sources of autografts and allografts.

2. Stem cell source

a. Autologous—patient receives own bone marrow or peripheral blood stem cells (PBSCs) harvested or collected before pretransplantation conditioning.

b. Allogeneic—patient receives bone marrow, PBSCs, or umbilical cord blood (UCB) from a healthy related or unrelated donor.

3. Factors affecting source of donor marrow

a. Primary disease to be treated

b. Availability of a histocompatible donor

c. Age and size of the patient

C. Allografting

1. Involves transplanting marrow PBSCs or UCB to a genetically different recipient.

a. The human leukocyte antigen (HLA) system is used to determine the best possible stem cell source for transplantation.

b. HLA is a protein—or marker—found on most cells in the body, including white blood cells (WBCs).

c. The immune system uses HLA markers to recognize "self" versus "non-self."

d. Half of the HLA antigens (HLA type) are inherited from each parent.

e. Eight HLA antigens are used in HLA typing allogeneic transplant recipients.

f. The most preferred situation is for hematopoietic stem cells (HSCs) to be donated by a 10-out-of-10 (10/10) antigen, HLA-matched sibling.

g. Partially matched family members or matched unrelated donors from a volunteer pool may also be used as donors (e.g., 6/10 match).

h. Within certain limitations, UCB may be used as a source of allogeneic stem cells in the related matched sibling and unrelated donor situations.

i. Allografts are indicated for some congenital abnormalities of bone marrow function or in disease involving marrow that is not amenable to cure with standard treatment (e.g., leukemias). Box 26.2 shows diseases treated with allogeneic transplantation.

j. Reduced intensity or nonmyeloablative HSCTs are used in the allogeneic transplantation setting when the patient is older, has preexisting comorbidities, and has a disease that will benefit from the GVT immunologic effect (Brown, 2018).

(1) The patient receives lower doses of chemotherapy plus immunotherapy often followed by a small dose of total-body irradiation (TBI) and then allogeneic transplantation of marrow or PBSCs.

(2) The objective is to induce an immunologic response known as the *GVT effect,* whereby the donor stem cells recognize the malignant cells and destroy them.

(3) This treatment is usually reserved for older patients (>60 years) or those with comorbidities (limited organ function); the risk of acute toxicities from the lowered

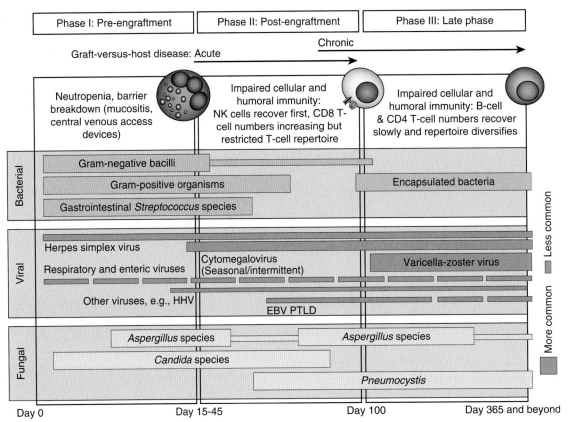

Fig. 26.1 Hematopoietic stem cell transplantation. (From Wikle Shapiro, T. (2017). In S. Newton, M. Hickey, & J. M. Brant (Eds.), *Mosby's Oncology nursing advisor: A comprehensive guide to clinical practice* (pp. 188). St. Louis: Elsevier.)

BOX 26.1   Sources of Marrow or Stem Cells

Allografts
- Matched sibling donor
  - Bone marrow
  - Peripheral blood stem cells
  - Umbilical cord blood
- Identical twin donor
  - Bone marrow
  - Peripheral blood stem cells
- Partially matched family member
  - Bone marrow
  - Peripheral blood stem cells

- Umbilical cord blood
- Matched unrelated donor
  - Bone marrow
  - Peripheral blood stem cells
  - Umbilical cord blood

Autografts
- Autologous bone marrow
- Autologous peripheral blood stem cells
- Autologous umbilical cord blood (rare)

---

doses of chemotherapy and radiotherapy is less.

2. Allografting requires the use of posttransplantation immunosuppression to prevent overwhelming graft-versus-host disease (GVHD), a condition in which donor T lymphocytes mount an immune response against the patient.

D. Autografting (Forman et al., 2016; Wikle Shapiro, 2017)

1. Autografting involves transplanting marrow or PBSCs back into the person from whom the blood cells originated.

2. Autologous bone marrow or PBSC transplantation is used as a method for treating a number of malignant disorders.

3. Using autologous marrow or PBSCs is not feasible in patients who have a deficiency of their functional bone marrow, as is the case with aplastic anemia, inborn errors of metabolism, and immunodeficiency states.

4. Autografting may be preferable to using an allogeneic source of stem cells (e.g., to avoid GVHD, in situations in which marrow contamination with malignant cells is unlikely, and when no

---

BOX 26.2 Diseases Treated with Allografting of Hematopoietic Stem Cells

Leukemias—Syndromes
Acute myelogenous leukemia
Acute lymphoblastic leukemia
Chronic myelogenous leukemia
Myelodysplastic syndromes
Acute myelofibroids

Immunodeficiencies
Severe combined immunodeficiency
Wiskott–Aldrich syndrome
Miscellaneous immunodeficiencies

Hematologic Disorders
β-Thalassemia
Sickle cell anemia
Congenital neutropenia
Osteopetrosis

Bone Marrow Failure
Severe aplastic anemia
Fanconi anemia
Reticular dysgenesis

Nonhematologic Genetic Disorders
Inclusion cell (I-cell) disease
Mucopolysaccharidosis
Adrenal leukodystrophy
Glycogen storage diseases
Miscellaneous metabolic disorders

Lymphoproliferative Disorders
Hodgkin disease
Non-Hodgkin lymphoma
Multiple myeloma
Chronic lymphocytic leukemia

---

evidence of an immunologic antitumor effect [GVT] with allogeneic transplantation exists).

5. Autologous stem cell transplantation (ASCT) is most frequently used for the treatment of multiple myeloma and lymphoma. ASCT is also utilized in the treatment of other malignancies such as lymphoma, neuroblastoma, and brain tumors in which the chance for cure is relatively low with standard or conventional doses of chemotherapy. In this case ASCT is considered a marrow or stem cell "rescue." Box 26.3 illustrates diseases treated with autologous transplantation.

6. In some autografting situations, it is debated whether a low (undetectable) level of tumor cells persisting in the infused cells may promote relapse. However, routine purging, even in diseases that involve bone marrow, is unproven.

BOX 26.3 Diseases Treated with Autografting of Hematopoietic Stem Cells

Lymphoproliferative Disorders
Hodgkin disease
Non-Hodgkin lymphoma
Multiple myeloma

Solid Tumors
Neuroblastoma
Ewing sarcoma
Hepatoblastoma
Testicular cancer
Osteosarcoma
Cerebral tumors

Others
Autoimmune diseases
Systemic lupus erythematosus
Rheumatoid arthritis
Juvenile-onset diabetes

Using PBSCs instead of bone marrow is known to lower the risk of tumor infusion.

7. PBSCs are almost exclusively used as an autografting source.

8. Autologous PBSC collection is generally performed after several cycles of chemotherapy.

9. Autologous HSCT can be effective in treating some autoimmune diseases because it allows for high doses of immunosuppressive therapy to be administered (Alchi et al., 2013).

10. Optimally, transplantation is performed as close to complete remission as possible, when the disease is "chemoresponsive," the patient has "minimal residual disease," or both (Wikle Shapiro, 2017).

E. In the patient receiving an allogeneic transplant, histocompatibility testing must be done to determine whether the patient and donor are genetically compatible (Kapadia & Greiner, 2018; National Marrow Donor Program [NMDP], 2018).

1. HLA testing—major histocompatibility complex encoded by genes (one pair from each parent) present on chromosome 6

a. Major loci of importance when using allogeneic stem marrow or PBSC donors are HLA-A, -B, -C, DRB1, and DQB1 (10 antigens). Only HLA-A, HLA-B, and DRB1 antigens (six antigens) are tested when using a UCB unit (Kapadia and Greiner, 2018).

b. The success of allogeneic transplantation is related to the degree of histocompatibility between the donor and recipient.

c. Patients have a one in four chance of having a 10/10 antigen–matched donor among their full siblings.

d. Patients without an HLA-matched sibling donor have approximately a 66% to 70% chance (depending on race or ethnicity) of finding an

HLA-matched unrelated volunteer donor or donated UCB donor from the National Marrow Donor Registry. Ethnic minority patients are less likely to find an HLA-compatible donor. Use of matched unrelated donors carries more risk because of higher incidence of GVHD and delay in immune reconstitution.

2. Further DNA testing of HLA-DR—performed to determine the degree of histocompatibility between donor and recipient

F. HSC recipient is prepared with dose-intense (marrow-ablative) therapy (Wikle Shapiro, 2017).

   1. The conditioning protocol is established based on the primary disease, patient's functional status, and type of transplant.

   2. The goals of a pretransplantation conditioning regimen are as follows:

      a. To eradicate remaining malignancy in the recipient

      b. To suppress the immune system of the recipient to allow for marrow engraftment (allografts only)

      c. To open spaces within the marrow compartment for newly infused PBSCs or marrow to engraft

   3. The conditioning regimen may include high-dose chemotherapy alone or in combination with total lymph node or TBI.

   4. Immunosuppressive therapy may also be used as part of the conditioning regimen in the allogeneic transplantation setting.

   5. Conditioning regimen is usually completed before marrow transplantation or infusion.

G. Marrow, PBSCs, or UCB from the donor (allogeneic) or the patient (autologous) is harvested and processed (Kitko, et al., 2018).

   1. Bone marrow harvesting is performed with the patient under general or regional anesthesia; most commonly used in pediatric transplantation.

      a. Two to four punctures are made in the posterior iliac crests bilaterally.

      b. Approximately 10 mL/kg of the recipient's body weight is aspirated from the donor.

      c. Marrow is then filtered to remove bone and fat particles.

      d. If a major ABO incompatibility exists between recipient and donor, the red blood cells (RBCs) are removed before infusion.

      e. Processed marrow is placed in a blood administration bag for cryopreservation (autologous) or immediate infusion (allogeneic).

      f. Matched, unrelated donor marrow or PBSCs are generally collected at the donor's closest NMDP collection center and then transported to the recipient's transplantation center for infusion. Further processing is generally performed at the recipient center

2. PBSCs are generally collected after stem cell mobilization with hematopoietic growth factors and/or chemotherapy (autologous only). Immunomodulators such as plerixafor may be used before stem cell collection.

   a. Cells are collected, usually via a large-bore intravenous catheter or a centrally placed pheresis catheter, using a special cell separator. After processing, autologous PBSCs are cryopreserved in small aliquots for future infusion.

   b. A minimum of 2.5×10^6 CD34+ cells are required to ensure successful engraftment. ⚠️

   c. With UCB, lower cell doses may be utilized.

   d. Patients undergo the conditioning regimen. Next, previously collected cells are thawed and reinfused. Fresh allogeneic PBSCs are infused as soon as possible, often not sooner than 24 hours after high-dose therapy is completed.

3. Stem cells from an umbilical cord may be used as a source, although UCB is generally reserved for patients weighing less than 60 kg. Studies are currently underway using multiple (>1) matched cord blood units for larger patients (Tiercy, 2014).

   a. Related and unrelated UCB cells are harvested at birth from volunteer maternal donors and are cryopreserved at a designated cord blood bank. Donated cord blood is accessible via the NMDP's Cord Blood Registry (NMDP, 2018; Shenoy, 2013).

   b. The cells are transported to the recipient's transplantation center, thawed, and infused on the day of transplantation.

4. Some centers are using a variety of experimental techniques to purge autologous marrow of possible tumor contaminants.

   a. Purging may be performed using monoclonal antibodies, chemotherapy, or physical means (centrifugation).

   b. Purging may damage the stem cells, thus increasing the risk of delayed engraftment or rejection.

H. Marrow HSCs are infused through a central venous catheter.

   1. Autologous marrow and PBSCs are thawed at the patient's bedside and reinfused via a central venous line.

   2. Freshly harvested marrow or PBSCs are brought to the patient's room and infused in a similar fashion to a unit of packed RBCs.

   3. If allogeneic cord blood is used, cells are thawed at the bedside and reinfused.

I. The patient is supported through the period of marrow aplasia (10–30 days). Preventive measures are instituted to decrease potential complications (e.g., infection, GVHD, sinusoidal obstructive syndrome [SOS]/veno-occlusive disease [VOD]). See Table 26.1 for preventive measures for bone marrow transplantation–associated

TABLE 26.1 Preventive Measures for Bone Marrow Transplantation–Associated Complications

Complication	Infection	Preventive and Treatment Measures	Nursing Implications
Graft-versus-host disease (GVHD), acute and chronic	• Results from engraftment of immunocompetent donor T lymphocytes reacting against immunocompetent recipient tissues (skin, gastrointestinal [GI] tract, liver) • Occurs in 30%–60% of all allogeneic bone marrow transplant recipients • Risk is increased when donor is not a 6/6 HLA antigen match or when a matched unrelated donor is used • May be either acute or chronic	• Depletion of T cells from marrow • Preventive immunosuppressive agents • Cyclosporine A (Gengraf, Sandimmune oral: Neoral) • FK 506 (tacrolimus) • High-dose steroids: • Antithymocyte globulin • Alemtuzumab (Campath) • Muromonab-CD3 (OKT-3/Ontak) • Thalidomide (Thalomid) • Monoclonal antibodies • Polyclonal antibodies • Mycophenolate mofetil (MMF) (Cellcept) • Methotrexate (Mexate) • Sirolimus (Rapamune) • Mesenchymal stem cells	• Monitor for delayed marrow engraftment. • Monitor for prolonged lymphopenia and neutropenia. • Evaluate cyclosporine or tacrolimus levels, and notify practitioner of significant abnormalities. • Monitor side effects of immunosuppressive agents. • Monitor for signs of infection. • Monitor weekly infection markers (viral polymerase chain reactions [PCRs], galactomannan). • Maintain skin integrity. • Maintain patient's functional capacity. • Monitor for signs of hemolytic-uremic syndrome.
Idiopathic pulmonary interstitial pneumonitis (infectious and noninfectious)	• Occurs most frequently in patients >30 yr with history of chest irradiation or previous bleomycin therapy; allogeneic transplantation, and CMV-positive with CMV-negative donor • Causative agents infectious • Cytomegalovirus • *Aspergillus* species • *Pneumocystis jiroveci* • Other infections 15% • Noninfectious cause • Diffuse alveolar hemorrhage (DAH) • Chemotherapy-related • GVHD • Radiation therapy	• Use of cytomegalovirus (CMV)—seronegative blood products • Use of filtered air system (HEPA) • Antimicrobial therapy • Ganciclovir (Cytovene) • Foscarnet (Foscavir) • Intravenous immunoglobulin • Trimethoprim and sulfamethoxazole • Aerosolized or intravenous (IV) pentamidine (NebuPent, Pentacarinat, Pentam 300) • Azoles (voriconazole, posaconazole) • Amphotericin B (Abelcet, AmBisome)	• Monitor for side effects of antimicrobial therapy. • Implement turning, coughing, and deep-breathing routine. • Encourage activity. • Provide transfusion therapy (DAH).
Hepatic sinusoidal obstruction syndrome	• Damage to the small sinusoids of the liver from pretransplantation conditioning regimen • Occurs in 5%–54% of patients; most common in patients undergoing matched, unrelated donor transplants and those with pretransplantation liver enzyme elevations or previous radiation to abdomen	• Defibrotide • Ursodiol (Actigall) • Heparin • Diuretics • Renal dose of dopamine • Strict fluid management	• Monitor liver function studies. • Monitor for weight gain. • Evaluate abdominal pain. • Use caution when administering drugs that are cleared via hepatic system because increased toxicity may occur. • Monitor renal function.

Adapted from Becze, E. (2011). Veno-occlusive disease is the most common hepatic complication in stem cell transplants. *ONS Connect 11*, 16-17; Ezzone, S. A. (Ed.). (2013). *Hematopoietic stem cell transplantation: a manual for nursing practice* (2nd ed.). Pittsburgh: Oncology Nursing Society.

TABLE 26.2 **Infectious Complications and Sites of Occurrence in Hematopoietic Stem Cell Transplantation Recipients**

Type	Organism, Disease	Common Site
First Month After Transplantation		
Viral	Herpes simplex virus (HSV)	Oral, esophageal, skin, gastrointestinal (GI) tract, and genital
	Respiratory syncytial virus (RSV)	Sinopulmonary
	Epstein–Barr virus (EBV)	Oral, esophageal, skin, GI tract
	Human herpesvirus type 6 (HHV6)	Pulmonary, central nervous system (CNS), GI tract
Bacterial	Gram-positive organisms (*Staphylococcus epidermidis*, *S. aureus*, streptococci)	Skin, blood, sinopulmonary
	Gram-negative organisms (*Escherichia coli, Pseudomonas aeruginosa, Klebsiella*)	GI tract, blood, oral, perirectal
Fungal	*Candida* (*C. albicans, C. glabrata, C. krusei*)	Oral, esophageal, skin
	Aspergillus fumigatus, A. flavus	Sinopulmonary, skin
1–4 Months After Transplantation		
Viral	Cytomegalovirus (CMV)	Pulmonary, hepatic, GI tract
	Enteric viruses (rotavirus, coxsackie virus, adenovirus)	Pulmonary, urinary, GI tract, hepatic
	RSV	Sinopulmonary
	Parainfluenza virus	Pulmonary
	BK human polyoma virus	Genitourinary
Bacterial	Gram-positive organisms	Sinopulmonary, skin, venous access devices
Fungal	*Candida* species	Oral, hepatosplenic, integument, venous access devices
	Aspergillus species	Sinopulmonary, CNS, skin
	Mucormycosis	Sinopulmonary
	Coccidioidomycosis	Sinopulmonary
	Cryptococcus neoformans	Pulmonary, CNS
Protozoa	*Pneumocystis jiroveci* (*carinii*)	Pulmonary
	Toxoplasma gondii	Pulmonary, CNS
4–12 Months After Transplantation		
Viral	CMV, echoviruses, RSV, varicella zoster virus (VZV), human polyoma virus	Integument, pulmonary, hepatic, genitourinary
Bacterial	Gram-positive organisms (*Streptococcus pneumoniae*),	Sinopulmonary, blood
	Haemophilus influenzae (pneumococci)	Sinopulmonary
Fungal	Aspergillosis	Sinopulmonary
	Coccidioidomycosis	Sinopulmonary
Protozoa	*P. jiroveci* (*carinii*)	Pulmonary
	Toxoplasma gondii	Pulmonary, CNS
12 Months After Transplantation		
Viral	VZV	Integument
	CMV	Pulmonary, hepatic
Bacterial	Gram-positive organisms (streptococci, *H. influenzae*, encapsulated bacteria)	Sinopulmonary, blood

Data from Ezzone, S. A. (Ed.). (2013). *Hematopoietic stem cell transplantation: a manual for nursing practice* (2nd ed., pp. 155-172). Pittsburgh: Oncology Nursing Society.

complication control practices. See Table 26.2 for infectious complications that occur following HSCT. ⚠

II. Role of bone marrow transplantation
   A. Cure—each patient is evaluated with curative intent.
   B. Disease control (palliation)—in some patients, notably those with multiple myeloma, autologous transplantation is used to increase the patient's progression-free survival.

ASSESSMENT

I. Pertinent medical history
   A. Diagnosis (see Boxes 26-2 and 26-3 for conditions commonly treated with HSCT) (Ezzone, 2013; Wikle Shapiro, 2017)
   B. Potential candidates for bone marrow transplantation—patients with malignancies at high risk for

recurrence after standard therapy; malignancies must demonstrate a response to either antineoplastic therapy or RT.

C. Factors that may increase the incidence of complications of marrow transplantation (Chadwalk and Greenstein, 2013; El-Ghammaz, 2017; Estey, 2013; Aranout, et al, 2014; Slack et al., 2013)

   1. Amount of previous cancer therapy, length of time since last therapy, response to past therapy, and length of disease-free interval

   2. Underlying kidney, lung, liver, or cardiac dysfunction

   3. Previous pretransplant or active infections and response to therapy

   4. Age—older patients (>17 years) more likely to develop complications

   5. Patients who are overweight or experiencing malnutrition at time of transplant

   6. Psychosocial dysfunction

II. Physical examination

  A. Pulmonary—respiratory rate, depth, and rhythm; lung expansion; adventitious breath sounds; oxygen saturation

  B. Renal—color and odor of urine and urinary output, edema, weight gain

  C. Mobility—muscle strength and endurance, range of motion, gait, activity level

  D. Nutrition—weight; skin turgor; amount, content, and patterns of nutritional intake

  E. Comfort level—pain rating, anxiety, ability to rest or engage

  F. Cardiovascular—heart rate and rhythm, heart sounds, blood pressure, perfusion

  G. Gastrointestinal (GI)—volume, color, consistency, and caliber of stool; abdominal pain; distention; bowel sounds

  H. Genitourinary—color of urine, suppleness of bladder, condition of perineum

  I. Integumentary—color and intactness of skin, condition of oral mucous membranes, dental evaluation, condition of perineum and rectum

  J. Neurologic—mental status, orientation, sensation, reflexes

III. Psychosocial examination

  A. Psychological evaluation

   1. Feelings on decision to undergo bone marrow transplantation

   2. Understanding of treatment aggressiveness, goals of therapy, chances of survival

   3. Number, type, effectiveness of coping mechanisms used in past stressful situations (before transplantation therapy) by patient and family members

   4. Perceptions of patient and family about isolation, prolonged hospitalization, living will, use of life support technology, and potential death or survival

   5. Caregiver's ability to comprehend role

B. Social evaluation

   1. Previous roles and responsibilities in the family and community

   2. Type, number, and history of use of support systems in the family and community

   3. Financial status—employment, insurance coverage, resources for daily living

   4. Eligibility for community resources

IV. Critical laboratory and diagnostic data unique to marrow transplantation (Ezzone, 2013)

  A. Hematologic—complete blood cell count, differential, platelet count, coagulation studies, type/crossmatch with marrow donor, donor chimerism, minimal residual disease markers, T-cell subsets with enumeration (Ezzone, 2013; Kim et al., 2013; Talekar and Olsen, 2018)

  B. Hepatic—liver transaminases (aspartate aminotransferase [AST], alanine aminotransferase [ALT]), lactic acid dehydrogenase (LDH), bilirubin, coagulation studies; liver duplex ultrasonography (Brown, 2018)

  C. Renal—electrolytes, blood urea nitrogen (BUN), serum creatinine, creatinine clearance; cyclosporine A, tacrolimus (FK-506), aminoglycoside, and vancomycin levels; viral urine cultures, BK virus polymerase chain reaction (PCR), electron microscopy, renal ultrasonography (Kapadia & Wikle Shapiro, 2018)

  D. Cardiovascular—electrocardiography (ECG), echocardiogram (echo) with cardiac ejection fraction or shorting fractions (in children), venography

  E. Pulmonary—chest radiography, computed tomography (CT) of chest or sinuses, pulmonary function tests (e.g., diffusing capacity of carbon monoxide [DLCO]), arterial blood gases [ABGs], oxygen saturation (pulse oximetry)

  F. Immune—antibody titers for cytomegalovirus (CMV) and herpesviruses (pretransplantation), Epstein–Barr virus (EBV) by quantitative PCR, hepatitis B surface antigen, immunoglobulin levels, HIV antibody, hepatitis C PCR, T-cell subsets (enumeration), CD45 RA/RO

  G. Infectious disease (Chadwick and Greenstein, 2013)—blood cultures for bacteria and fungi; urine and stool cultures for bacteria, fungi, and viruses; CMV quantitative PCR studies, adenovirus quantitative PCR studies, human herpesvirus type 6 (RNA) studies, herpesvirus titers and cultures, toxoplasmosis antigenemia studies, respiratory and sputum cultures for bacteria, fungi, viruses, *Legionella* antigen (urine), acid-fast bacilli (AFB); stool and urine for electron microscopy cultures, stool for *Clostridium difficile* toxin, stains for *Pneumocystis carinii* pneumonia (PCP), multiviral respiratory panel, galactomannan, beta D glucan.

V. Assess for unique complications after bone marrow transplantation

  A. GVHD (Table 26.3) (Bride, Patel, and Freedman, 2018; Nassereddine, 2017; Wikle Shapiro, 2017)

TABLE 26.3   Grading of Acute GVHD Extent of Organ Involvement

Organ	Stage	Parameters
Rash*		
Skin	I	< 25% BSA
	II	25%–50% BSA
	III	Rash on >50% BSA
	IV	Generalized erythroderma with bullous formation
Total Bilirubin		
Liver	I	2–3 mg/dL
	II	3–6 mg/dL
	III	6–15 mg/dL
	IV	>15 mg/dL

Volume of Diarrhea

		Adult	Pediatric
Gut	I	>500 mL/day	10–15 mL/kg/day
	II	>1000 mL/day	15–20 mL/kg/day
	III	>1500 mL/day	20–30 mL/kg/day
	IV	Adult and pediatric: severe abdominal pain with or without an ileus	

Overall Clinical Grade

Grade	Description
I	Stage I–II clinical skin GVHD
II	Stage III clinical skin GVHD *or*
	Stage I liver and/or stage I gut GVHD
	Only one system stage III or greater
III	Stage II–III liver and/or stage II–IV gut GVHD
	Only one system stage III or greater
IV	Stage IV clinical skin GVHD (with grade 2 or higher histology) *and*
	Stage IV clinical liver and/or gut GVHD

BSA, Body surface area; *GVHD,* graft-versus-host disease.
*Use rule of nines or burn chart to determine extent of rash.
Adapted from Dignan, F. L., Clark, A., Amrolia, P., et al. (2012). Diagnosis and management of acute graft-versus-host disease. Haemato-oncology Task Force of British Committee for Standards in Hematology; British Society for Blood and Marrow Transplantation. *British Journal of Hematology 158*(1), 30-45; Ezzone, S. A. (Ed.). (2013). *Hematopoietic stem cell transplantation: a manual for nursing practice* (2nd ed., pp. 103-154). Pittsburgh: Oncology Nursing Society.

1. Monitor condition of skin (erythema, rash), especially the face, palms of hands, and soles of feet
2. Evaluate changes in liver function study results
3. Monitor of amount, consistency, frequency, and color of stool
   a. Monitor viral and fungal infection
4. Monitor cyclosporin or tacrolimus levels
   B. Hepatic sinusoidal obstruction syndrome or hepatic veno-occlusive disease (Box 26.4) (Brown, 2018; Richardson et al., 2013, Wikle Shapiro, 2017)
   1. Weigh the patient daily; notify the medical practitioner of weight gain more than 5% of pretransplantation weight

2. Monitor the location of pain (right upper quadrant)
3. Evaluate for elevation in serum bilirubin level
4. Evaluate for bleeding, poor response to platelet transfusions, and abnormal coagulation factors
5. Evaluate for changes in mental status
6. Measure abdominal girth daily if possible veno-occlusive disease
7. Provide skin care for patients with hyperbilirubinemia
8. Evaluate level of abdominal pain
   C. Idiopathic pulmonary interstitial pneumonitis—infectious and noninfectious (Kapadia & Wikle Shapiro, 2018)
   1. Monitor temperature
   2. Assess for cough, chest pain, adventitious breath sounds, diminished oxygen saturation
   3. Evaluate activity tolerance

MANAGEMENT

I. Implement conditioning regimen ordered by the physician or other provider
II. Administer prophylactic antimicrobial therapy as ordered (CDC, 2000)
   A. Antibacterial prophylaxis with fluoroquinolones, third-generation cephalosporins amphotericin B by nebulation, caspofungin, fluconazole (Diflucan), posaconazole, voriconazole (Vfend) to prevent fungal infection (Xu, Shen, Tang, & Feng, 2013).
   B. Monitor therapeutic drugs levels of posaconazole and voriconazole.
   C. Trimethoprim–sulfamethoxazole (Septra, Bactrim), intravenously (IV) or inhaled pentamidine (Nebu-Pent, Pentacarinat, Pentam 300), or dapsone for prevention of PCP
   D. Acyclovir (Zovirax) for prevention of herpesvirus infection, ganciclovir (Cytovene), foscarnet

BOX 26.4   Risk Factors for the Development of Hepatic Sinusoidal Obstruction Syndrome

- Pretransplantation chemotherapy (conditioning regimens containing cyclophosphamide, with or without busulfan)
- Abdominal radiation
- Pretransplantation hepatotoxic drug therapy (e.g., gemtuzumab ozogamicin [Mylotarg])
- Elevated transaminases before conditioning regimen
- Human leukocyte antigen (HLA)–mismatched or unrelated allogeneic transplantation
- Viral hepatitis
- Metastatic liver disease
- Karnofsky score <90% before transplantation
- Second transplantation
- Older age recipient
- Female gender

(Foscavir), or cidofovir for prevention and treatment of CMV and other viral infections

E. Intravenous immunoglobulin G (IVIg) for prevention and treatment of CMV and other viral infections.

III. Administer hematopoietic growth factors as ordered.

IV. Administer immunosuppressive therapy to prevent and treat GVHD with cyclosporine, tacrolimus, sirolimus, mycophenolate, and antithymocyte globulin, systemic steroids, alemtuzumab (Campath), or others.

V. Administer ursodeoxycholic acid (Actigall), defibrotide, analgesics, vitamin K, fresh frozen plasma, and other blood products for the patients with VOD/SOS.

VI. Employ measures to prevent bladder toxicity—for patients receiving high-dose cyclophosphamide (Cytoxan), hemorrhagic cystitis is a potential complication (Kapadia & Wikle Shapiro, 2018).

A. Administer mesna (Mesnex), a uroprotectant, with high-dose cyclophosphamide

B. Provide IV hyperhydration

NONPHARMACOLOGIC MANAGEMENT

I. Maximize safety for the patient and family

A. Maintain aseptic techniques and the level of protective isolation identified by the HSCT program (see Table 26.1 for general guidelines)

B. Teach the patient and family strategies to decrease risk of infection, bleeding, and injury during period of aplasia after bone marrow, stem cell, or cord blood infusion

II. Minimize the incidence and severity of complications unique to bone marrow transplantation

A. Anxiety

1. Provide a thorough orientation to the inpatient and outpatient hematopoietic blood/bone marrow transplantation units and procedures

2. Implement strategies to encourage the patient and family to express concerns about bone marrow transplantation demands

3. Consult with an occupational therapist for diversional activities during isolation

4. Teach new anxiety-relieving strategies as desired or needed by patient and family

5. Assess caregiver's ability to implement care demands

B. Risk for infection—Figure 26.1 displays common opportunistic infections and time of occurrence after transplantation (Bride, et al., 2018; Wikle Shapiro, 2017)

1. Notify the provider of initial temperature greater than 101°F (38.3°C) or other symptoms indicative of infection

2. Teach the patient and family strategies to decrease risk of endogenous infections

a. Meticulous hand washing

b. Routine oral and perineal care

c. Skin care, including frequent baths for patients receiving thiotepa

3. Teach the patient and family strategies to decrease risk of exogenous infections

a. Restrict visitors with suspected or known infections

b. Limit visits by children (especially school-age children)

c. Place the patient on a low-microbial, stem cell transplantation (SCT) diet

d. Avoid invasive procedures (e.g., peripheral IV catheter, intramuscular injections, urinary catheterization, rectal examinations, rectal temperatures)

e. Recommend influenza vaccination for all close-contact individuals

f. Proper care of central venous catheter

g. Collect routine surveillance cultures for bacteria, fungi, and viruses, antigenemia/PCR studies, and *Aspergillus* antigen study

4. Transfuse irradiated, CMV-seronegative blood products or leukocyte-poor filtered blood products for all patients

C. Risk for injury

1. Encourage frequent voiding, accurate urine output, necessary after high-dose cyclophosphamide

2. If mesna not used with cyclophosphamide administration, provide continuous bladder irrigation (CBI) as ordered; administration of antispasmodics and analgesics for bladder spasms

3. Check urine specific gravity with each void on days of high-dose cyclophosphamide and 24 hours after the last dose as ordered

4. Monitor for cyclophosphamide-induced hyponatremia caused by syndrome of inappropriate antidiuretic hormone (SIADH) secretion

D. Alteration in oral mucous membranes

1. Encourage cryotherapy (ice chips) for patients receiving melphalan

2. Encourage good oral hygiene

E. Alteration in skin integrity

1. Instruct patient to bathe four times daily while receiving thiotepa because drug is excreted via the integumentary system and may lead to skin problems

2. Apply barrier creams to prevent perianal breakdown

F. Alteration in cardiovascular status

1. Monitor blood pressure and heart rate frequently with high-dose etoposide

2. Assess orthostatic hypotension with cyclophosphamide and high-dose etoposide

3. Assess decreased level of consciousness related to alcohol content in high-dose etoposide

G. Altered oral mucous membranes (see Chapter 40)

H. Nausea and vomiting (see Chapter 37)

IV. Interventions to enhance adaptation and rehabilitation

A. Implement a program of range-of-motion and isometric exercises during the isolation period, especially if the patient is taking high-dose steroids

B. Discuss potential changes in lifestyle and social interaction required immediately after discharge from the hospital

C. Provide long-term follow-up (Dandekar, 2018)

   1. Educate patient and family members on common outpatient problems after HSCT—fatigue, weight loss, sexual dysfunction, cataracts, chronic GVHD, chronic lung disease, herpes zoster virus, endocrinopathies, depression, isolation

   2. Ensure survivorship issues are addressed through long-term follow-up program

     a. Lifelong evaluation of allogeneic recipient for chronic GVHD

     b. Posttransplantation vaccinations

     c. Fertility issues

     d. Reentry into community and work

     e. Delayed organ dysfunction (pulmonary, cardiac, renal, adrenal dysfunction)

EXPECTED PATIENT OUTCOMES

I. The HSC recipient and family will demonstrate basic knowledge of the rationale for transplantation before undergoing the process.

II. The HSC recipient will remain free from preventive (nonopportunistic) infections throughout all phases of transplantation.

III. The HSC recipient can expect early identification and proactive, safe management of the transplant-specific complications of opportunistic infection, GVHD, and SOS/VOD.

IV. The HSC recipient and family will demonstrate basic knowledge of the late effects of hematopoietic transplantation.

REFERENCES

Alchi, B., Jayne, D., Labopin, M., Demin, A., Sergeevicheva, V., Alexander, T., … members, E.A.D.W.P. (2013). Autologous haematopoietic stem cell transplantation for systemic lupus erythematosus: data from the European Group for Blood and Marrow Transplantation registry. *Lupus, 22*(3), 245–253. https://doi.org/10.1177/0961203312470729.

Bride, K. L., Patel, N. S., & Freedman, J. L. (2018). In V. Brown (Ed.), *Hematopoietic stem cell transplantation for the pediatric hematologist/oncologist* (pp 257-265). Cham, Switzerland: Springer.

Brown, V. (Ed.), (2018). *Hematopoietic stem cell transplantation for the pediatric hematologist/oncologist.* Cham, Switzerland: Springer.

Dandekar, S. (2018). Life after HSCT: survivorship and long-term follow up issues. In V. Brown (Ed.), *Hematopoietic stem cell transplantation for the pediatric hematologist/oncologist* (pp. 385–4012). Cham, Switzerland: Springer.

El-Ghammaz, A. M. S., Ben Matoug, R., Elzimaity, M., & Mostafa, N. (2017). Nutritional status of allogeneic hematopoietic stem cell transplantation recipients: influencing risk factors and impact on survival. *Support Care Cancer, 25*(10), 3085–3093. https://doi.org/10.1007/s00520-017-3716-6.

Estey, E. H. (2013). Acute myeloid leukemia: 2013 update on risk-stratification and management. *Am J Hematol, 88*(4), 318–327. https://doi.org/10.1002/ajh.23404.

Ezzone, S. A. (Ed.), (2013). *Hematopoietic stem cell transplantation: a manual for nursing practice* (2nd ed, pp. 155–172). Pittsburgh: Oncology Nursing Society.

Forman, S., Negrin, R. S., Antin, J. H., & Appelbaum, F. (Eds.), (2016). *Thomas' hematopoietic cell transplantation.* (5th ed.). Malden, MA: Wiley-Blackwell.

Kapadia, M., & Greiner, R. (2018). How to select a donor for hematopoietic stem cell source: Related versus unrelated donors for allogeneic HSCT. In V. Brown (Ed.), *Hematopoietic stem cell transplantation for the pediatric hematologist/oncologist* (pp. 97–110). Cham, Switzerland: Springer.

Kapadia, M., & Wikle Shapiro, T. (2018). Pulmonary complications associated with HSCT. In V. Brown (Ed.), *Hematopoietic stem cell transplantation for the pediatric hematologist/oncologist* (pp. 301–329). Cham, Switzerland: Springer.

Kim, H. O., Oh, H. J., Lee, J. W., Jang, P. S., Chung, N. G., Cho, B., & Kim, H. K. (2013). Immune reconstitution after allogeneic hematopoietic stem cell transplantation in children: a single institution study of 59 patients. *Korean J Pediatr, 56*(1), 26–31. https://doi.org/10.3345/kjp.2013.56.1.26.

Kitko, C.-L., Gatwood, K., & Connelly, J. (2018). Preparing the patient for HCST: conditioning regimens and their scientific rationale. In V. Brown (Ed.), *Hematopoietic stem cell transplantation for the pediatric hematologist/oncologist* (pp. 139–174). Cham, Switzerland: Springer.

Nassereddine, S., Rafei, H., Elbahesh, E., & Tabbara, I. (2017). Acute graft versus host disease: a comprehensive Review. *Anticancer Res, 37*(4), 1547–1555. https://doi.org/10.21873/anticanres.11483.

National Marrow Donor Program (NMDP). (2018). Be the match. Accessed February 26, 2019. https://bethematch.org.

Richardson, P. G., Ho, V. T., Cutler, C., Glotzbecker, B., Antin, J. H., & Soiffer, R. (2013). Hepatic veno-occlusive disease after hematopoietic stem cell transplantation: novel insights to pathogenesis, current status of treatment, and future directions. *Biol Blood Marrow Transplant, 19*(1 Suppl). https://doi.org/10.1016/j.bbmt.2012.10.023 S88-90.

Shenoy, S. (2013). Umbilical cord blood: an evolving stem cell source for sickle cell disease transplants. *Stem Cells Transl Med, 2*(5), 337–340. https://doi.org/10.5966/sctm.2012-0180.

Slack, J. L., Dueck, A. C., Fauble, V. D., Sproat, L. O., Reeder, C. B., Noel, P., … Adams, R. H. (2013). Reduced toxicity conditioning and allogeneic stem cell transplantation in adults using fludarabine, carmustine, melphalan, and antithymocyte globulin: outcomes depend on disease risk index but not age, comorbidity score, donor type, or human leukocyte antigen mismatch. *Biol Blood Marrow Transplant, 19*(8), 1167–1174. https://doi.org/10.1016/j.bbmt.2013.05.001.

Tiercy, J. M. (2014). HLA-C incompatibilities in allogeneic unrelated hematopoietic stem cell transplantation. *Front Immunol, 5.* 216. https://doi.org/10.3389/fimmu.2014.00216.

Wikle Shapiro, T. (2017). Hematopoieticpp175-205 stem cell transplantation. In S. Newton, M. Hickey, & J. M. Brant (Eds.), *Mosby's Oncology nursing advisor: a comprehensive guide to clinical practice* (pp. 179–205). St. Louis: Elsevier.

Xu, S. X., Shen, J. L., Tang, X. F., & Feng, B. (2013). Newer antifungal agents for fungal infection prevention during hematopoietic cell transplantation: a meta-analysis. *Transplant Proc, 45*(1), 407–414. https://doi.org/10.1016/j.transproceed.2012.07.149.

27

Radiation Therapy

Susan Weiss Behrend

OVERVIEW

I. Timeline (Fig. 27.1) (Gianfaldoni et al., 2017; Heilmann, 2013; Slater, 2012)
   A. One of the earliest types of cancer treatment
   B. End of twentieth century: exponential clinical growth
      1. Computed tomography (CT) simulation, intensity-modulated radiation therapy (IMRT), reduced-dose inhomogeneity to target
      2. Field modulation and dose intensity
      3. 4D planning accounting for organ movement
      4. Fusion of positron emission tomography (PET) with CT
   C. Future
      1. Shortened treatment courses/hypofractionation
      2. Combined modality with immunotherapy
      3. Manipulate timing and dose of radiation therapy (RT) to counter cytoprotective response
      4. Continued clinical trials focus on sensitizers and protectors (Proud, 2014)
II. The radiation oncology multidisciplinary team (MDT)
   A. Radiation oncology nurse: role is to collaborate with MDT to coordinate clinical services and ensure continuity of care. Assess, plan, implement, and evaluate patient care pretreatment, during treatment, and posttreatment. Provide patient education.
   B. Radiation oncologist: physician specializing and certified in radiation oncology; responsible for planning, prescribing radiation course, and assessing patient's physical and psychosocial needs before treatment, during treatment, and in follow-up.
   C. Radiation therapists (RTTs): technically cross-trained to assist with treatment planning during simulation and to operate treatment delivery machines. Patients are escorted by the RTTs or other staff to the machines for safe positioning. RTTs interface with team members regarding patient care and assessment.
   D. Medical physicists and dosimetrists: determine actual tumor target volume to be treated; create specific plans to accomplish goal. Dosimetrists collaborate with radiation oncologists to establish the most suitable direction and size of the radiation beam. Physicists and dosimetrists provide dosimetric planning and distribution, provide safe application of therapeutic radiation treatment, and maintain local regional protection of vital organs and structures.
   E. Mold and cast technicians: trained to create custom assistive devices and lead blocks to ensure safe positioning and immobilization.
   F. Medical engineers: responsible for installation, calibration, and maintenance of machinery that delivers RT, simulation equipment, and all high-voltage accessories.
   G. Administrators: focus on the overall delivery of services, associated charges, reimbursement structures, and accountability.
   H. Social workers: coordinate care during RT treatment and provide supportive services for patients and caregivers.
III. Applied radiation physics
   A. Ionizing radiation is based on the ability of radiation to interact with atoms and molecules of tumor cells producing biologic effects.
   B. The atom is the basic unit of molecular structure.
      1. Radium, radon, and uranium are examples of unstable atoms that produce ionizing radiation.
      2. Stable atoms may produce ionizing radiation through excitation, ionization, and nuclear disintegration.
      3. Radiation produced by these processes can be classified as electromagnetic radiation or particulate radiation.
      4. The electromagnetic spectrum can be divided into five levels of decreasing wavelength: radio waves, infrared radiation, visible light, ultraviolet radiation, and ionizing radiation (Dieterich, et al., 2016).
   C. Teletherapy—external radiation delivered from high-energy equipment to the tumor target
      1. Two types of ionizing radiation externally administered are electromagnetic and particle sources

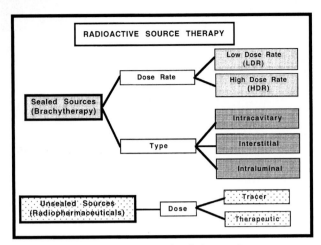

Fig. 27.1 The history of radiation oncology.

  a. Electromagnetic energy—produced by vibration of electromagnetic waves
  b. Waves—made up of electric and magnetic energy
  c. Ionizing radiation—electromagnetic energy: short wavelength, high energy
  d. X-rays and gamma rays—most widely used types of ionizing radiation, delivered from linear accelerators
  e. Ionizing radiation—radiation with enough energy to disrupt the atomic structure of the cells; a primary treatment modality using high-energy x-rays or particles.
  f. Particle radiation—emitted from protons, neutrons, and electrons found in and around the nucleus; delivered by linear accelerators or cyclotrons.
IV. Radiobiology
  A. Biological effects of radiation result in therapeutic outcomes
    1. Radiobiology—the science of the physical, chemical, and biological effects of ionizing radiation on living tissue.
    2. Radiobiologic effect—killing of tumor cells, halting further malignant growth, sparing of normal local and regional tissues and organs.
    3. Direct cellular damage—caused by damage to DNA chromosomal structures.
    4. Indirect cellular damage—occurs due to a series of chemical reactions that lead to the production of free radicals, causing toxic cellular changes.
    5. Cellular death—varies from the time of cellular division or in response to cellular degeneration (Hall, Giaccia 2019).
  B. Biological factors of RT
    1. Oxygen effect—well-oxygenated tumors are more responsive to radiation
    2. Relative biological effectiveness (RBE)—compares a test dose of radiation with a dose

of standard radiation that produces the same biologic response
    3. Dose rate—the rate at which a given radiation dose is delivered by a treatment machine
  C. Fractionation—treatment that takes the total dose of RT and divides it into equal fractions. A single dose of radiation has more of a biologic effect than the same dose fractionated (Hall, Giaccia 2019; Mitchell, 2013).
  D. Five Rs of radiobiology: provide the rationale for radiation fractionation
    1. Repair: DNA repair in response to sublethal or potentially lethal radiation damage. Fractionation of radiation allows normal tissues time to repair.
    2. Reassortment: radioresistant cells that synchronize into a more radiosensitive phase of the cell cycle after a fraction of radiation.
    3. Repopulation: tumor cell proliferation during radiation. Can be problematic with very-low-dose rates (VLDRs) or prolonged treatment.
    4. Reoxygenation: the importance of oxygen in mediating the cytotoxic effects of radiation due to free radical production. As tumor cells are killed with each fraction, formerly hypoxic cells become oxygenated.
    5. Radiosensitizing: ionizing RT is most effective on cells that are undifferentiated and undergoing active mitosis (Hall, Giaccia 2019).
V. Treatment planning and administration
  A. Consultation: initial comprehensive MDT assessment
  B. Immobilization: specialized casts and molds created
  C. Simulation: imaging determines treatment and target volume
  D. Localization: pinpointing the target and surrounding anatomic structures
  E. Calculation: medical physics dosimetry contours and creation of dose volume histograms; dose to target and tolerated dose to surrounding structures confirmed
  F. Verification: real-time setup on treatment machine
  G. Administration: actual treatment administration occurs (Behrend, 2018)
VI. Simulation
  A. Three-dimensional conformal radiotherapy (3D-CRT) treatment planning—occurs during simulation, requires complete CT data scan. Digital radiographs generated on local area networks (LANs) to image the target and critical local-regional structures and to determine treatment volume.
  B. CT simulator—single diagnostic treatment-planning machine that combines CT and virtual planning. CT simulation provides speed, accuracy, and efficiency of RT planning.
  C. The patient is positioned on the CT simulator table; tumor and normal structures are outlined on each

CT slice; computer creates a 3D transformation of the CT images into a digitally reconstructed radiograph (DRR).

D. The DRR can be manipulated for enhanced contrast. The radiation oncologist then draws virtual blocks directly onto the DRR to differentiate tumor from normal tissue. The mold room technician uses the DRR to construct customized blocks.

E. Virtual simulation—provides a fully documented beam arrangement. Patients are immobilized in a variety of ways, for example, hemi body foam torso casts and custom foam head supports with thermal plastic face masks (Videtic, Woody 2015).

VII. Target delineation

A. MRI simulation—provides accurate delineation of targets and critical normal structures, enhanced soft tissue views. CT scan is often coregistered with magnetic resonance imaging (MRI) scans to facilitate daily localization and position verification.

B. MRI advantageous in defining targets in the central nervous system, head and neck, and prostate (Mahase, Wernicke, Nori, 2015).

VIII. Planning/localization/imaging

A. Port films: mandatory radiographic images taken by linear accelerators to verify treatment fields.

B. Electronic portal imaging: assesses location and extent of disease, guides treatment planning and delivery, visualization of anatomy in tomographic planes.

1. Imaging is critical to define tumor volume, shape, and location of adjacent organs. CT scans provide tissue density used for dose calculations.

2. IMRT requires precise imaging of stationary and moving targets.

3. Image-guided radiation therapy (IGRT)—images obtained daily during treatment to account for variations in organ motion, patient, or plan setup (Behrend, 2018).

C. Imaging minimizes uncertainties in setup error, variations in target/organ motion.

1. Acquired images: CT, MRI, PET, single-photon emission computed tomography (SPECT), ultrasound (US), plane films, electronic portal images.

2. Processed images—derived from acquired anatomic image data: DRRs and volume-rendered images.

3. A PET scan is a nuclear medicine image that provides 3D mapping of functional processes in the body.

a. PET imaging most useful when fused with anatomic imaging; for example, PET/CT images or PET/MRI offers anatomic and metabolic information. PET images provide information for tumor staging, track tumor's response to treatment (Mahase, Wernicke, Nori, et al., 2015)

IX. Radiation dosing

A. RT dosing is based on medical physics and depends on:

1. Depth of the calculation points below the point of entry

2. Energy and penetrating power of the beam

3. Density of the tissue type to be penetrated

4. Distance from the radiation source to the skin

5. Size of the field on the skin surface and type and design of the collimator

B. Radiation-absorbed dose: energy deposited in a small fixed weight of tissue

1. Rad—unit of dose (radiation-absorbed dose or energy deposited in tissue)

2. Gray (Gy)—100 times larger (1 Gy = 100 rad)

3. One rad is the same as one-hundredth of a gray: 1 rad = 1/100 Gy = 1cGy

C. Dosimetry is the measurement of radiation dose, calculations, and measurements, and is required for determining the radiation dose delivered.

1. Dosimetry considers tissue compensation and variability of targets irradiated.

2. For RT to be delivered safely, effectively, and therapeutically, dosimetry measures RT doses through different anatomic structures and phantom material such as wax and gel bolus material (Kissick & Fakhraei 2016).

D. Field-modifying instruments: utilized as beam-modifying absorbers such as filters, wedges, or bolus material, which are placed in the path of a beam.

E. Tissue compensation: when radiation is projected along irregular or sloping surfaces, isodose curves bend. This distortion can cause nonuniformity of the dose to the target; has the potential to cause excessive irradiation of sensitive structures.

1. Wedges, bolus material, or compensators can eliminate this treatment administration challenge. Bolus tissue equivalent is made from gel or wax and acts as a tissue equivalent; placed directly on the skin to even irregular contours and to create a flat surface to normalize the path of the beam.

F. Compensators: provide required beam arrangements when treating irregular anatomic regions; made from metals, copper, brass, or lead; are placed at a distance from the target to provide a skin-sparing effect.

1. Compensate for missing wedges of tissue in the treatment field.

2. An example of a compensator is the use of copper during total-body irradiation (TBI) placed on the collimator to provide tissue heterogeneity and effective dose distribution (Khan, 2016).

X. Treatment delivery

A. IMRT

1. IMRT delivery of RT uses varied beam intensities called *beamlets*.

2. Manipulates radiation ray intensity within each beam, allows increased control of radiation dose to conform to irregularly shaped targets (Behrend, 2018).

B. IGRT
   1. IGRT ensures exact treatment field targeting reproducible alignment and immobilization.
      a. Required with IMRT to provide superior imaging techniques for enhanced target localization; patient alignment and quality assurance are image dependent during RT (Youl, Brock & Dawson, 2017).
      b. Examples of IGRT
         (1) Cone beam CT (CBCT): cone-shaped beam of x-rays with less exposure than conventional CT. Fast speed, yields sufficient data for exact 3D image reconstruction, verifies patient alignment and dose to target, with head and neck, lung, and pelvis targets.
         (2) Fiducial markers: used for prostate localization and dose escalation. Placed transrectally under US guidance to visualize the prostate gland and to plan localized radiation. The prostate gland moves internally; hence the fiducial gold seed markers pinpoint movement and assist with RT targeting. Markers are visualized during RT administration and serve as a fixed standard of reference (Bell, Eade, Kneebone, 2017).
      c. On-board imaging (OBI): the use of sophisticated imaging during RT administration to ensure accurate field setup. Imaging systems mounted on accelerators provide online verification, correction, and dynamic targeting with conformal treatment synchronized to patient movement.

C. Brachytherapy: the delivery of radioactive sources directly in or near the tumor.
   1. Common treatment modality for gynecologic, prostate tumors; also used to treat head and neck, ocular, central nervous system (CNS), and lung cancer.
   2. A single treatment modality or sequenced as part of external beam course of RT.
   3. Boosts to the tumor or surrounding bed can be given after or before surgery and/or systemic therapy (e.g. chemotherapy, immunotherapy).
   4. The advantage of brachytherapy is optimal RT dose to the tumor and sparing surrounding tissues and organs.
   5. Source placement varies; remains in place either temporarily or permanently.
      a. Temporary implants have high energies and long half-lives. Sources are inserted through catheters that are surgically placed in the tumor and administered through needles, seeds, and ribbons.
      b. Common radioactive sources are cesium-137 tubes, iridium-192 seeds contained in ribbons, and iodine-125 seeds.
   6. Delivery of brachytherapy is done with remote afterloading equipment for high dose rate (HDR) regimens. This radiation delivery system consists of a motor-driven transport system that robotically transfers radioactive material between a shielded safe and each treatment applicator. The source is connected to the end of a cable inside the afterloading unit, and the catheters are radiated one at a time until the designated dose is achieved.
      a. Gynecologic oncology
         (1) HDR cylinder used to treat cancers of the uterus and vagina.
         (2) HDR tandem and rings used to place the source for cervical cancer.
      b. For gynecologic and prostate cancers, combining EBRT with brachytherapy both treats bulky local disease and improves local control.

D. Treatment machines
   1. Linear accelerator (LINAC)
      a. Delivers high-energy RT using high-frequency electromagnetic waves to accelerate charged electrons through a linear tube pathway. The energy of the electrons increases during acceleration.
      b. The electron volt (eV) is the basic unit of energy in RT, and escalating energy levels are kilovolts (kV) and megavolts (MeV). Electrons produced by the LINAC strike a target and produce x-rays of varying energies in the range of 10 to 30 kV.
      c. Charged electrons are used to treat surface lesions and deep tumor targets. Energy of the LINAC varies from low (6 MeV), when electrons proceed straight down a short accelerator tube to strike the target and produce x-rays, to high (18 MeV). At high energies the accelerator structure is longer and must be angled to bend the electrons before striking the target.
      d. Collimation is an RT administration technique that shapes the radiation beam to the target. High atomic collimators can vary the field size from 4 × 4 cm to 40 × 40 cm and shape the beam into square or rectangular fields.
      e. The multileaf collimator (MLC) is a system of numerous lead leaves located in the LINAC and provides computerized customized blocking of critical anatomic organs and structures. The MLC is programmed to change the shape of the RT beams to match

the shape of the specific target. This is known as *dynamic beam shaping* and enhances critical tissue sparing (Khan, 2016).

2. Megavoltage external beam machines
   a. Low-energy megavoltage machines: administer 4 MeV to 6 MeV of energy; used to treat shallow or moderately deep tumors (e.g., breast, head and neck).
   b. Medium- to high-energy megavoltage machines: administer 10 MeV to 25 MeV of energy; treat deep-seated tumors of the thorax, abdomen, and pelvis.
      (1) Electron beams: deliver 6 MeV to 20 MeV of energy; effective for superficial cancers of the skin, lip, and chest wall, and for boosts to lymph nodes, head and neck cancers, and sparing of deep normal tissue.
      (2) Equipment usage guidelines, calibration checks, quality assurance, and realistic treatment loads regulated by the Nuclear Regulatory Commission (NRC) standards and published by the American Society of Therapeutic Radiation Oncology (ASTRO) (ASTRO, 2012).
      (3) Megavoltage machines are compact and have a rotating feature that provides 360-degree movement around the patient. Rotation offers options for beam angles to reach the target site. Safe rotation must consider sufficient distance to avoid collision with the stationary treatment couch.

3. Proton therapy—proton beams are positively charged particles with a heavy ion mass. They are accelerated at excessive speed with minimal deviation using megavoltage energy produced by proton accelerators. Proton beam therapy has specific indications that are supported by clinical evidence.
   a. Pediatric uses for treatment of the CNS are common due to low radiation dose and less risk for development of long-term radiation-related side effects such as compromised growth and development, and secondary malignancies in young adult cancer survivors (Lindrud-Doyle, 2015).
   b. Adult clinical indications are limited due to expense and efficacy (Swisher, Hahn, Bekelman, 2015). Therefore protons, if available, may be limited to treating diseases of the CNS, ocular, and skull-based tumors.
   c. Major advantage of protons is selective cell destruction. Proton energy distribution deposited more completely and precisely in designated tissue, which yields superior targeting and enhanced tumor control (Kooy & Adams, 2016).
   d. Proton facilities are costly and require ample land mass and specially trained personnel.

4. Stereotactic radiosurgery (SRS)
   a. A specialized radiation technique that delivers the total dose with one to five large, highly focused fractions of radiation to one or more intracranial targets.
   b. The goal of SRS is to administer directed ionizing radiation to the tumor and spare toxicity to surrounding normal tissues and structures.
   c. Indications: intracranial metastases, primary brain tumors, spinal metastases.
   d. Used to treat benign tumors such as acoustic neuromas, meningioma, pituitary adenoma, arteriovenous malformation, trigeminal neuralgia.

5. Stereotactic radiotherapy (SRT)
   a. SRT or fractionated SRT is an extension of SRS, delivered with more than one fraction utilizing nonrigid immobilization.
   b. Frames or thermoplastic masks may be used for CNS tumors; body frames are used for extracranial sites. SRT provides the precision of SRS and allows adjacent normal structures to repair sublethal damage.
   c. Specific clinical parameters must be met for SRT:
      (1) A small target/treatment volume with distinct circumferential lesions <4 cm
      (2) Distinctly defined target, precise radiation delivery with high conformity and exclusion of critically dose-limiting structures from the field such as the spinal cord and related structures (Bova & Friedman, 2016).

6. Stereotactic body radiation therapy (SBRT)
   a. The precise administration of large fractions; one to five fractions delivered to extracranial sites such as tumors of the lung, pancreas, and esophagus.
   b. When SBRT is administered, organ motion is accounted for with the use of pretreatment imaging, such as daily CT scans, which ensures accurate targeting of the RT beam when the target is precisely in the field (Behrend, 2015b).
      (1) SRS and SBRT are precise methods of delivering high doses of radiation to well-defined target volumes; not possible with conventional techniques.
      (2) Improved tumor control is achievable with the administration of large, highly focused deliberate fractions of radiation. Additionally, normal tissues and organs are spared long-term sequelae of treatment-related toxicity (Foster, Ramirez, & Timmerman, 2016).

c. Cyberknife image-guided radiosurgery
   (1) A frameless robotic radiosurgical system composed of a compact LINAC mounted on a robotic arm. The LINAC is directed by the robotic arm to deliver radiation to the tumor from multiple positions.
   (2) A cumulative radiation dose is delivered, and patient movement is accounted for with image guidance. The robotic arm compensates for movement and can reposition the LINAC throughout treatment.
   (3) The cyberknife provides noninvasive, surgical-like precision treatment for lesions of the brain, spine, and lungs. Treatment course varies from one to five fractions. Fractionated radiosurgery can be offered when the total dose of stereotactic RT is divided into smaller doses (Li, Mageras, Dong, Mohan 2016).

E. Positioning and immobilization
1. Critical components of RT delivery. Daily treatment must be reproducible and accurate. Patient positioning provides comfort and safety. Lethal dosing errors can occur if positioning and immobilization are not exact.
2. Immobilization devices
   a. Keep patients in a stationary position for daily treatment. Immobilizers help to minimize potential treatment setup errors, reduce the amount of radiation to normal tissues, and ensure the appropriate treatment to the target volume.
   b. Universally usable with all treatment planning systems. Radiation therapists assess immobilizer fit daily (account for weight change) to determine normal wear and tear and environmental changes that could affect the integrity of the immobilizing device.
3. Types of immobilization devices
   a. Head fixation devices—used during treatment of head, neck, and brain fields; made of thermoplastic mesh sheets attached to rigid frames. Warm water softens the system, so the mask is pulled down and molded to facial contours.
   b. Alpha cradle body cast—immobilization device used when pelvic and abdominal fields treated; reduce setup errors, allow for 3D conformal therapy treatment.
   c. Body supports—generic devices for positioning during treatment; provide comfort and stability during treatment: foam rubber wedges, lumbar supports, thigh and heel stirrups, prone face holders, and foot holders. Supports indexed by size, shape, and

elevation above treatment couch (Dieterich, et al., 2016).

F. Unsealed radionuclide sources
1. Oral and/or intravenous administration of radioactive substances.
2. A sealed-source radioisotope is encapsulated; an example is iodine-131 to treat benign and malignant thyroid conditions. Once ingested, the radioactive iodine emits beta and gamma radiation.
3. Beta radiation destroys thyroid tissue and thyroid cancer. Iodine not taken up by thyroid tissue is excreted through the kidneys into the urine. Strict guidelines exist for use of these sources in all patients. NRC guidelines must be followed to determine tolerated dose and management of radioactive waste.

G. Radiation safety
1. The major premise of radiation safety is to keep radiation exposure as low as reasonably achievable (ALARA). Recommended by the International Commission on Radiation Protection (ICRP) (1977), this standard assumed any exposure to ionizing radiation can increase the risk of developing cancer. This continues to be recommended by national and international radiation safety organizations. In the U.S., the NRC regulates brachytherapy and external beam therapy and radioactive materials, setting dose limits for workers, monitoring and labeling radioactive materials.
2. Guidelines for radiation safety and protection are based on principles of time, distance, and shielding (Dieterich, et al., 2016).
   a. A direct relationship exists between **TIME** and radiation exposure; the greater the time of exposure, the more radiation absorbed. Includes limiting time in the environment of the radioactive source or reducing time the source is exposed.
   b. The concept of **DISTANCE** relates to the inverse square law, whereby radiation intensity is reduced by the square of the distance from the source.
   c. **SHIELDING** provides a barrier between the individual and the radioactive source, preventing primary exposure through direct contact or secondary exposure through scatter radiation. Barriers to exposure include the use of gloves as protection from radioisotopes that are excreted through body fluids. Teletherapy vaults are shielded with lead, concrete, steel, or cast iron.
   d. Alarms and safety mechanisms are in place to prevent radiation beams from turning on if the room is not secure.

e. Areas where radioactive isotopes are used require labeling with radiation warning signs and notices indicating "radioactive material" and equipment with unsealed radioactive isotopes. The trefoil is the international radiation warning symbol, which indicates potential for contamination with radioactive material.

f. Personal monitoring devices measure and record radioactive exposure to personnel. Staff that may be exposed to gamma radiation at a rate of more than 200 micro sieverts per quarter are required to wear a ring badge and pocket ion chamber dosimeters. A radiation safety officer (RSO) is responsible for monitoring and reporting exposure results (ICRP, 1979).

g. Personnel must have full understanding of radiation protection and safety. Inadequate knowledge or fear may lead to suboptimal patient care. Nurses must understand effects of radiation, the risk of exposure, and the practices required to ensure safety for themselves and patients (Baeza, 2012).

h. The role of the RSO is to interface with regulatory bodies. Additionally, the RSO trains staff, monitors and documents exposure, develops quality assurance paradigms, purchases sealed sources, monitors leak testing, and conducts equipment maintenance checks.

i. Adhere to principles of time, distance, and shielding to reduce staff exposure to emitted radiation. Policies and procedures should guide care (Behrend, 2018).

ASSESSMENT

I. Pretreatment
  A. Assess understanding of goals of treatment, understanding of radiotherapy
  B. Knowledge and perceptions regarding treatment
  C. Factors influencing side effects
    1. Treatment factors: site, dose, field, type of radiotherapy, radiosensitivity of tissues
    2. Patient-related factors: nutrition, skin integrity, comorbidities
II. During and after treatment
  A. Assess for radiation-induced skin changes (see also Chapter 40)
    1. Radiation-induced skin changes are expected and commonly range from no reaction to mild changes; however, can rarely progress to moist, weeping, painful lesions that can severely affect physical and emotional quality of life. Enhanced treatment delivery systems now provide skin-sparing techniques that greatly minimize severity of skin changes.

2. Skin response to RT is dose dependent and reflects changes in the cellular components of all layers of the skin (epidermis, dermis, and vasculature).

3. The degree of skin reactions is dependent on the radiation treatment modality, beam energy, total radiation dose, daily fractionated dose, the size of the treatment field, and the variance in skin tolerance.

4. Assess patient-related risks: age, comorbidities, history of smoking, obesity, medications, and concomitant cancer treatment.

5. Assess anatomic areas of high risk: chest wall, supraclavicular, head and neck, face, and regions with skin folds.

6. Some chemotherapy and biotherapy agents increase skin radiosensitivity.

7. Acute skin-related side effects typically occur within the first 2 weeks of treatment and can become evident 1 to 3 months after initiation of treatment. Epidermal regeneration occurs within 3 to 5 weeks posttreatment. Complete healing can take up to 3 months. Chronic effects can manifest 3 months after initiation of treatment.

B. Assess fatigue (see also Chapter 36).
  1. Fatigue from cancer and associated treatment can be overwhelming, making it difficult for patients to follow daily treatment routines (Erickson, Spurlock, & Kramer, 2013).
  2. Can begin 2 to 3 weeks after the start of RT and persist from 1 to 4 months postcompletion; progressive symptom that occurs as a cumulative dose of radiation is administered; the degree of fatigue varies among patients.
  3. Assess during and after treatment, at each treatment visit, and in follow-up.
C. Assess other symptoms associated with radiotherapy.

MANAGEMENT

I. Manage patients along the continuum of care.
  A. Provide patients with educational plans, rationale for treatment, details of administration, toxicity profile, safety guidelines, and follow-up.
  B. Consider inviting patients and family members to visit the treatment room before initiation of actual course (Behrend, 2015a).
  C. Maximize safety during treatment.
    1. Prepare patient for radiotherapy to ease patient fears and ensure that a secure environment is provided during the treatment course (Forshaw, K, Hall, A, Boyes, 2017).
  D. Manage radiation-related toxicities

TABLE 27.1   Management of Skin Changes

Erythema

Characteristics	• Color range: red to pink to dusky • Warm, rash appearance may have surrounding edema • Skin can feel taut, reports of "awareness of skin" • Reaction confined to treatment field (beam entrance and exit sites) • Appears at 2–3 weeks of treatment
Management	• Reduce discomfort, maintain skin integrity • Cleanse with unscented, moisturizing soap • Pat dry/DO NOT RUB • Apply skin care products gently

Dry Desquamation

Characteristics	• Red or tan appearance • Dry, itchy, peeling, flaking • 2–3 weeks of treatment
Management	• Infection prevention • Cleanse with moisturizing, unscented soap • Avoid chlorinated water • Loose-fitting clothing • Warn against scratching; massage instead for comfort

Moist Desquamation

Characteristics	• The rate of repair of basal cells is inadequate for replacement of epidermis • Seen in skin folds • Moist, oozing serous fluid, crusting • Blistered, ulcerated, painful, edematous • Occurs 4–6 weeks into treatment
Management	• Infection prevention • Promote healing and lessen pain • Prevent irritation, friction, shearing • Cleanse with normal saline, pat dry, apply skin protection products • Moisture-vapor-permeable dressing • Hydrocolloid dressings • Hydrogels

Pruritus

Characteristics	• Drying of the skin surface with associated itching
Management	• Corticosteroid creams mixed with moisturizing lotions • Antifungal and steroid-based creams • Topical and systemic antihistamines • Cool compresses • Warn against scratching; massage for comfort instead

Hyperpigmentation

Characteristics	• Radiation activates melanin, which results in a skin-tanning effect
Management	• Skin care: clean and moisturize • Prepare patient for deepening skin color • Slow resolution posttreatment

Alopecia

Characteristics	• Loss of body hair • Rapidly growing hair • Hair shafts release from follicles • 2500 cGy–3000 cGy: hair growth slowed • 5500 cGy: hair loss is complete
Management	• Psychosocial patient support • Cleansing and moisturizing products for hair and scalp • Resource for prosthetics

Late Skin Effects of Radiation

Characteristics	• Chronic skin changes caused by RT can occur months to years after completing therapy. Endothelial cells and fibroblasts are the target cells for these late effects, which include: • Atrophy: thinning of skin • Fibrosis: scarring • Telangiectasia: narrowing of small superficial blood vessels • Hypopigmentation: loss of melanocytes • Necrosis: reduced blood flow • The incidence varies depending on treatment variables such as site, total dose, fraction size, or the use of brachytherapy. People treated with a high dose to the skin and large fractions are at greater risk of developing late skin effects.
Management	• Avoidance of mechanical, thermal, or chemical irritation • Trauma prevention • Sun protection • Skin lubrication

1. Provide skin care interventions (Table 27.1) based on evidence-based practice (EBP)—avoid interventions that lack evidence.
2. Provide site-specific management for radiation-induced toxicities (Table 27.2).
3. Reevaluate toxicities on an ongoing basis to ensure minimal toxicity and patient tolerance.

II. Considerations for specific procedures
   A. IGRT-specific guidelines
      1. Patient education should emphasize the use of specific equipment, additional time for IGRT, the purpose, and personnel involved (medical dosimetrists, engineers).
      2. This approach will enable patients to embrace the new technology and ensure thorough patient teaching (Behrend, 2018).
   B. Brachytherapy
      1. Coordinate pretreatment assessment and nursing care before and during brachytherapy administration and follow-up care.
      2. Administer preinsertion medication if tandem and ring placed.

TABLE 27.2 Management of Site-Specific Radiation Therapy Side Effects

Cerebral edema Headache/nausea/vomiting/seizures/ motor weakness/numbness, tingling of extremities/slurred speech/memory loss/dry eyes and mouth	Long-term neurologic deficits/brain radionecrosis	Oral Decadron/taper schedule/monitor for oral thrush/safety measures/fall risk/eye lubricant/salt and baking soda oral rinse
Mucositis/thick ropy saliva/xerostomia/ laryngitis/taste changes/dysphagia/ weight loss/dehydration/ myelosuppression if concomitant chemotherapy or biotherapy/hearing changes	Permanent loss of taste/permanent dry mouth/xerostomia/dental cavities/ damage to soft tissue or jaw bone/ secondary thyroid gland toxicity	Involve multidisciplinary team/nutrition/pain team/head and neck surgical team/dental oral surgeon management Salt/baking soda oral rinse/dental fluoride/ soft diet/encourage frequent high-caloric and -protein meals/parenteral nutrition loss/Compazine, Zofran, Kytril, IV hydration
Nausea/vomiting/diarrhea/weight loss/ decreased WBC, ANC, HGB/ thrombocytopenia/bleeding/possible dehydration/poor digestion Dysphagia/increased sputum production/ dyspnea/hemoptysis/hypoxia	Diarrhea/compromised digestion/less likely yet serious may experience ulcer bleeding/stenosis of bile ducts or intestines/liver or kidney failure Pneumonitis/esophageal narrowing	Frequent high-calorie meals/fluid intake/ electrolyte supplementation/weekly IV fluids/antiemetics with around-the-clock dosing/antidiarrheal agents Saline and bicarbonate mouthwash/cough suppressant/supplemental oxygen/ pulmonary fibrosis/oxygen conservation
Skin changes/pain/lymphedema Increased urinary frequency/urgency/ dysuria/hematuria/diarrhea/proctitis/ erectile dysfunction/vaginal bleeding and stenosis	Skin care/analgesia/physical therapy NSAIDS for pelvic cramping/alpha blockers for dysuria/balance of antidiarrhea medications stool bulking agents/vaginal dilator (after treatment-related acute inflammation 4–8 weeks post-RT) for vaginal stenosis	

3. Assist with insertion of tandem and ring, and insertion of urinary catheter.
4. Provide postbrachytherapy assessment and discharge teaching.

EXPECTED PATIENT OUTCOMES

I. Patient will be thoroughly educated about the trajectory of the radiotherapy course.
II. Patient will remain safe during radiation treatment procedures.
III. Radiation-related side effects will be anticipated, promptly identified, and managed to minimize treatment interruptions and lessen patient complications.

REFERENCES

ASTRO. (2012). *Safety Is No Accident: A Framework For Quality Radiation Oncology And Care.*

Baeza, M. (2012). Accident prevention in day-to-day clinical radiation therapy practice. *Ann ICRP, 41*(3-4), 179–187.

Behrend, S. (2015a). *Radiation Therapy, inPractice.* Pittsburgh: ONS PRESS.

Behrend, S. W. (2015b). Emergence of stereotactic body radiation therapy. *Oncology Nursing Forum, 42*(1), 103–104.

Behrend, S. (2018). Radiation Treatment Planning. In W. Yarbro (Ed.), *Cancer Nursing: Principles and Practice* (pp. 286–328). Boston: Jones and Bartlett.

Bell, L. J., Eade, T., Kneebone, A., et al. (2017). Initial experience with intra-fraction motion monitoring using Calypso guided volumetric modulated arc therapy for definitive prostate cancer treatment. *Journal of Medical Radiation Sciences*, 25–34.

Bova, F. J., & Friedman, W. A. (2016). Linac Radiosurgery System Requirements Procedures and Testing. In *Khan's Treatment Planning in Radiation Oncology* (4th ed., pp. 203-226) Philadelphia: Walters Kluwer.

Dietrich, S., Ford, E., Pavord, D., & Zeng, J. (2016). *Practical Radiation Oncology Physics* (1st ed.). A companion to Gunderson Tepper's *Clinical Radiation Oncology* (Chapter 10). Philadelphia: Elsevier.

Erickson, J., Spurlock, L. K., & Kramer, J. C. (2013). Self-care strategies to relieve fatigue in patients receiving radiation therapy. *Clin J Oncol Nurs, 17*, 319–324.

Forshaw, K., Hall, A. E, Boyes, A. W., Carey, M. L., & Martine, J. (2017) Patients' experience of Preparation for Radiation Therapy: A Qualitative Study. *Oncology Nursing Forum 44*(1).

Foster, R. D., Ramirez, E., & Timmerman, R. D. (2016). Stereotactic Ablative Radiotherapy. In *Khan's Treatment Planning in Radiation Oncology* (4th ed., pp. 227-243). Philadelphia: Walters Kluwer.

Gianfaldoni, S., Gianfaldoni, R., Wollina, U., Lotti, J., et al. (2017). *Open Access Maced J Med Sci., 5*(4), 521–525.

Hall, E. J., & Giaccia, A. J. (2019). *Radiobiology for the Radiologist* (Chapter 4). Philadelphia: Wolters Kluwer.

Heilmann, H. P. (2013). History of radiation oncology. In L. W. Brady & T. E. Yaeger (Eds.), *Encyclopedia of Radiation Oncology*. Berlin, Heidelberg: Springer.

International Commission on Radiological Protection, ICRP (1979) Limits for intakes of radionuclides by workers. *ICRP Publication 30*, Part 1. Ann. ICRP2 (3/4).

Khan, F. M., Gibbons, J. P., & Sperduto, P. W. (2016). *Treatment Planning in Radiation Oncology.* (4th ed., Chapter 1). Philadelphia: Walters Kluwer.

Kissick, M. W., & Fakhraei, S. (2016). Dosimetry introduction. In M. W. Kissick (Ed.), *Fakhraei Lectures on Radiation Dosimetry Physics: A Deeper Look into the Foundations of Clinical Protocols (111-128)*. Madison: Medical Physics Publishing.

Kooy, H. M., & Adams, J. A. (2016). Proton Beam Therapy. In *Khan's Treatment Planning in Radiation Oncology.* (4th ed.). Philadelphia: Walters Kluwer.

Li, G., Gig, S., Mageras, Dong L., & Mohan, R. (2016). Image-Guided Radiation Therapy. In *Khan's Treatment Planning in Radiation Oncology.* (4th ed., pp. 177-203). Philadelphia: Walters Kluwer.

Lindrud-Doyle, S. (2015). Proton Beam Therapy for Pediatric Malignancies. *Clinical Journal of Oncology Nursing, 19*(5), 521–524.

Mahase, S. S., Wernicke, A. G., Nori, D., & Parashar, B. (2015). Current and Emerging Roles of Functional Imaging in Radiation Therapy. *Discovery Medicine.*

McMenamin, E. (2014). Palliative radiotherapy and oncology nursing. *Seminars in Oncology Nursing, 30*, 242–252.

Mitchell, G. (2013). The rationale for fractionation in radiotherapy. *Clin J Oncol Nurs, 17*, 412–417.

NCCN (2018). *Clinical practice guidelines in oncology: cancer-related fatigue version 2.2018*-Retrieved February 20, 2018, from NCCN.org.

Proud, C. (2014). The promise of personalized treatment in radiation oncology? *Clin J Oncol Nurs, 18*, 185–189.

Slater, J. M. (2012). From X rays to ion beams: a short history of radiation therapy. In U. Linz (ed.) *Ion Beam Therapy, Biological and Medical Physics.* Springer Berlin Heidelberg.

Swisher-McClure, S., Hahn, S. M., & Bekelman, J. (2015). Proton beam therapy: the next disruptive innovation in healthcare? *Postgraduate Medical Journal, 91*, 241–243.

Videtic, G. & Woody N. (2015). Handbook of treatment planning in radiation oncology (2nd ed., Chapter 2) New York: Demos Medical Publishing, LLC.

Youl, M. Brock K.K., & Dawson, L.A. (2017) Image-guided radiation therapy. In W. Small, Tarbell, N.J., Yao, M (eds.), *Clinical Radiation Oncology: Indications, Techniques, and Results.* (3rd ed., pp. 83-98). Hoboken, John Wiley and Sons Inc.

28

Chemotherapy and Hormonal Therapy

Patti Davis and Anna Howard

OVERVIEW

I. Principles of cancer chemotherapy (Wellstein, 2018)
   A. Cancer chemotherapy remains an integral component of systemic therapy in both hematologic and solid tumors.
   B. The use of chemotherapy is based on concepts of cellular kinetics, which includes the cell cycle phases, cell cycle time, growth fraction, and tumor burden.
      1. Cell cycle—a highly regulated five-stage process of reproduction that occurs in both normal and malignant cells (Shields, Muehlbauer, & Shelburne, 2014)
         a. Gap 0 (G0), or resting phase
            (1) Cells are not dividing and are only susceptible to cell-cycle nonspecific chemotherapy; cellular activity continues but with a reduced rate of protein synthesis.
            (2) Entry into and out of the resting phase is influenced by growth factors and mitogen interaction with cell surface receptors.
         b. Gap 1 (G1): postmitotic phase, or interphase
            (1) Cells are activated to proliferate.
            (2) Enzymes for DNA synthesis are produced.
            (3) Protein and RNA synthesis occur.
         c. Synthesis (S)
            (1) Cellular DNA is replicated in preparation for DNA division.
         d. Gap 2 (G2), or premitotic phase
            (1) Further protein and RNA synthesis occurs.
            (2) Precursors of the mitotic spindle apparatus are produced.
            (3) Cells are ready for division or mitosis.
         e. Mitosis (M)—the shortest phase of the cell cycle in which cellular division occurs in five phases: prophase, prometaphase, metaphase, anaphase, and telophase. Some chemotherapies target microtubules during prophase.
         f. Cyclin complexes with cyclin-dependent kinases (CDKs) signal the cell to move through each phase of the cell cycle (Shields, et al., 2014)
            (1) CDK mutations can cause tumor development.
            (2) Anti-CDK/cyclin inhibitors are a new class of antineoplastic agents; the first approved agent was in 2015.
      2. Cell cycle time—the amount of time required for a cell to move from one mitosis to the next mitosis (Wellstein, 2018)
         a. The length of the total cell cycle varies with the specific type of cell.
         b. A shorter cell cycle time results in higher cell kill with exposure to cell cycle–specific agents.
      3. Growth fraction of tumor—the percentage of cells actively dividing at a given point in time
         a. A higher growth fraction results in a higher cell kill with exposure to cell cycle–specific agents.
         b. Tumors with a greater fraction of cells in G0 are more sensitive to cell cycle–nonspecific agents.
      4. Tumor burden—volume of cancer present
         a. Smaller: more sensitive to antineoplastic therapy.
         b. As the tumor burden increases, the growth rate slows and the number of cells actively dividing decreases.
         c. The higher the tumor burden, the greater heterogeneity of tumor cells, which in turn increases the likelihood of drug-resistant clone development.
   C. Approaches to chemotherapy (LeFebvre & Stiver, 2014; Wellstein, 2018)
      1. Single-agent chemotherapy
         a. Most common application is in the recurrent setting
         b. May be sequential based on regimen, toxicity, or response to therapy
            (1) Sequential—single chemotherapy agents administered one after the other (e.g., drug A until disease progression followed by drug B)
         c. Persistent use of single-agent chemotherapy increases the probability that drug-resistant clones will emerge.
      2. Combination chemotherapy—use of two or more antineoplastic agents to produce additive or synergistic results against tumor cells

a. Increases the number of cells exposed to cytotoxic effects if cells are in different cell cycle phases.

b. One agent modulates the toxicity of another agent.

c. Effective in large tumors containing a small number of proliferating cells; agents kill a high proportion of tumor cells and stimulate (recruit) remaining tumor cells to enter the proliferative phase; additional agents kill newly proliferating cells.

d. Emergence of drug resistance forestalled by combining agents.

e. May be given with target-specific agents (e.g., monoclonal antibodies)

f. Criteria for selection of antineoplastic agents for combination therapy
   (1) Cytotoxic activity when used alone to treat a specific cancer
   (2) Different, nonoverlapping toxicities
   (3) Toxicities that occur at different points of time from the treatment
   (4) Biological effects that result in enhanced cytotoxicity

3. Adjuvant chemotherapy—chemotherapy is delivered after the known cancer has been surgically removed or radiated

4. Neoadjuvant chemotherapy—chemotherapy delivered before surgery to provide optimal surgical removal or cosmesis

5. Concurrent chemotherapy and radiation—chemotherapy sensitizes tumor cells to radiation
   a. Useful in locally advanced cancers of esophagus, stomach, pancreas, cervix, anus, and head and neck
   b. Common chemotherapies used as radiosensitizers: 5-fluorouracil, cetuximab, cisplatin, mitomycin C, and temozolomide

6. Systemic chemotherapy—chemotherapy doses absorbed and distributed via the bloodstream to exert effects widely throughout the body. May be administered as oral or intravenous (IV) therapy.

7. Regional chemotherapy—method of delivering doses of chemotherapy to the specific site of the tumor—for example, the liver, bladder, peritoneal cavity, central nervous system (CNS), pleural space—while reducing the intensity of systemic toxicity.

8. High-dose chemotherapy—higher dose administered with supportive therapy or with an antidote to diminish toxicity (e.g., high-dose methotrexate with leucovorin rescue, ifosfamide with mesna).

9. Dose-dense chemotherapy—able to administer at more frequent intervals due to use of supportive therapy (e.g., colony-stimulating factors).

D. Factors influencing treatment response (LeFebvre & Stiver, 2014)

1. Characteristics of the tumor—location, size or tumor burden, growth rate or fraction, resistance (inherent or acquired), ratio of sensitivity of malignant cells and normal affected cells, genotype (e.g., molecular characteristics or hormone receptor status), or adequate blood supply with adequate drug uptake

2. Characteristics of the patient—physical status, performance status, age, comorbidities, physiologic deficits, prior therapies, psychosocial status, body mass index (BMI)

3. Administration or schedule—may influence efficacy or toxicity (Mancini & Modlin, 2011)

4. Routes—see Table 28.1

TABLE 28.1 Routes of Administration of Antineoplastic Agents

Route	Advantages	Disadvantages	Complications	Nursing Implications
Oral	Ease of administration Gives patient sense of control and independence Decreases time in health care facility and infusion center	Inconsistency of absorption Potential for drug–drug, food–drug, or herbal–drug interactions Compliance (over or under) Expensive Complex dosing and schedules Difficult to swallow	Drug-specific complications	Monitor patients' response via laboratory tests and follow-up via phone or appointment. Teach adherence with medication schedule. Teach patient techniques for handling drugs Caregivers should use gloves for handling chemotherapy; wash hands after handling (even when gloves used); bring unused oral chemotherapy back to the facility for

TABLE 28.1 Routes of Administration of Antineoplastic Agents—cont'd

Route	Advantages	Disadvantages	Complications	Nursing Implications
				disposal unless otherwise directed (e.g., lenalidomide/ thalidomide/ pomalidomide must be sent to Celgene for disposal). Don't crush tablets or open capsules unless specified in package insert.
Subcutaneous or intramuscular	Ease of administration IM = rapid absorption	Requires adequate muscle mass and tissue for absorption Inconsistent absorption	Infection Bleeding/bruising Pain or localized reaction at injection site Nerve damage Tissue necrosis	Evaluate platelet count before administration as needed. Use smallest-gauge needle possible. Prepare injection site with an antiseptic solution. Assess injection site for signs and symptoms of infection. Wear PPE. Rotate injection sites. Don't massage; use heat or ice packs on injection site
Intravenous	Consistent absorption; most common method of chemotherapy administration Required for vesicants (central access preferred for vesicants)	Sclerosing of veins over time	Infection Phlebitis Infiltration/ extravasation Pain Thrombosis	Use smallest catheter available. Always use safety device. Observe for signs and symptoms of infiltration Avoid areas of flection, lower extremities, and arms where lymph nodes have been removed. Peripheral IV site should not be older than 24 hours.
Intraarterial	Increased doses to tumor with decreased systemic side effects Common sites: liver, head and neck, bone Able to avoid extensive surgeries Patients with liver metastases may be surgical candidates after treatment	Requires surgical procedure or special radiography for catheter, port placement, or pump Not all patients are candidates Patients require specialized nursing care	Bleeding Embolism Pain Infection Catheter issues (migration or dislodgement) Occlusion Clots Device failure	Monitor for signs and symptoms of bleeding or occlusion. Monitor catheter site and affected limb.
Intrathecal or intraventricular	Delivers drug directly into cerebrospinal fluid	Requires lumbar puncture or surgical placement of reservoir or implanted pump Pump occlusion or malfunction	Increased intracranial pressure Headaches Confusion Lethargy	Observe site for signs of infection. Monitor reservoir or pump functioning. Assess patient for headache or signs of

Continued

TABLE 28.1   Routes of Administration of Antineoplastic Agents—cont'd

Route	Advantages	Disadvantages	Complications	Nursing Implications
		Requires additional education for nurse, patient, family Nurse Practice Act may vary for intrathecal or intraventricular chemotherapy administration Preservative-free medications used with epidural and intraspinal may be difficult to obtain	Nausea or vomiting Seizures Infection Malposition/migration of catheter	increased intracranial pressure. Evaluate platelet count before procedure. Vinca alkaloids are NEVER given intrathecally (IT) because of the potential for lethal neurotoxicity or necrosis. They should always be in an IV bag and never in a syringe to prevent accidental IT administration. Time-out should be performed before procedure.
Intraperitoneal	Direct exposure of intraabdominal surfaces to drug Decreases side effects due to lower doses of chemotherapy	Requires placement of Tenckhoff catheter or intraperitoneal port Only patients with minimal disease are candidates	Abdominal pain, distention Bleeding Ileus Intestinal perforation Infection Nausea Increased bladder irritation Dyspnea	Administer chemotherapy at room temperature. Place patient in semi-Fowler's Access with 19-g noncoring needle, 1–1.5 in. long. Check patency of catheter (note if no blood return) or port. Instill drug or solution according to protocol—infuse, dwell, and drain, or continuous infusion. Rotate patient side to side every 15 min for 1 hour postinfusion.
Intravesicular	Direct exposure of bladder surfaces to drug	Requires insertion of indwelling catheter	Urinary tract infection Cystitis Bladder contracture Urinary urgency Allergic drug reactions	Maintain sterile technique when inserting indwelling catheter. Follow provider's orders for positioning of patient and draining of agent.
Intrapleural	Sclerosing of pleural lining May prevent recurrence of malignant pleural effusion	Requires insertion of a thoracotomy tube Nurse Practice Act may not allow nurse to administer drug via intrapleural route Only physicians may administer	Pain Infection Pneumothorax	Monitor for complete drainage from pleural space before instillation of drug. Allow agent to remain for entire dwell time. Assess patient for pain, respiratory distress, anxiety.

Data from Menonna-Quinn, D. (2014). Administration considerations. In M. Polovich, M. Olsen, & K. LeFebvre (Eds.), *Chemotherapy and biotherapy guidelines and recommendations for practice* (4th ed., pp. 121–135). Pittsburg, USA: ONS; Wellstein, A. (2018). General Principles in the Pharmacotherapy of Cancer. In L. L. Brunton, R. Hilal-Dandan, & Knollmann (Eds.), *Goodman and Gilman's The Pharmacological Basis of Therapeutics*, 13th edition Chapter 66, eBook: McGraw-Hill; Chu, E., & DeVita, V. (2013). *Physicians' cancer chemotherapy drug manual 2013.* Burlington, MA: Jones & Bartlett Learning.

II. Role of chemotherapy in cancer care
   A. Cure—to have same life expectancy as if not diagnosed with cancer
   B. Control—to extend the length and quality of life when cure is not realistic
   C. Palliation—improve comfort when neither cure nor control is possible; relief of tumor-related symptoms
III. Types and classifications of chemotherapy (Table 28.2)—antineoplastic agents classified according to the phase of action during the cell cycle, mechanism of action,

TABLE 28.2 Classifications of Cancer Therapy Drugs

Alkylating Agents

Alkyl sulfonates	Aziridines	Triazenes and hydrazine
Busulfan (Myleran [PO]); Busulfex (IV)	Altretamine (Hexalen)	Dacarbazine (DTIC-DOME)
	Thiotepa (Thioplex)	Procarbazine (Matulane)
		Temozolomide (Temodar)

Nitrogen mustards	Nitrosoureas	Platinum analogs
Bendamustine (Treanda)	Carmustine (BCNU)	Carboplatin (Paraplatin)
Chlorambucil (Leukeran)	Lomustine (CNU)	Cisplatin (Platinol)
Cyclophosphamide (Cytoxan)	Streptozocin (Zanosar)	Oxaliplatin (Eloxatin)
Ifosfamide (Ifex)		
Melphalan (Alkeran)		
Mechlorethamine (Mustargen)		

Antimetabolites

Pyrimidine analogs	Folate antagonists	Purine analogs
Azacytidine (Vidaza)	Methotrexate (Folex)	Cladribine (Leustatin)
Capecitabine (Xeloda)	Pemetrexed (Alimta)	Clofarabine (Clolar)
Cytarabine (Cytosar)		Fludarabine (Fludara)
Cytarabine, liposomal (DepoCyt)		Mercaptopurine (Purinethol)
Decitabine (Dacogen)		Nelarabine (Arranon)
Floxuridine (FUDR)		Pentostatin (Nipent)
5-Fluorouracil (Adrucil)		Thioguanine (6-TG)
Gemcitabine (Gemzar)		

Antimicrotubule Agents

Epothilones	Taxanes	Miscellaneous
Ixabepilone (Ixempra)	Cabazitaxel (Jevtana)	Eribulin mesylate (Halaven)
	Docetaxel (Taxotere)	
	Paclitaxel (Taxol)	
	Paclitaxel, protein bound (Abraxane)	

Vinca Alkaloids

Vinblastine (Velban)	Vincristine (Oncovin)	Vindesine (Eldisine)
	Vincristine, liposomal (Marqibo)	Vinorelbine (Navvelbine)

Miscellaneous

Arsenic trioxide (Trisenox)	Dactinomycin (Actinomycin-D)	Omacetaxine (Synribo)
Asparaginase (Erwinase, Oncospar)	Hydroxyurea (Hydrea)	Trabectedin (Yondelis)
Bexarotene (Targretin)	Mitotane (Lysodren)	Tretinoin (Vesanoid)
		Pomalidomide (Pomalyst)
		Lenalidomide (Revlimid)

Topoisomerase I Inhibitors (Camptothecins)

Topotecan (Hycamtin)	Irinotecan (Camptosar)

Topoisomerase II Inhibitors

Anthracyclines	Anthracenedione	Epipodophyllotoxins
Daunorubicin (Cerubidine)	Bleomycin sulfate (Blenoxane)	Etoposide (VePesid)
Daunorubicin, liposomal (DaunoXome)	Mitomycin (Mutamycin)	Etoposide phosphate (Etopophos)
Doxorubicin (Adriamycin)	Mitoxantrone (Novantrone)	Teniposide (Vumon)
Doxorubicin, liposomal (Doxil)		
Epirubicin (Ellence)		
Idarubicin (Idamycin)		
Valrubicin (Valstar)		

Continued

TABLE 28.2 **Classifications of Cancer Therapy Drugs—cont'd**		
Hormones		
Antiestrogens	Aromatase Inhibitors	LH-RH Analogs and Antagonists
Fluvestrant (Faslodex)	Anastrazole (Arimidex)	Goserelin (Zoladex)
Megestrol acetate (Megace)	Exemestane (Aromasin)	Leuprolide (Lupron)
Tamoxifen citrate (Nolvadex)	Letrazole (Femara)	Degarelix (Firmagon)
Toremifene (Fareson)		
Miscellaneous Hormonal Agents	Antiandrogens	
Abiraterone acetate (Zytiga)	Bicalutamide (Casodex)	
Enzalutamide (Xtandi)	Flutamide (Eulexin)	
Estramustine (Emcyt)	Nilutamide (Nilandron)	

Data from Chemotherapy and Immunotherapy Guidelines and Recommendations for Practice (in press); Wellstein, A. (2018). General Principles in the Pharmacotherapy of Cancer. In L. L. Brunton, R. Hilal-Dandan, & Knollmann (Eds.), *Goodman and Gilman's The Pharmacological Basis of Therapeutics*, 13th edition Chapter 66, eBook: McGraw-Hill; Chu, E., & DeVita, V. (2013). *Physicians' cancer chemotherapy drug manual 2013.* Burlington, MA: Jones & Bartlett Learning.

biochemical structure, or physiologic action (Wellstein, Giaccone, Atkins, & Sausville, 2018)

A. Phase of action during the cell cycle
1. Cell cycle–specific agents
    a. Major cytotoxic effects are exerted on actively dividing cells at specific phases throughout the cell cycle.
    b. Agents are not active against cells in the resting phase (G0).
    c. Agents are schedule dependent and most effective if administered in divided doses or by continuous infusion.
    d. Cytotoxic effects occur during the cell cycle and are expressed when cell repair or division is attempted.
    e. Continuous infusion and multiple frequent doses of cell cycle–specific agents result in exposure of a greater number of cells and in a higher cell kill in tumors with short cell cycle times.
    f. Cell cycle–specific drugs include antimetabolites and plant alkaloids.
2. Cell cycle–nonspecific agents
    a. Major cytotoxic effects are exerted on cells at any phase in the cell cycle, including G0.
    b. Agents are dose dependent; most effective if administered by bolus doses, as the number of cells affected is proportional to the amount of drug given.
    c. Cytotoxic effects occur during the cell cycle and are expressed when cell division is attempted.
    d. Effective in treating tumors with slowly dividing cells.
    e. Cell cycle–nonspecific agents include alkylating agents, antitumor antibiotics, hormonal therapies, and nitrosoureas.
B. Biochemical structure, mechanism of action, or derivation

1. Alkylating agents (Wellstein, Giaccone, Atkins and Sausville 2018)
    a. Among the first antineoplastic drugs developed
    b. Mechanisms of action (MOAs)—interfere with DNA replication through cross-linking of DNA strands, DNA strand breakage, and abnormal base pairing of proteins, all interfering with normal DNA replication
    c. Most are cell cycle–nonspecific agents
    d. Major toxicities often directly related to the administered dose; pancytopenia, nausea and vomiting, mucosal/gastrointestinal (GI) toxicity, and neurotoxicity
        (1) General: peripheral granulocyte nadir approximately 6 to 10 days after administration with recovery about 14 to 21 days.
        (2) Nitrosoureas: peripheral granulocyte nadir is delayed; may appear about 4 to 6 weeks after dose.
    e. Seven major subgroups—nitrogen mustards, aziridines, alkyl sulfonates, DNA methylating agents, nitrosoureas, platinum compounds, and triazine compounds
    f. Special dosing considerations: carboplatin dose calculation using the Calvert equation is based on area under the curve (AUC), a measure of drug exposure, and the patient's renal function (Olsen, 2019)

Calvert equation = AUC × (eGFR + 25)
eGFR max for calculation = 125mL/hr
Adjusted weight may be used if BMI > 25

2. Antimetabolites (Wellstein, Giaccone, Atkins and Sausville 2018)
    a. Includes antifolates, pyrimidine analogs, and purine analogs

b. MOA—inhibit protein synthesis, substitute erroneous metabolites or structural analogs during DNA synthesis, and inhibit DNA synthesis

c. Most agents cell cycle specific (S phase)

d. Major toxicities in the hematopoietic and GI systems

3. Topoisomerase-targeting agents (Wellstein, Giaccone, Atkins and Sausville 2018)

   a. Topoisomerase I–directed agents—include the camptothecins

     (1) MOA: prevent realignment of DNA strands, maintain single-strand DNA breaks

     (2) Major toxicities affecting the hematopoietic and GI systems

   b. Topoisomerase II–targeting agents—anthracyclines, anthracenediones, actinomycins, and epipodophyllotoxins

     (1) MOA: prevent realigning of DNA strands, maintain double-strand DNA breaks

     (2) Major toxicities: hematopoietic, GI, cardiac (anthracyclines) systems

4. Microtubule-targeting agents (Wellstein, Giaccone, Atkins and Sausville 2018)

   a. MOA: prevents microtubule polymerization so the mitotic spindle cannot form; the cell cycle is stopped in metaphase; cells undergo apoptosis.

b. Include taxanes and vinca alkaloids, epothilone analogs

c. Most agents cell cycle specific, primarily late G2 and M phases

d. Major toxicities: hematopoietic, integumentary, neurologic, and reproductive systems

5. Differentiating agents (Wellstein, Giaccone, Atkins and Sausville 2018)

   a. Used in the treatment of acute promyelocytic leukemia (APL)

   b. Tretinoin, also known as *all-trans retinoic acid* or *ATRA*; oral agent

     (1) Produces maturation of primitive promyelocytes

     (2) Major toxicities: hepatotoxicity, differentiation syndrome (massive cytokine release from promyelocyte maturation may cause fever, dyspnea, pulmonary infiltrates, pericardial infiltrates)

   c. Arsenic trioxide, IV

     (1) MOA not well understood

     (2) Major toxicities: hepatotoxicity, QT prolongation, differentiation syndrome (although less common than tretinoin)

   d. Differentiation syndrome is prevented/treated with corticosteroids

IV. Hormonal therapy (Table 28.3)

TABLE 28.3 Hormonal Therapy

Hormone Category	Mechanism of Action	Uses	Side Effects
Adrenocorticoids	Lead to cell death—exact mechanism unknown	Lymphoma, acute lymphoblastic leukemia, chronic lymphocytic leukemia, and multiple myeloma	Hyperglycemia, insomnia, hypersensitivity, hypertension, osteoporosis, diabetes, and immune suppression
Androgens	Inhibit androgen binding to androgen receptors (AR); inhibit AR binding to DNA	Metastatic breast cancer, hypogonadism	Gynecomastia, headache, decreased libido
Antiandrogens	Drugs that prevent the effects of androgens	Castration-resistant prostate cancer	Hot flashes, loss of libido, impotence, and gynecomastia
Antiestrogens Pure antiestrogens	Function as an estrogen antagonist with no estrogen-agonist effects	Postmenopausal women with advanced breast cancer who had relapsed or progressed on prior endocrine therapy	Hot flashes, headache, dyspepsia, facial swelling, and vaginal discharge
Selective estrogen receptor modulators (SERMs)	Block estrogen activity (i.e., serve as estrogen antagonists) in some tissues (e.g., breast tissue) but also mimic estrogen effects (i.e., serve as estrogen agonists) in other tissues (e.g., endometrium)	Premenopausal and postmenopausal women with hormone-positive breast cancer	Hot flash, stroke, thromboembolic risk, uterine cancer, vaginal discharge, menstrual irregularities
Aromatase inhibitors (AIs)	Inhibits synthesis of estrogen by preventing conversion of estrogen precursors to estrogen	Postmenopausal and premenopausal breast cancer with ovarian suppression or ablation	Osteoporosis, hot flashes, elevated cholesterol, arthralgias, decreased libido, decreased vaginal lubrication

Continued

TABLE 28.3   Hormonal Therapy—cont'd

Hormone Category	Mechanism of Action	Uses	Side Effects
Gonadotropin-releasing hormone (GnRH) agonists	Bind to specific receptors on pituitary gonadotrophs responsible for gonadotropin secretion and synthesis Suppress ovarian production of estrogen in women Decrease testosterone production in males	Metastatic breast cancer; premenopausal; can be used with AI	Hot flashes, mood changes, weight gain, injection site reaction
GnRH antagonists	Compete with GnRH for receptors on gonadotroph cell membranes; inhibit GnRH-induced signal transduction and gonadotrophin secretion	Metastatic breast cancer, adjuvant therapy	Hot flashes, decreased libido, injection site reaction
Progestins	Exact mechanism unknown Thought to block the synthesis of luteinizing hormone in the pituitary gland without affecting ovarian sensitivity to gonadotrophins	Estrogen receptor positive, progesterone receptor positive metastatic breast cancer May be used as appetite stimulants due to side effects	Increased appetite, weight gain, diarrhea, rash

A. Overview
  1. First targeted therapy
  2. Used to treat breast, prostate, endometrial, and ovarian cancers
  3. Suppressing select hormones may inhibit cancerous cell growth of hormone-sensitive cancers

ASSESSMENT (NEUSS ET AL., 2017; OLSEN, 2019)

I. Pretreatment
  A. Cancer diagnosis information
    1. Pathology: cell type, cytogenetic findings (when relevant)
    2. Stage and grade of disease
    3. Risks and benefits of treatment
  B. Laboratory results
    1. Complete blood cell count with differential
    2. Comprehensive metabolic panel
    3. Electrolytes—including magnesium, potassium, and phosphorus
    4. Genetic/genomic considerations (e.g., HER2, KRAS, BRAF, EGFR, Alk rearrangement)
  C. Patient-related information
    1. Family and personal medical histories
    2. Comorbidities and preexisting conditions
    3. Thorough review of cardiac (including ejection fraction as indicated), pulmonary, GI, renal, reproductive, and neurologic functioning
    4. Behavioral and cognitive functioning
    5. Performance status
    6. Venous access—peripheral versus central
    7. Patient and family experience of prior therapies
      a. Side effects experienced and their severity
      b. Self-care measures and effectiveness in reducing side effects
    8. Understanding of the goal of therapy

II. Ongoing
  A. Performance status
  B. Vital signs
  C. Weight and height at least weekly when patient is in the health care setting
  D. Medication reconciliation
  E. Dietary intake, unintentional weight loss, use of nutraceuticals, supplements, complementary therapies that could interact with treatment
  F. Allergies or history of hypersensitivity or infusion reactions (note cycle of therapy)
    1. Taxane reactions occur most often in first or second infusion.
    2. Reactions to platinum agents occur most often during the fifth (oxaliplatin), sixth, or later infusion (carboplatin).
  G. Knowledge of, rationale for, and goals of treatment; schedule of agents to be given; potential side effects
  H. Psychosocial examination
    1. Previous responses to stressors and effective coping mechanisms
    2. Level of independence and responsibility, ability for self-care
    3. Support systems and personnel available to the patient and family
    4. Cultural, spiritual, and financial considerations
III. Management
  A. Interventions to maximize safe administration of chemotherapy (Neuss, et al., 2017; Olsen, 2019) ⚠
    1. Review of orders
      a. Compare orders with drug protocol or reference source, ensuring accuracy and completeness
      b. Orders to be regimen specific, preprinted, or electronic with a list of all agents and calculations in the regimen

c. Verbal orders not allowed except to hold or stop chemotherapy administration

d. Complete orders for IV treatment to include the patient's full name and a second identifier; date order is written; date medication is administered; diagnosis; regimen or protocol name, number, cycle number, and day when applicable; criteria to treat; number of cycles order is valid; allergies; full generic names of the agents; doses are written after abbreviation; trailing zeros and leading zero standards; dose calculation methodology; parameters for holding or modifying the treatment; route and rate of administration; supportive care agents or treatments; sequence; and time specifications (Neuss et al., 2017)

2. Determination of drug dosage
   a. Verification of actual height and weight on day of administration
   b. Calculation of body surface area (BSA) or appropriate dose calculation (e.g., AUC)
   c. Recalculation of drug dosage and checking against order

3. Review drugs to be administered and potential side effects and toxicities

4. Review and obtain orders for other medications: prehydration and posthydration IV fluids, antiemetics, premedications, if indicated, for hypersensitivity reactions

5. Verification of previous and current laboratory test values or need for dosage adjustment, if indicated

6. Verification that informed consent is documented according to practice or institution policies and procedures

7. Patient and caregiver teaching (e.g., chemotherapy administration procedures, antiemetic schedule, self-care measures for potential side effects)

8. Prepare drugs, as appropriate, following safe handling policies and procedures (NIOSH, 2016, USP, 2015, USP, 2017, Kerber & Polovich, 2014)
   a. Chemotherapies are hazardous drugs and may evidence one or more of the following characteristics:
      (1) Carcinogenic (cancer causing)
      (2) Teratogenic (fetal malformation or defects)
      (3) Associated with adverse reproductive outcomes
      (4) Genotoxic (damage genetic material)
      (5) Potential for other organ or system evidence of exposure or toxicity
   b. Employ safe handling of agents to minimize potential risks for occupational exposure to hazardous drugs:
      (1) Increased risk for malignancies

      (2) Embryofetal toxicities
      (3) Chromosomal damage
      (4) Other evidence of exposures (e.g., skin injury, alopecia, dermatitis)
   c. Mixing or compounding chemotherapy
      (1) Adhere to guidelines and recommendations from the Oncology Nursing Society (ONS), the Occupational Safety and Health Administration (OSHA), and the American Society of Health-Systems Pharmacists (ASHP)
         (a) ONS guidelines for safe handling of chemotherapy or hazardous drugs
         (b) National Institute for Occupational Safety and Health (NIOSH) Alert on Preventing Occupational Exposure to Antineoplastic and Other Hazardous Drugs in Health Care Settings, 2016
         (c) U.S. Pharmacopeia (USP), General Chapter 797 – "Pharmaceutical Compounding – Sterile Preparations," 2008
   d. USP, General Chapter 800 – "Hazardous Drugs – Handling in Healthcare Settings," 2017; potentially high risk for exposure if proper procedures and guidelines are not followed
   e. Correct use of personal protective equipment (PPE) can significantly reduce exposure to hazardous drugs
   f. All chemotherapy preparations, including opening capsules and crushing agents that can be administered as a powder, should take place in a primary engineering control (C-PEC) setting—biologic safety cabinet or a compounding aseptic containment isolator
      (1) Use vertical unidirectional air flow
      (2) Preparation area is vented to the outside (optimal) with exhaust emitted through a high-efficiency particulate air (HEPA) filter
      (3) Fan is operating continuously
      (4) Preparation area is housed in an area with negative pressure
      (5) C-PEC is inspected and serviced per manufacturer's recommendations; recertified if moved, repaired, with filter replacement, and every 6 months
      (6) Training essential to use techniques that minimize interference with air flow
   g. Wash hands and don PPE appropriate for use with chemotherapy
   h. Gather necessary supplies for compounding; limit items housed in the PEC to reduce both contamination of items and interference with air flow

i. Use closed-system transfer devices to reduce environmental contamination during drug preparation

j. Use double gloves for all handling; change every 30 minutes and whenever contamination occurs

k. Use closed-system transfer devices

l. Avoid overfilling syringes

m. Intravenous fluid (IVF)—spike and prime tubing before chemotherapy is added to minimize exposure

n. Damp-wipe outside of product (i.e., syringe, IVF) before placing in transport container; container should be identified as hazardous according to policy and procedures

o. Transport containers or bags—label to ensure awareness of contents; avoid contamination of the outside of the transport container or bags

p. Dispose contaminated compounding materials in a sealed container within the PEC; place into a puncture-proof container located adjacent to the PEC

q. Remove and discard outer gloves, followed by the gown and the inner gloves, taking care not to contaminate self

r. Wash hands with soap and water

9. Label drugs with the patient's full name and a second identifier (e.g., date of birth), generic drug name, route of administration, total dose, total volume, date of administration, sequence of drug administration (when applicable), drugs in divided doses need total number of doses (i.e., 1 of 2), date and time of preparation and expiration, warning sticker for handling requirements (Neuss et al., 2017)

10. Oral drugs to be labeled with patient's name and a second identifier, date and time of preparation and expiration, full generic drug name, dosage form and strength, quantity dispensed, number of pills per dose, administration schedule including how many times per day and any days off if applicable, instructions relating to food and other medication interactions, warning sticker for hazardous drug and for handling and/or storage requirements, and prescriber name (Neuss et al., 2017)

11. Before each chemotherapy administration, at least two practitioners approved by the health care setting to administer or prepare chemotherapy, verify and document the following: drug name, drug dose, infusion volume, or volume in syringe; rate of administration; expiration dates and/or times; appearance of drug; rate set on infusion pump, when applicable (Neuss et al., 2017)

12. Ensure appropriate supplies or pump is available
a. Emergency equipment
b. Agents for management of extravasation and/or anaphylaxis, as indicated
c. Spill kit
d. PPE

13. Don PPE or apply principles of safe handling throughout chemotherapy administration
a. Potential routes of exposure: absorption, inhalation, ingestion, injection
b. Guidelines regarding PPE
(1) Gloves—powder-free disposable gloves tested for use with hazardous drugs
(a) Double-glove for drug preparation, administration, and handling of contaminated waste.
(b) Inspect for defects before use; remove and discard immediately after use, damage, drug spill, or 30 minutes of wear.
(c) Do not reuse.
(2) Gowns—should be disposable, lint-free, low-permeability, with a solid front, long sleeves, tight cuffs, and back closure
(a) Discard if visibly contaminated, after handling hazardous drugs, or after leaving the area.
(b) Do not reuse.
(3) Respirators—NIOSH-approved protective respirator when aerosolization, if possible
(a) Check the material safety data sheet for appropriate respiratory protection.
(b) Surgical masks are not respirators; do not protect against vapors or aerosols.
(4) Eye and face protection—plastic face shield to be worn when splashing is possible; surgical masks do not provide protection for eye and face exposures.
(5) Chemotherapy precautions for handling body fluids and soiled linens.
(a) Precautions remain in effect for 48 hours after chemotherapy administration is complete.
(b) Laundry handling in the home setting: patients will wear gloves when handling soiled linen. Patients are to place their soiled clothes in a pillow case, washing twice in hot water using regular detergent. It is important to keep soiled clothing separate from other laundry.
(c) Skin exposure: remove soiled garment and wash the skin thoroughly with soap and water.

(d) Flush the toilet twice with the lid down to prevent particles from splashing; when a lid is not present, cover the toilet bowl with a plastic-backed pad (Polovich & Olsen, 2018).

(e) The following chemotherapies may have metabolites present in urine or feces for up to a week and require personal protection for this time period: carmustine, cisplatin, docetaxel, doxorubicin, etoposide, gemcitabine, methotrexate, mitoxantrone, teniposide, vincristine, and vinorelbine.

14. Venipuncture site selection criteria
    a. Select distal sites before proximal sites.
    b. Evaluate general condition of veins.
    c. Note type of medications to be infused.
    d. Avoid sites where damage to underlying tendons or nerves is more likely to occur—for example, antecubital region, wrist, dorsal surface of the hand; areas with recent venipuncture sites, sclerosed veins; or areas of previous surgery such as skin grafts, side of mastectomy, lumpectomy, node dissection, or partial amputation.

15. Monitor central or peripheral IV administration for presence of blood return before, during, and after administration of therapy.

16. Administer prechemotherapy hydration, antiemetics, other medications as ordered.

17. Administer chemotherapy drugs according to agency policy and procedures, following safe handling procedures in accordance with ASCO/ONS chemotherapy administration standards.

18. Administer agents designed to protect against specific toxic effects of chemotherapy (Jansen et al., 2014).
    a. Dexrazoxane (Zinecard)—to protect against cardiotoxicity in patients who require more than 300 mg/m^2 of doxorubicin (Pfizer, 2016)
    b. Amifostine (Ethyol)—to protect against renal toxicity from cisplatin therapy or xerostomia from radiation to the head and neck
    c. Mesna (Mesnex)—to protect against bladder toxicity from ifosfamide or high-dose cyclophosphamide
    d. Leucovorin—used as a rescue agent with methotrexate to prevent mucositis and other toxicities related to impaired methotrexate elimination

19. Assess the patient for signs of infiltration (burning, pain, swelling, redness).

20. Flush the IV tubing with appropriate solution after administering each agent and at completion of the infusion.

21. After drug administration, remove intact administration setup; the spike from the IVF containers should not be removed or tubing reused.

22. Remove of the needle or IV catheter.
    a. Apply gauze to the peripheral IV site.
    b. Apply gentle pressure to the site to reduce local bleeding.

23. Wash potentially contaminated surfaces; may include multiple steps depending on institution guidelines.
    a. Deactivate chemotherapy (bleach, peroxide, etc.)
    b. Decontaminate to remove chemotherapy residue (e.g., alcohol, water, bleach, or peroxide)
    c. Cleanse and disinfect with germicidal agents and disinfectants

24. Discard contaminated materials in the appropriate hazardous waste container.

25. Document medication administration, infusion site, patient education, and outcomes or response according to agency policy.

IV. Interventions to minimize risk of extravasation (Polovich & Schulmeister, 2014, Kreideh 2016; Piko et al., 2012)

A. Prevention is the best approach for avoiding extravasation injury.
    1. Chemotherapy administration should be limited to knowledgeable, clinically competent staff as defined per institutional policy. Competence is based on didactic education and clinical experience.
    2. Risk for extravasation should be assessed before treatment administration. Vigilance is always required during administration.
    3. Policies and procedures in the management of extravasations should be clearly delineated, readily accessible in all sites where vesicants may be administered, and periodically reviewed.

B. If extravasation is suspected, appropriate materials and antidotes should be obtained for the management of extravasation.
    1. Extravasation—infiltration or leakage of an IV antineoplastic agent into local tissues
        a. Irritants—agents that cause a local inflammatory reaction but do not cause tissue necrosis
        b. Vesicants—agents that have the potential to cause cellular damage or tissue destruction, or are inadvertently administered into the tissue; see Table 28.4 for a list of agents associated with extravasation and tissue injury
            (1) Observe for swelling, redness, lack of blood return, IV that slows or stops infusing, leaking around needle or catheter.
            (2) Instruct the patient to report pain, burning, or changes in sensations during chemotherapy administration.
            (3) Administer vesicants in larger veins of the arm, above the wrist and below the elbow.

TABLE 28.4	**Agents Associated with Extravasation or Tissue Injury**	
Vesicant	**Irritant**	**Vesicant or Irritant**
Amsacrine: none	Carboplatin: none	Bendamustine: none
Cisplatin: sodium thiosulfate	Carmustine:none	Bleomycin: none
Dacarbazine: none	Cyclophosphamide:none	Cabazitaxel: cold
Dactinomycin: cold	Gemcitabine: none	Dacarbazine
Daunorubicin: dexrazoxane, cold	Ifosfamide: none	Etoposide: none
Docetaxel: cold	Irinotecan: none	Fluorouracil: none
Doxorubicin: dexrazoxane, cold	Liposomal doxorubicin: none	Paclitaxel: cold
Epirubicin: dexrazoxane, cold	Methotrexate: none	Paclitaxel protein bound: none
Idarubicin: dexrazoxane, cold	Plicamycin: none	
Mechlorethamine: sodium thiosulfate, cold	Teniposide: none	
Melphalan: none	Topotecan: none	
Mitomycin: none		
Mitoxantrone: cold		
Oxaliplatin: dexamethasone (limited data), heat		
Streptozocin: none		
Trabectedin: cold		
Vinblastine: hyaluronidase, heat		
Vincristine: hyaluronidase, heat		
Vindesine: hyaluronidase, heat		
Vinorelbine: hyaluronidase, heat		

Medication: Antidote, cold versus heat therapy if indicated
Data from Wellstein, A. (2018). General principles in the pharmacotherapy of cancer. In L. L. Brunton, R. Hilal-Dandan, & Knollmann (Eds.), *Goodman and Gilman's The Pharmacological Basis of Therapeutics*, (13th ed., Chapter 66) eBook: McGraw-Hill; Chu, E., & DeVita, V. (2013). *Physicians & cancer chemotherapy drug manual 2013*. Burlington, MA: Jones & Bartlett Learning; Kreideh, F. Y., Mukadem, H. A., & El Saghir, N. S. (2016). Overview, prevention and management of chemotherapy extravasation. *World Journal of Clinical Oncology, 7*(1), 87–97.

Avoid areas of flexion or areas with minimal overlying tissue.

(4) Assess blood return on short-term/minibag infusions before, every 5 minutes during, and after the infusion is complete; limit administration to 30 to 60 minutes; do not administer through an IV pump; administer via gravity through a free-flowing primary IV line using a closed system transfer device (CSTD); remain with patient during the entire infusion

(5) Assess blood return on IV pushes every 2 to 5 mL when administering IV push and every 5 minutes for piggyback infusion.

(6) Assess blood return on continuous infusions before, during (per health care facility policy), and at completion; always infuse through a central access device.

c. If extravasation occurs or is suspected, do the following:

(1) Immediately discontinue infusion, leaving needle or IV catheter in place.

(2) Aspirate residual medication and blood from the IV tubing.

(3) Remove the IV needle or device.

(4) Assess symptoms or suspected site of extravasation.

(5) For most medications, treatment of extravasation is nonpharmacologic.

(a) Avoid applying pressure to the area to decrease spread of drug infiltrate.

(b) Administer antidote, if appropriate. Treatment for anthracycline extravasation with dexrazoxane is a 3-day regimen. It should begin as soon as possible, but within 6 hours of extravasation (Totect® (Dexrazoxane) [package insert]. Nashville, TN; (Cumberland Pharmaceuticals, 2017).

(c) Use heat or cold compresses as indicated for the agent extravasated (see Table 28.4).

(d) Elevate the affected extremity to decrease swelling.

(6) Notify the physician of extravasation; arrange follow-up.

(7) Document extravasation event to include date, time, needle size and type, site, method of administration, medications administered, sequence of antineoplastic agents, approximate amount of agent extravasated, patient-reported symptoms, nursing assessment of site, interventions, notification of physician, instructions given to patient, measurements and photographs, and follow-up measures.

V. Interventions to decrease the incidence and severity of complications of chemotherapy (Table 28.5)

TABLE 28.5   Specific Toxicities and Nursing Interventions for Selected Chemotherapeutic Agents

Toxicity	Chemotherapeutic Agents	Nursing Interventions
Hypersensitivity	Asparaginase Paclitaxel Bleomycin Carboplatin Cisplatin Docetaxel Etoposide Liposomal doxorubicin hydrochloride Oxaliplatin	Identify patients at risk—patients with previous allergic reactions to this or other medications; cycle of therapy. Assess for early signs of hypersensitivity—urticaria, pruritus, generalized uneasiness, hypertension, progressing to more severe reactions, including shortness of breath, chest pain, back pain, hypotension, bronchospasm, cyanosis, rigors, chills. Taxane reactions generally occur at onset of first and/or second infusion; platinum reactions generally occur after fifth infusion and during the infusion. Assess for signs of anaphylaxis-type reactions. Stop infusion if reaction is suspected. Administer oxygen to keep saturation 90% or greater. Administer medications to help resolve reaction (diphenhydramine, dexamethasone, Pepcid, epinephrine).
Pulmonary injury (pulmonary toxicity presenting as pneumonitis that may progress to pulmonary fibrosis)	Bleomycin Mitomycin Cyclophosphamide Methotrexate Cytosine arabinoside Carmustine Procarbazine	Monitor cumulative dose of bleomycin, which should not exceed 400 units; doses above this limit significantly increase risk of pulmonary toxicity. Avoid administering drugs with overlapping pulmonary toxicity together. Assess for signs of pulmonary toxicity—dry persistent cough, dyspnea, tachypnea, cyanosis, and basilar rales. Provide pulmonary toilet or adequate exercise. Higher levels of fraction of inspired oxygen (Fio_2) or use of granulocyte-colony stimulating factor (G-CSF) agents with bleomycin may increase pulmonary toxicity potential.
Renal toxicity	Cisplatin High-dose methotrexate	Monitor creatinine, blood urea nitrogen (BUN), and urinary output. Avoid use of other nephrotoxic agents. Provide adequate hydration or diuresis.
Ototoxicity	Carboplatin Cisplatin Oxaliplatin	Teach patient to report tinnitus. Monitor dose levels; risk increases with dosage >60–75 mg/m^2. Refer patient for audiography, if indicated.
Hemorrhagic cystitis	Cyclophosphamide Ifosfamide	Ensure adequate fluid intake >3000 mL/day unless contraindicated. Have the patient void every 2–4 hr during day and every 4 hr at night. Educate patient to report signs of cystitis. Administer mesna as ordered. Oral doses of cyclophosphamide should be given early in the day.
Cardiotoxicity manifested by electrocardiography (ECG) changes, congestive heart failure (CHF), cardiomyopathy, angina, dysrhythmias, tachycardia, bradycardia	Doxorubicin Daunorubicin Epirubicin Idarubicin Cyclophosphamide (high dose) 5-Fluorouracil	Monitor cumulative doses of anthracyclines; maximum cumulative dose is 550 mg/m^2 for doxorubicin—doses above this significantly increase risk for cardiotoxicity; maximal cumulative dose for doxorubicin is 450 mg/m^2 if patient received or is concurrently receiving radiation to mediastinum or cyclophosphamide.

Continued

TABLE 28.5   Specific Toxicities and Nursing Interventions for Selected Chemotherapeutic Agents—cont'd

Toxicity	Chemotherapeutic Agents	Nursing Interventions
	Capecitabine Mitoxantrone Trastuzumab Pertuzumab	Assess for signs of cardiotoxicity, including ECG changes; weight gain, pedal edema, chest pain, heart rate (irregular, too fast or too slow), shortness of breath, left ventricular ejection fraction (LVEF), and jugular vein distention (JVD). Mitoxantrone—risk is not as great as with daunorubicin and doxorubicin; risk is increased with cumulative doses >140 mg/m². HER-2 targeted agents should not be administered concomitantly with anthracyclines due to increased cardiotoxicity. They should be administered sequentially (e.g., regimen AC before TH).
Diarrhea	Irinotecan Panobinostat 5-Fluorouracil	Diarrhea may be managed with loperamide or atropine–diphenoxylate (Lomotil). Irinotecan: Give atropine prophylactically. Early and late diarrhea can be dose-limiting. Early diarrhea occurs within 24 hr of administration and is generally cholinergic; treatment may include atropine. Late diarrhea occurs >24 hr after dose and is managed with loperamide. Monitor electrolytes.
Peripheral neuropathy	Paclitaxel Cisplatin Carboplatin Oxaliplatin Bortezomib	Monitor for sensory and motor nerve changes and stocking–glove distribution of dysesthesia. Peripheral neuropathy appears in the distal extremities of hands and feet and progresses proximally. Dose modifications or delays may be utilized to minimize neuropathy. Loss of sense includes loss of proprioception, vibration, pain, temperature, and touch.
Hypotension	Etoposide	Rapid infusion may precipitate hypotension; administer over 30–60 min. Monitor blood pressure.
Neurotoxicity (central)	Ifosfamide Methotrexate Vincristine Cytarabine Intrathecal administration	Monitor creatinine, BUN, and albumin; risk of neurotoxicity increases with decreased renal function and low albumin level. Neurologic checks should be performed every 4 hr for patients at risk (e.g., high-dose ARA-C or ifosfamide). Have patients write their name and look for inconsistencies. Teach patients and families to report early signs of neurotoxicity.
Neurotoxicity (peripheral)	Paclitaxel Docetaxel Vincristine Vinorelbine Vinblastine Cisplatin Carboplatin Oxaliplatin	Assess for numbness and tingling of hands and feet, foot drop, decreased fine and gross motor abilities. Oxaliplatin—educate patients about cold sensitivity. Monitor for constipation as a potential early sign of neurotoxicity. Teach patient to report symptoms of neurotoxicity.
Nasopharyngitis	Cyclophosphamide	Infuse slowly over 30–60 min to decrease risk of nasopharyngitis (aka *wasabi nose*).

Data from Wellstein, A. (2018). General Principles in the Pharmacotherapy of Cancer. In L. L. Brunton, R. Hilal-Dandan, & Knollmann (Eds.), Goodman and Gilman's The Pharmacological Basis of Therapeutics, 13th edition Chapter 66, eBook: McGraw-Hill; Jansen, C., Davis, P., Katz, A., Douglas, T., Gilbert, C., Olsen, M., ⋯ Skinner, J., Robinson, C., Rogers, B., Wilson, B., & Shelton, B. (2014). Side effects of cancer therapy. In M. Polovich, M. Olsen, & K. LeFebvre (Eds.), *Chemotherapy and biotherapy guidelines and recommendations for practice* (4th ed., pp. 171–435). Pittsburg, USA: ONS.

EXPECTED PATIENT OUTCOMES

I. The patient can identify the chemotherapy agents and potential side effects related to the individual regimen they are receiving.

II. The patient will understand potential chemotherapy and hormonal therapy side effects and know when they should be reported.

REFERENCES

Chu, E., & DeVita, V. (2013). *Physicians' cancer chemotherapy drug manual 2013.* Burlington, MA: Jones & Bartlett Learning.

Connor, T.H., MacKenzie, B.A., DeBord, D.G., Trout, D.B., & O'Callaghan, J.P. (2016). NIOSH list of antineoplastic and other hazardous drugs in healthcare settings, 2016. By Cincinnati, OH: U.S. Department of Health and Human Services, Centers for Disease Control and Prevention, National Institute for Occupational Safety and Health, DHHS (NIOSH) Publication Number 2016-161 (Supersedes 2014-138).

Cumberland, Pharmaceuticals. (2017). *Totect® (Dexrazoxane) [package insert].* Nashville, TN: Cumberland Pharmaceuticals.

Jansen, C., Davis, P., Katz, A., Douglas, T., Gilbert, C., Olsen, M., … Skinner, J., Robinson, C., Rogers, B., Wilson, B., & Shelton, B. (2014). Side effects of cancer therapy. In M. Polovich, M. Olsen, & K. LeFebvre (Eds.), *Chemotherapy and biotherapy guidelines and recommendations for practice* (4th ed., pp. 171–435). Pittsburg, USA: ONS.

Kerber, Alice S., & Polovich, M. (2014). Nursing considerations in cancer treatment. In M. Polovich, M. Olsen, & K. LeFebvre (Eds.), *Chemotherapy and biotherapy guidelines and recommendations for practice* (4th ed., pp. 97–119). Pittsburg, USA: ONS.

Kreideh, F. Y., Mukadem, H. A., & El Saghir, N. S. (2016). Overview, prevention and management of chemotherapy extravasation. *World Journal of Clinical Oncology, 7*(1), 87–97.

LeFebvre, K., & Stiver, Wendy. (2014). Overview of cancer and cancer treatment. In M. Polovich, M. Olsen, & K. LeFebvre (Eds.), *Chemotherapy and biotherapy guidelines and recommendations for practice* (4th ed., pp. 1–16) (pp. 1–16). Pittsburg, USA: ONS.

Mancini, R., & Modlin, J. (2011). Chemotherapy administration sequence: a review of the literature and creation of a sequencing chart. *J Hematology and Oncology Pharmacy, 1*, 17–25.

Menonna-Quinn, D. (2014). Administration considerations. In M. Polovich, M. Olsen, & K. LeFebvre (Eds.), *Chemotherapy and biotherapy guidelines and recommendations for practice* (4th ed., pp. 121–135). Pittsburg, USA: ONS.

Neuss, M. N., Gilmore, T. R., Belderson, K. M., Billett, A. L., Conti-Kalchik, T., Harvet, B. E., & Polovich, M. (2017). 2016 Updated American Society of Clinical Oncology/Oncology Nursing Society Chemotherapy Administration safety standards, including standards for pediatric oncology. *Oncol Nurs Forum, 44* (1), 31–43. https://doi.org/10.1188/17.ONF.31-43.

Olsen, M., LeFebvre, K., & Brassil, K. (2019). *Chemotherapy and Immunotherapy Guidelines: Recommendations for Practice.* Pittsburgh: Oncology Nursing Press.

Pfizer. (2016). *Zinecard® (Dexrazoxane) [package insert].* New York, NY: Pfizer.

Piko, B., Laczo, I., Szatmari, K., Bassam, A. A., Szabo, Z., Ocsai, H. H., & Csotye, J. J. (2012). Overview of extravasation management and possibilities for risk reduction based on literature data. *Journal of Nursing Education and Practice, 3*(9), 93–105.

Polovich, M., & Olsen, M. M. (2018). *Safe handling of hazardous drugs* (3rd ed.). Pittsburg, USA: ONS.

Polovich, M., & Schulmeister, L. (2014). Infusion-related complications. In M. Polovich, M. Olsen, & K. LeFebvre (Eds.), *Chemotherapy and biotherapy guidelines and recommendations for practice* (4th ed., pp. 155–170). Pittsburg, USA: ONS.

Shields, S., Muehlbauer, P. M., & Shelburne, N. (2014). Principles of antineoplastic therapy. In M. Polovich, M. Olsen, & K. LeFebvre (Eds.), *Chemotherapy and biotherapy guidelines and recommendations for practice* (4th ed., pp. 25–50). Pittsburg, USA: ONS.

USP (2015). USP General Chapter 797 Pharmaceutical Compounding – Sterile Preparations. http://www.uspnf.com/notices/general-chapter-797-proposed-revision.

USP (2017). USP General Chapter 800 Hazardous Drugs – Handling in Healthcare Settings. http://www.usp.org/compounding/general-chapter-hazardous-drugs-handling-healthcare.

Wellstein, A. (2018). General principles in the pharmacotherapy of cancer. In L. L. Brunton, R. Hilal-Dandan, & Knollmann (Eds.), *Goodman and Gilman's The Pharmacological Basis of Therapeutics,* (13th ed., Chapter 66), *eBook*: McGraw-Hill.

Wellstein, A., Giaccone, G., Atkins, M. B., & Sausville, E. A. (2018). Cytotoxic drugs. In L. L. Brunton, R. Hilal-Dandan, & Knollmann (Eds.), *Goodman and Gilman's The Pharmacological Basis of Therapeutics,* (13th ed., Chapter 66), *eBook*: McGraw-Hill.

29

Biotherapies: Targeted Therapies and Immunotherapies

Kristine Deano Abueg and Brenda Keith

BIOTHERAPIES

Overview

I. The terms *biotherapy, immunotherapy,* and *targeted therapy* encompass a wide range of modalities, targets, and mechanisms. Sometimes referred to as *molecularly targeted drugs or therapies* or *precision medicines.*

A. Biotherapy—a broad range of treatments made from living organisms that mimic or augment the signals that normally control cell functions to reverse the deleterious effects of tumor genes. These substances may occur naturally in the body or may be made in the laboratory (NCI, 2018).

B. For the purposes of this chapter's discussion, biotherapies will be subdivided into two main categories: targeted therapies and immunotherapies.

1. Biotherapies that interfere with specific molecules involved with tumor growth and progression are referred to as *targeted therapies* (NCI, 2013). Examples include lapatinib and trastuzumab, which both target human epidermal growth factor receptor 2 (EGFR-2) implicated in tumor growth and metastases.

2. Biotherapies that use, stimulate, augment, or suppress the cells and cytokines of the immune system are referred to as *immunotherapy* or *biological response modifier therapy* and include checkpoint inhibitors, vaccines, and T-cell therapies (Eggert, 2017).

II. Mutations in tumor suppressor genes, oncogenes, and stability genes result in altered protein products, which disrupt the biological processes in which they are involved (Jeggo, et al., 2016).

A. Normal cell metabolism, growth, and proliferation are tightly controlled by circulating growth signals, regulatory cytokines, and cell signaling pathways.

B. Actions of altered gene products include the following:

1. Activation in the absence of appropriate growth signals

2. Bypassing cell signaling pathways

3. Bypassing or resistance to regulatory inhibition

C. Immunotherapies may be classified as targeted therapies in that they are designed to target specific molecules; for this chapter, targeted therapies and immunotherapies will be discussed separately.

III. Companion diagnostics evaluate molecular, genetic, and chemical characteristics of the tumor for appropriate application of the targeted therapy (Table 29.1).

A. Developed in parallel with the drug and have clinical utility after a drug's approval; included in the labeling

---

TABLE 29.1 Companion Diagnostics

SUMMARY OF SELECTED AGENTS WHOSE FDA INDICATION REQUIRES EXPRESSION OF SPECIFIC BIOMARKER

Agent	Biomarker
Erlotinib	EGFR
Cetuximab	EGFR, KRAS
Panitumumab	EGFR, KRAS
Afatinib	EGFR
Gefitinib	EGFR
Imatinib	BCR-Abl
	C-kit
	PDGFRB
Dasatinib	BCR-Abl
Nilotinib	BCR-Abl
Ponatinib	BCR-Abl
	T315I
Trastuzumab	HER2-neu
Pertuzumab	HER2-neu
Lapatinib	HER2-neu
Neratinib	HER2-neu
Trastuzumab emtansine	HER2-neu
Pembrolizumab	PD-L1
Olaparib	BRCA
Rucaparib	BRCA
Niraparib	BRCA
Trametinib–dabrafenib	BRAF
Alectinib (Alecensa)	ALK
Ceritinib (Zykadia)	ALK
Crizotinib (Xalkori)	ALK
Brigatinib (Alunbrig)	ALK,
Erlotinib	EGFR
Crizotinib	ALK
Vemurafenib	BRAF
Venetoclax	17p deletion

instructions for both the therapeutic product and the corresponding diagnostic test (FDA, 2016).

  B. According to the U.S. Food and Drug Administration (FDA), a companion assay can be used both to predict outcome and to monitor response. The FDA specifies three areas where a companion diagnostic is essential:

    1. Identification of patients most likely to benefit from a therapeutic product

    2. Identification of patients likely to be at increased risk of serious adverse reactions as a result of treatment with a particular therapeutic product

    3. Monitoring response to treatment by adjusting treatment (e.g., schedule, dose, discontinuation) to achieve improved efficacy or effectiveness (FDA, 2017).

TARGETED THERAPIES

Overview

  I. Targeted therapies interfere with molecules associated with cancer cell proliferation, growth, spread, and metabolism (Padma, 2015; Abramson, 2017). Specific targeted oncogenic mechanisms are as follows:

    A. Binding and inhibition of excess circulating growth factors: aberrant, excessive cell growth in cancer is often mediated by the interaction of excessive growth signals with overabundant receptors. Binding of growth factors or their receptors effectively "puts the brakes" on these pathways.

    B. Competing with aberrant cancer molecules for binding sites at specific activation points along the cell signaling pathway.

      1. Proliferation, differentiation, migration, metabolism, and apoptotic processes are tightly regulated by intracellular cell signaling pathways.

      2. Deregulation of cell signaling pathways leads to oncogene activation within a cell resulting in aberrant proliferation, invasion, metastases, and vascularization.

      3. Deregulation results from excessive production of constituent proteins or production of proteins that are activated independent of ligands.

      4. Inhibition or binding of the aberrant protein prevents the transmission of molecular "messages" down the cell signaling pathway. Doing so effectively shuts down the aberrant cell signaling pathway.

    C. Affecting regulatory proteins involved with apoptosis and the cell life cycle.

  II. Targeted therapy differs from standard chemotherapy in several ways. See Chapter 28.

    A. Act on specific molecular targets; most standard chemotherapies act on rapidly dividing normal and cancerous cells. Deliberately chosen or designed to interact with their target, whereas many standard chemotherapies were identified because they kill cells.

    B. Targeted therapies are cytostatic, meaning they block tumor cell proliferation; standard chemotherapy agents are cytotoxic (NCI, 2018).

    C. Targeted therapies fit with "lock and key" precision and specificity to target molecules, thus potentially causing fewer collateral side effects to off-target cells (Abramson, 2017).

  III. Efficacy and specificity of targeted therapy lies heavily on the appropriate identification and selection of target molecules; thus target molecules are selected on their ability to meet two specific criteria:

    A. Targeted tumor molecules should be critical to cell growth or survival.

    B. Ideal—targeted tumor molecules should be disproportionally overexpressed on cancer cells or in tumor environments and with low to minimal expression on normal cells.

      1. An example is EGFR-2 protein (HER2), which is present in normal cells but is expressed at high levels on the surface of cancer cells.

      2. Therapies targeting the HER2 pathway (trastuzumab, lapatinib, pertuzumab, and ado-trastuzumab emtansine) are associated with significant survival benefits in HER2-positive breast cancer.

    C. Target molecule may be highly expressed in normal and malignant cells; e.g., CD-20, which has a role in B-cell maturation and development; also expressed in B-cell lymphomas.

  IV. Targeted therapies are generally classified according to mechanism of action and then by their target molecule.

    A. Targets: target molecules include cell surface displayed antigens (TAAs), circulating growth factors, and intracellular cell signal molecules.

    B. Mechanisms: either engineered monoclonal antibodies that bind with target molecules or small-molecule inhibitors that interact directly with the target molecule.

  V. Target molecules can be classified by their role in cancer cell growth, migration, and metabolism. Major classes of target molecules are described here.

    A. Circulating growth factors in serum that stimulate growth (e.g., vascular endothelial growth factor [VEGF]).

    B. Cluster of differentiation molecules: membrane-bound antigens used for identification and classification for immunophenotyping of cells (e.g., CD20 in lymphoma).

    C. Extracellular portion of membrane-bound tyrosine kinases (also referred to as *tyrosine kinase receptor* [TKR]): receive and initiate cell signaling pathways either upon binding to a growth factor found in serum or upon interaction (dimerization) with another TKR. Examples include VEGF receptor and endothelial growth factor receptor.

D. Intracellular protein kinase chains that communicate signals from the membrane-bound TKR to the DNA.
   1. The most important protein kinases are the serine/threonine and tyrosine kinases
   2. Examples include the protein kinases RAS, RAF, MET, and ERK.
E. Cell cycle kinases that control the mitotic cell cycle (e.g., CDK4, CDK6) (Finn, Aleshin, & Slamon, 2016).
F. Intracellular enzymes that control DNA repair and cellular apoptosis. Main examples include proteasome inhibitors and poly (ADP-ribose) polymerase (PARP) inhibitors.
G. Angiogenesis proteins that promote vascular development in tumor environments.

VI. Monoclonal antibodies (Table 29.2): engineered proteins that bind to only one specific target substance with exceptional specificity, thereby interfering with the action of that target substance (Padma, 2015).
   A. Nomenclature of targeted therapies reveals their mechanism, derivation, and components (Table 29.3).

TABLE 29.2 Monoclonal Antibodies

Target	Antibody	Composition	Indications	Class-Associated Adverse Events
Unconjugated monoclonal antibodies				

Monoclonal-antibody mechanisms of action:
- Complement-dependent cytotoxicity (CDC) occurs upon MoAB-antigen binding initiating the complement cascade and ultimately triggering the release of chemotactic factors ending in membrane lysis.
- Antibody-dependent cell-mediated cytotoxicity (ADCC): antibody-mediated binding to membrane-bound target antigens triggering immune cell–mediated lysis.
- Antibody-dependent cellular phagocytosis (ADCP), wherein circulating macrophages engulf and digest antibody-coated cells.
- Decreases action of target molecule in cell signals, thereby inhibiting tumor growth, proliferation, and migration.

Target	Antibody	Composition	Indications	Class-Associated Adverse Events
CD19 and CD3	Blinatumomab (Blincyto)	Murine	• ALL	Infusion reactions Neurologic symptoms
CD20	Obinutuzumab (Gazyva)	Humanized IgG1	• CLL • Follicular lymphoma	Infusion reactions, neutropenia, lymphopenia, asthenia, severe mucocutaneous reactions, hepatitis B reactivation
	Ofatumumab (Arzerra)	Human IgG1	• CLL	
	Rituximab (Rituxan)	Chimeric IgG1	• NHL • CLL	
	Rituximab and hyaluronidase human (Rituxan Hycela)	Chimeric IgG1	• Follicular lymphoma • CLL	
CD38	Daratumumab (Darzalex)	Human IgG1	• Multiple myeloma	Upper respiratory infection, infusion reactions, diarrhea, fatigue, cough, pyrexia
CD52	Alemtuzumab (Campath)	Humanized IgG1	• Chronic lymphocytic leukemia (off-label)	Infusion reactions, opportunistic infections, cytopenia
EGFR	Necitumumab (Portrazza)	Human IgG1	• Squamous NCLC	Rash, asthenia, infection, diarrhea, radiation dermatitis, cytopenias
EGFR/ HER1	Cetuximab (Erbitux)	Chimeric IgG1	• CRC • Head and neck	
EGFR/HER1	Panitumumab (Voctibix)	Human IgG2	• CRC	
HER2	Pertuzumab (Perjeta)	Humanized	• HER2 + breast cancer	Alopecia, diarrhea, cytopenias, fatigue
HER2	Trastuzumab (Herceptin)	Humanized IgG1	• HER2 + breast cancer; gastric cancer	Fever, chills, headache, diarrhea
PDGFR-a	Olaratumab (Lartruvo)	Human IgG1	• Sarcoma	Cytopenias, hyperglycemia, decreased electrolytes, nausea, fatigue, musculoskeletal pain, mucositis, alopecia, vomiting, diarrhea, decreased appetite, abdominal pain, neuropathy, headache

TABLE 29.2 Monoclonal Antibodies—cont'd

Target	Antibody	Composition	Indications	Class-Associated Adverse Events
EGFR/ HER1	Cetuximab (Erbitux)	Chimeric IgG1	• KRAS wild type CRC, squamous head and neck cancer	Infusion reactions, rash, nail changes, diarrhea, opportunistic infections
SLAMF7	Elotuzumab (Empliciti)	Humanized IgG1	• Multiple myeloma	Fatigue, diarrhea, pyrexia, constipation, cough, peripheral neuropathy, nasopharyngitis, upper respiratory tract infection, decreased appetite, pneumonia
GD2	Dinutuximab (Unituxin)	Chimeric IgG1	• (Pediatric) neuroblastoma	Pain, pyrexia, thrombocytopenia, lymphopenia, infusion reactions, hypotension, hyponatremia, increased alanine aminotransferase, anemia, vomiting,
Unconjugated monoclonal antibodies (without immune activation)				
VEGF	Bevacizumab (Avastin) inhibition of VEGF interaction with its receptors	Humanized IgG1	Colon, renal, cervical, NSCLC, glioblastoma, ovarian	Hypertension, bleeding, proteinuria
VEGFR2	Ramucirumab (Cyramza) Inhibition of angiogenesis via binding of VEGFR	Human IgG1	Gastric, NSCLC, colon, rectal	Hypertension, diarrhea, headache
RANKL	Denosumab (Xgeva) inhibits osteoclast formation, function and survival	Human IgG2	• Skeletal event prevention • Hypercalcemia	
IL-6	Siltuximab (Sylvant) Inhibition of IL-5 manifested in Castleman disease	Chimeric	Castleman disease	
Conjugated monoclonal antibodies (in addition to all actions of monoclonal antibodies, delivery of cytotoxic chemotherapy or radiation)				
HER2	Ado-trastuzumab emtansine (Kadcyla) Chemotherapy conjugate: maytansine	Humanized IgG1	Breast	Thrombocytopenia, neuropathy, elevated LFTs
CD30	Brentuximab vedotin (Adcetris) Chemotherapy conjugate: monomethyl auristatin E	Chimeric IgG1	Lymphoma	Cytopenias, neutropenia, GI
CD33	Gemtuzumab ozogamicin Chemotherapy conjugate: antitumor antibiotic ozogamicin	Humanized IgG4	Acute myeloid leukemia	Hemorrhage, infection, fever, GI, headache, elevated LFTs, rash, mucositis
CD20	Ibritumomab tiuxetan (Zevalin) Conjugate: radioisotope yttrium-90	Murine IgG1	Low-grade or follicular B-cell NHL	
CD22	Inotuzumab ozogamicin (Besponsa) Chemotherapy conjugate: antitumor antibiotic ozogamicin	Humanized IgG4	B-cell precursor acute lymphoblastic leukemia	
Nect-4	Enfortumab vedotin			

ADCC, Antibody-dependent cellular cytotoxicity; *ADCP,* antibody-dependent cellular phagocytosis; *CD,* clusters of differentiation; *CDC,* complement-dependent cytotoxicity; *CLL,* chronic lymphocytic leukemia; *EGFR,* epidermal growth factor receptor; *GD2,* glycolipid disialoganglioside; *HER,* humanized epidermal growth factor receptor; *IgG,* immunoglobulin; *IL-6,* interleukin 6; *NHL,* non-Hodgkin lymphoma; *PDGFR-α,* platelet-derived growth factor receptor alpha; *RANKL,* receptor activator of nuclear factor kappa-B ligand; *SLAMF7,* signaling lymphocytic activation molecule family member 7; *VEGF,* vascular endothelial growth factor; *VEGFR2,* vascular endothelial growth factor receptor 2.

TABLE 29.3   Nomenclature

SMALL-MOLECULE TARGETED THERAPIES NOMENCLATURE:
PREFIX + SUBSTEM(S) + STEM

STEM = -IB (EXCEPT HISTONE DEACETYLASE INHIBITORS AND BCL-2)

Substem	Substem + stem	Target	Example
-tini-	-tinib	Tyrosine kinase inhibitors	afatinib, axitinib, bosutinib, dasatinib, erlotinib, gefitinib, sunitinib
-rafe-	-rafenib	RAF tyrosine kinase RAF/RAS/MEK pathway	dabrafenib, regorafenib, sorafenib, vemurafenib
-metin-	-metinib	MEK tyrosine kinase RAF/RAS/MEK pathway	cobimetinib, trametinib
-den-	-denib	Isocitrate dehydrogenase 2 (IDH2) enzyme inhibitor	enasidenib
-par-	-parib	PARP inhibitors of mammalian polyadenosine 5'-diphosphoribose polymerase enzyme	olaparib, rucaparib
-lis-	-lisib	PI3 kinase inhibitors (PI3K)	idelalisib
-deg-	-degib	Sonic hedgehog pathway inhibitors	sonidegib, vismodegib
-cicl-	-ciclib	Cyclin-dependent kinase (CDK) 4 and 6	palbociclib
-zo-	-zomib	Proteosome inhibitors	bortezomib, carfilzomib, ixazomib
-inostat	NA	Histone deacetylase inhibitors (HDAC)	vorinostat, belinostat, panobinostat
-toclax	NA	BCL-2 inhibitors	venetoclax

MONOCLONAL ANTIBODY TARGETED THERAPIES NOMENCLATURE
PREFIX + SUBSTEM 1 TARGET LOCATION + SUBSTEM 2 MONOCLONAL ANTIBODY DERIVATION + STEM

Substem 1	Substem Target Location	Example
-tu-	Target located on tumor	Tras**tu**zumab (targeted HER2, a cell surface–bound antigen)
-ci-	Target located in circulatory system	Beva**ci**zumab (targeting VEGF, growth factor found in circulation)
-li-	Target located on immune system	Ip**ili**mumab (targeted CTLA-4, protein found on T cells)

Substem 2	Monoclonal Antibody Derivation	Example
-**xi**mab	Chimeric human-mouse	Cetu**xi**mab Chimeric antibody with a tumor target (EGFR)
-**zu**mab	Humanized mouse	Bevaci**zu**mab Humanized mouse antibody with a circulatory system target (VEGF-A)
-**(m)u**mab	Fully human	Panitum**u**mab Fully human antibody with a tumor target (EGFR)
-**mo**mab	Mouse (murine)	Ibritum**o**mab Mouse based antibody targeting CD-20

CONJUGATED MOABS LIST THE BOUND TOXIN (CHEMOTHERAPY OR RADIOISOTOPE)

Substem 1	Substem 2	Bound Toxin	Example
-tu-	-zu-	emtansine	Trastuzumab–emtansine (monoclonal antibody targeting the HER2 cell surface–bound molecule attached to the chemotherapy emtansine
-tu-	-mo-	tiuxetan	Ibritumomab tiuxetan (monoclonal antibody targeting CD-20 on lymphoma cells delivering ytrium-90 radiotherapy)

Adapted from Abramson, R. (2017). Overview of targeted therapies for cancer. My Cancer Genome https://www.mycancergenome.org/content/molecular-medicine/overview-of-targeted-therapies-for-cancer; Wujcik, D.J. (2017) Personalized Medicine. Accessed 04/08/2018: http://media.oncologynurseadvisor.com/documents/303/ona_navsum_2017_wujcik-webvers_75667.pdf; Carter, P.S. (2015) Antibody Drug Nomenclature: Accessed 04/08/2018 http://www.antibodysociety.org/wordpress/wp-content/uploads/2015/12/Carter-IBC-INN-talk-Dec-2015-FINAL.pdf.

B. Monoclonal antibodies (MoABs) are constructed of two major components, or regions.
   1. The Fab component consists of hypervariable complementary determining regions (CDRs) that form highly specific antigen-binding sites. This region links to target antigens.
   2. The Fc component links to corresponding Fc receptors on immune effector cells and initiates complement-dependent cytotoxicity (CDC).

C. Construction of MoABs—derived from mice that have been injected with purified target proteins.

D. MoABs classified as either unconjugated or conjugated.
   1. Unconjugated = consists of unbound MoAB, primary action due to target protein disruption and/or cell lysis via antibody-dependent cellular toxicity (ADCC) or CDC.

2. Conjugated = consists of the MoAB chemically linked to chemotherapy or radiation (aka antibody–drug conjugates [ADCs]).

E. Mechanisms of monoclonal antibodies.

1. Due to MoAB's large size, accessible targets are generally located outside cells (in serum) or on the cell surface (NCI, 2018).

2. Binds with target proteins, thereby altering its specific intracellular signaling, function of growth factor receptors, and function of adhesion molecules. Through means of antibody engineering, MoABs bind to a targeted antigen with exceptional specificity (Padma, 2015).

3. ADCC: antibody-mediated binding to membrane-bound target antigens triggering immune cell–mediated lysis.

   a. Immediate effect of ADCC: antibody-coated cells are flagged for immune-mediated destruction (lysis) by cytotoxic effector cells.

   b. Delayed effect of ADCC: debris from lysed tumor cells taken up by circulating antigen-presenting cells (APCs), in turn stimulating memory cells and resulting in prolonged immune response to tumor antigen.

4. CDC occurs upon MoAB–antigen binding, initiating the complement cascade and triggering the release of chemotactic factors ending in membrane lysis.

5. Antibody-dependent cellular phagocytosis (ADCP) wherein circulating macrophages engulf and digest antibody coated cells.

6. ADCs (aka conjugated monoclonal antibodies) facilitate highly specific delivery of cytotoxic agents to the intended cancer cell target (MoABs conjugated to radioisotopes or toxins or chemotherapy) in addition to actions of unconjugated MoABs (Abramson, 2017).

7. Bispecific antibodies simultaneously address different antigens or epitopes, interfering with multiple surface receptors or ligands. An example of an approved bispecific antibody is blinatumomab.

8. Checkpoint inhibitors (CPIs) are monoclonal antibodies that target regulatory immune proteins; because their action primarily involves immune function, a full discussion can be found under the immunotherapy section rather than in the targeted therapy section.

VII. Small-molecule inhibitors (Table 29.4)

TABLE 29.4 Small-Molecule Inhibitors

Primary Therapeutic Target	Small-Molecule Inhibitors	Side Effects	Administration Considerations
ALK	Alectinib (Alecensa) RET	Fatigue, edema, constipation	
	Ceritinib (Zykadia) IGF-1R, InsR, ROS1	Diarrhea, fatigue, abdominal pain	With food
	Crizotinib (Xalkori) HGFR, ROS1,		With food
	Brigatinib (Alunbrig) ROS1, IGF-1R, FLT-3, EGFR	Nausea, diarrhea, fatigue, cough	With/without food
BCR-ABL	Bosutinib (Bosulif) Src family	Diarrhea, nausea, myelosuppression, rash,	With food
	Imatinib mesylate (Gleevec) PDGF, SCF, c-Kit (CD117)	Edema, nausea, vomiting, muscle cramps, musculoskeletal pain	With food
	Dasatinib (SPRYCEL SRC family, c-KIT, EPHA2, PDGFRb)	Myelosuppression, fluid retention, diarrhea, headache, skin rash	With/without food
	Nilotinib (Tasigna)	Myelosuppression, rash, nausea, headache	Without food
BCR-ABL; T3151 (VEGFR, PDGFR, EPH receptors, SRC kinases, Kit, RET, TIE2, FLT3)	Ponatinib (Iclusig)	Myelosuppression, rash, nausea, headache, hypertension	With/without food
BCL-2	Venetoclax (Venclexta)	Myelosuppression, diarrhea, nausea, upper respiratory tract infection, fatigue	With food

Continued

TABLE 29.4 Small-Molecule Inhibitors—cont'd

Primary Therapeutic Target	Small-Molecule Inhibitors	Side Effects	Administration Considerations
BRAF V600E	Dabrafenib (Tafinlar) (administer with trametinib)	Pyrexia, rash, chills, headache, arthralgia, nausea	Without food
	Vemurafenib (Zelboraf)	Arthralgia, rash, alopecia, fatigue, photosensitivity reaction	With/without food
BTK	Acalabrutinib (Calquence)	Anemia, thrombocytopenia, headache, neutropenia, diarrhea, fatigue, myalgia, bruising	With/without food
	Ibrutinib (Imbruvica)	Myelosuppression, diarrhea, muscle pain	With/without food
CDK 4 and 6	Abemaciclib (Verzenio)	Diarrhea, neutropenia, nausea, abdominal pain, infections	With/without food
	Palbociclib (Ibrance)	Neutropenia, infections, leukopenia, fatigue, nausea	With/without food
	Ribociclib (Kisqali)	Neutropenia, nausea, fatigue, diarrhea, leukopenia,	With/without food
EGFR	Erlotinib (Tarceva)	Rash, diarrhea, anorexia, fatigue, dyspnea, cough, nausea, and vomiting.	Empty stomach
	Afatinib (Gilotrif) HER2, HER4	Diarrhea, rash/acneiform dermatitis, stomatitis, paronychia, dry skin, decreased appetite, nausea	Empty stomach
	Gefitinib (Iressa) Reversible inhibitor	Skin reactions, diarrhea	With/without food
	Osimertinib (Tagrisso)	Diarrhea, rash, dry skin, fatigue	With/without food
HER1/EGFR and HER2	Lapatinib (Tykerb)	Diarrhea, palmar-plantar erythrodysesthesia, nausea, rash, vomiting, fatigue	At least 1 hour before or 1 hour after a meal
	Neratinib (Nerlynx) Irreversible inhibitor EGFR, HER4	Diarrhea, nausea, abdominal pain, fatigue, vomiting, rash, stomatitis, decreased appetite, muscle spasms, dyspepsia, AST or ALT increase	With food
Multiple kinases (VEGFR-1,-2,-3; FGFR-1, -2,-3,-4; PDGFRa, KIT, and RET)	Lenvatinib (Lenvima)	Hypertension, fatigue, diarrhea, arthralgia/myalgia, decreased appetite, weight decreased, nausea, stomatitis, headache	With/without food
Multiple tyrosine kinases (EGFR, VEGFR families, RET, BRK, TIE2, members of the EPH receptor and Src kinase families)	Vandetanib (Caprelsa)	Diarrhea/colitis, rash, acneiform dermatitis, hypertension, nausea, headache	With/without food
VEGFR-1, VEGFR-2, VEGFR-3	Axitinib (Inlyta)	Diarrhea, hypertension, fatigue, decreased appetite, nausea, dysphonia, palmar-plantar erythrodysesthesia (hand–foot) syndrome,	With or without food
VEGF, EGFR (RET, VEGFR-1, -2, -3, Kit, PDGFR-a and b, FGFR-1, -2, TIE2, DDR2, TrkA, Eph2A, RAF-1, BRAF, BRAF V600E, SAPK2, PTK5, Abl, CSF1R)	Regorafenib (Stivarga)	Pain (including gastrointestinal and abdominal pain), asthenia/fatigue, diarrhea, decreased appetite/food intake, hypertension, infection	Take with a low-fat breakfast
Multiple tyrosine kinases (MET, VEGFR-1,-2, and -3, AXL, RET, ROS1, TYRO3, MER, KIT, TRKB, FLT-3, and TIE-2)	Cabozantinib (Cabometyx) Tablet form (Cometriq) Capsule form	Diarrhea, fatigue, nausea, decreased appetite, hypertension, palmar-plantar erythrodysesthesia	At least 2 hours before and at least 1 hour after meals

TABLE 29.4 Small-Molecule Inhibitors—cont'd

Primary Therapeutic Target	Small-Molecule Inhibitors	Side Effects	Administration Considerations
MEK 1 and MEK2	Cobimetinib (Cotellic) Reversible inhibitor	Diarrhea, photosensitivity reaction, nausea, pyrexia, vomiting, elevated liver function tests	With or without food
	Trametinib (Mekinist)	Pyrexia, rash, diarrhea, lymphedema	With or without food
PARP	Niraparib (Zejula)	Myelosuppression, palpitations, nausea, constipation	With or without food
	Olaparib (Lynparza)	Myelosuppression, fatigue, nausea, infection	With or without food
	Rucaparib (Rubraca)	Nausea, fatigue (including asthenia), vomiting, anemia, dysgeusia, AST/ALT elevation, constipation, decreased appetite, diarrhea, thrombocytopenia, neutropenia, stomatitis, nasopharyngitis/URI, rash, abdominal pain/distention, dyspnea	With or without food
PI3K	Copanlisib (Aliqopa)	Hyperglycemia, diarrhea, hypertension, myelosuppression, nausea	IV
	Idelalisib (Zydelig)	Diarrhea, fatigue, nausea, cough, pyrexia, abdominal pain, pneumonia, rash	With/without food
proteasome inhibitor	Bortezomib (Velcade)	Nausea, diarrhea, myelosuppression, peripheral neuropathy, fatigue, neuralgia, constipation, vomiting, rash, pyrexia, anorexia	IV/SQ
	Carfilzomib (Kyprolis)	Anemia, fatigue, thrombocytopenia, nausea, pyrexia, dyspnea, diarrhea, headache, cough, edema peripheral	IV
	Ixazomib (Ninlaro)	Diarrhea, constipation, thrombocytopenia, peripheral neuropathy, nausea, peripheral edema, vomiting, back pain	1 hour before or at least 2 hours after food
IDH2 enzyme	Enasidenib (Idhifa)	Nausea, vomiting, diarrhea, elevated bilirubin	With/without food
mTOR	Everolimus (Afinitor)	Stomatitis, infection, rash, fatigue	With/without food
	Temsirolimus (Torisel)	Rash, asthenia, mucositis, nausea, edema, anorexia, anemia, hyperglycemia, hyperlipidemia, hypertriglyceridemia, elevated transaminases	IV
Multiple tyrosine kinases (VEGFR-1, -2, -3; PDGFR a & b; FGR-1 and -3, Kit, Itk, Lck, c-Fms)	Pazopanib (Votrient)	Diarrhea, hypertension, hair color changes (depigmentation), nausea, anorexia, vomiting	At least 1 hour before or 2 hours after a meal
JAK1 and JAK2	Ruxolitinib (Jakafi)	Myelosuppression, bruising, dizziness, headache	With/without food
Smoothened (a protein involved in Hedgehog pathway signal transduction)	Sonidegib (Odomzo)	Muscle spasms, alopecia, dysgeusia, fatigue, nausea, musculoskeletal pain, diarrhea	Empty stomach, at least 1 hour before or 2 hours after a meal
	Vismodegib (Erivedge)	Muscle spasms, alopecia, dysgeusia, weight loss, fatigue, nausea, diarrhea	With/without food
Multiple intracellular (c-CRAF, BRAF, mutant BRAF) and cell surface kinases (KIT, FLT-3, RET, RET/PTC, VEGFR-1, -2, -3)	Sorafenib (Nexavar)	Diarrhea, fatigue, infection, alopecia, hand–foot skin reaction, rash, weight loss	Without food

Continued

TABLE 29.4 Small-Molecule Inhibitors—cont'd

Primary Therapeutic Target	Small-Molecule Inhibitors	Side Effects	Administration Considerations
Multiple tyrosine kinases (PDGFRa&b, VEGFR-1, -2, -3, KIT, FLT3, CSF1R, RET)	Sunitinib malate (Sutent)	Fatigue/asthenia, diarrhea, mucositis/ stomatitis, nausea, decreased appetite/ anorexia, vomiting, abdominal pain	With/without food

ALK, Anaplastic lymphoma kinase; *ALL*, acute lymphoblastic leukemia; *AML*, acute myelogenous leukemia; *BCL-2*, B-cell lymphoma 2; *BCR-ABL*, breakpoint cluster region-Abelson; *BRAF*, B-raf proto-oncogene, serine/threonine kinase; *BRK*, breast tumor kinase; *BTK*, Bruton tyrosine kinase; *CD*, clusters of differentiation; *CDK*, cyclin-dependent kinase; *c-Fms*, transmembrane glycoprotein receptor tyrosine kinase; *CLL*, chronic lymphocytic leukemia; *CML*, chronic myelogenous leukemia; *c-CRAF*, C-raf proto-oncogene, serine/threonine kinase; *CSF1R*, colony stimulating factor 1 receptor; *EPHA2*, ephrin receptor A2; *FGFR*, fibroblast growth factor receptor; *FLT3*, Fms-like tyrosine kinase 3; *GIST*, gastrointestinal stromal tumor; *GVHD*, graft-versus-host disease; *HER1/EGFR*, human epidermal growth factor receptor 1/epidermal growth factor receptor; *HER2/HER4*, human epidermal growth factor receptor 2 or 4; *HCC*, hepatocellular carcinoma; *HGFR*, hepatocyte growth factor receptor; *IDH2*, isocitrate dehydrogenase 2; *IGF-1R*, insulin-like growth factor-1 receptor; *InsR*, insulin receptor; *Itk*, interleukin-2 receptor-inducible T-cell kinase; *JAK1/JAK2*, Janus-associated kinases; *KIT*, stem cell factor receptor; *Lck*, lymphocyte-specific protein tyrosine kinase; *MET*, mesenchymal-epithelial transition factor receptor; *MEK1/MEK2*, mitogen-activated extracellular signal regulated kinase 1 or 2; *NHL*, non-Hodgkin lymphoma; *PARP*, poly (ADP-ribose) polymerase; *Ph +*, Philadelphia chromosome-positive; *PDGF*, platelet-derived growth factor; *PDGFR*, platelet-derived growth factor receptor; *PI3K*, phosphatidylinositol 3-kinase; *PNET*, pancreatic neuroendocrine tumor; *PTK5*, protein tyrosine kinase 5; *RCC*, renal cell cancer; *RET*, rearranged during transfection; *RET/PTC*, rearranged in transformation/papillary thyroid carcinomas; *RON*, recepteur d'origine nantais; *ROS1*, c-ros oncogene 1; *SCF*, stem cell factor; *SLL*, small lymphocytic lymphoma; *SAPK2*, stress-activated protein kinase 2; *TRKB*, tropomyosin receptor kinase B; *TYRO3*, tyrosine-protein kinase receptor Byk; *TIE2*, tyrosine kinase with immunoglobulin-like and EGF-like domains 2; *VEGFR*, vascular endothelial growth factor receptor.

A. Generally, orally available, synthetic chemicals of smaller molecular size than MoABs.
1. Due to molecular size, able to penetrate cell membranes and target intracellular molecules (Abramson, 2017).
2. May interact with multiple targets simultaneously or act on a single target. Multiple-target inhibitors generally associated with greater toxicity.
3. Bioavailability significantly affected by metabolic and absorption factors: changes in stomach acidity and drug–drug/drug–food interactions, specifically p-glycoprotein and cytochrome p450 (Abueg, 2014).

B. Mechanism of small-molecule inhibitors is defined by the action of the target molecule.

C. Interferes with the enzymatic activity of the target protein (Abramson, 2017) associated with cancer cell proliferation, metastasis, or angiogenesis (Padma, 2015).

D. Unlike monoclonal antibodies, small-molecule inhibitors do not stimulate immune response.

VIII. Types of small-molecule inhibitors
A. Tyrosine kinase inhibitors (TKIs) are agents that target receptor tyrosine kinases (RTKs).
B. RTKs:
1. Key enzymes in the regulation of various cellular processes. Adenosine triphosphate (ATP) attaches to a binding site on the intracellular portion of the cell, continuing the cellular instructions to various pathways into the nucleus of the cell (Eggert, 2017).
2. Considered the starting point for many cellular signaling pathways.
3. Catalyze the transfer of a phosphate group from ATP to a hydroxyl group of a serine or threonine.
4. RTK downstream signaling pathways are mainly mitogen-activated protein kinase (MAPK), phosphatidylinositol 3-kinase (PI3K), Src, and other signaling pathways such as Janus-associated kinase (JAK) (Segaliny et al., 2015).
5. Function as part of a complex network system rather than in isolation. Extensive cross-talk or interaction between pathways occurs, a process known as *RTK coactivation* (Tan et al., 2017). Specific pathways are dysfunctional in certain cancers.

C. TKIs:
1. Block the binding site on the intracellular portion of a receptor.
2. Enter the cell membrane and bind at the ATP binding site, which prevents cellular instructions to specific pathways such as proliferation, apoptosis, metabolism, differentiation, or cell survival.
3. Some block one pathway; others interrupt more than one pathway (e.g., dual or multiple).

D. Mammalian target of rapamycin (mTOR) inhibitors target mTOR.
1. mTOR is a protein kinase that plays a key role in cell growth, proliferation, and regulation.
2. mTOR forms two distinct types of multiprotein complex, termed *mTOR complexes 1 and 2.*
3. mTOR signaling switched on by several oncogenic signaling pathways; hyperactive in most cancers.
4. Inhibition of mTOR signaling is another means of anticancer therapy (Xie et al., 2016).

5. Example: everolimus, which binds to intracellular proteins causing mTOR pathway inhibition, resulting in reduced levels of hypoxia-inducible factor, VEGF, and other proteins necessary for tumor cell progression and survival (Martelli, et al., 2018).

E. Proteasome inhibitors block proteasome, which is a large protein complex that breaks down proteins in the cell nucleus when they are no longer needed (NCI, 2015).

1. The ubiquitin–proteasome pathway (UPP) is the major pathway for intracellular protein degradation.

2. More than 80% of cellular proteins are degraded through this pathway.

3. Defects in the UPP pathway are associated with several diseases, including cancer, particularly multiple myeloma (Kubiczkova, et al., 2014).

F. PARP inhibitors block the PARP enzyme in cells.

1. Repair damaged DNA at single-strand DNA breaks. After the DNA is repaired, PARP leaves the site of damage. If single-strand DNA damage is unrepaired, double-strand breaks in DNA may occur, leading to death of the cell.

2. Responsible for repair of double-stranded DNA breaks, which is controlled by the *BRCA* genes. This process of repairing double-stranded DNA is known as *homologous recombination repair.*

3. When there is a mutation in *BRCA*, a second mechanism, controlled by PARP, becomes essential in the repair of DNA damage. However, this type of repair, nonhomologous end joining (NHEF), may lead to DNA alterations resulting in cancer, which explains why mutations in *BRCA1* and *BRCA2* increase cancer risk, particularly breast and ovarian cancers.

4. The addition of PARP inhibitors increases the single-strand breaks that cannot be repaired and may sensitize tumor cells to the effects of DNA-damaging chemotherapy.

5. PARP inhibitors may trap PARP on DNA, preventing PARP release from the site of damage.

6. *BRCA*-mutated cells are sensitive to PARP inhibition (Lord & Ashworth, 2017).

7. PARP inhibitors are used primarily in the management of patients with epithelial ovarian cancer who have known mutations (germline or somatic) in *BRCA* (Markman, 2018).

8. Examples: olaparib and rucaparib both used in *BRCA*-mutated epithelial ovarian cancer.

G. CDK4 and CDK6 are cyclin-dependent kinases

1. Control the transition between the G1 and S phases of the cell cycle. The S phase is the period during which the cell synthesizes new DNA.

2. Cancer progression is typified by the loss of cell cycle checkpoint control.

3. CDK4/6 inhibitors lead to cell cycle arrest in the G1 phase by preventing phosphorylation of retinoblastoma protein (Rb).

4. Estrogen receptor–positive breast cancer dependent on CDK4 for proliferation (de Groot et al., 2017).

5. Examples: palbociclib and ribociclib, which are used in the treatment of hormone receptor–positive, HER2-negative metastatic breast cancer.

IX. Adverse events (AEs) of targeted therapies are classified along dimensions that affect their management.

A. "On-target, off-tumor" AEs result from drug activity against normal tissue that displays similar or identical molecules as the primary target. Examples are listed next.

1. EGFR is highly expressed in normal skin and gastrointestinal cells. Introduction of anti-EGFR therapies will block normal EGFR-based cell signaling in those organs, resulting in dermatologic and gastrointestinal toxicity.

2. Cardiomyopathy in trastuzumab-treated patients results from on-target, off-tumor attachment on myocytes that express HER2-neu.

B. Selected targeted therapy AEs are biomarkers of efficacy.

1. Examples: hypertension as an early predictor of response rate in bevacizumab-treated colorectal cancer, or rash as a predictive biomarker in response to anti-EGFR therapies (Liu, 2013)

2. Early identification and management are preferable to early dose reduction or treatment discontinuation (Abueg, 2017; Liu and Kurzrock, 2015)

C. Targeted therapies can be prescribed as long-term maintenance regimens such that AEs should be managed as potentially chronic conditions (Dy & Adjei, 2013)

X. AEs of targeted therapy vary according to the mechanism and target. Highlights of key AEs relative to targeted therapies are discussed next.

A. Monoclonal antibodies are associated with infusion reactions, including hypersensitivity reactions and cytokine release syndromes (see Chapter 52).

B. EGFR-targeted therapies are frequently associated with cutaneous reactions such as rash, hair, and nail changes, as well as diarrhea resulting from EGFR therapy's impact on intestinal mucosa (Tables 29.5 and 29.6).

1. Inhibition of EGF suppresses cutaneous cell growth and cellular migration, frequently manifesting as papulopustular rash (Eaby-Sandy & Lynch, 2014).

2. Rash management should focus on supportive care to alleviate associated symptoms (pruritic, pain), psychosocial coping, and prevention of superinfection (Lacouture, 2016).

TABLE 29.5	**Management of Acneiform Rash**	
Description and assessment	• Rash peaks within first 2 weeks; diminishes within 6–8 weeks. • Severity influenced by therapeutic regimen, dose intensity, and certain patient characteristics. • Rash associated with MoABs is generally more frequent and severe, likely to be pruritic, pustular, and may require aggressive intervention. • Risk factors associated with TKIs are nonsmokers, fair skin, age over 70. • Occurrence and/or severity of rash may fluctuate during course of EGFR TKI therapy. • Assess patients weekly for signs of rash during the first 6 weeks of treatment with an EGFR TKI and every 6–8 weeks thereafter.	
Nonpharmacologic management	Moisturize entire body at least twice daily.	Use thick, alcohol-free, perfume-free emollient; creams and ointments preferred over lotions, as lotions contain alcohol.
	Culture swabs of skin discharge.	To determine presence of bacteria.
	Minimize sun exposure.	Use broad-spectrum physical sunscreen with SPF of at least 25. Wear protective clothing, including a wide-brimmed hat. Zinc oxide- or titanium dioxide-containing sunscreens preferred.
	Hydrate the skin.	Maintain oral hydration. Avoid hot showers and products that dry out the skin (e.g., benzoyl peroxide), as they can aggravate the rash.
	Referral to dermatologist.	Recommended for patients who experience severe (grade 3 or 4) skin-related toxicities.

EGFR, epidermal growth factor receptor; *IV*, intravenous; *MESTT*, Multinational Association for Supportive Care in Cancer Epidermal Growth Factor Receptor Inhibitor Skin Toxicity Tool; *MoABs*, monoclonal antibodies; *SPF*, sun protection factor; *TKI*, tyrosine kinase inhibitor.

TABLE 29.6	**Other Dermatologic Adverse Events**	
Toxicity	**Causative Agents**	**Symptoms/Notes**
Hand–foot skin reaction (HFSR)	Multikinase angiogenesis inhibitors (e.g., sorafenib, sunitinib, pazopanib)	Painful sensation in palms and soles, burning, tingling, swelling, redness, hypersensitivity to hot objects
Xerosis	EGFR inhibitors, multikinase inhibitors, mTOR inhibitors	Abnormally dry skin, most pronounced along extremities during first 3 months of treatment; pain, skin fragility
Nail changes	EGFR inhibitors	Nail changes in nail bed (onycholysis), nail fold (paronychia), nail matrix; fissures on fingertips or toes
Skin or hair depigmentation	Selected multikinase inhibitors (e.g., pazopanib, cabozantinib, sunitinib)	No specific treatment is available to alleviate the condition
Pruritus	EGFR inhibitors, VEGFR inhibitors, mTOR inhibitors, CD20 MoABs	An intense itching sensation; often associated with xerosis; onset can be concurrent with rash

Adapted from Macdonald, J., Macdonald, B., Golitz, L., LoRusso, P., & Sekulic, A. (2015). Cutaneous adverse effects of targeted therapies, part I: inhibitors of the cellular membrane. *Journal of the American Academy of Dermatology, 72*(2), 203-215; Bryce, J., & Boers-Doets, C. B. (2014). Non-rash dermatologic adverse events related to targeted therapies. *Semin Oncol Nurs, 30*(3), 155–168. https://doi.org/10.1016/j.soncn.2014.05.003.

3. EGFR rash frequently appears acnelike but should not be treated as such. See Chapter 40 for additional details on appropriate management.

C. Cardiac toxicities manifest in multiple fashions, including left ventricular ejection fraction (LVEF) dysfunction, hypertension, and arrhythmias (Tables 29.7 and 29.8).

1. LVEF decreases can result from anti-HER2 therapies' binding of the EGFR-1 tyrosine kinase, which plays a role in cardiac development and physiology, an on-target, off tumor AE, and is also observed in vascular endothelial growth factor (VEGFR) therapies.

2. Hypertension is frequently observed with anti-VEGFR therapies due to the rarefication of blood vessels, an on-target, off-tumor response; this is dose dependent and generally occurs within 3 to 4 weeks of starting therapy (Escalante et al., 2016).

3. Drug-induced QTc interval prolongation recorded via electrocardiogram (ECG) is a common risk associated with multiple TKI classes (e.g., BRAF inhibitors, VEGF agents, and BCR-ABL inhibitors).

D. Fluid retention (i.e., peripheral edema, pulmonary edema) observed in patients treated with BCR-ABl agents.

TABLE 29.7 Assessment and Management of Hypertension in VEGF-Treated Patients

Initial assessment	• Prior medical history: age >60, preexisting cardiovascular disease, diabetes mellitus, previously documented left ventricular hypertrophy, elevated body mass index, smoking, obesity, sedentary lifestyle, stress, diet, medications, and family history of cardiovascular disease • Physical examination: blood pressure, large body habitus, headaches, peripheral edema, evidence of cardiovascular compromise • Labs: serum creatinine, urinalysis with protein, lipid profile. • Assess for signs and symptoms of hypertension (headaches, dizziness, nosebleeds, flushing, peripheral edema, blurred vision, dyspnea) • Assess vital signs, heart and lung sounds, presence of JVD • CBC, urine analysis to evaluate for proteinuria, electrolytes, creatinine, BUN

Ongoing assessment while on therapy

• Physical examination: headaches, dizziness, nosebleeds, flushing, peripheral edema, blurred vision, dyspnea, vital signs, heart and lung sounds, presence of JVD

• CBC, urine analysis to evaluate for proteinuria, electrolytes, creatinine, BUN

Grading of hypertension	Grade 1	Grade 2	Grade 3	Grade 4
	Adult: Systolic BP 120–139 mm Hg or diastolic BP 80–89 mm Hg	Adult: Systolic BP 140–159 mm Hg or diastolic BP 90–99 mm Hg if previously WNL; change in baseline medical intervention indicated; recurrent or persistent (≥24 hr); symptomatic increase by >20 mm Hg (diastolic) or to >140/90 mm Hg; monotherapy indicated initiated	Adult: Systolic BP ≥160 mm Hg or diastolic BP ≥100 mm Hg; medical intervention indicated; more than one drug or more intensive therapy than previously used indicated	Adult and pediatric: Life-threatening consequences (e.g., malignant hypertension, transient or permanent neurologic deficit, hypertensive crisis); urgent intervention indicated

Pharmacologic management	• Address preexisting hypertension before initiation of treatment with targeted therapy; for preexisting hypertension, BP target for initiating VEGF inhibitor treatment should be <140/90 mm Hg, or lower if proteinuria present • Antihypertensive agents should be prescribed immediately upon detection of hypertension • Treatment of VEGF inhibitor-related hypertension (ACE inhibitors, beta blockers, calcium channel blockers)
Nonpharmacologic management	• Monitor BP throughout treatment with more frequent assessments during first cycle; decrease monitoring to every 2–3 weeks until BP is stable • Educate patients and families in monitoring for symptoms of hypertension and hypotension • Consider collaboration with cardiologist • Educate patients in healthy lifestyle changes (smoking cessation, regular exercise, limited alcohol intake, weight loss, stress management, diet modifications [low salt, low fat])

ACE, Angiotensin-converting enzyme; *BMI,* body mass index; *BP,* blood pressure; *BUN,* blood urea nitrogen; *CBC,* complete blood count; *JVD,* jugular venous distension; *VEGF,* vascular endothelial growth factor.

TABLE 29.8 Cardiotoxicity

Assessment	• Assess for risk factors (previous anthracycline exposure, hypertension, low baseline LVEF, older age) • Assess for signs and symptoms of cardiac toxicity • Obtain baseline LVEF via echocardiogram or MUGA • CBC, BUN, creatinine, electrolytes, electrocardiogram

Grading: left ventricular systolic dysfunction	Grade 3	Grade 4
	Symptomatic due to drop in ejection fraction responsive to intervention	Refractory or poorly controlled heart failure due to drop in ejection fraction; intervention such as ventricular assist device, intravenous vasopressor support, or heart transplant indicated

Pharmacologic management	• Consideration of ACE inhibitors or beta-blockers
Nonpharmacologic management	• Educate patients to report symptoms promptly • Collaboration with cardiologist • Educate patients in healthy lifestyle changes (smoking cessation, dietary modifications [low salt, low fat], regular exercise, limited alcohol intake, weight loss, stress management

ACE, Angiotensin-converting enzyme; *CBC,* complete blood count; *BUN,* blood urea nitrogen; *EF,* ejection fraction; *LVEF,* left ventricular ejection fraction; *MUGA,* multigated acquisition scan.

Data from Tajiri, K., Aonuma, K., & Sekine, I. (2017). Cardiovascular toxic effects of targeted cancer therapy. *Jpn J Clin Oncol,* 47(9), 779–785. https://doi.org/10.1093/jjco/hyx071.

E. Mucositis is commonly observed with mTOR, oral EGFR, and oral VEGFR inhibitors (Table 29.9).

F. Diarrhea is commonly observed with anti-EGFR monoclonal antibodies (Table 29.10).

1. Diarrhea common in patients treated with an EGFR TKI. EGF is responsible for maintaining mucosal integrity.

2. The underlying mechanism is poorly understood but is believed to be due to excessive chloride secretion, which leads to a secretory form of diarrhea.

3. May involve gut motility dysfunction or possibly inflammation; more common in patients receiving TKIs (Liu & Kurzrock, 2015).

TABLE 29.9	Oral Mucositis
Assessment	• Inspect oral mucosa, dentition, surrounding gums. • Assess symptoms (ranging from mild tingling to painful ulcers). • Mucositis-related mTOR inhibitors characterized by distinct ulcers, aphthous in appearance, oval, gray-white center, surrounded by erythematous halo. Lesions are clustered or coalescing, usually <1 cm in diameter. Localized to lips, lateral tongue, soft palate. May be accompanied by mouth pain, dysgeusia, or dysphagia without any evidence of clinically visible oral lesions. Patients with oral lesions are more likely to develop concurrent skin rashes and hand–foot syndrome.
Pharmacologic management	• Steroid-based mouthwashes may be of benefit in patients receiving everolimus based on the hypothesis that stomatitis due to that agent may arise from an inflammatory process. • Preventive care with 10 mL alcohol-free dexamethasone mouthwash (0.5 mg/5 mL oral solution) 4 times a day (swish for 2 minutes and spit) for 8 weeks significantly minimized or prevented all grades of mucositis in women receiving everolimus for advanced breast cancer. • Treatments for mTOR inhibitor stomatitis: • Topical analgesics for pain • Mucoadhesive gels or viscous solutions that coat the oral cavity (to protect oral mucosa) • Prophylactic antibiotics (to avoid secondary infections) • Steroid-based mouth rinses, topical steroids, topical antiinflammatory agents (to reduce inflammation/immune response) • Systemic analgesics/corticosteroids for moderate to severe stomatitis
Nonpharmacologic management	• Referral to dentist before initiation of therapy and during treatment to prevent serious sequelae. • Education about oral hygiene: frequent brushing with soft bristles every 2–3 hours for mild stomatitis; every 1–2 hours for more severe symptoms), using mild toothpaste (children's) or toothpaste without sodium lauryl sulfate; flossing and rinsing with saline or sodium bicarbonate after every meal to get rid of food particles; nonalcoholic mouthwashes. • Diet instructions: soft, moist, nonirritating foods; drink fluids. • Lip balms to help reduce mouth and lip dryness.

TABLE 29.10	Diarrhea from EGFR Therapies
Assessment	• Baseline bowel history beginning 6 weeks before starting EGFR treatment • Complete medication list (prescription, over-the-counter, laxatives and stool softeners, opioids or recent opioid withdrawal, recent antibiotic therapy, herbals, vitamins) • Type of diet • Other clinical and medical conditions • Travel history • Signs and symptoms of dehydration (orthostatic hypotension, dry mouth, excessive thirst, dizziness, feelings of weakness, decreased urination, weight loss) • Abdominal assessment (tenderness, distention) • Frequency and characteristics of stools, nocturnal stools, incontinence, cramping • Nausea/vomiting • Laboratory tests (CBC, stool test for occult blood, metabolic panel, stool cultures for enteric pathogens, *Clostridium difficile*, and ova and parasites)
Pharmacologic management	Loperamide • An opioid that decreases intestinal motility by directly affecting the smooth muscle of the intestine; few, if any, systemic effects due to minimal absorption • As diarrhea from targeted therapies is usually secretory, loperamide is the first drug of choice

TABLE 29.10	**Diarrhea from EGFR Therapies—cont'd**

	• Initial dose for grade 1 or 2 diarrhea is 4 mg followed by 2 mg every 4 hours or after every unformed stool (maximum daily dose of 16–20 mg) until there have been no episodes of diarrhea for 12 hours. If diarrhea persists over 48 hours, loperamide may be continued or discontinued, with use of other agents such as octreotide or tincture of opium
	Octreotide
	• Decreases the secretion of several hormones, prolongs intestinal transit time, increases absorption of fluid and electrolytes
	• Given subcutaneously at titrated doses from 100–150 micrograms (mcg) three times daily up to 500 mcg three times a day
	Deodorized tincture of opium
	• Contains the equivalent of 10 mg/mL of morphine
	• Recommended dose is 10–15 drops every 3–4 hours
	Short-term opioid treatment
	• Codeine 30 mg/day, which can be increased up to 60 mg four times a day, may be beneficial; although it should be stopped if the EGFR TKI treatment is discontinued
	Budesonide
	• Reduces inflammation
Nonpharmacologic management	• Instruct patients to report any change in bowel activity, especially if duration >48 hours or accompanied by fever or is grade 3 or 4
	• Dietary instructions: low fat, low fiber; minimal intake of fruit, red meat, alcohol, spicy food, caffeine
	• Dietary modifications: foods that build stool consistency (low in fiber; pectin containing), foods high in potassium, foods at room temperature to minimize peristalsis, increased fluids
	• Consider referral to dietitian upon initiating EGFR treatment
	• Consider referral to gastroenterologist if diarrhea does not improve despite discontinuation of EGFR therapy
	• Isotonic solutions 1–1.5 L/day; limit hypotonic fluids (water, tea, fruit juice) to 0.5 L/day
	• Maintain skin integrity: cleanse rectal area after each stool, apply topical skin barrier; sitz baths may help with anal discomfort

ADL, activities of daily living; *CBC,* complete blood count; *EGFR,* epidermal growth factor receptor.

Assessment

I. Pertinent personal history
  A. Assessment of current medications, including prescription and nonprescription, especially those that may be contraindicated with targeted therapies
    1. CYP450 substrates, inhibitors, and inducers
    2. Drugs that affect gastric pH (proton pump inhibitors, antacids)
    3. Warfarin and other coumarin-derived anticoagulants
    4. Aspirin, nonsteroidal antiinflammatory drugs (NSAIDs)
    5. Medications that may alter mentation or cognition
    6. Immunosuppressants
    7. Antihypertensive therapy
    8. Herbals, vitamins, other over-the-counter medications
    9. Laxatives, especially those used chronically
  B. Other concurrent anticancer therapies (radiation, hormonal, chemotherapy, targeted therapy, biotherapy, immunotherapy)
    1. Comorbidities may be exacerbated by side effects of targeted therapies
    2. Assess for history of, tolerance of, and response to prior therapies
  C. Disease status
    1. Site of cancer, stage of cancer, histology

    2. Drug-specific companion testing to determine sensitivity to targeted therapy, including single mutation assays and genomic panel assays
  D. Knowledge of goals of therapy, line of treatment, agents to be given
  E. Treatment details (e.g., diagnostic, curative, palliative, supportive, or investigational)
    1. Treatment plan, including duration and sequencing of therapy
    2. Requirements of treatment such as length of hospitalization, follow-up clinic visits, laboratory- and diagnostic test requirements, financial obligations
    3. Expected side effects and self-care skills required
II. Assessment of AE-specific risk factors
  A. Rash (see Table 29.5)
    1. Bacterial culture swabs of skin discharge should be considered to determine the presence of bacteria (Lacouture, 2016).
    2. Patients should be assessed weekly for signs of rash during the first 6 weeks of treatment with an EGFR TKI, every 6 to 8 weeks thereafter (Vogel and Paul, 2016).
    3. Patients with fair skin have an increased sensitivity to the damaging effects of ultraviolet (UV) sunlight and are more susceptible to developing severe

EGFR inhibitor–associated skin rash (Eaby-Sandy and Lynch, 2014).

B. Hypertension (see Table 29.7)

1. Risk factors: age over 60, high body mass index, smoking, obesity, sedentary lifestyle, stress, diet, proteinuria, baseline blood pressure (BP) $\geq 140/90$, abnormal electrolytes, elevated creatinine, and blood urea nitrogen (Walker, 2017)

2. Assess for signs and symptoms of hypertension, which may or may not be present. Some patients have headaches, dizziness, nosebleeds, or flushing. Peripheral edema, blurred vision, and dyspnea may be seen with uncontrolled hypertension. Assess vital signs, heart and lung sounds, and for the presence of jugular venous distension. Obtain a complete blood count and urine analysis to evaluate for proteinuria, electrolytes, creatinine, and blood urea nitrogen (Walker, 2017).

C. LVEF cardiotoxicity: previous anthracycline exposure, hypertension, a low-baseline LVEF, and older age (Tajiri et al., 2017) (see Table 29.8).

D. Diarrhea (see Table 29.10)

1. Baseline bowel history before initiation of EGFR inhibitor therapy. Obtain information about the patient's bowel habits for the 6-week period before starting treatment (Hofheinz et al., 2017).

2. Assess for signs and symptoms of dehydration: orthostatic hypotension, dry mouth, excessive thirst, dizziness, weakness, decreased urination, and weight loss.

III. Physical examination: thorough physical assessment by body system before initiation of therapy (to serve as baseline for comparison) and at regular intervals during therapy to evaluate tolerance and response. The reader is directed to symptom-specific sections of this book for detailed assessment guidance.

A. Assess respiratory function, heart rate, respiratory rate, cough, and peripheral edema for evidence of cardiopulmonary compromise.

B. Monitor BP throughout treatment; more frequently during the first cycle of treatment.

C. Monitor abdominal pain, ascites, and jaundice as evidence of liver dysfunction.

D. Monitor weight loss as a potential sign of hypophysitis.

E. Review skin for evidence of rash as a sign of allergic reaction, baseline and ongoing skin integrity, infection, autoimmune skin toxicity, and loss of skin turgor as a sign of dehydration.

F. Monitor lung sounds, cough, and peripheral edema suggestive of cardiopulmonary compromise with HER2 and MEK therapies.

G. Monitor level of consciousness, confusion, mental acuity, and evidence of seizures in patients at risk for cytokine release syndrome.

H. Assess for status of preexisting comorbidities with emphasis on diabetes

IV. Psychosocial examination

A. Assessment of baseline mental status

B. Assessment of cultural factors and health-related beliefs

C. Assessment of current social structure, including support systems, primary caregiver, housing and living arrangements, employment/work status

D. Assessment of type, number, and effectiveness of previous coping strategies used by patient and family

E. Determination of response to illness and emotional state

F. Assessment for ability to perform self-care activities

G. Assessment for patient adherence, especially oral targeted therapies, barriers

H. Consideration of financial status—need for referral to social worker or access to patient assistance programs (community and/or pharmaceutical sponsored)

Management

I. Pharmacologic

A. Cardioprotective treatments such as dexrazoxane may be added to address LVEF decline, allowing patients to continue treatment with HER2 inhibitors (see Chapter 33).

B. Angiotensin-converting enzyme inhibitors, beta blockers, and calcium channel blockers for VEGF inhibitor–related hypertension included, although currently there are no available guidelines recommending specific antihypertensives (Escalante et al., 2016).

C. Topical antiinfectives (clindamycin gel), steroids (e.g., hydrocortisone 2.5%, alclometasone), oral antibiotics (minocycline, doxycycline, or antibiotics covering skin flora), and emollients for maculopapular rash associated with EGFR inhibitors (Lacouture, 2016. Vogel and Paul, 2016).

D. Loperamide (escalated to octreotide as indicated) with oral hydration with electrolytes at the first episode of watery stool for therapy-induced diarrhea (Fischer-Cartlidge, 2014).

E. Antiinflammatory steroid-based mouthwashes with everolimus (Staves & Ramachandran, 2016).

F. Analgesics (topical and systemic) to ameliorate pain symptoms related to stomatitis.

G. Antiinfectives (antifungals, antibiotics) to treat or prevent superinfection (Fischer-Cartlidge, 2014). Concomitant antifungals with mTOR inhibitors can result in decreased drug clearance of the mTOR inhibitor, with resultant increase in mTOR inhibitor–related toxicities.

H. Premedication with corticosteroid, acetaminophen, antihistamine to prevent infusion reactions and hypersensitivity reactions.

I. For patients experiencing dyspepsia, suggest use of short-acting antacids or H2 blockers as alternatives to proton pump inhibitors.

II. Nonpharmacologic measures

A. Early identification and management of side effects is preferred over dose reduction or modifications.

B. Monitor for tolerance during infusions, assessing for risk of cytokine release especially in initial infusions, and for allergic reaction in subsequent infusions.

C. Education on adherence, symptoms to report, healthy habits.

D. Education to manage and report symptoms.

E. Patients should record consistency and frequency of stools, preceding foods, and treatments.

F. Multidisciplinary collaboration with interprofessional teams (Abueg, 2017): dieticians, dermatologists, gastroenterologists, pulmonologists, ophthalmologists, cardiologists, rheumatologists, and internal medicine practitioners should be consulted for appropriate for management of organ-specific disorders.

G. Focused education related to oral self-medication starting at initiation of drug therapy, including regularly scheduled assessments to evaluate compliance and tolerance.

Expected Patient Outcomes

I. Patients will be educated about the mechanism, dose, route, frequency, expected AEs, and emergent AEs related to targeted therapies emphasizing proper self-administration for oral agents, as applicable.

II. Patients will be monitored for AEs related to targeted therapies in a manner that promotes safety; early intervention of AEs will attempt to avoid treatment discontinuation.

IMMUNOTHERAPY

Overview

I. Immunotherapy—use of immunologic cells and pathways to reduce tumor burden (Bayer, et al., 2017; Brahmer, et al., 2018).

A. Immunotherapy utilizes antibodies, T cells, B cells, and cytokines to orchestrate direct immune-mediated cytotoxicity against tumor.

B. Immunotherapy capitalizes on the immune system's unique specificity and memory abilities.

C. Specificity refers to the ability to distinguish between healthy tissue and tumor by recognizing unique tumor-associated antigen.

D. Memory refers to the ability to recall previous encounters with an antigen. Memory cells (activated T and B cells) can more rapidly respond to tumor recurrence, leading to more lasting results.

II. Immunotherapy boosts the body's natural defenses by using substances to improve or restore immune function. Types of immunotherapy include monoclonal antibodies, oncolytic virus therapy, T-cell therapy, nonspecific immunotherapies, and cancer vaccines (American Society of Clinical Oncology [ASCO], 2018).

III. Immunotherapy is used to enhance normal immune function and to overcome a tumor's acquired ability to escape immune eradication (Beatty & Gladney, 2015).

IV. Tumor escape occurs when the immune system fails to recognize an in situ tumor, resulting from either deficient host immunity (from age- or disease-related alterations) or suppressive tumor microenvironments.

V. The suppressive tumor microenvironment includes upregulated expression of checkpoint molecules, inhibitory cytokines, and neo-antigens that mimic self-proteins.

VI. Classes of immunotherapy—immunotherapy can be classified by the specific immune system pathway utilized (Bayer, et al., 2017; McGettigan & Rubin, 2017; Michot, et al., 2016). See Table 29.11.

A. Cytokines such as interleukin-2 and interferon are naturally occurring chemicals that stimulate and regulate the immune system (see Chapter 8).

B. Passive or adoptive immuno-oncology: use of exogenously grown or manufactured immunologic substances that target predefined tumor antigens by immunologic cytotoxicity (e.g., monoclonal antibodies and T-cell therapy).

1. Monoclonal antibodies (discussed earlier under targeted therapy)

   a. Effect tumor kill by ADCC, CDC, and ADCP.

   b. MoABs can be mass-produced to target tumor antigens theoretically shared by all patients harboring specific tumor markers. Examples include trastuzumab targeting the HER2 protein on HER2-positive cancers and cetuximab targeting the EGFR receptor on head and neck and colon cancers.

2. Checkpoint inhibitors interfere with regulatory proteins exploited by tumors to evade immune activity.

   a. On healthy cells, checkpoint molecules inhibit T cells' cytotoxicity, thus preventing autoimmune reactions. Malignant tumors can cloak themselves in these checkpoint molecules, thus evading immune elimination and allowing unchecked tumor growth.

   b. CPIs restore T-cell recognition of tumor and promote antitumor response.

   c. Note: The underlying mechanism of checkpoint inhibitors are monoclonal antibodies; however, their action primarily involves immune function; thus a full discussion on CPIs follows later rather than in the targeted therapy section earlier.

3. Adoptive cellular therapy capitalizes on the cytotoxic and memory functions of T cells to effect tumor kill (Yang & Rosenberg, 2016)

   a. T-cell therapy is manufactured for individual patients using their own T cells harvested either from their tumor or their peripheral blood.

   b. T cells harvested from a patient's tumor (tumor infiltrating lymphocytes [TILs]) already recognize tumor-associated antigen. TILs are harvested, expanded into large quantities in culture, and reinfused back into the same patient.

   c. T cells harvested from peripheral blood are not yet tumor specific and must be reprogrammed with tumor antigen receptors. Chimeric

TABLE 29.11 Classifications of Immunotherapies

Class	Mechanism of Action	Description of Agents	
		Checkpoint Targets	**Agents**
Checkpoint inhibitors	Inhibition of regulatory proteins leading to restoration of immune activity. Key targeted proteins include PD-1/PD-L1 and CLTA-4/B7–1/B7–2.	Anti-CTLA4 Anti-PD1 Anti-PD-L1 TIGIT	Ipilimumab (Yervoy) Pembrolizumab (Keytruda) Nivolumab (Opdivo) Atezolizumab (Tecentriq) Avelumab (Bevancio) Durvalumab (Imfinzi) ASP8374 (investigational)
		Chimeric Antigen Receptor	**Agents**
Chimeric antigen receptor therapy	Personalized T-cell therapy using host T cells that have been genetically modified to target tumor-specific antigen.	CD-19	Tisagenlecleucel (Kymriah) Axicabtagene (Yescarta) Investigational agents and associated antigens Anti-HER2 CAR-T Anti-GD2 CAR-T Anti-GPC3 CAR-T
		TIL infusion	**Agents**
Tumor infiltrating lymphocytes	Personalized T-cell therapy using the host's own tumor infiltrating cells that have been expanded ex vivo and reinfused to patient	LN-145	Head and neck, melanoma, cervical
		Oncolytic virus and gene modification	**Agents**
Oncolytic vaccine therapy	Injection of attenuated virus that selectively targets cancer cells, releasing cellular contents. Genetically modified to stimulate immune response to tumor antigens.	HSV-1 and GM-CSF	T-Vec (Imlygic, talimogene laherparepvec

antigen receptor therapy (CAR-T) uses DNA vector processes to attach tumor antigen receptors to T cells. These are expanded into large quantities in culture and reinfused back into the same patient.

A. Active immunotherapy (vaccination) conditions the host immune system to generate its own sustained response to current and future tumor growth (Fukuhara, et al., 2016).

1. Oncolytic viral therapy is the injection of attenuated viruses into tumor, resulting in tumor lysis and presentation of tumor-associated antigen (TAAs) to circulating T cells and B cells.

2. Dendritic cell vaccines are personalized therapies based on a patient's own extracted antigen-presenting cells engineered to recognize TAA.

III. Adverse events of immunotherapy vary according to the type of immunotherapy used. (Brahmer, et al., 2018; Gordon, et al., 2017; Michot, et al., 2016; Puzanov, et al., 2017; Smith & Venella, 2017; Spain, et al., 2016)

A. Checkpoint inhibitors are primarily associated with immune-related adverse events (irAEs) (Table 29.12).

1. Most checkpoint inhibitor ARs due to autoimmune attack on normal cells by activated T cells.

2. Common (>20%) irAEs include skin rash, hepatic toxicity, fatigue, pneumonitis, gastrointestinal toxicity.

3. Less common (<20%) irAEs include neurologic, endocrine, ocular, pancreatic enzymes, and hematological symptoms.

4. CTLA-4 is generally associated with more severe AEs than PD-1 therapies.

B. Vaccines are associated with injection site pain and flulike symptoms.

C. Adoptive T-cell therapy, particularly CAR-T, is associated with cytokine release syndrome, tumor lysis syndrome, neurologic symptoms, and decreased B cells (B-cell aplasia).

D. Monoclonal antibodies associated with infusion reactions and target-specific toxicities (discussed earlier)

E. Immunotherapy AEs are different from chemotherapy AEs in terms of timing, pathophysiology, and management.

1. Immunotherapies activate memory function of immune cells; thus AEs may appear and/or persist for the duration of the immune cell lifespan; can occur/recur after therapy cessation.

2. Combining chemotherapy and immunotherapy or combining two or more immunotherapies can increase the risk of AEs and broaden the range of potential AEs.

3. As with targeted therapies, "on-target, off-tumor" AEs result from immune activity against normal tissue that coincidentally expresses the target

TABLE 29.12   Major Adverse Events of Checkpoint Inhibitors

Body System	Presenting Symptoms
Dermatologic	Vitiligo, pruritus, maculopapular rash
Endocrine	Hyperthyroidism, hypothyroidism, hypophysitis (alterations in TSH, T4, T3, ACTH; significant fatigue, appetite, somnolence)
Gastrointestinal	Colitis (abdominal pain with endoscopic evidence of inflammation), diarrhea (increase in frequency of stools)
Hepatic	Liver dysfunction (elevated ALT, AST, total bilirubin), hepatitis
Pneumonitis	Persistent dry cough, ground-glass opacities on imaging, fine inspiratory crackles
Fatigue	Loss of stamina, shortness of breath, malaise, muscle weakness
Musculoskeletal	Arthralgia, polyarthritis
Pancreas	Elevations on lipase and amylase

From Michot, J. M., Bigenwald, C., Champiat, S., Collins, M., Carbonnel, F., Postel-Vinay, S., & Lambotte, O. (2016). Immune-related adverse events with immune checkpoint blockade: a comprehensive review. *Eur J Cancer, 54,* 139–148. https://doi.org/10.1016/j.ejca.2015.11.016; Brahmer, J.R., Lacchetti, C., Schneider, B.J., et al. (2018). Management of immune-related adverse events in patients treated with immune checkpoint inhibitor therapy: American Society of Clinical Oncology Clinical Practice Guideline. *Journal of Clinical Oncology,* Feb14. Available at: http://ascopubs.org/doi/abs/10.1200/JCO.2017.77.6385.

antigen. Examples include cytotoxic T cells cross-reacting against CD-19+ B cells in patients treated with CAR-T cell therapy resulting in B-cell aplasia.

Assessment

I. Pertinent personal and family history (Brahmer et al., 2018; Puzanov et al., 2017)
  A. Documentation: family and medical history and comorbidities.
  B. Note history of preexisting autoimmune disease such as rheumatoid arthritis, myasthenia gravis, myositis, autoimmune hepatitis, systemic lupus erythematosus, inflammatory bowel disease, Wegener granulomatosis, Sjögren syndrome, Guillain–Barré syndrome, multiple sclerosis, vasculitis, or glomerulonephritis.
  C. Record all medications, including prescriptions, over-the-counter medications, homeopathic preparations, herbal supplements, and vitamins.
  D. Assess for preexisting use of immunosuppressive agents such as chronic corticosteroids, as these may counteract immunotherapy activity.
  E. Assess for tolerance of prior lines of therapy and residual adverse drug reactions.
II. Disease history, stage, and molecular characteristics
  A. Review molecular assays (e.g., fluorescence in situ hybridization [FISH], immunohistochemical [IHC]) that indicate expression levels of target proteins such as PDL-1 and CD-19.

  B. Review extent of disease as discussed in pathology reports, biopsies, and imaging.
  C. Higher disease burden is correlated with higher risk of severe cytokine release syndrome in patients treated with CAR T-cell therapy (Teachey et al., 2016).
III. Knowledge of, rationale for, and goals of treatment, agent to be given.
  A. Assess patient's expectations of efficacy and tumor response.
  B. Assess patient's attitude toward tumor response monitoring and pseudoprogression.
    1. Pseudoprogression is due to infiltrating T cells causing initial growth of tumor size followed by shrinkage.
    2. Pseudoprogression is not accompanied by clinical worsening of disease.
    3. Pseudoprogression occurs in a small subset of patients treated with checkpoint inhibitors.
  C. Assess patient's awareness that immunotherapy AEs may present at any time after drug initiation (i.e., rash may appear months after drug cessation).
IV. Laboratory and diagnostic data (Teachey et al., 2016; Spain et al., 2016)
  A. Complete blood count with differential with emphasis on long-term trends.
  B. Liver function tests (aspartate aminotransferase [AST], alanine aminotransferase [ALT], total bilirubin)
  C. Thyroid function tests, especially with checkpoint inhibitors (thyroid-stimulating hormone [TSH], T4, T3)
  D. Amylase and lipase for evidence of pancreatic dysfunction
  E. Complete metabolic panel, including electrolytes and kidney function, to check for autoimmune activity and tumor lysis syndrome
  F. Inflammatory marker elevation: cytokines including interleukin-6, lactate dehydrogenase, C-reactive protein, and ferritin
V. Physical examination
  A. Complete physical examination in all patients should include the following elements
    1. Assess respiratory function, heart rate, respiratory rate, cough, and peripheral edema for evidence of cardiopulmonary compromise.
    2. Monitor abdominal pain, ascites, and jaundice as evidence of liver dysfunction.
    3. Monitor weight loss as a potential sign of hypophysitis.
    4. Review skin for evidence of rash as sign of allergic reaction or autoimmune skin toxicity and for loss of skin turgor as sign of dehydration.
    5. Monitor lung sounds and cough as evidence of pneumonitis.
  B. Specific immunotherapy classes should focus on high-risk, drug-specific assessments.

1. Checkpoint inhibitors: colitis, rash, pneumonitis-associated shortness of breath, and endocrinopathy-associated fatigue and malaise.

C. CAR-T: fever, tachycardia, arrhythmia, and neurologic changes; peripheral edema indicative of cytokine release syndrome. Assess for preexisting comorbidities with emphasis on diabetes and other autoimmune disorders.

VI. Psychosocial examination

A. Assess for coping skills and evidence of coping dysfunction.

B. Assess for stressors brought on by irAEs.

C. Assess for socioeconomic burdens imposed by long-term therapy.

Management

I. Pharmacologic (Table 29.13)

A. Provide symptomatic relief for irAEs, cytokine release, and infusion reactions (Brahmer et al., 2018; Gordon et al., 2017, Michot et al., 2016, Puzanov et al., 2017; Smith & Venella, 2017; Spain et al., 2016)

1. Oral and topical antihistamines can be effective to control skin reactions.

2. Loperamide (Imodium) can be effective first-line agents for mild diarrhea.

B. Autoimmune disorders resulting from checkpoint inhibitor therapy are primarily treated with short courses of topical or oral corticosteroids until symptoms resolve to baseline or ≤ grade 1 (Brahmer et al., 2018; Gordon et al., 2017; Michot et al., 2016; Puzanov et al., 2017; Smith & Venella, 2017; Spain et al., 2016)

1. If symptoms do not respond, intensify immunosuppressant therapy with prednisone/methylprednisolone 1 to 2 mg/kg/day, or infliximab.

2. Corticosteroids should be tapered over 4 to 6 weeks.

3. Other agents used (depending on specific irAE) include infliximab, vedolizumab, omalizumab, gamma-aminobutyric acid (GABA) agonists, mycophenolate (liver dysfunction).

C. Autoimmune thyroid disease is treated with thyroid hormone (levothyroxine) and/or short course of high-dose steroids (1 mg/kg prednisone or equivalent) (Brahmer et al., 2018; Gordon et al., 2017, Michot et al., 2016, Puzanov et al., 2017; Smith & Venella, 2017; Spain et al., 2016)

D. CAR-T AEs require intensive supportive care.

1. Tumor lysis syndrome should be managed with hydration, allopurinol, and Kayexalate as indicated by electrolyte laboratory tests.

2. Neurologic symptoms resulting from CAR-T therapy are managed with antiepileptics.

3. Cytokine release syndrome resulting from CAR-T therapy is "managed with immunosuppressive agents titrated to control symptoms without interfering with the efficacy of T cells" (Smith & Venella, 2017; Brudno & Kochenderfer, 2016).

TABLE 29.13   General Algorithm for Management of Treatment-Related Adverse Events of Checkpoint Inhibitors

Less than grade 1 At first appearance of symptoms	• Proactively monitor for symptoms and signs of adverse events • Assume symptoms are immune related unless proven otherwise • Rule out nonimmune-related causes • Grade symptoms using standardized assessment scale
Grade 1 or grade 2	• Increase monitoring • Treat symptoms • Consider holding immunotherapy • Monitor for resolution to ≤ grade 1
Grade 2	• Initiation of corticosteroids • Monitor for resolution to ≤ grade 1 • Monitor tolerance to corticosteroids • If not responding, intensification of corticosteroids or addition to alternative immunosuppressive therapy according to affected organ
Grade 3 or grade 4	• Prepare for potential discontinuation of immunotherapy • Consult with interdisciplinary team for management of affected organ/system • Intensify high-dose corticosteroid and consider addition of alternative immunosuppressive therapy

Data from Michot, J. M., Bigenwald, C., Champiat, S., Collins, M., Carbonnel, F., Postel-Vinay, S., & Lambotte, O. (2016). Immune-related adverse events with immune checkpoint blockade: a comprehensive review. *Eur J Cancer, 54,* 139–148. https://doi.org/10.1016/j.ejca.2015. 11.016; Brahmer, J.R., Lacchetti, C., Schneider, B.J., et al. (2018). Management of immune-related adverse events in patients treated with immune checkpoint inhibitor therapy: American Society of Clinical Oncology Clinical Practice Guideline. *Journal of Clinical Oncology,* Feb14. Available at: http://ascopubs.org/doi/abs/10.1200/JCO.2017. 77.6385; Puzanov, I., Diab, A., Abdallah, K., Bingham, C. O., 3rd, Brogdon, C., Dadu, R., . . . Society for Immunotherapy of Cancer Toxicity Management Working, G. (2017). Managing toxicities associated with immune checkpoint inhibitors: consensus recommendations from the Society for Immunotherapy of Cancer (SITC) Toxicity Management Working Group. *J Immunother Cancer, 5*(1), 95. https://doi.org/10.1186/s40425-017-0300-z.

4. Supportive care treatments include pain medications, antiemetics, vasopressors, aggressive hydration, oxygenation, antianxiolytics, and antipyretics.

5. More severe cases require immunosuppression with corticosteroids such as tocilizumab, which targets the IL-6 receptor counteracting inflammation, methylprednisolone, or dexamethasone.

II. Nonpharmacologic

A. Before starting immunotherapy

1. Providers should familiarize themselves with updated guidelines and recommendations for the care of immunotherapy-related toxicities, including review of National Comprehensive Cancer Network (NCCN) and ASCO guidelines.

2. Assure patient verbalizes monitoring instructions after infusion, has printed instructions, and has 24/7 contact information for treatment team.

3. Educate patient on importance of effective contraception for at least 5 months after final dose of immunotherapy.

4. Patients should be advised to carry wallet cards that describe specific immunotherapy, expected irAEs, and health care contact team.

5. Review drug-specific side effect profile before every administration and assess for those symptoms.

B. Patient education (Brahmer et al., 2018; McGettigan & Rubin, 2017; Smith & Venella, 2017)

1. Educate patients about the immunotherapy component of their therapy, including normal role of the immune system and mechanism of their immunotherapy agent.

2. Educate patients about nature of AEs of immunotherapies, emphasizing the following:
   a. Multiple organ systems can be affected simultaneously.
   b. Autoimmune disorders can result from immune system activation from immunotherapy.
   c. Organs that share the same antigen as the target may be affected by immunotherapy.
   d. Onset of irAEs can occur/recur any time after treatment initiation or after treatment has stopped.
   e. Combination therapy increases risk of AEs.

3. Educate patients that nononcology providers should consult with oncology team when any new symptoms occur because these may require immune-specific interventions not typical in nononcology patients.

C. Monitor for safety during therapy

1. Assume a high level of suspicion that symptoms are treatment related unless definitive evidence supports an alternative cause.

2. Monitor laboratory values before each infusion and at all follow-up visits.

3. Assess symptoms and grade severity using a standardized grading scale such as the Common Terminology Criteria for Adverse Events (CTCAE).
   a. In general, patients experiencing grade 1 AEs should be carefully monitored during treatment.
   b. Moderate or grade 2 AEs will generally require dose interruption or delay until symptoms resolve.
   c. Severe or grade 3 and higher AEs generally require treatment cessation and intensive long-term management to prevent deleterious autoimmune sequelae.

4. Monitor for early signs of cytokine release syndrome, including fever, tachycardia, hypotension, respiratory distress, peripheral edema, and altered level of consciousness.

5. Rule out other potential causes for common symptoms.
   a. Assess recent dietary pattern, community sources of infection, and assess for *Clostridium difficile* for patients experiencing diarrhea.
   b. Assess for allergen contact in patients experiencing rash.
   c. Assess community sources of infection, seasonal allergies in patients experiencing cough.

D. Manage emergent AEs appropriately.

1. Review treatment plan for emergency medication orders before infusion.

2. Educate patient about worrisome signs of symptoms that require immediate reporting.

3. Assure availability of safety equipment.

4. Monitor for signs of emergent AEs.
   a. Cytokine release syndrome: fever, hypotension, seizure, pancytopenia, tachycardia, tachypnea, respiratory distress, peripheral edema, and altered level of consciousness.
   b. Infusion reactions: fever/chills/rigors, pruritus, edema, flushing/headache, hyper-/hypotension, shortness of breath, cough, wheezing, change in level of consciousness, diaphoresis, arthralgia.

5. Stop infusion immediately if evidence of infusion reaction.
   a. Assess for cardiopulmonary status.
   b. Infusions may be restarted or slowed with mild reactions.
   c. Infusions may be discontinued permanently with severe reactions.
   d. Monitor for tolerance of corticosteroids and other immunosuppressive agents used for irAEs. Prepare for possible rechallenge with immunotherapies if irAEs resolve to ≤grade 1.

E. Collaborate with interprofessional teams (Abueg, 2017)

1. Dermatologists, gastroenterologists, pulmonologists, ophthalmologists, cardiologists, rheumatologists, and internal medicine practitioners should be consulted for appropriate for management of organ-specific disorders.

2. Because irAEs can present at any time after initiation of drug and persist after cessation, nurses should assure that primary care providers are aware of long-term risk and associated signs of immune dysfunction.

Expected Patient Outcomes

I. Patients will be properly educated about the mechanism, dose, route, frequency, expected AEs, and emergent AEs related to immunotherapies.

II. Patients will be monitored for AEs related to immunotherapies in a manner appropriate for the specific immunotherapy drug classification.

REFERENCES

Abramson, R. (2017). Overview of targeted therapies for cancer. *My Cancer Genome.* https://www.mycancergenome.org/content/molecular-medicine/overview-of-targeted-therapies-for-cancer.

Abueg, K. (2014). Bioavailability of tyrosine kinase inhibitors: an added component of assessment. *Clinical Journal of Oncology Nursing, 18*(6), 714–716.

Abueg, K. (2017). Interprofessional management of toxicities related to cancer precision medicine. *Seminars In Oncology Nursing, 33*(4), 376–383.

American Society of Clinical Oncology (ASCO). (2018). *Understanding immunotherapy.* https://www.cancer.net/navigating-cancer-care/how-cancer-treated/immunotherapy-and-vaccines/understanding-immunotherapy.

Bayer, V., Amaya, B., Baniewicz, D., Callahan, C., Marsh, L., & McCoy, A. S. (2017). Cancer immunotherapy: an evidence-based overview and implications for practice. *Clinical Journal of Oncology Nursing, 21*(2), 13–21.

Beatty, G. L., & Gladney, W. L. (2015). Immune escape mechanisms as a guide for cancer immunotherapy. *Clinical Cancer Research, 21,* 687–692. https://doi.org/10.1158/1078-0432.CCR-14-1860.

Brahmer, J.R., Lacchetti, C., Schneider, B.J., et al. (2018). Management of immune-related adverse events in patients treated with immune checkpoint inhibitor therapy: American Society of Clinical Oncology Clinical Practice Guideline. *Journal of Clinical Oncology,* Feb14. Available at: http://ascopubs.org/doi/abs/10.1200/JCO.2017.77.6385.

Brudno, J. N., & Kochenderfer, J. N. (2016). Toxicities of chimeric antigen receptor T cells: recognition and management. *Blood, 127*(26), 3321–3330. https://doi.org/10.1182/blood-2016-04-703751.

Bryce, J., & Boers-Doets, C. B. (2014). Non-rash dermatologic adverse events related to targeted therapies. *Semin Oncol Nurs, 30*(3), 155–168. https://doi.org/10.1016/j.soncn.2014.05.003.

Califano, R., Tariq, N., Compton, S., Fitzgerald, D. A., Harwood, C. A., Lal, R., & Nicolson, M. (2015). Expert consensus on the management of adverse events from EGFR tyrosine kinase inhibitors in the UK. *Drugs, 75*(12), 1335–1348. https://doi.org/10.1007/s40265-015-0434-6.

Common Terminology Criteria for Adverse Events (CTCAE). (November 27, 2017). Version 5.0. Published https://ctep.cancer.gov/protocoldevelopment/electronic_applications/docs/CTCAE_v5_Quick_Reference_5x7.pdf. accessed March 17, 2017.

de Groot, A. F., Kuijpers, C. J., & Kroep, J. R. (2017). CDK4/6 inhibition in early and metastatic breast cancer: a review. *Cancer Treat Rev, 60,* 130–138. https://doi.org/10.1016/j.ctrv.2017.09.003.

De Jesus-Gonzalez, N., Robinson, E., Moslehi, J., & Humphreys, B. D. (2012). Management of antiangiogenic therapy-induced hypertension. *Hypertension, 60*(3), 607–615. https://doi.org/10.1161/HYPERTENSIONAHA.112.196774

Dy, G. K., & Adjei, A. A. (2013). Understanding, recognizing, and managing toxicities of targeted anticancer therapies. *CA: A Cancer Journal for Clinicians, 63*(4), 249–279. https://doi.org/10.3322/caac.21184.

Eaby-Sandy, B., & Lynch, K. (2014). Side effects of targeted therapies: rash. *Semin Oncol Nurs, 30*(3), 147–154. https://doi.org/10.1016/j.soncn.2014.06.001.

Eggert, J. (2017). Precision medicine: biologics and targeted therapies. In J. Eggert (Ed.), *Cancer basics* (2nd ed.). Pittsburgh, PA: Oncology Nursing Society.

Escalante, C. P., Lu, M., & Marten, C. A. (2016). Update of targeted therapy-induced hypertension: basics for non-oncology providers. *Curr Hypertens Rev, 12*(2), 112–120.

Finn, R. S., Aleshin, A., & Slamon, D. J. (2016). Targeting the cyclin-dependent kinases (CDK) 4/6 in estrogen receptor-positive breast cancers. *Breast Cancer Res, 18*(1), 17. https://doi.org/10.1186/s13058-015-0661-5.

Fischer-Cartlidge, E. A. (2014). Assessment and management of gastrointestinal toxicities and lab abnormalities related to targeted therapy. *Semin Oncol Nurs, 30*(3), 183–189. https://doi.org/10.1016/j.soncn.2014.05.006.

Food & Drug Administration (FDA). (2016). *Principles for codevelopment of an in vitro companion diagnostic device with a therapeutic product.* https://www.fda.gov/downloads/MedicalDevices/DeviceRegulationandGuidance/GuidanceDocuments/UCM510824.pdf.

Food & Drug Administration (FDA). (2017). *Companion testing* https://www.fda.gov/MedicalDevices/ProductsandMedicalProcedures/InVitroDiagnostics/ucm407297.htm.

Fukuhara, H., Ino, Y., & Todo, T. (2016). Oncolytic virus therapy: a new era of cancer treatment at dawn. *Cancer Sci, 107*(10), 1373–1379. https://doi.org/10.1111/cas.13027.

Gordon, R., Kasler, M. K., Stasi, K., Shames, Y., Errante, M., Ciccolini, K., & Fischer-Cartlidge, E. (2017). Checkpoint inhibitors: common immune-related adverse events and their management. *Clin J Oncol Nurs, 21*(2 Suppl), 45–52. https://doi.org/10.1188/17.CJON.S2.45-52.

Hofheinz, R. D., Segaert, S., Safont, M. J., Demonty, G., & Prenen, H. (2017). Management of adverse events during treatment of gastrointestinal cancers with epidermal growth factor inhibitors. *Crit Rev Oncol Hematol, 114,* 102–113. https://doi.org/10.1016/j.critrevonc.2017.03.032.

Jeggo, P. A., Pearl, L. H., & Carr, A. M. (2016). DNA repair, genome stability and cancer: a historical perspective. *Nat Rev Cancer, 16* (1), 35–42. https://doi.org/10.1038/nrc.2015.4.

Kubiczkova, L., Pour, L., Sedlarikova, L., Hajek, R., & Sevcikova, S. (2014). Proteasome inhibitors - molecular basis and current perspectives in multiple myeloma. *J Cell Mol Med, 18*(6), 947–961. https://doi.org/10.1111/jcmm.12279.

Lacouture, M. (2016). Management of dermatologic toxicities associated with targeted therapy. *Journal of the Advanced Practitioner in Oncology, 7*(3), 331–334.

Lacouture, M. E., Maitland, M. L., Segaert, S., Setser, A., Baran, R., Fox, L. P., & Trotti, A. (2010). A proposed EGFR inhibitor dermatologic adverse event-specific grading scale from the MASCC skin toxicity study group. *Support Care Cancer, 18* (4), 509–522. https://doi.org/10.1007/s00520-009-0744-x

Liu, H.-B., Wu, Y., Lv, T.-F., et al. (2013). Skin rash could predict the response to EGFR tyrosine kinase inhibitor and the prognosis for patients with non-small cell lung cancer: a systematic review and meta-analysis. *PLoS ONE, 8*(1). https://doi.org/10.1371/journal.pone.0055128.

Liu, S., & Kurzrock, R. (2015). Understanding toxicities of targeted agents: implications for anti-tumor activity and management. *Semin Oncol, 42*(6), 863–875. https://doi.org/10.1053/j.seminoncol.2015.09.032.

Lord, C. J., & Ashworth, A. (2017). PARP inhibitors: synthetic lethality in the clinic. *Science*, *355*(6330), 1152–1158. https://doi.org/10.1126/science.aam7344.

Macdonald, J. B., Macdonald, B., Golitz, L. E., LoRusso, P., & Sekulic, A. (2015). Cutaneous adverse effects of targeted therapies: part I: inhibitors of the cellular membrane. *J Am Acad Dermatol*, *72*(2), 203–218. quiz 219-220. https://doi.org/10.1016/j.jaad.2014.07.032.

Martelli, A. M., Buontempo, F., & McCubrey, J. A. (2018). Drug discovery targeting the mTOR pathway. *Clin Sci (Lond)*, *132*(5), 543–568. https://doi.org/10.1042/CS20171158.

McGettigan, S., & Rubin, K. M. (2017). PD-1 inhibitor therapy: consensus statement from the faculty of the melanoma nursing initiative on managing adverse events. *Clin J Oncol Nurs*, *21*(4), 42–51. https://doi.org/10.1188/17.CJON.S4.42-51. Suppl.

Michot, J. M., Bigenwald, C., Champiat, S., Collins, M., Carbonnel, F., Postel-Vinay, S., & Lambotte, O. (2016). Immune-related adverse events with immune checkpoint blockade: a comprehensive review. *Eur J Cancer*, *54*, 139–148. https://doi.org/10.1016/j.ejca.2015.11.016.

National Cancer Institute (NCI). (2013). *Biological therapies for cancer*. https://www.cancer.gov/about-cancer/treatment/types/immunotherapy/bio-therapies-fact-sheet.

National Cancer Institute (NCI). (2015). *NCI dictionary of cancer terms*. https://www.cancer.gov/publications/dictionaries/cancer-terms.

National Cancer Institute (NCI). (2018). *Targeted cancer therapies*. https://www.cancer.gov/about-cancer/treatment/types/targeted-therapies/targeted-therapies-fact-sheet.

Padma, V. V. (2015). An overview of targeted cancer therapy. *Biomedicine (Taipei)*, *5*(4), 19. https://doi.org/10.7603/s40681-015-0019-4.

Pessi, M. A., Zilembo, N., Haspinger, E. R., Molino, L., Di Cosimo, S., Garassino, M., & Ripamonti, C. I. (2014). Targeted therapy-induced diarrhea: a review of the literature. *Crit Rev Oncol Hematol*, *90*(2), 165–179. https://doi.org/10.1016/j.critrevonc.2013.11.008.

Puzanov, I., Diab, A., Abdallah, K., Bingham, C. O., 3rd, Brogdon, C., Dadu, R. . . . Society for Immunotherapy of Cancer Toxicity Management Working, G. (2017). Managing toxicities associated with immune checkpoint inhibitors: consensus recommendations from the Society for Immunotherapy of Cancer (SITC) Toxicity Management Working Group. *J*

Immunother Cancer, *5*(1), 95. https://doi.org/10.1186/s40425-017-0300-z.

Segaliny, A. I., Tellez-Gabriel, M., Heymann, M. F., & Heymann, D. (2015). Receptor tyrosine kinases: characterisation, mechanism of action and therapeutic interests for bone cancers. *J Bone Oncol*, *4*(1), 1–12. https://doi.org/10.1016/j.jbo.2015.01.001.

Smith, L. T., & Venella, K. (2017). Cytokine release syndrome: inpatient care for adverse events of CAR-T cell therapy. *Clinical Journal of Oncology Nursing*, *21*(2), 29–34. https://doi.org/10.1188/17.CJON.S2.29-34.

Spain, L., Diem, S., & Larkin, J. (2016). Management of toxicities of immune checkpoint inhibitors. *Cancer Treat Rev*, *44*, 51–60. https://doi.org/10.1016/j.ctrv.2016.02.001.

Staves, K., & Ramchandran, K. (2016). Prevention and treatment options for mTOR inhibitor-associated stomatitis. *The Journal of Community and Supportive Oncology*, *15*(2), 74–81.

Tajiri, K., Aonuma, K., & Sekine, I. (2017). Cardiovascular toxic effects of targeted cancer therapy. *Jpn J Clin Oncol*, *47*(9), 779–785. https://doi.org/10.1093/jjco/hyx071.

Tan, A. C., Vyse, S., & Huang, P. H. (2017). Exploiting receptor tyrosine kinase co-activation for cancer therapy. *Drug Discov Today*, *22*(1), 72–84. https://doi.org/10.1016/j.drudis.2016.07.010.

Teachey, D. T., Lacey, S. F., Shaw, P. A., Melenhorst, J. J., Maude, S. L., Frey, N., & Grupp, S. A. (2016). Identification of predictive biomarkers for cytokine release syndrome after chimeric antigen receptor T-cell therapy for acute lymphoblastic leukemia. *Cancer Discov*, *6*(6), 664–679. https://doi.org/10.1158/2159-8290.CD-16-0040.

Vogel, W., & Paul, J. (2016). Management strategies for adverse events associated with EGFR TKIs in non-small cell lung cancer. *Journal of the Advanced Practitioner in Oncology*, *7*(7), 723–735.

Walker, D. (2017). Hypertension. In S. Newton, M. Hickey, & J. Brant (Eds.), *Mosby's Oncology Nursing Advisor: a comprehensive guide to clinical practice* (2nd ed.). St. Louis, MO: Elsevier.

Xie, J., Wang, X., & Proud, C. (2016). mTOR inhibitors in cancer therapy. *F1000Research*, *5*(F1000 Faculty Review), 1-11. https://doi.org/doi:10.12688/f1000research.9207.1

Yang, J. C., & Rosenberg, S. A. (2016). Adoptive T-cell therapy for cancer. *Adv Immunol*, *130*, 279–294. https://doi.org/10.1016/bs.ai.2015.12.006.

30

Support Therapies and Access Devices

Dawn Camp-Sorrell

BLOOD COMPONENT THERAPY

Overview

I. Use of blood component therapy in cancer care has increased because of the following reasons (Connell, 2016; National Comprehensive Cancer Network [NCCN], 2017; Schmidt, Refaai, & Blumberg, 2016):
   A. Advancement of surgical oncology techniques
   B. Use of more aggressive single-modality and multi-modality cancer therapy and the resulting bone marrow suppression
   C. Development of donor programs, hemapheresis technology, and hematopoietic stem cell transplantation therapies, all of which serve to increase the available range of blood component therapies
   D. Less use of erythropoietin due to potential for disease progression

II. Types of blood component therapy (Table 30.1)

III. Sources of blood components (Basu & Kulkami, 2014; Connell, 2016)
   A. Homologous blood component—blood collected from screened donors for transfusion to another individual
   B. Autologous blood—blood collected from the intended recipient
      1. Self-donation usually made before elective surgery
      2. Red blood cell (RBC) salvage during surgery by use of automated "cell saver" device or manual suction equipment
   C. Directly donated blood—blood component collected from a donor designated by the intended recipient

IV. Benefits of transfusion (Basu & Kulkami, 2014; Connell, 2016; NCCN, 2017; Schiffer et al., 2017; West, Gea-Banacloche, Stroncek, & Kadri, 2017)
   A. RBCs—correction of anemia
      1. Hemoglobin should increase 1 g/dL or hematocrit by 3% with 1 unit
      2. Improvement of symptoms (e.g., fatigue, weakness, shortness of breath [SOB])
   B. Platelets—correction of thrombocytopenia
      1. Increase of 30 to 60 × 103/mL with 1 unit of apheresis platelets
      2. Decrease in signs of bleeding
   C. Plasma—correct clotting factor deficiencies, expand blood volume, provide osmotic diuresis
   D. White blood cells (WBCs)—increase of WBCs and decrease of infection risk
   E. Cryoprecipitate—corrects dilution of clotting factors secondary to massive hemorrhage, extensive transfusion, liver failure, or consumption coagulopathy secondary to disseminated intravascular coagulation (DIC) by raising fibrinogen level by 5 to 10 mg/dL
   F. IgG—maintain antibody levels, prevent infection, confer passive immunity

V. Potential complications of blood component therapy (Brand, 2016; Carson, Triulzi, & Ness, 2017; Cohen et al., 2017; Connell, 2016; DeLisle, 2018; Elemary et al., 2017; Henneman et al., 2017; Kim, Xia, Chang, & Pritts, 2016; Lozano & Cid, 2016; NCCN, 2017; Schiffer et al., 2017; Schmidt et al., 2016; West et al., 2017)
   A. Acute reactions: occurring with 24 hours of the transfusion ⚠
      1. Hemolytic reactions: usually due to ABO incompatibility
      2. Febrile nonhemolytic reactions: often a reaction to passively transfused cytokines
      3. Allergic reactions: hypersensitivity reaction to donor plasma proteins
      4. Anaphylaxis: reaction from antibody to donor plasma proteins (IgA, complement 4 or haptoglobin)
      5. Transfusion-associated circulatory overload (TACO): rapid infusion causing fluid to accumulate leading to pulmonary edema
      6. Hypothermia
      7. Bacteremia or sepsis
      8. Coagulation problems in massive transfusion (e.g., with hemorrhage)
      9. Metabolic derangement such as hypocalcemia or hyperkalemia
      10. Transfusion-related acute lung injury (TRALI): reaction caused by WBC antibodies in the transfused product reacting with patient's WBCs
      11. Urticaria reaction
   B. Delayed—develops at least 48 hours, months, or (rarely) years later

TABLE 30.1 Types of Blood Component Therapy

Blood Component	Indication	Consideration
Whole blood	Replacement of blood volume Replacement of RBCs	Rarely used, except in extreme loss of volume
RBCs (packed)	Correction of anemia, for replacement of RBCs	Volume overload
Leukocyte-reduced RBCs	Prior febrile reactions to packed RBCs Reduction of alloimmunizations Reduction of immunomodulatory effects	May use a leukocyte filter to further reduce risk of reaction
Washed or plasma-poor RBCs	Prior urticarial reaction, IgA deficiency	Increased viscosity of blood; thin with normal saline before transfusion
Frozen packed RBCs	Rare blood types, autologous donations	Used in patients with a history of severe RBC reactions
Platelets, pooled	Control or prevent bleeding; platelet count <10,000–20,000/mm^3 or patient is bleeding or preoperative	Few RBCs present; ABO compatibility not required
Single-donor platelets	Reduction of alloimmunization, lower risk of infection, exposure to one donor	Lack of adequate increase in platelet count
Leukocyte-reduced platelets	Prior febrile reaction to platelets Reduction of alloimmunization	Febrile reactions; poor increase in platelet count
HLA-matched platelets	Poor response to prior platelet transfusion because of alloimmunization	Obtain posttransfusion platelet count if HLA-matched platelets are used
Granulocytes	Documented refractory infection from bacteria or fungi not responsive to therapy, with severe neutropenia, not expected to recover for several days to 1 week	Long-term therapeutic effect questionable Transfuse within 24 hours after collection
Fresh frozen plasma	Increase in the level of clotting factors in patient with documented coagulation deficiency; expand blood volume, provide osmotic diuresis	Plasma compatibility preferred with recipient; when thawed, must transfuse within 24 hr; watch for fluid overload All coagulation factors present
Cryoprecipitate	Increase in levels of factors VIII and XIII, fibrinogen, fibronectin, and von Willebrand factor due to massive hemorrhage, extensive transfusion liver failure or consumption coagulopathy due to DIC	Plasma compatibility preferred; when thawed, must transfuse within 6 hr; if pooled, within 4 hr
Factor VIII	Hemophilia A or low AT III levels	In patients with volume overload problems, plasma cannot be used
Factor IX	Hemophilia B deficiency	Need replacement of factor; treated by injection of purified factor IX
Colloid solutions	Expand blood volume	ABO compatibility not required
Plasma substitutes	Chiefly 5% and 25% albumin and PPF	Provide volume expansion and colloid replacement without risk of hepatitis or HIV
Serum immune globulins	To provide passive immunity protection (e.g., against cytomegalovirus) or treat hypogammaglobulinemia	Avoid transfusion for patient with allergic reactions to plasma

AT, Antithrombin; *HIV,* human immunodeficiency virus; *HLA,* human leukocyte antigen; *IgA,* immunoglobulin A; *PPF,* plasma protein fraction; *RBCs,* red blood cells.

1. Hemolytic reactions causing immune destruction of transfused RBCs, which are attacked by the recipient's antibodies
2. Iron overload from frequent RBC transfusions
3. Refractory to blood products
4. Posttransfusion purpura: antibody destroys transfused and patient's own platelets
5. Transfusion-associated graft-versus-host disease (GVHD): rare occurrence due to engraftment of viable donor T cells from blood component in a susceptible recipient; blood cells irradiated to prevent
6. Alloimmunization—patient develops alloantibodies against the donor's antigens
7. Transmission of virus (e.g., hepatitis, HIV, herpes, cytomegalovirus [CMV], West Nile, Zika)

C. Transfusion of the incorrect product to the incorrect patient

Assessment

I. Factors that increase the likelihood for receipt of blood component therapy (Connell, 2016; NCCN, 2017; MacLennan, 2016; Schiffer et al., 2017; West et al., 2017)
   A. Cancer treatment (e.g., surgery, stem cell transplantation)
   B. Cancer that has invaded the bone marrow
   C. Drugs that suppress bone marrow production
   D. Chronic bacterial, fungal, or viral infection

E. Older age

F. Malnutrition, including deficiencies in folate, vitamin B_{12}, and iron

G. Chronic immune deficiency

H. Comorbidities—heart disease, diabetes, renal failure, liver disease

I. Acute blood loss

II. Evaluation of laboratory data (Basu & Kulkami, 2014; Brand, 2016; Carson et al., 2017; Connell, 2016; MacLennan, 2016; NCCN, 2017; Schiffer et al., 2017)

A. ABO type and Rh factor

B. Hemoglobin—transfusion guideline less than 7 g/dL or if symptomatic

C. Platelet count: transfusion guidelines
1. Less than 10,000/mm^3, with or without bleeding
2. Less than 20,000/mm^3, with active bleeding
3. Less than 50,000/mm^3 and scheduled for surgical procedure

D. Neutrophils—less than 500/mm^3, with an infection unresponsive to antibiotic therapy

E. International normalized ratio (INR) greater than 1.69 and partial thromboplastin time (PTT) and prothrombin time (PT) prolonged

F. DIC—laboratory assessment, if indicated: fibrinogen less than 150 mg/dL, fibrin/fibrinogen degradation products (FDPs) greater than 40, D-dimer assay elevated

G. Immunoglobulin G (IgG) level decreased

H. Autoantibodies—clinically significant; form from prior transfusions

Management

I. Medical management

A. Prevent and manage transfusion reactions (Cohen et al., 2017; Connell, 2016; DeLisle, 2018; Henneman et al., 2017)
1. Premedicate patient with antipyretics and antihistamines, usually acetaminophen and diphenhydramine, especially for previous reaction. Steroid may be added as premedication for severe reactions previously.
2. If a reaction occurs:
   a. Stop infusion and keep intravenous (IV) line open with normal saline (NS) solution.
   b. Report reaction to the provider and the transfusion service or blood bank.
   c. Recheck identifying tags and numbers on the blood component at the bedside.
3. Treat symptoms as ordered:
   a. Diphenhydramine—administer 25 to 50 mg intravenously.
   b. Hydrocortisone—have 50 to 100 mg IV available for severe reactions.
   c. Meperidine (Demerol)— 25 to 50 mg IV for uncontrolled rigors
   d. Acetaminophen—administer 650 to 1000 mg by mouth (PO).
   e. Oxygen—administer if indicated.

f. Diuretic—administer for fluid overload or reduce intravascular volume.

g. Epinephrine or solumedrol—administer for allergic/anaphylactic reaction.

h. Vasopressor support—administer if indicated for hypotension

4. Send blood bag, attached administration set, and labels to the blood bank or service.

5. Collect blood and urine samples.

B. Employ pharmacologic management as indicated (Connell, 2016)
1. Recombinant factor VIIa for patients with existing coagulopathy
   a. Activates factor X to factor Xa; activated factor Xa converts prothrombin to thrombin, then acts to convert fibrinogen to fibrin, forming a hemostatic plug
   b. Approved for treatment of bleeding episodes in hemophilia A or B patients with inhibitors to factor VIII or factor IX
   c. Potential use in those with DIC, liver disease, and thrombocytopenia refractory to human leukocyte antigen (HLA)–matched platelets
2. Vitamin K—essential for activating factors II, VII, IX, and X because its deficiency impairs the function of clotting factors
3. Artificial plasma indicated for treatment of shock, acute liver failure, acute respiratory distress syndrome (ARDS), severe hyponatremia, renal dialysis

II. Nursing Management

I. Maximize patient safety ⚠ (Basu & Kulkami, 2014; Brand, 2016; Cohen et al., 2017; Connell, 2016; Kim et al., 2016; Lozano & Cid, 2016; Schmidt et al., 2016)

A. Obtain, store, and administer blood components according to institutional protocol.

B. Ensure bacterial and viral screening of blood components.

C. Check blood component type with medical order, identification numbers with another registered nurse with patient identification information before administration.

D. Examine blood product for clots, bubbles, particulates, and discoloration.

E. Ensure that medications or IV fluids are never added to blood products.

F. Restrict transfusion to those who have clear indications for such therapy, and only transfuse the minimum number of units necessary.

G. Obtain transfusion informed consent.

H. Administer CMV-negative products to patients who do not have the virus.

II. Monitor for complications of blood component therapy (DeLiesle, 2018; Henneman et al., 2017; NCCN, 2017)

A. General signs/symptoms—fever, chills, muscle aches and pain, back pain, chest pain, headache, and warmth or redness at site of infusion or along vessel

B. Respiratory—SOB, tachypnea, apnea, cough, wheezing, rales, air embolism

C. Cardiovascular—bradycardia or tachycardia, hypotension or hypertension, facial flushing, cyanosis of extremities, cool clammy skin, distended neck veins, and edema

D. Integumentary—rash, hives, swelling, urticaria, posttransfusion purpura, diaphoresis

E. Gastrointestinal (GI)—nausea, vomiting, abdominal cramping, and pain

F. Renal—dark, concentrated, red- to brown-colored urine

G. Delayed complications—hemolytic transfusion reaction, GVHD (from nonirradiated blood), iron overload, alloimmunization, infections (hepatitis, HIV, CMV, bacterial contamination)

III. Decrease incidence and severity of transfusion reaction (Cohen et al., 2017; Connell, 2016; DeLisle, 2018; Elemary et al., 2017; Kim et al., 2016; NCCN, 2017; West et al., 2017)

A. Attach appropriate filter, blood component set, or both to the blood product

1. Use leukocyte reduction filter to reduce the number of leukocytes transfused to the patient in a unit of RBCs

2. Administer irradiated blood components to all allogeneic hematopoietic stem cell transplantation (HSCT) recipients and others to prevent transfusion of leukocytes

B. Use 22-gauge (preferably 20-gauge) or larger needle for infusion when transfusing RBCs and platelets

C. Infuse component over time, according to institutional guidelines

1. Packed RBCs—infuse slowly initial 15 minutes, then remainder over 1 to 3 hours per unit; no longer than 4 hours per unit from the time issued from the blood bank

2. Platelets—infuse random-donor or single-donor platelets over 15 to 30 minutes or according to volume

3. Granulocytes—infused slowly over 2 to 4 hours

4. Fresh frozen plasma—each unit administered slowly or as tolerated

5. Cryoprecipitate—infused rapidly over 15 minutes or less

6. Concentrated factor VIII or factor IX—infused rapidly over 15 minutes or less

D. Monitor for transfusion reaction—fever/chills, SOB, dyspnea, hives, wheezing, flank/back pain, hematuria, hypotension, tachycardia, chest pain, headache

E. Prevent and manage infusion reactions according to protocol (see earlier)

F. Document transfusion reaction

1. Date and time noted

2. Signs and symptoms observed

3. Actions taken

G. Monitor patient for approximately 2 hours after transfusion to ensure that an acute reaction does not occur

IV. Educate patient and family

A. Educate about the purpose of the transfusion or blood component therapy

B. Review of procedure for administration of blood component therapy

C. Educate about the signs/symptoms of transfusion reaction that should be reported

V. Monitor for response to blood component therapy

A. Monitor changes in laboratory values

B. Assess for changes in symptoms (e.g., reduction in fatigue or SOB)

C. Monitor for signs and symptoms of bleeding

VI. Patients who refuse blood component therapy (Elemary et al., 2017; NCCN, 2017)

A. Discuss reasons for refusal, such as religious beliefs that prohibit the use of blood products or personal preference

B. Techniques for minimization of blood loss or minimize transfusions

1. Minimize routine blood testing

2. Use pediatric blood collection tubes

3. Suppress menstrual cycles in patients with thrombocytopenia

4. Minimize GI bleeding with proton pump inhibitors and bowel management

5. Administer iron component therapy for iron deficiency

6. Ensure growth factor therapy when indicated

7. Avoid anticoagulation, including heparin flushes or alteplase use

8. Use vitamin supplementation such as folic acid, vitamin B, and vitamin K

ACCESS DEVICES—VENOUS, ARTERIAL, PERITONEAL, INTRAVENTRICULAR, EPIDURAL OR INTRATHECAL, AND PLEURAL

Overview

I. Access devices are essential in the care of patients with cancer because of the following (Camp-Sorrell & Matey, 2017; Conley, Buckley, Magarace, Hsieh, & Pedulla, 2017; Schiffer et al., 2013; Wang, Lin, Chou, Lin, & Huang, 2017):

A. Combination IV therapy in the treatment of cancer

B. Administering therapies into multiple body systems

C. Supportive therapy (nutritional support, antibiotics, blood component therapy)

D. Increased laboratory monitoring required with aggressive therapy

E. Use of pleural, arterial, peritoneal, epidural, intrathecal, and intraventricular therapy

II. Types of venous access devices
  A. Short-term or intermediate-term peripheral catheters—to infuse fluids, medications, blood products, and peripheral total parenteral nutrition (TPN) and to obtain blood specimens (Adams, Little, Vinsant, & Khandelwal, 2016; Bertoglio et al., 2017; Carr, Higgins, Cooke, Rippey, & Rickard, 2017)
    1. Description—single-lumen or multilumen catheters
    2. Insertion—peripherally in forearm or antecubital fossa into the cephalic, basilic, or median cubital vein
    3. Types
      a. Peripheral catheters—inserted into a peripheral vein; change as indicated
      b. Midline catheters—inserted into peripheral vein terminating in the axillary vein in the upper arm; used for therapy for up to 6 weeks or longer
  B. Nontunneled venous short-term catheters (Fang, Yang, Song, Jiang, & Liu, 2017; Simon & Summers, 2017)
    1. Description: immediate access; removal when clinically indicated; available in single or multilumen (up to five-lumen design)
    2. Insertion of nontunneled catheters centrally in jugular vein, subclavian vein, superior vena cava (SVC), or inferior vena cava
  C. Long-term venous catheters—maintained for months to years
    1. Overview—distal tip lies in the lower third of the SVC
      a. Power-injectable designs available to deliver power injection flow rates required for contrast-enhanced injections; withstand high infusion pressures
      b. Available with pressure-activated safety valve (PASV) located in the catheter hub; designed to permit fluid infusion and decrease risk of blood reflux
      c. Catheter tip must be confirmed before initial use—by ultrasound (during placement if used), fluoroscopy, or chest x-ray
      d. Available with open or closed distal tip
    2. Tunneled (Blanco-Guzman, 2018; Fang et al., 2017)
      a. Description—single-lumen or multilumen catheters
        (1) Dacron cuff attached to the catheter, becoming embedded into the subcutaneous (SC) tissue after tunneling
          (a) Stabilizes the catheter
          (b) Minimizes the risk of ascending infections up the tunnel
        (2) Antimicrobial cuff available at the exit site to prevent ascending microbes; releases antimicrobial activity for approximately 4 to 6 weeks

      b. Insertion—percutaneous insertion using the internal jugular in the interventional radiology (IR) or surgery under ultrasound or fluoroscopy
        (1) Once vein is cannulated, the guidewire is advanced into the vein.
        (2) Catheter is tunneled through the SC tissue to exit on the anterior chest, typically above the nipple line midway between the sternum and clavicle.
    3. Implanted port (Blanco-Guzman, 2018; Conley et al., 2017; Fang et al., 2017; Tabatabaie et al., 2017; Wang et al., 2017)
      a. Description—single- or double-port device
        (1) Port body with reservoir inside covered with self-sealing septum
        (2) Port body with an attached or nonattached catheter
        (3) Port is accessed with a straight or angled noncoring needle
      b. Types—anterior chest or peripheral (basilic, cephalic, or median cubital veins)
      c. Insertion in IR or surgery using ultrasound or fluoroscopy guidance
    4. Peripherally inserted central catheters (PICCs) (Fang et al., 2017; Kang et al., 2017)
      a. Description—single, double, or triple lumen
        (1) Approved for use up to 12 months; however, evidence supports longer duration if device is functioning without complication
        (2) Securement device stabilizes external portion at the antecubital fossa or just above the elbow
        (3) Insertion at the bedside or IR typically under ultrasound guidance
        (4) Inserted peripherally into the cephalic, accessory cephalic, basilic, or median cubital
III. Types of nonvenous access devices
  A. Arterial catheters (Camp-Sorrell & Matey, 2017; Homma, Onimaru, Matsuura, Robbins, & Fujii, 2016)
    1. Descriptions—for short- or long-term chemotherapy administration
      a. Smaller internal diameters and thicker walls because of higher vascular arterial pressure
      b. Delivers high concentrations of drug directly to the tumor with decreased systemic exposure
      c. One-way valve to prevent retrograde blood flow
      d. Intraarterial therapies are considered regional treatment, with the arterial catheter directly threaded into the artery that feeds the tumor
    2. Insertion in IR or surgery
      a. Catheter inserted into the artery for perfusion, usually hepatic artery, similar to venous

placement; hypogastric, femoral, and brachial arteries used

    b. Port or pump surgically placed in SC pocket over a bony prominence

  3. Types—temporary percutaneous, implanted arterial port, implanted pump

B. Peritoneal catheters—for administration of chemotherapy into the peritoneal cavity or for the treatment of ascites (Camp-Sorrell & Matey, 2017; Maleux et al., 2016; Woodley-Cook, Tarulli, Tan, Rajan, & Simons, 2016)

  1. Descriptions

    a. A single-lumen catheter; may have multiple fenestrated holes to permit increased distribution of chemotherapy

    b. Temporarily or permanently implanted into the peritoneal cavity

  2. Insertion in IR or surgery

    a. Catheter placed through the anterior abdominal wall at the level of the umbilicus with tip directed toward cul-de-sac of the pelvis

    b. Tunnel—catheter tunneled in the SC tissue side of the midline or abdomen

    c. Port—placed in SC pocket over a bony prominence, usually a lower rib

  3. Types—temporary catheter, tunneled catheter, implanted port

C. Intraventricular reservoir (Ommaya reservoir)—for access to the ventricular system as an alternative to repeated lumbar punctures; provides direct access to cerebrospinal fluid (CSF) (Camp-Sorrell & Matey, 2017)

  1. Description—dome-shaped with catheter attached

  2. Insertion— in IR or surgery, reservoir surgically placed under the scalp, and the catheter threaded into the lateral ventricle

D. Epidural and intrathecal catheters—for administration of opioid analgesics and anesthetic mediations, chemotherapy, CSF sampling, and antispasmodic agents intrathecally (Camp-Sorrell & Matey, 2017)

  1. Description

    a. Epidural—catheter placed in the epidural space

    b. Intrathecal—catheter inserted below the dura where CSF circulates

  2. Insertion in IR or surgery; at the bedside for short-term use

    a. Catheter inserted into the epidural space, usually at L2–3, L3–4, or L4–5 or intrathecal space, usually at L2–3, L3–4, or L4–5

    b. Tunneled in the SC tissue; exits the waist or side of the abdomen after catheter inserted into epidural or intrathecal space

    c. Pump implanted into a created SC pocket and placed over a bony prominence with catheter inserted into the epidural or intrathecal space

  3. Types—temporary catheter, tunneled catheter, implanted port

E. Intrapleural catheters: for administration of intrapleural medication and to drain the pleural cavity (Camp-Sorrell & Matey, 2017; Penz, Watt, Hergott, Rahman, & Psallidas, 2017)

  1. Description—single lumen with drainage side holes inserted through the chest wall into the pleural cavity between the visceral and parietal pleura

  2. Insertion: in IR or surgery, exception with temporary short term at bedside

  3. Types—nontunneled for short-term use, tunneled for long-term use

IV. Complications associated with access devices (Table 30.2) (Adams et al., 2016; Bell & O'Grady, 2017; Blanco-Guzman, 2018; Kramer, Smith, & Souweidane, 2014; Lau, Kosteniuk, Macdonald, & Megyesi, 2018; Maleux et al., 2016; Sayed et al., 2018; Simon &

TABLE 30.2 Interventions for Mechanical Complications of Access Devices

Complication	Prevention	Restoration of Problem
Occlusion	Maintain flushing routine, flush with pulsatile (push-pause) method to cause swirling action in device. Always flush with normal saline before and after drug administration, blood withdrawal, and administration of blood products. Avoid incompatible drugs.	Change patient position, roll on to right or left side, sit up, lie flat. Change intrathoracic pressures: have patient inhale fully and hold breath or exhale fully and hold breath. Attempt pulsatile method using normal saline-filled syringe (avoid using high force or high pressure) or administer fibrinolytic agent per provider order. If occlusion the result of clotted blood, tPA may be instilled with a provider order. If drug precipitate, determine type of drug, check with pharmacist for drug to dissolve precipitate such as the following: • Lipids dissolve with ethyl alcohol 70% • Drugs dissolve with sodium bicarbonate (1 mEq/mL) or hydrochloric acid (0.1 N)

Continued

TABLE 30.2	Interventions for Mechanical Complications of Access Devices—cont'd	
Complication	**Prevention**	**Restoration of Problem**
Pinch-off syndrome	Proper placement by surgeon	Surgical removal is performed, as indicated, to avoid fracture.
Catheter dislodgement	Avoid pulling on the catheter Use securement device Teach patient to avoid manipulation of catheter or port and prevent trauma to catheter	Refer to physician for resuturing if tip of the catheter remains in the vessel Remove device, as indicated
Catheter migration	Protect device from trauma Anchor device appropriately with securement device Monitor length of catheter (tunnel, midline, PICC) to ensure placement intact Radiography ordered for long-term catheters to confirm placement	Refer to physician for repositioning catheter using fluoroscopy Remove device, as indicated
Catheter pinholes, tracks, cuts	Avoid use of scissors or sharp objects near the catheter Clamp properly over reinforced area on catheter	Repair using appropriate repair kit
Erosion of port through subcutaneous tissue	Avoid placing port at sites of actual or potential tissue damage (in radiation field) Avoid trauma or pressure over port	Device removal
Port–catheter separation	High-pressure infusions or flushing with 1- or 3-mL syringes when clogged	Remove device
Dislodgement of port access needle	Secure needle in place Avoid tension on the needle or tubing	Remove needle, and reaccess port using a sterile noncoring needle

Summers, 2017; Tabatabaie et al., 2017; Woodley-Cook et al., 2016)

A. Infection—presence of redness, pain, swelling, warmth, or drainage at exit site or along tunnel or pocket
   1. Preventive measures
      a. Most infections occur at the insertion or access site, hub of catheter, or both. Catheters coated with chlorhexidine, silver sulfadiazine, or antibiotics are recommended to decrease infection in short-term, nontunneled venous catheters.
      b. Hubs can be coated with antiinfective agents such as chlorhexidine.
      c. Use antiseptic before accessing needleless connectors or hubs.
      d. Removal of catheter based on clinical judgment and need for the device.
   2. Dressing changes (Camp-Sorrell & Matey, 2017; Conley et al., 2017; Schiffer et al., 2013)
      a. Gauze—changed every other day or prn (as needed) if soiled or nonocclusive
      b. Transparent—changed every 7 days or prn if soiled or nonocclusive
      c. Exit site cleansed with chlorhexidine solution
      d. Use of needleless connectors and protective caps to minimize risk of infections recommended
   3. Bundle care to include the following:
      a. Frequent hand washing before and after use
      b. Optimal catheter site selection
      c. Maximal sterile barrier precautions on insertion of device

      d. Alcohol hub decontamination before each access
      e. Review line necessity daily with prompt removal of unnecessary lines

B. Occlusion—inability to infuse fluid, or difficulty infusing, or inability to withdraw blood or fluid from a body cavity—that is, peritoneal fluid (Camp-Sorrell & Matey, 2017; Conley et al., 2017; Hajjar, 2017; Tabatabaie et al., 2017)
   1. Occlusion—occurs in up to 40% of patients within 1 to 2 years of device placement
      a. Fibrin sheath—may form at the catheter tip, causing a one-way valve effect, allowing infusion of IV fluids into the patient but causing withdrawal occlusion. Most common cause of thrombotic occlusion and the most common cause of partial occlusion.
      b. Intraluminal blood clot—may cause complete obstruction by forming around the catheter surface.
      c. Mural thrombus—a clot that adheres to the vessel wall, forming a thrombus, and occludes the tip of the catheter.
      d. Deep vein thrombosis (DVT)—occludes the vein, typically in the upper extremity. Most commonly found in the subclavian; can be axillary, brachial, and brachiocephalic veins.
   2. Precipitation—occurs when incompatible medications or solutions are simultaneously infused, or sequentially infused without adequate flushing in between

3. Mechanical withdrawal occlusions
   a. Pinch-off syndrome—catheter becomes pinched between the clavicle and the first rib, with possible catheter fracture (Camp-Sorrell & Matey, 2017).
   b. When complete fracture occurs, the distal portion of the catheter can travel to the jugular vein, superior vena cava, heart cavities, or lung.
4. Use device-specific flushing procedures according to current guidelines to prevent occlusion (Camp-Sorrell & Matey, 2017; Conley et al., 2017; Schiffer et al., 2013)

C. Catheter tip migration—regional discomfort, pain, swelling, or difficulty in using device or catheter fracture or tear

D. Air embolism—presence of sudden-onset pallor or cyanosis, SOB, cough, or tachycardia

E. Pneumothorax—presence of SOB, chest pain, or tachycardia
   1. Follow-up imaging after placement
   2. Close monitoring of patient; chest radiography to assess for pneumothorax

F. Arterial injury—bleeding at exit or entrance site caused by puncture of artery near access site; close monitoring of patient after placement

G. Phlebitis—mechanical or chemical irritation that may cause injury to vein; close monitoring of exit site (Kang et al., 2017)

H. Extravasation—(see Chapter 28)

I. Arrhythmia—caused by line placement in right atrium or ventricle; reposition catheter

V. Infusion systems are essential in patients with cancer because of need to administer chemotherapy, opioids, antibiotics, antifungals, and nutritional therapy in a variety of settings, including the patient's home. Three basic infusion systems exist (Table 30.3) (Armstrong, Byron, & Hamill, 2017; Camp-Sorrell & Matey, 2017; Chambers, Pabia, Sawyer, & Tang, 2017; Kim, Peterfreund, & Lovich, 2017; Mandel, 2017; Salman et al., 2017)

Assessment (Blanco-Guzman, 2018; Camp-Sorrell & Matey, 2017; Conley et al., 2017; Simon & Summers, 2017)

I. Identify potential candidates for access devices and informed consent obtained
II. Physical examination
   A. Evaluate potential device insertion site
   B. Evaluate condition of skin over potential insertion site
   C. Assess patency of access device
   D. Evaluate patient for potential infection, because most devices would not be placed in the presence of a bloodstream infection
   E. Assess for coagulopathies and low platelet, as ordered, to assess for bleeding potential
   F. Assess current medications, especially for anticoagulants and aspirin
III. Psychosocial examination
   A. Ability of patient or family to care for the access device when applicable
   B. Knowledge of procedures for use of access device for therapy
   C. Concerns expressed about implications of insertion of device
   D. Anxiety related to the procedure

Management

I. Medical management
   A. Manage access device infection

TABLE 30.3 Infusion Systems

Infusion System	Use	Method	Infusion rates/Volume	Mechanism	Alarms	Comments	Complications
Peristaltic	Blood products; IV medications; TPN, IVF, chemotherapy	C/I	Wide range; low to high rates and volume; dual chamber for simultaneous infusions	Linear/rotary peristaltic to propel fluid forward	Visual and audible	Smart pump technology	Occlusion; kinked tubing; pump malfunction
Syringe	Concentrated drugs or antibiotics; chemotherapy	I	Small volume; rate regulated by size of syringe	Motor-driven gear mechanism propels fluid by forcing plunger of syringe	Audible	Smart pump technology; lightweight; portable	Kinked tubing; pump malfunction
Elastomeric	Antibiotics, chemotherapy	I	Small volume	Infusion pressure when filled causes membrane to deflate	None	Lightweight; portable	Empty reservoir due to runaway rate

C/I, Continuous and intermittent; *IV*, intravenous; *TPN*, total parenteral nutrition.

1. Administer antibiotics, as indicated
   a. Vancomycin recommended for empiric therapy until organism identified
   b. Adjustment of antibiotics based on culture results
   c. Consider the use of antibiotic lock therapy in patients diagnosed with catheter-related infection, or at a high risk of infection, or myelosuppressed.
2. Remove access device, as indicated
3. Complicated infection, tunnel, or port pocket infection
4. Endocarditis, osteomyelitis, or septic thrombosis
5. Totally occluded catheter from thrombosis or precipitation
6. Septic shock
7. Recurrent line infection despite adequate antibiotic therapy
8. Therapy completed
   B. Ensure accurate device placement
   1. Obtain radiographic confirmation before accessing the device initially to ensure correct placement
   2. Dye study can be ordered if the device needs to be reassessed because of lack of blood draw or inability to infuse
   C. Maintain catheter patency
   1. Administer anticoagulant or fibrinolytic, as indicated
   2. Upper extremity DVT—anticoagulation therapy while device in place, may need to continue anticoagulation for a time after removal
   3. Tissue plasminogen activator (tPA) administered, as indicated, to restore patency

Nursing Management

I. Maximize patient safety ⚠
   A. Maintain aseptic technique when entering or manipulating the device
   B. Teach patient and family emergency procedures if the device is damaged
   C. Obtain radiographic confirmation of device placement before initial use (radiographic imaging not necessary for peripheral and midlines)
   D. Teach family and patient how to care for and maintain access device according to agency policy and procedure
   1. Evaluate understanding of care, including return demonstration
   2. Provide visual aids in the teaching process
II. Minimize risks for complications of access devices (Camp-Sorrell & Matey, 2017; Chambers, Abaid, & Gauhar, 2017; Homma et al., 2016; Kiehela, Hamunen, & Heiskanen, 2017; Kramer et al., 2014; Maleux et al., 2016)
   A. Obtain cultures, as indicated
   1. Blood cultures drawn peripherally and through device
   2. Culture exit or entrance site and body fluid such as urine, peritoneal, or spinal fluid

Expected Patient Outcomes

I. The patient will progress toward the achievement of normal blood counts, normalized coagulation profile, and replete IgG levels.
II. The patient and family will be aware of blood product indications and when to report side effects.
III. The patient will receive access device therapy safely.
IV. The patient and family will identify potential problems of their individual access device, provide self-care when indicated, and know when to notify the health care team for complications.

REFERENCES

Adams, D. Z., Little, A., Vinsant, C., & Khandelwal, S. (2016). The midline catheter: a clinical review. *The Journal of Emergency Medicine, 51*, 252–258. https://doi.org/10.1016/j.jemermed.2016.05.029.

Armstrong, M., Byron, S., & Hamill, C. (2017). The role and safe use of the ambulatory syringe pump in palliative and end-of-life care. *International Journal of Palliative Nursing, 23*(3), 108–110. https://doi.org/10.12968/ijpn.2017.23.3.108.

Basu, D., & Kulkarni, R. (2014). Overview of blood components and their preparation. *Indian Journal of Anaesthesia, 58*, 529–537. https://doi.org/10.4103/0019-5049.144647.

Bell, T., & O'Grady, N. P. (2017). Prevention of central line-associated bloodstream infections. *Infectious Disease Clinics of North America, 31*, 551–559. https://doi.org/10.1016/j.idc.2017.05.007.

Bertoglio, S., van Boxtel, T., Goossens, G. A., Dougherty, L., Furtwanger, R., Lennan, E., … Stas, M. (2017). Improving outcomes of short peripheral vascular access in oncology and chemotherapy administration. *The Journal of Vascular Access, 18*(2), 89–96. https://doi.org/10.5301/jva.5000668.

Blanco-Guzman, M. O. (2018). Implanted vascular access device options: a focused review on safety and outcomes. *Transfusion, 58*(suppl 1), 558–568. https://doi.org/10.1111/trf.14503.

Brand, A. (2016). Immunological complications of blood transfusions. *Presse Medicale. 45*, https://doi.org/10.1016/j.LPM.2016.06.024 (7-8 Pt2 e313-324.

Camp-Sorrell, D., & Matey, L. (Eds.), (2017). *Access device standards of practice for oncology nursing*. Pittsburgh: Oncology Nursing Society.

Carr, P. J., Higgins, N. S., Cooke, M. L., Rippey, J., & Rickard, C. M. (2017). Tools, clinical prediction rules, and algorithms for the insertion of peripheral intravenous catheters in adult hospitalized patients: a systematic scoping review of literature. *Journal of Hospital Medicine 12*(10), epub, https://doi.org/10.12788/jhm.2836.

Carson, J. L., Triulzi, D. J., & Ness, P. M. (2017). Indications for and adverse effects of red-cell transfusion. *New England Journal of Medicine, 377*, 1261–1272. https://doi.org/10.1056/NEJMra1612789.

Chambers, D. M., Abaid, B., & Gauhar, U. (2017). Indwelling pleural catheters for nonmalignant effusions: evidence-based answers to clinical concerns. *The American Journal of the Medical Sciences, 354*, 230–235. https://doi.org/10.1016/j.amjms.2017.03.003.

Chambers, C. R., Pabia, M., Sawyer, M., & Tang, P. A. (2017). Baxter elastomeric pumps: feasibility of weight estimates. *Journal of Oncology Pharmacy Practice, 23*, 429–435. https://doi.org/10.1177/1078155216656928.

Cohen, R., Escorcia, A., Tasmin, F., Lima, A., Lin, Y., Lieberman, L., ... Cserti-Gazdewich, C. (2017). Feeling the burn: the significant burden of febrile nonhemolytic transfusion reactions. *Transfusion, 57*, 1674–1683. https://doi.org/10.1111/trf.14099.

Conley, S. B., Buckley, P., Magarace, L., Hsieh, C., & Pedulla, L. V. (2017). Standardizing best nursing practice for implanted ports. *Journal of Infusion Nursing, 40*, 165–174. https://doi.org/10.1097/NAN.0000000000000217.

Connell, N. T. (2016). Transfusion medicine. *Primary Care, 43*, 651–659. https://doi.org/10.1016/j.pop.2016-07.004.

DeLisle, J. (2018). Is this a blood transfusion reaction? Don't hesitate; check it out. *Journal of Infusion Nursing, 41*(1), 43–51. https://doi.org/10.1097/NAN.0000000000000261.

Elemary, M., Seghatchian, J., Stakiw, J., Bosch, M., Sabry, W., & Goubran, H. (2017). Transfusion challenges in hematology oncology and hematopoietic stem cell transplant – literature review and local experience. *Transfusion and Apheresis Science, 56*, 317–321. https://doi.org/10.1016/j.transci.2017.05.022.

Fang, S., Yang, J., Song, L., Jiang, Y., & Liu, Y. (2017). Comparison of three types of central venous catheters in patients with malignant tumor receiving chemotherapy. *Patient Preference and Adherence, 11*, 1197–1204. https://doi.org/10.2147/PPA.S142556.

Hajjar, K. A. (2017). Central venous catheter thrombosis and the fibrin sleeve: unraveling the mystery. *European Journal of Haematology, 98*(4), 318–319. https://doi.org/10.1111/ejh.12642.

Henneman, E. A., Andrzejewski, C., Gawlinski, A., McAfee, K., Panaccione, T., & Dziel, K. (2017). Transfusion-associated circulatory overload: evidence-based strategies to prevent, identify, and manage a serious adverse event. *Critical Care Nurse, 37*(5), 58–66. https://doi.org/10.4037/ccn2017770.

Homma, A., Onimaru, R., Matsuura, K., Robbins, K. T., & Fujii, M. (2016). Intra-arterial chemoradiotherapy for head and neck cancer. *Japanese Journal of Clinical Oncology, 46*(1), 4–12. https://doi.org/10.1093/jjco/hyv151.

Kang, J., Chen, W., Sun, W., Ge, R., Li, H., Ma, E., ... Liu, W. (2017). Peripherally inserted central catheter-related complications in cancer patients: a prospective study of over 50,000 catheter days. *Journal of Vascular Access, 18*(2), 153–157. https://doi.org/10.5301/jva.50000670.

Kiehela, L., Hamunen, K., & Heiskanen, T. (2017). Spinal analgesia for severe cancer pain: a retrospective analysis of 60 patients. *Scandinavian Journal of Pain, 17*, 140–145. https://doi.org/10.1016/j.sjpain.2017.04.073.

Kim, U. R., Peterfreund, R. A., & Lovich, M. A. (2017). Drug infusion systems: technologies, performance, and pitfalls. *Anesthesia and Analgesia, 124*, 1493–1505. https://doi.org/10.1213/ANE.0000000000001707.

Kim, Y., Xia, B. T., Chang, A. L., & Pritts, T. A. (2016). Role of leukoreduction of packed red blood cell units in trauma patients: a review. *International Journal of Hematology Research, 2*(2), 124–129. epub 10.17554/j.issn.2409-3548.2016.02.31.

Kramer, K., Smith, M., & Souweidane, M. M. (2014). Safety profile of long-term intraventricular access devices in pediatric patients receiving radioimmunotherapy for central nervous system malignancies. *Pediatric Blood and Cancer, 61*, 1590–1592. https://doi.org/10.1002/pbc.25080.

Lau, J. C., Kosteniuk, S. E., Macdonald, D. R., & Megyesi, J. F. (2018). Image-guided ommaya reservoir insertion for intraventricular chemotherapy: a retrospective series. *Acta Neurochirurgica, 160*, 539–544. https://doi.org/10.1007/s00701-017-3454-z.

Lozano, M., & Cid, J. (2016). Platelet concentrates: balancing between efficacy and safety? *Presse Medicale, 45*, e289–e298. https://doi.org/10.1016/ j.LPM.2016.06.020.

MacLennan, S. (2016). Focus on fresh frozen plasma – facilitating optimal management of bleeding through collaboration between clinicians and transfusion specialists on component specifications. *Presse Medicale, 45*, e299–e302. https://doi.org/10.1016/ j.LPM.2016.06.021.

Maleux, G., Indesteege, I., Laenen, A., Verslype, C., Vergote, I., & Prenen, H. (2016). Tenckhoff tunneled peritoneal catheter placement in the palliative treatment of malignant ascites: technical results and overall clinical outcome. *Radiology and Oncology, 50*(2), 197–203. https://doi.org/10.1515/raon-2016-0002.

Mandel, J. E. (2017). Understanding infusion pumps. *Anesthesia and Analgesia*, Aug 30, epub. https://doi.org/10.1213/ANE.0000000000002396.

National Comprehensive Cancer Network (NCCN). (2017). *Cancer and chemotherapy-induced anemia guidelines, version 2* (p. 2018). http://www.nccn.org/professionals/physician_gls/pdf/anemia.pdf.

Penz, E., Watt, K. N., Hergott, C. A., Rahman, N. M., & Psallidas, I. (2017). Management of malignant pleural effusion: challenges and solutions. *Cancer Management and Research, 9*, 229–241. https://doi.org/10.2147/CMAR.S95663.

Salman, D., Biliune, J., Kayyali, R., Ashton, J., Brown, P., McCarthy, T., ... Nabhani-Gebara, S. (2017). Evaluation of the performance of elastomeric pumps in practice: are we under-delivering on chemotherapy treatments? *Current Medical Research and Opinion, 33*, 2153–2159. https://doi.org/10.1080/03007995.2017.1374936.

Sayed, D., Monroe, F., Orr, W. N., Phadnis, M., Khan, T. W., Braun, E., ... Nicol, A. (2018). Retrospective analysis of intrathecal drug delivery: outcomes, efficacy, and risk for cancer-related pain at a high volume academic medical center. *Neuromodulation*, Feb 14, epub. https://doi.org/10.1111/ner.12759.

Schiffer, C. A., Bohlke, K., Delaney, M., Hume, H., Magdalinski, A. J., McCullough, J. L., ... Anderson, K. C. (2017). Platelet transfusion for patients with cancer: American Society of Clinical Oncology clinical practice guideline update. *Journal of Clinical Oncology, 36*, 283–299. https://doi.org/10.1200/JCO.2017.76.1734.

Schiffer, C. A., Mangu, P. B., Wade, J. C., Camp-Sorrell, D., Dope, D. G., El-Rayes, B. F. , et al. (2013). Central venous catheter care for the patient with cancer: American Society of Clinical Oncology clinical practice guideline. *Journal of Clinical Oncology*, 1–15, https://doi.org/e-pub. 10.1200/JOP.2012.000780.

Schmidt, A. E., Refaai, M. A., & Blumberg, N. (2016). Past, present and forecast of transfusion medicine: what has changed and what is expected to change? *Presse Medicale, 45*, e253–e272. https://doi.org/10.1016/ j.LPM.2016.06.017.

Simon, E. M., & Summers, S. M. (2017). Vascular access complications: an emergency medicine approach. *Emergency Medical Clinics of North America, 35*, 771–788. https://doi.org/10.1016/j.emc.2017.06.004.

Tabatabaie, O., Kasumova, G. G., Eskander, M. F., Critchlow, J. F., Tawa, N. E., & Tseng, J. F. (2017). Totally implantable venous access devices: a review of complications and management strategies. *American Journal of Clinical Oncology*, 40(1), 94–105. https://doi.org/10.1097/COC.0000000000000361.

Wang, Y. C., Lin, P. L., Chou, W. H., Lin, C. P., & Huang, C. H. (2017). Long-term outcomes of totally implantable venous access devices. *Supportive Care in Cancer*, 25, 2049–2054. https://doi.org/10.1007/s00520-017-3592-0.

West, K. A., Gea-Banacloche, J., Stroncek, D., & Kadri, S. S. (2017). Granulocyte transfusions in the management of invasive fungal infections. *British Journal of Haematology*, 177, 357–374. https://doi.org/10.1111/bjh.14597.

Woodley-Cook, J., Tarulli, E., Tan, K. T., Rajan, D. K., & Simons, M. E. (2016). Safety and effectiveness of percutaneously inserted peritoneal ports compared to surgically inserted ports in a retrospective study of 87 patients with ovarian carcinoma over a 10-year period. *Cardiovascular and Interventional Radiology*, 39, 1629–1635. https://doi.org/10.1007-s00270-016-1433-z.

Pharmacologic Interventions

Tia Wheatley and Rowena N. Schwartz

ANTIMICROBIALS (BOW, 2015; NATIONAL COMPREHENSIVE CANCER NETWORK, 2018a; SHELTON, 2018; WINGARD, 2016; ZITELLA, 2014)

Overview

I. Rationale and indications
   A. For treatment of active infections
      1. Neutropenia, immunodeficiency associated with primary cancer, immune suppression, and mucosal barrier injury increase risk of infection in cancer patients.
         a. Splenectomy and functional asplenia
         b. Immunosuppressive agents, including but not limited to corticosteroids, purine analog (e.g., cladribine), alemtuzumab, anti-CD20 monoclonal antibodies (e.g., rituximab), and temozolomide
      2. Due to compromised immune function, patients with cancer may not exhibit typical signs and symptoms of infection.
      3. Prompt treatment of suspected infection is required to prevent sepsis and life-threatening sequelae.
   B. For prophylaxis use to prevent infection in high-risk populations (examples follow)
      1. Patients with anticipated absolute neutrophil count <500 cells/microL for >7 days, including but not limited to:
         a. Hematopoietic stem cell transplantation
         b. Chemotherapy induction for acute myeloid leukemia
      2. Patients receiving immunosuppressive therapy (see earlier)
      3. Patients with prior infections or active infection at time of treatment

II. Types of antimicrobial drugs (Table 31.1)
   A. Agents: antibacterial agents, antifungal agents, antiviral agents, vaccinations

B. Initial evaluation
   1. Fever may be the earliest and/or only warning sign of infection. ⚠️
      a. Antipyretics, including acetaminophen, aspirin, and nonsteroidal antiinflammatory agents, should be avoided in individuals at risk for infection and/or neutropenia, as they may mask fever. Evaluate concurrent medication use (including over-the-counter [OTC] medications) before therapy to assure discontinuation of antipyretics; patient/caregiver education about avoiding antipyretics is essential.
      b. Temperature threshold for neutropenic patients is defined as a single oral temperature 38.3°C (101°F) or a sustained temperature of 38°C (100.4°F) over 1 hour.
      c. Assure patient and caregiver have thermometer to measure temperature.
      d. For accurate results, axillary temperatures should be avoided. Rectal temperatures should also be avoided to prevent potential injury to the rectal mucosa.
      e. Fever is one sign of infection; patients with symptoms of infection without fever should be considered to have an infection (e.g., productive cough, burning on urination, diarrhea, redness or swelling of the skin or mucosa, pain).
   2. History and physical examination
      a. Evaluate patient and family history of infection.
      b. Evaluate presence of patient risk factors for infection, including comorbidities, concurrent medications, and prior history of exposures and infections.
      c. Assess for signs and symptoms of organ-specific infection or inflammation.
      d. Laboratory and radiology evaluation
         (1) Complete blood count with differential, blood chemistry, liver function, renal

TABLE 31.1 Antimicrobials Used for the Immunocompromised Patient

Antibacterials

Penicillins

- Natural or semisynthetic antibiotics produced by or derived from fungus *Penicillium*
- β-lactam antibiotics structurally and pharmacologically related to other β-lactam antibiotics, including cephalosporins
- Penicillins are divided into groups, including natural penicillins (e.g., penicillin G), penicillinase-resistant penicillins (e.g. oxacillin), aminopenicillins (e.g., ampicillin), and extended-spectrum penicillins (e.g., piperacillin)
- Extended-spectrum penicillins have wider activity than the other groups of penicillins, and are available in the United States only in fixed combinations with β-lactamase inhibitors (e.g., clavulanate or tazobactam)

Drug	Coverage Summary	Dose	Comments
Piperacillin-tazobactam (Zosyn)	Gram-positive aerobic bacteria Gram-negative aerobic bacterial Anaerobic bacteria	4.5 h IV every 6 hr Consider dose reduction with renal dysfunction	First-line therapy for neutropenic fever May produce false-positive galactomannan Should not be used for meningitis Common adverse effects: Hypersensitivity/rash, drug fever, diarrhea

Cephalosporins

- Cephalosporins are semisynthetic β-lactam antibiotics that are pharmacologically related to penicillins.
- Cephalosporins are divided into "generations" based on the spectra of activity. First-generation cephalosporins are usually active against gram-positive cocci but have limited activity against gram-negative bacteria (e.g., cefazolin). Second-generation cephalosporins are usually active against bacteria susceptible to first-generation cephalosporins and most strains of *Haemophilus influenza* (e.g., cefaclor). Third-generation cephalosporins are less active against some gram-positive organisms but have increased activity against gram-negative bacteria compared with first and second generations (e.g., ceftriaxone). Fourth-generation has expanded spectrum against gram-negative bacteria, often including *P. aeruginosa* (e.g., cefepime). Fifth-generation cephalosporin has activity against both gram-positive and gram-negative bacteria, including activity against methicillin-resistant *S. aureus* (MRSA) (e.g., ceftaroline fosamil)

Drug	Coverage Summary	Dose	Comments
Ceftazidime (Fortaz, Tazicef) (third-generation cephalosporin)	Gram-negative bacteria Poor gram-positive activity (breakthrough streptococcal infections reported)	2 g IV every 8 hr (for febrile neutropenia) Dose adjustment needed for renal dysfunction	Limited activity against gram-positive bacteria and increasing resistance of gram-negative bacteria; not routinely used as empiric monotherapy in febrile neutropenia in most institutions. Increased resistance reported. Often considered second-line therapy for neutropenic fever due to limitation in coverage compared with other agents. Ceftazidime/avibactam is a combination product. Avibactam inactivates β-lactamases. Common adverse effects: Hypersensitivity/rash, drug fever, diarrhea
Cefepime (Maxipime) (fourth-generation cephalosporin)	Gram-positive bacteria Gram-negative bacteria	2 g IV every 8 hr (for febrile neutropenia) Dose adjustments needed for renal dysfunction	Option for initial empiric therapy for febrile neutropenic patient. Not active against *Enterococcus* species. Not active against most anaerobes.
Ceftaroline fosamil (Teflaro)	Gram-positive bacteria MRSA Gram-negative bacteria	600 mg IV every 12 hr Dose adjustments needed for renal dysfunction	Indicated for community-acquired pneumonia and skin/skin structure infections.

TABLE 31.1 Antimicrobials Used for the Immunocompromised Patient—cont'd

Carbapenem
- Broad-spectrum activity against many gram-positive, gram-negative, and anaerobic organisms.

Doripenem	Gram-positive bacteria	500 mg IV q 8 hr	
Imipenem/cilastatin sodium	Gram-negative bacteria	500 mg IV q 6 hr	Increasing resistance seen in many institutions.
	Anaerobic organisms	Dose adjustment needed for renal dysfunction	Lowers seizure threshold.
Meropenem	Preferred against extended-spectrum beta-lactamase and serious *Enterobacter* infections	1–2 gram IV q 8 hr Dose adjustment needed for renal dysfunction	Effective for meningitis, nosocomial pneumonia, and intraabdominal infections. Carbapenemase-producing bacteria have been documented.

Fluoroquinolones
- Broad-spectrum antimicrobial agents
- Coverage is dependent on agent
- Avoid for empiric therapy if patient treated with fluoroquinolone prophylaxis

Ciprofloxacin (Cipro)	Gram-negative bacteria, including *P. aeruginosa* Atypical bacteria Limited gram-positive bacteria	PO 500–750 mg PO every 12 hr (with amoxicillin or clavulanic acid for low-risk febrile neutropenia) IV 400 mg IV every 8–12 hr Dose adjustments needed for renal dysfunction	Role in prevention of infection in immunocompromised host. Not as effective as others in the class for respiratory infection. Used in combination with amoxicillin/clavulanate for patients with low-risk febrile neutropenia. Should be used with caution in pediatric patients (tendon rupture).
Levofloxacin (Levaquin)	Gram-positive bacteria Gram-negative bacteria Atypical bacteria Limited anaerobic bacteria	PO 500–750 mg PO every 24 hr (prophylaxis of neutropenic fever) IV 500–750 mg IV every 24 hr Dose adjustment needed for renal dysfunction	Use as prophylaxis may increase gram-negative resistance.
Moxifloxacin (Avelox)	Gram-positive bacteria Limited gram-negative bacteria (limited activity against *Pseudomonas*) Atypical bacteria Anaerobic bacteria	400 mg PO every 24 hr 400 mg IV every 24 hr No dose adjustment needed for renal dysfunction	

Aminoglycosides
- Activity is primarily against gram-negative organisms
- Historically used as double coverage with another anti-*Pseudomonas* agent in neutropenic febrile patient; role has changed to use as double coverage based on sensitivities of identified agent and empirically in seriously ill or hemodynamically unstable patient with suspected infection.

Amikacin	Gram-negative bacteria	Weight-based dosing (extended interval) Dose modification based on renal dysfunction	Nephrotoxicity and ototoxicity limit use. Good activity against *Pseudomonas*. Used for double coverage of gram-negative infections. Dose is adjusted based on pharmacokinetic parameters.
Gentamicin	Gram-negative bacteria Gram-positive bacteria (synergy with beta-lactams)		
Tobramycin	Gram-negative bacteria		

Continued

TABLE 31.1   Antimicrobials Used for the Immunocompromised Patient—cont'd

Gram-Positive Antibacterial Agents

Vancomycin	Gram-positive bacteria No activity in VRE	15 mg/kg IV q 12 hr PO dosing is used for treatment of *C. difficile*: 125 mg PO every 6 hr Dose modifications required in renal dysfunction (based on drug serum concentrations)	Often added to cover gram-positive infection in patients with febrile neutropenia, although with increased incidence of resistance recommend limiting routine use. Doses adjusted based on drug serum trough concentrations.
Linezolid (Zyvox)	Gram-positive bacteria, including VRE and MRSA	IV: 600 mg IV every 12 hr PO: 600 mg PO every 12 hr	Hematologic toxicity (e.g., thrombocytopenia) seen most commonly with use >2 weeks. Serotonin syndrome may occur, use with caution with SSRI. Active against VRE.
Daptomycin (Cubicin)	Gram-positive bacteria	6 mg/kg/d IV Dose adjusted for renal function	Active against vancomycin-resistant enterococci, although not FDA approved for this indication. May cause rhabdomyolysis; monitor creatine phosphokinase (CPK) weekly. **Not active** against pulmonary infections due to inactivation by pulmonary surfactant.

Miscellaneous

Trimethoprim/ sulfamethoxazole (TMP/SMX) (Bactrim, Septra)	Activity against gram-negative and gram-positive bacteria (not active for *Pseudomonas*) *Pneumocystis jiroveci*	PO (prophylaxis for pneumocystis): single-strength tablet once daily, double-strength tablet three times weekly IV (treatment): 15 mg/kg daily in divided doses every 6–8 hr based on trimethoprim Dose adjustment required for renal dysfunction	Used as prophylaxis and treatment of *P. jiroveci* (commonly used with temozolomide therapy). Assure adequate kidney function, and maintain hydration throughout therapy (drug can precipitate in tubule). Monitor for myelosuppression.

Antifungals
Azoles

Fluconazole (Diflucan)	*Candida* (except *C. glabrata* and *C. krusei*)	100–400 mg IV/PO daily Dose adjustment required in renal dysfunction	Not active against molds. Prolongation of QTc, monitor other medications. Drug–drug interactions are common. Used as prophylaxis in high-risk patient populations (e.g., transplantation, acute leukemia).
Isavuconazonium (Cresemba)	Invasive aspergillosis and mucormycosis	Loading dose: 372 mg IV/PO q 8 hr × 6 doses followed by 372 mg IV/PO daily	Drug–drug interactions are common. Contraindicated in familial short QT syndrome.
Itraconazole (Sporanox)	*Candida* Aspergillosis Rare molds Dimorphic fungi *C. neoformans*	PO: 400 mg PO daily Loading doses used in some clinical situations	The capsule and oral solution formulation are not bioequivalent and therefore not interchangeable. Do not use with gastric acid–lowering agents, as they may inhibit absorption. Contraindicated in patients with significant cardiac systolic dysfunction.

10

TABLE 31.1 Antimicrobials Used for the Immunocompromised Patient—cont'd

Posaconazole (Noxafil)	*Candida* *Aspergillus* sp. *Zygomycetes* sp. Rare molds Dimorphic fungi *C. neoformans*	Prophylaxis: PO: 300 mg PO BID × 1 day, then 300 mg PO daily IV: 300 mg IV q 12 hr × 1 day then 300 mg IV daily Off-label use for treatment is a higher dose	Absorption related to stomach pH; avoid acid suppressants. Take with fatty food, nutritional substitute, or acidic beverage to increase absorption. Effective as prophylaxis in patients with acute myeloid leukemia and chronic graft-versus-host disease
Voriconazole (Vfend)	*Candida* *Aspergillus* Dimorphic fungi *C. neoformans*	IV: 6 mg/kg IV twice daily × two doses; then 4 mg/kg IV twice daily PO: 400 mg PO q 12 hr × 2 then dose based on weight q 12 hr Dose adjustment for renal function in IV formulation only	Poor activity against *Zygomycetes*. Used as empiric therapy in febrile neutropenia. Evidence suggests dose adjustments by weekly troughs increases efficacy. Target concentration for TDM = 1–5.5 mg/L.

Amphotericin B

Amphotericin B deoxycholate	*Candida* *Aspergillus* (not *Aspergillus terrus*) *Zygomycetes* *Cryptococcus* Dimorphic fungi	Dose: 0.5–1.5 mg/kg IV once daily	Nephrotoxicity, electrolyte wasting, and infusion reaction limit use. Alternative formulations have replaced this in clinical practice. Prehydration with normal saline and premedication with acetaminophen and diphenhydramine are necessary.
Liposomal amphotericin B (AmBisome)		3–5 mg/kg IV once daily	Less renal and infusional toxicity than deoxycholate.
Amphotericin B lipid complex (Abelcet)		5 mg/kg IV once daily	Less renal and infusional toxicity than deoxycholate.

Echinocandins

Anidulafungin (Eraxis)	*Candida*; *C. auris* may be resistant	200 mg IV on day 1, then 100 mg IV daily	First-line therapy for candidemia and invasive candidiasis.
Caspofungin (Cancidas)	*Aspergillus*	70 mg IV once daily × 1 dose; then 50 mg IV once daily Dose reduction for patients with liver dysfunction	Empiric therapy for febrile neutropenia when fungal coverage is needed. Poor CNS penetration.
Micafungin (Mycamine)		Prophylaxis: 50–100 mg IV once daily Treatment: 100–150 mg IV once daily	

Select Antivirals

Acyclovir	HSV VZV	Dose is based on clinical situation. Dosing is based on ideal body weight when weight-based dosing is used.	Effective as prophylaxis for patients who are HSV-positive Fluid hydration is necessary if high doses are used.
Famciclovir	HSV VZV	Prophylaxis: 250 mg PO BID Treatment: dose dependent on virus	
Ganciclovir	HSV VZV CMV	Treatment doses and regimens are dependent on clinical situation	Effective preemptive therapy for CMV in high-risk patients. Myelosuppression. Limited data for HHV-6 and HHV-8.
Valacyclovir	HSV VZV	Prophylaxis: 500 mg PO BID or TID Treatment: 1 gram PO TID	Metabolized to acyclovir. Improved bioavailability compared with acyclovir.

Continued

TABLE 31.1	Antimicrobials Used for the Immunocompromised Patient—cont'd			
Valganciclovir	HSV VZV CMV	Prophylaxis: 900 mg PO once daily Preemptive therapy CMV: 900 mg PO twice daily × 2-wk minimum and until negative test; then taper dose for maintenance		Metabolized to ganciclovir. Myelosuppression. Prophylaxis used for patients with previous CMV reactivation. Limited data for HHV-6 and HHV-8.
Cidofovir	HSV VZV CMV Adenovirus	Treatment: 5 mg/kg IV every week × two doses; then taper per clinical guidelines		Significant renal toxicity requires aggressive pre- and posthydration. Ocular toxicity. Myelosuppression. Give probenecid to prevent renal reabsorption. Second-line therapy for CMV. First-line therapy for adenovirus.

CMV, Cytomegalovirus; *HHV-6,* human herpes virus 6; *HSV,* herpes simplex virus; *IV,* intravenous; *PO,* by mouth; *TDM,* therapeutic drug monitoring *VZV,* varicella zoster virus.

Adapted from National Comprehensive Cancer Network. (2017a). *Prevention and treatment of cancer-related infections (v1.2018)* http://www.nccn.org/professionals/physician_gls/pdf/infections.pdf.

function, lactate dehydrogenase (LDH), lactic acid, urinalysis

(2) Chest x-ray or computed tomography (CT) scan with respiratory signs/symptoms

(3) Ultrasound for abdominal or pelvic infections if suspected.

(4) Magnetic resonance imaging (MRI) for suspected joint or neurologic infections if suspected.

e. Obtain cultures (gold standard for diagnosis)

(1) Blood cultures

(a) One set should be obtained peripherally and one from central lines if patient has a central venous catheter.

(b) Two peripheral culture sets should be drawn if no central venous catheter is in place.

(c) Consider use of a phlebotomy team for peripheral blood cultures to reduce possible contamination, false positives (Snyder, et al., 2012).

(d) Central venous catheter blood cultures are required to rule out catheter colonization (Snyder, et al., 2012).

(2) Urine cultures if urinary tract infection is suspected

(3) Sputum cultures

(4) Stool cultures, if diarrhea is present

(5) Wound and drainage cultures, if appropriate

C. Initiation of empiric antimicrobial therapy

1. Initiation of empiric antibiotics should be started as soon after presentation as possible after cultures are obtained. Empiric antimicrobial therapy should not be delayed to determine therapy based on results of cultures, although adjustment of empiric therapy may be warranted based on culture results.

2. Selection of antibiotics is based on the following:

a. Patient risk assessment, clinical status, organ dysfunction, comorbidities, identified disruption of mucosal barriers (e.g., mucositis, wounds), medications (e.g., prophylactic antibiotics, anticancer therapies), and allergies

b. Site(s) of suspected infection (if known)

c. Antimicrobial action (bactericidal preferred to bacteriostatic), coverage, and institutional/local susceptibilities of pathogens

3. Low-risk patients with febrile neutropenia

a. Individuals considered low risk if the expected duration of neutropenia is <7 days. This risk assessment is based on the chemotherapy regimen (e.g., many standard regimens used to treat solid tumors) and patient-specific factors.

b. Antimicrobial prophylaxis is not routinely warranted at this time. May consider viral prophylaxis in patients with prior herpes simplex virus (HSV).

c. Empiric antimicrobial therapy includes intravenous (IV) monotherapy that covers *Pseudomonas aeruginosa,* including imipenem/cilastatin, meropenem, piperacillin/tazobactam, and cefepime. Local institutional bacterial susceptibilities should be considered.

d. Oral therapy that covers *Pseudomonas,* including ciprofloxacin + amoxicillin/clavulanate, ciprofloxacin + clindamycin, moxifloxacin, or levofloxacin (Levaquin). Note, this option is not recommended in patients receiving quinolones for prophylaxis.

4. Intermediate- or high-risk febrile neutropenic patients
    a. Many factors are considered to determine intermediate or high risk, including type of anticancer agent, intensity of therapy, anticipated neutropenia, and patient-specific factors.
    b. Antimicrobial prophylaxis may be considered based on regimen and patient risk factors.
    c. Empiric antimicrobial therapy may include IV monotherapy that covers *P. aeruginosa*, including imipenem/cilastatin, meropenem, piperacillin/tazobactam, and cefepime. Local institutional bacterial susceptibilities should be considered for treatment decisions.
    d. Combination IV antibiotic for empiric therapy not routinely recommended but may be considered in select patients (e.g., clinically unstable patients or a history of resistant infections). Options to double-coverage gram-negative bacteria include the addition of an aminoglycoside agent to those noted earlier.
    e. The use of vancomycin as part of the empiric therapy of a febrile neutropenic patient may be considered in select clinical situations (e.g., clinical instability, clinically apparent, serious IV catheter–related infections). The routine use of vancomycin has led to increased occurrence of vancomycin-resistant pathogens and should be avoided.
D. Modification of empiric antimicrobial therapy
    1. Antibiotic therapy should be modified based on the results of cultures.
    2. Antibiotic therapy should be modified if patient symptoms do not resolve or worsen.
    3. Duration of antimicrobial therapy is sufficient for the resolution of the fever without exposure to unnecessary antimicrobial side effects.
        a. Recovery of neutrophil count (absolute neutrophil count [ANC] $\geq$500 cells/mm^3)
        b. Clinical status (e.g., afebrile for 2–3 days)
        c. Identification of pathogen (e.g., positive culture)
        d. Low-risk patients that are clinically stable with negative cultures but the ANC remains <500, consider discontinuation of antibiotics after a total of 5 to 7 days
    4. If fever and/or clinical status is unresponsive to initial antibiotic therapy, the risk of a nonbacterial cause(s), bacterial organisms resistant to antimicrobial therapy (e.g., methicillin-resistant *Staphylococcus aureus*, vancomycin-resistant *Enterococcus*), inadequate serum and/or tissue concentrations of antimicrobials, or drug fever should be considered.
    5. Antiviral therapy should be considered if patient has a history of positive titers or positive history of an outbreak during chemotherapy (e.g., herpes simplex, herpes zoster).
    6. Antifungal coverage may be appropriate to add to initial antimicrobial regimen
        a. Consider in patients at risk for fungal infections (e.g., concurrent corticosteroids, history of fungal infection, exposure, duration of antibiotics including prophylaxis, uncontrolled diabetic)
        b. One third of febrile neutropenic patients who do not respond to 1 week of antimicrobial therapy have a systemic fungal infection.
        c. Most common organisms include *Candida* and *Aspergillus.*
    7. Consider consultation with infectious disease specialist for complex situations.
III. Potential adverse effects of antimicrobial therapy (see Table 31.1)
    A. Antimicrobial adverse effects may be class specific (e.g., hypersensitivity with β-lactam antibiotics), agent specific, and/or dose-related
    B. Suprainfection secondary to overgrowth of microorganisms not covered
    C. Renal toxicity—acute renal tubular necrosis, nephritis, electrolyte imbalances
    D. Hematologic—thrombocytopenia, neutropenia, anemia
    E. Hepatotoxicity—elevated liver function tests
    F. Cardiovascular—phlebitis, hypotension, arrhythmias, prolonged QTc interval
    G. Gastrointestinal (GI)—nausea, vomiting, anorexia, diarrhea, colitis, *Clostridium difficile* infection
    H. Neurotoxicity—seizures, dizziness, ototoxicity
    I. Dermatologic—rash, Stevens–Johnson syndrome, thrush, esophagitis, vaginitis
    J. Fluid and electrolyte imbalances—hypokalemia, hypernatremia, hypomagnesemia, dehydration, fluid volume overload
    K. Hypersensitivity reactions

Assessment

I. Assessment for presence of risk factors
    A. Disruption of skin and mucosal barriers
    B. Altered immune function
        1. Patients with hematologic malignancies have an 8.7 times higher risk for developing an infection due to bone marrow dysfunction compared with patients with solid tumor malignancies.
        2. Advanced or refractory disease.
        3. Concurrent corticosteroids (including inhaled steroids).
        4. Select chemotherapy (e.g., purine antimetabolites).
    C. Comorbidities
        1. Diabetes
        2. HIV disease
        3. Renal or hepatic disease
        4. GI disease

5. Pulmonary disease
6. Graft-versus-host disease
D. Tumor invasion, necrosis, and/or obstruction
E. Cancer treatment (chemotherapy, radiation, surgery)
   1. Surgical disruption of skin
   2. Bone marrow suppression
   3. Invasive procedures (e.g., insertion of central venous catheters, indwelling urinary catheters, nasogastric tubes)
   4. Immunosuppressive agents, corticosteroids, and T-cell–depleting agents
   5. Stem cell transplantation
   6. Stomatitis or mucositis
   7. Blood transfusion
   8. Neutropenia with ANC less than 1500/mm^3
   9. Previous antibiotic therapy
F. Patient characteristics
   1. Malnutrition
   2. Age
   3. Frequent hospitalizations
   4. History of infectious disease
   5. Recent travel

II. History of drug allergies or drug reaction or intolerance
III. Physical examination
A. Oral mucosa
B. Central line insertion site
C. Abdomen
D. Lungs
E. Cardiovascular
F. Skin
IV. Medication reconciliation, including use of OTC medications
V. Evaluation of diagnostic and laboratory data
VI. Antimicrobial stewardship tasks and functions performed by nurses (Olans, Olans, & Witt, 2017)
A. Appropriately triage and place patients in appropriate isolation precautions.
B. Gather information about patient allergies, past medical history, and medication reconciliation.
C. Obtain cultures before starting antibiotics. Monitor and report results to treating physician in a timely manner. Adjust treatment plan based on laboratory and radiology reports.
D. Administer antimicrobials and monitor for adverse events. Review patient's response to therapy, and communicate changes in status to physician and pharmacist.
E. Monitor patient's clinical progress and capacity to transition from IV to oral medications.
F. Communicate and manage transition to outpatient services, skilled nursing facilities, and/or long-term care facilities.
G. Educate patients/families, perform discharge teaching, infection prevention practices.
VII. Assessment of patient's and family's adherence to protective measures

A. Maintain good personal hygiene, including frequent hand washing
B. Perform frequent oral care
C. Avoid exposure to communicable diseases and environmental contaminates
D. Maintain vaccination schedule
   1. Patients receiving chemotherapy and/or immunosuppressive medications should not receive live vaccines due to the risk of infection (Hibberd, 2018).
   2. Inactivated vaccines may be administered >2 weeks before chemotherapy; live virus vaccines should be given >4 weeks before chemotherapy (Hibberd, 2018).
   3. Posttransplant immunization schedule
      a. Inactivated vaccines are administered at least 6 months posttransplant and include pneumococcal, diphtheria/tetanus/pertussis (DTaP), *Haemophilus influenzae* type B, hepatitis B virus (HBV), meningococcus, and influenza
      b. Live virus vaccines: measles/mumps/rubella (MMR) and zoster (shingles vaccine) are administered at least 24 months posttransplant
      c. Live virus vaccines should not be given while the patient is taking immunosuppressant medications for graft vs. host disease
      d. CD34 markers may be used as a means of timing vaccine administration posttransplant
E. Proper food handling, preparation, and storage

Management

I. Manage elevated body temperature and prevent infection
II. Provide patient and family education
A. Risk factors, signs, and symptoms for infection (see Assessment)
B. Rationale for antimicrobial drug therapy and taking antimicrobials as scheduled
C. When and how to notify health care provider
   1. Body temperature greater than 100.4°F
   2. Signs or symptoms of infection
   3. Hypersensitivities to antimicrobial medication
D. Protective measures
III. Prevent and monitor adverse effects of antimicrobial therapy (see Table 31.1)
IV. Monitor therapeutic response to antimicrobial therapy
A. Monitor temperature, pulse, respirations, and blood pressure
B. Monitor cultures
C. Discussion about rationale for immediate evaluation of fever ⚠
D. Assess changes in laboratory values or fluid volume status
E. Revaluate medications (e.g., antimicrobial) and adjust to individual patient needs

ANTIINFLAMMATORY AGENTS (MARTIN, 2014; NCCN, 2018)

Overview

I. Rationale and indications

A. To reduce inflammation, manage fevers, and treat pain (e.g., bone pain)

1. Although the inflammatory process is a protective mechanism, in certain situations it may cause harm and pain to the patient.

2. Inhibition of cyclooxygenase leads to decreased prostaglandin production, which can decrease the adverse effects of inflammation

II. Types of nonopioids and antiinflammatory agents

A. Nonsteroidal antiinflammatory drugs (NSAIDs) and salicylates (Table 31.2)

B. Corticosteroids (Table 31.3)

C. Acetaminophen

III. Principles of medical management

A. Treatment of mild to moderate musculoskeletal or surgical pain

TABLE 31.2 Analgesics

NONSTEROIDAL ANTIINFLAMMATORY DRUGS (NSAIDS)

Agent	Adult Oral Dosages (maximum is per 24 hr)	Notable Drug Information
Diclofenac (various)	Initial: 25–50 mg PO Usual: 25–50 mg PO q 8 hr Maximum: 150 mg PO	GI side effects; take with food. Patch available (q 12 hr) Gel available (q 4 hr) BBW: Cardiovascular thrombotic events, gastrointestinal bleeding, ulceration and perforation.
Etodolac (Lodine, Lodine XL)	Initial: 200–400 mg PO Usual: 200–400 mg PO q 6–8 hr Maximum: 1000 mg PO	GI side effects, fluid retention BBW: Cardiovascular thrombotic events, gastrointestinal bleeding, ulceration and perforation.
Fenoprofen (generic)	Initial dose: 200 mg PO Usual: 200 mg PO q 4–6 hr (pain), 400–600 mg PO q 4–6 hr (osteoarthritis) Maximum: 3200 mg PO	Prescription required; dizziness, GI side effects BBW: Cardiovascular thrombotic events, gastrointestinal bleeding, ulceration and perforation.
Ibuprofen PO (generic)	Initial dose: 200–400 mg PO Usual: 200–400 mg PO q 4–6 hr; higher doses of 200–800 mg q 8 hr PO Maximum: 3200 mg PO	200 mg available OTC; GI side effects BBW: Cardiovascular thrombotic events, gastrointestinal bleeding, ulceration, and perforation.
Ibuprofen IV (Caldolor) (antipyretic)	Initial dose: 400 mg Usual: 400 mg IV q 4–6 prn Maximum: 3200 mg	Patient should be well hydrated before administration BBW: Cardiovascular thrombotic events, gastrointestinal bleeding, ulceration, and perforation.
Indomethacin (generic)	Initial: 25 mg PO Usual: 25 mg PO q 8–12 hr Maximum: 200 mg PO	Renal toxicity, GI side effects Note: Extended-release product available for once-daily dosing, suppository for rectal dosing, intravenous BBW: Cardiovascular thrombotic events, gastrointestinal bleeding, ulceration, and perforation.
Ketoprofen (various)	Initial dose: 25 mg PO Usual: 25–75 mg PO q 6–8 hr Maximum: 300 mg PO	GI side effects, headache, dizziness Note: Extended-release product available for once-daily dosing BBW: Cardiovascular thrombotic events, gastrointestinal bleeding, ulceration, and perforation.
Ketorolac (Toradol)	Oral: Initial: 10–20 mg PO Usual: 10 mg PO q 4–6 hr Maximum: 40 mg PO Parenteral: Initial: 30–60 mg IM or 15–30 mg IV (single dose only) Usual: 15–30 mg IV q 6 hr Maximum: 60–120 mg IV	Use lower doses in older adults. Maximum of 5 days is recommended. A nasal spray of ketorolac is also available. BBW: Cardiovascular thrombotic events, gastrointestinal bleeding, ulceration and perforation, hypersensitivity reactions, contraindicated in advanced renal impairment, risk of bleeding.
Naproxen (generics) [OTC]	Initial: 250 mg PO Usual Dose: 250–500 mg PO q 12 hr Maximum: 1000 mg PO	BBW: Cardiovascular thrombotic events, gastrointestinal bleeding, ulceration and perforation.
Piroxicam (Feldene)	20 mg daily (max. 40 mg)	Long half-life allows for once-daily dosing; use with caution in older patients; causes fluid retention. Not indicated for pain.

Continued

TABLE 31.2 Analgesics—cont'd

NONSTEROIDAL ANTIINFLAMMATORY DRUGS (NSAIDS)

Agent	Adult Oral Dosages (maximum is per 24 hr)	Notable Drug Information
Sulindac (Clinoril)	Initial: 150 mg PO Usual: 150–200 mg PO q 12 hr (for indications) Maximum: 400 mg PO	Indication for osteoarthritis, rheumatoid arthritis, AS. BBW: Cardiovascular thrombotic events, gastrointestinal bleeding, ulceration and perforation. May be associated with less renal toxicity. Not approved for pain. Indication for arthritis, ankylosing spondylitis, and bursitis/tendinitis of shoulder.
Tolmetin (Tolectin)	Initial: 400 mg PO Frequency: 200–600 mg PO q 8 hr (for indications) Maximum: 1800 mg PO	Fewer GI side effects; take on empty stomach. Not indicated for pain. Indication for osteoarthritis and rheumatoid arthritis. BBW: cardiovascular risk, gastrointestinal risk.
NSAIDs: Cox-2 Selective Agent		
Celecoxib (Celebrex)	Initial: 400 mg PO Usual: 100–200 mg PO q 12 hr Maximum: 400 mg PO	GI safety advantages yet to be demonstrated with chronic use. Fewer GI and platelet side effects; mostly hepatic metabolism by CYP-2C9 (drug interactions). BBW: Serious cardiovascular risk, serious gastrointestinal risk.
Salicylates		
Acetylsalicylic acid (ASA), aspirin	Initial: 325 mg PO Usual: 325–650 mg PO q 4–6 hr Maximum: 4000 mg PO Rectal: 300–600 mg prn q 4 hr for no more than 10 days	Do not combine with NSAIDs (exception is with low dose for cardiovascular use of 81 mg PO daily); potent antiplatelet effects; tinnitus at high doses.
Choline magnesium trisalicylate (Trilisate)	Initial: 1500 mg PO Usual: 1500 mg PO q 12 hr Maximum: 3000 mg PO	Has no antiplatelet effect; tinnitus.
Salsalate (Disalcid; various generics)	Initial: 750 mg PO Usual: 750 mg PO q 8–12 hr Maximum: 3000 mg PO	Has no antiplatelet effect. No indication for pain. Indication for osteoarthritis, rheumatoid arthritis, and related rheumatic disorders. BBW: Cardiovascular thrombotic events, gastrointestinal bleeding, ulceration and perforation.

AS, ankylosing spondylitis; *BBW*, black box warning; *GI*, gastrointestinal; *NSAIDs*, nonsteroidal antiinflammatory drugs; *OTC*, over the counter.

TABLE 31.3 Corticosteroids

Corticosteroids	Equivalent Oral Dose*	Duration of HPA Suppression
Short-Acting (8–12 hr)		
Cortisone	25 mg	1.25–1.5 days
Hydrocortisone	20 mg	1.25–1.5 days
Intermediate-Acting (12–36 hr)		
Methylprednisone (e.g., Medrol)	4 mg	1.25–1.5 days
Prednisolone	5 mg	1.25–1.5 days
Prednisone	5 mg	1.25–1.5 days
Long-Acting		
Dexamethasone (Decadron)	0.75 mg	2.75 days

*Equivalent dosages are general approximations.

B. Management of bone pain, often in combination with other analgesics
C. Antipyretic—NSAIDS and acetaminophen
IV. Potential adverse effects of NSAIDS (Table 31.4)
   A. GI effects (e.g., nausea, dyspepsia, ulceration)
   B. Renal toxicity
   C. Decrease platelet function
   D. Cardiac toxicity
   E. Confusion, especially in older adults

Assessment

I. Indications for patient use and considerations
   A. Musculoskeletal pain
      1. Older age
      2. History of arthritis, neuromuscular disease, or diabetes

TABLE 31.4 Adverse Effects of Nonsteroidal Antiinflammatory Drugs (NSAIDs) and Corticosteroids

Adverse Effects	Nursing Implications
NSAIDs	
Gastrointestinal	
Ulceration, bleeding, gastritis, dyspepsia, abdominal pain, constipation, PUD	Administer with food or milk.
	Note guaiac stool.
Risks increase with age, chronic use, concomitant corticosteroid use and history of PUD; misoprostol (Cytotec) can be used to prevent NSAID-induced ulcers.	Assess for signs and symptoms of GI bleeding.
Pancreas	
Pancreatitis reported with sulindac	Monitor serum amylase and lipase levels and urinary amylase level results.
	Monitor for signs and symptoms of pancreatitis (e.g., sudden and intense epigastric pain, nausea and vomiting, low-grade fever, jaundice).
Hepatic	
Increased ALT, AST, bilirubin levels; risks for hepatotoxicity include alcoholism, chronic active hepatitis, history of hepatitis, cirrhosis, and CHF	Monitor liver enzymes, bilirubin laboratory results.
	Assess health history for risk factors.
Central Nervous System	
Dizziness, drowsiness, lightheadedness or vertigo, somnolence, mental confusion	Neurologic examination for alertness and orientation.
	Advise clients and families to avoid driving or other hazardous activities that require mental alertness until CNS effects can be determined.
	Implement measures for client safety as needed (e.g., assist with ambulation, fall precautions).
Malaise, fatigue	Avoid alcohol and other CNS depressants.
	Assess level of fatigue.
	Provide for rest periods.
Headache	Monitor CBC laboratory test results.
	Assess level of headache and administer pain medications as needed.
Cardiovascular	
CHF, peripheral edema, fluid retention, hypertension	Monitor fluid status, lung sounds, pitting edema, vital signs, and daily weights.
Renal	
Acute renal failure, elevated BUN and serum creatinine levels and proteinuria; risks include age, chronic renal disease, CHF, muscle breakdown (e.g., significant exercise) and dehydration.	Maintain hydration during use.
	Monitor urine intake and output.
	Monitor BUN, creatinine, urinalysis laboratory test results, and blood pressure.
	Assess for edema. Monitor weight.
	Assess health history for risk factors.
Hematologic	
Neutropenia, leukopenia, decrease platelet function, decreased hemoglobin and hematocrit levels; *exception:* choline magnesium trisalicylate (Trilisate)	Monitor CBC results with differentials clinically necessary.
	Assess and implement measures to manage infection, bleeding, and fatigue (see Chapter 30).
	Monitor platelet levels.
	No IM shots.
	Implement bleeding precautions per institution protocol.

Continued

TABLE 31.4   Adverse Effects of Nonsteroidal Antiinflammatory Drugs (NSAIDs) and Corticosteroids—cont'd

Adverse Effects	Nursing Implications
Special Senses Visual disturbance, blurred vision, photophobia, ocular cataracts, glaucoma, ear pain, tinnitus	Stress the importance of regular eye examinations and hearing tests. Educate client about reporting blurred vision, eye pain, ear pain, and tinnitus to health care provider and about darkening room or wearing sunglasses if photophobic.
Hypersensitivity Asthma and anaphylaxis	Monitor for hypersensitivity reactions—changes in respiratory status, itching, hives, fever, pain, changes in pulse rate, decrease in blood pressure, decrease in urinary output. Assess breath sounds; elevate HOB to ease breathing. Administer oxygen as needed. Administer bronchodilators, antihistamines, agents as needed.
Respiratory Dyspnea, hemoptysis, bronchospasm, shortness of breath	NSAIDs are contraindicated in clients with ASA allergy, nasal polyps, bronchospastic disease. Perform respiratory assessment; monitor breath sounds. Examine sputum for color and consistency. Elevate HOB to ease breathing. Administer bronchodilators and oxygen, as needed.
Dermatologic and Skeletal Rash, erythema, urticarial, photosensitivity, osteoporosis, poor wound healing, skin thinning, growth arrest	Observe for rash and monitor wounds for prolonged healing time or changes in wound bed. Advice clients to use sunblock, wear protective clothing, protect skin, avoid prolonged exposure to sunlight. Monitor height.
Pituitary Adrenal insufficiency caused by prolonged use and rapid withdrawal	Monitor blood glucose and electrolyte laboratory test results. Monitor vital signs and presence of peripheral edema.
Infectious Disease Immunosuppressive with increased risk of infections—bacterial, fungal, viral; activation of tuberculosis and spread of herpes conjunctivitis	Observe for signs of cortisol insufficiency, such as fever, orthostatic hypotension, syncopal episodes, disorientation, myalgia, and arthralgia. Cultures, dermatologic examination. Administer antimicrobial drugs and antipyretics as needed. Be aware that signs and symptoms of infection may be masked by NSAIDs.
Corticosteroids ***Cushing Syndrome with Long-Term Use*** Contral obesity, moon face, buffalo hump, easy bruising, acne, hirsutism, striae, skin atrophy	Assess patient's body image concerns. Provide opportunity for client to share concerns and discuss coping strategies. Educate regarding care of skin and safety precautions.
Electrolyte and Metabolic Imbalances Hyperglycemia, hypernatremia, hypokalemia, and hypocalcemia, leading to edema, hypertension, diabetes, osteoporosis	Monitor laboratory results (blood glucose, electrolytes, calcium), vital signs, body weight. Assess for edema.

TABLE 31.4 Adverse Effects of Nonsteroidal Antiinflammatory Drugs (NSAIDs) and Corticosteroids—cont'd

Adverse Effects	Nursing Implications
Neuromuscular and Skeletal Arthralgia, myalgia, fatigue, muscle weakness, myopathy, osteoporosis, muscle wasting, fractures	Monitor muscle strength. Administer pain medication as needed. Encourage regular exercise to promote bone development. Implement safety measures to prevent falls and injuries.
Ocular Effects Cataracts and glaucoma	Regular eye examinations. Educate client to report any eye pain or blurred vision to health care provider. Those with open-angle glaucoma should avoid corticosteroids.
Suppression of Pituitary-Adrenal Function With long-term use, sudden withdrawal may cause acute adrenal insufficiency and dependence, fever, myalgia, arthralgia, malaise; unable to respond to stress. This may occur with chronic use, or with frequent courses over time (e.g., myeloma).	Monitor blood pressure for hypotension. Monitor electrolytes for hyponatremia. Assess for dehydration, fatigue, diarrhea, anorexia. Monitor vital signs and muscle and joint pain; administer pain medication. Educate regarding stressful situations, both physiologic and emotional, and when to contact a health care professional for assistance.
Psychiatric Disturbances Paranoia, psychosis, hallucinations Insomnia	Observe for and report any mental status changes. Suicide precautions if needed Refer to mental health professional as needed. Take in morning if clinically appropriate.
Gastrointestinal Peptic ulcers, GI bleeding	Assess for epigastric pain 1–3 hr after meals. Assess for nausea or vomiting, and observe for hematemesis. Monitor CBC and guaiac stools or emesis.
Miscellaneous Immunosuppression Poor wound healing, menstrual irregularities, arrest of growth	Increase risk of infection, including fungal infections, viral infections, and opportunistic infections. Counsel patients about appropriate hygiene to minimize risk of fungal infections, including mouth care. Assess any wounds for prolonged healing. Monitor CBC with differential; assess and manage effects of low white blood cell, red blood cell, and platelet counts. Monitor height.

ALT, Alanine aminotransferase; *ASA,* acetylsalicylic acid; *AST,* aspartate aminotransferase; *BUN,* blood urea nitrogen; *CBC,* complete blood cell count; *CHF,* congestive heart failure; *CNS,* central nervous system; *GI,* gastrointestinal; *HOB,* head of bed; *IM,* intramuscular; *NSAIDs,* nonsteroidal antiinflammatory drugs; *PUD,* peptic ulcer disease.

3. Bone metastasis
4. Treatment with high-dose vinblastine, paclitaxel (>250mg/m²)
B. Sepsis with persistent high fever
C. Patients at risk for toxicities with NSAIDs
   1. Age older than 65 years
   2. History of GI ulcers
   3. Renal insufficiency
   4. Cardiovascular disease
   5. Concurrent aspirin or anticoagulant use
   6. History of ulcerative colitis

III. Physical examination
   A. Vital signs (e.g., fever)
   B. Assessment and reassessment of pain—onset, duration, intensity, description, location, aggravating and relieving factors, functional or quality-of-life impairment
IV. Medication reconciliation
   A. The antiplatelet effects of NSAIDs require caution be taken with any anticoagulants and other antiplatelet medications (e.g., clopidogrel)
V. Evaluation of diagnostic and laboratory data
   A. Complete blood cell count (e.g., platelet count)

B. Renal and hepatic function
C. Erythrocyte sedimentation rate
D. C-reactive protein
E. Coagulation studies
F. Radiologic imaging (e.g., x-ray, CT scan, MRI)

Management

I. Patient and family education
   A. Rationale and medication schedule for antiinflammatory drug therapy
   B. Adverse effects and strategies to prevent and manage them
   C. Adverse effects to report to health care team ⚠️
II. Monitor for adverse effects of antiinflammatory drug therapy (see Table 31.4)
III. Decrease the incidence and manage the adverse effects of antiinflammatory drug therapy (see Table 31.4) ⚠️
   A. Establish patient's allergies before administering NSAIDs.
   B. Review patient's current medications for potential drug interactions.
   C. Counsel patient and caregiver to assure communication of all medication changes during and after therapy, including addition of complementary and/or alternative medication or dietary strategies, or discontinuation of therapies.
   D. Review the use of complementary therapy that may alter the metabolism of NSAIDs and/or potentiate the toxicities associated with NSAIDs (e.g., bleeding).
   E. NSAIDs are contraindicated in patients with aspirin allergy or hypersensitivity to acetylsalicylic acid (ASA), nasal polyps, and bronchospastic disease.
   F. NSAIDs' effect on renal blood flow may decrease clearance of medications eliminated via the kidneys and result in increased drug exposure and toxicities (e.g., decrease clearance of pemetrexed and methotrexate, increase renal toxicity with cisplatin).
   G. NSAIDs are antipyretics; may mask a fever in an individual with infection. Agents should be avoided in patients receiving myelosuppressive therapy when neutropenic.
   H. NSAIDs decrease platelet function; should be avoided when patient is thrombocytopenic.
IV. Monitor for therapeutic response to antiinflammatory drug therapy
   A. Assess patient for adequate symptom relief (e.g., pain).
   B. Assess patient for infection because the antipyretic and antiinflammatory actions of NSAIDs may mask signs and symptoms of infection. ⚠️
   C. Maintain hydration to protect kidney for patients taking NSAIDs.
   D. Avoid the concomitant use of NSAIDs and medications known to decrease platelets (e.g., chemotherapy) or increase risk of bleeding (e.g., anticoagulants and antiplatelet medications).

ANTIEMETIC AGENTS (BASCH ET AL., 2011; FEYER & JORDAN, 2011; HAINSWORTH, 2008; HESKETH, 2008; HESKETH, KRIS, BASCHE, & LYMAN, 2017; NCCN, 2018B)

Overview (see also Chapter 37)

I. For prevention and treatment of chemotherapy-induced nausea and vomiting (CINV)
II. For causes of nausea and vomiting in addition to CINV
III. Types of nausea and vomiting
   A. Chemotherapy induced (see Chapter 37)
      1. Risk factors
         a. Emetogenic potential of chemotherapy agent)
         b. Dose, route, frequency, and cycle of chemotherapy
         c. Radiation field (e.g., whole body, upper abdomen, craniospinal)
         d. Patient characteristics
   B. Types of antiemetic drugs (Table 31.5)
      1. Mechanism via interference of neurotransmission of nausea to the vomiting center via trough disruption of signaling pathways. Some agents target a single neurotransmitters, whereas some block multiple neurotransmitters (e.g., olanzapine).
         a. Major neurotransmitter targets
            (1) Serotonin (5-HT3 antagonists; e.g., ondansetron)
            (2) Neurokinin (NK1 antagonists; e.g., aprepitant)
            (3) Dopamine (D2 antagonists; e.g., prochlorperazine)
            (4) Histamine (H1 antagonists; e.g., promethazine)
            (5) Acetylcholine (muscarinics; e.g., scopolamine)
            (6) Cannabinoid (cannabinoid agonists; e.g., dronabinol)
         b. Corticosteroids are effective in preventing acute CINV and management of delayed CINV. The mechanism of this effect is not fully understood.
         c. The use of nonpharmaceutical approaches to prevent and/or manage CINV complements the use of pharmacologic strategies.
IV. Principles of medical management
   A. Goal—prevention of nausea and vomiting
   B. Use lowest effective antiemetic dose(s) before chemotherapy to prevent CINV
   C. Select appropriate antiemetics (see Table 31.5) based on evidence for optimal prevention of CINV based on patient-specific factors and treatment-specific factors (e.g., emetogenic potential of the chemotherapy regimen)
   D. Administer antiemetics prophylactically to cover onset, peak, and duration period of each chemotherapeutic agent and for breakthrough CINV

TABLE 31.5 Antiemetic Therapy: Select Pharmacologic Agents

Name	Route Dose/Schedule (Adult)	Adverse Effects of Class	Nursing Implications
Serotonin Receptor Antagonists (5HT3 antagonists)			
Ondansetron	IV 8–16 mg IV before chemotherapy (daily) PO 16–24 mg PO before chemotherapy (daily) Oral is as effective as parenteral route if dosed appropriately	Headache Cardiovascular Constipation	Assess for headache with higher doses and consider acetaminophen for headache. Increase QTc, evaluate potential drug and disease interactions. Assess for number and consistency of stools. Administer stool softeners (docusate) and stimulants (senna) to prevent constipation as appropriate. Increase fluids and fiber in diet. Encourage exercise as tolerated.
Granisetron	IV Dose: 0.01 mg/kg (maximum 1 mg) before chemotherapy (once daily maximum) PO Dose: 2 mg PO before chemotherapy (once daily maximum) Transdermal patch (Sancuso) Dose: 3.1 mg/24 hr applied 24–48 hr before first dose Subcutaneous (Sustol): Extended-release product containing 10 mg/0.4 mL in single dose (administered no more frequently than every 7 days)	Transient increases in serum AST, GPT	Monitor liver function test results. Administration: Give higher doses over at least 30 minutes to prevent dizziness, headache, hypotension.
Dolasetron	PO Dose: 100 mg PO before chemotherapy		Consider ECG for tachycardia or new onset of shortness of breath.
Palonosetron	IV Dose: 0.25 mg before chemotherapy PO Available as a fixed combination product with netupitant (see later)		Do not use short-acting 5HT3 antagonist concurrently in patients receiving palonosetron (within 3–5 days of treatment).
Neurokinin Antagonists			
Aprepitant	PO Dose: 125 mg on day 1 before chemotherapy; then 80 mg daily on days 2 and 3 IV (injectable emulsion) Dose: 130 mg IV once before chemotherapy	Constipation	Assess for number and consistency of stools. Administer stool softeners (docusate) and stimulants (senna) to prevent constipation. Increase fluids and roughage in diet.
Fosaprepitant	IV Dose: 150 mg IV once before chemotherapy	Diarrhea Hiccups Fatigue	Monitor for stool number and consistency. Monitor for hiccups. If persistent, then consider chlorpromazine (Thorazine), or a muscle relaxer may be considered. Possibly related to dexamethasone. Likely from chemotherapy administration and not the drug itself.

Continued

TABLE 31.5 Antiemetic Therapy: Select Pharmacologic Agents—cont'd

Name	Route Dose/Schedule (Adult)	Adverse Effects of Class	Nursing Implications
Fosnetupitant (combined with palonosetron)	IV (Akynzeo) Dose: 235 mg fosnetupitant (available as a combination with 0.25 mg palonosetron IV) once before chemotherapy		Administered over 30 min as infusion.
Netupitant (combined with palonosetron)	PO (Akynzeo) Dose: 300 mg (available as combination with palonosetron 0.5 mg PO) once before chemotherapy		Headache and fatigue.
Rolapitant	PO Dose: 180 mg PO once before chemotherapy		Dizziness, decreased appetite.

Dopamine receptor antagonists
- Dopamine antagonists include phenothiazines (e.g., prochlorperazine) and butyrophenones (e.g., droperidol). Agents such as metoclopramide and olanzapine target multiple receptors, including dopamine receptors.
- Class-related side effects include sedation, dystonia, akathisia, constipation.

Name	Route Dose/Schedule (Adult)	Adverse Effects of Class	Nursing Implications
Droperidol	IV Dose: 0.625 mg every 6 hr as needed	Sedation	Assess level of sedation. Patient should avoid tasks that require alertness until drug response is established. Patient should avoid alcohol and other CNS depressants.
Haloperidol		Dystonia Akathisia	Monitor for and be prepared to treat EPSs with diphenhydramine 25 mg IV or PO.
Metoclopramide (mechanism includes combination of dopamine receptor antagonist, serotonin receptor antagonist and enhances response to acetylcholine in gastrointestinal tract)	PO Dose: 10 mg as needed q 4–6 hr prn	Hypotension Prolongation of QT interval	Monitor VS. Monitor ECG and check for the QTc level each time. Do not administer if 500 msec or over. If patient complains of shortness of breath or skipped heartbeats, notify health care provider. Black box warning or sudden depth due to prolonged QT interval.
		Extrapyramidal symptoms (EPSs) (e.g., akathisia, acute dystonic reactions); increased incidence in patients <40 years	Assess for EPS reactions. May use lower doses if EPSs occur Dystonia: anticholinergic agents (e.g., diphenhydramine) to treat Akathisia presenting as restlessness: manage with benzodiazepines (e.g., lorazepam)
		Diarrhea (high doses)	Assess number and consistency of stools. Administration: Do not administer to patients with prior hypersensitivity to procaine or procainamide, epilepsy or pheochromocytoma, or if stimulation of GI motility is contraindicated (e.g., mechanical obstruction, GI bleeding).

TABLE 31.5 Antiemetic Therapy: Select Pharmacologic Agents—cont'd

Name	Route Dose/Schedule (Adult)	Adverse Effects of Class	Nursing Implications
Olanzapine (mechanism of action includes antagonist of receptors, including dopamine, serotonin, histamine and acetylcholine-muscarine)	PO Doses of 10 mg po daily at bedtime are recommended for acute and delayed nausea (set duration). This drug is not used as a prn medication.	CNS including fatigue, drowsiness and sleep disturbances Caution in elderly patients with dementia-related psychosis Drug interactions with agents such as benzodiazepines and other antiemetics.	Assess other medications that may increase side effects. Initiate with lower doses than stated in guidelines. Assess medications before initiation of olanzapine.
Prochlorperazine	IV Dose: 10 mg every 4–6 hr scheduled or as needed PO Dose: 10 mg every 4–6 hr as scheduled or needed PR Dose: 25 mg every 12 hr as needed	Sedation Blurred vision EPSs (e.g., akathisia)	Have patients avoid tasks that require alertness until drug response is established. Have patients avoid alcohol and other CNS depressants. Assess vision and impact on safety. Monitor for and be prepared to treat EPSs with diphenhydramine 25 mg IV or PO.
Promethazine (in addition to dopamine receptor antagonism, promethazine competes with histamine at the histamine receptor)	IV Dose: 12.5–25 mg every 4 hr as scheduled or needed PO Dose: 12.5–25 mg every 4 hr as scheduled or needed	Dry mouth Orthostatic hypotension Anticholinergic crisis with overuse Rash (promethazine) Photosensitivity (promethazine) Respiratory depression (promethazine)	Have patient suck on ice chips or sugar-free hard candy. Counsel about care when standing from sitting. Give diphenhydramine for treatment for anticholinergic crisis. Monitor for new rash with therapy. Patients should avoid sun exposure. Particular caution for patients taking concomitant respiratory depressants. (e.g. opiates)
Corticosteroids			
Dexamethasone	Dose: 4–20 mg PO have been used, dependent in part on the combination of antiemetic	Dyspepsia Hiccups Euphoria and insomnia Fluid retention Hyperglycemia Hypokalemia	Take with food or milk. Monitor weight. Assess for prolonged hiccups. Assess emotional status and ability to sleep. Counsel to take doses before noon if possible. Monitor intake and output and weight. Assess for edema. Monitor blood pressure in at-risk patients. Monitor blood sugar and electrolyte results. Assess for effects of low potassium.
Methylprednisolone	IV 125 mg before chemotherapy	Burning with infusion	Slow IV infusion to prevent perineal itching/burning. Similar side effects as seen with dexamethasone.
Cannabinoid			
Dronabinol	PO 5–10 mg every 3 or 6 hr	Sedation and dizziness Dry mouth	Patient should suck on ice chips or hard candy. Encourage frequent intake of fluids.

Continued

TABLE 31.5 Antiemetic Therapy: Select Pharmacologic Agents—cont'd

Name	Route Dose/Schedule (Adult)	Adverse Effects of Class	Nursing Implications
		Euphoria or dysphoria	Assess emotional status (more common in older adult patients).
		Orthostatic hypotension	Monitor VS and BP lying and sitting or standing for orthostatic changes. Educate patient to rise slowly from lying or sitting position.
Benzodiazepine			
Lorazepam	IV 0.5–2.0 mg every 4–6 hr PO 0.5–2.0 mg every 4–6 hr	CNS side effects (sedation, disorientation, dizziness, weakness)	Assess patient's level of consciousness and risk for oversedation. Patient should avoid tasks that require alertness until drug response is established. Patient should avoid alcohol and other CNS depressants. Implement measures for patient safety, such as fall precautions.
		Autograde amnesia	Assess memory. Minimize patient education while patients are taking benzodiazepines unless caregiver present.
		Hypotension	Monitor VS.

AST, Aspartate transaminase; *BP,* blood pressure; *CNS,* central nervous system; *ECG,* electrocardiography; *GI,* gastrointestinal; *GPT,* glutamic-pyruvic transaminase; *IV,* intravenous; *PO,* by mouth; *PR,* per rectum; *prn,* as needed; *VS,* vital signs.
Adapted from National Comprehensive Cancer Network. (2018b). *Antiemesis (v 2.2018).* http://www.nccn.org/professionals/physician_gls/pdf/antiemesis.pdf.

E. Assess patient for risk of delayed emesis and prophylactic therapy, if indicated

F. Follow-up assessment—48 to 72 hours after chemotherapy; modify plan if indicated

V. Prophylaxis of nausea and vomiting (Hesketh, et al., 2017; NCCN, 2018b)

A. Based on recommendations from National Comprehensive Cancer Network (NCCN) based on single day of chemotherapy. Duration of therapy is based on the entire chemotherapy regimen, and this provides a guide for clinicians.

B. Examples of highly emetogenic IV chemotherapy: acute and delayed emesis prevention

1. NK1 RA + 5-HT3 RA + dexamethasone before chemotherapy followed by NK1 RA (if needed) and dexamethasone

2. If long-acting NK1 RA used before chemotherapy, no NK1 RA needed after

3. Olanzapine + palonosetron + dexamethasone before therapy followed by olanzapine

4. Olanzapine + NK1 RA + 5HT3 RA + dexamethasone before therapy followed by olanzapine + NK1 RA (if needed) + dexamethasone

5. If long-acting NK1 RA used before chemotherapy, no NK1 RA is needed after

C. Examples of moderately emetogenic agents

1. 5HT3 RA + dexamethasone chemotherapy followed by dexamethasone or 5HT3 RA monotherapy.

2. Olanzapine + palonosetron + dexamethasone before therapy followed by olanzapine

3. NK1 RA + 5HT3 RA + dexamethasone before therapy followed by NK1 RA (if needed) ± dexamethasone

a. If long-acting NK1 RA used before chemotherapy, no NK1RA is needed after.

D. Low-emetogenic agents: treatment options include dexamethasone or metoclopramide or prochlorperazine, or single-agent short-acting 5HT3 antagonist. The regimen should be modified based on the patient response

E. No emetogenic risk: no routine prophylaxis is recommended. Antiemetics are appropriate based on patient response and/or risk factors.

VI. Agents for breakthrough nausea and vomiting (Basch et al., 2011; Feyer & Jordan, 2011; Hainsworth, 2008; Hesketh, 2008; NCCN, 2018b)

A. The decision for appropriate antiemetics for management of any breakthrough CINV is determined, in part, by the agents given to prevent CINV. For example, if palonosetron is given before chemotherapy, the use of another 5HT3 antagonist is not warranted for the management of breakthrough CINV for the initial few days after palonosetron (a long-acting 5HT3 RA).

1. Dopamine antagonists: prochlorperazine, droperidol, promethazine
2. Dexamethasone
3. Lorazepam
4. Ondansetron
5. Metoclopramide
6. Cannabinoids
   a. Dronabinol
   b. Nabilone
7. Cannabis (medical marijuana) may be legal in some locations and has been used for management of symptoms, including CINV

VII. Potential adverse effects (Hesketh, 2008) (see Table 31.5)

Assessment

I. Patient history
   A. Identify risk factors, concomitant medications, prescribed chemotherapy regimen
   B. Fluid status and dietary intake
   C. Onset of symptoms, accompanying symptoms, and relieving factors
   D. Symptom effects on functional status and quality of life
II. Physical examination
   A. Examination of the oral cavity, abdomen, and skin
   B. Number, volume, and characteristics of emetic episodes
   C. Intake and output
      1. Fluid balance (assess for signs of dehydration)
      2. Weight
      3. Concentrated urine or low urine output
      4. Dietary intake and ability to drink fluids
   D. Hematemesis
   E. Orthostatic hypotension
III. Effectiveness of prescribed antiemetic regimen
IV. Evaluation of diagnostic and laboratory data
   A. Serum electrolyte values
   B. Renal and hepatic function
   C. Abdomen radiograph (kidney, ureter, bladder [KUB]) if obstruction suspected

Management

I. Interventions to manage nausea and vomiting
   A. Follow recommended guidelines for antiemetic chemotherapy prophylaxis
   B. Assess patient's nausea and vomiting status during and after chemotherapy administration; telephone follow-up in outpatient setting on days 2 and 3 of cycle
   C. Ensure patient understands rationale for medication adherence and administration schedule for nausea management at home
II. Interventions to manage fluid deficit
   A. Encourage adequate oral (PO) intake
   B. Provide IV hydration if patient is unable to maintain adequate oral intake
   C. Monitor weight
III. Patient and caregiver education
   A. Rationale for antiemetic drug therapy
   B. Manage adverse effects of antiemetic regimen, refractory nausea and vomiting
   C. Adverse effects to report to health care team
      1. Weight loss
      2. Unable to keep down fluids or antiemetic medications
      3. Concentrated urine
   D. Dietary interventions—take antiemetics before meals so they are effective during and after the meal
IV. Interventions to decrease the incidence, monitor response, and manage antiemetic drug therapy adverse effects (see Table 31.5)
   A. Implement strategies to maximize patient safety
   B. Monitor for response to antiemetic therapy after chemotherapy and before each consecutive treatment
      1. Assess for mental status changes, dizziness, sedation; implementing safety measures (e.g., fall precautions), as needed
      2. Modify antiemetic strategy as needed for delayed CINV

ANALGESICS (NCCN, 2018)

Overview

I. Rationale and indications (see Chapter 44)
   A. >50% of patients will experience pain during their disease trajectory
      1. Pain can be related to the disease, cancer treatment, or both.
      2. Patients may also suffer from chronic nonmalignant pain (e.g., back injury).
   B. Analgesics are used to manage both nociceptive and neuropathic pain
   C. Types of cancer-related pain (see Chapter 44)
      1. Acute: self-limiting pain
      2. Chronic: pain lasts longer than 3 months
      3. Refractory: pain that is resistant to prescribed interventions
      4. Breakthrough: pain occurs despite adequate control of background pain; commonly associated with chronic pain
II. Types of analgesics
   A. Opioids
   B. Nonopioid analgesics (see Antiinflammatory Agents section)

C. Adjuvants (see Psychotropic Drugs: Anxiolytics and Sedative-Hypnotics)

III. Principles of medical management
  A. Selection of appropriate analgesia is based on pharmacokinetic factors and patient's physical needs, age, history of analgesia usage, and organ function.
  B. The most appropriate dose is the one that controls pain through a 24-hour period.
  C. If opioids are used, patients should have long-acting and breakthrough options available when pain is constant.
  D. As doses are titrated to effective levels, long-acting and breakthrough doses should be increased; breakthrough dose should be 10% to 20% of the 24-hour long-acting dose.
  E. Prophylaxis for constipation with a stool softener and bowel stimulant should be considered for all patients started on opioid analgesics, and the regimen should be optimized to assure regular bowel movements.
  F. The effectiveness and the side effect profile should be reassessed (see Chapter 34).

G. Tolerance occurs in patients who take opioids regularly; that is, they require higher doses to achieve the same amount of analgesia.
H. Physical dependence occurs in all patients who take opioids regularly; a withdrawal syndrome will occur if the opioid is abruptly stopped.
I. Psychological dependence is addiction that occurs when patients crave the opioid, use the drug compulsively, and continue use despite harm.

IV. Routes of administration
  A. Oral
    1. Often most convenient and preferred route
    2. Immediate- and extended-release dosing available
  B. Transdermal
  C. Parenteral: IV, subcutaneous, intrathecal
  D. Topical
  E. Buccal, transmucosal, or nasal for rapid-onset opioids
  F. Rectal

V. Potential adverse effects
  A. Adverse effect profile of opioid analgesics (Table 31.6)
  B. Drug interactions with multidrug regimens

TABLE 31.6 Side Effects of Opioid Analgesics

Side Effects	Nursing Implications
Gastrointestinal	
Nausea, vomiting	Consider changing to another opioid, as some agents are associated with less nausea (e.g., hydromorphone). Monitor nausea and number of vomiting episodes and effect on comfort and fluid balance; administer antiemetic drug therapy as needed. Assure nausea and vomiting not related to constipation.
Constipation	Assess bowel elimination patterns and compare with patient's normal pattern; administer stool softeners and/or stimulant cathartics prophylactically.
Narcotized bowel	Increase fluid and dietary fiber intake; abdominal assessment; report decreased or absent bowel sounds and increased abdominal pain.
Cardiovascular	
Arteriolar vasodilation and reduced peripheral resistance; decrease in blood pressure; tachycardia, bradycardia	Monitor vital signs, blood pressure for orthostatic hypotension. Provide for patient safety if blood pressure is low.
Respiratory	
Depressant effect on brainstem reduces respiratory rate, minute volume, tidal exchange; irregular and periodic breathing; respiratory arrest	Monitor level of sedation; respiratory rate and depth; arterial blood gases; vital signs, O_2 saturations; have available narcotic antagonist and measures for respiratory assistance as appropriate for clinical setting.
Decreased cough reflex	Monitor coughing ability postoperatively; use aspiration precautions.
Central Nervous System	
Drowsiness, alteration in mood and mental clouding; visual and auditory hallucinations, euphoria, dizziness, disorientation, paranoia; lethargy, inability to concentrate, apathy; seizures, uncontrollable twitching, myoclonus	Neurologic assessment at baseline to facilitate ongoing assessment. Optimize sleep hygiene, including management of pain during night. Provide for patient safety. Institute fall precautions, as needed. Avoid meperidine use. Monitor closely for any preseizure activity for individuals taking meperidine; monitor for twitching. Level of sedation may indicate degree of respiratory depression.

TABLE 31.6 Side Effects of Opioid Analgesics—cont'd

Side Effects	Nursing Implications
	Methylphenidate (Ritalin), 5–10 mg, PO BID or TID, may be helpful for somnolence or mental clouding from opioids.
Pupil	
Miosis	Monitor pupil size and response to light (contraction).
Smooth Muscle	
Contraction of gallbladder, bile duct, sphincter of Oddi	Monitor for signs of gastric upset; if present, evaluate liver and pancreatic function tests.
Genitourinary	
Urinary retention	Monitor urine output, palpate bladder, catheterize (straight or indwelling), as needed. This is often a transitory side effect seen with initiation and increasing of dose.
Dermatologic	
Skin rash, cutaneous vasodilation	Monitor skin integrity. Administer antihistamines for allergic reactions. Consider change in opioid. Educate patient to avoid scratching. Provide cool environment.

BID, Twice daily; *PO,* by mouth; *TID,* three times daily.

C. Dependence
   1. Physical dependence is universal; it is physiologic.
   2. Opioid withdrawal
      a. Doses of opioids should not be abruptly withdrawn to avoid opioid withdrawal. A sign of physical dependence, not psychological addiction.
      b. Symptoms of withdrawal
         (1) Nausea and vomiting
         (2) Diarrhea
         (3) Perspiration
         (4) Tachycardia
         (5) Chills
         (6) Restless legs syndrome
         (7) Dysphoria
         (8) Anxiety or paranoia
         (9) Insomnia
D. Other sedative or hypnotic drugs—potentiate sedative properties of opioids and combination opiate substances
E. Adverse drug interactions
   1. Drugs that lower seizure threshold—increased risk of seizures with concomitant administration
   2. Concomitant drugs that alter mental status equilibrium
   3. Drugs that alter hepatic metabolism, renal excretion
   4. Drugs that alter bioavailability, absorption, or pharmacokinetics of the administered drug
F. Organ alterations
   1. Surgical resections, including gastrectomy, jejunectomy, and duodenectomy, may increase transit time, decrease absorption, or both.
   2. Feeding tubes inserted at various points in the GI tract may not be the appropriate point of absorption of an individual drug.
   3. Pharmacologically induced changes in gut motility.
      a. Tube feedings or fluids administered through tubes may increase transit time and decrease absorption
      b. Laxatives
      c. Muscarinics (e.g., atropine)
      d. Prokinetic agents (e.g., metoclopramide)
   4. Renal insufficiency—may slow rate of elimination of drug, metabolites, or both, leading to increased potential for toxicities
   5. Hepatic insufficiency—may increase amount of drug available to body because of decreased first-pass effect, altered enzyme pathways, other metabolic pathways
   6. Central nervous system (CNS)—brain metastases, underlying seizure disorders may predispose to CNS toxicity
   7. Urinary—benign prostatic hypertrophy may contribute to urinary retention
   8. Respiratory—underlying restrictive or obstructive disease may potentiate respiratory compromise from opioids
   9. Cardiovascular—coronary artery disease, congestive heart failure
   10. Opioid considerations
      a. Codeine—a prodrug metabolized by p450; some patients lack the enzyme to convert it to the active analgesic form and it is ineffective; others may experience drug accumulation

b. Meperidine—retention of normeperidine, the active metabolite, may cause seizures

c. Hydromorphone (metabolites exist but clinical significance is unknown)

d. Tramadol—risk of serotonin syndrome with antidepressants

e. Morphine—metabolites can accumulate and cause oversedation

G. Transdermal considerations

1. Occlusive dressings increase absorption; moisture content can affect skin adherence

2. Heat

3. Ulcerations

4. Fat-to-lean body ratio—transdermal preparations not recommended in cachectic patients; longer time to onset in obese patients

Assessment

I. Identify patients at risk for pain

A. Assess and reassess pain—onset, duration, intensity, description, location, aggravating and relieving factors

1. Reassessment after pharmacologic intervention should occur 1 hour after oral analgesic administration and 15 minutes after parenteral analgesic administration

B. History of past and current analgesia regimens and their effectiveness

C. Psychological manifestations

1. Anxiety and/or depression

2. Cognitive behavioral changes

3. Social isolation

D. Patient and caregiver history: history of addiction or opioid use disorder

E. Assessment of patient's and caregiver's spiritual and cultural beliefs

II. Physical examination

A. Presence of inflammation or infection

B. Sensory examination

C. Musculoskeletal examination

D. Psychological examination

E. Patient safety

1. Respiratory depression

2. Sedation

3. Potential for addiction or opioid use disorder

III. Medication reconciliation

IV. Evaluation of diagnostic and laboratory studies

A. Radiographic studies (e.g., bone scan, CT, MRI)

B. Nerve blocks and nerve conduction studies

C. Toxicology screen

Management

I. Manage pain effectively and safely

II. Provide patient and caregiver education

A. Rationale for taking analgesic medications, including schedule of administration—long-acting and break-through agents; scheduled and as-needed agents

B. Adverse effects and strategies for management

1. Reinforce the need for stool softeners when taking opioids to prevent constipation

2. Take medications with food to prevent GI upset

3. Antihistamines for pruritus

C. Adverse effects to report to health care team

1. Respiratory depression or sedation

2. Analgesics not effective in managing pain

3. Constipation not relieved with stool softeners

D. Signs of physical dependence, addiction, and opioid withdrawal

III. Prevent/manage adverse effects of medication regimen (see Table 31.6)

A. Review of patient's medications for possible drug interactions

B. Presence of comorbidities (e.g., renal, cardiac, respiratory, or hepatic disease)

IV. Patient response to analgesia

A. Assessment of pain control

B. Assessment for adverse effects, toxicity, and drug interactions

C. Assessment of patient safety and medication tolerance

V. Revaluate pharmaceutical plan and adjust according to individual patient needs

PSYCHOTROPIC DRUGS: ANXIOLYTICS AND SEDATIVE-HYPNOTICS (COHEN & WHITE, 2018; MATTHEWS, 2018; NCCN, 2017d)

Overview

I. Rationale and indications

A. Psychosocial care is a standard of quality cancer care and should be included as routine for cancer treatment, including survivorship

B. Anxiety (see Chapter 50)

1. Commonly referred to as *distress,* as it is a less stigmatizing, more acceptable term

2. Estimated to occur in up to close to 50% of patients at some time throughout their cancer trajectory

3. Risk factors for anxiety

a. History of anxiety disorder or traumatic experience

b. Medical factors: type of treatment, pain, site, and stage of disease

c. Psychological factors: coping ability, emotional maturity, diagnosis

d. Social factors: younger patients, patients without strong familial support, and less educated patients have a higher incidence of distress and anxiety

e. Stimulants: caffeine, steroids

f. Medication withdrawal: barbiturates, benzodiazepines

4. Anxiolytics in patients with cancer

a. To reduce anxiety associated with cancer and its management
b. To eliminate functional impairment
c. To manage comorbid anxiety
d. To reduce pain associated with anxiety
e. To manage alcohol or narcotic withdrawal
f. To prevent or manage anticipatory nausea or vomiting or treat CINV

C. Sleep disturbance (see Chapter 46)
1. An estimated one third to one half of cancer survivors experience some degree of sleep disturbance
2. Pharmacologic risk factors for sleep disturbances
   a. Cancer treatment and side effects, medications used to treat side effects (e.g., opioids, antiemetics, anxiolytics, steroids for symptom management)
   b. Caffeine, alcohol, or other stimulant consumption

D. Management of anxiety (Traeger et al., 2012)
1. Rule out other (treatable) medical conditions with similar symptoms
2. Manage participating factors (e.g., pain, shortness of breath, drug-induced anxiety)
3. Employ nonpharmacologic strategies (e.g., relaxation, meditation)

E. Pharmacologic therapy
1. Selective serotonin reuptake inhibitors (SSRIs):
   a. Start at low dose and increase to optimal dose
   b. May induce anxiety symptoms early in therapy
   c. Abrupt discontinuation may precipitate withdrawal syndrome
   d. Effect may not be seen for the first 2 to 4 weeks
2. Serotonin-norepinephrine reuptake inhibitors (SNRIs)
   a. Start at low dose and increase to optimal dose
   b. May induce anxiety symptoms early in therapy
   c. Abrupt discontinuation may precipitate withdrawal syndrome
   d. Effect seen in 2 to 4 weeks
3. Benzodiazepines (Table 31.7)
   a. Considered second line for anxiety, but may be useful for short-term mitigation.
   b. Does not treat cognitive symptoms of anxiety (e.g., worry).
   c. Concerns for use include physical dependence and withdrawal effects. It is important to gradually decrease dose over time to avoid discontinuation syndrome.

TABLE 31.7 Comparison of Benzodiazepines

Drug	Comparative Oral Dose (mg)	Metabolic Pathway	Half-Life of Parent Drug (hr)
Short Acting			
Midazolam (Versed)	None		0.5–1
Triazolam (Halcion)	0.25–0.5 mg	CYP3A4 (no active metabolite)	1–4
Intermediate Acting			
Alprazolam (Xanax)	0.5	CYP3A4 (active metabolite)	6–20
Clonazepam (Klonopin)	0.25	CYP3A4 (no active metabolite)	20–40
Lorazepam (Ativan)	1	Glucuronidation (no active metabolite)	10–20
Oxazepam (Serax)	15 mg	(no active metabolite)	10–20
Temazepam (Restoril)	30 mg	Glucuronidation, CYP2C19, and CYP3A4 (no active metabolite)	10–20
Long Acting			
Chlordiazepoxide (Librium)	10 mg	(active metabolite)	5–30
Diazepam (Valium)	5	CYP2C19 and CYP3A4 (active metabolite)	20–50

From Lexi-Comp Online: *Lexi-drugs online,* and package inserts for agents.
CYP pathway: Knowledge of the particular enzymes involved in the metabolism of medications is important to assess potential drug–drug interactions and to modify the dose(s) or agents appropriately. If a medication is metabolized by one or multiple CYP enzymes extensively, any modification of those enzymes may result in change of the exposure to the medication. For example, drugs that inhibit an enzyme important in the metabolism of other medications may result in decreased metabolism and increased exposure of the medication. A drug that induces an enzyme important in the metabolism of other medications may result in increased metabolism and decreased exposure of the medication. A drug that is identified as a substrate for an enzyme is potentially vulnerable to changes in enzyme activity. If you have questions or concerns about the potential for drug–drug interactions while caring for a patient, consider collaboration with a pharmacist.

4. Tricyclic antidepressants
5. Other agents, including buspirone, mirtazapine, gabapentin, atypical antipsychotics (e.g., risperidone, olanzapine)
   a. Gabapentin and pregabalin are not Food and Drug Administration (FDA) approved for anxiety disorders
   b. Atypical antipsychotics have been used in treatment of anxiety disorders

II. Management of sleep disorders
  A. Pharmacologic options for sleep disorders
    1. Antihistamines (e.g., diphenhydramine, doxylamine)
     a. Tolerance to the sedative effects may develop within 10 days of frequent use
     b. Paradoxical excitation may occur in some individuals
    2. Antidepressants (e.g., trazadone, mirtazapine, doxepin)
    3. Melatonin
     a. OTC products are not standardized
     b. Common dose ranges from 0.3 to 5 mg
    4. Ramelteon (Rozerem)
     a. Receptor agonist with high affinity for two melatonin receptors
     b. Treatment for sleep latency
    5. Benzodiazepines (see Table 31.7)
     a. Reduce time to sleep onset and prolong the first two stages of sleep
     b. Reduce time in deep sleep and rapid eye movement (REM) sleep
     c. Can produce rebound insomnia when discontinued
    6. Nonbenzodiazepines—receptor agonists with effects similar to benzodiazepines
     a. Zolpidem (Ambien) indicated for sleep latency, maintenance, and middle-of-the-night awakenings (dependent on product)
     b. Zaleplon (Sonata) indicated for sleep latency
     c. Zopiclone (Imovane)
     d. Eszopiclone (Lunesta) indicated for sleep latency and maintenance
    7. Suvorexant (Belsomra)

III. Principles of medical management of anxiety and sleep disturbances (NCCN, 2017)
  A. Selection of therapy
    1. Psychotherapy
    2. Pharmacologic (see Table 31.7)
     a. Half-life
     b. Sedative properties
     c. Psychomotor and memory impairment
     d. Dose–response profiles
     e. Duration of therapy
     f. Routes of administration
     g. Compromised organ function
     h. Age-related alterations
     i. Cost

IV. Potential adverse effects
  A. CNS effects
  B. Potential for addiction, dependency, and abuse
  C. Rebound insomnia for short-acting agents
  D. Complex sleep-related behaviors (e.g., sleepwalking)
  E. Motor incoordination
  F. Behavioral changes, delirium
  G. Respiratory suppression
    1. Sedation
    2. Dizziness
    3. Lightheadedness
    4. Cognitive impairment
    5. Particularly in older adults
    6. Caution should be used in patients with pulmonary disease (e.g., chronic obstructive pulmonary disease [COPD])

V. Drug interactions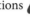
  A. Alcohol
    1. Concomitant consumption of alcohol and these medications should be avoided.
  B. Inhibitors or inducers of hepatic enzymes

Assessment

I. Identify patients at risk for distress or sleep disturbances
  A. Assess for signs and symptoms of anxiety and sleep disorders
  B. Patient screening tools
    1. NCCN Distress Thermometer (scores of 4 or higher are associated with higher levels of distress)
    2. Sleep diaries or questionnaires; Insomnia Severity Index
  C. Patient and family history

II. Physical examination
  A. Alterations in functional performance
  B. Concurrent medication or cancer-related symptoms

III. Medication reconciliation
  A. Sudden withdrawal from sedatives can lead to increase in anxiety
  B. Medications used to treat cancer-treatment side effects can lead to sleep disturbance (e.g., opioids, antiemetics, steroids)
  C. Medication interactions can increase adverse side effects of anxiolytics and sedative-hypnotics

IV. Evaluate diagnostic and laboratory data
  A. Hepatic and renal function
  B. Toxicology screen

V. Patient safety
  A. Assess for signs of psychomotor or cognitive impairment
  B. Assess for signs of dependency or abuse

Management

I. Manage sleep disturbances, pain, and emotional distress
II. Patient and caregiver education

A. Rationale for use of sedative-hypnotic or anxiolytic drug therapy and taking them as scheduled or only when needed

B. Adverse effects of anxiolytics and sedative-hypnotic medications and strategies to manage them
1. Pharmacologic interventions for sleep disturbances classified by Oncology Nursing Society as "benefit balanced with harm" due to potential harmful side effects and medication interactions
2. Safety considerations due to decreased motor coordination, excessive drowsiness
3. Potential for addiction, dependency, or abuse
4. Avoid concurrent use with opioids or alcohol
5. Side effects more pronounced in older patients

C. Adverse effects to report to health care team
1. Signs of medication withdrawal, addiction, tolerance, or dependence
2. Cognitive impairment

III. Monitor for adverse effects of sedative-hypnotic or anxiolytic drugs

IV. Decrease the incidence and manage the adverse effects of sedative-hypnotic or anxiolytic drugs
A. Assess baseline data (e.g., vital signs; CNS—orientation, alertness, affect; respiratory effort, rate, depth)
B. Review patient's medical history for existing or previous conditions
C. Review patient's medications for potential drug interactions ⚠

V. Monitor for response to psychotropic drugs
A. Psychiatry or psychology consultation as needed
B. Assess level of anxiety and amount of restful sleep

VI. Reevaluate pharmaceutical plan and adjust according to individual patient needs

VII. Refer to psychosocial services (e.g.: social work, mental health professional, counseling) or chaplain as needed

ANTIDEPRESSANTS (COHEN & WHITE, 2018; NCCN, 2017d)

Overview

I. Rationale and indications
A. For treatment of pain (adjuvant therapy)
B. For treatment of depression
C. Definition and incidence of depression (see Chapter 50)
1. Sad, empty, irritable mood accompanied by somatic or cognitive changes that affect daily functioning
2. Major depressive disorder—depressive symptoms lasting most of day, every day, for at least 2 weeks; may have suicidal thoughts, recurrent thoughts of dying ⚠
3. Often difficult to identify in cancer patients because symptoms can mimic treatment side effects (e.g., fatigue, weight loss, changes in appetite)
4. Occurs in about 25% of patients with cancer, leading to poor quality of life and functional status,

higher use of health care services, and nonadherence with treatment

D. Pharmacologic risk factors for depression
1. Poor pain control
2. Medications used in cancer treatment

E. Purposes of antidepressants
1. To treat clinical unipolar or bipolar depression or anxiety
2. To treat depression associated with chronic pain
3. As adjuvant pharmacologic pain management in pain conditions, including postherpetic neuralgia, migraine and chronic tension headaches, sundowner syndrome
4. To treat insomnia

II. Types of antidepressants (Table 31.8)
A. SSRIs
1. Toxicities include nausea, constipation, diarrhea, dry mouth, dizziness, nervousness and insomnia, and sexual dysfunction.
2. Frequency of adverse effects is agent specific.

B. SNRIs
1. Toxicities include anxiety, nausea/vomiting, dizziness, constipation, insomnia, diaphoresis and increased blood pressure (agent specific), sexual dysfunction, and discontinuation syndrome.

C. Tricyclic antidepressants (TCAs)
1. Often used later in therapy (second and third line) secondary to side effects and risk with overdosage. Overdosages may be lethal; contraindicated in older adults.
2. Common side effects include anticholinergic effects of blurred vision, dry mouth, constipation, antihistamine effects (including sedation and weight gain), and alpha-adrenergic inhibition (including postural hypotension, reflex tachycardia, and priapism).

D. Monoamine oxidase inhibitors (MAOIs)
1. Dietary modifications to avoid tyramine.
2. Drug–drug interactions can result in hypertensive crisis. A required washout period for the drug is dependent on the drug's half-life.
3. Toxicity includes hypertensive crisis and serotonin syndrome.

E. Bupropion

F. Nefazodone

G. Trazodone—may also be used as a sleep aid

H. Mirtazapine—may increase appetite

I. Vilazodone

J. Levomilnacipran

K. Vortioxetine

L. Lithium

III. Principles of medical management
A. Selection of therapy
1. Efficacy (prior history)
2. Comorbidities
3. Side effect profile of patient
4. Concern with risk of overdose

TABLE 31.8 Antidepressants Classification and Indications

Medication	Classification	Indications
Amitriptyline	TCA (tetracyclic antidepressant)	Depression
Amoxapine	TCA	Depression
Bupropion	NDRI	Major depressive disorder
		Seasonal affective disorder
		Smoking cessation (bupropion SR [Zyban])
Citalopram	SSRI	Depression
Clomipramine	TCA	Obsessive compulsive disorder (OCD)
Desipramine	TCA	Depression
Desvenlafaxine	SSNI	Major depressive disorder
Doxepin	TCA	Depression
		Insomnia
Duloxetine	SSNI	Major depressive disorder
		General anxiety disorder
		Diabetic peripheral neuropathy
		Chronic musculoskeletal pain
Escitalopram	SSRI	Major depressive disorder
		General anxiety disorder
Fluoxetine	SSRI	Major depressive disorder
		OCD
		Bulimia nervosa
		Panic disorder
		Depressive episodes associated with bipolar I disorders (with olanzapine)
Fluvoxamine	SSRI	OCDs
Imipramine	TCA	Depression
Isocarboxazid	MAOI	Depression
Maprotiline	TCA	Depression
Milnacipran		Fibromyalgia
Mirtazapine	5HT and α2-adrenergic antagonist	Depression
Nefazodone	Mixed 5HT	Depression
Nortriptyline	TCA	Depression
Paroxetine	SSRI	General anxiety disorder
		Posttraumatic stress disorder
		Major depression disorder
		OCDs
		Panic disorder
		Social anxiety disorders
		Premenstrual dysphoric disorder
Phenelzine	MAOI	Depression
Protriptyline	TCA	Depression
Selegiline	MAOI	Major depressive disorder
Sertraline	SSRI	Panic disorder
		Posttraumatic stress disorder
		Social anxiety disorder
		Premenstrual dysphoric disorder
Tranylcypromine	MAOI	Major depressive disorder
Trazodone	Mixed 5HT	Depression
		Major depressive disorder
Trimipramine	TCA	Depression
Venlafaxine	SSNI	Major depressive disorder
		General anxiety disorder
		Panic disorder
		Social anxiety disorder
Vilazodone	Mixed 5HT	Major depressive disorder

5-HT, serotonin; *MAOI,* monoamine oxidase inhibitor; *NDRI,* norepinephrine and dopamine reuptake inhibitor; *SNRI,* serotonin-norepinephrine reuptake inhibitors; *SSRI,* Selective serotonin reuptake inhibition.

5. Optimizing side effects for efficacy (e.g., increasing appetite with weight loss)
6. Patient preference
IV. Potential adverse effects (Table 31.9)
   A. Drug–drug interactions
   B. Dietary restrictions

Assessment

I. Identification of patients at risk for depression
   A. Patient screening tools
      1. Patient Health Questionnaire
      2. NCCN Distress Thermometer (scores of 4 or higher have clinical significance)
      3. Suicide Risk Assessment
      4. Hospital Anxiety and Depression Scale
   B. Alcohol or substance abuse
   C. Assessment of unrelieved or chronic pain and fatigue
II. Physical examination
III. Medication reconciliation
   A. Several interactions between antidepressant and cancer treatment medications exist (e.g., antidepressants and tamoxifen)
   B. Antidepressant therapeutic effect can take up to 3 weeks; ensure patient adherence
   C. Withdrawal symptoms can occur with abrupt discontinuation
IV. Evaluate diagnostic and laboratory data
V. Assess patient's and family's understanding of depression as an illness

Management

I. Manage effects of depression, pain, and fatigue
II. Patient and caregiver education
   A. Rationale for use of antidepressant drug therapy and taking antidepressants as scheduled; time necessary for therapeutic response to agent; potential for withdrawal effects with abrupt cessation; continue therapy for 6 months after improvement in symptoms to avoid relapse of depression; gradually taper dose at discontinuation
   B. Adverse effects to report to health care team
      1. Suicidal ideation and worsening symptoms
      2. Presence of unwanted side effects with prescribed antidepressant therapy (weight gain, dizziness, sedative effects, palpitations)
      3. Serotonin syndrome (hyperreflexia, tremors, tachycardia, nausea, diarrhea, agitation, confusion)
III. Monitor for adverse effects of antidepressants
IV. Decrease the incidence and manage the adverse effects of antidepressants
V. Monitor for therapeutic response to antidepressants
   A. Monitor patient for emotional changes, suicidal ideation
   B. Obtain psychiatric or psychological consultation as needed

C. Monitor patient for response to pain management interventions
D. Assess for adverse effects, toxicity, and drug–drug interactions
VI. Reevaluate pharmaceutical plan and adjust according to individual patient needs
VII. Refer to psychosocial services or chaplain as needed

ANTICONVULSANTS (ARMSTRONG, ET AL., 2016; OLSEN, LEFEBVRE, & BRASSIL, 2019; SANTOMASSO, ET AL., 2018; TRADOUNSKY, 2013)

Overview

I. Rationale and indications
   A. Epilepsy
      1. Disturbance of electrical activity in the brain
      2. Classified by where they occur in the brain (the focus), the patient's level of awareness, and the presence of motor movements
   B. For prophylaxis and treatment of seizure activity
      1. Intracranial causes—primary brain tumors, primary CNS lymphoma, or metastatic cancer
      2. Drug-induced causes (treatments that lower the seizure threshold)
         a. Chemotherapy: asparaginase, busulfan, carmustine, cisplatin, cyclophosphamide, dacarbazine, docetaxel, etoposide, 5-FU, gemcitabine ifosfamide, thalidomide, and vinca alkaloids (Olsen, LeFebvre, & Brassil, 2019)
         b. Antibiotics
         c. Antidepressants
         d. Opioids
         e. Chimeric antigen receptor (CAR) T-cell therapies (Santomasso, et al., 2018)
         f. Intrathecal chemotherapy
      3. Metabolic abnormalities
         a. Electrolyte imbalance (hypernatremia, hyponatremia, hypercalcemia, syndrome of inappropriate antidiuretic hormone secretion [SIADH])
         b. Hyperglycemia or hypoglycemia
      4. Other causes of seizures in patients with cancer
         a. Cerebral edema (e.g., increased intracranial pressure)
         b. Stroke (e.g., hemorrhage)
         c. CNS infections (e.g., meningitis)
         d. Posterior reversible encephalopathy syndrome (PRES)
         e. Radiation toxicity
   C. As adjuvant pharmacologic therapy for neuropathic pain (e.g., peripheral neuropathy)
II. Types of anticonvulsants (Table 31.10)
   A. Diagnose appropriate seizure activity
   B. Diagnose appropriate pain syndrome

TABLE 31.9 Antidepressants Toxicity Comparison

Drug	Initial Dose	Anticholinergic	Sedation	Orthostatic Hypotension	Conduction Abnormalities	GI Distress	Weight Gain	Comments
Tricyclic Antidepressants								
Amitriptyline (generic)	25–50 mg q HS	4+	4+	3+	3+	1+	4+	Higher doses are used in the management of depression.
Desipramine (generic)	25–75 mg q HS	1+	2+	2+	2+	–	1+	Dose increases should be made in 25-mg increments.
Imipramine (generic)	25–75 mg q HS	3+	3+	4+	3+	1+	4+	Also used for chronic pain.
Nortriptyline (generic)	25–50 mg q HS	2+	2+	1+	2+	0	2+	Lower doses recommended for older patients.
Selective Serotonin Reuptake Inhibitors								
Citalopram	20 mg q AM	0	0	0	0	3+	1+	Significant sexual dysfunction
Escitalopram	10 mg q AM	0	0	0	0	3+	1+	Significant sexual dysfunction
Fluoxetine	10–20 mg q AM	0	0	0	0	3+	1+	CYP2B6 and 2D6 inhibitor (do not use with tamoxifen); significant sexual dysfunction
Fluvoxamine	50 mg q day	0	1+	0	0	3+	–	
Paroxetine	10–20 mg q AM	1+	1+	0	0	3+	2+	CYP2B6 and 2D6 inhibitor (do not use with tamoxifen); significant sexual dysfunction
Sertraline	20–50 mg once daily	0	0	0	0	3+	1+	CYP2B6 and 2D6 inhibitor (do not use with tamoxifen); significant sexual dysfunction
Mixed-Action Agents								
Bupropion	150 mg q AM; BID (SR tab)	0	0	0	1+	1+	0	Contraindicated with seizures, bulimia, or anorexia; low incidence of sexual dysfunction
Duloxetine	40–60 mg once daily	1+	1+	0	1+	3+	0	Also used for neuropathy
Venlafaxine	37.5 mg once daily (XR tab)	1+	1+	0	1+	3+	0	Frequency of hypertension increases with dose; often used for hot flashes from tamoxifen
Desvenlafaxine	50 mg once daily	0	1+	1+	0	3+	0	—
Mirtazapine	15 mg q HS	1+	3+	1+	1+	0	3+	Doses >15 mg/day less sedating; low incidence of sexual dysfunction; reported to increase appetite
Trazodone	50 mg TID	0	4+	3+	1+	1+	2+	Often used for insomnia (50–150 mg q HS)

AM, Morning; *BID,* twice daily; *HS,* at bedtime; *q,* every; *SR,* sustained-release; *TID,* three times a day; *XR,* extended-release.

Adapted from Lacy, C. F., Armstrong, L. L., Goldman, M. P., Lance, L. L. (2011). *Drug information handbook* (20th ed.; pp. 1143–1147). Hudson, OH: Lexi-Comp.

TABLE 31.10   Anticonvulsant Medications

Drug (common brand name)	Dose	Target Serum Concentrations	Side Effects
Brivaracetam (Briviact)	Dose: 50–100 mg BID		Fatigue, hypersomnia, weakness
Carbamazepine (Tegretol)	Adults: 400 mg PO daily	4–12 mcg/mL	Dose-related: Diplopia, drowsiness, nausea Others: Hyponatremia Aplastic anemia Leukopenia Rash
Clonazepam (Klonopin)	Initiate at 0.5 mg PO 1–3 times daily, titrate to effectiveness	Not established	Dose-related: Ataxia Memory impairment Sedation
Eslicarbazepine (Aptiom)	Initial: 400 mg PO daily Dose: 1200 mg PO daily (maximum dose)		Dizziness, drowsiness, nausea, vomiting, headache, diplopia, fatigue, ataxia, tremor
Ezogabine (Potiga)	Initial: 100 mg PO TID Dose: 600 – 1200 mg PO daily in divided doses.		Urinary retention, dizziness, fatigue, confusion, disorientation, hallucinations, diplopia Chronic use: Bluish pigmentation of skin, nails and retina
Felbamate (Felbatol)	Initial: 1200 mg PO Dose: 1200–3600 mg/day in 3 or 4 divided doses	30–60 mcg/mL	Dose-related: Anxiety Insomnia Nausea Anorexia Other: Aplastic anemia (monitor CBC) Liver dysfunction (monitor LFT)
Gabapentin (Neurotin)	Initial: 300 mg PO (may start lower in select patients, or higher in select situations) Dose: 900–3600 mg/day PO in 3–4 divided doses	2–20 mcg/mL	Dose-related: Sedation Dizziness ataxia Other: Weight gain Peripheral edema
Lacosamide (Vimpat)	Initial: 100 mg PO per day in divided doses and titrate Dose: 200–400 mg/day PO	Not established	Dose-related: Ataxia Dizziness Diplopia Nausea Headache Other: PR interval prolongation (baseline ECG and monitor as needed) Increase LFT
Lamotrigine (Lamictal)	Dose: 150–500 mg/day PO in 2–3 divided doses. Dose may be lower if used in combination with valproic acid. Note: Initiated at lower dose and titrated based on overall therapy.	4–20 mcg/mL	Dose-related: Ataxia Drowsiness Headache Insomnia Sedation Diplopia Other: Rash

Continued

TABLE 31.10   Anticonvulsant Medications—cont'd

Drug (common brand name)	Dose	Target Serum Concentrations	Side Effects
Levetiracetam (Keppra)	Initiate at 500–1000 mg/day PO and titrate as needed (divided dose) Dose:1000–3000 mg/day PO	12–46 mcg/mL	Dose-related: Somnolence Dizziness Other: Depression Rash Psychosis (rare, more common in elderly)
Oxcarbazepine (Trileptal)	Initial: 300 mg PO twice daily and titrate. Dose: 600–1200 mg/day PO	3–35 mcg/mL	Dose-related: Dizziness Somnolence Ataxia Nausea Other: Hyponatremia (chronic side effect) Rash 23%–30% cross-sensitivity to carbamazepine
Perampanel (Fycompa) CIII	Initial: 2 mg PO q HS Dose: 4–12 mg PO daily		Dizziness, somnolence, headache, fatigue
Phenobarbital (generic)	Maintenance dose: 1–4mg/kg/day PO as a single or divided daily dose	15–40 mcg/mL	Dose-related: Ataxia, drowsiness, sedation Others: attention deficit, cognitive impairment, hyperactivity
Phenytoin (Dilantin) Fosphenytoin (Cerebyx) Note: Phenytoin prodrug only available IV	Initial: 3–5 mg/kg Loading dose of 15–20 mg/kg may be used. Dose: 300–600 mg PO daily (based on serum level)	10–20 mcg/mL (total) Unbound phenytoin: 0.5–3 mcg/mL Note: Phenytoin is highly protein bound, and unbound phenytoin should be measured in patients with low serum albumin	Dose related: Ataxia, nystagmus, dizziness, headache, sedation, lethargy, Other: Rash Blood dyscrasia Folate deficiency Hirsutism Allergy, Hepatotoxicity
Pregabalin (Lyrica)	Initial: 150 mg PO Dose: 300 mg PO/day (split doses)	Not established	Dose related: Dizziness, somnolence, dry mouth, vision changes Other: Pedal edema Increase CPK Thrombocytopenia Weight gain
Rufinamide (Banzel)	Approved as adjunctive treatment of seizures with Lennox–Gastaut syndrome in children 4 yr or older.		Somnolence, dizziness, gait disturbances, ataxia QT shortening (up to 20 msec)
Tiagabine (Gabitril)	Initial: 4–8 mg/day Dose: 80 mg	0.02–0.2 mcg/mL	Dose related: Dizziness, fatigue, difficulty concentrating, nervousness depression
Topiramate (Topamax)	Initial: 25–50 mg PO daily Dose: 200–1000 mg PO per day	5–20 mcg/mL	Dose related: Difficulty concentrating, psychomotor slowing, speech and language problems. Other: Metabolic acidosis, acute angle glaucoma, kidney stones

TABLE 31.10 Anticonvulsant Medications—cont'd

Drug (common brand name)	Dose	Target Serum Concentrations	Side Effects
Valproic acid	Initial: 15 mg/kg Dose: 60 mg/kg (3000–5000 mg)	50–100 mcg/mL	Dose related: GI upset, sedation, unsteadiness, tremor, thrombocytopenia Other: Liver dysfunction (monitor LFT) Pancreatitis Alopecia
Vigabatrin (Sabril)	Initial: 500 mg PO twice daily Dose: 1500 mg PO twice daily	0.8–36 mcg/mL	Dose related: Visual field defects, fatigue, sedation, tremor, blurred vision, weight gain Other: Peripheral neuropathy anemia
Zonisamide (Zonegran)	Initial: 100 mg PO daily Dose: 300–400 mg PO per day	10–40 mcg/mL	Dose related: Sedation, dizziness, cognitive impairment, nausea Other: Rash (sulfa drug) metabolic acidosis

From Weller, M., Stupp, R., & Wick, W. (2012). Epilepsy meets cancer: When, why and what to do about it? *Lancet Oncology, 13,* 375-382; Rogers, S. J., & Cavazos, J. E. (2014). *Epilepsy. Pharmacotherapy: A pathophysiologic approach* (9th ed.), (pp. 855-882). New York: McGraw-Hill.

C. Selection of appropriate pharmacologic therapy (see Table 31.10)
  1. Neurology consultation should be considered.
  2. Determine etiology of seizure to best manage long term, if needed.
    a. Seizure should not be presumed to be from tumor.
    b. Evaluation of other causes should be undertaken.
  3. No substantial differences between efficacy of medications.
    a. Agent selection is determined by comorbidities, adverse effects, drug–drug interactions, cost, etc.
  4. Therapeutic selection is based on drug interactions and tolerance.
IV. Potential adverse effects (see Table 31.10)

Assessment

I. Identify patients at risk for seizure activity—older adults and pediatric patients at higher risk
II. Identify patients at risk for neuropathic pain
III. Physical examination
  A. Neurologic examination
    1. Mental status—general appearance, level of consciousness, mood and affect, thought content and intellectual capacity, behavior
    2. Cranial nerve assessment
    3. Sensory and motor function, gait
    4. Assessment of reflexes
    5. Presence of aura with seizure onset
IV. Medication reconciliation

A. Medications that lower the seizure threshold
B. Benzodiazepine withdrawal
C. Some anticonvulsants are enzyme inducers, which can accelerate metabolism of other drugs and reduce serum levels
V. Evaluation of diagnostic and laboratory data
  A. Anticonvulsant serum levels
  B. Serum electrolyte values
  C. Cerebrospinal fluid (CSF) culture
  D. Electroencephalogram (EEG), CT, MRI

Management

I. Ensure patient safety in the event of a seizure
  A. Institute seizure precautions
    1. Padded side rails, bed in lowest position
    2. Suction setup to maintain airway
    3. Safe environment free of physical hazards
  B. Assess for injuries after completion of the seizure activity
    1. Vital signs
    2. Neurologic examination
II. Patient and caregiver education
  A. Rationale for use of anticonvulsant drug therapy and taking as scheduled
  B. Adverse effects and strategies to manage adverse effects
  C. Adverse effects to report to health care team
  D. Emphasize patient safety
    1. Do not restrain patient during seizure
    2. Turn patient's head to side if vomiting

3. Avoid putting anything in patient's mouth during seizure
4. Patients should not drive or operate machinery
5. High-risk patients should wear a medical alert bracelet at all times

III. Monitor for adverse effects of anticonvulsants
IV. Decrease the incidence and manage the adverse effects of anticonvulsants
  A. Assessment of baseline data (e.g., neurologic status)
  B. Review of patient's medical history for existing or previous conditions
  C. Review of patient's medications for potential drug–drug interactions
  D. Conducting patient and family teaching (e.g., good oral hygiene, avoiding driving or other potentially hazardous activity that requires mental alertness)
V. Monitor for a therapeutic response to anticonvulsant drug therapy
  A. Assessment of neurologic status and pain level
  B. Assessment for adverse effects, toxicity, and drug interactions

MYELOID GROWTH FACTORS (BENNETT, DJULBEGOVIC, NORRIS, & ARMITAGE, 2013; CAMP-SORRELL, 2018; NCCN, 2017e)

Overview

I. Rationale and indications
  A. Myeloid growth factors (MGFs)—biological agents that stimulate the proliferation and activation of mature myeloid cells (e.g., neutrophils, erythrocytes, and platelets)
  B. Mature myeloid cells are often destroyed by chemotherapy and radiation treatment
    1. Nearly all chemotherapy treatments will cause a degree of myelosuppression, which can be a dose-limiting toxicity
    2. MGF use is supported in high-risk patients: previous chemotherapy regimen, presence of comorbidities (e.g., diabetes, cardiac or kidney disease), poor nutritional status, advanced disease, tumor-related bone marrow involvement
  C. Cancer-related indications
    1. Reduce incidence, length, and severity of neutropenia (ANC less than 500/mm^3) and febrile neutropenia (neutropenia plus a temperature of more than 38.5°C) in high-risk patients
      a. Febrile neutropenia is a serious side effect of treatment and is associated with significant morbidity and mortality
      b. High-risk cancer types: bladder, breast, esophageal, lymphoma, kidney, melanoma, multiple myeloma, ovarian/testicular, sarcoma, myelodysplastic syndromes, leukemia

2. Mobilization of hematopoietic stem cells before stem cell collection and for supportive care after transplant
      a. Granulocyte colony stimulating factor (G-CSF) is routinely used after autologous and cord blood transplantation to support neutrophil engraftment
    3. Treatment of malignancy and treatment-related anemia
II. Types of growth factors in clinical use
  A. White blood cell growth factors
    1. G-CSF (filgrastim, pegfilgrastim, Tbo-filgrastim, and biosimilar products)
      a. Filgrastim
      b. Tbo-filgrastim is not licensed as a biosimilar in the United States and does have different FDA-approved clinical indications from filgrastim
      c. Filgrastim-sndz is licensed in United States as biosimilar (reference product: filgrastim)
      d. Pegfilgrastim
      e. Pegfilgrastim-jmdb is licensed as a biosimilar (reference product: pegfilgrastim)
    2. GM-CSF (sargramostim)
      a. Receptors exist on myeloid cell lines.
      b. Major effect stimulates the proliferation and differentiation of the cells destined for the neutrophil and macrophage lines.
      c. Granulocyte-macrophage colony stimulating factor (GM-CSF) enhances functional activities of neutrophils and monocytes or macrophages, leads to enhanced activity in clearing bacterial and fungal organisms.
      d. GM-CSF stimulates production of secondary cytokines such as tumor necrosis factor (TNF), interleukin-1 (IL-1), and macrophage colony-stimulating factor (M-CSF).
    3. Erythropoietin (epoetin alfa and darbepoetin alfa)
III. Principles of medical management
  A. G-CSF and GM-CSF
    1. Prevention of febrile neutropenia with G-CSF or GM-CSF is more effective than treatment of febrile neutropenia with G-CSF or GM-CSF.
    2. Prevention of neutropenia by using G-CSF or GM-CSF is indicated in patients with 20% or greater risk of febrile neutropenia as determined by chemotherapy regimen or patient-specific factors.
    3. Risk of neutropenia determined primarily by chemotherapeutic regimen (review NCCN guidelines for list of regimens with ≥20% risk of febrile neutropenia).
    4. The intent of treatment may be a consideration for the use of white blood cell growth factor (WBC-GF); dose modification may be an appropriate option for individuals that are not receiving treatment for curative intent.

5. Risk is increased in select patients, including:
   a. Prior chemotherapy or radiation therapy
   b. Persistent neutropenia
   c. Bone marrow involvement of the tumor
   d. Recent surgery or open wounds
   e. Liver dysfunction
   f. Renal dysfunction
   g. Age (>56 years)
6. G-CSF shown to decrease days on antibiotics and hospital stay by 1 day, but it does not decrease mortality.
7. Pegfilgrastim at least as effective as filgrastim in prevention of febrile neutropenia.
8. Filgrastim is used to mobilize stem cells from the bone marrow to be collected peripherally before allogeneic or autologous stem cell transplantation.
9. Pegfilgrastim has limited use in stem cell mobilization at this time.
   a. Increased age (>65 years)
   b. Extensive previous treatments (chemotherapy and radiation therapy)
   c. Hematologic malignancy
   d. Multiple comorbidities (e.g., diabetes, COPD)
   e. Some data suggest it may be a more effective agent, but this has not been shown in randomized controlled trials.
B. Erythropoiesis-stimulating agents (ESA) or erythropoietin (EPO) (epoetin alfa, epoetin alfa-epbx, darbepoetin)
   1. EPO causes an increase in hemoglobin (>2 g/dL) more effectively than placebo in patients with anemia caused by chemotherapy.
   2. Concern has been raised by multiple clinical trials suggesting a decrease in progression-free and overall survival in patients receiving EPO during chemotherapy, radiotherapy, or no active treatment. EPO is not recommended for treatment of chemotherapy induced anemia (CIA) in the curative setting. ⚠️
   3. ESA shortened overall survival and/or increased the risk of tumor progression in studies of patients with breast, non–small cell lung cancer (NSCLC), head and neck cancer, lymphoid, and cervical cancers.
   4. EPO should not be given to patients with hemoglobin greater than 10 g/dL
   5. Treatment goals
   6. Important to evaluate iron stores before use
      a. EPO also decreases the number of red blood cell (RBC) transfusions required to treat anemia.
      b. The FDA eliminated the need for a risk evaluation and migration strategy (REMS) before administration of ESAs.
      c. EPO is not recommended in select patient populations.

d. EPO shown to increase the risk of venous thromboembolism as well. ⚠️
   (1) Cancer patients not receiving active treatment
   (2) Cancer patients receiving chemotherapy with a curative intent
e. To prevent RBC transfusions
f. To ensure that the starting dose and maintenance dose are lowest to prevent RBC transfusion.
g. Iron is an important component of RBCs.
h. Patients who are iron-deficient will not respond to EPO.

IV. Potential adverse effects
   A. Side effects (Table 31.11)

Assessment

I. Identify patients at risk for the following:
   A. Neutropenia—ANC less than 500/mm^3
      1. Patients older than 65 years old
      2. Female gender
      3. Poor nutritional status
      4. Comorbidities (COPD, diabetes, cardiovascular disease)
      5. Prior chemotherapy and/or radiation
      6. Tumor involvement in the bone marrow
      7. Presence of open sores or unhealed wounds
   B. Anemia—hemoglobin level less than 10 g/dL
   C. Thrombocytopenia—platelet count less than 75,000 cells/mm^3
II. Physical examination
   A. Neutropenia—assess for signs of infection or inflammation of the lungs, skin, oral cavity, venous access devices, GI tract
   B. Anemia—assess for signs of irritability, fatigue, pallor, headaches, hypotension
   C. Thrombocytopenia—assess for signs of easy bruising, nosebleeds, bleeding gums, blood in the urine or stool, petechiae, headaches, changes in mental status
III. Medication reconciliation
   A. Date of last chemotherapy cycle
   B. Cell nadir occurs 7 to 14 days after chemotherapy treatment
IV. Evaluation of diagnostic and laboratory data
   A. Complete blood count with differential

Management

I. Manage neutropenia or infection, thrombocytopenia or bleeding, and anemia or fatigue
II. Patient and family education
   A. Rationale for medication indication and schedule
      1. High-risk patients need to return to clinic 24 to 72 hours after the completion of chemotherapy for G-CSF administration

TABLE 31.11   Growth Factors

Drug	Indications	Toxicities	Management
White Blood Cell Growth Factors			
Filgrastim (Neupogen)	Use to decrease risk of infection, as manifested by febrile neutropenia, in patients with nonmyeloid malignancies receiving myelosuppressive chemotherapy. Myeloid recovery after induction or consolidation chemotherapy in AML. Myeloid recovery in patients with nonmyeloid malignancies undergoing myeloablative chemotherapy followed by marrow transplantation. Mobilization of hematopoietic progenitor cells into the peripheral blood for collection by leukapheresis. Patients with severe chronic neutropenia.	Bone pain	Monitor level of pain; administer acetaminophen for bone pain. Monitor CBC for increase in neutrophils. *Precautions:* Contraindicated in patients with known hypersensitivity to *Escherichia coli*–derived products; do not shake vial vigorously if giving subcutaneous injection.
Filgrastim-sndz (Zarxio) (biosimilar)	Use to decrease risk of infection, as manifested by febrile neutropenia, in patients with nonmyeloid malignancies receiving myelosuppressive chemotherapy. Myeloid recovery after induction or consolidation chemotherapy in AML. Myeloid recovery in patients with nonmyeloid malignancies undergoing myeloablative chemotherapy followed by marrow transplantation. Mobilization of hematopoietic progenitor cells into the peripheral blood for collection by leukapheresis. Patients with severe chronic neutropenia.	See filgrastim.	See filgrastim.
Pegfilgrastim (Neulasta)		Bone pain	Monitor level of pain; administer acetaminophen for bone pain. See filgrastim.
		Adult respiratory distress syndrome (rare)	Assess respiratory status (breath sounds, rate, pattern and depth of respirations, oxygen saturation); notify physician of worsening symptoms.
		Splenic rupture	Abdominal assessment and pain; notify physician. Monitor CBC laboratory test results for return of neutrophils. *Precautions:* Contraindicated in patients with known hypersensitivity to *E. coli*–derived proteins; do not administer sooner than 24 hr after chemotherapy, and in the case of pegfilgrastim must be no sooner than 14 days before chemotherapy.
Sargramostim (Leukine) GM-CSF	AML after induction chemotherapy Autologous peripheral blood progenitor cell mobilization and collection Autologous peripheral blood progenitor cell and bone marrow transplantation Allogeneic bone marrow transplantation	Low dose: bone pain, local skin reaction, fever, flulike syndrome, headache, arthralgias, myalgias	Monitor level of pain. Management of flulike symptoms with antipyretics if appropriate based on ANC, fluids, rest, comfort measures for symptoms.

TABLE 31.11 Growth Factors—cont'd

Drug	Indications	Toxicities	Management
	Allogeneic or autologous bone marrow transplantation: treatment of delayed neutrophil recovery or graft failure Acute exposure to myelosuppressive doses of radiation	High dose: capillary leak syndrome, pericardial effusions, third spacing of fluids Phlebitis with peripheral IV administration	High dose: closely monitor VS, fluid, edema, I&O, electrolytes, and CBC. Monitor injection site for pain, redness or induration.
Tbo-filgrastim (Granix) Not a biosimilar in the U.S.	Reduce the duration of severe neutropenia in patients with nonmyeloid malignancies receiving myelosuppressive anticancer drugs.	See filgrastim.	See filgrastim.

Red Blood Cell Growth Factors

Drug	Indications	Toxicities	Management
Erythropoietin (Epogen, Procrit)	Anemia due to chronic kidney disease. Anemia due to zidovudine in patients with HIV infection Anemia due to chemotherapy in patients with cancer (nonmyeloid malignancies) Reduction of allogeneic read blood cell transfusions in patients undergoing elective, noncardiac, nonvascular surgery. LIMITATIONS: Not indicated in cancer patients who are not receiving myelosuppressive chemotherapy. Not indicated in cancer patient when the anticipated outcome is cure. Not indicated in patients with cancer receiving myelosuppressive chemotherapy in whom the anemia can be managed by transfusion. Not indicated in patients scheduled for surgery who are willing to donate autologous blood. Not indicated in patients undergoing cardiac or vascular surgery. Not indicated as a substitute for RBC transfusions in patients who require immediate correction of anemia.	Hypertension Thrombotic events Seizures Headaches Skin rashes, urticaria; transient rash at injection site	Monitor blood pressure. Assess for possible emboli in lower extremities or lungs. Assess for seizure activity; implement seizure precautions as needed. Assess level of headache; administer pain medication as needed. Assess skin before the start of treatment and during treatment; rotate injection sites. Monitor CBC laboratory test results for increase in red blood cell count.
Darbepoetin, (Aranesp)	Anemia due to chronic kidney disease. Anemia due to chemotherapy in patients with cancer. LIMITATIONS: Not indicated in cancer patients who are not receiving myelosuppressive chemotherapy. Not indicated in cancer patient when the anticipated outcome is cure. Not indicated in patients with cancer receiving myelosuppressive chemotherapy in whom the anemia can be managed by transfusion. Not indicated as a substitute for RBC transfusions in patients who require immediate correction of anemia.	Hypertension Fatigue Edema Vascular access thrombosis and thrombotic events	Contraindicated in patients with uncontrolled hypertension; closely monitor blood pressure of all patients; rotate injection sites; monitor blood counts. Assess level of fatigue; provide for periods of rest between activities; educate about energy-conserving strategies. Assess skin for edema; elevate lower extremities; protect skin from damage; intake and output; assess breath sounds. Assess for possible emboli in lower extremities or lungs and in vascular access devices; report positive evidence to physician.

Continued

Drug	Indications	Toxicities	Management
		Fever, pneumonia, dyspnea, sepsis	Monitor VS; monitor respiratory status (e.g., breath sounds; rate, depth, ease, and pattern of respirations; dyspnea, shortness of breath; oxygen saturation); administer antipyretics and antimicrobials as needed.
		Seizures	Assess for seizure activity; implement seizure precautions as needed.
		Nausea, vomiting, diarrhea, dehydration	GI assessment and effect of nausea, vomiting, and diarrhea on comfort, fluid balance, perineal skin; intake and output; administer antiemetic and antidiarrheal drugs as needed; encourage fluids if tolerated; monitor signs of dehydration (dry skin and mucous membranes, concentrated urine, thirst, fever). Monitor CBC laboratory test results for increase in red blood cell count.

CBC, complete blood cell count; *GI,* gastrointestinal; *GM-CSF,* granulocyte-macrophage colony-stimulating factor; *HIV,* human immunodeficiency virus, *IV,* intravenous; *VS,* vital signs.

2. Subcutaneous injection route and potential for multiple injections (e.g., stem cell mobilization)
B. Adverse effects and strategies to manage them
  1. Common side effects include bone pain, mild fever, pain at injection site, and changes in blood pressure
  2. Patients should take NSAIDs or nonopioid analgesics to control pain
C. Adverse effects to report to health care team
  1. Changes in respiratory status (e.g., dyspnea)
  2. Swelling or redness in lower extremities, which may indicate a blood clot
  3. Pain not relieved by NSAIDs or nonopioid analgesics
III. Monitor for adverse effects of MGFs (see Table 31.11)
IV. Decrease the incidence and manage the adverse effects of MGFs (see Table 31.11)
  A. Assess baseline data (e.g., vital signs, neurologic status)
  B. Review patient's medical history for existing or previous conditions
  C. Review patient's medications for potential drug interactions
  D. Conduct patient and family teaching (e.g., on side effects and self-management; medication administration)
V. Monitor for response to MGFs
  A. Monitor laboratory results (e.g., complete blood count)
  B. Assess activity level, presence of infection, and/or bleeding
  C. Assess for adverse effects, toxicity, and drug interactions

EXPECTED PATIENT OUTCOMES

I. The patient and caregiver will verbalize understanding of prevention, early detection, or treatment of infection during neutropenia
II. Patient and caregiver will exhibit adherence to protective measures and good personal hygiene
III. Patient and caregiver will verbalize understanding of therapy rationale and medication schedule
IV. Patient and caregiver will list potential adverse effects of medication and when to call health care team

REFERENCES

Armstrong, T. S., Grant, R., Gilbert, M. R., Lee, J. W., & Norden, A. (2016). Epilepsy in glioma patients: mechanisms, management, and impact of anticonvulsant therapy. *Neuro-Oncology, 18*(6), 779–789. https://doi.org/10.1093/neuonc/nov269.

Bennett, C. L., Djulbegovic, B., Norris, L. B., & Armitage, J. O. (2013). Colony-stimulation factors for febrile neutropenia during cancer therapy. *New England Journal of Medicine, 368,* 1131–1139. https://doi.org/10.1056/NEJMct1210890.

Bow, E. (2015). Treatment and prevention of neutropenic fever syndromes in adult cancer patients at low risk for complication. *UpToDate, Topic 13951, Version 21.0.* Retrieved from: https://www.uptodate.com/contents/treatment-and-prevention-of-neutropenic-fever-syndromes-in-adult-cancer-patients-at-low-risk-for- complications?search = cancer%20infection& source = search_result&selectedTitle = 1~150 &usage_type = default.

Camp-Sorrell, D. (2018). Chemotherapy toxicities and management. In C. H. Yarbro, D. Wujcik, & B. H. Gobel (Eds.), *Cancer nursing: principles & practice* (pp. 497–554). Burlington: Jones & Bartlett Learning.

Hesketh, P. J. (2017). Prevention and treatment of chemotherapy-induced nausea and vomiting in adults. *UpToDate, Topic 1151, Version 78.0.* Retrieved from https://www.uptodate.com/contents/prevention-and-treatment-of-chemotherapy-induced-nausea-and-vomiting-in-adults?search = chemotherapy%20induced%20nausea%20and%20vomiting&source = search_result&selectedTitle = 1~73&usage_type = default&display_rank = 1.

Hesketh, P. J., Kris, M. G., Basche, K., & Lyman, G. H. (2017). Antiemetics: American Society of Clinical Oncology Clinical Practice Guideline Update. *Journal Clinical Oncology, 35*, 3240–3261. https://doi.org/10.1200/JCO.2017.74.4789.

Hibberd, P. L. (2018). Immunizations in adults with cancer. *UpToDate, Topic 3899, Version 26.0.* Retrieved from https://www.uptodate.com/contents/immunizations-in-adults-with-cancer?search = oncology%20AND%20vaccines&source = search_result&selectedTitle = 3~150&usage_type = default&display_rank = 3.

Martin, V. R. (2014). Arthralgias and myalgias. In C. H. Yarbro, D. Wujcik, & B. H. Gobel (Eds.), *Cancer symptom management* (pp. 13–25). Burlington: Jones & Bartlett Learning.

Matthews, E. E. (2018). Sleep disorders. In C. H. Yarbro, D. Wujcik, & B. H. Gobel (Eds.), *Cancer nursing: Principles & practice* (pp. 1051–1072). Burlington: Jones & Bartlett Learning.

National Comprehensive Cancer Network [NCCN]. (2017). *Distress management (v2.2017).* Retrieved from: https://www.nccn.org/professionals/physician_gls/pdf/distress.pdf.

National Comprehensive Cancer Network. (2017a). *Prevention and treatment of cancer-related infections. (v1.2018).* Retrieved from: https://www.nccn.org/professionals/physician_gls/pdf/infections.pdf.

National Comprehensive Cancer Network. (2017c). *Adult cancer pain. (v 2.2017).* Retrieved from: https://www.nccn.org/professionals/physician_gls/pdf/pain.pdf.

National Comprehensive Cancer Network [NCCN]. (2017d). *Distress management (v2.2017).* Retrieved from https://www.nccn.org/professionals/physician_gls/pdf/distress.pdf.

National Comprehensive Cancer Network [NCCN]. (2017e). *Myeloid growth factors (v. 2.2017).* Retrieved from https://www.nccn.org/professionals/physician_gls/pdf/myeloid_growth.pdf.

National Comprehensive Cancer Network. (2018a). *Adult cancer pain. (v1.2018).*

National Comprehensive Cancer Network. (2018b). Antiemesis. (v 2.2018). Retrieved from: https://www.nccn.org/professionals/physician_gls/pdf/antiemesis.pdf

Olans, R. D., Olans, R. N., & Witt, D. J. (2017). Good nursing is good antibiotic stewardship. *American Journal of Nursing, 117*(8), 58–63. https://doi.org/10.1097/01.NAJ.0000521974.76835.e0.

Olsen, M., LeFebvre, K. B., & Brassil, K. (2019). *Chemotherapy and immunotherapy guidelines and recommendations for practice.* Pittsburgh, PA: Oncology Nursing Society.

Santomasso, B. D., Park, J. H., Salloum, D., Riviere, I., Flynn, J., Mead, E., Halton, E., Wang, X., Senechal, B., Purdon, T., Cross, J. R., Liu, H., Vachha, B., Chen, X., DeAngelis, L. M., Li, D., Bernal, Y., Gonen, M., Wendel, H. G., Sadelain, M., & Brentjens, R. (2018). Clinical and biological correlates of neurotoxicity associated with CAR T-cell therapy in patients with B-cell acute lymphoblastic leukemia. *Cancer Discovery, 8*(8), 959–971. https://doi.org/10.1158/2159-8290.CD-17-1319.

Shelton, B. K. (2018). Infection. In C. H. Yarbro, D. Wujcik, & B. H. Gobel (Eds.), *Cancer nursing: principles & practice* (pp. 817–850). Burlington: Jones & Bartlett Learning.

Snyder, S. R., Favoretto, A. M., Baeta, R. A., Derzon, J. H., Madison, B. M., Mass, D., … Liebow, E. B. (2012). Effectiveness of practices to reduce blood culture contamination: a laboratory medicine best practices systematic review and meta-analysis. *Clinical Biochemistry, 45*, 999–1011.

Tradounsky, G. (2013). Seizures in palliative care. *Canadian Family Physician, 59*, 951–955.

Wingard, J. R. (2016). *Prophylaxis of infection during chemotherapy-induced neutropenia in high-risk adults. UpToDate, Topic 1153, Version 26.0.* Retrieved from: https://www.uptodate.com/contents/prophylaxis-of-infection-during-chemotherapy-induced-neutropenia-in-high-risk-adults?source =psee_link#H875811313.

Zitella, L. J. (2014). Infection. In C. H. Yarbro, D. Wujcik, & B. H. Gobel (Eds.), *Cancer symptom management* (pp. 131–157). Burlington: Jones & Bartlett Learning.

32

Complementary, Alternative, and Integrative Modalities

Roberta Bourgon

OVERVIEW

I. Definitions: therapies that may be used to enhance the efficacy of conventional (allopathic, biologic, scientific, orthodox, Western) medicine therapy, alleviate side effects of conventional treatment, and improve the patient's sense of well-being and quality of life or both

A. Complementary: therapies that fall outside of conventional medicine, such as acupuncture, herbal/botanical medicine, mind–body therapies, neutraceuticals, and energy medicine.

B. Alternative: nonconventional therapies used in place of what is offered conventionally. Patients may choose these therapies if there is nothing offered conventionally, if they have exhausted the conventional treatment options, and/or if what is offered conventionally is not within their belief system or culture.

C. Integrative medicine, integrative health care, and integrative oncology: refer to combining evidence-based complementary therapies with conventional treatment regimens.

D. Complementary and alternative medicine (CAM): describes the entire domain of therapies that fall outside of conventional medicine.

E. Other complementary and integrative modality definitions are listed in Box 32.1.

II. Current trends in the U.S.

A. CAM use prevalent among cancer patients— estimated 12.5% to 73% (Berretta et al., 2017).

B. CAM use is most associated with younger age, higher income and higher education, and those that receive family pressure to do so (Latte-Naor, 2018; NCCIH, 2017a).

C. A growing number of conventional medicine providers are offering complementary therapies, which has resulted in the increasing utilization of integrative oncology approaches.

1. In palliative care and hospice settings, mind and body practices, including massage therapy, aromatherapy, music therapy, and acupuncture, are common therapies used to treat pain and anxiety (Zeng, Wand, Ward, & Hume, 2017).

2. Many academic and private cancer treatment centers offer a range of complementary services with the establishment of the Society for Integrative Oncology to advance evidence-based, comprehensive, integrative health care to improve the lives of people dealing with cancer (www.integrativeonc.org).

3. Many National Cancer Institute (NCI)–designated cancer centers offer information regarding integrative medicine and CAM services on their websites and directly to patients, with acupuncture, massage, mediation, yoga, and consultations regarding nutrition, dietary supplements, and herbs being the most commonly offered (Yun, 2017).

III. Classification of CAM therapies

A. The National Center for Complementary and Integrative Health (NCCIH) lists two subgroups of complementary health approaches (NCCIH, 2017b)

1. Natural products, including herbs, vitamins, minerals, and probiotics.

2. Mind and body practices, including but not limited to yoga, chiropractic and osteopathic manipulation, meditation, massage therapy, acupuncture, relaxation techniques, tai chi, qi gong, healing touch, hypnotherapy, and movement therapies.

B. Other complementary therapies include whole medical systems health approaches and biologically based practices.

IV. Natural products (Table 32.1)

A. Herbal/botanical medicine

1. Supplement use is estimated in over 50% of cancer patients, and one third do not disclose this use to the health care team (Berretta, 2017).

2. These substances are usually safe but can pose significant risk to the patient due to interactions with conventionally prescribed medications.

3. Many conventional chemotherapeutic agents used today have their roots in botanical medicine (e.g., taxanes: Pacific yew [*Taxus brevifolia*]), vinca alkaloids: periwinkle (*Cantharanthus roseus*), camptothecin: xishu (*Camptotheca acuminate*), podophyllotoxin

BOX 32.1 Complementary, Alternative, and Integrative Modality Definitions

Alternative medical systems are therapies based upon complete systems of theory and practice that have evolved apart from, and in many cases that predate, conventional medical approaches used in the U.S. Examples of such systems are Ayurveda, traditional Chinese medicine, homeopathy, traditional medicine of indigenous cultures, naturopathy, and Tibetan medicine, to name a few.

Energy therapies are defined as therapies that use energy fields. Two such therapies are commonly used: 1) biofield therapies, which are aimed at affecting the energy fields that surround and penetrate the human body to restore health. The existence of such energy fields has not been scientifically verified. Examples of such therapies include reiki, qi gong, therapeutic touch; 2) electromagnetic-based therapies, which use electromagnetic fields such as pulsed fields, magnetic fields, or alternating or direct current fields to affect changes in the body. Examples include magnet therapy and pulsed magnetic fields.

Exercise therapies utilize health-enhancing systems of movement and exercise and include practices such as the yoga asanas and tai chi.

Manipulative and body-based methods involve the movement and/or manipulation of one or more parts of the body to influence the health of the whole body. These therapies include chiropractic, therapeutic massage, osteopathy, and reflexology.

Mind–body interventions employ a variety of techniques to enhance the mind's ability to affect the body, its overall function, and perception of symptoms. These therapies include meditation, hypnosis, art therapy, music therapy, biofeedback, guided imagery, relaxation techniques, cognitive behavioral therapy, support groups, and aromatherapy.

Nutritional therapeutics include the use of nutrients, nonnutrients, bioactive food components used as chemopreventive agents, and specific foods or diets used as cancer prevention of treatment strategies. These therapies include the macrobiotic diet, Gerson therapy, ketogenic diet, Kelley/Gonzalez regimen, vitamins, and minerals.

Pharmacologic and biologic treatments include the off-label use of certain drugs, hormones, complex natural products, vaccines, and other biological interventions not yet accepted in mainstream medicine. Examples include metformin, intravenous (IV) vitamin C, low-dose naltrexone, laetrile, antineoplastons, 714X, hydrazine sulfate, alpha lipoic acid, DCA, melatonin, etc.

- **Subcategory:** Complex natural products are an assortment of plant samples (botanicals), extracts of crude natural substances, and unfractionated extracts from marine organisms used for healing and treatment of disease. Examples include herbs and herbal extracts (mistletoe or *Viscum album*, mixtures of tea polyphenols, mushroom extracts, etc.).

Spiritual therapies are therapies that focus on deep, often religious, beliefs and feelings, including a person's sense of peace, purpose, connection to others, and beliefs about the meaning of life. Examples include intercessory prayer, spiritual healing, etc.

Adapted from Office of Cancer Complementary and Alternative Medicine (2012). Categories of CAM Therapies. Available at https://cam.cancer.gov/health_information/categories_of_cam_therapies.htm

TABLE 32.1 Natural Products

Botanical/Supplement	CyP isoform Affected	Effects on CYP450	In vitro or Animal Data	Human Data	Specific Effects Relevant to Oncology
Allium sativum (garlic)	2E1, 2C9, 2C19, 3A4,	Inhibition	•	•	Docetaxel
Andrographis paniculata (andrographis)	3A4, 2D6	Inhibition	•		
Angelica sinensis (dong quai)	1A2, 2D6, 2C9, 2E1,3A4	Inhibition	•		
Arctium lappa (burdock)	3A4, 2C19	Inhibition	•		
Arctostaphylos uva ursi (uva ursi)	3A4	Inhibition		•	
Boswellia serrata (frankincense)	1A2, 2D6, 2C8,2C9, 2C19, 3A4	Inhibition	•		
Camellia sinensis (green tea)	3A4 (considered minor)	Inhibition	•		Use with bortezomib (directly blocked the apoptotic effect) In vivo human trials failed to demonstrate effects on 2D6, 1A2, 2C9, and 3A4 at recommended doses.
Centella asiatica (gotu kola)	2C9, 2D6, 3A4	Inhibition		•	
Cimicifuga racemosa (black cohosh)	3A4, 2D6	Inhibition	•	•	Human data failed to show inhibition or induction of 3A4. It was a potent modulator of 2D6 in in vivo (human) studies; however, failed to demonstrate effect when coadministered with tamoxifen.

Continued

TABLE 32.1 **Natural Products—cont'd**

Botanical/Supplement	CyP isoform Affected	Effects on CYP450	In vitro or Animal Data	Human Data	Specific Effects Relevant to Oncology
Cinnamomum burmani (cinnamon)	2D6	Inhibition	•		
Cucruma longa (turmeric)	2C9, 2C19, 2D6, 3A4	Inhibition	•		
Echinacea purpurea (echinacea)	2C19, 2D6, 3A4	Inhibition	•		Docetaxel
Ginkgo biloba (ginkgo)	2C9, 2C19, 2E1, 3A4	Inhibition	•	•	
Glycyrrhiza glabra (licorice)	3A4, 2D6	Inhibition	•		
Hypericum perforatum (St. John's wort)	3A4, 2E1, 2C19 1A2, 2C9	Inhibition	•	•	Irinotecan Imatinib Docetaxel
Hydrastis canadensis (goldenseal)	2C9, 2D6, 3A4	Inhibition	•	•	
Matricaria recutita (chamomile)	1A2, 2C9, 2C19, 2D6, 3A4, 4A9/11, 2E1	Inhibition	•	•	
Mentha piperita (peppermint)	3A4	Inhibition	•	•	
Panax quinquefolius (American ginseng)	2C9, 2C19, 2D6, 3A4	Inhibition	•	•	Human trials at recommended doses did not demonstrate induction of 3A4 by Panax ginseng.
Piper methysticum (kava kava)	3A4, 2E1, 1A2	Inhibition	•	•	Human data confirm that kava is a potent inhibitor of 2E1 but does not seem to inhibit 3A4 or 2D6 at recommended doses.
Rhodiola rosea (rhodiola)	2D6, 3A4	Inhibition	•		
Schisandra chinensis/ sphenantherea (schizandra)	3A4	Inhibition	•		Impact on drugs transported by P-glycoprotein
Silybum marianum (milk thistle)	3A4, 2C8, 2C9, 2C19, 2D6, 2E1	Inhibition	•		Human data did not support the effects in vitro at daily recommended doses and in fact failed to show clinically relevant effects on 3A4, 1A2, 2D6, and 2E1.
Uncaria tomentosa (cat's claw)	3A4	Inhibition	•		
Tanacetum parthenium (feverfew)	2C9, 2C19, 2D6, 3A4	Inhibition		•	
Valeriana officinalis (valerian root)	3A4	Inhibition	•		
Zingiber aromaticum (ginger)	2C9, 2C19, 2D6, 3A4	Inhibition	•	•	

(etoposide): mayapple or wild mandrake (*Podophyllum peltatum*).

4. Herbal/botanical medicine and dietary supplements are not Food and Drug Administration (FDA) approved or well regulated in U.S. as in other countries; access to safe and effective herbal/botanical medicine not guaranteed.

V. Mind–body modalities

A. Include art and color therapy, eye movement desensitization and reprocessing (EMDR), guided imagery, meditation, music therapy, neurolinguistics programming, tai chi, and yoga (Table 32.2)

VI. Manipulative and body-based practices

A. Modalities include acupuncture, acupressure, Alexander technique, cranial osteopathy, dance therapy,

TABLE 32.2 Mind–Body Modalities

Art therapy—different art mediums (drawing, coloring, painting, sculpting, and multimedia) to assist the patient in restoring, maintaining, or improving physical, mental, emotional, and spiritual well-being.	• Based on the concept that the creative process helps people resolve inner conflict and process issues, reduce stress, increase self-esteem and self-awareness, and achieve insight. • Requires a master's degree in art therapy; may require licensure, credentials, or both, depending on the state.
Color therapy (chromotherapy)—uses electronic instrumentation and color receptivity to integrate nervous system and body–mind.	• Based on premise that color conveys energy at different frequencies and the human body responds to these vibrational frequencies. • May be used to increase well-being and is used to treat acute and chronic ailments.
Eye movement desensitization and reprocessing (EMDR)—a psychotherapy technique based on the concept that distressing events are associated with specific rapid eye movements.	• The therapist helps the patient recall distressing events, eliciting the associated rapid eye movements, and then redirects the eye movements through stimulation or distraction, thereby breaking the connection that is causing distressing thoughts and feelings to persist.
Guided imagery—a structured process that uses live or recorded scripts describing different scenarios or detailed images to guide the patient through a process.	• May lead the patient through progressive muscle relaxation or visualization of a treatment process (e.g., visualization of chemotherapy entering the body and seeking out cancer cells to remove them from the body). • Techniques—use of a coach who narrates the imagery, an audio recording, or a video recording.
Meditation—a method of quieting the mind to facilitate inner peace; numerous forms of meditation, ranging from simple focused breathing to transcendental meditation; practices share characteristics and often involve focused breathing and a relaxed yet alert state that promotes control over thoughts and feelings.	• Studies have shown that a relaxed state of mind may decrease perceived stress, relieve muscle tension, enhance sense of well-being, boost immune response. • Mindfulness-based stress reduction (MBSR) is a technique whereby patients are trained to develop awareness of experiences moment by moment and in the context of all senses. • Yoga nidra meditation teaches patients to explore sensations, emotions, and thoughts, and then to dissociate from them. • Transcendental meditation uses a *mantra* (a word, sound, phrase) to direct focus, prevent distraction. • Some states require therapists to have a master's degree, certification, or both
Music therapy—an applied psychotherapy that uses making or listening to music to explore behavioral, emotional, or spiritual disruption and to assist the patient in resolving these issues.	• Music interventions may have beneficial effects on anxiety, pain, fatigue, and quality of life in people with cancer.
Neurolinguistic programming (NLP)—a systematic approach to changing thought patterns, thereby changing perceptions.	• One example is the use of a "gratitude journal." The patient is instructed to record daily entries in a journal, specifically recalling positive aspects of his or her life to promote a positive outlook over time. The concept is that one gets more of whatever one focuses on.
Tai chi—an ancient Chinese practice of movements coordinated with breathing techniques. Qi gong and tai chi have been found to have positive effects on cancer-specific quality of life, fatigue, immune function, and cortisol levels in patients with cancer.	• Derived from martial art form. • Enhances coordination and balance, and promotes physical, emotional, and spiritual well-being. • Contraindications: none have been reported, but clearance from a provider to engage in exercise/physical activity is recommended.
Yoga—strength and flexibility achieved using specific postures and controlled breathing; found to improve psychological outcomes (e.g., depression, anxiety, and distress), quality-of-life measures, sleep issues, fatigue, gastrointestinal symptoms, and overall health-related quality-of-life measures in patients with cancer (Danhauer, 2017; Kiecolt-Glaser, 2014; Pan, 2017). In cancer survivors, yoga has been found to improve sleep quality and insomnia (Mustian, 2013).	• Has evolved into mainstream practice with multiple variations, ranging from restorative (gentle) yoga to promote well-being in frail patients to power yoga, which uses a vigorous, fitness-based approach. • Has a meditative component that brings harmony to body, mind, and spirit. • Contraindications: patients with glaucoma, hypertension, those with sciatica, those with movement restrictions, and those currently pregnant need to be cautious while practicing yoga and should modify or avoid certain poses. The risk for injury due to strain/sprain is possible if one is not cautious.

Feldenkrais method, lymphatic therapy, and traditional Chinese medicine (Table 32.3)

VII. Whole medical systems (Baliga, 2013)

    A. Therapeutic approaches include Ayurveda, chiropractic medicine, homeopathy, and osteopathic medicine (Table 32.4).

VIII. Biologically based practices

    A. Therapies that use substances found in nature to treat illness and promote wellness, including biofeedback; herbal therapy; hydrotherapy; nutritional counseling; and energy work, energy therapy, and biofield therapy (Table 32.5).

TABLE 32.3 Manipulative and Body-Based Practices

Acupuncture—an ancient Oriental technique associated with traditional Chinese medicine (TCM), used to restore or promote health and well-being using fine-gauge needles inserted into specific points on the body to stimulate or disperse the flow of energy. Acupuncture shown to have therapeutic benefit for management of cancer-related fatigue, chemotherapy-induced nausea and vomiting, and leukopenia in cancer patients.	• Used in conjunction with methods such as massage, herbal remedies, and nutritional counseling. • May be a safe and effective treatment for chronic lymphedema related to breast cancer treatment. • Used for pain and chemotherapy-related nausea and vomiting with mostly favorable results. • Avoid at the site of tumor or metastasis, at the site of tumor nodules or skin ulcerations, on broken skin, or a site of active infection or radiation burn. • Avoid over any open surgical wound, in limbs with lymphedema, over areas of instability of the spine (e.g., multiple myeloma), or in any areas with considerable anatomic distortion from surgery. • Contraindicated in patients who are neutropenic or severely thrombocytopenic.
Acupressure—the use of finger or hand pressure over specific points on the body to relieve symptoms or to influence specific organ function.	• May be used to release tension, reestablish the natural flow of energy, or both. • Contraindicated in patients with bleeding disorders or thrombocytopenia and in those taking anticoagulant medications such as warfarin (Coumadin). • Should not be done over body areas with tumor, lymphadenopathy, or both.
Alexander technique.	• Uses movement and touch to restore balance in the body and neuromuscular function, thus allowing the body to regain a relaxed, healthy posture.
Aromatherapy—uses essential oils extracted from herbs and other plants.	• Treats physical imbalances and restores psychological and spiritual well-being. • Essential oils are inhaled, applied topically, or ingested. • Currently no standardization of practice; a wide range of quality in essential oils, as processing is not regulated. • Topical application of essential oils to be avoided unless they are prepared by a trained specialist.
Cranial osteopathy—uses gentle manipulation of the skull to reestablish natural configuration and movement.	• Disorders manifested throughout the body can be improved by realigning the skull.
Dance therapy—dance and music combined to facilitate uplifting of the mind, body, and spirit through natural body movement.	
Feldenkrais method—a somatic education system that teaches movement and gentle manipulation to increase body awareness and improve body function.	• Used to improve posture and promote flexibility and freedom of movement.
Lymphatic therapy—the use of vigorous massage to stimulate flow of lymphatic fluid.	• Intended to move lymph fluid and release toxins stored in the lymphatic system; refreshes the immune system. • Manual, gentle lymphatic drainage used to prevent and treat lymphedema after breast cancer surgery.
Massage—the use of manual pressure and strokes on muscle tissue. Conflicting results exist for the effectiveness of massage therapy in patients with cancer.	• Used to reduce emotional and physical tension, increase circulation, and relieve muscular pain. • Can provide comfort and increased body awareness. • Contraindicated in or near areas of infection, tumors, incisions or indwelling devices, or in presence of contagious disease, contagious rashes, or open sores; patients who are thrombocytopenic (platelet count less than 50,000). • Patients with peripheral neuropathy (grade 3 or greater) should not receive massage over the affected areas. • Patients with suspected/known bone metastasis should not receive pressure or jostling over the areas of concern. • Patients who have received radiation therapy to lymph nodes in the armpit, groin, neck, or jaw, or those who have had removal of these nodes; excessive pressure on the limb or area being drained by those lymph nodes is to be avoided except for those trained in lymphatic drainage. ⚠

TABLE 32.3 Manipulative and Body-Based Practices—cont'd	
	• Neutropenic precautions (including gloves and a mask) should be used with any patients who are neutropenic. Patients with severe neutropenia (white blood cell [WBC] <1500) should not receive massage.
	• Massage therapists should wear gloves when massaging patients receiving high-dose methotrexate, cytarabine (Ara-C) and cyclophosphamide, as agents are eliminated through skin.
	• Massage should not be performed on patients receiving anthracyclines (or other agents) to avoid increasing peripheral circulation and worsening the risk of hand/foot syndrome.
	• Avoid massage in affected limb with presence of a known deep vein thrombosis (DVT) and on medications that potentially increase risks of clotting or are at increased risk of clotting due to their disease process.
Neuromuscular therapy—massage therapy that uses moderate pressure on muscles, nerves, and trigger points to decrease pain and tension.	
Physical therapy—used to correct mechanical body ailments and restore normal musculoskeletal functioning.	• Procedures designed to relieve pain, reduce swelling, strengthen muscles, and restore range of motion • Includes a combination of massage, electrostimulation, ultrasonography, and prescribed exercises.
Qi gong—Chinese meditative practice that combines physical postures with focused intention and breathing techniques to release, cleanse, strengthen, and circulate energy.	• Used for stress reduction and to enhance the body's natural healing abilities. • May increase vitality and awareness of internal energy that furthers the mind–body connection. • Can be performed in a standing or sitting position.
Shiatsu—a Japanese form of body work like acupressure.	• Uses finger and palm pressure to manipulate energetic pathways to improve the flow of energy. • Pressure applied to specific points in a continuous rhythmic sequence. • Used to calm an overactive sympathetic nervous system, improve circulation, relieve muscle tension, and alleviate stress. • Patient is fully clothed during treatment, unlike other massage techniques, and no oil is applied to the body. • May not be safe in cancer patients, who are at increased risk of blood clots, because the type of manipulations may dislodge a blood clot.
Trigger point therapy—a method of compression of specific points in muscle tissue to relieve pain and tension.	• May be used with therapeutic massage and passive stretching. • Treatment goals aimed at decreasing swelling and stiffness and increasing range of motion. • Like physical therapy, exercises assigned to be performed at home between treatment sessions.

TABLE 32.4 Whole Medical Systems	
Ayurveda—taken from the Sanskrit, *ayus,* which means "life or lifespan," and *veda,* which means "knowledge."	• Ayurveda—based on the principle that maintaining balance in the body, mind, and consciousness is used to preserve health and treat illness • Specific interventions—driven by the individual's *prakriti* (nature), which is determined by the three *gunas* (ways of being: *tamas, rajas, sattva*); human physiology believed to be the result of the combination of the three *doshas* (*pitta, kapha,* and *vatta*) in each individual; energy (or *prana*) flows through the body through channels or *nadis;* disruption in the flow of energy results in disease. • Interventions—aimed at rebalancing the *doshas* and restoring the flow of energy; may include proper diet, hydration, and lifestyle (e.g., following a set sleep–wake routine, detoxification or cleansing techniques, specific massage techniques [*marma* therapy], specific movements, or spoken words [*mantras*])

Continued

TABLE 32.4   Whole Medical Systems—cont'd

Chiropractic medicine—emphasizes structural alignment of the spine.	• Adjustments made through manipulation of the spine and joints to reestablish normal central nervous system (CNS) functioning. • Interventions include massage, nutrition, and specialized kinesiology. • Chiropractic medicine contraindicated in patients with bone metastasis, spinal cord compression, thrombocytopenia, or venous thrombosis.
Homeopathy—based on the precept of healing through the administration of specific substances.	• Substances are chosen according to the following beliefs: • Like cures like. • The more a remedy is diluted, the greater is the potency. • Illness is specific to the individual. • This form of medicine is based on the belief that symptoms are an indication that the body is attempting to rid itself of disease. • Treatment based on the whole person as opposed to focusing on symptoms. • No known interactions with drugs, herbs, foods, laboratory tests, diseases, or conditions.
Osteopathic medicine—focuses on the relationship between the structure and function of the body; osteopaths are fully licensed to diagnose, treat, and prescribe in conventional medicine.	• Recognizes that structure and function are subject to a range of disorders. • Uses physical manipulation to facilitate self-healing in the individual, as well as conventional medical therapies.

Traditional Chinese medicine (TCM)—originated in China and evolved over thousands of years.	• Includes key concepts:
	  • Yin-yang—concept of two opposing complementary forces that are brought into balance to maintain healthy body and mind.
	  • Meridians—pathways or channels that run throughout the body through which *qi* (energy, pronounced "chee") or energy flows; disruption in flow of qi results in disease; acupuncture and other techniques used to direct, redirect, or unblock the flow of qi.
	  • Five elements—fire, earth, metal, water, and wood, which correspond to various organs and tissues in the body.
	  • Eight principles—used in TCM to analyze symptoms; principles include cold-heat, interior-exterior, excess-deficiency, yin-yang.
	  • Interventions—include use of herbs, acupuncture, and other methods [e.g., moxibustion, cupping, mind–body therapy] to enhance health and treat illness.

TABLE 32.5   Biologically Based Practices

Biofeedback—a technique for teaching the patient to recognize, observe, and learn to control biological responses to stress	• Monitors are used to give feedback to the patient about vital signs (blood pressure, heart rate, and respiratory rate), and the patient is taught to relax through visualization and focused breathing, among other methods. • By conscious effort, patients learn to bring about change in vital functions.
Herbal therapy—the use of herbs and their chemical properties to treat specific conditions or to improve general health and well-being	• Herbal preparations are used in alcohol extractions, liquid extractions, salves, teas, capsules, oils, liquids, or in their raw forms and are taken internally, inhaled, or applied directly to the body. Therapeutic-aims: restoration of health, supporting the body's mechanisms of immunity, elimination, detoxification, and homeostasis. • The use of herbal medicines should be monitored by a knowledgeable provider, members of the health care team, or both. Caution should be used with herbs that are known to affect the CYP3A4267 pathway because of the potential for herb–drug interactions (e.g., St. John's wort).

TABLE 32.5 **Biologically Based Practices—cont'd**	
Hydrotherapy—the application of water to the body in its various forms (ice, water, steam) and at an extreme temperature (hot or cold) to restore and maintain health Nutritional counseling—the use of diet, nutritional supplements, or both to prevent and manage illness or to enhance and maintain health	• Treatments include water baths, steam baths, saunas, and application of hot or cold compresses. • Contrast hydrotherapy (alternating application of hot and cold). • Registered dieticians often involved in care of patients going through cancer treatment, but many different practitioners make dietary recommendations. Important to know who is making recommendations and for what therapeutic goal. • Diet therapies may or may not be appropriate. • The recommendation of dietary supplements is like that with herbal medications. It is important to know who is making the recommendations and with what educational background. The health care team (nurses, physicians, pharmacists, etc.) needs to be aware of what someone is taking, and someone knowledgeable in how these supplements interplay with conventional therapies should be monitoring their use.
Energy work, energy therapy, biofield therapy—a broad category of work aimed at influencing the major energy centers (*chakras*) of the body and the flow of a patient's internal and external energy; energy work can be used to treat physical symptoms and emotional or spiritual distress or enhance well-being	• Reiki—an energy healing modality whereby the practitioner uses his or her hands to direct the flow of energy to various parts of the body to facilitate healing and relaxation; hands are placed on the body in specific patterns without deep pressure to redirect or restore energy flow. • Therapeutic touch—a technique for balancing the flow of energy in the body through transfer of human energy, based on the concept that disruption in energy flow leads to disease and restoring that flow can lead to health, growth, order, and wholeness. • Healing touch—an energy healing technique that uses the nursing process. • Magnetic therapy—use of magnets to influence magnetic fields to positively affect the nervous system, organs, and tissues to stimulate healing.

ASSESSMENT

I. Use of CAM—may negatively interfere or interact with conventional cancer treatment; nursing assessment to include questions directed at determining patient use of CAM and discussion regarding the risks and benefits, as needed ⚠️
II. Relevant patient demographics and clinical information
   A. Demographics—age, gender, education, residence, economic status, ethnic and cultural identity
   B. Clinical information—should include comorbidities, allergies, medications (including CAM), and cancer disease information: type, stage, cancer treatments
III. Initial and ongoing patient assessment of CAM—should include a comprehensive assessment
   A. Disturbances or imbalances in the following areas:
      1. Physical well-being
      2. Nutritional status, functional performance status
      3. Psychosocial status, emotional and mental well-being
      4. Sexual functioning
      5. Age-related developmental issues
      6. Spiritual well-being
      7. Energy field disturbances
   B. Identification of risk in the areas of the following:
      1. Environmental factors
      2. Cultural practices
      3. Family dynamics
      4. Socioeconomic status
      5. Health behaviors
   C. Patient values and preferences
      1. Meaning of health and well-being
      2. Religious and spiritual practices
      3. Cultural practices
      4. Lifestyle patterns

MANAGEMENT

I. Interventions to increase patient knowledge about CAM and its effects on conventional therapy.
   A. Encourage open communication about conventional therapy options and CAM
      1. Support informal dialogue initiated by nurses, patients, and their caregivers
         a. Success depends on building rapport, ensuring a culturally sensitive and nonjudgmental social and professional environment.

b. Nurses must recognize quick dismissals of CAM may shut down further communication.

c. CAM therapies used by patient, who is guiding the use of the therapies, if known, should be documented.

d. Disclosure of CAM use is an ongoing process that is shaped by patient's health concerns and rapport with the health care team.

2. Explain conventional therapies in a way that patients can understand.

3. Review and discuss chemotherapeutic agents and potential effects of CAM therapy. Suggest avoidance of all herbs/supplements with the newer classes of drugs (PD-1 inhibitors, PDL-inhibitors, CAR-T cell, PARP inhibitors, Bruton's tyrosine kinase inhibitors, etc.) until more information is available.

4. Try to comprehend why conventional medicine may not satisfy patient (e.g., lack of psychosocial support, poor symptom control, inconvenience, lack of understanding)

5. Explore patient rationales for using CAM or contemplating CAM use (e.g., accessibility, fear of side effects, social pressure, agency and empowerment)

6. Emphasize and support the patient's right to choose among therapeutic options
   a. Therapeutic objectives for patient may not be the same as the health care team.

B. Ability to differentiate CAM practices that interfere with conventional medicine from those that complement it
   1. Validate the appropriate use of CAM and explain how some CAM practices may interfere with conventional medicine (e.g., cause antagonistic or other undesirable biophysical results, delay in or termination of conventional treatment) (Table 32.6).

II. Incorporation of compatible CAM practices into conventional interventions to increase health care provider's knowledge about CAM, its effects on conventional therapy, and resources
A. Support the need for a well-informed health care team
   1. Familiarity with CAM resources available in the institution, community, and Internet
   2. Knowledge about CAM sources (including health food vendors)
   3. Recognition that patients are important sources of information about CAM
   4. Awareness that CAM may reflect cultural preferences and is an integral component of a patient's family and social identity
   5. Ability to effectively discuss CAM from a scientific, evidence-based perspective
      a. Recognition that failure to offer objective information about safety and efficacy compromises patient-initiated dialogue about CAM

TABLE 32.6 Potential CAM Drug Interactions with Chemotherapeutic Agents

Chemotherapeutic Agent	Cytochrome Enzymes Utilized for Metabolism	Expected Effect on the Drug
Cyclophosphamide	2C8, 2B6, 3A4, 2C9, 2C19	Increased
Ifosfamide	3A4, 3A5	Decreased
Dacarbazine	1A2	Increased
Paclitaxel	2C8, 3A4	Decreased
Docetaxel	3A4	Decreased
Vinblastine	3A4	Decreased
Vincristine	3A4	Decreased
Navelbine	3A4	Decreased
Etoposide	3A4	Decreased
Irinotecan	3A4, 3A5	Decreased
Topotecan	3A4	Decreased
Tamoxifen	3A4, 1A2	Decreased
Arimidex	3A4, 1A2, 2C8–9, 2C19	Decreased
Aromasin	3A4, 1A2, 2C8–9, 2C19	Decreased
Femara	3A4, 1A2, 2C8–9, 2C19	Decreased
Iressa	3A4	Decreased

b. Offer appropriate referrals to trusted trained professionals, as indicated

EXPECTED PATIENT OUTCOMES

I. The patient will disclose and discuss the use of CAM therapies and verbalize understanding of potential cancer therapy interactions.

REFERENCES

Baliga, M. S., Meera, S., Vaishnav, L. K., Rao, S., & Palatty, P. L. (2013). Rasayana drugs from the Ayurvedic system of medicine as possible radioprotective agents in cancer treatment. *Integrative Cancer Therapeutics, 12*(6), 455–463. https://doi.org/10.1177/1534735413490233.

Berretta, M., Pepa, C. D., Tralongo, P., Fulvi, A., Martellotta, F., Lleshi, A., & Facchini, G. (2017). Use of complementary and alternative medicine (CAM) in cancer patients: an Italian multicenter survey. *Oncotarget, 8*(15), 24401–24414. https://doi.org/10.18632/oncotarget.14224.

Latte-Naor, S., Sidlow, R., Sun, L., Li, Q. S., & Mao, J. J. (2018). Influence of family on expected benefits of complementary and alternative medicine (CAM) in cancer patients. *Supportive Care in Cancer.* https://doi.org/10.1007/s00520-018-4053-0.

National Center for Complementary and Integrative Health (NCCIH). (2017a). The use of complementary and alternative medicine in the United States. In *Retrieved from* https://nccih.nih.gov/research/statistics/2007/camsurvey_fs1.htm.

National Center for Complementary and Integrative Health (NCCIH). (2017b). Complementary, alternative, or integrative health: what's in a name? Retrieved from, https://nccih.nih.gov/health/integrative-health.

Yun, H., Sun, L., & Mao, J. J. (2017). Growth of integrative medicine at leading cancer centers between 2009 and 2016: a systematic analysis of NCI-designated comprehensive cancer center websites. *Journal of the National Cancer Institute Monograph, 2017*(52). https://doi.org/10.1093/jncimonographs/lgx004.

Zeng, Y., Wang, C., Ward, K., & Hume, A. (2017). Complementary and alternative medicine for management of symptoms in hospice & palliative care (S780). *Journal of Pain and Symptom Management, 53*(2), 454. https://doi.org/10.1016/j.jpainsymman.2016.12.291.

33

Cardiovascular Symptoms

Deborah Kirk Walker

LYMPHEDEMA

Overview

I. Definition—obstruction of the lymphatic system that causes accumulation of lymph fluid in interstitial spaces.

II. Pathophysiology—occlusion or damage to the venous side of capillaries, decreases reabsorption of lymphatic fluid made up of protein, water, fats, and wastes from cells, thereby causing swelling or lymphedema (Hespe, Nores, Huang, & Mehrara, 2017).
   A. Primary lymphedema—genetic or familial abnormalities present at birth.
   B. Secondary lymphedema—damage or destruction of the lymphatic system.

III. Incidence
   A. Varies per cancer diagnosis, increased with lymph node dissection and disease involvement of the lymph system.
   B. May occur within days of a traumatic event and last a lifetime if the event is permanent (i.e., lymph node dissection).

IV. Risk factors (Lasinski, 2013; NCI, 2015; Zhu et al., 2014)
   A. Noncancer related
      1. Poor nutrition
      2. Genetics (Ridner, 2013)
      3. Thrombophlebitis
      4. Skin inflammation or chronic disorders of the skin
      5. Obesity/elevated body mass index (BMI)
   B. Cancer diagnosis related
      1. Tumor invasion and/or advanced disease
      2. Infection—affected extremity, concurrent illness
      3. Air travel with suboptimal cabin pressure, long-distance travel, prolonged immobilization
      4. Traumatic injury to affected extremity
      5. Excessive physical use of affected extremity; prolonged standing (lower extremity)
   C. Treatment related
      1. Surgical lymph node dissection, number of lymph nodes removed, type of surgery, seroma formation after surgery, or delayed wound healing
      2. Radiation therapy—location and formation of scars or fibrosis

Assessment (Wanchai, Beck, Stewart, & Armer, 2013)

I. History
   A. Past medical history—illnesses, type of cancer, history of thrombus
   B. Current medications
   C. Past surgical history
   D. Treatment history
   E. Attributes of each symptom—onset, location, duration, characteristics, aggravating symptoms, relieving factors, treatment
      1. Cause, location, and duration of swelling

II. Physical examination
   A. Tightness of clothing, shoes, wristwatch, jewelry
   B. Visible puffiness
   C. Pain, stiffness, weakness, numbness, paresthesia of affected extremity
   D. Redness, warmth of affected extremity
   E. Tends to occur distal to proximal
   F. Thickening, pitting, and erythema of skin; peau d'orange changes
   G. Increased pigmentation/superficial veins, stasis dermatitis
   H. Induration with nonpitting edema
   I. Secondary cellulitis
   J. Decreased range of motion, feeling of heaviness of affected extremity

III. Psychosocial assessment
   A. Interventions to assess quality of life, psychosocial distress, and disability (Fu & Kang, 2013; Ki et al., 2016; Li et al., 2016)

IV. Assessment tools (Bernas, 2013; Ridner, 2013)
   A. Objective screening tools
      1. Circumference measurements.
         a. Arm measured 5 and 10 cm above and below the olecranon process and compared with the other extremity
         b. Leg measured at the level of the calf
      2. Water displacement method to measure limb volume
         a. Limitations due to difficulty using in clinic setting and does not indicate lymphedema location.

TABLE 33.1 Staging and Grading of Lymphedema

Stage 1: Mild, spontaneously reversible. Slight heaviness of extremity; skin smooth textured with pitting edema; may have pain and erythema.

Stage 2: Moderate, irreversible. May have tissue fibrosis; skin stretched, shiny, with nonpitting edema.

Stage 3: Severe, lymphostatic elephantiasis, irreversible. Skin discolored, stretched, firm; rare in breast cancer.

Grade 1 – swelling, pitting edema; 5%–10% difference in size at greatest point or mass of limbs.

Grade 2 – obvious obstruction, taut skin; 10%–30% difference in size at greatest point or mass of limbs.

Grade 3 – limb starts to look disfigured; interferes with activities of daily living (ADLs); more than 30% difference in size at greatest point or mass of limbs

Grade 4 – often progresses to malignancy; disabling and may need removal of affected extremity; 5%–10% difference in size or mass of limbs.

---

3. Perometer, using infrared light to measure fluid volume of the limb.
4. Bioelectrical impedance uses electrical currents through the regions to determine volume.
   B. Subjective screening tools
   1. Selected based on goal of assessment (i.e., screening, referrals, response to treatment)
      a. Examples of selected tools—the Functional Assessment of Cancer Therapy questionnaire with breast cancer and arm function subscales (FACT B+4), the Lymphedema and Breast Cancer Questionnaire (LBCQ), and the Morbidity Screening Tool.
V. Clinical staging/grading
   A. Staging of lymphedema by examination evaluates the progression of the disease. Grading evaluates severity of signs and symptoms (Table 33.1) (NCI, 2015).
VI. Imaging and laboratory tests (Bernas, 2013)
   A. Lymphoscintigraphy—radioactive mapping of lymphatic vessels.
   B. Ultrasound for evaluation of tissue and fluid.
   C. Computed tomography (CT), magnetic resonance imaging (MRI), or positron emission tomography (PET) scan are not approved for evaluation of lymphedema but can be used to evaluate soft tissue or a possible mass.

Management

I. Treat suspected infections with early antibiotic treatment.
II. Manage acute and chronic pain.
III. Use interventions in conjunction with other modalities to reduce symptoms associated with lymphedema.
   A. Recommended for practice

1. Complete decongestive therapy—standard of care.
2. Compression bandaging, compression garment.
   B. Likely to be effective for practice
   1. Axillary reverse mapping (ARM)
   2. Exercise
   3. Prevention and early intervention protocols
      a. Early evaluation
      b. Referrals to lymphedema specialist, advocacy groups, National Lymphedema Network
   4. Weight management
   C. Other considerations
   1. Avoid prolonged standing.
   2. Elevate affected extremity.
   3. Avoid extreme heat—may worsen the swelling (e.g., hot tubs).
   4. Skin care program with proper bathing, drying, lubrication.
   5. Compression garments when flying.
IV. Patient education
   A. Signs and symptoms to report (e.g., high risk for infection).
   B. Need for lifelong follow-up.
   C. A low-sodium, high-fiber, weight-control diet.
   D. Importance of skin care to maintain skin integrity and prevent infections.
   E. Education to eliminate safety hazards to prevent injury.
   F. Maintain healthy weight.
   G. Limit time in extreme temperatures.
   H. Wear loose-fitting clothes.

EDEMA

Overview

I. Definition—fluid accumulation in interstitial spaces.
II. Pathophysiology (Trayes, Studdiford, Pickle, & Tully, 2013)—the movement of fluid from the vascular space into the interstitial space by an alteration in one or more of the following:
   A. Increased capillary pressure—when volume of blood is expanded or with obstruction; extrinsic sodium and water retention by the kidneys caused by renal failure, reduction of cardiac output or systemic vascular resistance can cause edema. Stimulation of the renin–angiotensin system causes an increase in pressure in the vascular bed (forcing fluid into interstitial spaces) (i.e., heart disease, renal disease, cirrhosis, deep venous thrombosis [DVT]).
   B. Increased capillary permeability—from vascular injury (i.e., burns, radiation, drug reactions, infection); treatment with interleukin-2 or vascular endothelial growth factors.
   C. Obstruction of lymph system—see Lymphedema.
   D. Decreased plasma oncotic pressure—results in increased fluid in the tissues; albumin causes retention of fluid in the vascular bed. When albumin is

decreased, fluid leaks into interstitial spaces (i.e., proteinuria, hepatic failure, malabsorption, protein malnutrition).
  E. Raised hydrostatic pressure—fluid driven from the capillaries into the interstitial spaces (i.e., venous obstruction, fluid retention, prolonged standing).
III. May be associated with the following (Bonita & Pradhan, 2013; Ryberg, 2013; Trayes, Studdiford, Pickle & Tully, 2013).
  A. Lymphatic obstruction by tumor or DVT.
  B. Cancer—common with kidney, liver, ovarian.
  C. Systemic conditions—heart failure, nephrotic syndrome, liver failure, thyroid disease, obstructive sleep apnea.
  D. Medications may include hormones, nonsteroidal antiinflammatory drugs (NSAIDs), calcium channel blockers, tricyclic antidepressants, steroids, interleukin-2 (IL-2) therapy, corticosteroids, beta blockers.
  E. Chemotherapy (i.e., cisplatin, docetaxel, gemcitabine)
  F. Monoclonal antibodies (i.e., bevacizumab)
  G. Targeted therapies (i.e., imatinib mesylate)
  H. Antiangiogenesis agents (i.e., thalidomide)
  I. Allergic response or septic shock, which leads to histamine release
  J. Poor nutrition, hypoproteinemia, hypoalbuminemia
  K. Iatrogenic causes—plasma expanders, intravenous (IV) fluid overload, blood component therapy
  L. Burns, trauma, sepsis
  M. Allergic reactions
  N. Malignant ascites
IV. Incidence
  A. Unknown because the problem is underreported.
  B. May be increasing because of longer survival rates.
V. Risk factors (Bonita & Pradhan, 2013; Ryberg, 2013; Trayes, Studdiford, Pickle & Tully, 2013)
  A. Preexisting cardiac, renal, liver disease, thyroid disease.
  B. Cancer (i.e., kidney, liver or ovarian cancers).
  C. Cancer treatments (i.e., cisplatin, docetaxel).
  D. Decreased mobility.
  E. Long-distance travel.
  F. Prior history of edema.
  G. Certain medications.
  H. DVT.
  I. Hypertension.

Assessment (Bonita & Pradhan, 2013; Ryberg, 2013; Trayes, Studdiford, Pickle & Tully, 2013)
I. History
  A. Past medical history—cardiac, renal, liver disease, thyroid disease, DVT, popliteal cyst, trauma
  B. Past surgical history
  C. Treatment history
  D. Medication history

  E. Attributes of each symptom—onset, location, duration, characteristics, aggravating symptoms, relieving factors, treatment
    1. Timing of edema
    2. Does it change with position
    3. Unilateral/bilateral
II. Physical examination
  A. Tightness of clothing, shoes, jewelry, watch.
  B. Pain or stiffness.
  C. Weight gain.
  D. Shortness of breath, dyspnea on exertion, orthopnea, paroxysmal nocturnal dyspnea, rales.
  E. Frequent or decreased urination.
  F. Presence of S_3 or S_4 heart sound.
  G. Increased jugular venous pressure.
  H. Increased blood pressure and tachycardia.
  I. Ascites, hepatomegaly.
  J. Dependent edema (extremities, sacrum).
  K. Skin thickening/skin tightness.
  L. Decreased peripheral pulses.
  M. Changes in skin integrity, temperature, color, texture, signs of infection or trauma.
III. Psychosocial
  A. Interventions to relieve symptoms and improve quality of life
IV. Laboratory and diagnostic tests
  A. Serum albumin and protein may be decreased.
  B. Creatinine, blood urea nitrogen (BUN) may be increased with kidney disease.
  C. Liver function tests may be increased with cirrhosis.
  D. Thyroid studies should be performed to rule out thyroid disease.
  E. Brain natriuretic peptide (BNP) will be elevated with edema that may be caused by heart failure.
  F. Chest x-ray (CXR)—evidence of fluid overload, increased size of heart shadow.
  G. Echocardiogram—decreased ejection fraction (EF) in heart failure.
  H. Ultrasound to rule out a DVT or thrombophlebitis if edema is unilateral.
  I. Urinalysis for protein.

Management (Trayes, Studdiford, Pickle & Tully, 2013)
I. Treat the underlying cause (i.e., congestive heart failure [CHF], nephrotic syndrome, liver failure/cirrhosis, thrombophlebitis, lymphedema, DVT).
  A. Diuretics.
  B. Angiotensin-converting enzyme (ACE) inhibitors or, if not tolerated, angiotensin receptor blockers (ARBs).
  C. Beta blockers.
  D. Analgesics as needed.
II. Elevate extremities above level of heart.
III. Compression stockings.
IV. Maintain lubrication of skin.

V. Bed rest to promote diuresis; reposition every 2 hours.
VI. Fluid restriction.
VII. Treatment of underlying cause.
VIII. Monitor intake and output, electrolytes, serum albumin.
IX. Protect extremity from injury. ⚠
X. Walk or other exercise.
XI. Protect from extreme temperatures. ⚠
XII. Provide patient education.
   A. Low-sodium, well-balanced diet, protein in diet for those with hypoalbuminemia.
   B. Employ appropriate skin care strategies.
   C. Avoid prolonged standing or sitting with legs crossed.
   D. Avoid hepatotoxic drugs and alcohol.
   E. Fluid restriction may be warranted.
   F. Walk or exercise to maintain muscle strength and joint range of motion.
   G. Perform daily weights and report greater than a 3- to 4-pound gain.
   H. Educate patient and family regarding risks for electrolyte disturbance and possible interventions if symptoms occur.
   I. Wear support hose with instruction on how to apply them appropriately.

MALIGNANT PERICARDIAL EFFUSION

Overview

I. Definition—accumulation of fluid in the pericardial sac that affects cardiac function, resulting in decreased cardiac output.
II. Pathophysiology (Burazor, Imazio, Markel, & Adler, 2013).
   A. Malignant pericardial effusions may develop from:
      1. Metastatic disease that has moved into the cardiac space through local advancement, spread by blood or lymph systems or obstruction from adenopathy (i.e., most common lung or breast cancer; can occur in lymphoma, renal cell, angiosarcoma, clear cell sarcoma, melanoma, mesothelioma, gastric cancer, ovarian cancer, primary cardiac myxoma, prostate cancer, squamous cell carcinoma of the head and neck, or multiple myeloma)
      2. Treatment complications from radiation fibrosis causing damage to structure; chemotherapy causing damage to endothelial cells or cardiomyocytes, or both
      3. Infection in an immunocompromised patient
III. May be associated with the following (Burazor et al., 2013; Petrofsky, 2014):
   A. Primary tumors of the pericardium; mesothelioma most common.
   B. Direct tumor invasion of the myocardium; more common with lung tumors, thymoma, esophageal tumors, lymphoma.
   C. Obstruction of mediastinal lymph nodes by tumor.

D. Infection (bacterial, viral, fungal).
E. Fibrosis secondary to radiation therapy (RT).
F. Drug induced.
G. Autoimmune disease.
IV. Incidence (Burazor et al., 2013).
   A. Once diagnosed, prognosis is poor.
   B. Varies by malignant process involved.
V. Risk factors (Burazor et al., 2013; Petrofsky, 2014)
   A. Coexisting cardiac disease, systemic lupus erythematosus, bacterial endocarditis.
   B. RT of 3000 cGy to more than 33% of heart or fraction sizes of more than 300 cGy/day.
   C. High-dose chemotherapy or biotherapy agents that cause capillary permeability.
      1. Chemotherapy (i.e., cytosine arabinoside, cyclophosphamide, busulfan, doxorubicin, gemcitabine)
      2. Biological agents (i.e., interferon, IL-2, IL-11, granulocyte-macrophage colony-stimulating factor)
      3. Targeted agents (i.e., imatinib, dasatinib)
      4. Arsenic trioxide
      5. All-trans retinoic acid
   D. Rare causes include hemorrhagic tamponade from direct injury or infectious etiology.
   E. Malignancies (i.e., lung cancer, breast cancer, melanoma, lymphoma, leukemia)
   F. Thoracic lymphatic obstruction (i.e., from lymphadenopathy related to HIV disease or malignancies of the lymphatic system, hematologic malignancies, lymphangioleiomyomatosis, extramedullary multiple myeloma, or thymic cancer)

Assessment (Burazor et al., 2013; Petrofsky, 2014)

I. History
   A. Past medical history—cardiac, renal, liver disease, trauma
   B. Past surgical history
   C. Medication and treatment history
   D. Attributes of each symptom—onset, location, duration, characteristics, aggravating symptoms, relieving factors, treatment.
      1. Sudden onset, location of discomfort, nonproductive cough.
      2. Slowly developing effusions compensate for progressive reduction in cardiac output as the effusion occurs. May not demonstrate symptoms until more than 1000 mL of fluid is in the pericardial sac.
      3. Most common symptom with malignancy-related pericardial disease is dyspnea.
      4. Excessive yawning has been associated with pericardial effusion.
II. Physical examination
   A. Symptoms reflect chronicity.
      1. Slowly developing effusions may have little or no symptoms.
      2. Rapidly developing effusions may be symptomatic at 50 to 80 mL (normal pericardial fluid volume = 15–50 mL).

B. Fatigue, malaise, weakness.

C. Dyspnea at rest and with exertion.

D. Dull, nonpositional chest pain and distant, muffled heart sounds are a late finding.

E. Nonproductive cough.

F. Tachycardia, hypotension, jugular vein distention, decreased peripheral pulses.

G. Anxiousness, restlessness.

H. Nausea and vomiting.

I. Pericardial friction rub more likely to occur with radiation-induced or nonmalignant effusions.

J. Point of maximal impulse shifted to left.

K. Moderately increased central venous pressure (15–18 cm of H_2O or 8–12 mm Hg).

L. 2 to 3+ pedal edema with slowly developing effusions; may be absent with rapid development of effusion.

M. Narrowing pulse pressure, pulsus paradoxus greater than 13 mm Hg.

N. Cool, clammy extremities.

O. Hepatomegaly/splenomegaly.

III. Imaging and laboratory tests (Burazor et al., 2013; Petrofsky, 2014)

A. CXR indicating cardiac enlargement, widened mediastinum, "water bottle" shape of heart, pulmonary infiltrates.

B. Electrocardiogram (ECG) changes including low-voltage QRS, tachycardia, nonspecific ST-T changes; electrical alternans is a rare finding.

C. Echocardiogram is a definitive test for effusion and cardiac function.

D. CT of chest especially helpful with large tumor burden.

E. May evaluate pericardial fluid for lactate dehydrogenase, protein, and tumor markers.

F. Cardiac catheterization may be indicated if the diagnosis is in question.

G. Troponins may be elevated.

H. White blood cell count will be elevated with infection.

I. C-reactive protein elevated with inflammation.

J. BNP elevated with fluid overload.

Management (Burazor et al., 2013; Petrofsky, 2014)

I. Chemotherapy may be indicated if tumor responsive (i.e., lymphoma, leukemia, breast cancer).

II. Administer sclerosing agents into pericardial space as indicated (e.g., talc, bleomycin).

III. Oxygen therapy.

IV. Diuretics probably not beneficial.

V. Pain management.

VI. Nursing management.

A. Drain of pericardial fluid such as percutaneous pericardiocentesis.

B. Radiation may be indicated, but not common.

C. Elevate head of bed to relieve dyspnea.

D. Minimize activities to conserve energy.

E. May elect no treatment with close follow-up if asymptomatic.

F. Consult palliative care

VII. Nonpharmacologic

A. Interventions for patient education.

1. Preparation for pericardial drainage.

2. Energy conservation methods.

3. Relaxation techniques.

4. Activity modification to conserve energy.

CARDIOVASCULAR TOXICITY RELATED TO CANCER THERAPY

Overview

I. Definition—damage to the cardiac muscle, conduction system, coronary arteries, valves, and/or pericardium related to cancer therapies that may cause alterations in cardiac function (Curigliano et al., 2016).

II. Types of cardiovascular toxicities (CVT) associated with cancer therapies (Curigliano et al., 2016; Jain, Russell, Schwartz, Panjrath, & Aronow, 2017)

A. Left ventricular dysfunction (LVD)

B. Heart failure (HF)

C. Hypertension (HTN) treatment induced

D. Ischemia

E. Rhythm disturbances

1. Conduction damage

2. QT prolongation

F. Venous thromboembolism (VTE) with or without arterial thromboembolism (ATE)

G. Myopericarditis

III. Drug classes associated with CVT (Curigliano et al., 2016; Jain et al., 2017)

A. Alkylating agents—associated with acute myopericarditis, pericardial effusions, arrhythmias, HTN, thromboembolism, and heart failure (i.e., cyclophosphamide).

B. Angiogenesis inhibitors—bradycardia, thromboembolism, and HTN may be seen (i.e., thalidomide, lenalidomide, pomalidomide)

C. Anthracyclines—may cause toxicity from injury of free radicals that result in myocardial cell loss, fibrosis, and loss of contractility resulting in left ventricular dysfunction (LVD), HF, myopericarditis (i.e., doxorubicin, daunorubicin, epirubicin, idarubicin, mitoxantrone)

D. Antiandrogens—can cause hyperlipidemia, thromboembolism, QT prolongation

E. Antiangiogenic antibodies—may cause HTN, ischemia (i.e., bevacizumab)

F. Antiestrogens—can cause thromboembolism, HTN

G. Antimetabolites—can cause coronary artery spasm resulting in angina, arrhythmia, myocardial infarction, cardiac arrest, and sudden death; coronary artery thrombosis and apoptosis of myocardial cells (i.e., 5FU, capecitabine, gemcitabine).

H. Antimicrotubule agents—may cause early HF, arrhythmias, ischemia (i.e., paclitaxel, docetaxel, etoposide, vincristine, vinblastine).

I. Checkpoint inhibitors—myopericarditis, atrial fibrillation, ventricular arrhythmias, HF (i.e., nivolumab, pembrolizumab, ipilimumab)

J. HER2/neu blockers—inhibits certain pathways critical to cardiac function, which may increase the risk for HF (i.e., trastuzumab, pertuzumab)

K. Histone deacetylase inhibitors—may cause QT prolongation or thromboembolism (i.e., vorinostat)

L. Miscellaneous drugs—such as arsenic trioxide (QT prolongation), tretinoin (HF, hypotension), bleomycin (myopericarditis)

M. mTOR inhibitors—HTN, angina, DVT/pulmonary embolism (PE) (i.e., everolimus, temsirolimus)

N. Platinum agents—HTN, hypotension, dyslipidemia, early atherosclerosis, coronary artery disease, Raynaud syndrome, thromboembolic events, HF, angina, acute myocardial infarction (AMI), autonomic cardiovascular dysfunction, myocarditis, pericarditis, cardiomyopathy, arrhythmias, atrial fibrillation, complete atrioventricular block

O. Proteasome inhibitors—may cause HF and ischemia (i.e., bortezomib, carfilzomib)

P. Tyrosine kinase inhibitors (TKIs)–may cause HF, QT prolongation, HTN, ischemia, thromboembolism (i.e., dasatinib, lapatinib, imatinib, sunitinib)

IV. Incidence (Bonita & Pradham, 2013; Curigliano et al., 2016; Jain et al., 2017)

A. Acute reactions—infrequent; reversible.
    1. Occur within 24 hours of drug administration.
    2. Usually self-limiting and cease when the drug is stopped.
    3. May not require discontinuation of the drug.

B. Early onset within 1 year after treatment—infrequent.

C. Late onset after 1 year of completing therapy.
    1. Occurs with cumulative doses of drugs.
    2. Dilated cardiomyopathy can occur.

V. RT

A. Incidence (Bonita & Pradham, 2013; Curigliano et al., 2016; Jain et al., 2017).

B. Acute reactions—infrequent; reversible.
    1. Occur within 24 hours of drug administration.
    2. Usually self-limiting and cease when the drug is stopped.
    3. May not require discontinuation of the drug.

C. Early onset within 1 year after treatment—infrequent.

D. Late onset after 1 year of completing therapy.
    1. Occurs with cumulative doses of drugs.
    2. Dilated cardiomyopathy can occur.

VI. Risk factors (Carver, Szalda, & Ky, 2013; Csapo & Lazar, 2014)

A. Preexisting heart disease, HTN, hyperlipidemia.

B. History of smoking.

C. Age younger than 15 years or advanced age >65.

D. Certain cardiotoxic drugs.
    1. Doses that place patient at risk:
        a. Doxorubicin >550 mg/m^2
        b. Liposomal doxorubicin >900 mg/m^2
        c. Epirubicin >720 mg/m^2
        d. Mitoxantrone >120 mg/m^2
        e. Idarubicin >90 mg/m^2

E. Exceeding recommended total doses of chemotherapy or high dose in short period.

F. Radiation treatment field which includes the heart.

G. Acute cardiac event during treatment.

H. Combination chest radiation with anthracycline.

I. Other: female, obesity, comorbid disease, previous cancer treatment that had cardiotoxicity.

Assessment (Carver, Szalda & Ky, 2013; Csapo & Lazar, 2014)

I. History

A. Past medical history—preexisting cardiac disease, electrolyte imbalances, renal or liver disease, dyslipidemia, diabetes

B. Past surgical history

C. Medication history

D. Treatment history—prior chemotherapy and radiation

E. Attributes of each symptom—onset, location, duration, characteristics, aggravating symptoms, relieving factors, treatment.
    1. Palpitations, chest pain

II. Physical examination

A. Orthostatic symptoms, arrhythmias, jugular vein distention, bilateral pedal edema, presence of S_3 or S_4, murmurs with valvular abnormalities, decreased cardiac ejection fraction
    1. Tachycardia—early sign in anthracycline toxicity.

B. Shortness of breath, dyspnea, orthopnea, nonproductive cough

C. Exercise intolerance, fatigue

D. Weight gain

E. Syncope

III. Psychosocial assessment

A. Interventions used to relieve symptoms and improve quality of life

IV. Imaging and laboratory tests (Cao, Zhu, Wager, & Meng, 2017; Curigliano et al., 2016)

A. ECG changes.
    1. Premature atrial contractions, premature ventricular contractions.
    2. Nonspecific ST-T wave changes.

B. Echocardiogram or multigated acquisition scan (MUGA scan).
    1. Monitor left ventricular function—usually decreased EF.
        a. Decreased EF to less than 45% or decrease of more than 5% over baseline requires consideration for discontinuing the drug or holding

treatment and monitoring the EF until improvement. Resuming drug is individualized.
2. Pericardial effusion.
3. Left ventricular hypertrophy.
C. MRI—gold standard for evaluation of left ventricular volumes, mass, and function; however, it is cost prohibitive.
D. BMI/waist circumference.
E. Laboratory changes that may affect cardiac function
1. Laboratory tests affecting cardiac function—potassium, magnesium, calcium, renal function, thyroid, lipid levels
a. Electrolytes should be monitored, especially with drugs that may prolong the QT interval.
2. Cardiac biomarkers of early myocardial damage—troponins, BNP

Management (Bonita & Pradhan, 2013; Cardinale, Bacchiani, Beggiato, Colobo & Cipolla, 2013; Carver, Szalda, & Ky, 2013; Curigliano et al., 2016; Jain et al., 2017)

I. Interventions to treat cardiotoxicity with pharmacologic methods are based on underlying event (Curigliano et al., 2016).
A. Lipid-lowering agents if indicated for hyperlipidemia.
B. Beta blockers and ACE inhibitors.
1. Can be used for left ventricular dysfunction.
C. ARBs concurrent with anthracyclines help prevent cardiac damage.
D. ACE inhibitors and calcium channel blockers to treat hypertension.
E. Minimize risk of QT prolongation.
1. Avoid drug-to-drug interactions.
2. Monitor and treat electrolyte disturbances.
F. Administer cardiac protective iron chelating agents, such as dexrazoxane (Zinecard), to prevent doxorubicin-induced cardiotoxicity in patients with metastatic breast cancer who require more than 300 mg/m^2 of drug; liposomal doxorubicin to decrease cardiotoxicity.
G. Anticoagulate patients at risk for venous thromboembolism
II. Nursing management (Curigliano et al., 2016; Jain et al., 2017)
A. Cardiovascular risk assessment before treatment starts
B. Screening of cardiovascular function at appropriate intervals
C. Valvular surgery may be indicated with radiation-induced valvular disease
D. Management of underlying disease—both cancer and cardiac
E. Radiation management to reduce exposure to cardiac structure
F. Prevent cardiotoxicity
1. Document total cumulative dose of drug; discontinue when maximum dose is achieved.
a. Doxorubicin: 550 mg/m^2

b. Daunorubicin (Cerubidine, DaunoXome): 600 mg/m^2
c. Mitoxantrone (Novantrone): 160 mg/m^2
d. High-dose cyclophosphamide: 144 mg/kg for 4 days
G. Monitor baseline and interval ECG or MUGA scan.
H. Monitor vital signs and weight.
I. Monitor exposure of radiation therapy to minimize cardiac toxicity.
J. Patient education.
1. Signs and symptoms to report.
2. Well-balanced diet, with a focus on any restrictions.
3. Importance for medically approved exercise program.

THROMBOTIC EVENTS

Overview

I. Definition—venous thrombus or arterial embolus interfering with venous drainage or obstructing arterial blood flow.
II. Pathophysiology (Falanga, Russo, Milesi, & Vignoli, 2017; Myers, 2015).
A. A thrombus may form in the setting of stasis, endothelial injury, and/or a hypercoagulable state (Virchow triad).
1. The thrombus is composed of red blood cells, fibrin, and platelets; fills the vessel lumen, causing partial or complete obstruction of blood flow; or may shed emboli, causing PE or cerebrovascular accident.
2. The thrombus may float freely in the blood vessel, leading to embolization where it lodges in a blood vessel, causing partial or complete obstruction of blood flow.
B. Tumor cells may be associated with procoagulant activities.
1. Tumor cells deposit fibrin in tissues, acting late in clotting cascade, providing a surface for prothrombinase assembly.
2. Microvasculature becomes hyperpermeable, allowing clotting proteins to leak into extravascular space.
3. Procoagulants released from cancer cells initiate the clotting cascade.
III. Risk factors (Falanga et al., 2017, NCCN, 2019)
A. Active cancer
1. Some sites are higher risk (i.e., stomach, brain, pancreas, bladder)
2. Advanced stage higher risk
B. Lymphadenopathy
C. Presence of venous access device
D. Comorbidities (i.e., infections, HF, renal disease)
E. Poor performance status; prolonged immobilization
F. Older age
G. Cancer treatments

1. Cytotoxic agents
2. Hormonal therapies (i.e., tamoxifen)
3. Antiangiogenic agents—thalidomide
4. Erythropoietic-stimulating agents

H. Smoking

I. Obesity

J. Surgery

K. Hospitalizations—especially prolonged

L. Prior personal history of VTE; familial/acquired hypercoagulability/thrombophilia

M. Laboratory abnormalities
   1. Prechemotherapy platelet count >350,000/mcL
   2. Prechemotherapy white blood cell count >11,000/mcL
   3. Hgb <10g/dL

N. Blood transfusions

IV. Incidence rates vary in persons with cancer by disease. Ranging from 8% to 19% depending on tumor type (NCCN, 2019).

A. High risk: cancers of the lung, gastrointestinal tract, pancreatic, prostate, ovary.

B. Leukemias, multiple myeloma, Hodgkin and non-Hodgkin lymphoma.

C. Advanced disease or metastatic disease.

Assessment (Falanga et al., 2017; NCCN, 2019)

I. History

A. Past medical history—including history of VTE

B. Family history of any blood disorders, thrombus

C. Past surgical history

D. Medication history

E. Treatment history—prior chemotherapy and radiation

F. Attributes of each symptom—onset, location, duration, characteristics, aggravating symptoms, relieving factors, treatment

G. Pain in calf with walking, dull ache, tight feeling

II. Physical examination

A. Venous occlusion.
   1. Tenderness over involved vein, palpable venous cord.
   2. Unilateral edema of involved extremity.
   3. Distention of superficial collateral veins.

B. Arterial embolus.
   1. Severe pain in the involved extremity.
   2. Extremity coolness, pallor.
   3. Absent or decreased pulse.

C. Pulmonary embolus.
   1. Chest pain.
   2. Dyspnea, shallow respirations, tachypnea.
   3. Sudden onset of anxiety.
   4. Cardiopulmonary arrest.
   5. Decreased pulse oximetry.
   6. Decreased breath sounds with pleural friction rub.

D. Clotting abnormalities.
   1. Easy bruising.
   2. Bleeding from mucous membranes, in urine or stool.

III. Imaging and laboratory tests (NCCN, 2019)

A. Complete blood count and platelet count—thrombocytosis.

B. Abnormal venous ultrasound (US) or venogram with VTE.

C. Liver function tests, BUN, creatinine.

D. Abnormal arteriogram with arterial embolus.

E. Abnormal spiral CT or ventilation-perfusion (V-Q) scan with PE.

F. Prothrombin time (PT), partial thrombin time (PTT), international normalized ratio (INR), abnormal clotting factors, D-dimer.

G. Consider evaluation for hypercoagulable states such as protein C, protein S, antithrombin III, factor V Leiden, prothrombin gene mutation, homocysteine, antiphospholipid antibodies.

H. Magnetic resonance venography for pelvic and iliac veins and vena cava—can be cost prohibitive.

Management (NCCN, 2019)

I. Prevent thrombotic events in high-risk patients.

A. Anticoagulation prophylaxis is not recommended in patients receiving standard chemotherapy.

B. Consider prophylaxis in patients with high risk.
   1. Low-molecular weight heparin (LMWH).
   2. Unfractionated heparin
   3. Acetylsalicylic acid (aspirin, ASA), 81 mg
   4. Anticoagulants: warfarin (adjust INR 2-3), rivaroxaban, apixaban

II. Treat acute emboli

A. LMWH.

B. Unfractionated heparin IV/subcutaneous.

C. Direct oral anticoagulation if LMWH is contraindicated.

D. Oxygen for PE.

E. Pain management.

III. Prevent thrombotic events in high-risk patients.

A. Ambulate frequently, leg exercises if bedridden.

B. Elevate foot with knee flexed.

C. Employ intermittent pneumatic compression device.

D. Refer to physical therapy and/or occupational therapy

IV. Treatment of acute embolus.

A. Place inferior vena cava filter if pharmacologic management is contraindicated.

B. Arterial embolectomy.

C. Thrombolysis consider on case-by-case basis.

D. Monitor laboratory parameters—PT, PTT, INR.

V. Provide patient education.

A. Medication administration.

B. Preventive measures.

C. Bleeding precautions if patient taking anticoagulant.

D. Dietary restrictions—avoid foods high in vitamin K.

E. Smoking cessation.

F. Activity restrictions.

EXPECTED PATIENT OUTCOMES

I. Patient will maintain moderate activity, muscle strength, and joint range of motion.

II. Patient will perform self-care activities by performing regular skin care and maintain stable weight and decrease edema.

III. Patient will have an acceptable level of pain control, maintain an adequate level of functioning of the affected lymphedema area, and protect the affected extremity from trauma.

IV. Patient will maintain cardiac output, tissue perfusion, and EF within 5% of baseline with normal vital signs and oxygenation level and no signs of fluid overload.

V. Patient will verbalize abnormalities to report to health care provider.

REFERENCES

Bernas, M. (2013). Assessment and risk reduction in lymphedema. *Seminars in Oncology Nursing, 29*(1), 12–19. https://doi.org/10.1016/j.soncn.2012.11.003.

Bonita, R., & Pradhan, R. (2013). Cardiovascular toxicities of cancer chemotherapy. *Seminars in Oncology, 40*(2), 186–198. https://doi.org/10.1053/j.seminoncol.2013.01.004.

Burazor, I., Imazio, M., Markel, G., & Adler, Y. (2013). Malignant pericardial effusion. *Cardiology, 124*(4), 224–232. https://doi.org/10.1159/000348559.

Cao, L., Zhu, W., Wager, E. A., & Meng, Q. H. (2017). Biomarkers for monitoring chemotherapy-induced cardiotoxicity. *Critical Reviews in Clinical Laboratory Sciences, 54*(2), 87–101. https://doi.org/10.1080/10408363.2016.1261270.

Cardinale, D., Bacchiani, G., Beggiato, M., Alessandro, C., & Cipolla, C. M. (2013). Strategies to prevent and treat cardiovascular risk in cancer patients. *Seminars in Oncology, 40*(2), 186–198. https://doi.org/10.1053/j.seminoncol.2013.01.008.

Carver, J. R., Szalda, D., & Ky, B. (2013). Asymptomatic cardiac toxicity in long-term cancer survivors: defining the population and recommendations for surveillance. *Seminars in Oncology, 40*(2), 229–238. https://doi.org/10.1053/j.seminoncol.2013.01.005.

Csapo, M., & Lazar, L. (2014). Chemotherapy-induced cardiotoxicity: pathophysiology and prevention. *Clujul Medical, 87*(3), 135–142. https://doi.org/10.15386/cjmed-339.

Curigliano, G., Cardinale, D., Dent, S., Criscitiello, C., Aseyev, O., & Lenihan, & Cipolla, C. (2016). Cardiotoxicity of anticancer treatments: epidemiology, detection, and management. *CA: A Cancer Journal for Clinicians, 66*, 309–325. https://doi.org/10.3322/caac.21341.

Falanga, A., Russo, L., Milesi, V., & Vignoli, A. (2017). Mechanisms and risk factors of thrombosis in cancer. *Critical Reviews in Oncology/Hematology, 118*, 79–83.

Fu, M., Deng, J., & Armer, J. M. (2014). Putting evidence into practice: cancer-related lymphedema: evolving evidence for treatment and management from 2009-2014. *Clinical Journal of Oncology Nursing, 18*(6), 68–79. https://doi.org/10.1188/14.CJON.S3.68-79.

Fu, M. R., & Kang, Y. (2013). Psychosocial impact of living with cancer-related lymphedema. *Seminars in Oncology Nursing, 29*(1), 50–60. https://doi.org/10.1016/j.soncn.2012.11.007.

Hespe, G. E., Nores, G. N., Huang, J. J., & Mehrara, B. J. (2017). Pathophysiology of lymphedema – is there a chance for medication treatment? *Journal of Surgical Oncology, 115*, 96–98. https://doi.org/10.1002/jso.24414.

Jain, D., Russell, R. R., Schwartz, R. G., Panjrath, G. S., & Aronow, W. (2017). Cardiac complications of cancer therapy: pathology, identification, prevention, treatment, and future directions. *Current Cardiology Reports, 19*(36), 1–12. https://doi.org/10.1007/s11886-017-0846-x.

Ki, E. Y., Park, J. S., Lee, K. H., & Hur, S. Y. (2016). Incidence and risk factors of lower extremity lymphedema after gynecologic surgery in ovarian cancer. *International Journal of Gynecological Cancer, 26*(7), 1327–1332. https://doi.org/10.1097/IGC.0000000000000757.

Lasinski, B. B. (2013). Complete decongestive therapy for treatment of lymphedema. *Seminars in Oncology Nursing, 29*(1), 20–27. https://doi.org/10.1016/j.soncn.2012.004.

Li, L., Yuan, L., Chen, X., Wang, Q., Tian, J., Yang, K., & Zhou, E. (2016). Current treatments for breast cancer-related lymphoedema: a systematic review. *Asian Pacific Journal of Cancer Prevention, 17*, 4875–4883. https://doi.org/10.22034/APJCP.2016.17.11.4875.

Myers, D. D. (2015). Pathophysiology of venous thrombosis. *Phlebology: The Journal of Venous Disease, 30*(1), 7–13. https://doi.org/10.1177/0268355515569424.

National Cancer Institute. (2015). *Lymphedema (PDQ) Health Professional Version.* Retrieved https://www.cancer.gov/about-cancer/treatment/sideeffects/lymphedema/lymphedema-hp-pdq/#link/_8_toc.

NCCN (2019). *Guidelines Cancer-Associated Venous Thromboembolic Disease [v1.2019].* Retrieved from https://www.nccn.org/professionals/physician_gls/pdf/vte.pdf.

Petrofsky, M. (2014). Management of malignant pericardial effusion. *Journal of Advanced Practitioner Oncology, 5*(4), 281–289.

Ridner, S. H. (2013). Pathophysiology of lymphedema. *Seminars in Oncology Nursing, 29*(1), 4–11. https://doi.org/10.1016/j.soncn.2012.002.

Ryberg, M. (2013). Cardiovascular toxicities of biological therapies. *Seminars in Oncology, 40*(2), 168–177. https://doi.org/10.1053/j.seminoncol.2013.01.002.

Trayes, K. P., Studdiford, J. S., Pickle, S., & Tully, A. S. (2013). Edema: diagnosis and management. *American Family Physician, 88*(2), 102–110.

Wanchai, A., Beck, M., Stewart, B. R., & Armer, J. M. (2013). Management of lymphedema for cancer patients with complex needs. *Seminars in Oncology Nursing, 29*(1), 61–65. https://doi.org/10.1016/j.soncn.2012.001.

Zhu, Y., Xie, Y., Liu, F., Guo, Q., Shen, P., & Tian, Y. (2014). Systemic analysis on risk factors for breast cancer related lymphedema. *Asian Pacific Journal of Cancer Prevention, 15*(16), 6535–6541. https://doi.org/10.7314/APJCP.2014.15.16.6535.

Cognitive Symptoms

Catherine E. Jansen

CANCER AND CANCER TREATMENT-RELATED COGNITIVE IMPAIRMENT

Overview

I. Definition—functional decline in one or more cognitive domains may include attention and concentration, executive function, information processing speed, language, motor function, visuospatial skill, learning, and/or memory (Jansen, 2017).

II. Pathophysiology is not fully understood, and therefore likely multifactorial (Allen, Myers, Jansen, Merriman, & Von Ah, 2018; Jansen, 2017).

A. Direct effects of central nervous system (CNS) tumors, surgical removal of CNS tumors, and cranial irradiation, which can result in structural and functional damage specific to tumor location (Edelstein, Richard, & Bernstein, 2017).

B. Direct effects of chemotherapy on neuroprogenitor cells and oligodendrocytes.

C. Cytokine dysregulation stimulated by cancer, chemotherapy, and/or immunotherapy can lead to inflammation and oxidative stress, as well as altered neurotransmitter metabolism and neural function.

D. Changes in hormonal levels (e.g., estrogen, testosterone) from surgery, hormonal therapies, and/or chemotherapy may alter cognition.

III. Risk factors (Ahles & Root, 2018; Allen et al., 2018; Castel et al., 2017)

A. Disease-related factors
1. Primary CNS cancers: prevalence 90%
2. Non-CNS cancers: prevalence estimated up to 40% before treatment
3. Advanced, metastatic, or terminal disease

B. Treatment-related factors: chemotherapy, hormonal therapy, immunotherapy, surgery, and/or radiation to the CNS and including
1. Dose intensity, cumulative effect, and/or multimodality therapy
2. Treatment toxicities (e.g., anemia, fatigue, nausea, organ dysfunction)

3. Concomitant or supportive medications (e.g., anticholinergics, antiemetics, benzodiazepines, corticosteroids, opioids)

C. Individual characteristics that may increase risk for cognitive impairment
1. Age (cognitive decline occurs with aging)
2. Sensory deficits (e.g., hearing, vision)
3. Comorbidities (e.g., cardiovascular disease, hypertension, diabetes)
4. Genetic polymorphisms (e.g., apolipoprotein E4 [APOE] allele, catechol-O-methyltransferase [COMT] val allele)
5. Psychological factors (e.g., anxiety, depression, stress)

Assessment (Allen et al., 2018; Jansen, 2017)

I. History and physical examination
A. Presence of cognitive complaints—difficulties with retaining new information, handling complex tasks, altered perception, and/or impaired communication.
B. Medical history—cancer history (e.g., disease trajectory), current and prior cancer treatments, systemic cancer and/or treatment effects, presence of significant comorbidities, current medications.
C. Neurologic assessment for presence of any focal deficits and refer for further evaluation and/or neuropsychological testing as indicated.

II. Psychosocial assessment
A. Changes in emotional and behavioral affect (e.g., anxiety, depression, distress).
B. Lifestyle factors (e.g., alcohol or drug use, diet, exercise), nutritional deficiencies (e.g., thiamine, vitamin E), work history.
C. Impact of cognitive impairment on social interactions and ability to function.

III. Imaging and laboratory tests (Allen et al., 2018; Jansen, 2017; NCCN 2019)
A. Complete blood cell count (CBC) with differential to rule out anemia.
B. Electrolytes, including calcium, to rule out electrolyte imbalance(s).

C. Liver, renal, and thyroid function tests to determine any organ dysfunction.

D. Vitamin B_{12} and folate levels to evaluate for nutritional deficiencies.

E. Computed tomography (CT) or magnetic resonance imaging (MRI) to rule out structural abnormalities in patients with focal neurologic deficits or at high risk for recurrence or metastatic disease to the CNS.

Management

I. Medical management (Allen et al., 2018, NCCN, 2019, Von Ah, Jansen, & Allen, 2014)

A. Cognitive training—structured repetitive tasks aimed at improving a specific cognitive skill (e.g., attention, memory).

B. Exercise (e.g., aerobics, resistance training, tai chi, yoga).

C. Effectiveness not established for the use of psychostimulants (e.g., dexmethylphenidate, methylphenidate, modafinil), acetylcholinesterase inhibitors (e.g., donepezil), and/or N-methyl-D-aspartate (NMDA) receptors (e.g., memantine). However, a psychostimulant trial may be considered if nonpharmacologic interventions are not effective.

II. Nursing management (Allen et al., 2018, NCCN, 2019, Von Ah, Jansen, & Allen, 2014)

A. Reinforce cognitive and exercise training plans.

DELIRIUM

Overview

I. Definition—disturbance in level of attention and awareness, often accompanied by changes in other cognitive domains and characterized by an acute onset (hours to days) with fluctuations in symptom(s) severity throughout the day (Lawlor & Bush, 2015).

A. Hypoactive delirium: characterized by the presence of psychomotor retardation, sedation, lethargy, and/or decreased awareness of surroundings.

B. Hyperactive delirium: characterized by the presence of restlessness, hypervigilance, agitation, hallucinations, and/or delusions.

II. Pathophysiology (Bush, Tierney, & Lawlor, 2017; Lawlor & Bush, 2015; Maldonado, 2017)

A. Indirect effects of cancer, cancer treatment(s), and/or concomitant medications that result in organ failure, metabolic or electrolyte imbalance, infection, and/or paraneoplastic syndromes.

B. Substance intoxication or withdrawal (e.g., alcohol, benzodiazepines).

C. Alteration in neurotransmitter synthesis, function, and/or activity secondary to systemic disturbances.

III. Risk factors (Lawlor & Bush, 2015; Maldonado, 2017)

A. Disease related

1. Primary or metastatic CNS disease.
2. Non-CNS cancers: prevalence 25% to 40%.

3. Advanced or terminal-stage cancers: prevalence 45% to 88%.

4. Paraneoplastic syndromes (e.g., syndrome of inappropriate antidiuretic hormone secretion [SIADH]).

B. Treatment-related—current chemotherapy, immunotherapy, radiation to CNS, surgery (e.g., postoperative effects in elderly)

1. Concomitant or supportive medications (e.g., analgesics, antidepressants, antiemetics, antihistamines, antiinfectives, antivirals, corticosteroids).

2. Treatment toxicities (e.g., dehydration, electrolyte and/or metabolic abnormalities [e.g., calcium, glucose, sodium], neuropsychiatric complications [e.g., encephalopathy, hallucinations, delusions]).

C. Other pertinent contributing factors—alcohol or drug (e.g., barbiturates, benzodiazepines, selective serotonin reuptake inhibitors, opioids) withdrawal, dehydration, hypoxia, organ dysfunction, systemic infections and sepsis, unrelieved pain.

D. Individual characteristics—advanced age, baseline dementia, reduced mobility and/or functional performance status, nutritional deficiencies, sensory impairments (e.g., visual, hearing), sleep–wake disturbances.

Assessment (Lawlor & Bush, 2015; Maldonado, 2017; Oh, Fong, Hshieh, & Inouye, 2017)

I. History and physical examination (involve caregivers)

A. Medical history—cancer history (e.g., disease trajectory), current cancer treatments, recent febrile illness, history of organ failure, presence of risk factors for delirium.

B. Review current medications and identify those known to cause delirium or that have high anticholinergic potential.

C. Attention to neurologic status (acute change in mental status with a fluctuating course, inattention, disorganized thinking, altered level of consciousness, agitation, restlessness, hallucinations, or delusions).

II. Imaging and laboratory tests targeted to evaluate for suspected etiology

A. Electrolytes, including calcium, magnesium, phosphate.

B. CBC with differential.

C. Urinalysis and culture if indicated

D. Arterial blood gas if hypoxic.

E. Liver, renal, and thyroid function tests.

F. Lumbar puncture can be considered if etiology not obvious.

Management

I. Medical management (Bush et al., 2017; Lawlor & Bush, 2015; Maldonado, 2017; Oh et al., 2017)

A. Identify and treat reversible causes (e.g., dehydration, infection, metabolic imbalance, pain).

B. Minimize, taper, or discontinue medications that may contribute to delirium.

C. Consider low-dose antipsychotic (e.g., haloperidol 0.25–0.5 mg every 30 minutes, not to exceed 5 mg in 24 hours) for management of severe agitation.

II. Nursing management (Bush et al., 2017; Maldonado, 2017; Oh et al., 2017)

A. Minimize sensory deficits (eyeglasses, hearing aid).

B. Promote uninterrupted sleep.

C. Encourage ambulation.

D. Avoid excessive sensory stimulation and/or restraints.

E. Provide frequent reorientation and reassurance.

F. Incorporate environmental strategies (e.g., well-lit room with familiar objects, visible clock/calendar, caregiver continuity).

Expected Patient Outcomes

I. Patient's cognitive complaints will be acknowledged, and modifiable causes for cognitive symptoms will be identified and treated.

II. Caregivers will understand the nature of cognitive symptoms and potential outcomes.

III. The patient's symptoms will be managed to promote safety and prevent harm.

IV. Screen for reversible factors that may contribute to cognitive impairment.

V. Assess for cognitive problems that may interfere with patient's ability to independently perform activities of daily living and self-care strategies (including medication management).

REFERENCES

Ahles, T. A., & Root, J. C. (2018). Cognitive effects of cancer and cancer treatments. *Annual Review of Clinical Psychology, 14,* 425–451. https://doi.org/10.1146/annurev-clinpsy-050817-084903.

Allen, D., Myers, J., Jansen, C., Merriman, J., & Von Ah, D. (2018). Assessment and management of cancer- and cancer-treatment related cognitive impairment. *Journal for Nurse Practitioners, 14* (4), 217–224.

Bush, S. H., Tierney, S., & Lawlor, P. G. (2017). Clinical assessment and management of delirium in the palliative care setting. *Drugs, 77*(15), 1623–1643.

Castel, H., Denouel, A., Lange, M., Tono, M. C., Dubois, M., & Joly, F. (2017). Biomarkers associated with cognitive impairment in treated cancer patients: potential predisposition and risk factors. *Frontiers in Pharmacology, 8,* 138.

Edelstein, K., Richard, N. M., & Bernstein, L. J. (2017). Neurocognitive impact of cranial radiation in adults with cancer: an update of recent findings. *Current Opinion in Supportive and Palliative Care, 11*(1), 32–37.

Jansen, C. E. (2017). Cognitive changes. In J. Eggert (Ed.), *Cancer basics* (2nd ed., pp. 381–395). Pittsburgh, PA: Oncology Nursing Society.

Lawlor, P. G., & Bush, S. H. (2015). Delirium in patients with cancer: assessment, impact, mechanisms and management. *Nature Reviews Clinical Oncology, 12*(2), 77–92.

Maldonado, J. R. (2017). Acute brain failure: pathophysiology, diagnosis, management, and sequelae of delirium. *Critical Care Clinics, 33*(3), 461–519.

National Comprehensive Cancer Network. (2019). *NCCN clinical practice guidelines in oncology: survivorship [v.1.2019].* Retrieved from (2019). https://www.nccn.org/professionals/physician_gls/pdf/survivorship.pdf.

Oh, E. S., Fong, T. G., Hshieh, T. T., & Inouye, S. K. (2017). Delirium in older persons: advances in diagnosis and treatment. *Journal of the American Medication Association, 318*(12), 1161–1174.

Von Ah, D., Jansen, C., & Allen, D. H. (2014). Evidence-based interventions for cancer- and treatment-related cognitive impairment. *Clinical Journal of Oncology Nursing, 18*(Suppl. 6), 607–615.

35

Endocrine Symptoms

Marianne Davies

I. Overview: endocrine organs—thyroid, parathyroid, adrenal, pituitary gland, hypothalamus, pineal, thymus, pancreas, ovaries, testes. Dysfunction can occur due to acute or latent toxicity from cancer therapies or cancer occurrence in affected gland.
   A. Thyroid gland: secretes triiodothyronine (T_3) and thyroxine (T_4) in response to thyroid-stimulating hormone (TSH) released by the pituitary gland. T_3 and T_4 regulate body temperature, heart rate, and other metabolic processes. Dysfunction includes thyroiditis, hypothyroidism, hyperthyroidism, Graves disease, and goiters.
   B. Parathyroid gland: secretes parathyroid hormone (PTH). PTH regulates serum calcium and vitamin D. Dysfunction includes hypoparathyroidism and hyperparathyroidism.
   C. Adrenal gland: produces mineralocorticoids (aldosterone), glucocorticoids (cortisol and corticosterone), and androgens. Dysfunction includes primary or secondary adrenal insufficiency and Cushing syndrome.
   D. Pituitary gland: produces adrenocorticotropic hormone (ACTH), gonadotropic hormones (luteinizing hormone [LH], follicle-stimulating hormone [FSH]), human growth hormone (hGH), prolactin, and TSH. Pituitary stores vasopressin (antidiuretic hormone [ADH]) and oxytocin. Dysfunction includes hypophysitis, hypopituitarism, and central diabetes.

II. Etiology and risk factors
   A. Disease-related: carcinoma of the thyroid, parathyroid, pituitary, or adrenal gland.
   B. Treatment-related factors:
      1. Surgical resection—thyroid, parathyroid, adrenal, or pituitary gland.
      2. External radiation therapy to the head and/or neck (doses of 18 Gy or more) (Alba, 2016; Appelman-Dijkstra, 2014; Chemaitilly, 2014; Christakis, 2017; Mostoufi-Moab, 2016).
      3. Radioiodine (I-131) therapy (Albano, 2017; Fard-Esfahani, 2014).
      4. Systemic therapy (Barroso-Sousa, 2018; Faje, 2016; Konda, 2017; Lee, 2017; Morganstein, 2017; Torino, 2013)

         a. Immune modulatory therapy: immune checkpoint inhibitors, interferon-alfa, interleukin-2, lenalidomide, thalidomide
         b. Tyrosine kinase inhibitors
         c. High-dose chemotherapy preparation for stem cell transplantation
         d. Supportive care medications: denosumab, bisphosphonates, glucocorticoids

III. Assessment (Barroso-Sousa, 2018; Sznol, 2017)
   A. See Table 35.1.

IV. Management (Cukier, 2017; Davies, 2017; Brahmer et al., 2018)
   A. Endocrinopathy
      1. Refer to the Risk Evaluation and Mitigation Strategy (REMS) program for select medications (interferon alpha-2b, ipilimumab, lenalidomide, pazopanib, sunitinib, thalidomide) (NCCN, 2018).
      2. Review Puzanov et al. (2017) for toxicities related to checkpoint inhibitor therapy.
      3. For severe symptomatic endocrinopathy secondary to immune checkpoint inhibitor—steroids to suppress autoimmune response. Methylprednisolone 1 to 2 mg/kg/day, with slow taper over weeks, based on response.
      4. Consider consultation with endocrinologist.
      5. Signs and symptoms of endocrinopathy may mimic therapy intolerance, so ongoing assessment and early diagnosis of thyroid, parathyroid, pituitary, and adrenal dysfunction is critical. Undiagnosed and untreated dysfunction may lead to other metabolic alterations (reduced drug metabolism) and trigger other life-threatening consequences. In many cases, cancer treatments may be continued as endocrine hormones can be safely replaced. However, with severe dysfunction, cancer treatments may need to be held temporarily or permanently discontinued.
      6. Patient education about potential symptoms; when to notify health care team
      7. Patients with endocrine dysfunction should carry card or bracelet to alert emergency medical personnel.

TABLE 35.1 Endocrinopathy Assessment

Endocrine Organ Dysfunction	Presentation	Physical Examination	Diagnostic Tests
Hyperthyroidism/ thyrotoxicosis	Anxiety, emotional lability, agitation, weakness, dyspnea, palpitation, heat intolerance, increased perspiration	Weight loss, tremor, hyperactivity, rapid speech, lid lag, warm and moist skin, hair thinning, tachycardia, irregular pulse, hyperreflexia, proximal muscle weakness	Low TSH; high (or normal) free T_4 and T_3 concentrations Thyrotoxic storm: rare Ultrasound (US), CT scan, or MRI of neck: rarely needed.
Hypothyroidism	Fatigue, weakness, depression, dyspnea, constipation, cold intolerance, myalgias, arthralgias	Weight gain, dry coarse skin, skin thickening, hoarseness, decreased hearing, slow speech, delayed relaxation of tendon reflexes, bradycardia, periorbital edema, enlargement of tongue, diastolic hypertension	Primary: normal-high TSH; low free T_4 and T_3 concentrations. Secondary (due to central dysfunction, i.e.. hypophysitis): low or normal TSH; low free T_4
Hyperparathyroidism	"Moans, groans, stones, and bones....with psychiatric overtones" (Linert, 2008), fatigue, anorexia, weakness, depression, cognitive or neuromuscular dysfunction, bone pain, polyuria, polydipsia; If severe: nausea, emesis, confusion, lethargy, stupor	Hypertension, bradycardia Renal colic If severe: asymptomatic bone fractures Severe: parathyroid crisis/storm	Hypercalcemia, elevated PTH, normal or elevated 1,25D concentration; hypercalciuric, decreased eGFR, decreased serum phosphate and magnesium. Abdominal US or CT: kidney stones ECG: shortened QT interval If severe: decreased bone density
Hypoparathyroidism	Fatigue, anxiety, depression, irritability *Acute hypocalcemia:* tetany (perioral numbness, paresthesia of hands and feet, muscle cramps, laryngospasm, imbalance, seizures) *Chronic hypocalcemia:* coarse hair, dry skin, brittle nails, pruritis	Acute: hypotension, heart failure Chronic: skeletal abnormalities, dental abnormalities, cataracts	Hypocalcemia, low PTH level, normal 25[OH]D; normal or low 1,25D concentration Acute hypocalcemia: prolonged QT interval, arrhythmia Skeletal survey to rule out lytic bone lesions
Hypopituitarism, hypophysitis	Fatigue, anorexia, visual changes, headache, myalgias, polyuria, polydipsia	Hypotension, tachycardia, weight loss	Secondary adrenal insufficiency: normal or low morning ACTH, low or undetectable cortisol level, hyponatremia. Alteration in LH, FSH, prolactin estradiol (females) and testosterone (males). Central hypothyroidism Type 1 diabetes: hyponatremia MRI of brain with pituitary cuts.
Adrenal insufficiency	Anorexia, nausea, emesis, abdominal pain, fatigue, myalgias, arthralgias, dizziness, syncope, lethargy, impaired memory, irritability, confusion	Hypotension, postural hypotension Adrenal crisis (life-threatening): hypovolemic shock, coma	Electrolyte disturbances. Low basal morning serum cortisol (<3 mcg/dL [80nmol/L]), suboptimal response to short ACTH (cosyntropin) stimulation test, low ACTH, hyponatremia, hypoglycemia [hold opioids for at least 8 hours before testing, as opioids can suppress pituitary–adrenal axis] Abdominal CT or MRI: rarely required.
Diabetes insipidus	Polyuria, polydipsia		Serum and urine osmolarity after 8–12 hours without fluid intake: fluid deprivation test.

25[OH]D, serum 25-hydroxyvitamin D; *1,25D*, 1,25-dihydroxyvitamin D; *ACTH*, adrenocorticotropic hormone; *FSH*, follicle-stimulating hormone; *LH*, luteinizing hormone; *PTH*, parathyroid hormone; T_3, total triiodothyronine; T_4, total thyroxine; *TPO*, antithyroid peroxidase; *TSH*, thyroid stimulating hormone

8. Monitor closely with frequent assessment in the elderly, as symptoms may be more profound.

B. Hyperthyroidism management (Lee, 2017; Ross, 2016)

1. Secondary to immune checkpoint inhibitors

   a. Patients at low risk for cardiovascular events: symptomatic treatment with beta blockers

   b. Patients at high risk for cardiovascular events (i.e., history of coronary artery disease, cardiac arrhythmia, heart failure): methylprednisolone 1 to 2 mg/kg daily until severity of toxicity is resolved to baseline.

   c. Monitor TSH and free T_4 every 2 to 3 weeks, as most cases progress to hypothyroidism

   d. Monitor TSH and T_4 laboratory results, report any abnormalities

   e. Promote adequate hydration

   f. Manage fatigue (Chapter 36)

2. Secondary to other causes

   a. Antithyroid agents: methimazole, propylthiouracil (PTU)

   b. Radioactive iodine

   c. Surgery

C. Hypothyroidism management (Barroso-Sousa, 2018; Jonklaas, 2014; Lee, 2017).

1. Patients will require lifetime repletion.

   a. Mild hypothyroidism (TSH <10 U/L): if asymptomatic, observation only

   b. Levothyroxine: start 0.8 to 1.6 mcg/kg/day, take with water, empty stomach.

   c. Older patients and those with coronary artery disease should start on lower dose (25–50 mcg/day).

   d. Monitor TSH and T_4 levels. It takes 4 to 6 weeks to reach steady-state concentration before dose adjustments are made. Adjust dosing to patient symptoms and T_4 level; TSH cannot be used to monitor, as it is suppressed in patients taking levothyroxine supplements.

   e. Monitor TSH and T_4 levels every 4 to 6 weeks until stable, then every 6 months.

   f. Monitor for potential drug interactions that may interfere with absorption or metabolism of levothyroxine. (e.g., estrogen, selective estrogen receptor modulators [SERMs], carbamazepine, ciprofloxacin, fluorouracil, furosemide, metformin, methadone, phenytoin, phenobarbital, ferrous sulfate, sucralfate, aluminum hydroxide gel, calcium carbonate, sertraline, raloxifene, lansoprazole, omeprazole).

   g. Patients treated with brain, head, and neck irradiation should have TSH and free T_4 measured yearly

   h. Promote rest, hydration.

   i. Manage gastrointestinal motility (constipation).

D. Hyperparathyroidism management (Bilezikian, 2014)

1. Assess kidney function for estimated glomerular filtration rate (eGFR), as at risk for developing kidney stones.

2. Avoid factors that aggravate hypercalcemia (diuretics, dehydration, high-calcium diet).

3. Parathyroidectomy may be necessary.

4. Cinacalcet 30 mg BID if not candidate for surgery.

5. Encourage adequate hydration to minimize risk of nephrolithiasis.

6. Provide comfort measures to alleviate bone pain.

7. Provide written and verbal information on low-calcium/high-phosphate diet).

8. Promote rest resulting from muscle weakness.

9. Monitor fluid balance (intake and output) and serum electrolytes (potassium, calcium, phosphates, and magnesium).

E. Hypoparathyroidism management: treatment depends on severity of condition. (Leidig-Bruckner, 2016)

1. Medication management

   a. Acute (corrected calcium ≤7.5 mg/dL, tetany, seizures, prolonged QT interval): will require emergency intervention with intravenous (IV) calcium gluconate

   b. Mild to moderate and chronic (corrected calcium ≥7.5 mg/dL): oral calcium 1 to 2 g calcium carbonate in divided doses and calcitriol 0.25 mcg twice daily (vitamin D), titrated weekly to low-normal calcium levels

   c. Monitor serum calcium, albumin, magnesium, and phosphate levels after surgery. Monitor urine, serum calcium, phosphate levels weekly after supplementation initiated.

2. Educate on diet (increase in calcium-rich foods; lower phosphate intake)

3. Monitor for side effects from oral calcium supplements

4. Educate patient about how to take phosphate binders

F. Hypophysitis management: focused on treating resultant secondary organ dysfunction.

1. Secondary adrenal insufficiency: glucocorticoid repletion

2. Secondary hypothyroidism: thyroid repletion after glucocorticoid deficiency is treated to avoid precipitating adrenal crisis

3. Severe hypophysitis; high-dose steroids (methylprednisolone 0.5–1.0 mg/kg/day or equivalent)

4. Secondary hypogonadism: testosterone

5. Type 1 diabetes insipidus: basal-bolus insulin; desmopressin acetate (subcutaneous, nasal, oral) dosed to achieve urine concentrations lasting 8 to 24 hours and prevent nocturia

6. Monitor serum sodium to prevent hyponatremia

7. Fluid management

8. Assess for altered mental status

9. Monitor for risk of decreased cardiac output

G. Adrenal insufficiency management

1. Short-acting glucocorticoid: hydrocortisone repletion 7 to 10 mg/m^2/day, divided doses (10 mg in morning and 5 mg in afternoon) (glucocorticoid and mineral corticoid activity).
2. Long-acting glucocorticoid: dexamethasone 0.5 mg/day or prednisone 5 mg/day.
3. Mineral corticoid (primary adrenal insufficiency): fludrocortisone 0.1 mg/day. Consider lower dose (0.05 mg/day) if patient is already on hydrocortisone.
4. Patients should be instructed in "minor sick-day" stress dosing of steroid repletion. May be required to increase glucocorticoids to two to three times the dosing.
5. Adrenal crisis: IV hydrocortisone 50 to 100 mg every 6 to 8 hours
6. during critical illness and emergencies; aggressive fluid replacement.
7. Patients should carry supplies for emergency stress dosing and should carry card or bracelet to alert emergency personnel.
8. Patients should alert health care providers of history, as stress doses of steroids may be necessary for critical illness and surgical procedures.
9. Assess for altered nutritional status.
10. Monitor for risk of decreased cardiac output.

V. Expected Patient Outcomes

A. Patient will continue treatments with proper management of endocrinopathies.
B. Patient and caregivers will verbalize understanding of symptoms to report to health care provider that may be associated with endocrinopathies.

REFERENCES

Alba, J. R., Basterra, J., Ferrer, J. C., Santonja, F., & Zapater, E. (2016). Hypothyroidism in patients treated with radiotherapy for head and neck carcinoma: standardised long-term follow-up study. *Journal of Laryngology & Otology*, 130(5), 478–481. https://doi.org/10.1017/S0022215116000967.

Albano, D., Bertagna, F., Panarotto, M. B., & Giubbini, R. (2017). Early and late adverse effects of radioiodine for pediatric differentiated thyroid cancer. *Pediatric Blood and Cancer*, 64(11) https://doi.org/10.1002/pbc.26595.

Appelman-Dijkstra, N. M., Malgo, F., Neelis, K. J., Coremans, I., Biermasz, N. R., & Pereira, A. M. (2014). Pituitary dysfunction in adult patients after cranial irradiation for head and nasopharyngeal tumours. *Radiotherapy Oncology*, 113(1), 102–107. https://doi.org/10.1016/j.radonc.2014.08.018.

Barroso-Sousa, R., Ott, P. A., Hodi, F. S., Kaiser, U. B., Tolaney, S. M., & Min, L. (2018). Endocrine dysfunction induced by immune checkpoint inhibitors: practical recommendations for diagnosis and clinical management. *Cancer*, 124(6), 1111–1121. https://doi.org/10.1002/cncr.31200.

Bilezikian, J. P., Brandi, M. L., Eastell, R., Silverberg, S. J., Udelsman, R., Marcocci, C., & Potts, J. T. Jr. (2014). Guidelines for the management of asymptomatic primary hyperparathyroidism: summary statement from the Fourth International Workshop. *Journal of Clinical Endocrinology & Metabolism*, 99(10), 3561–3569. https://doi.org/10.1210/jc.2014-1413.

Brahmer, J. R., Lacchetti, C., Schneider, B. J., Atkins, M. B., Brassil, K. J., Caterino, J. M., ... National Comprehensive Cancer, N (2018). Management of immune-related adverse events in patients treated with immune checkpoint inhibitor therapy: American Society of Clinical Oncology clinical practice guideline. *Journal of Clinical Oncology*, 36(17), 1714–1768. https://doi.org/10.1200/JCO.2017.77.6385.

Chemaitilly, W., & Hudson, M. M. (2014). Update on endocrine and metabolic therapy-related late effects observed in survivors of childhood neoplasia. *Current Opinion in Endocrinology, Diabetes and Obesity*, 21(1), 71–76. https://doi.org/10.1097/MED.0000000000000029.

Christakis, I., Silva, A. M., Williams, M. D., Garden, A., Grubbs, E. G., Busaidy, N. L., & Zafereo, M. (2017). Postoperative local-regional radiation therapy in the treatment of parathyroid carcinoma: the MD Anderson experience of 35 years. *Practical Radiation Oncology*, 7(6), e463–e470. https://doi.org/10.1016/j.prro.2017.05.009.

Cukier, P., Santini, F. C., Scaranti, M., & Hoff, A. O. (2017). Endocrine side effects of cancer immunotherapy. *Endocr Relat Cancer*, 24(12), T331–T347. https://doi.org/10.1530/ERC-17-0358.

Davies, M., & Duffield, E. A. (2017). Safety of checkpoint inhibitors for cancer treatment: strategies for patient monitoring and management of immune-mediated adverse events. *Immuno Targets and Therapy*, 6, 51–71. https://doi.org/10.2147/ITT.S141577.

Eastell, R., Brandi, M. L., Costa, A. G., D'Amour, P., Shoback, D. M., & Thakker, R. V. (2014). Diagnosis of asymptomatic primary hyperparathyroidism: proceedings of the Fourth International Workshop. *Journal of Clinical Endocrinology & Metabolism*, 99(10), 3570–3579. https://doi.org/10.1210/jc.2014-1414.

Faje, A. (2016). Immunotherapy and hypophysitis: clinical presentation, treatment, and biologic insights. *Pituitary*, 19(1), 82–92. https://doi.org/10.1007/s11102-015-0671-4.

Fard-Esfahani, A., Emami-Ardekani, A., Fallahi, B., Fard-Esfahani, P., Beiki, D., Hassanzadeh-Ra, A., & Eftekhari, M. (2014). Adverse effects of radioactive iodine-131 treatment for differentiated thyroid carcinoma. *Nuclear Medicine Communications*, 35(8), 808–817. https://doi.org/10.1097/MNM.0000000000000132.

Jonklaas, J., Bianco, A. C., Bauer, A. J., Burman, K. D., Cappola, A. R., Celi, F. S., ... American Thyroid Association Task Force on Thyroid Hormone, R (2014). Guidelines for the treatment of hypothyroidism: prepared by the American Thyroid Association task force on thyroid hormone replacement. *Thyroid*, 24(12), 1670–1751. https://doi.org/10.1089/thy.2014.0028.

Konda, B., Nabhan, F., & Shah, M. H. (2017). Endocrine dysfunction following immune checkpoint inhibitor therapy. *Current Opinion in Endocrinology, Diabetes and Obesity*, 24(5), 337–347. https://doi.org/10.1097/MED.0000000000000357.

Lee, H., Hodi, F. S., Giobbie-Hurder, A., Ott, P. A., Buchbinder, E. I., Haq, R., & Min, L. (2017). Characterization of thyroid disorders in patients receiving immune checkpoint inhibition therapy. *Cancer Immunology Research*, 5(12), 1133–1140. https://doi.org/10.1158/2326-6066.CIR-17-0208.

Leidig-Bruckner, G., Bruckner, T., Raue, F., & Frank-Raue, K. (2016). Long-term follow-up and treatment of postoperative permanent hypoparathyroidism in patients with medullary thyroid carcinoma: differences in complete and partial disease. *Hormone and Metabolic Research, 48*(12), 806–813. https://doi.org/10.1055/s-0042-118181.

Morganstein, D. L., Lai, Z., Spain, L., Diem, S., Levine, D., Mace, C., & Larkin, J. (2017). Thyroid abnormalities following the use of cytotoxic T-lymphocyte antigen-4 and programmed death receptor protein-1 inhibitors in the treatment of melanoma. *Clinical Endocrinology (Oxf), 86*(4), 614–620. https://doi.org/10.1111/cen.13297.

Mostoufi-Moab, S., Seidel, K., Leisenring, W. M., Armstrong, G. T., Oeffinger, K. C., Stovall, M., & Sklar, C. A. (2016). Endocrine abnormalities in aging survivors of childhood cancer: a report from the childhood cancer survivor study. *J Clin Oncol, 34*(27), 3240–3247. https://doi.org/10.1200/JCO.2016.66.6545.

National Comprehensive Cancer Network (NCCN) (2018). *NCCN clinical practice guidelines in oncology: REMS.* https://www.nccn.org/rems/

Ospina, N. S., Al Nofal, A., Bancos, I., Javed, A., Benkhadra, K., Kapoor, E., & Murad, M. H. (2016). ACTH stimulation tests for the diagnosis of adrenal insufficiency: systematic review and meta-analysis. *Journal of Clinical Endocrinology & Metabolism, 101*(2), 427–434. https://doi.org/10.1210/jc.2015-1700.

Park, S., Jeon, M. J., Song, E., Oh, H. S., Kim, M., Kwon, H., & Kim, W. G. (2017). Clinical features of early and late postoperative hypothyroidism after lobectomy. *Journal of Clinical Endocrinology & Metabolism, 102*(4), 1317–1324. https://doi.org/10.1210/jc.2016-3597.

Piper, H. G., Bugis, S. P., Wilkins, G. E., Walker, B. A., Wiseman, S., & Baliski, C. R. (2005). Detecting and defining hypothyroidism after hemithyroidectomy. *American Journal of Surgery, 189*(5), 587–591. discussion 591 https://doi.org/10.1016/j.amjsurg.2005.01.038.

Puzanov, I., Diab, A., Abdallah, K., Bingham, C. O., 3rd, Brogdon, C., Dadu, R., … Society for Immunotherapy of Cancer Toxicity Management Working, G (2017). Managing toxicities associated with immune checkpoint inhibitors: consensus recommendations from the Society for Immunotherapy of Cancer (SITC) Toxicity Management Working Group. *Journal of Immunotherapy of cancer, 5*(1), 95. https://doi.org/10.1186/s40425-017-0300-z.

Ross, D. S., Burch, H. B., Cooper, D. S., Greenlee, M. C., Laurberg, P., Maia, A. L., & Walter, M. A. (2016). 2016 American thyroid association guidelines for diagnosis and management of hyperthyroidism and other causes of thyrotoxicosis. *Thyroid, 26* (10), 1343–1421. https://doi.org/10.1089/thy.2016.0229.

Surks, M. I., Ortiz, E., Daniels, G. H., Sawin, C. T., Col, N. F., Cobin, R. H., & Weissman, N. J. (2004). Subclinical thyroid disease: scientific review and guidelines for diagnosis and management. *Journal American Medical Association, 291*(2), 228–238.

Sznol, M., Postow, M. A., Davies, M. J., Pavlick, A. C., Plimack, E. R., Shaheen, M., & Robert, C. (2017). Endocrine-related adverse events associated with immune checkpoint blockade and expert insights on their management. *Cancer Treatment Reviews, 58*, 70–76. https://doi.org/10.1016/j.ctrv.2017.06.002.

Torino, F., Barnabei, A., Paragliola, R., Baldelli, R., Appetecchia, M., & Corsello, S. M. (2013). Thyroid dysfunction as an unintended side effect of anticancer drugs. *Thyroid, 23*(11), 1345–1366. https://doi.org/10.1089/thy.2013.0241.

36

Fatigue

Jeannine M. Brant

OVERVIEW

I. Definition—cancer-related fatigue is defined as an unusual, persistent, and subjective sense of tiredness; not proportional to activity; interferes with usual functioning (National Cancer Comprehensive Network, 2018)

II. Physiology (Berger, Mooney, et al., 2015; Tariman & Dhorajiwala, 2016)
   A. The physiology of cancer-related fatigue is not well understood.
   B. Common underlying mechanisms
      1. Elevated proinflammatory cytokines, interleukins, tumor necrosis factor
      2. 5-Hydroxytryptophan dysregulation
      3. Hypothalamic–pituitary–adrenal axis dysfunction
      4. Circadian rhythm disturbances
      5. Increased vagal tone
   C. Fatigue is often seen with other symptoms related to cancer and its treatment—pain, distress, and sleep disturbances have been found to cluster with fatigue (Miaskowski et al., 2017)

III. Risk factors (Berger, Mooney, et al., 2015; Wang et al., 2014)
   A. Disease-related factors
      1. Fatigue precedes and accompanies most malignancies and is dependent on the stage and duration of illness
      2. 70% to 80% of patients with cancer report fatigue at some point
      3. 29% of survivors in complete remission continue to experience fatigue, which may persist long-term
      4. Comorbidities and underlying diseases may increase fatigue
      5. Disease-related anemia with a decrease in hemoglobin and hematocrit levels causes fatigue
   B. Treatment-related factors (Berger, Mitchell, Jacobsen, & Pirl, 2015)
      1. Occurs in 80% of patients undergoing chemotherapy or radiation therapy. Highest risks include:
         a. Receiving opioids during treatment
         b. Poor performance status
         c. Weight loss >5% in 6 months
         d. Concurrent chemoradiation

      2. Targeted or immunotherapy, hormone therapy, surgery
      3. Treatment-related toxicities: anemia, hypothyroidism, endocrinopathies
      4. Medications—opioids, hypnotics, anxiolytics, antihistamines, antiemetics
         a. Drugs crossing the blood–brain barrier may cause neurotoxic effects, leading to fatigue.
         b. Nausea, vomiting, diarrhea, and anemia, and end products from tumor death are thought to contribute to fatigue.
         c. Some cancer treatment may cause hypothyroidism, potentiating fatigue even more in these individuals.
         d. Treatments aimed at suppressing hormone-dependent cancers may cause fatigue, as seen in breast and prostate cancers.
         e. Immobilization, anxiety, pain control, anesthesia, and infection.
         f. Preoperative fatigue may affect postoperative fatigue.

ASSESSMENT

I. National Comprehensive Cancer Network (NCCN) guidelines screening for fatigue
   A. Screen for the presence of fatigue at initial visit and at appropriate intervals during and after treatment
      1. Patient self-report—the gold standard, 0 to 10 scale, with 0 being "no tiredness" and 10 being "worst possible tiredness"
      2. Family and caregiver insight of the effect that fatigue has on the patient
   B. Comprehensive assessment for patients with moderate to severe fatigue (Cope, 2014)
      1. Focused history and physical examination
      2. Other contributing factors that may play into the fatigue (e.g., pain, nutritional issues, sleep disturbances, medications)
      3. Disease status, length and types of treatments, current comorbidities, or other health issues that may contribute to or potentiate fatigue

4. Assessment of the degree of fatigue by evaluating onset, patterns, alleviating factors, duration, and the impact it has on overall functioning
5. Impact of fatigue on quality of life (QOL) and function—patients may report fatigue to be more of a distressing symptom than other symptoms
6. Signs of anemia, such as low hemoglobin level
7. Electrolyte disturbances
8. Low levels of iron, vitamin B_{12}, folate, ferritin
9. Hypothyroidism and low hormone levels, endocrine dysfunction
10. Low vitamin D levels

MANAGEMENT (TABLE 36.1)

I. Medical management (Mitchell et al., 2014)
   A. Treat the malignancy or the underlying cause
   B. Pharmacologic interventions are inferior to nonpharmacologic modalities (Mustian et al., 2017).
   C. Erythropoiesis-stimulating agents (ESAs)
      1. May improve fatigue if anemia is severe
      2. Benefits should be balanced with risks: elevated risk of thromboembolic complications, decreased survival
   D. Blood transfusion for severe anemia
   E. Low-dose dexamethasone 4 mg twice daily for 2 weeks
      1. Some benefits, but larger trials are lacking
      2. Risks should be carefully weighed with benefits
      3. May be more appropriate in patients at the end of life
   F. Psychostimulants (Qu et al., 2016)
      1. Methylphenidate may be beneficial
      2. Modafinil lacks evidence
   G. Antidepressants—effectiveness not established, further trials are needed

TABLE 36.1 Interventions Recommended for Cancer-Related Fatigue in Adults*

Address treatable contributors to fatigue
Manage concurrent symptoms
Physical activity/exercise
Rehabilitation
Psychoeducation
Meditation, mindfulness-based stress reduction, and cognitive behavioral stress management
Relaxation
Cognitive behavioral therapy for fatigue, depression, and pain
Cognitive behavioral therapy for sleep
Yoga

*Interventions identified as likely to be beneficial by the National Comprehensive Cancer Network (NCCN), The Oncology Nursing Society (ONS), Canadian Partnership Against Cancer and Canadian Association of Psychosocial Oncology (CPAC/CAPO), and American Society of Clinical Oncology (ASCO).
From Berger, A. M., Mitchell, S. A., Jacobsen, P. B., & Pirl, W. F. (2015). Screening, evaluation, and management of cancer-related fatigue: Ready for implementation to practice? *CA Cancer J Clin, 65*(3), 190-211. https://doi.org/10.3322/caac.21268.

1. Paroxetine—some evidence in fatigue in women with hot flashes and in patients receiving interferon
2. Venlafaxine—may improve fatigue in women who have hot flashes
   H. Evidence is lacking for the management of fatigue with nutritional supplements and herbal remedies; ginseng has limited evidence
II. Nursing management (Mitchell et al., 2014)
   A. Recommend exercise and physical activity
      1. Strongest evidence in the management of cancer-related fatigue
      2. Encourage exercise tailored according to patient's ability
      3. Type of exercise does not appear to influence fatigue outcomes (Tomlinson, Diorio, Beyene, & Sung, 2014)
   B. Offer psychoeducational interventions—likely to be effective (see Table 36.1)
      1. Energy conservation and activity management may be beneficial
      2. Management of concurrent symptoms
   C. Provide education to patient and family (Du et al., 2015)
      1. Discuss the potential for fatigue at the time of diagnosis and at treatment initiation
      2. Provide information to the patient and family about therapies known to cause fatigue
      3. Provide information about interventions used to treat fatigue, focusing on nonpharmacologic modalities
      4. Educate the patient and family about the management of fatigue based on strategies that are recommended for practice or likely to be effective
         a. Restoration of attention—reducing environmental demands (information, stimuli, distractions) to conserve attention for priority needs
         b. Sleep and rest—having the patient maintain adequate sleep and rest
   D. Facilitate patient and family coping
      1. Encourage the patient and family to discuss fatigue and its impact on activities of daily living (ADLs)
      2. Consult with psychosocial services when fatigue may be related to psychological and social factors such as depression, stress, or difficulty coping with the disease
      3. Acknowledge the potential for fatigue to interfere with sexuality

EXPECTED PATIENT OUTCOMES

I. The patient and caregiver will report fatigue to the health care team and discuss its impact on function and overall health.
II. The patient and caregiver will identify nonpharmacologic strategies to manage fatigue.

REFERENCES

Berger, A. M., Mitchell, S. A., Jacobsen, P. B., & Pirl, W. F. (2015). Screening, evaluation, and management of cancer-related fatigue: ready for implementation to practice? *CA Cancer J Clin*, 65(3), 190–211. https://doi.org/10.3322/caac.21268.

Berger, A. M., Mooney, K., Alvarez-Perez, A., Breitbart, W. S., Carpenter, K. M., Cella, D., & Smith, C. (2015). Cancer-related fatigue, Version 2.2015. *J Natl Compr Canc Netw*, 13(8), 1012–1039.

Cope, D. G. (2014). Fatigue. In D. Camp-Sorrel, & R. A. Hawkins (Eds.), *Clinical manual for the oncology advanced practice nurse* (3rd ed., pp. 1407–1414). Pittsburgh, PA: ONS Press.

Du, S., Hu, L., Dong, J., Xu, G., Jin, S., Zhang, H., & Yin, H. (2015). Patient education programs for cancer-related fatigue: a systematic review. *Patient Educ Couns*, 98(11), 1308–1319. https://doi.org/10.1016/j.pec.2015.05.003.

Miaskowski, C., Barsevick, A., Berger, A., Casagrande, R., Grady, P. A., Jacobsen, P., & Marden, S. (2017). Advancing symptom science through symptom cluster research: expert panel proceedings and recommendations. *J Natl Cancer Inst*, 109(4). https://doi.org/10.1093/jnci/djw253.

Mitchell, S. A., Hoffman, A. J., Clark, J. C., DeGennaro, R. M., Poirier, P., Robinson, C. B., & Weisbrod, B. L. (2014). Putting evidence into practice: an update of evidence-based interventions for cancer-related fatigue during and following treatment. *Clin J Oncol Nurs*, 18, 38–58. https://doi.org/10.1188/14.cjon.s3.38-58 Suppl.

Mustian, K. M., Alfano, C. M., Heckler, C., Kleckner, A. S., Kleckner, I. R., Leach, C. R., & Miller, S. M. (2017). Comparison of pharmaceutical, psychological, and exercise treatments for cancer-related fatigue: a meta-analysis. *JAMA Oncol*, 3(7), 961–968. https://doi.org/10.1001/jamaoncol.2016.6914.

National Cancer Comprehensive Network. (2019). *Cancer-related fatigue, v.1.2019*. Retrieved from (2019). https://www.nccn.org/professionals/physician_gls/pdf/fatigue.pdf.

Qu, D., Zhang, Z., Yu, X., Zhao, J., Qiu, F., & Huang, J. (2016). Psychotropic drugs for the management of cancer-related fatigue: a systematic review and meta-analysis. *Eur J Cancer Care (Engl)*, 25(6), 970–979. https://doi.org/10.1111/ecc.12397.

Tariman, J. D., & Dhorajiwala, S. (2016). Genomic variants associated with cancer-related fatigue: a systematic review. *Clin J Oncol Nurs*, 20(5), 537–546. https://doi.org/10.1188/16.cjon.537-546.

Tomlinson, D., Diorio, C., Beyene, J., & Sung, L. (2014). Effect of exercise on cancer-related fatigue: a meta-analysis. *Am J Phys Med Rehabil*, 93(8), 675–686. https://doi.org/10.1097/phm.0000000000000083.

Wang, X. S., Zhao, F., Fisch, M. J., O'Mara, A. M., Cella, D., Mendoza, T. R., & Cleeland, C. S. (2014). Prevalence and characteristics of moderate to severe fatigue: a multicenter study in cancer patients and survivors. *Cancer*, 120(3), 425–432. https://doi.org/10.1002/cncr.28434.

37

Gastrointestinal Symptoms

Rita Wickham

XEROSTOMIA

Overview (AAOM Clinical Practice Statement [AAOM], 2016; Buglione et al, 2016; Dyasanoor & Saddu, 2014; Epstein & Jensen, 2015; Michaelsen, Gronhoj, Michaelsen, Friborg, & von Buchwald, 2017; Millsop, Wang, & Fazel, 2017; Vigarios, Epstein, & Sibaud, 2017; Villa & Akintoye, 2018)

I. Definition: subjective sensation of mouth dryness, secondary to abnormal salivary gland function (true xerostomia), or without objective signs of hyposalivation.

II. Salivary glands (parotid, submaxillary, sublingual and other) secrete clear and watery saliva with two major components: ptyalin (digestive enzyme) and mucin (protective, lubricating). Saliva is antimicrobial, has mechanical cleansing action, controls pH, removes food debris, lubricates oral cavity, maintains oral mucosa, and remineralizes teeth.

III. Causes and risk factors for true xerostomia are summarized in Table 37.1.

  A. Radiotherapy (RT) ± chemotherapy (CT) for head and neck cancer (HNC) that includes salivary glands.

    1. 50% to 60% develop salivary gland hypofunction, sticky saliva, and dry mouth

    2. Reduced saliva flow alters physiologic, biochemical, and antimicrobial functions

    3. Negatively affects chewing, swallowing, smell, taste, and other oral functions

    4. May be accompanied by burning or painful mouth, halitosis, glossitis (smooth, erythematous tongue), cracked lips, dysphagia

    5. Consequences—oral infections (bacterial, viral, yeast), dental caries, worsened nutritional state, and decreased overall health status and quality of life (QOL)

  B. Transient or prolonged xerostomia related to cumulative RT dose and volume of salivary gland tissue in treatment field

  C. Other medications and concomitant diseases

  D. Lifestyle influences—alterable risk factors

    1. Alcohol, caffeine

    2. Cigarette smoking, nicotine

    3. Drugs that decrease salivary flow

Assessment (Carvalho, Medeiros-Filho, & Ferreira, 2018; Epstein & Jensen, 2015; McLaughlin & Mahon, 2014; Millsop et al, 2017)

I. Focused history—ask patient about:

  A. Dry mouth—severity, onset, aggravating and alleviating factors

  B. Difficulty chewing or eating (especially crunchy or hard, spicy, or acidic foods)

  C. Difficulty swallowing (observe swallowing)

  D. Altered taste

  E. Change in/difficulty in wearing dentures

  F. Difficulty speaking (note voice quality)

  G. Other medical conditions associated with xerostomia

  H. Social history (cigarettes, alcohol, caffeine-containing beverages)

  I. Thoroughly review prescription (Rx) and over-the-counter (OTC) medications/products

II. Physical examination—use penlight to thoroughly examine mouth for signs of xerostomia

  A. Lips and corner of mouth—dryness, cracking, swelling, or ulceration

  B. Tongue—any lines or fissures, loss of papillae

  C. Mucous membranes/gingiva—are they dry, shiny, smooth

  D. Saliva, consistency/quality—foamy, thick, ropy, scant saliva; little/none mouth floor

  E. Teeth—plaque, detritus, two or more cavities

  F. Mucosal debris on palate

  G. Dental mirror or tongue blade may stick to tongue or buccal mucosa

III. Psychosocial assessment

  A. Ask about changes in social aspects and enjoyment of eating because of dry mouth

  B. Ask about altered taste for sweet, sour, and bitter that decrease pleasure of eating; thick saliva is highly concentrated in sodium that adversely affects tastes

  C. Ask about noticeable changes in speaking and discomfort from oral burning or pain

IV. Imaging and laboratory tests

  A. Sialometry (measure of saliva flow, evaluated after overnight or after 2-hour fast): with patient sitting upright, normal salivary flow rate stimulated—1.5 to 2.0 mL/min, unstimulated—0.3 to 0.4 mL/min; less than 0.12 to 0.16 mL/min abnormal

  B. Other, if indicated by concomitant disease

TABLE 37.1 Some Causes of Xerostomia

Drug-Related	Disease-Related	Other
Agents with anticholinergic properties • Antihypertensives/antiarrhythmics (e.g., lisinopril, metoprolol, atenolol) • Antidepressants (desipramine, fluoxetine, venlafaxine) • Antipsychotics (e.g., haloperidol, olanzapine) • Antiallergy/antipuritics (e.g., azelastine, desloratadine) • Anticonvulsants (e.g., pregabalin, sodium valproate) • Antihistamines • Antiparkinsons • Antivirals (maraviroc, didanosine, saquinavir) Anticholinergic/antimuscarinic agents • Hyoscyamine, scopolamine, atropine • Darifenacin (urinary incontinence) Other • Diuretics • Opioids • Nicotine • Sedatives • Antineoplastic agents (everolimus, temsirolimus, bevacizumab, sorafenib, immune checkpoint inhibitors, fluorouracil [5-FU]- and taxane-based regimens	Diabetes mellitus Autoimmune causes: • Autoimmune thyroid disease • Sjögren syndrome (primary or secondary) • Rheumatoid arthritis • Systemic lupus erythematosus • Scleroderma • Primary biliary cirrhosis Viral infectious causes: • Hepatitis C • Human immunodeficiency virus (HIV) • Cytomegalovirus • Epstein–Barr virus Granulomatosis causes: • Amyloidosis • Sarcoidosis • Wegener granulomatosis	Radiotherapy to the head and neck Stem cell transplantation Chronic graft-versus-host disease (GVHD) Anxiety or depression Aging Lifestyle factors: • Tobacco use • Alcohol use • Caffeinated beverage consumption • Dehydration • Heavy snoring • Mouth breathing • Upper respiratory tract infections

Management (AAOM, 2016; Carvalho et al, 2018; Mercadante, Al Hamad, Lodi, Porter, & Fedele, 2017; Millsop et al, 2017; Riley, Glenny, Hua, & Worthington, 2017; Villa & Akintoye, 2018)

I. Medical management
  A. Oral sialogogues—systemic agents to increase saliva secretion (weak evidence).
    1. Evidence mixed for benefits of HNC survivors and use of pilocarpine (Salagen) and cevimeline (Evoxac)
    2. Pilocarpine—contraindicated in chronic cardiovascular or pulmonary disease, uncontrolled asthma, narrow-angle glaucoma, or taking beta blockers
    3. Cevimeline has fewer side effects but is more expensive
    4. Use for 1 to 2 weeks before evaluating efficacy
  B. Topical products temporarily decrease mouth dryness (Millsop et al., 2017)
    1. Mucin-based saliva substitutes (e.g., Aquoral, Biotene Mouthwash, Moi-Stir, NeutraSal, SalivaMAX, Salivart, and Xero-Lube) resemble natural saliva, increase salivary viscosity, well tolerated.

II. Nursing management
  A. Teach patients strategies that may decrease oral dryness and associated symptoms
    1. Take frequent sips of water (also helps maintain hydration)
    2. Suck ice cubes or sugarless Popsicles to help keep the mouth cool and moist
    3. Moisten foods with liquids, milk, or gravy
    4. Avoid crunchy, spicy, acidic, or hard foods
    5. Bland mouth rinses (1 teaspoon salt, 1 teaspoon baking soda, 1 L of water); lessen oral dryness and neutralize pH
    6. Remind patient about good oral hygiene—toothpastes, mouthwashes, and gels (may be salivary stimulants); regular dental visits with frequent cleaning and topical fluoride application to prevent dental caries
    7. Advise patient to seek prompt medical treatment if infection develops
  B. Lifestyle modifications
    1. Limit alcohol intake; after consuming alcohol, drink glass of water or brush teeth
    2. Eliminate or limit caffeine-containing beverages
    3. Encourage/support smokers to join smoking cessation program

DYSPHAGIA (ORAL)

Overview (Alterio et al, 2017; Arrese, Carrau, & Plowman, 2017; Carucci & Turner, 2015; Cederholm et al, 2015; Denaro, Merlano, & Russi, 2013; Gallegos, Brito-de la Fuente, Clav, Costa, & Assegehegn, 2017; King, Dunlap, Tennant, & Pitts, 2016; Sasegbon & Hamdy, 2017; http://patients.gi.org/topics/dysphagia/)

I. Definition—impaired or impossible swallowing of ingested food, medications, liquids, or saliva
   A. Swallowing is a highly coordinated, rapid process; food is masticated and combined with saliva, moved from mouth to pharynx, to esophagus, and finally the stomach.
   B. Oropharyngeal dysphagia (OD) occurs at start of swallowing and is a symptom of a problem in the mouth or in the pharynx.
      1. OD usually causes reflexive coughing and a sense of choking with swallowing
      2. Other possible symptoms are voice change, frequent throat clearing, and earache
   C. Esophageal dysphagia (ED) caused by esophageal disease is relatively uncommon. Patient feels like food is sticking in their neck or upper chest a few seconds after they start to swallow.
II. Depending on the underlying cause, dysphagia may progress slowly or rapidly and advance from difficulty in swallowing solids, to swallowing liquids, and finally saliva.
III. Major complications: aspiration, pneumonia, weight loss and protein-calorie malnutrition (PCM), dehydration, airway obstruction that increases morbidity and mortality ⚠
IV. Oropharyngeal dysphagia—causes and risk factors
   A. Stroke (most frequent cause of OD)
   B. Degenerative neurologic disease (e.g. Parkinson disease, multiple sclerosis, Alzheimer disease or other dementia) trauma, central nervous system (CNS) tumor, reduced level of consciousness
   C. Infections that cause oropharyngeal inflammation and ulceration
   D. Congenital skeletal abnormalities or stenosis may cause mechanical dysphagia
   E. Iatrogenic—related to treatment (surgical, drugs, RT, etc.), other medications
   F. HNC the most common cancer-related cause of OD
      1. Mechanical dysphagia—onset may precede diagnosis of large (T3–T4) base of tongue, supraglottic, or pharyngeal tumors
      2. Mechanical dysphagia—may occur postsurgery from inflammation and edema
      3. OD develops in 30% to 50% of HNC patients treated with intensive RT (± CT or targeted agent); ≈33% improve, 50% do not, and 20% worsen over time

4. Early RT-related damage to base of tongue, pharynx, larynx, or epiglottis causes inflammation, edema, and painful acute OD (Fig. 37.1)
5. RT with concomitant CT/targeted therapy increases incidence and strongly predicts severe (grade 3) acute dysphagia
6. Late RT-induced OD causes nonspecific fibrosis and/or atrophy and can occur months to years later, even in patients without significant acute dysphagia
7. >50% of HNC patients with OD have silent aspiration; swallowed substances pass through vocal cords into trachea without inducing cough or other overt OD signs
8. <50% report symptoms unless a health care professional specifically asks about swallowing problems
9. High risk for RT-related OD: baseline weight loss, malnutrition, xerostomia, smoking, large local tumor, oropharyngeal or nasopharyngeal tumor, and anticholinergic medications

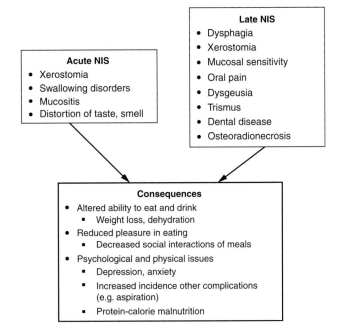

Fig. 37.1 Impact of radiotherapy ± chemotherapy-induced symptoms on nutrition of head and neck cancer patients. Head and neck cancer patients may experience xorostomia, dysphagia, and mucositis (and other manifestations) during chemotherapy or radiotherapy. This constellation of nutritional impact symptoms (NIS) often occurs during or immediately after treatment (acute NIS) and progresses to chronic NIS. Patients' ability and enjoyment of eating are compromised, and they seek out nutritional strategies. NIS is not merely bothersome but can affect QOL during treatment and have long-term effects on survivorship or palliation. (Adapted from Bressan V., et al. (2017). The life experience of nutrition impact symptoms during treatment for head and neck cancer patients: a systematic review and meta-synthesis. Supportive Care in Cancer, 25, 1699-1712. doi:10.1007/s00520-017-3618-7.)

V. Esophageal dysphagia (Kruger, 2014)
   A. Esophageal drug-related injury (e.g., oral bisphosphonates, nonsteroidal antiinflammatory drugs [NSAIDs], potassium chloride, theophylline, etc.)
   B. Gastroesophageal reflux disease (GERD), obesity, metabolic syndrome, esophageal obstruction, and mucosal injury
   C. Esophageal motility disorder or infection
   D. Intrinsic or extrinsic tumor—esophageal carcinoma or hilar lymphadenopathy secondary to lung cancer (both likely advanced disease; treated palliatively)

Assessment (Arrese et al, 2017; Belafsky et al, 2008; Brodsky et al, 2016; Bressan et al, 2017; Cheney, Siddiqui, Litts, Kuhn, & Belafsky, 2015; Espitalier et al, 2018; Gallegos et al, 2017; Holmes, 2016; Jansson-Knodell, Codipilly, & Leggett, 2017; Miles et al, 2013; NCI CTCAE, 2018; Verdonschot et al, 2017; Wirth et al, 2016; Zuniga, Ebersole, & Jamal, 2018)

I. Primary assessment goals
   A. Evaluate the patient's ability to swallow without respiratory complications
   B. Determine whether patient is ingesting sufficient calories and water
   C. Collaborative assessment—nurse, physician, speech-language pathologist (SLP), dietician, etc.

II. History—ask patient about:
   A. Cancer diagnosis and past/current treatment (RT, CT, targeted agents)
   B. Other disease states associated with dysphagia
   C. Recent history of recurrent pneumonia
   D. Ask patient if they do not want to eat or if they cannot eat to differentiate anorexia, chronic disease-related malnutrition from dysphagia, starvation-related malnutrition
   E. Swallowing quality
      1. What happens when you try to swallow? How often does this happen?
      2. Is it difficult for you to swallow solids, liquids, or both?
      3. Cough, choking, or drooling during or after eating
      4. How long it takes to eat a meal (compared with usual)
      5. Estimate severity of dysphagia:
         a. Eating Assessment Tool 10 (EAT-10)—reliable, valid, and easy to use, patient-reported screen to self-report dysphagia symptoms and aspiration risk and identify need for further evaluation (Fig. 37.2)
         b. National Cancer Institute Common Terminology Criteria for Adverse Events addresses several gastrointestinal (GI) symptoms, including dysphagia (Table 37.2)
   F. Patient report of pain or discomfort; weakness of lips, tongue, or jaw; "lump in throat"
   G. Impact of dysphagia on nutrition

To what extent are the following scenarios problematic for you?					
Circle the appropriate response	0 = No problem		4 = Severe problem		
1. My swallowing problem has caused me to lose weight.	0	1	2	3	4
2. My swallowing problem interferes with my ability to go out for meals.	0	1	2	3	4
3. Swallowing liquids takes extra effort.	0	1	2	3	4
4. Swallowing solids takes extra effort.	0	1	2	3	4
5. Swallowing pills takes extra effort.	0	1	2	3	4
6. Swallowing is painful.	0	1	2	3	4
7. The pleasure of eating is affected by my swallowing.	0	1	2	3	4
8. When I swallow food sticks in my throat.	0	1	2	3	4
9. I cough when I eat.	0	1	2	3	4
10. Swallowing is stressful.	0	1	2	3	4

Fig. 37.2 Eating Assessment Tool (EAT-10). (From Belafsky, P. C., Mouadeb, D. A., Rees, C. J., Pryor, J. C., Postma, G. N., ... & Leonard, R. J. (2008). Validity and reliability of the Eating Assessment Tool (EAT-10). *Annals of Otolaryngology, Rhinology, and Laryngology, 117,* 919-924.)

TABLE 37.2 Common Terminology Criteria for Adverse Events (CTCAE): GI Symptoms

	1	2	3	4	5
Dysphagia	Symptomatic; able to eat regular diet	Symptomatic; altered eating/swallowing	Severely altered eating/swallowing; tube feeding, TPN, or hospitalization indicated	Life-threatening consequences; urgent intervention indicated	Death
Mucositis – Oral	Asymptomatic or mild symptoms; intervention not indicated	Moderate pain or ulcers, do not interfere with PO intake; modified diet indicated	Severe pain; interferes with PO intake	Life-threatening consequences; urgent intervention indicated	Death
Nausea	Loss of appetite without alteration in eating habits	Oral intake decreased, no significant weight loss, dehydration, or malnutrition	Inadequate PO caloric or fluid intake; tube feeding, TPN, or hospitalization indicated	-	-
Vomiting	Intervention not indicated	Outpatient IV hydration; medical intervention indicated	Tube feeding, TPN, or hospitalization indicated	Life-threatening consequences	Death
Ascites	Asymptomatic; clinical or diagnostic observations only; intervention not indicated	Symptomatic; medical intervention indicated	Severe symptoms; invasive intervention indicated	Life-threatening consequences; urgent operative intervention indicated	Death
Constipation	Occasional or intermittent symptoms; occasional use of stool softener laxative, dietary modification, or enema	Persistent symptoms with regular use of laxatives or enemas indicated	Symptoms interfere with activities of daily living; obstipation with manual evacuation indicated	Life-threatening consequences (e.g., obstruction, toxic megacolon)	Death
Diarrhea	Increase <4 stools per day over baseline	Increase 4–6 stools per day over baseline	Increase >7 stools per day over baseline Incontinence Hospitalization	Life threatening consequences; urgent intervention indicated	Death

H. OD/ED increases risk for dehydration, secondary risk for aspiration pneumonia due to lessened oropharyngeal clearing and infection ⚠️

III. Physical examination

A. Observe patient for unilateral facial droop (stroke), drooling, choking or coughing with swallowing, and gurgling voice quality

B. Oral examination for associated xerostomia, mucositis, candida, or other infections

C. Observe patient's ability to chew, hold food in mouth, and use tongue to effectively propel food to the back of the mouth and the oropharynx

D. Auscultate lungs because of potential for aspiration

E. Weigh patient two to three times a week; follow fluid balance and nutritional status

F. SLP or trained nurse can do bedside screens for dysphagia

1. Two-step water swallow test.

a. One small (1–5 mL) sip—observe for coughing/choking ± voice changes (e.g., wet/gurgly voice quality): rules aspiration in (risk for false negative because of silent aspiration)

b. Consecutive large (90–100 mL) sips, no clinical signs: rules aspiration out

2. Cough reflex test useful to identify silent aspiration. Nebulized citric acid, which induces cough, administered by face mask. Coughing or choking signals aspiration (absence of such symptoms does not exclude silent aspiration).

IV. Psychosocial assessment—ask patient about

A. Changes in mood (e.g., feeling depressed, anxious, embarrassed, frustrated, or angry)

B. If they eat alone—social isolation is common because of chewing and swallowing difficulties, coughing while eating, taking much longer to finish a meal than others

C. If they have less or no enjoyment or disinterest in eating

V. Imaging and laboratory tests

A. "Gold standard" diagnostic tests for OD—either functional endoscopic evaluation of swallowing (FEES) or video fluoroscopy swallowing study (VFSS).

1. FEES—fiber-optic nasoendoscopic evaluation; easy to do, greater sensitivity

2. VFSS—dynamic examination; evaluates safety, efficacy, character of swallowing; better quantification of pharyngeal residue; helps assess therapeutic strategies

Management (Beck, Kjaersgaard, Hansen, & Poulsen, 2017; Dai et al, 2014; Gallegos et al, 2017; Krisciunas et al, 2017; Wirth et al, 2016)

I. Medical management: antifungal and antibiotic agents, analgesics, or other medications may be indicated for accompanying problems
   A. Enteral feedings by a nasogastric feeding tube (NGT) or a percutaneous endoscopic gastrostomy (PEG) are preferred over parenteral nutrition because of cost-effectiveness and lower infection rates. Interventions for ED related to esophageal cancer.
      1. Self-expanding metal stent (SEMS)
      2. RT alternative for some patients
II. Nursing management
   A. No evidence that "dysphagia rehabilitation," "swallowing therapy," or "active e-stim" effectively improves symptoms of dysphagia
   B. SLP and the dietician/nutritionist—central to formulating OD management plan
      1. Consistency of foods, fluids that can be safely swallowed must be determined before starting nutritional support.
      2. Modifying solids, semisolids may increase palatability and ability to be swallowed.
      3. Low-quality evidence for thickened liquids (e.g., Thick-It, Thick & Easy, nectar) to maintain adequate hydration and prevent aspiration
   C. If a patient has been unable to orally consume ≥60% of their estimated daily nutritional need for 1 week, an alternative feeding method should be started.
   D. Review patient medications and explore strategies to maintain adherence (e.g., alternative formulations that are easier to swallow, whether pills can be crushed and taken with applesauce, or if they cannot because of slow-release).

MUCOSITIS (ORAL)

Overview (Bonomi & Batt, 2015; Cinausero et al, 2017; De Sanctis et al, 2016; Kwon, 2016; Marcussen et al, 2017; Kwon, 2016; Maria, Eliopoulos, & Muanza, 2017; Peterson et al, 2016; Villa & Sonis, 2015)

I. Mucositis—CT- or RT-induced, painful inflammation and ulceration of the mucous membranes lining the GI tract.
II. Oral/oropharyngeal mucositis (OM) affects the keratinized mucosa of the dorsal tongue, gingiva, and/or hard palate; mucositis can also develop in the small intestine (GI mucositis) or the rectal mucosa (proctitis).

III. OM severity ranges from superficial erythema and soreness to full-thickness mucosal ulcerations with major pain; delayed, interrupted, or discontinued treatment; systemic infection; hospitalization; impaired oral nutrition; and economic burden.
IV. Mucositis is a systemic effect from CT or targeted therapy, and a local effect of RT.
   A. Incidence: 20% to 40% of patients receiving standard-dose CT, 60% to 100% of those undergoing hematopoietic stem cell transplantation (HSCT), and almost all patients receiving RT for HNC (>50% with grade 3 or 4).
   B. Involves epithelial mucosa, submucosal cells and tissues, and basal membrane.
V. Pathogenesis—time course differs, depending on mucosal location and therapy, and CT or RT
   A. Initiation—within seconds of injury to highly proliferative, normal cells (mucosa, submucosa, and basal stem) and supporting connective tissues, DNA damage and other cellular responses lead to tissue changes.
   B. A primary damage response; transcription factors upregulate an innate immune response and activate expression of genes and multiple pathways, production of cytokines and modulators associated with the progression of mucositis
   C. Mucositis becomes clinically apparent in the ulceration phase—loss of mucosal integrity, painful lesions, submucosal breach with bacterial colonization and secondary infection
   D. Healing occurs after chemotherapy or radiotherapy stopped; submucosa and mesenchyme signal the mucosa to reepithelialize. The mucosa appears normal, but residual angiogenesis means increased risk for future mucositis episodes.
VI. Targeted therapies can cause stomatitis: not well documented, different pathogenesis (Cinausero et al, 2017; Lo Muzio, Arena, Troiano, & Villa, 2018; Peterson, Boers-Doets, Bensadoun, & Herrstedt, 2015; Peterson et al, 2016).
   A. Stomatitis—oral tissue inflammatory condition unrelated to CT or RT; targeted therapy—associated oral sensitivity or pain (without lesions), xerostomia, taste change.
   B. Usually occurs in the first cycle. Superficial aphthous ulcers (herpes simplex–like)—single or multiple small (≤0.5 cm) superficial, discrete, well-demarcated ulcers with erythematous borders and covered with grayish-white pseudomembrane.
   C. Ulcers develop within 5 days on inner aspect of lips, the ventral and lateral tongue surfaces, and soft palate; usually resolve in 1 week.
   D. Reported with mTOR inhibitors (e.g., everolimus, temsirolimus, and ridaforolimus), some epidermal growth factor receptor (EGFR) inhibitors (e.g., bevacizumab and erlotinib), and tyrosine kinase inhibitor (TKIs) (e.g., sorafenib gefitinib, lapatinib, and sunitinib).

VII. Clinical manifestations of OM
- A. Cycled or conditioning CT regimens: mild erythema starts 3 to 4 days after CT; ulcers thereafter; peak intensity days 7 and 14; usually resolves in next week
- B. RT for HNC (fractionated: 2 grays [Gy]/day, total 10 Gy/week)
  1. Oral mucosal erythema and soreness start around the end of week 1.
  2. Cumulative dose 20 to 30 Gy: frank ulcers, pain worsens, and oral intake decreases.
  3. Continued RT (to total 60–70 Gy): increased cumulative damage; difficult-to-control pain.
  4. OM typically resolves 2 to 4 weeks after RT completion, may persist longer.
- C. Progressive ulcerative OM: more diffuse, ulcers may coalesce and be accompanied by:
  1. Thick secretions that induce coughing, aspiration ⚠, and disturb sleep
  2. Pain that necessitates opioid analgesics
  3. Impaired speaking, eating, drinking, and swallowing.
  4. High risk—gram-negative bacterial or yeast infections and septic complications

VIII. Causes and risk factors
- A. CT—drugs with highest risk for OM: cyclophosphamide, doxorubicin, vincristine, etoposide, ifosfamide, methotrexate, docetaxel, paclitaxel, cisplatin, carboplatin, oxaliplatin, irinotecan, 5-fluorouracil (5-FU), leucovorin, and vinorelbine
  1. CT has cumulative effect—risk rises with repeated cycles
  2. High-dose CT, as with conditioning regimens for allogeneic stem cell transplant
  3. Methotrexate to prevent acute graft-versus-host disease (GVHD) increases risk
- B. RT for HNC
- C. Combined CT-RT increases risk to greater degree
- D. Baseline nutritional status below average—body mass index (BMI) <18.5
- E. Unintentional pretherapy weight loss (>5% over 1 month or >10% last 6 months)
- F. Poor oral hygiene, periodontal disease
- G. Persistent smoking or alcohol use
- H. Xerostomia
- I. Impaired renal function (high serum creatinine) may increase risk

Assessment (Bonomi & Batt, 2015; De Sanctis et al, 2016; Gangadharan et al, 2017; Gussgard, Hope, Jokstad, Tenenbaum, & Wood, 2015; Kanagalingam et al, 2018; Kushner et al, 2008; NCI-CTCAE, 2018)

I. History—ask patient about:
- A. Current cancer therapy regimen, particularly CT or RT for HNC; previous OM
- B. Usual oral hygiene, dentures, dental visits
- C. Any changes in eating, swallowing, coughing, or choking
- D. Screen for PCM; >50% of HNC or GI cancer patients secondary to cancer or treatment. PCM severe if patient has ≥2:
  1. Weight loss: >2% in 1 week, 5% in 1 month, or 7.5% in 3 months
  2. Obvious noticeable muscle wasting
  3. Loss of subcutaneous fat
  4. Nutritional intake <50% of recommended for ≥2 weeks
  5. Significantly reduced functional capacity or bedridden
- E. Use OM grading scale on consistent basis to document progression/resolution
  1. National Cancer Institute Common Terminology Criteria for Adverse Events (NCI-CTCAE)
  2. Patient-Reported Oral Mucositis Symptom (PROMS) Scale (Fig. 37.3)
- F. Oral pain/discomfort: severity/intensity, adequacy of current analgesic
- G. Mouth dryness

II. Physical examination
- A. Recommended: regularly assess OM—at least once a week (instruct patient to report worsening OM symptoms between examinations).
- B. Use a penlight to examine mouth for redness, swelling, discrete or confluent ulceration, white patches; note saliva—thick and sticky. Remove dentures to assess.
- C. Auscultate lungs because of potential for aspiration.

III. Psychosocial assessment—ask patient:
- A. Does sore mouth interfere with eating, drinking, talking; make them feel depressed
- B. If they no longer enjoy the social interaction of eating with others
- C. If they eat alone because it takes much longer to finish a meal than others because of difficulty chewing, swallowing, coughing, or pain while eating

IV. Imaging and laboratory tests: none specific to OM

Management (Alfieri et al, 2016; Bonomi & Batt, 2015; Chaveli-Lopez & Bagan-Sebastian, 2016; Chen, Seabrook, Fulford, & Rajakumar, 2017; Kakoei et al, 2018; Kanagalingam et al, 2018; Lalla et al, 2014; Moslemi et al, 2016; Rapone et al, 2016; Soliman & Shehata, 2015; Zecha et al, 2016, ONS, 2017b)

I. Medical management
- A. Palifermin (keratinocyte growth factor)—Food and Drug Administration (FDA)–approved for patients with hematologic malignancy receiving high-dose CT/total body irradiation (TBI), followed by autologous HCST; 60 microgram/kg per day 3 days before and after conditioning regimen (very costly) to reduce incidence and severity of OM

Items	Anchors (100 cm visual analogue scale)	
Mouth pain	No pain	Worst possible pain
Difficulty speaking because of mouth sores	No trouble speaking	Impossible to speak
Restriction of speech because of mouth sores	No restriction of speech	Complete restriction of speech
Difficulty eating hard foods (hard bread, potato chips, etc.) because of mouth sores	No trouble eating hard foods	Impossible to eat hard foods
Difficulty eating soft foods (Jello, pudding, etc.) because of mouth sores	No trouble eating soft foods	Impossible to eat soft foods
Restriction of eating because of mouth sores	No restriction of eating	Complete restriction of eating
Difficulty drinking because of mouth sores	No trouble drinking	Impossible to drink
Restriction of drinking because of mouth sores	No restriction of drinking	Complete restriction of drinking
Difficulty swallowing because of mouth sores	Not difficult to swallow	Impossible to swallow
Change in taste	No change in taste	Complete change in taste

Fig. 37.3 Patient-Reported Oral Mucositis Symptom (PROMS) Scale. (From Kushner, J. A., Lawrence, H. P., Shoval, I., Kiss, T. L., Devins, G. M., Lee, L., & Tenenbaum, H. C. (2008). Development and validation of a patient-reported oral mucositis symptom (PROMS) scale. *Journal of the Canadian Dental Association, 74*(1), 59a-59j.)

B. Supportive care drugs—analgesics (opioids and adjuvants) to relieve severe pain
  1. >97% of patients with ulcerative OM require opioid analgesics (usually morphine equivalent) by week 4. Opioid doses increase to week 7, usually needed for 6 weeks after treatment completion.
C. Adding adjuvant analgesics may be opioid sparing
  1. Add gabapentin to analgesic regimen.
  2. Doxepin 0.5% mouthwash or PO doxepin: ≤40% of patients achieve sufficient OM pain control—use as adjunct.
  3. Simple or niosomal amitriptyline mouthwash, or benzydamine (NSAID mouthwash 15 mL, swish 30 seconds, and spit) provide temporary pain relief.
D. Low-level laser therapy (administered to discrete areas of OM, biweekly to daily) reduces OM prevalence, severity, duration, and associated pain.
E. Many controlled studies of cryotherapy; significantly reduces OM severity.
  1. Instruct patient to hold ice chips in mouth for 5 minutes before CT or RT, during CT/RT, and up to 30 minutes afterward.
  2. Very helpful: 5-FU and high-dose melphalan; inconclusive results—methotrexate, etoposide, cisplatin, mitomycin, edatrexate, and vinblastine.
  3. Contraindicated with oxaliplatin because of risk for laryngopharyngeal dysesthesia.
II. Nursing management
A. Preventive oral care—pretreatment dental examination and instruction (oral and written) for oral hygiene regimen.
B. Remind patients about helpful dietary tips for painful OM: avoid spicy food, hot foods and drinks, eat soft or moistened foods.

C. Topical protective/coating agent—benzocaine (Orabase, Oratect Gel, Hurricane) ± analgesic (e.g., viscous lidocaine, magic mouthwash) may give some temporary relief.
D. Use of normal saline, salt and baking soda (0.5 teaspoon each in 1 cup of warm water), or plain water rinses.

NAUSEA AND VOMITING

Overview (Andrews & Sanger, 2014; da Silva, Sousa, Guimaraes, Slullitel, & Ashmawi, 2015; Dranitsaris et al, 2017; Feyer, Jahn, & Jordan, 2014; Kaye et al, 2017; Molassiotis et al, 2016; NCCN, 2018; Navari, 2018; Sharkey, Darmani, & Parker, 2014; Singh & Kuo, 2016; Walsh et al, 2017)

I. Definitions
  A. Nausea—uniquely unpleasant sensory and emotional experience; feeling epigastric or upper abdominal queasiness or need to vomit.
  B. Retching—spasmodic inspiratory movements with glottis closed and abdominal muscle contractions, no expulsion of stomach contents.
  C. Vomiting—autonomic and motor reflex, coordinated contraction of abdominal muscles and diaphragm with forceful expulsion of gastric contents from mouth.
  D. Nausea usually precedes vomiting, but either can occur alone.
II. Physiology of nausea and vomiting (N&V)
  A. N&V reflexes protect against accidental ingestion of toxic substances, cause oral expulsion and GI dysrhythmia with slowed passage of stomach contents to the intestine, hepatic circulation, and bloodstream.

B. Chemotherapy-induced N&V (CINV), radiotherapy-induced N&V (RINV), and postsurgical N&V (PONV) incorrectly identified as harmful and induce N&V.

C. The "vomiting center" (VC), a group of neurons in the medulla in the brainstem, is the final common pathway for vomiting from any cause.

D. Neurotransmitters and neuroreceptors in peripheral and central pathways carry signals to the VC.

   1. The GI tract—primarily via the vagus nerve (and stretch receptors in obstruction).

   2. The chemotherapy trigger zone (CTZ) is near the VC and receives chemical signals from the bloodstream and cerebrospinal fluid (CSF).

   3. The cerebral cortex and limbic region add subjective and emotional responses.

   4. The vestibular apparatus (middle ear) plays the major role in motion sickness.

   5. The endocannabinoid system, activated by peripheral or central emetic stimuli, modulate N&V via cannabinoid-1 (CB1) receptors in the brain.

   6. Multiple GI tract, brain neurotransmitters, and receptors have roles in N&V and thus antiemetic selection (Table 37.3).

   7. Understanding of nausea is poor. A unique nausea "threshold" may rapidly respond to intrinsic cognitive, GI, CNS and autonomic influences, and emotional centers.

III. CINV, which is best understood, involves two major pathways:

A. Emetogenic CT damages GI mucosal cells and releases serotonin (5HT) from enterochromaffin cells. 5HT binds to and activates $5HT_3$ receptors on vagus nerve, initiating emetic signal and acute CINV during the first 24 hours after CT.

B. Substance P (SP) and neurokin-1 (NK_1) receptors are abundant in the brain. Emetic stimuli cause SP binding at NK_1 receptors in the CTZ, amplifying the emetic message—particularly during delayed CINV that may persist for a few to many days.

C. If antiemetics inadequate for CINV, patients may experience breakthrough CINV.

TABLE 37.3 Antiemetics Based on Neurotransmitters and Neuroreceptor Binding

Neurotransmitter	Binds to	SITE OF ACTION CNS	GI	Effect	Medication	Examples	Uses
Serotonin (5HT)	5HT3	?	✓	Agonist: increases N&V	5HT3 RA	ondansetron granisetron palonosetron olanzapine	CINV PONV*
	5HT4	?	✓	Antagonist: decreases GI motility	5HT4 agonist	metoclopramide chlorpromazine	Delayed CINV Gastroparesis
Substance P (SP)	NK1	✓		Agonist: increases N&V	NK1 RA	aprepitant/fosaprepitant netupitant (combined with palonosetron – NEPA) rolapitant (half-life 180 hr)	CINV PONV*
Dopamine (D)	D2	✓	?	Agonist: increases N&V	D2 RA	droperidol, haloperidol prochlorperazine metoclopramide olanzapine, mirtazapine	CINV CINV: rescue PONV Palliative
Unknown	NA	?	?			dexamethasone	CINV PONV Palliative
Cannabinoid (CB)	CB1	✓		Poorly understood		Dronabinol (Marinol, Syndros)	Rescue CINV
Acetylcholine (Ach)	M		✓	Agonist: increases N&V	M antagonist (anticholinergic)	hyoscine (Scopolamine) glycopyrrolate	Bowel obstruction PONV
Histamine	H1			Agonist: increases N&V	H1 antagonist (antihistamine)	cyclizine chlorpromazine prochlorperazine olanzapine	Bowel obstruction
Unknown	NA					gabapentin	PONV

*Smaller doses used for PONV than CINV.

D. Anticipatory nausea (AN)—conditioned response to poorly controlled CINV; 8% to 14% of patients have AN before subsequent CT; can become more intense over successive CT cycles.

E. AN and CINV can lead to refractory CINV not responsive to standard antiemetics.

IV. Risk factors

A. Iatrogenic

1. CT emetogenicity: highly emetogenic (HEC: >90%, e.g., cisplatin, anthracycline–cyclophosphamide combination, mechlorethamine); moderately emetogenic (MEC: 30%–90%, e.g., carboplatin, cyclophosphamide, doxorubicin, oxaliplatin); low emetogenic (10%–30%, e.g., cetuximab, docetaxel, paclitaxel); and minimal emetogenic (<10%, e.g., fludarabine, rituximab, vincristine).

2. RT: total body RT (TBI >90%), upper abdominal or hemibody (60%–90%), cranium, lower thorax, pelvis (30%–60%), breast and extremities (<30%).

3. Concurrent CT-RT.

4. Inhalational anesthesia (PONV).

5. Opioids (tolerance usually develops within 1–2 weeks).

B. Patient-related

1. Female gender: greater incidence, lower response rates to antiemetics than men

2. Younger individuals (age 5-60) at greater risk

3. CINV with prior chemotherapy (strong predictor for CINV and PONV)

4. Anticipatory nausea and vomiting; prechemotherapy anxiety or expectations

5. No history of significant alcohol consumption

6. History of hyperemesis with pregnancy; history of motion sickness

7. Pharmacogenomic differences, particularly in 5HT3 receptor antagonist (RA) metabolism

C. Disease-related (often multifactorial)

1. Partial, intermittent, or complete bowel obstruction

2. Metabolic imbalance: hypercalcemia, hyponatremia, hyperglycemia, uremia

3. Gastric stasis secondary to ascites or hepatomegaly

4. Increased intracranial pressure with brain tumors or meningeal disease

5. Paraneoplastic neuropathy

6. Obstipation

7. Dyspepsia or gastritis

Assessment (Collis & Mather, 2015; Glare, Miller, Nikolova, & Tickoo, 2011; NCI-CTCAE, 2018; Navari, 2018; Rha, Sohn, Kim, Kim, & Lee, 2018)

I. Assessment goals may vary, depending on start of CT or RT (identify and incorporate risk factors into management plan) or from another problem (reversible cause vs. palliation)

II. History

A. Ask about N&V separately

1. Onset, pattern over time, frequency (intermittent or constant)

2. Severity (e.g., 0–10 scale or verbal descriptor scale [none, mild, moderate, severe], NCI-CTCAE)

3. Any associated symptoms (e.g., bloating, early satiety, sense of stomach fullness)

4. Review risk factors (see earlier) with patient, especially past or current CT, antiemetics used and effectiveness, any folk remedies successfully used.

III. Physical examination

A. Nausea may induce parasympathetic manifestations: pallor, perspiration, tachycardia, feeling dizzy and weak

B. Assess for signs of dehydration, orthostasis

C. Abdominal assessment (e.g., for ascites, large stool in colon); weight

IV. Psychosocial assessment

A. Ask patient if nausea (or vomiting) affects work, roles and responsibilities, and mood.

B. Ask if inadequate control of N&V has had negative effects on their partner or other family members.

V. Imaging and laboratory tests

A. Imaging only to identify underlying treatable cause

B. Laboratory—chemistries: serum electrolyte disturbances, hepatic and renal function, serum calcium intake and output

Management (Chelkeba et al, 2017; Enblom, Steineck, & Borjeson, 2017; Herrstedt et al, 2017; Hesketh, Bohlke, & Kris, 2017; Malamood, Roberts, Kataria, Parkman, & Schey, 2017; Marx et al, 2017; Mehra et al, 2018; Murray-Brown & Dorman, 2015; NCCN, 2018; Ruhlmann et al, 2017; Walsh et al, 2017; Zaini et al, 2018; ONS, 2017a)

I. Medical management

A. Principles of antiemetic management

1. Goal: prevention for the entire expected period of N&V

2. CINV or RINV: select antiemetics based on emetogenicity of regimen

3. Consider additional risk factors (see earlier) that may increase likelihood of N&V

4. N&V from other causes: antiemetic selected on suspected etiology

5. If N&V persist, add another antiemetic

6. Use PO antiemetics when possible (nauseated patients may not be able to take)

7. Use adjunct agents (e.g., H2 blocker to prevent dyspepsia/nausea, or lorazepam to decrease anxiety) as needed

TABLE 37.4   Guideline Recommendations – Standard of Care Antiemetics for CINV/RINV

	ASCO		NCCN		MASCC	
	Acute	**Delayed**	**Acute**	**Delayed**	**Acute**	**Delayed**
HEC	NK1 RA + 5HT3 RA + dex + olanzapine	dex + olanzapine d 2–4	NK1 RA + 5HT3 RA + dex **or** olanzapine + palonosetron + dex		NK1 RA + 5HT3 RA + dexamethasone	dex + NK1 RA **or** NK1 RA
MEC	5HT3 RA + dex ± NK1 RA	5HT3 RA + dex d 1 dex d 2–3	5HT3RA + dex **or** NK1 RA + 5HT3 RA + dex	Varies by d 1 antiemetics	5HT3 RA + dex	dex d 2–3
LEC	5-HT3 RA **or** dex	None recommended	dex **or** metoclopramide **or** prochlorperazine **or** 5HT3 RA	None recommended	dex **or** 5HT3 RA **or** D2 RA	None recommended
minimal	No routine prophylaxis		No routine prophylaxis		No routine prophylaxis	
HER	No guideline		5HT3 RA (ondansetron or		5HT3 RA + dex	
MER	recommendations		granisetron) + dex		5HT3 RA ± dex	
LER			None recommended		dex – prophylaxis or rescue **or** 5HT3 RA – prophylaxis or rescue	
minimal					Rescue – dex **or** D2 RA **or** 5HT3 RA	

B. CINV/RINV standard-of-care antiemetics (Table 37.4)
 1. 5HT$_3$ RAs: ondansetron (oral – PO, intravenous – IV), granisetron (PO, IV, transdermal, depot injection), palonosetron (IV)
 2. NK$_1$ RAs: aprepitant/fosaprepitant (PO/IV), netupitant (fixed PO dose with palonosetron), rolapitant (IV)
 3. Corticosteroid: dexamethasone (antiemetic mechanism unknown)
 4. Olanzapine—binds to multiple receptors involved in N&V (5HT3, dopamine, histamine, and muscarinic); clinically significant decreases in nausea.
C. Other antiemetics (e.g., adjunct, rescue, palliative, opioid)
 1. Cannabinoid agonists: dronabinol (Marinol, Syndros), nabilone (Cesamet)—rescue
 2. Dopamine (D2) RAs: metoclopramide (prokinetic—avoid in patients with GI obstruction), haloperidol, prochlorperazine, chlorpromazine—for palliative care, rescue antiemetics
 3. Mirtazapine—use for nausea, early satiety, cachexia, and weight loss, not sedating
 4 Antisecretory drugs (e.g., hyoscine or octreotide)—not antiemetics but useful for colic, GI obstruction
 5. Benzodiazepines (e.g., lorazepam, alprazolam [Xanax]); not antiemetics—decrease anxiety
II. Nursing management—adjuncts to antiemetics
A. Ask patient about any nondrug measures that have been helpful for past nausea or N&V
B. Ginger—reverses cisplatin-induced delayed gastric emptying, may alleviate or relieve GI dysmotility, muscarinic and histaminergic antagonistic properties
C. Dietary strategies (e.g., smaller, more frequent meals; increase water intake; or avoid coffee)—scant evidence
D. Relaxation techniques

ASCITES

Overview (Eitan et al, 2018; Flaherty, 2015; Knight et al, 2018; Maeda, Kobayashi, & Sakamoto, 2015; Stukan, 2017)
 I. Ascites—abnormal accumulation of fluid in the peritoneal cavity, occurs with some cancers (≈90% of cases occur with benign diseases, most in end-stage cirrhosis).
A. Normally, 5 to 20 mL of peritoneal fluid lubricate organ and bowel surfaces; 50 to 100 mL/hour diffuses from serum to peritoneum, back to circulation (via lymphatics)
B. Malignant ascites (MA) incidence
 1. Ovarian cancer ≈38% of women have MA at diagnosis
 2. Pancreatobiliary (21%), unknown primary (20%), gastric cancer (18%)
 3. Can occur in tumors that metastasize to the liver or peritoneum (e.g., gastric, colon, pancreas, lung, adrenal, bladder, and breast)
 II. Pathogenesis of MA is not fully understood; most likely multifactorial.
A. Almost always exudative (exerts osmotic pressure), leads to fluid overproduction, accumulation that exceeds peritoneum's resorptive capacity
 1. Cancer cells lining the peritoneum produce inflammatory cytokines; cause large molecules to amass and exert osmotic pressure with subsequent MA.
 2. Tumor-expressed vascular endothelial growth factor (VEGF) induces angiogenesis; alters vascular and peritoneal membrane permeability, with increased MA accumulation.

3. Some tumors seed malignant cells within the peritoneal cavity (carcinomatosis); these increase osmotic pressure and MA.
    4. Liver metastases may cause ascites secondary to portal hypertension.
  B. Any or a combination of these events overwhelms the capacity to drain peritoneal fluid and leads to refractory MA (persists or recurs after drainage)
III. Symptoms of refractory ascites are often more distressing than the underlying cancer
  A. Abdominal distension and pain
  B. Nausea, anorexia, vomiting, early satiety, and weight change
  C. Fatigue
  D. Dyspnea
IV. Patients with refractory MA have symptoms that reflect advanced cancer as well as MA. Prognoses for those with nonovarian cancer is 1 to 6 months, and for those with ovarian cancer is 10 to 24 months (27% are alive at 5 years).

Assessment (Brown & Neville-Webbe, 2016; Day, Mitchell, Keen, & Perkins, 2013; Eitan et al, 2018; Knight et al, 2018; NCI-CTCAE, 2018; Sangisetty & Miner, 2012; Stukan, 2017)

I. History
  A. Does the patient have suspected cancer or a confirmed diagnosis?
  B. Ask patient about presence of MA symptoms (e.g., abdominal fullness or feeling bloated, increased waist size, discomfort or pain, changed appetite or nausea, feeling short of breath, or change in activity).
  C. Ascites Symptom Mini-Scale (Fig. 37.4)—assesses ovarian cancer–related MA symptoms; useful to monitor worsening symptoms and relief after MA drainage.
  D. NCI-CTCAE
II. Physical examination
  A. Physical examination cannot identify small MA (≤100 mL) in asymptomatic patients
  B. Ascites of ≥1500 mL is clinically evident
  C. Larger ascites: abdomen may appear distended; could be obscured in an obese person

  D. Palpate/percuss abdomen for fluid wave, shifting dullness, bulging flanks, everted umbilicus, and stretched skin
III. Psychosocial assessment
  A. Ask patient if they feel depressed or anxious, or have difficulty thinking or concentrating (do not usually improve with drainage of ascites).
  B. If they report shortness of breath, ask if they feel anxious or fearful.
  C. Embarrassed because they "look pregnant," have problem finding clothes that fit.
  D. Ask if MA has altered their mobility, independence, family, and social activities.
IV. Imaging and laboratory tests
  A. Ultrasound of the abdomen—screen for MA; can detect ≥100 cc of fluid.
  B. CT or magnetic resonance imaging (MRI) of abdomen to identify primary malignancy; position emission tomography (PET) occult metastases.
  C. Ascites cytology analysis—diagnostic gold standard to identify/rule out tumor; protein concentration, ascites character—exudative vs. transudative, bacteria.
  D. Tumors that do not shed into peritoneum require biopsy to confirm diagnosis.
  E. Coagulation screen may be done before paracentesis.
  F. Chemistry panel, complete blood count (CBC): hypoalbuminemia, liver/renal dysfunction, anemia, infection.

Management (Brown & Neville-Webbe, 2016; Flaherty, 2015; Korpi et al, 2018; Maleux et al, 2016; Sangisetty & Miner, 2012; Stukan, 2017)

I. Management aims: relieve symptoms, improve QOL, treat primary cause—if feasible.
II. Medical management
  A. Diuretics (spironolactone and furosemide, titrated as needed) may be used for MA secondary to liver metastases and portal hypertension; possible adverse effects are systemic volume depletion, electrolyte abnormalities, renal dysfunction, and N&V.
  B. Adjunct or palliative chemotherapy or targeted therapy (systemic or intraperitoneal) indicated for some patients.

Symptom	Not at all				Very much
Shortness of breath	1	2	3	4	5
Distended abdomen	1	2	3	4	5
Decreased mobility	1	2	3	4	5
Fatigue	1	2	3	4	5
Loss of appetite	1	2	3	4	5

Fig. 37.4 The Ascites Symptom Mini-Scale. (From Eitan, R., Raban, O., Tsoref, D., Jakobson-Setton, A., Sabah, G., Salman, L., ... & Ben-Haroush, A. (2018). Malignant ascites: validation of a novel ascites symptom mini-scale for use in patients with ovarian cancer. *Int J Gynecol Cancer, 28*(6), 1162–1166. https://doi.org/10.1097/IGC. 0000000000001276.)

C. Paracentesis—fine tube inserted into peritoneum under ultrasound guidance; connected to collection bag, ascites freely drained, and catheter removed.
   1. Safe, well tolerated; 80% to 93% symptom relief (e.g., decreased abdominal distension and discomfort, dyspnea, nausea, anorexia, fatigue, and mobility).
   2. Low risk of complications (pain, hypotension, peritonitis, loculation of ascites, bowel perforation, and development of adhesions).
D. Volume that can safely be removed depends on type of ascites
   1. Exudative MA (peritoneal carcinomatosis)—up to 9 liters
   2. Transudative (liver metastases with portal hypertension)—rapid, large-volume drainage may cause hemodynamic instability (IV fluids may prevent hypotension).
E. MA may reaccumulate rapidly; average symptom relief 10 days (range 4–45 days).
F. Permanent subcutaneously tunneled abdominal catheter alternative to intermittent paracentesis for some patients.
   1. Tenckhoff (peritoneal dialysis) double-cuffed, PleurX single-cuffed, or Aspira double-cuffed vacuum system catheters.
   2. Low risk for manageable complications: exit-site infection, ascites leakage at catheter exit, catheter occlusion, fibrin sleeve formation at catheter tip that impedes drainage, or catheter dislodgment.
   3. Patient can drain catheter at home—not to dryness, but to symptom relief when needed. Vendors provide dressing and drainage supplies.
   4. Vacuum system catheters—maximum drainage (1000 mL) in ≥15 minutes; usual drainage every other day, 1 to 2 liters.
   5. Permanent catheters can be used for intraperitoneal chemotherapy.

CONSTIPATION

Overview (Candy et al., 2015; Dzierzanowski & Ciałkowska-Rysz, 2015; Erichsen, Milberg, Jaarsma, & Friedrichsen, 2016; Wickham, 2017; Williams, Mowlazadch, Sisler, & Williams, 2015)

I. Constipation arbitrarily defined as <3 bowel movements (BMs) per week
   A. Patients who have fewer than 3 BMS/week do not view themselves as constipated; rather, they define constipation as hard stools accompanied by straining.
   B. Constipation is one of the most frequent symptoms in patients receiving therapy.
   C. Disease progression may be accompanied by worsening bowel symptoms, along with increased fatigue and impaired ability to communicate.

D. Constipation can progress to impaction, stool packing in distal colon and rectum, with overflow diarrhea.
II. Physiology—extended bowel transit time allows greater absorption of water in feces through the bowel wall, results in hard and dry stools that are difficult to pass
III. Potential etiologic factors (often multicausal)
   A. Organic
      1. Cancer related (e.g., GI tumor, pelvic tumor mass, spinal cord involvement, GI obstruction, autonomic dysfunction, brain tumor, radiation fibrosis)
      2. Metabolic causes (dehydration, hypercalcemia, hypokalemia, hyponatremia, hypothyroidism, uremia, diabetes)
      3. Other diseases (diabetes, Parkinson disease, chronic obstructive pulmonary disease, heart disease)
      4. Other GI: small-bowel bacteria overgrowth, diverticulitis, anorectal fissures
      5. Female gender
   B. Functional
      1. Environmental/cultural (lack of privacy, comfort, or assistance with toileting; cultural sensitivities regarding BMs)
      2. Dietary: insufficient fluid intake, low-fiber diet
      3. Pain with defecation (anorectal pain, bone pain, other cancer pain)
      4. Other (advanced age, inactivity, decreased mobility, confined to bed, depression, sedation, progressive cachexia)
      5. Weakness/fatigue (proximal or central myopathy)
      6. Lower performance status is related to a higher likelihood of constipation
   C. Drug related (polypharmacy is more significant than single drugs)
      1. Opioids—constipation increases with longer use
      2. Anticholinergics (antihistamines, belladonna, antiparkinsonian drugs, antipsychotics, antispasmodics, monoamine oxidase [MAO] inhibitors, tricyclic antidepressants)
      3. Chemotherapy agents (alkylating agents, vinca alkaloids)
      4. 5-HT3 receptor antagonist antiemetics
      5. NSAIDs, anticonvulsants (carbamazepine), antihypertensives (beta blockers, calcium channel blockers, central-acting antiarrhythmics, diuretics)
      6. Metal ion–containing agents (aluminum, antacids, bismuth, calcium, iron supplements, lithium, sucralfate)

Assessment (Andrews & Morgan, 2013; Candy et al., 2015; Erichsen et al, 2016; NCI-CTCAE, 2018; Rhondali et al, 2013; Wickham, 2017)

I. History—ask patient:
   A. What they consider "normal" BMs and "constipation" (agree on definitions)

B. What is their usual BM pattern

C. Ask them to rate from 0 (no constipation) to 10 (worst constipation)

    1. Simple yes/no question may miss almost a third of constipated patients

    2. Rating of ≥3 indicates constipation and further workup

D. NCI-CTCAE

E. What are their BMs like (e.g., small or large; rocks or marbles; soft, hard, or liquid; color, odor, blood, or mucus)

F. Do they have hemorrhoids or other rectal problems?

G. Do they have abdominal fullness or bloating, nausea, diarrhea, or a constant feeling of having to move their bowels with an empty colon (tenesmus)?

H. Do they take laxatives or use suppositories or enemas? Which, how much, how often? How much do laxatives help?

I. Other medications

J. Activity level: altered mobility, fatigue or weakness—may interfere with usual BMs

K. Current diet and appetite, fiber intake (can patient consume fiber 30 grams per day with sufficient fluids to maximize bulk effects and avoid exacerbating constipation)

L. Medical conditions affecting laxative selection (e.g., vocal cord paralysis precludes mineral oil, or impaired renal function contraindicates magnesium salts)

II. Physical examination

  A. Abdomen

    1. Inspect abdomen for symmetry, distention, bulges, visible peristalsis

    2. Auscultate all quadrants for normal, hyperactive, or absent bowel sounds

    3. Palpate for masses to distinguish stool (indents) from tumors (do not)

    4. Percuss for gas or fluid with ascites; tympany and distention

  B. Rectal examination (avoid in neutropenic or thrombocytopenic patient); ensure privacy and consider cultural norms

    1. Poor anal sphincter tone—may indicate spinal cord problem

    2. Hard, dry stool in the rectum (fecal impaction)—patient may need disimpaction before starting oral laxative therapy

    3. Hemorrhoids or fissures—stool softener may be indicated

III. Psychosocial assessment

  A. Ask patient if constipation affects their comfort, activities of daily living, mood

  B. Does the patient avoid taking opioid analgesics because some pain is better than feeling constipated?

  C. Does constipation add to anxiety or depression?

IV. Imaging and laboratory tests

  A. Tests to identify contributing factors (e.g., hypercalcemia or diabetes) or risks from interventions (e.g., blood urea nitrogen [BUN], creatinine to assess renal function, white blood cells [WBCs] and platelets to identify risks with manual disimpaction).

  B. Flat plate of abdomen radiograph may distinguish severe constipation, fecal impaction, and obstruction.

Management (Andrews & Morgan, 2013; Dzierzanowski & Ciałkowska-Rysz, 2015; Garcia & Shamliyan, 2018; https://www.ons.org/practice-resources/pep/constipation)

I. Medical management

  A. Oral (PO) laxatives

    1. Stimulant—senna or bisacodyl

    2. Osmotic—lactulose (prescription agent), polyethylene glycol, sorbitol—indigestible and nonabsorbable sugars

    3. Directly stimulate bowel wall neurons that induce forceful peristalsis and release water and electrolytes into the intestine

    4. First-line laxatives, particularly for opioid-induced constipation (OIC); administer proactively and titrate doses to effect

  B. PO stool softeners—docusate (Colace, Surfak), mineral oil

    1. Lower surface tension, soften and lubricate stools

    2. Ineffective for established constipation and OIC; less effective than psyllium

    3. Must increase fluid intake to soften stools; contraindicated in advanced cancer

  C. PO bulking agents: soluble—psyllium (e.g., Metamucil), insoluble—methylcellulose (e.g., Citrucel)

    1. Worsen slow-transit opioid– or anticholinergic-related constipation

    2. Avoid in patients with advanced disease; insufficient PO fluids may lead to fecal impaction or GI obstruction

  D. Peripheral opioid antagonist (methylnaltrexone subcutaneous); only patients with OIC who do not respond to maximized laxative doses

  E. Rectally administered agents

    1. Suppository: bisacodyl, glycerin (hyperosmotic, lubricant)

    2. Enemas: phosphate (Fleet), microenema, mineral oil

    3. Preferred for rapid and predictable evacuation of stool from rectum and distal colon, such as patients with fecal impaction

II. Nursing management

  A. Meager evidence that most nondrug measures (e.g., recommending trying to have BM same time each morning) are helpful for cancer patients.

  B. Dietary fiber, increasing oral fluids, and exercise depend on performance status and prognosis; may or may not be useful (or possible).

1. Fiber may increase number of BMs but not change stool consistency, laxative use, or painful BMs.
2. Dietary fiber might be effective for mild or moderate but not severe constipation in relatively healthy patients.
3. Fiber can worsen early satiety, increase constipation in patients with limited fluid intake.
4. Cachectic patients may be unable to consume sufficient food and liquids for effective gut transit and feces consistency.

DIARRHEA

Overview (Andreyev et al, 2014; Cherny, 2008; Cinausero et al, 2017; Liu et al, 2018; McQuade, Stojanovska, Abalo, Bornstein, & Nurgali, 2016; Pessi et al, 2014; Sweetser, 2012; Yeung, 2016)

I. Diarrhea is the passage of more than three unformed stools in 24 hours.
   A. Objective definition: passing stools of >200 g or >200 mL per 24 hours.
II. Diarrhea key manifestation of GI tract mucositis (GIM) after CT or RT to abdomen/pelvis.
   A. Prevalence and severity of GIM depends on drug/regimen, dose, and administration schedule, and can be classified as:
      1. Nonpersistent (existing for <4 weeks) or persistent (lasting >4 weeks); may persist for years posttreatment
      2. Early onset (<24 hours after administration) or late onset (>24 hours after administration)
      3. Uncomplicated (grade 1–2, usually manageable at home) or complicated (grade 3–4, generally requires hospitalization)
   B. Drugs commonly causing GIM: 5-fluorouracil (5FU)—folinic acid (leucovorin), irinotecan, capecitabine, gemcitabine, methotrexate, cyclophosphamide, cisplatin, oxaliplatin, carboplatin, doxorubicin, paclitaxel, docetaxel, cabazitaxel, thalidomide
      1. Example: GIM occurs in 89% of patients receiving FOLFIRI (5FU + leucovorin + irinotecan) and 50% with FOLFOX (5FU + oxaliplatin).
   C. RT-induced GIM can occur after RT to the anus, rectum, cervix, uterus, prostate, urinary bladder, or testes; total body irradiation conditioning for HSCT increases GIM throughout the GI tract.
      1. Small-bowel complications related to volume of small intestine in the RT field.
      2. RT-related GIM is usually grade 1 or 2.
   D. List of targeted therapies causing diarrhea growing; includes EGF-TKIs, monoclonal antibodies (MoABs), mammalian target of rapamycin (mTOR) inhibitors, mitogen-activated protein kinases (MAPK) signaling cascade inhibitors.
      1. Usually mild, but grade 3 diarrhea sometimes occurs.
      2. Mechanisms may differ by class, not identified.
      3. GIM is more frequent with combination therapies (Cinausero et al., 2017).
III. Other causes of diarrhea
   A. Fecal impaction with overflow diarrhea
   B. Paraneoplastic, secondary to a neuroendocrine tumor
   C. GVHD
   D. *Clostridium difficile* (*C. diff*) diarrhea, secondary to antibiotics, prolonged NGT, GI surgery, repeated enemas, or chemotherapy
   E. Enteral tube feedings
   F. Unrelated to cancer
      1. Lactose intolerance, food poisoning
      2. Viral gastroenteritis
      3. Inflammatory bowel disease or irritable bowel syndrome
      4. Excessive dosing (laxatives, magnesium-based antacids, nutritional supplements, antibiotics, proton pump inhibitors, selective serotonin reuptake inhibitors, NSAIDs).
IV. The hallmarks of diarrhea from any cause are GI tract water and electrolyte imbalance
   A. Damaged villi less able to absorb fluid and nutrients from small bowel into circulation
   B. Nonabsorbable nutrients exert osmotic pressure to pull water into the intestine
   C. Greater numbers of immature secretory cells increase GI secretion
   D. These factors exceed colon's capacity to absorb water from feces, diarrhea results
V. Pathogenesis of CT- and RT-induced GIM
   A. CT and RT diarrhea/GIM occur by the same mechanisms as oral mucositis
      1. Injury to rapidly dividing GI epithelium and submucosa initiates GIM cascade. The small intestine (single-cell-layer mucosa) is particularly vulnerable.
      2. Transcription factors generate messengers to activate immune response and upregulate proinflammatory cytokines.
      3. Signal amplification activates other pathways, with inflammation and apoptosis of GI epithelial stem cells.
      4. Ulceration phase: superficial and submucosal GI damage causes shift in bacteria when WBCs decreasing; increased risk for secondary infection.
      5. Healing occurs after chemotherapy or radiotherapy complete. Although mucosa epithelium regenerates, residual damage increases the risk for future GIM.
VI. Diarrhea can range from bothersome to life threatening. Severe GIM can lead to:
   A. Treatment interruptions, dose reductions, or early discontinuation
   B. Hospitalization and readmission, and significant economic burden

C. Profound dehydration, electrolyte imbalance, and hypovolemia; severe CT-induced GIM may lead to 4 to 6 liters of diarrhea stools/day.

D. Other possible complications—hemorrhoids, perianal skin breakdown, malnutrition, cachexia and weight loss, fatigue, declining immune function, and renal failure.

Assessment (Andreyev et al, 2014; Barr & Smith, 2014; McQuade et al, 2016; NCI CTCAE, 2018; Pessi et al, 2014; Sweetser, 2012)

I. History
  A. Thoroughly documented bowel history is crucial for timely follow-up interventions
    1. Is the patient at risk for or experiencing CT- or RT-related diarrhea now?
    2. What "normal" bowel habit was before cancer diagnosis
    3. If bowel habit changed since diagnosis.
    4. What BMs are like now: frequency, color, watery, bloody, mucus-filled, amount, odor, stool consistency. Abdominal and rectal (or stoma) pain.
    5. Sense of diarrhea: does patient wake at night because they have to move their bowels, do they have any steatorrhea (stools with excessive fat—are often pale, foamy, foul-smelling, float in toilet bowl, and flush poorly), do they have urgency to move bowels or any BM incontinence (urgent GI consult indicated)?
    6. Associated abdominal symptoms: cramping, abdominal pain, bloating, passing gas
  B. Current cancer treatment, if any; which and last treatment.
  C. Review medications (Rx and OTC)—any of these started in last 10 to 14 days?
  D. Associated symptoms of dehydration
    1. Any change in urinating (less frequently or smaller amounts, urine color, odor)
    2. More thirsty than usual?
    3. Sudden, rapid weight loss (1-liter weighs 1 kg)
    4. Any dizziness, falling down, or fainting (orthostasis)?
    5. Any change in their thinking (mental status)?
  E. Dietary factors
    1. Recent changes (e.g., more fiber or roughage, fried or fatty foods)
    2. Fluids: fruit juices, coffee, alcohol
  F. Particularly worrying symptom constellation:
    1. Abdominal cramps not relieved by loperamide
    2. Unable to eat
    3. Worsening fatigue or weakness
    4. Chest pain
    5. N&V not controlled by antiemetics
    6. Dehydration with decreased urine output, fever (temperature >38.5°C)
    7. GI bleeding
    8. Previous admission for diarrhea
  G. NCI-CTCAE Severity of diarrhea

VII. Physical examination—assess degree of patient's dehydration
  A. General appearance (ill, listless)
  B. Mucous membranes (dry, normal), skin turgor
  C. Circulatory: any delayed capillary refill time, tachycardia, orthostasis (blood pressure [BP] decreases <40 mm Hg systolic and/or 20 mm Hg diastolic in <15 seconds after standing)
  D. Any acute abdominal processes, such as hyperactive bowel sounds
  E. Rectal examination: assess for perineal skin irritation, rectal tenderness, blood, and stool consistency (any hard, dry stool in rectum [fecal impaction]; loose stool may flow around stool (overflow) and reported as diarrhea.
III. Psychosocial assessment
  A. Ask patient if diarrhea interferes with social activities, such as going out to dinner with friends, because of concerns of uncontrollable diarrhea.
  B. Ask patient if they feel depressed, anxious, or embarrassed because of diarrhea.
  C. Ask if diarrhea has caused change/limited usual home or work activities
IV. Imaging and laboratory tests
  A. Flat plate of abdomen, abdominal ultrasound, abdominal CT if indicated
  B. Fecal occult blood testing
  C. Stool culture for C. difficile (patients who develop unexplained diarrhea after 3 days of hospitalization; positive in 15%–20%)
  D. CBC, serum chemistries, and electrolytes

Management (Andreyev et al, 2014; Barr & Smith, 2014; Churgay & Aftab, 2012; Mardas, Madry, & Stelmach-Mardas, 2017; McQuade et al, 2016; Yeung, 2016; https://www.ons.org/practice-resources/pep/diarrhea)

I. Medical management
  A. Opioid antidiarrheals
    1. Loperamide—first-line for CT GIM (minimal systemic absorption, does not cross the blood–brain barrier into the CNS). Patients must call oncology provider if eight 2-mg tablets in 24 hours has no effect on diarrhea.
    2. Deodorized tincture of opium—second-line opioid antidiarrheal agent; inhibits peristalsis, increases GI transit time, promotes fluid reabsorption.
  B. Octreotide—synthetic somatostatin analog, inhibits gut hormones, increases gut transit time. Second line if unresponsive to loperamide after 48 hours.
II. Nursing management
  A. Rehydration—first priority to manage acute GIM/diarrhea (grade 1–2 at home)
    1. Approximate fluid deficit (excludes electrolyte imbalance): patient's usual weight minus present weight (e.g., 70 kg − 68 kg = 2 kg = 2-liter deficit)

2. Continue maintenance fluids and replace ongoing losses with PO commercial (Pedialyte or similar) or homemade oral rehydration solution (ORS): mix 0.5 teaspoon of salt, 6 teaspoons of sugar, and 1 liter of water.
3. Hospitalization, IV rehydration necessary if PO rehydration not feasible or sufficient, grade 3 to 4 diarrhea.

B. Patient/family teaching; patients hesitant to take medicines and "bother" clinicians. Patients and caregivers need verbal, written information; verbalize understanding.
   1. Before CT started, emphasize diarrhea/GIM can potentially become life threatening, and optimal management is critically important.
   2. Provide regimen-based information sheet: treatment schedule, possible adverse effects, including need for IV fluids and other treatment measures for diarrhea.
   3. Use large font, simple language. Confirm patient, caregiver comprehension.
   4. Send patient home with antidiarrheal tablets; instruct them to keep pills with them in case diarrhea starts when they go out.
   5. Encourage patient to self-medicate and keep a record of use.
   6. Reiterate/reinforce information at every clinical visit throughout treatment.

C. Dietary modifications may help decrease diarrhea symptoms.
   1. Avoid foods: spicy, fatty, greasy, or fried; vegetables (especially cruciferous, gas-forming); high fiber, high sugar, and stone fruits (e.g., apricots, cherries, peaches)
   2. Avoid beverages that may worsen diarrhea: caffeine, alcohol, fruit juices, high-osmolar dietary supplements, lactose-containing dairy products, hot liquids
   3. Avoid foods, beverages sweetened with sorbitol or xylitol, and tobacco
   4. Do: eat low-fat, high-potassium diet; 6 to 8 small meals and snacks per day; drink room-temperature clear liquids.
   5. BRAT diet (bananas, rice, apples, toast) may reduce the frequency of stools.

EXPECTED PATIENT OUTCOMES

I. Patient's nutritional status will be maintained or improved.
II. Patient verbalizes understanding of how to titrate laxatives (per instructions) to comfort and to notify nurse when self-care measures not effective.
III. Patient maintains adequate hydration status or informs oncology team if unable to do so.
IV. Patient promptly reports any OM complications (e.g., eating, swallowing, or choking).

V. Patient takes prescribed antiemetics, as ordered, for entire expected period of N&V.
VI. Patient will not experience AN or refractory CINV.
VII. Patient will remain hydrated and not experience uncontrolled diarrhea.

REFERENCES

Alfieri, S., Ripamonti, C. I., Marceglia, S., Orlandi, E., Iacovelli, N. A., Granata, R., … Bossi, P. (2016). Temporal course and predictive factors of analgesic opioid requirement for chemoradiation-induced oral mucositis in oropharyngeal cancer. *Head & Neck*, 38(suppl 1), E521–E527. https://doi.org/10.1002/hed.24272.

Alterio, D., Gerardi, M. A., Cella, L., Spoto, R., Zurlo, V., Sabbatini, A., Fodor, C., … Jereczek-Fossa, B. A. (2017). Radiation-induced acute dysphagia. *Strahlentherapie Und Onkologie*, 193, 971–981. https://doi.org/10.1007/s00066-017-1206-x.

American Academy of Oral Medicine (AAOM). (2016). AAOM Clinical Practice Statement: subject: clinical management of cancer therapy-induced salivary gland hypofunction and xerostomia. *Oral Surgery, Oral Medicine, Oral Pathology, Oral Radiology*, 122, 310–312. https://doi.org/10.1016/j.oooo.2016.04.015.

Andrews, A., & Morgan, G. (2013). Constipation in palliative care: treatment options and considerations for individual patient management. *International Journal of Palliative Nursing*, 266(19), 268–273. https://doi.org/10.12968/ijpn.2013.19.6.266.

Andrews, P. L. R., & Sanger, G. J. (2014). Nausea and the quest for the perfect anti-emetic. *European Journal of Pharmacology*, 722, 108–121. https://doi.org/10.1016/j.ejphar.2013.09.072.

Andreyev, J., Ross, P., Donnellan, C., Lennan, E., Leonard, P., Waters, C., … Ferry, D. (2014). Guidance on the management of diarrhoea during cancer chemotherapy. *Lancet Oncology*, 15, e447–e460. https://doi.org/10.1016/S1470-2045(14)70006-3.

Arrese, L. C., Carrau, R., & Plowman, E. K. (2017). Relationship between the Eating Assessment Tool-10 and objective clinical ratings of swallowing function in individuals with head and neck cancer. *Dysphagia*, 32, 83–89. https://doi.org/10.1007/s00455-016-9741-7.

Barr, W., & Smith, A. (2014). Acute diarrhea in adults. *American Family Physician*, 89(3), 180–189.

Beck, A. M., Kjaersgaard, A., Hansen, T., & Poulsen, I. (2017). Systematic review and evidence based recommendations on texture modified foods and thickened liquids for adults (above 17 years) with oropharyngeal dysphagia - an updated clinical guideline. *Clinical Nutrition*, 1–12.

Belafsky, P. C., Mouadeb, D. A., Rees, C. J., Pryor, J. C., Postma, G. N., Allen, J., & Leonard, R. J. (2008). Validity and reliability of the Eating Assessment Tool (EAT-10). *Annals of Otolaryngology, Rhinology, and Laryngology*, 117, 919–924. https://doi.org/10.1177/000348940811701210.

Bonomi, M., & Batt, K. (2015). Supportive management of mucositis and metabolic derangements in head and neck cancer patients. *Cancers*, 7, 1743–1757. https://doi.org/10.3390/cancers7030862.

Bressan, V., Bagnasco, A., Aleo, G., Catania, G., Zanini, M. P., Timmins, F., & Sasso, L. (2017). The life experience of nutrition impact symptoms during treatment for head and neck cancer patients: a systematic review and meta-synthesis. *Supportive Care in Cancer, 25*, 1699–1712. https://doi.org/10.1007/s00520-017-3618-7.

Brodsky, M. B., Suiter, D. M., González-Fernández, M., Michtalik, H. J., Frymark, T. B., Venediktov, R., & Schooling, T. (2016). Screening accuracy for aspiration using bedside water swallow tests: a systematic review and meta-analysis. *Chest, 150*, 148–163. https://doi.org/10.1016/j.chest.2016.03.059.

Brown S. & Neville-Webbe H. (2016). Management of malignant ascites in the acute oncology setting. *The Oncologist.*

Buglione, M., Cavagnini, R., Di Rosario, F., Maddalo, M., Vassalli, L., … Magrini, S. M. (2016). Oral toxicity management in head and neck cancer patients treated with chemotherapy and radiation: xerostomia and trismus (part 2). Literature review and consensus statement. *Critical Reviews in Oncology/Hematology, 102*, 47–54. https://doi.org/10.1016/j.critrevonc.2015.08.010.

Candy, B., Jones, L., Larkin, P. J., Vickerstaff, V., Tookman, A., & Stone, P. (2015). Laxatives for the management of constipation in people receiving palliative care. *Cochrane Collaboration, 5*, 1–36. https://doi.org/10.1002/14651858.CD003448.pub4.

Carucci, L. R., & Turner, M. A. (2015). Dysphagia revisited: common and unusual causes. *Radiographics, 35*, 105–122. https://doi.org/10.1148/rg.351130150.

Carvalho, C. G., Medeiros-Filho, J. B., & Ferreira, M. C. (2018). Guide for health professionals addressing oral care for individuals in oncological treatment based on scientific evidence. *Supportive Care in Cancer.* https://doi.org/10.1007/s00520-018-4111-7. First Online: February 22, 2018.

Cederholm, T., Bosaeus, I., Barazzoni, R., Bauer, J., Van Gossum, A., Klek, S., … Singer, P. (2015). Diagnostic criteria for malnutrition - an ESPEN consensus statement. *Clinical Nutrition, 34*, 335–340. https://doi.org/10.1016/j.clnu.2015.03.001.

Chaveli-Lopez, B., & Bagan-Sebastian, J. V. (2016). Treatment of oral mucositis due to chemotherapy. *Journal of Clinical and Experimental Dentistry, 8*, e201–e209.

Chelkeba, L., Gidey, K., Mamo, A., Yohannes, B., Matso, T., & Melaku, T. (2017). Olanzapine for chemotherapy-induced nausea and vomiting: systematic review and meta-analysis. *Pharmacy Practice (Granada), 15*(1), 877. https://doi.org/10.18549/PharmPract.2017.01.877.

Chen, J., Seabrook, J., Fulford, A., & Rajakumar, I. (2017). Icing oral mucositis: oral cryotherapy in multiple myeloma patients undergoing autologous hematopoietic stem cell transplant. *Journal of Oncology Pharmacy Practice, 23*, 116–120. https://doi.org/10.1177/1078155215620920.

Cheney, D. M., Siddiqui, M. T., Litts, J. K., Kuhn, M. A., & Belafsky, P. C. (2015). The ability of the 10-item Eating Assessment Tool (EAT-10) to predict aspiration risk in persons with dysphagia. *Annals of Otology, Rhinology & Laryngology, 124*, 351–354. https://doi.org/10.1177/0003489414558107.

Cherny, N. I. (2008). Evaluation and management of treatment-related diarrhea in patients with advanced cancer: a review. *Journal of Pain and Symptom Management, 36*, 413–423. https://doi.org/10.1016/j.jpainsymman.2007.10.007.

Churgay, C. A., & Aftab, Z. (2012). Gastroenteritis in children: part II. Prevention and management. *American Family Physician, 85*, 1066–1070.

Cinausero, M., Aprile, G., Ermacora, P., Basile, D., Vitale, M. G., Fanotto, V., … Sonis, S. T. (2017). New frontiers in the pathobiology and treatment of cancer regimen-related mucosal injury. *Frontiers in Pharmacology, 8*, 354. https://doi.org/10.3389/fphar.2017.00354. Jun 8.

Collis, E., & Mather, H. (2015). Nausea and vomiting in palliative care. *British Medical Journal, 351*, h6249. https://doi.org/10.1136/bmj.h6249.

da Silva, H. B. G., Sousa, A. M., Guimaraes, G. M. N., Slullitel, A., & Ashmawi, H. A. (2015). Does previous chemotherapy-induced nausea and vomiting predict postoperative nausea and vomiting? *Acta Anaesthesiologica Scandinavica, 59*, 1145–1153. https://doi.org/10.1111/aas.12552.

Dai, Y., Li, C., Xie, Y., Liu, X., Zhang, J., Zhou, J., … Yang, S. (2014). Interventions for dysphagia in oesophageal cancer (review). *Cochrane Database of Systematic Reviews.* (Issue 10). https://doi.org/10.1002/14651858.CD005048.pub4 Art. No.: CD005048.

Day, R., Mitchell, T., Keen, A., & Perkins, P. (2013). The experiences of patients with ascites secondary to cancer: a qualitative study. *Palliative Medicine, 27*, 739–746. https://doi.org/10.1177/0269216313480400.

Denaro, N., Merlano, M. C., & Russi, E. G. (2013). Dysphagia in head and neck cancer patients: pretreatment evaluation, predictive factors, and assessment during radio-chemotherapy, recommendations. *Clinical and Experimental Otorhinolaryngology, 6*, 117–126. https://doi.org/10.3342/ceo.2013.6.3.117.

De Sanctis, V., Bossi, P., Sanguineti, G., Trippa, F., Ferrari, D., Bacigalupo, A., … Lalla, R. V. (2016). Mucositis in head and neck cancer patients treated with radiotherapy and systemic therapies: literature review and consensus statements. *Critical Reviews in Oncology/Hematology, 100*, 147–166. https://doi.org/10.1016/j.critrevonc.2016.01.010.

Dranitsaris, G., Molassiotis, A., Clemons, M., Roeland, E., Schwartzberg, L., Dielenseger, P., … Aapro, M. (2017). The development of a prediction tool to identify cancer patients at high risk for chemotherapy induced nausea and vomiting. *Annals of Oncology, 28*, 1260–1267. https://doi.org/10.1093/annonc/mdx100.

Dyasanoor, S., & Saddu, S. C. (2014). Association of xerostomia and assessment of salivary flow using modified Schirmer test among smokers and healthy individuals: a preliminary study. *Journal of Clinical and Diagnostic Research, 8*, 211–213. https://doi.org/10.7860/JCDR/2014/6650.3846.

Dzierzanowski, T., & Ciałkowska-Rysz, A. (2015). Behavioral risk factors of constipation in palliative care patients. *Supportive Care in Cancer, 23*, 1787–1793. https://doi.org/10.1007/s00520-014-2495-6.

Eitan, R., Raban, O., Tsoref, D., Jakobson-Setton, A., Sabah, G., Salman, L., … Ben-Haroush, A. (2018). Malignant ascites: validation of a novel ascites symptom mini-scale for use in patients with ovarian cancer. *Int J Gynecol Cancer, 28*(6), 1162–1166. https://doi.org/10.1097/IGC.0000000000001276.

Enblom, A., Steineck, G., & Borjesond, S. (2017). Complementary and alternative medicine self-care strategies for nausea in patients undergoing abdominal or pelvic irradiation for cancer: a longitudinal observational study of implementation in routine care. *Complementary Therapies in Medicine, 34*, 141–148. https://doi.org/10.1016/j.ctim.2017.08.003.

Epstein, J. B., & Jensen, S. B. (2015). Management of hyposalivation and xerostomia: criteria for treatment strategies. *Compendium Continuing Education Dentistry, 36*, 600–603.

Erichsen, E., Milberg, A., Jaarsma, T., & Friedrichsen, M. (2016). Constipation in specialized palliative care: factors related to constipation when applying different definitions. *Supportive Care in Cancer, 24*, 691–698. https://doi.org/10.1007/s00520-015-2831-5.

Espitalier, F., Fanous, A., Aviv, J., Bassiouny, S., Desuter, G., ... Crevier-Buchman, L. (2018). International consensus (ICON) on assessment of oropharyngeal dysphagia. *European Annals of Otorhinolaryngology, Head and Neck Diseases, 135*, S17–S21. https://doi.org/10.1016/j.anorl.2017.12.009.

Feyer, P., Jahn, F., & Jordan, K. (2014). Radiation induced nausea and vomiting. *European Journal of Pharmacology, 722*, 165–171. https://doi.org/10.1016/j.ejphar.2013.09.069.

Flaherty, A. M. C. (2015). Management of malignancy-related ascites. *Oncology Nursing Forum, 42*, 96–99. https://doi.org/10.1188/15.ONF.96-99.

Gallegos, C., Brito-de la Fuente, E., Clav, P., Costa, A., & Assegehegn, G. (2017). Nutritional aspects of dysphagia. *Advances in Food and Nutrition Research, 81*, 271–318. https://doi.org/10.1016/bs.afnr.2016.11.008.

Garcia, J. M., & Shamliyan, T. A. (2018). Management of opioid-induced constipation in patients with malignancy. *The American Journal of Medicine (in press)..* https://doi.org/10.1016/j.amjmed.2018.02.038.

Glare, P., Miller, J., Nikolova, T., & Tickoo, R. (2011). Treating nausea and vomiting in palliative care: a review. *Clinical Interventions in Aging, 6*, 243–259. https://doi.org/10.2147/CIA.S13109.

Gussgard, A. M., Jokstad, A., Hope, A. J., Wood, R., & Tenenbaum, H. (2015). Radiation-induced mucositis in patients with head and neck cancer: should the signs or the symptoms be measured? *Journal of the Canadian Dental Association, 81*, f11.

Herrstedt, J., Roila, F., Warr, D., Celio, L., Navari, R. M., Hesketh, P. J., ... Aapro, M. S. (2017). 2016 Updated MASCC/ESMO consensus recommendations: prevention of nausea and vomiting following high emetic risk chemotherapy. *Supportive Care in Cancer, 25*, 277–288. https://doi.org/10.1007/s00520-016-3313-0.

Hesketh, P. J., Bohlke, K., & Kris, M. G. (2017). Antiemetics: American Society of Clinical Oncology clinical practice guideline update summary. *Journal of Oncology Practice, 13*, 825–830. https://doi.org/10.1200/JCO.2017.74.4789.

Holmes, S. (2016). A service evaluation of cough reflex testing to guide dysphagia management in the postsurgical adult head and neck patient population. *Current Opinion in Otolaryngology & Head and Neck Surgery, 24*, 191–196. https://doi.org/10.1097/MOO.0000000000000256.

Jansson-Knodell, C. L., Codipilly, D. C., & Leggett Wallisch, C. L. (2017). Making dysphagia easier to swallow: a review for the practicing clinician. *Mayo Clinic Proceedings, 92*, 965–972. https://doi.org/10.1016/j.mayocp.2017.03.021.

Kakoei, S., Pardakhty, A., Hashemipour, M. A., Larizadeh, H., Kalantar, B., & Tahmasebi, E. (2018). Comparison the pain relief of amitriptyline mouthwash with benzydamine in oral mucositis. *Journal of Dentistry (Shīrāz, Iran), 19*(1), 34–40.

Kanagalingam, J., Wahid, M. I. A., Lin, J.-C., Cupino, N. A., Liu, E., Kang, J.-H., ... Moon, H. (2018). Patient and oncologist perceptions regarding symptoms and impact on quality-of-life of oral mucositis in cancer treatment: results from the Awareness Drives Oral Mucositis PercepTion (ADOPT) study. *Journal of Supportive Care in Cancer, 26*(7), 2191–2200. https://doi.org/10.1007/s00520-018-4050-3.

Kaye, A. D., Cornett, E. M., Chalabi, J., Naim, N. Z., Novitch, M. B., Creel, J. B., ... Urman, R. D. (2017). Pharmacology of antiemetics: update and current considerations in anesthesia practice. *Anesthesiology Clinics, 35*, e41–e54. https://doi.org/10.1016/j.anclin.2017.01.003.

King, S. N., Dunlap, N. E., Tennant, P. A., & Pitts, T. (2016). Pathophysiology of radiation-dysphagia in head and neck cancer. *Dysphagia, 31*, 339–351. https://doi.org/10.1007/s00455-016-9710-1.

Korpi, S., Salminen, V. V., Piili, R. P., Paunu, N., Luukkaala, T., & Lehto, J. T. (2018). Therapeutic procedures for malignant ascites in a palliative care outpatient clinic. *Journal of Palliative Medicine, 21*(6), 836–841. https://doi.org/10.1089/jpm.2017.0616.

Knight, J. A., Thompson, S. M., Fleming, C. J., Bendel, E. C., Neisen, M. J., Neidert, N. B., ... Woodrum, D. A. (2018). Safety and effectiveness of palliative tunneled peritoneal drainage catheters in the management of refractory malignant and non-malignant ascites. *Cardiovascular and Interventional Radiology, 41*, 753–761. https://doi.org/10.1007/s00270-017-1872-1.

Krisciunas, G. P., Castellano, K., McCulloch, T. M., Lazarus, C. L., Pauloski, B. R., Meyer, T. K., ... Langmore, S. E. (2017). Impact of compliance on dysphagia rehabilitation in head and neck cancer patients: results from a nulti-center clinical trial. *Dysphagia, 32*, 3279. https://doi.org/10.1007/s00455-016-9760-4. 3236.

Kruger, D. (2014). Assessing esophageal dysphagia. *Journal of the American Academy of Physician Assistants, 27*(5), 23–30. https://doi.org/10.1097/01.JAA.0000446227.85554.fb.

Kushner, J. A., Lawrence, H. P., Shoval, I., Kiss, T. L., Devins, G. M., Lee, L., & Tenenbaum, H. C. (2008). Development and validation of a patient-reported oral mucositis symptom (PROMS) scale. *Journal of the Canadian Dental Association, 74*, 59a–59j.

Kwon, Y. (2016). Mechanism-based management for mucositis: option for treating side effects without compromising the efficacy of cancer therapy. *OncoTargets and Therapy, 9*, 2007–2016. https://doi.org/10.2147/OTT.S96899.

Lalla, R. V., Bowen, J., Barasch, A., Elting, L., Epstein, J., Keefe, D. M., & Elad, S. (2014). MASCC/ISOO clinical practice guidelines for the management of mucositis secondary to cancer therapy. *Cancer, 120*, 1453–1461. https://doi.org/10.1002/cncr.28592.

Liu, J., Nicum, S., Reichardt, P., Croitoru, K., Illek, B., Schmidinger, M., ... Jayson, G. C. (2018). Assessment and management of diarrhea following VEGF receptor TKI treatment in patients with ovarian cancer. *Gynecologic Oncology, 150*(1), 173–179. https://doi.org/10.1016/j.ygyno.2018.03.058.

Lo Muzio L., Arena, C., Troiano, G., & Villa, A. (2018). Oral stomatitis and mTOR inhibitors: a review of current evidence in 20,915 patients. *Oral Diseases, 24*, 144–171. https://doi.org/10.1111/odi.12795.

Maeda, H., Kobayashi, M., & Sakamoto, J. (2015). Evaluation and treatment of malignant ascites secondary to gastric cancer. *World Journal of Gastroenterology, 21*, 10936–10947. https://doi.org/10.3748/wjg.v21.i39.10936.

Malamood, M., Roberts, A., Kataria, R., Parkman, H. P., & Schey, R. (2017). Mirtazapine for symptom control in refractory gastroparesis. *Drug Design, Development and Therapy, 11*, 1035–1041. https://doi.org/10.2147/DDDT.S125743.

Maleux, G., Indesteege, I., Laenen, A., Verslype, C., Vergote, I., & Prenen, H. (2016). Tenckhoff tunneled peritoneal catheter placement in the palliative treatment of malignant ascites: technical results and overall clinical outcome. *Radiology and Oncology, 50*, 197–203. https://doi.org/10.1515/raon-2016-0002.

Mardas, M., Madry, R., & Stelmach-Mardas, M. (2017). Link between diet and chemotherapy related gastrointestinal side effects. *Contemporary Oncology (Pozn), 21*, 162–167. https://doi.org/10.5114/wo.2017.66896.

Maria, O. M., Eliopoulos, N., & Muanza, T. (2017). Radiation-induced oral mucositis. *Frontiers in Oncology. 7*, https://doi.org/10.3389/fonc.2017.00089. article 89.

Marx, W., Ried, K., McCarthy, A. L., Vitetta, L., Sali, A., McKavanagh, D., & Isenring, L. (2017). Ginger—mechanism of action in chemotherapy induced nausea and vomiting: a review. *Critical Reviews in Food Science and Nutrition, 57*, 141–146. https://doi.org/10.1080/10408398.2013.865590.

McLaughlin, L., & Mahon, S. M. (2014). Taste dysfunction and eating behaviors in survivors of head and neck cancer treatment. *MEDSURG Nursing, 23*, 165–171. https://doi.org/10.1188/12.CJON.171-178.

McQuade, R. M., Stojanovska, V., Abalo, R., Bornstein, J. C., & Nurgali, K. (2016). Chemotherapy- induced constipation and diarrhea: pathophysiology, current and emerging treatments. *Frontiers in Pharmacology, 7*, 414. https://doi.org/10.3389/fphar.2016.00414.

Mehra, N., Ganesan, P., Ganesan, T. S., Veeriah, S., Boopathy, A., Radhakrishnan, V., ... Sagar, T. G. (2018). Effectiveness of olanzapine in patients who fail therapy with aprepitant while receiving highly emetogenic chemotherapy. *Medical Oncology, 35*, 12. https://doi.org/10.1007/s12032-017-1074-3.

Mercadante, V., Al Hamad A., Lodi, G., Porter, S., & Fedele, S. (2017). Interventions for the management of radiotherapy-induced xerostomia and hyposalivation: a systematic review and meta-analysis. *Oral Oncology, 66*, 64–74. https://doi.org/10.1016/j.oraloncology.2016.12.031.

Miles, A., Moore, S., McFarlane, M., Lee, F., Allen, J., & Huckabee, M. L. (2013). Comparison of cough reflex test against instrumental assessment of aspiration. *Physiology & Behavior, 118*, 25–31. https://doi.org/10.1016/j.physbeh.2013.05.004.

Millsop, J. W., Wang, E. A., & Fazel, N. (2017). Etiology, evaluation, and management of xerostomia. *Clinics in Dermatology., 35*, 468–476. https://doi.org/10.1016/j.clindermatol.2017.06.010.

Molassiotis, A., Lee, P. H., Burke, T. A., Dicato, M., Gascon, P., Roila, F., & Aapro, M. (2016). Anticipatory nausea, risk factors, and its impact on chemotherapy-induced nausea and vomiting: results from the Pan European Emesis Registry study. *Journal of Pain and Symptom Management, 51*, 987–993. https://doi.org/10.1016/j.jpainsymman.2015.12.317.

Moslemi, D., Nokhandani, A. M., Otaghsaraei, M. T., Moghadamnia, Y., Kazemi, S., & Moghadamnia, A. A. (2016). Management of chemo/radiation-induced oral mucositis in patients with head and neck cancer: a review of the current literature. *Radiotherapy and Oncology, 120*, 13–20. https://doi.org/10.1016/j.radonc.2016.04.001.

Murray-Brown, F., & Dorman, S. (2015). Haloperidol for the treatment of nausea and vomiting in palliative care patients (review). *The Cochrane Collaboration.* (Issue 11). https://doi.org/10.1002/14651858.CD006271.pub3 Art. No.: CD006271.

National Cancer Institute. *Common terminology criteria for adverse events* (NCI CTCAE [version 5], 2018). https://ctep.cancer.gov/protocoldevelopment/electronic_applications/ctc.htm.

NCCN. (2018). *Clinical practice guidelines in oncology.* Antiemesis Version 1. https://www.nccn.org/professionals/physician_gls/default.aspx#supportive.

Navari, R. M. (2018). Managing nausea and vomiting in patients with cancer: what works. *Oncology, 32*(3), 121–125. 131, 136.

Oncology Nursing Society (ONS). (2017a). Putting evidence into practice. Chemotherapy-induced nausea and vomiting—adult. https://www.ons.org/practice-resources/pep/chemotherapy-induced-nausea-and-vomiting/.

Oncology Nursing Society (2017b). Putting evidence into practice (PEP): what's new in mucositis. Last update May 10th, 2017. Available at https://www.ons.org/practice-resources/pep/mucositis.

Pessi, M. A., Zilembo, N., Haspinger, E. R., Molino, L., Di Cosimo, S., Garassino, M., & Ripamonti, C. I. (2014). Targeted therapy-induced diarrhea: a review of the literature. *Critical Reviews in Oncology/Hematology, 90*, 165–179. https://doi.org/10.1016/j.critrevonc.2013.11.008.

Peterson, D. E., Boers-Doets, C. B., Bensadoun, R. J., & Herrstedt, J. (2015). Management of oral and gastrointestinal mucosal injury: ESMO clinical practice guidelines for diagnosis, treatment, and follow-up. *Annals of Oncology, 26*(Suppl 5), v139–v151. https://doi.org/10.1093/annonc/mdv202.

Peterson, D. E., O'Shaughnessy, J. A., Rugo, H. S., Elad, S., Schubert, M. M., Viet, C. T., ... Meiller, T. F. (2016). Oral mucosal injury caused by mammalian target of rapamycin inhibitors: emerging perspectives on pathobiology and impact on clinical practice. *Cancer Medicine, 5*, 1897–1907. https://doi.org/10.1002/cam4.761.

Rapone, B., Nardi, G. M., Di Venere, D., Pettini, F., Grassi, F. R., & Corsalini, M. (2016). Oral hygiene in patient with oral cancer undergoing chemotherapy and/or radiotherapy after prosthesis rehabilitation: protocol proposal. *Oral & Implantology, 9*(Suppl 1), 90–97. https://doi.org/10.11138/orl/2016.9.1S.090.

Rha, S. Y., Sohn, J., Kim, G. M., Kim, H. R., & Lee, J. (2018). The benefit of pro re nata antiemetics provided with guideline-consistent antiemetics in delayed nausea control. *Cancer Nurs, 41*(2), E49–E57. https://doi.org/10.1097/NCC.0000000000000484.

Rhondali, W., Nguyen, L., Palmer, J. L., Kang, D.-H., Hui, D., & Bruera, E. (2013). Self-reported constipation in patients with advanced cancer: a preliminary report. *Journal of Pain and Symptom Management, 45*, 23–32. https://doi.org/10.1016/j.jpainsymman.2012.01.009.

Riley, P., Glenny, A. M., Hua, F., & Worthington, H. V. (2017). Pharmacological interventions for preventing dry mouth and salivary gland dysfunction following radiotherapy. *Cochrane Database of Systematic Reviews, Issue, 7*, CD012744. https://doi.org/10.1002/14651858.CD012744.

Ruhlmann, C. H., Jahn, F., Jordan, K., Dennis, K., Maranzano, E., Molassiotis, A., ... Feyer, P. (2017). 2016 updated MASCC/ESMO consensus recommendations: prevention of radiotherapy-induced nausea and vomiting. *Supportive Care in Cancer, 25*, 309–316. https://doi.org/10.1007/s00520-016-3407-8.

Sasegbon, A., & Hamdy, S. (2017). The anatomy and physiology of normal and abnormal swallowing in oropharyngeal dysphagia. *Neurogastroenterology & Motility. 29*. https://doi.org/10.1111/nmo.13100.

Sangisetty, S. L., & Miner, T. J. (2012). Malignant ascites: a review of prognostic factors, pathophysiology and therapeutic measures. *World Journal of Gastrointestinal Surgery, 4*(4), 87–95. https://doi.org/10.4240/wjgs.v4.i4.87.

Sharkey, K. A., Darmani, N. A., & Parker, L. A. (2014). Regulation of nausea and vomiting by cannabinoids and the endocannabinoid system. *European Journal of Pharmacology, 722*, 134–146. https://doi.org/10.1016/j.ejphar.2013.09.068.

Singh, P., & Kuo, B. (2016). Central aspects of nausea and vomiting in GI disorders. *Current Treatment Options in Gastroenterology, 14*, 444–451. https://doi.org/10.1007/s11938-016-0107-x.

Soliman, G. H., & Shehata, O. S. (2015). Efficacy of cryotherapy on oral mucositis prevention among patients with head and neck cancers who undergoing radiotherapy. *IOSR Journal of Nursing and Health Science, 4*(4), 53–61.

Stukan, M. (2017). Drainage of malignant ascites: patient selection and perspectives. *Cancer Management and Research, 9*, 115–130. https://doi.org/10.2147/CMAR.S100210.

Sweetser, S. (2012). Evaluating the patient with diarrhea: a case-based approach. *Mayo Clinic Proceedings, 87*, 596–602. https://doi.org/10.1016/j.mayocp.2012.02.015.

Verdonschot, R. J. C. G., Baijens, L. W. J., Vanbelle, S., van de Kolk, I., Kremer, B., & Leue, C. (2017). Affective symptoms in patients with oropharyngeal dysphagia: a systematic review. *Journal of Psychosomatic Research, 97*, 102–110. https://doi.org/10.1016/j.jpsychores.2017.04.006.

Vigarios, E., Epstein, J. B., & Sibaud, V. (2017). Oral mucosal changes induced by anticancer targeted therapies and immune checkpoint inhibitors. *Supportive Care in Cancer, 25*, 1713–1739. https://doi.org/10.1007/s00520-017-3629-4.

Villa, A., & Akintoye, S. O. (2018). Dental management of patients who have undergone oral cancer therapy. *Dental Clinics of North America, 62*, 131–142. https://doi.org/10.1016/j.cden.2017.08.010.

Villa, A., & Sonis, S. T. (2015). Mucositis: pathobiology and management. *Current Opinion in Oncology, 27*, 159–164. https://doi.org/10.1097/CCO.0000000000000180.

Walsh, D., Davis, M., Ripamonti, C., Bruera, E., Davies, A., & Molassiotis, A. (2017). 2016 updated MASCC/ESMO consensus recommendations: management of nausea and vomiting in advanced cancer. *Supportive Care in Cancer, 25*, 333–340. https://doi.org/10.1007/s00520-016-3371-3.

Wickham, R. J. (2017). Managing constipation in adults with cancer. *Journal of the Advanced Practitioner in Oncology, 8*, 149–161.

Williams, A. R., Mowlazadeh, B., Sisler, L., & Williams, P. D. (2015). Self-reported assessment of symptoms and self-care within a

cohort of U.S. veterans during outpatient care for cancer. *Clinical Journal of Oncology Nursing, 19*, 595–602. https://doi.org/10.1188/15.CJON.595-602.

Wirth, R., Dziewas, R., Beck, A. M., Clave, P., Hamdy, S., Heppner, H. J., … Volkert, D. (2016). Oropharyngeal dysphagia in older persons – from pathophysiology to adequate intervention: a review and summary of an international expert meeting. *Clinical Interventions in Aging, 11*, 189–208. https://doi.org/10.2147/CIA.S97481.

Pedersen, A. M. L., … Dawes, C. (2017). A guide to medications inducing salivary gland dysfunction, xerostomia, and subjective sialorrhea: a systematic review. *Drugs in R & D, 17*, 1–28.

Yeung, S.-C. J. (2016). Diarrhea. In K. H. Todd & C. R. Thomas Jr., (Eds.), *Oncologic Emergenc Medicine* (pp. 319–326). Switzerland: Springer International Publishing.

Zaini, S., Guan, N. C., Sulaiman, A. H., Zainal, N. Z., Huri, H. Z., & Shamsudin, S. H. (2018). The use of antidepressants for physical symptoms in cancer. *Current Drug Targets, 19*. https://doi.org/10.2174/1389450119666180226125026. online ahead of print.

Zecha, J. A. E. M., Raber-Durlacher, J. E., Nair, R. G., Epstein, J. B., Elad, S., Hamblin, M. R., … Bensadoun, R.-J. (2016). Low-level laser therapy/photobiomodulation in the management of side effects of chemoradiation therapy in head and neck cancer: part 2: proposed applications and treatment protocols. *Supportive Care in Cancer, 24*, 2793–2805. https://doi.org/10.1007/s00520-016-3153-y.

Zuniga, S. A., Ebersole, B., & Jamal, N. (2018). Utility of Eating Assessment Tool-10 in predicting aspiration in patients with unilateral vocal fold paralysis. *Otolaryngol Head Neck Surg, 159*(1), 92–96. https://doi.org/10.1177/0194599818762328.

38

Genitourinary Symptoms

Sally Maliski

URINARY INCONTINENCE

Overview

I. Physiology (see Chapter 15)
- A. Definition
  1. Urinary incontinence—involuntary loss of urine to the extent it becomes a problem
  2. Stress—involuntary loss of urine during laughing, coughing, sneezing, or other physical activities that increase abdominal pressure
  3. Urge—involuntary loss of urine with an abrupt and strong desire to void
  4. Reflex—involuntary loss of urine with no sensation of urge or bladder fullness
  5. Functional—state in which an individual experiences incontinence because of difficulty in reaching or inability to reach the toilet before urination
  6. Total—continuous loss of urine without distention or awareness of bladder fullness
  7. Urinary retention—chronic inability to void followed by involuntary voiding (overflow incontinence) due to overdistention of the bladder (Society of Urologic Nursing and Associates, 2017)
- B. Mechanisms
  1. Storage problems
     a. Involuntary contracting of bladder during filling
     b. Reduced compliance of bladder wall
     c. Sensory urgency
     d. Loss of bladder neck and proximal urethra support (Chang, Hung, Hu, & Chu, 2018)
     e. Intrinsic sphincter dysfunction
  2. Emptying problems
     a. Loss of or impaired contractility
     b. Urethral or prostatic obstruction

II. Risk factors
- A. Disease related
  1. Loss of ability to inhibit bladder or rectal contractions (Society for Urology Nursing and Associates, 2017)
  2. Loss of sphincter competency (Society for Urology Nursing and Associates, 2017)
     a. Impaired or lost sensation of the bladder
     b. Obstruction of the bladder
     c. Immobility commonly associated with chronic degenerative disease
     d. Loss of functional ability
     e. Previous transurethral resection of the prostate, anastomotic stricture, stage of disease, surgical technique, experience of the surgeon (Society for Urology Nursing and Associates, 2017)
- B. Treatment related
  1. Surgical intervention that disrupts neural pathways.
  2. Inflammatory reaction from radiation therapy (RT) on bladder and bowel
  3. Chemotherapy agents that cause neurotoxic side effects
  4. Fistula formation as a complication of disease, surgery, or RT
  5. Cryosurgery, which may cause urinary incontinence, urethral sloughing, bladder neck obstruction (Society for Urology Nursing and Associates, 2017)
  6. Medications, including anticholinergics, diuretics, narcotics, sedatives, hypnotics, tranquilizers, and laxatives
  7. Complications associated with indwelling catheter (Society of Urologic Nursing and Associates, 2017; Jahn, Beutner, & Langer, 2012)

Assessment

I. History
- A. Personal history
- B. Cognitive ability
- C. Neurologic disease or symptoms
- D. Motivation to self-care in toileting
- E. Manual dexterity and mobility
- F. Living arrangements
- G. Identification of caregiver and degree of caregiver involvement
- H. Prescription and nonprescription medications
- I. Impact of incontinence on self-esteem and interpersonal relationships

II. Past and present patterns of elimination
- A. Precipitants of incontinence—caffeine and alcohol consumption, physical activity
  1. Surgery, trauma, recent illnesses
- B. Daily fluid intake

C. Urinary tract symptoms

D. Duration of incontinence

E. Frequency and amount of continence and incontinence

F. Previous treatments and its effects

G. Bladder diary for 3 days (Society for Urology Nursing and Associates, 2017)

III. Physical findings

A. Presence of abdominal masses

B. Palpation of full bladder

C. Pelvic organ prolapse

D. Fecal impaction to be ruled out

E. Neurologic assessment

F. Presence of incontinence, odor, perineal skin irritation or breakdown

IV. Diagnostic testing

A. Urinalysis and culture and sensitivity

B. Cough stress test

C. Presence and amount of postvoiding residual urine

D. Urodynamic and imaging studies

E. Cystoscopy to identify site of obstruction (Society of Urologic Nursing and Associates, 2017)

Management

I. Medical Management

A. Interventions to promote urinary continence

1. Anticholinergics

2. Tricyclic antidepressants

3. Potassium channel openers (Society for Urology Nursing and Associates, 2017)

4. Electrostimulation (Society for Urology Nursing and Associates, 2017)

5. Urology consultation

II. Nursing management

A. Supportive techniques

1. Assess and minimize barriers to toileting

2. Daily assessment of perianal skin

3. Instruct patient to clean area after every voiding or bowel movement

4. Apply moisture barrier ointment or skin barrier

5. Use of absorbent pads or briefs (Society for Urologic Nursing and Associates, 2017)

6. Use of penile compression devices for males and pessaries for females (Society for Urologic Nursing and Associates, 2017)

7. Use of external condom and internal catheters (Jahn et al., 2012)

B. Behavioral techniques

1. Establish a routine schedule for voiding (habit training)

2. Ask the patient on a regular basis about voiding (prompt voiding)

3. Teach the patient to suppress the urge to void (bladder retraining)

4. Teach the patient how to perform Kegel exercises

5. Have the patient decrease fluid intake in the evening

6. Have the patient reduce intake of caffeine-containing beverages and other bladder irritants

OSTOMIES AND URINARY DIVERSIONS

Overview

I. Urinary diversions

A. Surgically created to divert the urine stream away from the original lower urinary tract

1. Performed in situations in which the bladder is removed—that is, radical cystectomy or radical cystoprostatectomy for cancer of the bladder

2. Involves removal of the bladder, pelvic lymph nodes, prostate (in men) and uterus, fallopian tubes, ovaries, and anterior vaginal wall, possibly urethra (in women)

3. Sexual dysfunction common because of neural damage from surgery (Yarbro, Wujik, & Gobel, 2018)

B. Types of urinary diversions (Thalmann, 2017)

1. Ileal conduit

a. Created from segment of small bowel; as the proximal end is sutured closed the distal end is brought out through the abdominal wall; a stoma is created, and the ureters are implanted into the small-bowel segment

b. Urine produced almost continuously

c. Requires an external collection device

d. High risk for urinary tract infections and stone formation (Society for Urology Nursing and Associates, 2017)

C. Continent diversions (Pearce & Daneshmand, 2018)

1. Reservoir constructed from ileum or large intestine

2. Construction of the reservoir via a one-way-flap valve (Society for Urology Nursing and Associates, 2017)

3. External collection device not needed

a. Patient will need to catheterize through the stoma every 4 to 6 hours

D. Orthoptic neobladder (Kretschmer, Grimm, Buchner, Stief, & Karl, 2016)

1. A surgically constructed bladder created from the intestine and attached to urethra

2. Intermittent catheterization needed for urinary retention

3. Voiding by relaxation of urinary sphincters and simultaneous Valsalva maneuver

4. Contraindications to neobladder—cancer extending into urethra, history of inflammatory bowel disease, radiation, or previous bowel resection (Society for Urology Nursing and Associates, 2017)

II. Risk factors

A. Pelvic radiation

B. Chemotherapy

C. Bladder cancer with muscle invasion (Society for Urology Nursing and Associates, 2017)

III. Effects of treatment
   A. Pelvic exenteration
   B. Pelvic and abdominal radiation
   C. Mucosal damage when the stoma is in the field of radiation (Society for Urology Nursing and Associates, 2017)

Assessment

I. Pertinent personal history
   A. Type of surgery and stoma
   B. Previous pelvic or abdominal radiation or chemotherapy treatments
   C. Changes in patterns of urinary elimination
   D. Recurrent or chronic urinary tract infections
   E. Difficulty in catheterizing a continent diversion
   F. Diet habits and fluid consumption

II. Physical findings
   A. Characteristics of stoma and peristomal skin
   B. Presence of leakage of urine from a continent diversion

Management

I. Nursing management
   A. Interventions regarding care of urinary diversion
      1. Teach patient how to care for urinary diversion
         a. Stoma placement
         b. Scars, bony prominences, skin creases, belt line, or hernia to be avoided
      2. Select appliance based on type of effluent, abdominal contour, manual dexterity, patient preference, cost
      3. Change appliance every 5 days and as needed
      4. Ensure barrier clears stoma by {⅛} inch; protect exposed skin with barrier paste
      5. Gently remove pouch by pushing down on skin while lifting up on the pouch
      6. Cleanse peristomal skin with water and pat dry
      7. Assess stoma and skin around stoma with each appliance change
      8. Empty pouch when one-third to one-half full and before chemotherapy
      9. Protect stoma from injury (Society for Urology Nursing and Associates, 2017)
      10. Monitor volume, color, and consistency of effluent
      11. Monitor functioning of new urinary diversion starting 3 to 5 days after surgery
      12. Catheterize new continent diversions 3 to 4 weeks after surgery (Society for Urology Nursing and Associates, 2017)
         a. Ureteral stents are irrigated every 6 to 8 hours several weeks postoperatively
         b. As urinary output from continent diversion increases, urine output from ureteral stents decreases
      13. Catheterize through the stoma to drain urine from the reservoir every 4 to 6 hours
      14. Recommend referral to the wound, ostomy, continence nurse if needed
   B. Interventions to promote body image and self-esteem
      1. Acknowledge normalcy of emotional response to change in urinary function
      2. Encourage patient to verbalize positive or negative feelings
      3. Assist patient in incorporating changes into activities of daily living, social life interpersonal relationships, and occupational activities
      4. Help patient identify ways to cope that have been useful in the past
      5. Refer patient and caregivers to support groups and provide resources

RENAL DYSFUNCTION

Overview

I. Pathophysiology (see Chapter 15)
II. Risk factors
   A. Effects of disease
      1. Compression of ureters by metastatic tumor causing obstruction, resulting in hydronephrosis (Society for Urology Nursing and Associates, 2017)
      2. Compression of blood vessels by mass or tumor may cause venous occlusion
         a. Reduction of blood flow may impair kidney function
      3. Inability of kidneys to concentrate urine occurs in hypercalcemia of malignancy
         a. Kidneys are attempting to excrete calcium in blood, leading to diuresis and electrolyte disturbances
         b. Hypercalcemia of malignancy occurs more commonly in breast cancer with metastases, multiple myeloma, squamous cell cancer of the lung and head and neck, renal cell cancer, lymphomas, and leukemia (Thomas, 2014; Yarbro Wujik, & Gobel, 2018)
      4. Advanced prostate or cervical cancer renal problems are related to postrenal obstructive uropathy (Yarbro et al., 2018)
   B. Treatment related
      1. Radiation to renal structures may lead to permanent fibrosis and atrophy
      2. Precipitation of uric acid or calcium phosphate crystallization from tumor lysis
      3. Fluid and electrolyte imbalances caused by chemotherapy agents
      4. Nephrotoxic agents cause a direct effect

Assessment

I. Pertinent personal history to identify risk factors
   A. Advanced age
   B. Diuretics, cardiac and nephrotoxic medications
   C. Type of malignancy

D. Comorbidities such as hypertension, diabetes insipidus, diabetes mellitus

E. Previous pelvic or abdominal radiation or chemotherapy treatments

F. Renal stones

G. Preexisting renal impairment

II. Physical findings

A. Cardiovascular—arrhythmias, rapid thready pulse, orthostatic hypotension

B. Neurologic—lethargy, confusion

C. Poor skin turgor, dry mucous membranes

D. Gastrointestinal (GI)—nausea, vomiting, polydipsia, splenomegaly

E. Genitourinary—nocturia, polyuria, oliguria, flank pain, dysuria

III. Laboratory data

A. Serum creatinine and blood urea nitrogen (BUN) levels reflect renal function

B. Creatinine clearance study before implementing nephrotoxic chemotherapy

C. Elevation of serum uric acid and calcium levels and a decrease in potassium and magnesium levels may suggest renal impairment (Thomas, 2014; Yarbro et al., 2018)

Management

I. Medical management

A. Pharmacologic interventions

1. Saline hydration with appropriate diuretic (Thomas, 2014)

2. Oral or intravenous (IV) sodium bicarbonate to maintain alkaline urine

3. Amifostine and sodium thiosulfate for cisplatin nephrotoxicity (Thomas, 2014)

4. Replace electrolytes as needed

5. Administer diuretics as needed

II. Nursing management

A. Interventions to incorporate patient and family in care

1. Teach about maintaining adequate hydration and safe weight-bearing activity

2. Teach signs and symptoms of electrolyte imbalance and fluid volume excess and the appropriate time to seek medical attention

3. Explain properties of medications prescribed

B. Monitor for signs and symptoms of renal toxicity

1. Verify baseline renal function

2. Monitor intake and output closely

a. Maintain a greater intake than output unless contraindicated

b. Monitor for obstructive diuresis after the removal of obstruction

c. Strain urine for stones if indicated

3. Monitor vital signs and postural blood pressure

4. Monitor relevant laboratory data

5. Record daily weights

6. Maximize mobility (Yarbro et al., 2018)

III. Interventions to incorporate patient and family in care

A. Teach about maintaining adequate hydration and safe weight-bearing activity

B. Teach signs and symptoms of electrolyte imbalance and fluid volume excess, and the appropriate time to seek medical attention

C. Explain properties of medications prescribed

Expected Patient Outcomes

I. The patient will maintain adequate hydration, urinary output, and urinary continence.

II. The patient will verbalize understanding of behavioral techniques to decrease urinary incontinence.

III. The patient will be able to care for the urinary diversion device.

IV. The patient will verbalize coping skills and signs of acceptance for urinary diversion device.

REFERENCES

Chang, L. W., Hung, S. C., Hu, J. C., & Chu, K. Y. (2018). Retzius sparing robotic-assisted prostatectomy associated with less bladder neck descent and better early continence outcomes. *Anticancer Research*, 38(1), 345–351.

Jahn, P., Beutner, K., & Langer, G. (2012). Types of indwelling urinary catheters for long-term bladder drainage in adults. *Cochrane Database Systematic Reviews*. 10, CD004997 https://doi.org/10.1002/14651858.CD004997.pub3CD004997.

Kretschmer, A., Grimm, T., Buchner, A., Stief, C. G., & Karl, A. (2016). Prognostic features for quality of life after radical cystectomy and orthotopic neobladder. *International Brazilian Journal of Urology*, 42(6), 1109–1120. https://doi.org/10.1590/S1677-5538.IBJU.2015.0491.

Pearce, S. M., & Daneshmand, S. (2018). Continent cutaneous diversion. *Urology Clinics of North America*, 45(1), 55–65. https://doi.org/10.1016/j.ucl.2017.09.004.

Society for Urologic Nursing and Associates. (2017). *Urologic nursing: scope and standards: Society for Urologic Nursing and Associates.*

Thalmann, G. N. (2017). Quality improvement in cystectomy with enhanced recovery (QUICCER). *British Journal of Urology*, 119(1), 4–5. https://doi.org/10.1111/bju.13553.

Thomas, N. (Ed.), (2014). *Renal nursing* (4th ed.). Edinburgh: Elsevier.

Yarbro, C. H., Wujik, D., & Gobel, B. H. (2018). *Cancer nursing: principles and practice* (8th ed.). Sudbury, MA: Jones & Bartlett.

39

Hematologic and Immune Symptoms

Eileen Galvin

OVERVIEW

I. Definition—*myelosuppression,* a reduction in bone marrow function that results in a reduced production of red blood cells (RBCs), white blood cells (WBCs), and platelets (Plt) into the peripheral circulation (Rodlin et al., 2017).

II. Physiology (Aliper, et al., 2014; Flowers, 2013, Kurtin & Bilotti, 2013; Lyman, 2014; Manea, 2014; Morrison & Scadden, 2014; Rodlin et al., 2017; Zhu et al., 2017)

A. The bone marrow is the primary source for development of the components of blood (hematopoiesis), including myeloid and lymphoid progenitor cells.

1. Myeloid cells include granulocytes (neutrophils, eosinophils, basophils, monocytes), RBCs, and platelets.

2. Lymphoid cells include B and T lymphocytes.

B. Risk factors for myelotoxicity are broadly categorized into three types: disease related, patient related, and treatment related.

C. Chemotherapy-induced myelosuppression is the most common dose-limiting adverse event in cancer treatment.

1. Each antineoplastic agent varies with respect to the onset and duration of cytopenias, depending on pharmacokinetic variables: dose, frequency, route of administration, absorption, distribution, metabolism, and excretion.

D. Treatment-related myeloid cytopenias, neutropenia and thrombocytopenia, are most common.

1. Neutropenia—absolute neutrophil count (ANC) below 1500/mm^3 places the patient at increased risk of infection and sepsis.

2. Thrombocytopenia—platelet count below the normal range; places the patient at increased risk of bleeding

3. Anemia—hemoglobin below 10 g/dL places the patient at increased risk of fatigue and tissue hypoxia

E. The severity of myeloid cytopenias is based on common grading criteria (Table 39.1).

F. Treatment-related lymphopenia is less common.

1. Lymphopenia, a reduction in the number of B or T lymphocytes, places the patient at risk for opportunistic infections.

NEUTROPENIA

Overview

I. Definition—a decrease in the number of circulating neutrophils in the blood evidenced by ANC less than the lower limit of normal (LLN) (see Table 39.1)

A. Lifespan—1 to 3 days (as little as 6 hours in stress situations)

B. How to calculate ANC: Total WBC × Total Neutrophil count (% segmented neutrophil count + % bands) = ANC. Example:

1. WBC = 3.1 1000/μL

2. Neutrophils (25%) + bands (10%) = 35%

3. ANC = 3100 × 0.35 = 1085/mm^3 = grade 2 neutropenia

II. Physiology (Aliper, 2014; Lyman, et al., 2014, Kurtin, 2012; Morrison, 2014)

A. Chemotherapy-induced neutropenia (CIN) is one of the most common dose-limiting toxicities associated with systemic treatment for cancer.

B. Neutrophils divide rapidly and are susceptible to the cytotoxic effects of chemotherapy.

C. Chemotherapy and radiation therapy may also damage the bone marrow microenvironment, including the stroma and cytokine milieu.

1. Radiation to bone marrow–producing regions—pelvis, ribs, sternum, skull, metaphyses of the long bones—may cause prolonged cytopenias.

III. Risk factors (Flowers et al., 2013; National Comprehensive Cancer Network, 2018) (Table 39.2)

A. Host-related factors

B. Treatment-related factors

1. Type and dose of chemotherapy

2. Location of radiation therapy

Assessment

See Table 39.3.

Management (see Table 39.3)

I. Medical management (Aliper et al., 2014; Flowers et al, 2013; Kurtin & Bilotti, 2013; Lyman et al., 2014; NCCN, 2015; Pherwani et al., 2015; Thomas et al, 2015; Vioral & Wentley, 2015; Yu et al., 2015)

TABLE 39.1   Overview of Neutropenia

Neutropenia	A decrease in the number of circulating neutrophils in the blood evidenced by an absolute neutrophil count (ANC) less than 1000/µl	Grade 1: ANC < LLN—1500/mm³ Grade 2: ANC < 500–1000/mm³ Grade 3: ANC <1000–500/mm³ Grade 4: ANC <500/mm³
Febrile neutropenia (FN)	ANC <1000/mm³ and a single temperature of >38.3°C (101°F) or a sustained temperature of ≥38°C (100.4°F) for more than 1 hour	

From CTC-AE version 4, Leiding, J. W. (2017). Neutrophil evolution and their diseases in humans. *Frontiers in Immunology. 8*(1009). https://doi.org/10.3389/fimmu.2017.01009; Lyman, G., Esteban, A., & Pettengell, R. (2014). Risk factors for febrile neutropenia among patients with cancer receiving chemotherapy: a systematic review. *Critical Reviews in Oncology /Hematology, 90*(3), 190–199; Nesher, L., & Rolston, K. V. (2014). The current spectrum of infection in cancer patients with chemotherapy related neutropenia. *Infection, 42*(1), 5–13.

TABLE 39.2   Risk Factors Associated with Chemotherapy-Induced Myeloid Toxicity

Host-Related Factors	Disease- and Treatment-Related Factors
Age greater than 65 years	High tumor burden/extensive disease
Female gender	History of chemotherapy or radiation
Body surface area <2 m²	Preexisting cytopenias
ECOG performance scale (PS) ≥2	Bone marrow involvement with tumor
Malnutrition	Type of chemotherapy
Decrease immune function	Dose intensity of chemotherapy
Comorbidities: COPD, diabetes, renal impairment, and liver disease	Elevated lactate dehydrogenase level
	Neutropenia lasting more than 4 days after an episode of FN
Open wounds or recent surgery	Concurrent mucositis, colitis, or typhlitis
	ICU admission
	DIC
Active infection or preexisting fungal infections	Cross-reactive protein level greater than 100 mg/L at day 5 of treatment for FN
Drug–drug interactions	Bleeding severe enough to require transfusion
	Arrhythmia or electrocardiographic changes requiring treatment
	Hypoalbuminemia
	Hyperbilirubinemia, hematologic malignancy, hospitalization

COPD, chronic obstructive pulmonary disease; *DIC,* disseminated intravascular coagulation; *ECOG,* Eastern Cooperative Oncology Group; *FN,* febrile neutropenia; *ICU,* intensive care unit.

TABLE 39.3   Assessment and Recommendations for Prevention and Management of Chemotherapy-Induced Neutropenia and Febrile Neutropenia

Assessment	• See Table 39.2 for a description of risk factors for CIN due to disease-related, host-related, and treatment-related factors • Review of current/previous cancer therapy; chemotherapy, radiation therapy, and multimodal therapy • Previous neutropenia or neutropenic fevers • Hematopoietic growth factor use • Review of bone marrow biopsy report, if available, to determine bone marrow involvement or hypocellularity • Evaluate vital signs; fever most common manifestation of infection, rigors (should be treated immediately), hypotension or tachypnea, evaluate characteristic signs of infection (erythema, induration, drainage, and cough), assess for change in mental status.
Laboratory data	• CBC with differential, calculation of ANC, culture and sensitivity of urine, blood, stool, sputum, CSF, wound, and drainage tubes
Radiology	• Chest radiography (PA and lateral) • Patient and caregiver education for infection prevention appropriate to the level of risk
Prevention	• Prophylactic use of colony-stimulating factors is recommended when: • Risk of CTC-AE grades 3–4 or FN is >20% in the setting of potentially curable disease or where dose intensity is necessary for optimal clinical outcomes • Risk of CTC-AE 3–4 CIN or FN is 10%–20% in patients with high-risk profile (see Table 27.1) • FDA-approved agents: • Filgrastim (Neupogen: see dosing guidelines at www.neupogen.com) • Filgrastim-sndz (Zarxio: see dosing guidelines at http://www.zarxio.com) • Pegfilgrastim (Neulasta: see dosing guidelines at www.neulasta.com)
Management of CIN	• Consider prophylactic antibiotics for patients with hematologic malignancies at very high risk for FN—fluoroquinolone ± glycopeptide, antifungal, antiviral • Implement primary prevention as noted earlier • Establish a plan for close monitoring of blood counts in initial phase of treatment where risk is greatest • Review reportable signs and symptoms with patients and caregivers, including who to contact and how to do so

TABLE 39.3 Assessment and Recommendations for Prevention and Management of Chemotherapy-Induced Neutropenia and Febrile Neutropenia—cont'd

	• Subsequent treatment may require dose modification, dose delay, or administration of G-CSF agents as secondary prophylaxis • Low-risk patients with anticipated early recovery can be managed in an outpatient setting • Most common AEs associated with G-CSF agents include bone pain, myalgia, arthralgia, and fever • Bone pain can be effectively managed with naproxen 225 mg and loratadine 10 mg q12h at the onset of bone pain and continue until resolved (generally 48–72 hr)
Management of FN	• Considered a medical emergency • Prompt intervention is critical to avoid morbidity and mortality • Rapid assessment for risk of clinical deterioration • Implement institutional standard of care for FN, including obtaining cultures (blood and urine), PA and lateral chest x-ray, viral and VRE swabs if indicated, and prompt administration of IV antibiotics (cefepime most common first-line agent) • Unstable patients should be transported by emergency medical services equipped with ACLS capabilities • Patients at very high risk for poor-prognosis FN may require ICU admission

AE, adverse event; *ACLS*, advanced cardiac life support; *ANC*, absolute neutrophil count; *CBC*, complete blood count; *CIN*, chemotherapy-induced neutropenia; *CSF*, cerebrospinal fluid; *CTC-AE*, Common Terminology Criteria for Adverse Events; *FDA*, U.S. Food and Drug Administration; *FN*, febrile neutropenia; *G-CSF*, granulocyte colony-stimulating factor; hypotension, systolic blood pressure <90 mm Hg; *ICU*, intensive care unit; *IV*, intravenous; *PA*, posteroanterior; tachypnea, respiratory rate >24; *VRE*, vancomycin-resistant enterococci.

TABLE 39.4 General Factors Associated with Poor-Prognosis FN

Hypotension—systolic blood pressure (SBP) less than 90 mm Hg
Tachypnea—respiratory rate (RR) greater than 24 breaths/min
Serum albumin— less than 3.3 g/dL
Serum bicarbonate level—less than 21 mmol/L
High procalcitonin level—greater than 2.0 ng/mL
Cross-reactive protein level—greater than 20 mg/L at baseline
Circulating soluble triggering receptor (sTREM-1) —greater than100 pg/mL
High pentraxin 3 (PTX3) levels at the onset of FN

A. Intensive care unit (ICU) admission for patients with febrile neutropenia (FN) at high risk for poor prognosis (Table 39.4)
II. Nursing management (Kurtin, 2012)
   A. Interventions to minimize the occurrence of infection
      1. Use strict hand washing technique
      2. Encourage patient to bathe daily, taking care to maintain meticulous personal hygiene, including oral and perineal care
      3. Restrict presence of vases with fresh flowers or other sources of stagnant water
      4. Limit visitors to those without communicable illness, especially children
      5. Change water in pitchers, denture cups, and nebulizers daily
   B. Use aseptic technique for all nursing interventions, including all indwelling catheters (e.g., venous access devices; urinary, biliary, or feeding tubes), wounds, or invasive procedures; specific institutional guidelines to be referred to for management of central catheters
III. Interventions to monitor for complications
   A. Establish a plan for monitoring blood counts based on the patient's individual risk profile (see Table 39.2)
   B. Monitor for nadir (the lowest point of the blood cell levels after cancer treatment)
      1. Nadir becomes apparent as immature cells in the marrow are destroyed and become absent in the bloodstream
      2. Usually 7 to 14 days after chemotherapy, with variability for combined modality treatments, nitrosourea agents, and radiation to the pelvis
      3. Occasional occurrence after biotherapy
      4. Usually after multimodal treatment; nadir occurring sooner and more severely than from single-modality therapy
   C. Cancer treatment may be delayed for an ANC less than 1000 to 1500/mm^3
   D. Monitor for signs and symptoms of infection
IV. Interventions to incorporate patient and family in care
   A. Teach about personal hygiene measures to minimize the occurrence of infection—examples: wiping the perineal area from front to back after voiding and after a stool; daily bathing
   B. Teach about infection precautions and how to minimize the risk of infection—example: strict hand washing
   C. Teach about subcutaneous administration of hematopoietic growth factors
   D. Teach about the symptoms for which to call the physician or nurse, such as temperature higher than 100.5°F (38.1°C), productive cough, painful urination, or sore throat

ANEMIA

Overview

I. Definition—a disorder characterized by a reduction in the amount of hemoglobin in 100 mL of blood (CTC-AE version 4) (Table 39.5)
   A. Patients at increased risk of fatigue, tachycardia, tachypnea, chest pain, dyspnea, and syncope
   B. Risk related to severity of anemia (Table 39.6)
II. Physiology (Aliper et al., 2014; Morrison & Scadden, 2014)

A. Erythrocytes are developed from the myeloid stem cells in bone marrow.
B. Function of RBCs is to carry oxygen to all cells in the body.
C. Anemia is a common finding in patients with cancer, with an incidence ranging from 30% to 90% (Gilreath, Stenehjem, & Ro, 2014).
III. Risk factors (Bertlotti et al., 2017; Li et al., 2017; Russell et al., 2017) (see Table 39.6)
   A. Patient-related factors
   B. Disease-related factors
   C. Treatment-related factors

Assessment

See Table 39.7.

TABLE 39.5 Definition of Anemia

Anemia	A disorder characterized by a reduction in the amount of hemoglobin in 100 mL of blood A hemoglobin value below 10 g/dL places the patient at increased risk of fatigue and tissue hypoxia Red blood cell (RBC) lifespan is 120 days Normal value gender specific: Female – hemoglobin (Hgb): 11.5–15.5 g/dL; hematocrit (Hct): 35%–46% Male – Hgb: 13.5–17.5 g/dL; Hct: 40%–51%	Grade 1: Hgb < LLN—10.0 g/dL Grade 2: Hgb < 10.0–8.0 g/dL Grade 3: Hgb <8.0 g/dL, transfusion indicated Grade 4: Hgb <6.2–4.9 g/dL, life-threatening consequences; urgent intervention indicated

Common Terminology Criteria for Adverse Events version 4

TABLE 39.6 Risk Factors Associated with Chemotherapy-Induced Anemia

Host-Related Factors	Disease- and Treatment-Related Factors
See Table 39.2 Autoimmune hemolytic anemia Chronic GI blood loss Malnutrition with deficiencies of folic acid, vitamin B12 Chronic renal insufficiency Rare genetic disorders that affect RBC production – thalassemia	Invasion of tumor cells in the bone marrow or cancers involving the bone marrow; multiple myeloma, lymphoma, leukemia, or myelodysplastic syndrome Erythroid leukemia Type of chemotherapy Dose intensity of chemotherapy Drug-induced RBC aplasia (rare)

GI, Gastrointestinal; *RBC*, red blood cell.

TABLE 39.7 Assessment and Recommendations for Management of Chemotherapy-Induced Anemia

Assessment	• Previous cancer treatment history: chemotherapy, radiation therapy, or multimodal therapy. • Current medications that could alter RBC function. • Social history of alcohol and illicit drug use. • Assess for bleeding from nose, rectum, ears, oral cavity; assess blood in stool, urine, and vomitus.
Laboratory data Prevention	• Assess menstrual bleeding and the number of sanitary napkins or tampons used. • Assess for changes that indicate intracranial bleeding: level of consciousness, restlessness, headache, seizures, pupil changes, ataxia. • CBC with platelets and differential. • Evaluation of contributing factors for anemia: iron deficiency, folate deficiency, vitamin B12 deficiency, GI blood loss, hemolysis screening, thyroid function, testosterone level, serum Epo level. • Identification of patients at high risk for anemia and the secondary effects. • Consideration of individual characteristics of the patient such as underlying comorbidities affected by anemia; cardiovascular and pulmonary diseases.
Treatment of CIA	• Patient and caregiver education for conservation of energy, planning of activities, and reportable signs and symptoms. • Establish a plan of care for monitoring blood counts and follow-up. • Maintain a current type and screen for patients requiring frequent transfusions.
Transfusion of PRBCs	• Evaluation of symptoms of anemia with consideration of individual patient characteristics. • Treat the underlying cause(s). • Weigh the risks and benefits of each treatment approach (PRBC transfusion, ESA administration).

TABLE 39.7 Assessment and Recommendations for Management of Chemotherapy-Induced Anemia—cont'd

| | • Requires informed consent.
| | • Asymptomatic patients; transfuse to maintain hemodynamic stability.
| | • Symptomatic with hemorrhage transfuse to maintain Hgb 8–10 g/dL
| | • Symptomatic with Hgb <10 g/dL: transfuse to maintain Hgb >10 g/dL
| | • Acute coronary syndromes with anemia: transfuse to maintain Hgb >10 g/dL
| | • Benefits
| | • Rapid increase in Hgb may improve fatigue in some patients
| | • Risks
| | • Viral transmission; HIV: 3.1/100,000, hepatitis C: 5.1/100,000, hepatitis B: 3.41–3.43/100,000
| | • TRALI: 0.81/100,000
| | • TACO: 1%–6%, higher in ICU and postoperative settings
| | • Febrile nonhemolytic reactions: 1.1%–2.15%
| | • Exacerbation of underlying cardiopulmonary disease, including CHF
| | • Iron overload and secondary organ toxicity
| | • FDA-approved agents: darbepoetin alfa (Aranesp), epoetin alfa (Epogen, Procrit)
| | • Not indicated in patients receiving chemotherapy for curative intent
| | • Requires informed consent
| ESAs | • Goal is to administer the lowest dose necessary to avoid PRBC transfusion not to exceed Hgb of 10 g/dL
| | • If Hgb rises greater than 1 g/dL in any 2-week period, dose reductions are required: see prescribing information (https://www.fda.gov/Drugs/DrugSafety/ucm109375.htm)
| | • Benefits
| | • Avoidance of transfusions
| | • Risks
| | • Inferior survival and decreased time to progression, most notably with target Hgb >12 g/dL
| | • Thrombosis: increased risk with history of coagulopathy, obesity, coronary artery disease, thrombocytosis, hypertension, hospitalization

CBC, complete blood count; *CHF,* congestive heart failure; *CIA,* chemotherapy-induced anemia; *ESA,* erythropoietin-stimulating proteins; *FDA,* Food and Drug Administration; *GI,* gastrointestinal; *HIV,* human immunodeficiency virus; *ICU,* intensive care unit; *PRBC,* packed red blood cells; *RBC,* red blood cell; *TACO,* transfusion-associated circulatory overload; *TRALI,* transfusion-related acute lung injury.

Management (see Table 39.7)

I. Medical management (Aliper et al., 2014; Berlotti et al, 2017; Flowers et al, 2013; Kurtin & Bilotti, 2013; Li et al., 2017; Lyman et al., 2014; Morrison & Scadden, 2014; Pherwani et al, 2015; Russell et al., 2017; Uhl et al., 2017; Warnock, 2016; Yu et al., 2015; Zhu et al., 2017).

  A. Prevent anemia

    1. Packed RBC transfusions as indicated (see Chapter 30)

    2. Erythropoietin-stimulating proteins (ESAs) as indicated; use with caution in patients with curative goals of treatment (see Table 39.7)

II. Nursing management (Kurtin, 2012) ⚠

  A. Interventions to minimize secondary effects of anemia

    1. Cancer treatment generally held for Hgb less than 7.5 g/dL with the exception of known bone marrow disorders

    2. Packed red blood cell (PRBC) transfusions based on World Health Organization (WHO) guidelines for transfusion

  B. Strategies to incorporate patient and family in care ⚠

    1. Teach the caregiver and patient about energy conservation and reportable signs and symptoms

    2. Teach the caregiver and patient about signs of transfusion reactions

    3. Teach about safety measures to decrease the potential for injury caused by syncope or dyspnea during periods of anemia

THROMBOCYTOPENIA

Overview

I. Definition—decrease in the circulating platelets below the LLN based on institutional laboratory measures (Table 39.8) (CTC-AE version 4)

II. Physiology (Aliper et al., 2014; Morrison & Scadden, 2014)

  A. Megakaryocytes develop and form the myeloid stem cells in bone marrow.

  B. Each megakaryocyte produces millions of platelets each day and can be measured in peripheral blood.

  C. The function of platelets is to maintain vascular hemostasis, prevent blood loss through platelet adhesion to block small breaks in blood vessels, and initiate clotting mechanisms.

III. Risk factors (Aliper et al., 2014; Bertlotti et al, 2017; Li et al., 2017; Morrison & Scadden, 2014; Russell et al., 2017; Uhl et al., 2017) (Table 39.9)
   A. Patient-related factors
   B. Disease-related factors
   C. Treatment-related factors

Assessment

See Table 39.10.

TABLE 39.8 Overview of Thrombocytopenia

Thrombocytopenia	A finding based on laboratory test results that indicate a decrease in number of platelets in a blood specimen	Grade 1: Plt < LLN–75,000/mm^3
		Grade 2: Plt < 75,000–50,000/mm^3
	Patients with thrombocytopenia at an increased risk of bleeding	Grade 3: Plt < 50,000–25,000/mm^3
	Lifespan: 10–12 days (as little as 24 hours in stressful situations)	Grade 4: Plt < 25,000/mm^3

CTC-AE version 4

TABLE 39.9 Risk Factors Associated with Chemotherapy-Induced Thrombocytopenia

Host-Related Factors	Disease- and Treatment-Related Factors
See Table 39.2	Invasion of tumor cells in the bone marrow or cancers involving the bone marrow; multiple myeloma, lymphoma, leukemia, or myelodysplastic syndrome
Underlying platelet disorders; idiopathic thrombocytopenic purpura, thrombotic thrombocytopenic purpura	
Coagulation abnormalities	Megakaryocytic leukemia
Splenomegaly	Hypercoagulation; paraneoplastic syndromes, DIC, and thrombosis
Hypocoagulation; vitamin K deficiency from malnutrition or from liver disease, which alters the development of prothrombin and several clotting factors	Endotoxins released from bacteria during an infection can damage platelets and later platelet aggregation
	Drug interactions
	Platelet count usually decreases in 7–14 days after administration of chemotherapy or sooner with multimodal treatment

DIC, Disseminated intravascular coagulation.

TABLE 39.10 Assessment and Recommendations for Management of Chemotherapy-Induced Thrombocytopenia

Assessment	• Previous cancer treatment history: chemotherapy, radiation therapy, or multimodal therapy.
	• Current medications that could alter platelet production.
	• Social history of alcohol and illicit drug use.
	• Assess for bleeding from nose, rectum, ears, oral cavity; assess blood in stool, urine, and vomitus.
	• Assess menstrual bleeding and the number of sanitary napkins or tampons used.
Laboratory data	• Assess for changes that indicate intracranial bleeding: level of consciousness, restlessness, headache, seizures, pupil changes, ataxia.
Prevention	• Assess skin for ecchymosis, purpura, oozing of puncture sites, and petechiae.
	• Assess for conjunctiva hemorrhage and sclera injection.
	• Platelet count.
	• Coagulation values: fibrinogen, prothrombin time, partial thromboplastin time, platelet antibodies.
	• Identification of patients at high risk for thrombocytopenia and bleeding.
	• Consideration of individual characteristics of the patient, including proximity to treatment center, concomitant anticoagulation therapy or antiplatelet drugs, prior response to platelets, concurrent inflammatory process or infection, central nervous system (CNS) disease.
	• Patient and caregiver education for conservation of energy, planning of activities, and reportable signs and symptoms.
Treatment of CIT	• Establish a plan of care for monitoring blood counts and follow-up.
	• Maintain a current type and screen for patients requiring frequent transfusions.
	• Progestational agents may decrease menstrual bleeding.
Transfusion of platelets	• Withholding anticoagulation therapy for platelet count less than 50,000/μL.
	• Evaluation of symptoms of thrombocytopenia with consideration of individual patient characteristics.
	• Treat the underlying cause(s).
	• Weigh the risks and benefits of each treatment.
	• Requires informed consent

TABLE 39.10 Assessment and Recommendations for Management of Chemotherapy-Induced Thrombocytopenia—cont'd

	• World Health Organization (WHO) bleeding grades; grade 1 – petechiae, ecchymosis, occult blood in body secretions, mild vaginal spotting; grade 2 – evidence of gross hematuria not requiring red blood cell (RBC) transfusion over routine needs: epistaxis, hematuria, hematemesis; grade 3 – hemorrhage of one or more units of packed red blood cells (PRBCs) per day; grade 4 – life-threatening hemorrhage, defined as massive bleeding causing hemodynamic compromise or bleeding into a vital organ (intracranial, pericardial, or pulmonary hemorrhage). • Platelets less than 10,000/µL – threshold for therapeutic platelet transfusion. Patients with history of bleeding or active infection may require higher threshold for transfusion. Surgical or invasive procedure needs to maintain platelets greater than 50,000 µL. Neurosurgical procedures – platelets need to be maintained greater than 10,000 µL • Random donor platelets (RDP) – common dose is 4–6 random donor units (pooled from multiple units of whole blood). • Single-donor platelets (SDP) – larger volume –1 unit = 60 mL; 6 units = 360 mL. Single-donor apheresis platelets = 200 mL, takes 1.5–2 hours to process and costs more than twice the cost of RDP transfusion.
Benefits	• Improvement in bleeding symptoms
Risks	• RDP exposes results in patient exposure to more donors • Refractory to platelet transfusions (alloimmunization) • Transfusion reaction or transmitted disease • Delay in administering treatment on time or dose delays; dose reductions • Internal bleeding; intracranial, gastrointestinal (GI), or respiratory tract bleeding • Death

Management

I. Medical management (Aliper et al., 2014; Berlotti et al, 2017; Kaufman et al., 2015; Kurtin & Bilotti, 2013; Li et al., 2017; Morrison & Scadden, 2014; NCCN, 2017a, Pherwani et al., 2015; Russell et al., 2017; Uhl et al., 2017; Warnock, 2016; Yu et al., 2015; Zhu et al., 2017) (see Table 39.10)
   A. Prevention of thrombocytopenia
      1. Identification of patients at high risk for thrombocytopenia and bleeding
         a. WHO bleeding grades
            (1) Grade 1—petechiae, ecchymosis, occult blood in body secretions, mild vaginal spotting
            (2) Grade 2—evidence of gross hemorrhage not requiring RBC transfusion over routine needs: epistaxis, hematuria, hematemesis
            (3) Grade 3—hemorrhage of one or more units of PRBCs per day
            (4) Grade 4—life-threatening hemorrhage, defined as either massive bleeding causing hemodynamic compromise or bleeding into a vital organ (e.g., intracranial, pericardial, or pulmonary hemorrhage)
II. Nursing management (Robinson et al., 2014)
   A. Interventions to minimize the occurrence of bleeding
      1. Avoid the use or overinflation of a blood pressure cuff or use of a tourniquet when the platelet count is less than 20,000/mm^3
      2. Avoid invasive procedures such as enema, taking rectal temperature, administering suppositories, bladder catheterization, venipuncture, finger stick, use of nasogastric tubes, administering subcutaneous or intramuscular injection

      3. Preparation of the environment to avoid trauma (e.g., padding side rails, arranging furniture to eliminate sharp corners, clearing walkways)
      4. Apply firm direct pressure to venipuncture site for 5 minutes
   B. Encourage patient to wear shoes during ambulation to maintain skin integrity
   C. Encourage patient to avoid sharp objects such as a straight-edge razor
   D. If bleeding not controlled, apply absorbable gelatin sponges or liquid thrombin
   E. For nosebleeds, place patient in high Fowler position and apply pressure to the nose
   F. Apply ice packs to decrease the bleeding
   G. Implement a bowel elimination regimen to prevent constipation
   H. Use soft toothbrushes to avoid gingival trauma
   I. Instruct patient to avoid physical activity that may lead to trauma
   J. Monitor platelet levels
   K. Cancer treatment usually withheld for platelet count less than 50,000 to 100,000/mm^3
   L. Platelet transfusion based on WHO guidelines for transfusion
III. Implementation of strategies to incorporate patient and family in care
   A. Teach the patient and caregiver bleeding precautions
   B. Teach the patient and caregiver signs of bleeding that should be called to the attention of the physician or nurse
   C. Teach about safety measures to decrease the occurrence of bleeding when performing activities of daily living, including fall prevention

INFECTION

Overview

I. Definition—when the body or a part of the body is invaded by a microorganism or virus and an infection develops, depending on three factors (Goldman et al., 2017; Kyi et al., 2014; Nesher & Rolston, 2014; Rolston, 2017) (Table 39.11)

  A. Infectious diseases an important factor in morbidity and mortality in cancer patients

II. Physiology

  A. Susceptibility to cancer-related infections results from the nature of the malignancy and cancer treatments.

    1. Impairment of host defense mechanisms—skin and mucosal barriers (mucositis, dermatologic reactions, invasive procedures), neutropenia, immunosuppression

    2. Increased susceptibility to infections with variable risk throughout the cancer diagnosis

    3. Prolonged immunosuppression, which increases the risk of opportunistic infections (viruses, fungi, mycobacteria, rare bacterial strains) and more severe consequences of common pathogens

  B. Most important physical barrier against invasion of organism—skin, mucosal barriers

  C. WBCs, particularly neutrophils, an important defense against infection

III. Risk factors (Goldman et al., 2017; Kyi et al., 2014; Nesher & Rolston, 2014; Rolston, 2017) (Table 39.12)

  A. Patient-related factors

  B. Disease- and treatment-related factors

Assessment

See Table 39.13.

TABLE 39.11   Overview of Infection

Infection	When the body or a part of the body is invaded by a microorganism or virus and an infection develops, depending on susceptibility to cancer-related infections, physical barriers against invasion of an organism, skin and mucosal barriers, and WBCs, specifically, neutrophils, an important defense against infection.	WBC important in defense against infection: Impairment of host defense mechanisms—skin and mucosal barriers (mucositis, dermatologic reactions, invasive procedures), neutropenia, immunosuppression Increased susceptibility to infections with variable risk throughout the cancer diagnosis Prolonged immunosuppression, which increases the risk of opportunistic infections (viruses, fungi, mycobacteria, rare bacterial strains) and more severe consequences of common pathogens

WBC, White blood cell.

TABLE 39.12   Risk Factors Associated with Chemotherapy-Induced Infection

Patient-Related Factors	Disease- and Treatment-Related Factors
See Table 39.2	Immunodeficiency associated with primary malignancy
Disruption of mucosal barriers	High tumor burden
Splenectomy or functional asplenia	Corticosteroids and other lymphotoxic agents
Comorbid conditions	Cytotoxic chemotherapy
Malnutrition; hypoalbuminemia	T- and B-cell suppressants, steroids, purine analogs, alemtuzumab
Hypogammaglobulinemia	
Remission status	Radiation therapy
HIV	Solid organ transplantation
Barriers breached – vascular access device (VAD), mucositis, surgery	Hematopoietic stem cell transplantation; graft-versus-host disease (GVHD)

TABLE 39.13   Assessment and Recommendations for Management of Chemotherapy-Induced Infection

History	• Previous cancer treatment history: chemotherapy, radiation therapy, or multimodal therapy • Review of infection history • Review of known allergies to medications, especially antibiotics • Review of immunosuppressive therapy
Physical examination	• Complete physical examination to isolate potential source of infection; skin, mucosa, lungs, sinus, perirectal, abdomen, wounds, indwelling catheters • Assessment of mental status for orientation, confusion, memory recall, alertness • Assessment for rapidity of onset of symptoms • Assessment of vital signs every 4–8 hours; fever, hypotension or tachypnea (RR >24) indicative of high risk for clinical deterioration • Assessment of urine or stool for color, consistency or clarity, odor, presence of blood

TABLE 39.13 Assessment and Recommendations for Management of Chemotherapy-Induced Infection—cont'd

Laboratory data	• CBC with differential, culture and sensitivity testing of urine, blood, stool, sputum, wounds, drainage bags or tubes, rectal swabs for VRE, oral swabs for viruses, stool for *Clostridium difficile*, skin or wound swabs for bacterial, viral, fungal infections, skin punch biopsy to isolate fungal infections.
Radiology	• Chest radiography (PA and lateral) • Additional radiology testing based on suspected source
Prevention	• Institute preventive antimicrobial treatments for patients at high risk for opportunistic viral, fungal, and bacterial infections • Isolate source if possible
Treatment	• Administer antibiotics according to organism isolated • Administer WBC line growth factors, as appropriate (see Neutropenia)
Risks	• Delay in treatment or ineligibility for selected treatment because of infection history • Pneumonia and acute respiratory distress • Septic shock • Resistance to antibiotics or superinfection • Death

CBC, complete blood count; *PA,* posteroanterior; *RR,* Respiratory rate; *VRE,* vancomycin-resistant enterococcus; *WBC,* white blood cell.

Management

I. Medical management (Goldman et al., 2017; Kyi et al., 2014; Nesher & Rolston, 2014; Rolston, 2017) (see Table 39.13)
   A. Identification of patients at risk
   B. Institute preventive antimicrobial treatments for patients at high risk for viral, fungal, or opportunistic bacterial infections
   C. Isolation of the source, if possible
   D. Administration of antibiotics according to organism isolated
   E. Administration of WBC line growth factors, as appropriate (see Neutropenia)

II. Nursing management (NCCN, 2017b)
   A. Interventions to minimize infections ⚠
      1. Use strict hand washing before and after all contact with patient
      2. Promote and encourage meticulous personal and oral hygiene, perineal care
      3. Avoid unnecessary invasive procedures such as giving enemas, taking rectal temperatures, bladder catheterization, and venipuncture
      4. Administer vaccinations such as flu vaccine (Pneumovax) to prevent communicable infections

TABLE 39.14 Risk Factors Associated with Cancer-Related Hemorrhage

Disease-Related Factors	Treatment-Related Factors
Cerebral hemorrhage may occur with severe thrombocytopenia or with brain metastases Myeloproliferative disorders such as polycythemia vera, myelofibrosis, and thrombocytopenia may cause hemorrhage DIC may result from prostate cancer or acute promyelocytic leukemia Paraneoplastic syndromes may stimulate bleeding Splenomegaly may cause bleeding	Bone marrow or hematopoietic stem cell transplantation may cause a diffuse alveolar hemorrhage characterized by cough, dyspnea, and hypoxemia DIC may occur as a result of cancer treatment High-dose chemotherapy such as with cyclophosphamide (Cytoxan) and ifosfamide may cause hemorrhagic cystitis or myocardial hemorrhage Ibrutinib All types of surgical procedures pose a risk for hemorrhage, especially if tumor is embedded within arteries or veins

DIC, Disseminated intravascular coagulation.

      5. Use of aseptic technique when performing nursing interventions
      6. Ensure adequate hydration and a high-calorie, high-protein diet
   B. Interventions to locate source of infection
      1. Obtain appropriate cultures such as blood, sputum, stool, urine, and wounds, as indicated
      2. Educate the patient and caregiver about signs and symptoms of infection and when to call the physician or nurse ⚠
      3. Have chest radiography performed as ordered
      4. Report critical changes in patient assessment parameters to physician ⚠

HEMORRHAGE

Overview

I. Definition—the occurrence of abnormal internal or external discharge of blood
II. Physiology
   A. Hemostasis is the process of a solid clot forming in the blood from a fluid component.
   B. Coagulation is the mechanism of forming a stable fibrin clot.
   C. Hemorrhage occurs in cancer patients from alterations in hemostasis or coagulation mechanisms.
III. Risk factors (Caron et al., 2017, Johnstone & Rich, 2017; Russell et al., 2017) (Table 39.14)
   A. Disease related
   B. Treatment related

Assessment

See Table 39.15.

TABLE 39.15	**Assessment and Recommendations for Management of Cancer-Related Hemorrhage**
History	• Previous cancer treatment history: chemotherapy, radiation therapy, or multimodal therapy • Ascertain recent traumatic events • Review of the cancer • Evidence of metastasis to the brain or bone marrow • Leukemia, especially nonlymphocytic leukemia, may cause hemorrhage as a result of a paraneoplastic process
Physical examination	• Review past medical history for occurrence of peptic or gastric ulcer disease or esophageal varices
Laboratory data	• Assess for signs of hemorrhage complications; weak/irregular pulse, pale skin, cold/moist skin
Treatment	• Assess all stool, urine, and sputum for blood • Assess vital signs • Assess for neurologic deficits such as reduced level of alertness or orientation • CBC, coagulation factors, occult stool test, bleeding time • Administration of appropriate blood products • Administration of oxygen • Administration of vasopressors – may control severe bleeding • Lavage with iced saline through nasogastric tube – may control bleeding
Risks	• Viral infection from numerous blood transfusions • Shock • Transfusion reaction • Death

CBC, Complete blood count.

Management

I. Medical management (Johnstone & Rich, 2017; Russell et al., 2017) (see Table 39.15)

II. Nursing management (NCCN, 2017a)

A. Interventions to minimize the bleeding

1. Apply occlusive dressings to bleeding wounds after cleansing the area
2. If applicable, elevate the body part above the heart level and apply firm pressure over the area
3. Administer plasma and other blood components

B. Interventions to monitor for complications ⚠

1. Hemodynamic measurements—decrease in cardiac output and decrease in blood pressure (BP)
2. Strict intake and output records to detect negative fluid balance

3. Report critical changes in the patient's assessment parameters to the physician such as change in mental status, decrease in BP, increase in bleeding

FEVER AND CHILLS

Overview

I. Definition—elevation of body temperature above 100.4°F (38°C) to 101.3°F (38.5°C) orally (CTC-AE version 4)

A. Chills (shivering) occur as a body's response to heat loss when the body's temperature abruptly increases, as with fever or a drug reaction.

B. Involuntary contractions of the skeletal muscles occur with shivering.

C. The internal body temperature is maintained by shivering, which is a thermoregulatory mechanism.

D. Shivering is a subjective feeling of cold.

E. Fever is initiated by the release of endogenous pyrogens from phagocytic WBCs.

F. Vasodilation and sweating are physiologic mechanisms used to increase heat loss.

G. Vasoconstriction and shivering are the body's mechanisms for conserving or producing heat.

H. Production of fever occurs as a response to the elevation of the set point in the temperature-regulating center in the hypothalamus.

I. Shivering results in an increase in metabolic activity and oxygen consumption brought about by an increase in muscle tone.

J. Skin temperature drops because of vasoconstriction, which decreases heat loss.

K. Each degree of temperature Fahrenheit results in a 7% increase in metabolic rate and increases the demands on the heart.

TABLE 39.16	**Risk Factors Associated with Chemotherapy-Induced Fever and Chills**
Disease-Related Factors	**Treatment-Related Factors**
See Neutropenia and Infection sections Tumor involving the hypothalamus Paraneoplastic syndromes Pyrogens released by the tumor cells Tumors associated with tumor-induced fever; Hodgkin lymphoma, osteogenic sarcoma, lymphoma, liver metastasis	See Neutropenia and Infection sections Chemotherapy side effects causing drug fever or flulike syndrome (e.g., bleomycin, daunorubicin, thiotepa, methotrexate, dacarbazine, plicamycin) Blood transfusion reaction Biotherapy side effect from interferon, monoclonal antibody, or interleukin Steroid-induced adrenal insufficiency Drug-induced fever; vancomycin or amphotericin B Invasive procedure

II. Physiology
  A. The thermoregulatory center in the hypothalamus controls body temperature.
  B. Various heat loss mechanisms help return temperature to normal levels during fevers.
III. Risk factors (Kryzanowska et al., 2016) (Table 39.16)
  A. Disease related
  B. Treatment related

Management (Kryzanowska et al., 2016; NCCN, 2017b) (Table 39.17)

I. Medical management
  A. Interventions to locate the source of infection
    1. Obtain cultures from the blood, throat, urine, stool, sputum, and wounds when an infection is suspected, including cultures from all access devices
II. Nursing management
  A. Interventions to provide comfort
    1. Promote slow cooling of the skin and mucous membranes
    2. Tepid sponge baths
    3. Reduce amount of patient clothing
    4. Mechanical cooling blankets

    5. Reduction of the environmental temperature
    6. Avoid rapid reduction in body temperature that can cause chilling by providing warm blankets or heating pads at the first sign of chilling
    7. Change damp clothing immediately to prevent chilling
    8. Administer acetaminophen, aspirin, or ibuprofen to reduce fever, as ordered
      a. Acetaminophen—not to exceed 4000 mg in a 24-hour period; to be used with caution in patients with liver disease
      b. Aspirin—to be used with caution in patients with platelet disorders
      c. Ibuprofen—to be used with caution in patients with renal impairment
    9. Increase fluid intake to prevent dehydration
    10. Educate patient as to self-care measures for fever or chills, including medication management
  B. Interventions to minimize the occurrence of infection in common sites
    1. Encourage patient to cough and take deep breaths every 4 to 8 hours while awake
    2. Encourage patient to perform oral hygiene every 4 hours while awake
    3. Encourage patient to void frequently
    4. Instruct the patient to avoid the use of douches or tampons
    5. Encourage the patient to eat well-balanced meals and increase fluid intake

TABLE 39.17 Assessment and Recommendations for Management of Cancer-Related Fever and Chills

History	• Previous cancer treatment history: chemotherapy, radiation therapy, or multimodal therapy • Previous exposure to infections • Type of cancer and extent of disease • Previous blood transfusions • Current medications • History of hypersensitivity reactions
Physical examination	• Frequent assessment of vital signs • Complete physical examination to ascertain source of fever
Laboratory data	• Review laboratory data, additional analysis based on suspected cause (e.g., neutropenia-related fevers, drug reaction fevers, drug reactions, cholangitis)
Treatment	• Administer acetaminophen alternated with ibuprofen every 2 hours to decrease fever and drug toxicity; caution in patients with thrombocytopenia • Nonsteroidal antiinflammatory drugs (NSAIDs) for tumor-induced fever; caution in patients with thrombocytopenia and renal insufficiency • Treat the underlying cause
Risks	• Increase in fatigue, muscle weakness, myalgia, reduced quality of life • Dyspnea • Cardiopulmonary compromise • Death

EXPECTED PATIENT OUTCOMES

I. Patient will be free of major infectious complications because neutropenia is prevented or promptly managed.
II. Patient and caregiver accurately describe appropriate infection precautions.
III. Patient and caregiver accurately describe appropriate energy conservation strategies.
IV. Patient remains without complications as a result of hemorrhage.
V. Patient and caregiver accurately describe appropriate bleeding precautions.

REFERENCES

Aliper, A. M., Frieden-Korovkina, V. P., Buzdin, A., Roumiantsev, S. A., & Zhavoronkov, A. (2014). A role for G-CSF and GM-CSF in nonmyeloid cancers. *Cancer Medicine, 3*(4), 737–746.

Caron, F., Leong, D. P., Hillis, C., Fraser, G., & Siegal, D. (2017). Current understanding of bleeding with ibrutinib use: a systematic review and meta-analysis. *Blood Advances, 1*(12), 772–778.

Flowers, C. R., Seidenfeld, J., Bow, E. J., Karten, C., Gleason, C., Hawley, D. K., et al. (2013). Antimicrobial prophylaxis and outpatient management of fever and neutropenia in adults treated for malignancy: American Society of Clinical Oncology clinical practice guideline. *Journal of Clinical Oncology, 31,* 794–810.

Gilreath, J., Stenehjem, D., & Ro, G. (2014). Diagnosis and treatment of cancer-related anemia. *The American Journal of Hematology*, 89(2), 203–221.

Goldman, J. D., Gallaher, A., Jain, R., Stednick, Z., Menon, M., Boechkh, M., et al. (2017). Infusion-compatible antibiotic formulations for rapid administration to improve outcomes in cancer outpatients with severe sepsis and septic shock: the sepsis STAT pack. *Journal of the National Comprehensive Cancer Network*, 15, 457–464.

Johnstone, C., & Rich, S. (2017). Bleeding in cancer patients and its treatment: a review. *Annals of Palliative Medicine*, 0(0) Retrieved from http://apm.amegroups.com/article/view/17761.

Kaufman, R. M., Djulbegovic, B., Gernsheimer, T., et al. (2015). Platelet transfusion: A clinical practice guideline from the AABB. *Annals of Internal Medicine*, 162, 205–213.

Kryzanowska, M. K., Walker-Dilks, A. M., Morris, R., Gupta, R., Halligan, C. T., Kouroukis, K., et al. (2016). Approach to evaluation of fever in ambulatory cancer patients receiving chemotherapy: a systematic review. *Cancer Treatment Reviews*, 51, 35–45.

Kurtin, S. (2012). Myeloid toxicity of cancer treatment. *Journal of the Advanced Practitioner in Oncology*, 3, 209–224.

Kurtin, S., & Bilotti, E. (2013). Novel agents for the treatment of multiple myeloma: proteasome inhibitors and immunomodulatory agents. *Journal of the Advanced Practitioner in Oncology*, 4(5), 307–321.

Kyi, C., Hellmann, M. D., Wolchok, J. D., Chapman, P. B., & Postow, M. A. (2014). Opportunistic infections in patients treated with immunotherapy for cancer. *Journal for Immunotherapy of Cancer*, 2, 19. https://doi.org/10.1186/2051-1426-2-19.

Leiding, J. W. (2017). Neutrophil evolution and their diseases in humans. *Frontiers in Immunology*. 8(1009). https://doi.org/10.3389/fimmu.2017.01009.

Li, A., Davis, C., Wu, Q., Li, S., Kesten, M. F., Holmberg, L. A., et al. (2017). Management of venous thromboembolism during thrombocytopenia after autologous hematopoetic transplantation. *Blood Advances*, 1(12), 707–714.

Lyman, G., Esteban, A., & Pettengell, R. (2014). Risk factors for febrile neutropenia among patients with cancer receiving chemotherapy: a systematic review. *Critical Reviews in Oncology / Hematology*, 90(3), 190–199.

Manea, P. J. (2014). Optimizing the management of patients with myelofibrosis. *Clinical Journal of Oncology Nursing*, 18(3), 330–337.

Morrison, S. J., & Scadden, D. T. (2014). The bone marrow niche for haematopoietic stem cells. *Nature*, 505(7483), 327–334. https://doi.org/10.1038/nature12984.

National Comprehensive Cancer Network. (2017a). *Cancer and chemotherapy induced anemia, version 1.2018*. Retrieved from https://www.nccn.org/professionals/physician_gls/pdf/anemia pdf.

National Comprehensive Cancer Network. (2017b). *Prevention and treatment of cancer related infections, version 1.2018*. Retrieved from https://www.nccn.org/professionals/physician_gls/pdf/infections.pdf.

National Comprehensive Cancer Network. (2018). *NCCN clinical practice guidelines in oncology. Myeloid growth factors version 1.2018*. Retrieved from https://www.nccn.org/professionals/physician_gls/pdf/myeloid_growth.pdf.

Nesher, L., & Rolston, K. V. (2014). The current spectrum of infection in cancer patients with chemotherapy related neutropenia. *Infection*, 42(1), 5–13.

Pherwani, N., Ghayed, J. M., Holle, L. M., & Karpiuk, E. L. (2015). Outpatient management of febrile neutropenia associated with chemotherapy. Risk stratification and treatment review. *American Journal of Health-System Pharmacy*, 78(8), 619–631. https://doi.org/10.2146/ajhp140194.

Robinson, D., Schulz, G., Langley, R., Donze, K., Winchester, K., & Rodgers, C. (2014). Evidence-based practice recommendations for hydration in children and adolescents with cancer receiving intravenous cyclophosphamide. *Journal of Pediatric Oncology Nursing : Official Journal of the Association of Pediatric Oncology Nurses*, 31(4), 191–199. https://doi.org/10.1177/1043454214532024.

Rolston, K. V. I. (2017). Infections in cancer patients with solid tumors: a review. *Infectious Diseases and Therapy*, 6(1), 69–83.

Russell, L., Holst, L. B., Kieldsen, L., Stensballe, J., & Perner, A. (2017). Risks of bleeding and thrombosis in intensive care unit patients with haematological malignancies. *Annals of Intensive Care*, 7(1), 119. https://doi.org/10.1186/s13613-017-0341-y.

Thomas, J., Smith, T. J., Bohlke, K., Lyman, G. H., Carson, K. R., Crawford, J., et al. (2015). Recommendations for the use of WBC growth factors: american society of clinical oncology clinical practice guideline update. *Journal of Clinical Oncology*, 33(28), 3199–3212.

Uhl, L., Assmann, S. F., Hamza, T., Harrison, R. W., Gernsheimer, T., & Slicter, S. J. (2017). Laboratory predictors of bleeding and the effect of platelet and RBC transfusions on bleeding outcomes in the PLADO trial. *Blood*, 130, 1247–1258.

Vioral, A., & Wentley, D. (2015). Managing oncology neutropenia and sepsis in the intensive care unit. *Critical Care Nursing Quarterly*, 38(2), 165–174.

Warnock, C. (2016). Neutropenic sepsis: prevention, identification and treatment. *Nursing Standard*, 30(35), 51–60. https://doi.org/10.7748/ns.30.35.51.s48.

Yu, J. L., Chan, K., Kurin, M., Pasetka, M., Kiss, A., Sridhar, S. S., et al. (2015). Clinical outcomes and cost-effectiveness of primary prophylaxis of febrile neutropenia during adjuvant docetaxel and cyclophosphamide chemotherapy for breast cancer. *Breast Journal*, 21(6), 658–664. https://doi.org/10.1111/tbj.12501.

Zhu, C., Wang, Y., Wang, X., Bai, C., Su, D., Cao, B., et al. (2017). Profiling chemotherapy-associated myelotoxicity among Chinese gastric cancer population receiving cytotoxic conventional regimens: epidemiological features, timing, predictors and clinical impacts. *Journal of Cancer*, 8(13), 2614–2625. https://doi.org/10.7150/jca.17847.

40

Integumentary Symptoms

Kathy Waitman

OVERVIEW

I. Physiology
   A. The skin is composed of three layers—the epidermis, the dermis, and the subcutaneous tissue.
   B. Intact skin protects the body from harmful microbes, temperature changes, physical trauma, and radiation.
   C. Skin is the first line of defense by regulating thermal processes, protecting underlying structures, and excreting waste.
      1. The epidermis is the avascular outer layer, which serves as a barrier to prevent water loss and renews itself continuously through cell division.
      2. The dermis, the inner connective tissue layer, is highly vascular, with afferent sensory nerve receptors, which provides nutritional support to the avascular epidermal layer.
      3. The subcutaneous tissue is composed of adipose tissue, which serves as a cushion to trauma, an insulator to temperature changes, and an energy reservoir.
II. Risk factors
   A. Disease related (Table 40.1)
      1. Thrombocytopenia
      2. Cutaneous metastases or direct tumor extension (late manifestation in the course of the illness for solid tumors of the breast and lung, squamous cell carcinoma of the head and neck, malignant melanoma, lymphoma, Kaposi sarcoma)
      3. Primary cutaneous paraneoplastic syndromes—acanthosis nigricans, acquired ichthyosis, Paget disease, telangiectasia, hypertrichosis, lanuginosa acquisita, erythroderma (Coggshall et al., 2017)
      4. Primary malignant skin cancer (melanoma, basal cell carcinoma, squamous cell carcinoma, Kaposi sarcoma)
      5. Mycosis fungoides (slow, progressive, cutaneous T-cell lymphoma)
      6. Premalignant lesions (actinic keratosis, leukoplakia, dysplastic nevus syndrome)
      7. Desquamative skin reaction (radiation enhancement, radiation recall, combined modality therapy) as a result of chemotherapy in association with radiation therapy
      8. Fragile skin from steroid therapy
      9. Erythema multiforme (widespread, scattered, cutaneous vesicles) associated with multiple drugs
      10. Erythema nodosum (tender, subcutaneous, anterior leg nodules)—hypersensitivity reaction to penicillin or sulfonamides
      11. Graft-versus-host disease (skin reaction related to bone marrow transplantation) (Strong Rodrigues et al., 2018)
      12. Malnutrition—decreased protein stores
      13. Other effects—alopecia, pressure ulcers, (lymph) edema, pruritus, jaundice, incontinence, infection
         a. Chest tubes, Foley catheter, biliary catheters
         b. Feeding tubes—gastrostomy, jejunostomy
         c. Tubes for decompression and drains
   B. Treatment related (Chemocare, 2019; National Cancer Institute, 2015)
      1. Side effects of biological response modifiers and targeted therapy such as epidermal growth factor receptor (EGFR) inhibitors/chemotherapy/radiation therapy
      2. Extravasation of chemotherapy (anthracyclines, taxanes, antimetabolites)
      3. Reaction or sensitivity to tape or adhesive dressings (central and peripheral intravenous [IV] access)

ASSESSMENT

I. History (Gawkrodger & Ardern-Jones, 2017; Pereira et al., 2016)
   A. Presence of risk factors
   B. Patient's age
   C. General health status
   D. Exposure to infection
   E. Recent treatment and anticipated side effects
   F. Current drug therapy
   G. Past and current skin conditions
   H. Review of personal hygiene practices
   I. Nutritional status
   J. Smoking habits
   K. Incontinence of bowel or bladder
   L. Review of medication history and potential allergies
   M. Presence of underlying disease

TABLE 40.1   Etiologic Factors of Skin Reactions

Skin Reaction	General Class of Reaction	Drug Class or Mechanism
Skin Reactions Found with Radiation Therapy Alone		
Acute radiation dermatitis	Immediate dermatitis occurring in radiated areas with erythema, pain, dermal swelling, itching, necrosis	May occur with all radiation therapy Mechanism is free radical damage to tissue
Chronic radiation dermatitis	Long-term effects of radiation therapy in port area with thinning of skin, scarring and contractures, telangiectasias, long-term skin sensitivity to irritants and environmental agents	May occur with all radiation therapy Mechanism is free radical damage to tissue Severity depends on port size and total dose
Skin Reactions Found with Chemotherapy and Radiation Therapy in Combination		
Radiation recall dermatitis	Occurs in previously irradiated skin within 1–2 weeks after chemotherapy; erythema, edema, superficial ulcerations, superficial skin sloughing	Drugs such as cetuximab, doxorubicin (Doxil, Adriamycin), docetaxel (Taxotere), gemcitabine (Gemzar), paclitaxel (Taxol), capecitabine, 5-FU
Skin Reactions Found with Chemotherapy alone		
Allergic or Immune Complex Reactions		
Activation of already existing immune complex reaction in collagen vascular diseases of systemic lupus erythematosus and progressive systemic sclerosis (scleroderma)	Chemotherapy drug activates immune complexes already circulating due to underlying collagen vascular disease process, causing circular, red, scaly rash	Many drugs
Contact allergy (activated T cells) and may not develop until 24–36 hours after contact with the allergen	Allergic response where drug touches skin (erythema, local swelling, desquamation, blistering, necrosis possible)	Chemicals found in poison ivy, oak, and sumac Nickel and cobalt in metal jewelry, clothing snaps, zippers, and metal-plated objects Latex in gloves and rubberized clothing Neomycin in antibiotic skin ointments Potassium dichromate, a tanning agent found in leather shoes and clothing
Erythema multiforme (antigen–antibody complexes)	Rash with typical target lesions involving extremities, including palms and soles, can progress to generalized	Many drugs
Immunoglobulin E (IgE) mediated	Itching, redness, swelling within 1 hour after infusion begun; if life threatening, termed *anaphylaxis* and includes decreased blood pressure, decreased level of consciousness, airway and breathing compromise	Platinum derivatives (cisplatin, carboplatin)
Serum sickness (antigen–antibody complexes)	Flulike symptoms, which may progress to life threatening	Rituximab
Vasculitis (from antigen–antibody complexes	Generalized vascular inflammation with end organ damage	Methotrexate
Extravasation injury (drug leaks from IV site into surrounding tissue)	Varying severity depending on specific drug (swelling, redness, irritation, local tissue loss, necrosis)	Many drugs
Light-Related Reactions		
Photo enhancement	Drug given several days after sunburn causes sunburn to reappear in that area	Many drugs
Photosensitivity	Patient more sensitive to sun in solar-exposed areas and may develop severe sunburn	Antitumor antibiotics; many drugs
Phototoxicity	Allergic response on solar-exposed areas may be severe with edema, erythema, blistering; if very severe, may result in permanent hyperpigmentation	Many drugs

Continued

TABLE 40.1 Etiologic Factors of Skin Reactions—cont'd

Skin Reaction	General Class of Reaction	Drug Class or Mechanism
Nail Changes		
Beah lines	Transverse lines in nails, bands corresponding to when drug was given or time when critical illness occurred	Any chemotherapy agent or critical illness
Onycholysis	Nail lifts from base	Paclitaxel, docetaxel, cyclophosphamide, doxorubicin, 5-fluorouracil (5-FU), hydroxyurea, combination of vinblastine + bleomycin
Nail inflammation	Inflammatory changes around nail, including paronychia	EGFR (epidermal growth factor receptor) inhibitors (cetuximab, gefitinib), taxanes (docetaxel)
Pigment Changes of Skin, Mucous Membranes, Nails, Hair		
Drug secreted in sweat may induce pigmentation Flag sign	Under areas where adhesive tape applied and skin sweats	Docetaxel, thiotepa, ifosfamide
Generalized hyperpigmentation of all skin	Pigment loss of hair during time drug is given; all skin involved	Many drugs Busulfan (termed *busulfan tan*), pegylated liposomal doxorubicin, hydroxyurea, methotrexate Cyclophosphamide
Gums	Permanent hyperpigmentation of gums	Cisplatin, hydroxyurea, bleomycin
Hyperpigmentation in areas of pressure or injury	Injured skin only, although inciting injury may be mild	Tegafur (5-FU derivative)
Hyperpigmentation of palms, soles, nails	Circular areas of hyperpigmentation in these locations	Daunorubicin
Hyperpigmentation of solar-exposed skin	Sun-exposed areas only	Daunorubicin
Scalp hyperpigmentation Variety of pigmentary changes of skin and appendages	Circular hyperpigmented areas in scalp General types of pigmentary changes especially common with drugs listed	Various cytotoxic drugs (alkylating agents, tumor-directed antibiotics)
Various types of hyperpigmentation—serpentine, generalized, other	Generalized hyperpigmentation (all skin), of sun-exposed areas only, serpentine (follows underlying vein where drug infused), mucosa of tongue, nails, conjunctiva of eyes	5-FU
Rashes		
Generalized rash of hands and feet	Usually localized but can become more generalized	Tyrosine kinase signal transduction inhibitors (occurs with 50% of patients on higher doses of imatinib)
Acneiform rash	Papules and pustules similar to acne, although this rash contains *no* comedones; commonly involves face and also back, upper chest	EGFR inhibitors (cetuximab, gefitinib, nivolumab, ipilimumab, pembrolizumab)
Hand–foot syndrome, or acral erythema	Erythema of hands and feet, dysesthesias	Various chemotherapy drugs (capecitabine)
Toxicity to rapidly dividing cells	Alopecia, mouth ulcers, gastrointestinal (GI) tract ulcers, GI yeast overgrowth and other infections from decreased mucous production (mucous is protective), bone marrow effects of anemia, decreased platelets, decreased white blood cells (WBCs), decreased production of sperm and ova	Most chemotherapy drugs; probability of occurrence depends on how much the drug affects rapidly dividing cell groups
Xerosis (dry skin)	Common—can progress to chronic xerotic dermatitis and secondary infection	Many drugs

From DeHaven, C. (2007). *Chemotherapy and radiotherapy effects on the skin.* http://www.spsscs.org/feature-articles/chemotherapy-and-radiotherapy-effects-on-the-skin. Used with permission.

N. Patterns of pruritus, including circadian occurrence (pruritus typically increases at night), timing, onset, duration, impact on daily activities

O. Aggravating and alleviating factors

P. Patient's self-report

Q. Adjective lists describing pruritus—constant, intermittent, transient, burning, numbness

II. Physical examination (Gawkrodger & Ardern-Jones, 2017)

A. Skin—color, pigmentation, integrity, temperature, texture, turgor, presence of sloughing

B. Presence of petechiae, purpura, ecchymosis, jaundice

C. Presence of erythema, dry desquamation, moist desquamation

D. Presence and grade of rash (Common Toxicity Criteria for Adverse Events, [CTCAE])

E. Local inflammation at injection site (erythema, induration, blisters)

F. Ulcerations of mouth; dry, cracked mucous membranes and lips

G. Presence of alopecia

H. Presence of pruritus or jaundice

I. Integrity of tube sites, perirectal tissue, perineal tissue

J. Presence of pressure ulcers

K. Presence of pain

L. Vaginal discharge and erythema

III. Psychosocial examination

A. New diagnosis of a malignancy—pruritus may be the presenting symptom

B. Presence of stress and anxiety

IV. Laboratory data

A. Complete blood cell (CBC) count—elevated white blood cell (WBC) count, anemia, eosinophilia, polycythemia, thrombocytopenia

B. Blood chemistries—hyperglycemia, hyperuricemia, elevated blood urea nitrogen (BUN) or creatinine, abnormal liver function tests, bilirubin, alkaline phosphatase

C. Thyroid function tests—hypoactive or hyperactive thyroid

D. Other—low ferritin level, increased sedimentation rate, human immunodeficiency virus (HIV) antibody assay (if immunosuppression or lymphoma is a possibility)

E. Urinalysis—glycosuria

MANAGEMENT

I. Interventions to increase or maintain dietary and fluid intake

A. Offer small frequent meals with increased protein and calories

B. Moisten foods with liquids, sauces, and gravy

C. Have the patient increase fluid intake to 3 L/day if not medically contraindicated (e.g., water and calorie-dense fluids such as protein drinks, milk, juice)

D. Have the patient rinse the oral cavity with normal saline or a nonalcoholic mouthwash

II. Interventions to decrease inflammation of mucous membranes (see Chapter 28)

III. Interventions to teach self-care techniques and prevent complications

A. Teach the patient and caregiver to assess the skin every 4 hours

B. Teach patient and caregiver tube and drain management

C. Assist with turning and positioning every 2 hours

D. Massage uninjured areas gently

E. Use of an air mattress, specialty bed, or water mattress for high-risk persons

F. Instruct on gentle skin cleansing with mild pH-balanced skin cleanser

G. Rinse soap thoroughly off skin and pat skin dry

H. Moisturize and lubricate skin

I. Use of dry, clean, wrinkle-free linens and devices such as an egg crate mattress

J. Use of specialty beds

IV. Interventions to protect skin integrity

A. Teach

1. Risk factors and effects of treatments on skin

2. Use of protective film, skin barriers, or collection devices around drains and tubes with copious drainage

3. Use of sterile technique for invasive procedures such as insertion of tubes

4. Hand washing

5. Reportable signs and symptoms of infections

B. Keep patient's fingernails smooth and short

C. Recommend use of cotton clothing and avoidance of restrictive clothing

D. Report changes in skin color, integrity, pain, increased pruritus, drainage (amount, odor, color, consistency) to health care provider

V. Interventions for oral, perineal, and general hygiene

A. Use of soft toothbrush or oral sponges

B. Apply moisturizers to oral mucosa

C. Cleanse the perineal area with mild soap, rinsing thoroughly, patting the area dry, and applying a skin barrier after each bowel movement

D. Apply adhesive perineum pad or panty liner without deodorant to the undergarment

E. Gently cleanse skin with mild soap and tepid water and pat dry with soft cloth

F. Add emollients to bath water, skin lubricants to skin other than to irradiated sites

G. Oatmeal baths

H. Application of cool or warm compresses

I. Avoid alcohol-based skin lotions

J. Prophylactic medications

K. Medications to manage rash (Table 40.2)

VI. Interventions to adapt and cope with hair loss (see Chapter 36)

VII. Interventions for radiation-induced acute and chronic skin reactions (see Chapter 21)

TABLE 40.2   Pharmacologic Management of Pruritus

Pharmacologic Agent	Type of Pruritus	Comments
Diphenhydramine, cimetidine (H1 and H2 antagonists)	Urticaria, allergic drug reactions, advanced disease	May cause drowsiness
Corticosteroids/steroids	Inflammatory pruritus, local skin reactions, immune-mediated rash	Can be given orally or topically as a cream rubbed onto the pruritic skin
Naloxone and methylnaltrexone (opioid antagonists), butorphanol (kappa opioid receptor agonist)	Opioid-induced pruritus related to mu-receptor agonists	Pruritus in up to 50% of patients receiving opioids; if pruritus is caused by an opioid and symptom management has failed, consider switching to another opioid May reverse analgesic effect so use with caution
Capsaicin	Postherpetic neuralgia, psoriasis	Helpful for treating chronic and localized pruritus
Aprepitant (substance P neurokinin receptors)	Sezary syndrome, cutaneous T-cell lymphoma, metastatic cancer, erlotinib-induced itch	Clinical trials needed to verify efficacy
Mirtazapine	Cancer-related itch, nocturnal itch	Other antidepressants may help with itch

Adapted from Tey, H. L., & Yosipovitch, G. (2011). Targeted treatment of pruritus: a look into the future. *British Journal of Dermatology, 165*(1), 5-17.

EXPECTED PATIENT OUTCOMES

I. The patient will verbalize self-care skin techniques to maintain skin integrity.

II. The patient will report skin changes such as color, integrity, pain, increased pruritus, rash, or drainage (amount, odor, color, consistency) to the health care provider.

REFERENCES

Chemocare (2019). Skin Reactions. Available at http://chemocare.com/chemotherapy/side-effects/skin-reactions.aspx

Coggshall, K., Tello, T. L., North, J. P., & Yu, S. S. (2017). Merkel cell carcinoma: an update and review: pathogenesis, diagnosis, and staging. *Journal of the American Academy of Dermatology, 78*(3), 433–442. (2017). https://doi.org/10.1016/j.jaad.2017.12.

Gawkrodger, D., & Ardern-Jones, M. R. (2017). *Dermatology: an illustrated colour text* (6th ed.). Elsevier Ltd.

National Cancer Institute (2015). Skin and Nail Changes during Cancer Treatment. Available at https://www.cancer.gov/about-cancer/treatment/side-effects/skin-nail-changes

Pereira, M. P., Kremer, A. E., Mettang, T., & Ständer, S. (2016). Chronic pruritus in the absence of skin disease: pathophysiology, diagnosis and treatment. *American Journal of Clinical Dermatology, 17*(4), 337–348.

Strong Rodrigues, K., Oliveira-Ribeiro, C., de Abreu Fiuza Gomes, S., & Knobler, R. (2018). Cutaneous graft-versus-host disease: diagnosis and treatment. *American Journal of Clinical Dermatology, 19*(1), 33–50.

41

Musculoskeletal Symptoms

Kathy Waitman

OVERVIEW

I. Definitions
   A. Musculoskeletal alterations—affecting the body's joints, ligaments, muscles, nerves, tendons, and structures that support limbs, neck, and back.
   B. Impaired physical mobility (immobility)—a state in which the patient experiences or is at risk for a limitation in independent, purposeful physical movement of the body or one or more extremities (Joglekar, Ashghar, et al., 2015; Joglekar, Nau, and Mehzhir, 2015).
II. Physiology
   A. Sarcopenia is subclinical loss of skeletal muscle mass and is commonly observed in patients with malignancy (Joglekar, Ashghar, et al., 2015; Joglekar et al., 2015).
   B. Inactivity and limited use or disuse of muscle groups may decrease the muscles' ability to contract and may lead to decreased muscle size, muscle atrophy, and weakness.
   C. Motor impairment (spasticity, muscle weakness, paralysis, hemiparesis, ataxia) may occur in primary cancer (brain tumors, multiple myeloma) or as a secondary effect in metastatic disease (spinal cord compression), infections, and cancer therapy or in nonmalignant conditions.
III. Risk factors
   A. Skeletal system tumor
   B. Tumors of the brain and spinal cord
   C. Obstruction in lymphatic or systemic circulation
   D. Bone pain, stiffness, fatigue
   E. Spinal cord compression
   F. Sensory-perceptual alterations
   G. Nonmalignant conditions—herniated disks, vertebral fractures secondary to osteoporosis, ear infections
   H. Complications of bed rest
   I. Complications of cardiopulmonary disorders
   J. Dehydration
   K. Side effects of treatment, including corticosteroid therapy, radiation therapy, and chemotherapy/endocrine therapy
   L. Nerve and muscle damage from surgical intervention

M. Changes in physical activity level
N. Independent versus dependent personality
O. Presence or absence of social support
P. Depression or high or low stress level

ASSESSMENT

I. History
   A. Presence of risk factors
   B. Recent treatment and anticipated side effects
   C. Decreased activity level
   D. Functional status using a standardized tool (Tables 41.1 and 41.2)
   E. Presence of pain, muscle weakness, and fatigue
   F. Presence of dyspnea, activity intolerance
   G. Presence of vertigo, ringing in ears, or blurred vision
   H. Evaluation of fall risk
   I. History of alcohol or drug use
   J. Current exercise practice
   K. Current therapy
II. Physical examination
   A. Changes in muscle tone, strength, and muscle mass
   B. Unintentional weight loss
   C. Strength and motor function
   D. Mobility and sensory function
   E. Changes in sexual function
   F. Changes in bowel and bladder function/incontinence and loss of sphincter control
   G. Range of joint motion
   H. Positive Babinski sign and reflexes
   I. Alignment, balance, gait, and joint structure
   J. Difficulty changing position from sitting to standing
   K. Difficulty writing name
III. Psychosocial examination
   A. Depression
   B. Anxiety
   C. Lack of motivation
IV. Laboratory data (Khan, Dellinger, Waguespack, 2017)
   A. Electrolyte abnormalities (hyper or hypo)
      1. Calcium stabilizes blood pressure and controls skeletal muscle contraction. It's also used to build strong bones and teeth.
      2. Chloride is necessary to maintain proper balance of body fluids.

TABLE 41.1 Eastern Cooperative Oncology Group (ECOG) Performance Status

Grade	Performance Status
0	Fully active, able to carry on all predisease performance without restriction
1	Restricted in physically strenuous activity but ambulatory and able to carry out work of a light or sedentary nature (e.g., light housework, office work)
2	Ambulatory and capable of all self-care but unable to carry out any work activities; up and about more than 50% of waking hours
3	Capable of only limited self-care, confined to bed or chair more than 50% of waking hours
4	Completely disabled; cannot carry on any self-care; totally confined to bed or chair
5	Dead

From Oken, M. M., Creech, R. H., Tormey, D. C., Horton, J., Davis, T. E., McFadden, E. T., & Carbone, P. P. (1982). Toxicity and response criteria of the Eastern Cooperative Oncology Group. *American Journal of Clinical Oncology, 5,* 649-655.

TABLE 41.2 Karnofsky Performance Scale

Percentage of Normal Performance Status	Definitions
100	Normal; no complaints; no evidence of disease
90	Able to carry on normal activity; minor signs or symptoms of disease
80	Normal activity with effort; some signs or symptoms of disease
70	Cares for self; unable to carry on normal activity or do active work
60	Requires occasional assistance but is able to care for most of needs
50	Requires considerable assistance and frequent medical care
40	Disabled; requires special care and assistance
30	Severely disabled; hospitalization is indicated, although death is not imminent
10	Moribund; fatal process progressing rapidly
0	Dead

From Karnofsky, D. A., & Burchenal, J. H. (1949). The clinical evaluation of chemotherapeutic agents in cancer. In C. M. MacLeod (Ed.), *Evaluation of chemotherapeutic agents,* (p. 196). New York, NY: Columbia University.

3. Magnesium is a critical mineral that regulates many important functions (muscle contraction, heart rhythm, and nerve function)
4. Phosphate interacts closely with calcium
5. Potassium regulates heart function and helps maintain healthy nerves and muscles

6. Sodium maintains fluid balance, critical for normal body function, helps regulate nerve function and muscle contraction
B. Lumbar puncture results to evaluate for disease to central nervous system

MANAGEMENT

I. Manage electrolyte disturbances; replace as needed
II. Interventions to increase physical functioning (Martin, 2014)
  A. Have the patient perform active-range-of-motion (AROM) exercises on unaffected limbs at least three or four times per day and passive range of motion (PROM) on affected limbs
  B. Monitor progress from AROM to functional activities
  C. Maintain body alignment while the patient is in bed
  D. Change the patient's position every 2 hours
  E. Observe the patient before, during, and after activity or exercise
  F. Obtain appropriate assistive devices (e.g., splints, walker, cane, overhead trapeze)
  G. Consult with rehabilitation services for physical and occupational therapy
III. Interventions to decrease risk of further complications of immobility
  A. Establish a routine for activities of daily living (ADLs)
  B. Assist and supervise as needed
  C. Place the call light within reach when the patient is left alone
IV. Interventions to maximize safety for the patient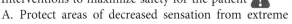
  A. Protect areas of decreased sensation from extreme heat and cold
  B. Teach the patient with decreased perception of extremities to check where the limb is placed when changing positions
  C. Place the bed in low position and the two side rails at the head of bed (HOB) up
  D. Clear pathways in room and hallways
  E. Use night lights or soft lighting at night to enhance vision
V. Interventions to enhance adaptation and rehabilitation
  A. Positive reinforcement for behaviors that contribute to positive outcomes
  B. Have the patient and family responsible for aspects of care according to capabilities
  C. Initiate and follow up with referrals to rehabilitation services
VI. Interventions to incorporate patient and family in care
  A. Instruct patient and family about signs and symptoms to report
  B. Discuss risk factors for impaired mobility

EXPECTED PATIENT OUTCOMES

I. Patient will gain an enhanced sense of balance and strengthen compensatory body parts to prevent skin breakdown and enhance increased venous return, prevent stiffness, and maintain muscle strength and stamina.

REFERENCES

Joglekar, S., Ashghar, A., Mott, S., Benjamin, E., Johnson, B., Button, A., et al. (2015). Sarcopenia is an independent predictor of complications following pancreatectomy for adenocarcinoma. *Journal of Surgical Oncology, 111*(6), 771–775. https://doi.org/10.1002/jso.23862.

Joglekar, S., Nau, P., & Mehzhir, J. (2015). The impact of sarcopenia on survival and complications in surgical oncology: a review of the current literature. *Journal of Surgical Oncology, 112*(5), 503–509. http:// doi.org/10.1002/jso.24095

Karnofsky, D. A., & Burchenal, J. H. (1949). The clinical evaluation of chemotherapeutic agents in cancer. In C. M. MacLeod (Ed.), *Evaluation of chemotherapeutic agents*, (p. 196). New York, NY: Columbia University.

Khan, M., Dellinger, R., & Waguespack, S. (2017). Electrolyte disturbances in critically ill cancer patients: an endocrine perspective. *Journal of Intensive Care Medicine, 33*(3), 147–158. https://doi.org/10.1177/0885066617706650.

Martin, V. R. (2014). Arthralgias and myalgias. In C. H. Yarbro, D. Wujcik, & B. H. Gobel (Eds.), *Cancer symptom management* (4th ed., pp. 13–23). Burlington, VT: Jones and Bartlett.

Oken, M. M., Creech, R. H., Tormey, D. C., Horton, J., Davis, T. E., McFadden, E. T., & Carbone, P. P. (1982). Toxicity and response criteria of the Eastern Cooperative Oncology Group. *American Journal of Clinical Oncology, 5*, 649–655.

42

Neurologic Symptoms

Kathy Waitman

OVERVIEW

I. Physiology/definitions
   A. Neuropathies—any functional disturbances, pathologic changes, or both in the peripheral nervous system (PNS): cranial, sensory, and motor nerves and portions of the autonomic nervous system
   B. Neuropathies of the central nervous system (CNS)—seizures, encephalopathy, cerebellar dysfunction, ophthalmologic toxicities and ototoxicities, mental status changes, and peripheral neuropathies with sensory and motor dysfunction
   C. Incidence and severity of neuropathies—may vary, depending on administration of immunosuppressive therapy, surgeries, diagnosis, or other treatments
   D. Toxicities—may be dose related from chemotherapy or other therapies, and reversible on discontinuation of therapy or exposure to poisons

II. Risk factors
   A. Disease related (Ibañez-Juliá, et al., 2018; Nobile-Orazio, Bianco, & Nozza, 2017)
      1. Effects of cancer
      2. Postherpetic neuralgia (PHN)
      3. Presence of infiltrative emergencies (e.g., spinal cord compression)
      4. Other diseases (e.g., history of hepatic or neurologic dysfunction)
      5. Preexisting neuropathies because of diabetes mellitus, human immunodeficiency virus (HIV) infection, preexisting vitamin B complex deficiency may include—tingling of fingers and toes, jaw pain, foot drop, muscular atrophy
   B. Treatment related (Eltobgy, et al., 2017; Flatters, Dougherty, & Colvin, 2017; Pachman, Watson, & Loprinzi, 2014; Grisdale & Armstrong, 2014)
      1. Side effects of chemotherapy and immunotherapy (e.g., cerebellar dysfunction, strokelike reaction, generalized weakness, gait disturbance, numbness of feet, loss of proprioception, vibratory sensation) (Table 42.1).
      2. Side effects of radiation therapy (e.g., ataxia, dysarthria, nystagmus, radicular pain) and preexisting peripheral neuropathy related to radiation therapy.
   C. Individual (Grisdale & Armstrong, 2014)
      1. Age—older than 60 years
      2. Social issues (malnutrition, alcohol abuse, repetitive actions)

ASSESSMENT (Table 42.2)

I. History (Grisdale & Armstrong, 2014)
   A. Presence of risk factors or other comorbidities such as diabetes, idiopathic neuropathy before chemotherapy
   B. Psychiatric and current social situation
   C. Acute herpes zoster
   D. Recent chemotherapy treatment and anticipated side effects
   E. Presence of weakness
   F. Presence of burning, numbness, tingling in feet and hands, perioral numbness, paresthesias—stocking–glove distribution
   G. Presence of paresthesia of hands and feet, constipation, loss of deep tendon reflex
   H. Presence of cerebellar involvement (e.g., tremors, loss of balance)
   I. Ability to perform activities of daily living (ADLs) and occupational and recreational activities
   J. Current medication therapy
   K. Presence of anxiety, low self-esteem
II. Physical examination
   A. Vital signs
   B. Baseline sensory, mobility, motor function, autonomic function, cranial nerve assessment, and cerebellar function
   C. Speech or language ability
   D. Sight-related changes (e.g., blurred vision, impaired color perception)
III. Psychological examination
   A. Anxiety management strategies
   B. Coping style and ability
IV. Laboratory data
   A. Nerve conduction studies (e.g., electromyography [EMG])
   B. Muscle or nerve biopsy

TABLE 42.1	**Chemotherapy Agents Associated with Peripheral Neuropathy**				
Antineoplastic Agent	**Associated Neuropathy**	**Antineoplastic Agent**	**Associated Neuropathy**	**Antineoplastic Agent**	**Associated Neuropathy**
Bortezomib	Sensory	Etoposide (VP-16)	Sensory Motor	Vinblastine	Sensory Motor Cranial Autonomic
Carboplatin	Sensory Cranial (rare) Autonomic	5-Fluorouracil	Motor (rare)	Vincristine	Sensory Motor Cranial Autonomic
Carmustine (BCNU)	Cranial Automatic	Hexamethylmelamine	Sensory Motor	Vindesine	Sensory Motor Cranial Autonomic
Cisplatin	Sensory Motor Cranial	Methotrexate	Sensory Motor Cranial	Vinorelbine	Sensory Motor Cranial Autonomic (mild)
Cytarabine (Ara-C)	Sensory Motor Cranial	Paclitaxel	Sensory Motor Autonomic (mild)		
Docetaxel	Sensory Motor Autonomic (mild)	Procarbazine	Sensory Motor		
Doxifluridine (5-dFUrd)	Sensory Motor	Teniposide (VM-26)	Sensory Motor		

TABLE 42.2	**Assessment of Neuropathy**
Function	**Procedure**
Cerebellar and proprioception	• Evaluate rapid alternating movement of hands. • Observe for accurate movement of extremities. • Evaluate balance using Romberg test: have patient stand with feet together, arms at side with eyes closed. A slight sway is normal. • Observe gait for stride and stance.
Sensory function	• Test for response to touch and pain. • Check vibration sense using a tuning fork. • Evaluate position sense: move a finger or great toe up and down while patient's eyes are closed; have patient identify position of the digit. • Assess for discrimination between sharp and dull sensations. • Evaluate the ability to distinguish the body part being touched. • Evaluate for stereognosis, the ability to distinguish a common object, such as a coin. • Evaluate for graphesthesia, the ability to identify a common letter or number drawn on the hand.
Deep tendon reflexes	• Test deep tendon reflexes (biceps, brachioradial, triceps, patellar, Achilles). • Check for clonus.

From Marrs, J., & Newton, S. (2003). Updating your peripheral neuropathy "know how." *Clinical Journal of Oncology Nursing, 7*(3), 299-303.

MANAGEMENT

I. Pharmacologic interventions for pain reduction (Grisdale & Armstrong, 2014)
   A. Mild analgesics—acetaminophen (Tylenol) and nonsteroidal antiinflammatory drugs
   B. Antidepressants—amitriptyline (Elavil), imipramine (Tofranil), nortriptyline (Pamelor), duloxetine (Cymbalta)
   C. Anticonvulsants (e.g., gabapentin [Neurontin], pregabalin [Lyrica], valproic acid [Depakote])
   D. Opioids
   E. Lidocaine 5% patch
   F. Glutamine
   G. Use of creams (e.g., application of capsaicin cream three or four times daily)
II. Interventions to increase participation in care

A. Assess knowledge of early signs and symptoms of neuropathies
B. Teach about side effects of chemotherapy
C. Teach about hand and foot care (use of massage and lotions)
D. Refer to occupational and rehabilitation services
E. Before chemotherapy, instruct patient about potential neurologic side effects
F. Instruct patient on how to maintain a safe environment both at home and at work
G. Give positive feedback and honest reassurance
H. Empower patient to communicate with physician and nurse about symptoms

III. Interventions to minimize diminished sensations
A. Have patient protect hands and feet from cold through use of gloves and socks
B. Have patient avoid excess stimulation of skin and avoid tight clothing
C. Have patient wear gloves for gardening activities
D. Teach about inspection of affected areas for burns, cuts, abrasions

IV. Interventions to promote self-care and decrease mobility impairment
A. Collaborate with physical and occupational rehabilitation services
B. Develop an exercise and muscle-strengthening program
C. Use assistive devices to assist with mobilization and fine motor needs
D. Assist in performance of ADLs as needed

V. Nonpharmacologic interventions to manage pain, anxiety, depression
A. Encourage exercise
B. Consider transcutaneous electrical nerve stimulation (TENS)
C. Offer acupuncture and acupressure
D. Encourage relaxation techniques—yoga, meditation, guided imagery
E. Refer for biofeedback
F. Encourage art and music therapy

EXPECTED PATIENT OUTCOMES

I. The patient will understand the risk for neuropathies and monitor for signs and symptoms to report to staff.

II. Patient verbalizes measures to maximize safety and manage self-care (i.e., maintains or increases mobility, verbalizes a satisfactory relief of pain, maintains regular bowel function).

III. The patient will maintain function to promote the ability to carry out ADLs, decrease pain, and improve quality of life.

REFERENCES

Eltobgy, M., Oweira, H., Petrausch, U., Helbling, D., Schmidt, J., Mehrabi, A., … Abdel-Rahman, O. (2017). Immune-related neurological toxicities among solid tumor patients treated with immune checkpoint inhibitors: a systematic review. *Journal of Expert Review of Neurotherapeutics, 17*(7), 725–736. https://doi.org/10.1080/14737175.2017.1336088.

Flatters, S. J., Dougherty, P. M., & Colvin, L. A. (2017). Clinical and preclinical perspectives on chemotherapy-induced peripheral neuropathy (CIPN): a narrative review. *British Journal of Anesthesia, 119*(4), 737–749. https://doi.org/10.1093/bja/aex229.

Grisdale, K. A. & Armstrong, T, S, (2014). In D. Camp-Sorrell and R. A. Hawkins (Eds.), Clinical manual for the oncology advanced practice nurse (3rd ed., pp. 1146-1147). Pittsburgh, PA: Oncology Nursing Society.

Ibañez-Juliá, M. J., Berzero, G., Reyes-Botero, G., Maisonobe, T., Lenglet, T., Slim, M., … Psimaras, D. (2018). Antineoplastic agents exacerbating Charcot Marie Tooth disease: red flags to avoid permanent disability. *Acta Oncologica, 57*(3), 403–411. https://doi.org/10.1080/0284186X.2017.1415462.

Marrs, J., & Newton, S. (2003). Updating your peripheral neuropathy "know how". *Clinical Journal of Oncology Nursing, 7*(3), 299–303.

Nobile-Orazio, E., Bianco, M., & Nozza, A. (2017). Advances in the treatment of paraproteinemic neuropathy. *Current Treatment Options Neurology, 19*(43). https://doi.org/10.1007/s11940-017-0479-9.

Pachman, D. R., Watson, J. C., & Loprinzi, C. L. (2014). Therapeutic strategies for cancer treatment related peripheral neuropathies. *Current Treatment Options in Oncology, 15*(4), 567–580. https://doi.org/10.1007/s11864-014-0303-7.

43

Nutrition Issues

Diane Cope

WEIGHT CHANGES AND BODY COMPOSITION

Overview

I. Definition
   A. Overnutrition or undernutrition (weight gain, weight loss, and changes in body composition) associated with cancer and cancer treatments, which may negatively affect cancer recurrence, survival, morbidity, and quality of life (QOL).
   B. Body composition is the relative proportions of protein, fat, water, and mineral components in the body.
II. Risk factors for weight gain
   A. Treatment related
      1. Multiagent chemotherapy regimens, regimens containing steroids, or both
      2. Effusions—pleural, pericardial, abdominal
      3. Edema
      4. Obstruction
      5. Inactivity
      6. Electrolyte imbalances
      7. Hormonal drugs, steroids, biological medications such as interleukin-2 (IL-2)
      8. Metabolic complications
      9. Adjuvant chemotherapy for breast cancer
III. Risk factors for weight loss (Arends, Bachmann, Baracos, et al., 2016)
   A. Disease related
      1. Increased risk with non-Hodgkin's lymphoma, lung, and gastrointestinal (GI) cancers
      2. Protein-calorie malnutrition caused by the metabolic effects of the tumor
      3. Tumor location—increased weight loss associated with upper respiratory and gastric tumors
      4. Alterations in ability to eat
      5. Disrupted absorption of nutrients
   B. Treatment related
      1. Surgery related
         a. Increased risk with head and neck, esophageal, gastric, pancreatic, or colorectal cancer surgeries
         b. Postprandial dumping syndrome associated with gastric resections
         c. Frequent tests usually needed in surgical oncology patients; may limit intake, require dietary restrictions, or both

   d. Increased calories expended, energy needs increased during perioperative period
      2. Radiation therapy
         a. Radiation field related with head and neck, lung, and GI cancers.
         b. Increased risk for anorexia, diarrhea, nausea, vomiting, mucositis, esophagitis, gastritis, xerostomia, and taste changes
      3. Chemotherapy
         a. Nausea and vomiting with prevalence of nausea estimated at 42% to 52% (Farrell, Brearley, Pilling, & Molassiotis, 2013).
         b. Indirect effects causing anorexia, fatigue, constipation, taste changes, anxiety, and depression
   C. Multifactorial
      1. Insensible losses (e.g., perspiration, gastric suction, surgical drains, fistulas, wounds)
      2. Acute or chronic diarrhea caused by drugs (e.g., antibiotics, chemotherapy), dietary alterations, infectious processes (e.g., Clostridium difficile), intestinal ischemia, fecal impaction, irritable bowel disease, laxative abuse, endocrine disorders, malabsorption, surgery, and radiation colitis
      3. Post–stem cell transplantation acute and chronic graft-versus-host disease (GVHD)
      4. Presence of concurrent symptoms related to cancer treatment, including anorexia, taste alterations, mucositis, pain, anxiety, depression, and fatigue
      5. Medication side effects, including antibiotics, opioids, biological, and targeted therapies

Assessment (Jager-Wittenaar & Ottery, 2017; White, Guenter, Jensen, Malone, & Schofield, 2012)

I. History
   A. Previous dietary patterns, food preferences, cultural preferences, food allergies, eating habits, and history of weight changes
   B. Patterns of weight changes: type, onset, duration, severity; early satiety; associated symptoms—nausea, food intolerances, taste abnormalities, mouth/throat pain, dysphagia, vomiting, diarrhea; other factors—precipitating, aggravating, alleviating factors

C. Current or recent treatment for cancer and experienced side effects

D. Assessment of patient for associated cultural, socioeconomic, emotional, and motivational factors that may affect weight loss or gain

E. Ability to carry out interventions to maintain weight

F. Use of food, nutritional supplements, and other remedies

II. Physical examination

A. Determine present weight, height, and amount of total weight loss or gain

B. Assess for dehydration, electrolyte imbalances, serum albumin

C. Assess mobility, skin tone and turgor, muscle strength

D. Evaluation and reassessment of nutritional status

1. Assess/screen each patient for changes in nutritional status at each contact (on admission to the hospital and at regular follow-up intervals, during each home visit, or at outpatient clinic visits).

Management

I. Interventions to increase calorie and nutritional value of oral intake

A. Teach patient or caregiver to do the following:

1. Take oral supplements to increase protein-calorie intake, between meals, bedtime

2. Limit liquids at mealtime because they may cause early satiety and nausea

3. Discuss taste changes, review liquids and foods that patient may be able to tolerate

4. Consume nutritionally dense/high-protein foods such as cottage cheese, puddings, and oatmeal

5. Eat frequent, small portions throughout the day

6. Maximize food intake during periods of greatest strength and appetite, usually early in the day

7. Increase kilocalorie (kcal) protein content of foods by adding protein powders, instant nonfat dry milk powder/instant breakfast powders to gravies, puddings, other foods

8. Maximize food preferences and access to favorite foods within dietary restrictions

9. Choose high-protein, high-calorie, healthy snacks between meals

10. Try cold, room-temperature, and soft foods to improve intake

II. Interventions to promote comfort while eating

A. Administer pain medications, if needed, 30 to 60 minutes before meals

B. Perform oral hygiene before and after meals

C. Try cold, room-temperature, and soft foods to improve intake

III. Patient and caregiver education

A. Assist patient/caregiver with calculating individualized calorie and protein requirements so realistic goals can be set for weight changes; may need to consult with a nutritionist

B. Use proper quantities of foods from the food groups that provide a balanced, nutritious diet for weight control

C. Have the patient engage in regular exercise, if able

D. Encourage consultation with a dietitian

TASTE ALTERATIONS

Overview

I. Definition—actual or perceived change in taste sensation or loss of taste

A. Hypogeusesthesia—a decrease in the acuity of the taste sensation

B. Dysgeusia—an unusual taste perception, perceived as unpleasant

C. Ageusia—an absence of the taste sensation, "mouth blindness"

II. Physiology

A. Taste is a chemical sense that is mediated through specialized epithelial cells located in the oral cavity, oropharynx, larynx, and upper third of esophagus

B. Receptor sites in taste buds on the tongue are innervated by cranial nerves, which send taste information about sweet, sour, salty, and bitter sensations to the medulla and cortex

C. Taste and smell are integrated functions

1. Air entering the nostrils ascends to the olfactory cleft, connects with olfactory receptors

2. During chewing and swallowing, air is pushed from the mouth into the nose, stimulating the olfactory receptor, carrying the signal via cranial nerve I to the cortex and subcortex II

III. Pathophysiology (Murtaza, Hichami, Khan, Ghiringhelli, & Khan, 2017)

A. Cell damage

1. Decrease in the number of normal cell receptors

2. Alteration of cell structure or receptor surface changes

3. Interruption of neural coding

B. Rapidly proliferating cancer cells release a number of cytokines/chemokines, initiating recruitment of macrophages and neutrophils and an inflammatory state, which may modulate areas of the brain involved in the control of taste and smell perception

C. Alteration in carbohydrate metabolism and taste perception may be a common mechanism between type 2 diabetes and cancer

D. Excretion of amino acid–like substances from the tumor cells changes taste bud sensations (sweet, sour, bitter, salty)

E. Zinc deficiency caused by oncolytic agents, which bind and chelate zinc, result in loss of taste

F. Invasion of tumor into the oral cavity or salivary glands

G. Oral infections such as candidiasis

H. Treatment related

1. Radiation therapy: changes in salivation production and consistency may precede mucositis or xerostomia (Nguyen, Reyland, & Barlow, 2012; Sroussi, Epstein, Bensadoun, et al., 2017)
   a. Destruction of the taste buds occurs by 3–4 weeks, commonly affecting all taste modalities, and return to baseline 6–12 months after treatment, or never return to normal
   b. Saliva may become thick or tenacious early, and membranes may become dry at about day 10–14 during radiation treatment; condition may continue for 2–4 months after completion of radiation therapy (RT); beverages or foods that are slightly tart or carbonated may help thin secretions
2. Surgical interventions: specific surgical sites—oral cavity, tongue, salivary glands, pathway of the olfactory nerve, tracheostomy
3. Chemotherapy
   a. Certain drugs have a greater effect on taste sensation than others—for example, cisplatin (Platinol), ironotecan (Camptosar), cyclophosphamide (Cytoxan), dacarbazine (DTIC-Dome), dactinomycin (actinomycin D, Cosmegen), mechlorethamine (nitrogen mustard, Mustargen), methotrexate (Mexate), vincristine (Oncovin), and fluorouracil (5-FU, 5-fluorouracil)

IV. Risk factors
   A. Poor oral hygiene
   B. Nutritional deficiencies—zinc, copper, nickel, niacin, vitamins A and C
   C. Age-induced degeneration of the taste buds
   D. Learned aversions
      1. Taste changes that develop when a food is associated with unpleasant symptoms such as nausea, vomiting, and pain
      2. Seem to develop most rapidly to new or novel foods

Assessment

I. History
   A. Presence of hypogeusesthesia, ageusia, or dysgeusia
   B. History of risk factors, including degree and duration of taste alterations
   C. Subjective description of changes in taste and impact of taste alterations on nutritional status and usual lifestyle patterns
   D. Constant or intermittent metallic and bitter taste; increased or decreased threshold for the sweetness sensation; increased threshold for salty and sour tastes; decreased threshold for bitter taste; and aversion to meats, coffee, chocolate

II. Physical examination
   A. Oral assessment
   B. Weight

C. Presence of other physical problems associated with altered intake
   1. Evaluate oral cavity and throat for presence of erythema, desquamation, dryness or excess saliva, and ulceration
   2. Assess for signs and symptoms of secondary oral infection

III. Laboratory findings associated with compromised nutritional status
   A. Decreased levels of albumin, transferrin, and total lymphocytes
   B. Decreased levels of zinc, copper, and nickel
   C. Decreased levels of niacin and vitamin A

Management (Kalaskar, 2014)

I. Interventions to minimize risk of occurrence and severity of taste alterations
   A. Institute measures to increase sensitivity of taste buds, decrease food aversion, increase salivation, and compensate for oral dryness
      1. Experiment with spices and flavorings to enhance taste
      2. Use the aroma of foods to stimulate taste
      3. Increase fluid intake with meals
      4. Encourage oral hygiene before and after meals
      5. Add sweeteners to foods and marinate meats in sweet juices
      6. Substitute other sources of protein for poorly tolerated protein sources such as meats
      7. Have patient avoid the sight and smell of unpleasant foods
      8. Have patient consume candies such as lemon drops or chew gum to change taste before meals and before chemotherapy treatment to reduce metallic taste and stimulate saliva
      9. Increase water or juices at frequent intervals—for example, several times per hour
      10. Spray water, saline, or artificial saliva on the mucous membranes
      11. Have patient suck on smooth, flat, tart candies or lozenges to stimulate saliva
      12. Have patient avoid alcohol, commercial mouthwashes, and smoking
      13. Humidify environmental air
      14. Offer foods that are moist or have gravy or sauces and discourage intake of dry foods such as toast or crackers

II. Interventions to monitor for complications related to taste alterations
   A. Weigh patient at regular intervals
   B. Maintain a daily diet record
   C. Teach patients the importance of diligent oral care and inspection, and ensure that they are aware of conditions for which they should contact the health care team

III. Interventions to include patient and caregiver in care (see Anorexia, Planning and Implementation sections)

Expected Patient Outcome

I. Patient will utilize appropriate interventions to decrease risk of taste alterations to achieve and maintain optimal nutrition.

ANOREXIA

Overview

I. Definition—loss of appetite accompanied by decreased oral intake; usually accompanied by other symptoms that exacerbate decreased food intake and progressive weight loss, with approximately 80% incidence in patients with cancer from diagnosis to advanced stages

II. Sequelae of anorexia (Berry, Blonquist, Mayak, 2018)
   A. Decreased calorie and protein intake with subsequent loss of fat and muscle mass, weight loss, weakness, fatigue.
      1. May lead to cachexia, which may affect prognosis by making patient less tolerant of therapy, causing dose or schedule changes that may diminish treatment effectiveness
   B. Abnormalities of carbohydrate, protein, and fat metabolism
   C. Visceral and lean body mass depletion—muscle atrophy, visceral organ atrophy, hypoalbuminemia, anemia
   D. Compromised humoral and cellular immune function—impaired neutrophil function (chemotaxis, fungicidal, bactericidal) and delayed bone marrow production
      1. Protein-calorie malnutrition interferes with the delivery of oncologic therapy and increases the severity of side effects of treatment

III. Physiology
   A. Food intake is regulated by long- and short-term mediators involved in transmission of signals between neurotransmitters in the peripheral and central nervous systems
      1. Short-acting mediators in gut are responsible for satiety signals and maintenance of food intake based on energy expenditure and maintenance of body weight.
         a. Increased food intake and reduction of fat utilization stimulated by ghrelin, a gut hormone.
      2. Long-acting mediators consist of insulin and leptin.
         a. Insulin regulates nutrient storage and energy balance
         b. Leptin regulates adipose energy reserves, with low leptin levels increasing hypothalamic signals that stimulate feeding, decrease appetite-suppressing signals

IV. Pathophysiology (Ezeoke & Morley, 2015)
   A. Multifactorial
   B. Tumor-related peripheral or central effects

1. Peripheral
   a. Substances released by the tumor such as proinflammatory cytokines, lactate, and parathormone-related peptide
   b. Tumors causing dysphagia or altering gut function
   c. Tumors altering nutrients such as zinc deficiency
   d. Tumors causing hypoxia
   e. Increased peripheral tryptophan leading to increased central serotonin
   f. Alterations in release of peripheral hormones that alter feeding such as peptide tyrosine and ghrelin
2. Central
   a. Tumors causing alterations in neurotransmitters, neuropeptides, and prostaglandins that modulate feeding
3. Psychological factors
   a. Anxiety, depression, fear, or distress
4. Social factors
   a. Loss of pleasure previously associated with food
   b. Changes in eating environment
   c. Changes in companionship during eating
5. Physiologic factors
   a. Presence of concurrent symptoms, including nausea or vomiting, early satiety, diarrhea, constipation, pain, dysphagia, mucositis, ascites, taste/smell alterations
   b. Metabolic disturbances: hypercalcemia, hypokalemia, uremia, hyponatremia
   c. Medication side effects associated with opioids, antibiotics, and iron
   d. Treatment-related effects from chemotherapy, RT, surgery, and biotherapy

V. Risk factors (O'Leary, 2016)
   A. Advanced cancer
   B. Pulmonary and cardiac comorbidities
   C. Older age
   D. Multimodal treatment
   E. Solid tumors, especially lung and GI cancers

Assessment

I. History
   A. Previous dietary patterns, food preferences, eating habits, bowel patterns, and history of anorexia with patient and family
   B. Patterns of anorexia—onset, frequency, severity; associated symptoms—food intolerances, early satiety, nausea, taste abnormalities, mouth or throat pain, dysphagia; other factors—precipitating, aggravating, alleviating factors
   C. Previous self-care strategies
   D. Current or recent treatment for cancer and side effects
      1. Ability to implement interventions to relieve anorexia
      2. Use of food and nutritional supplements

3. Use of alternative or complementary nutritional products

II. Physical examination

A. Determine present weight and amount of total weight loss

B. Assess for dehydration, electrolyte imbalances, or both—dry mouth, poor skin turgor, decreased urinary output

C. Assess for associated ethnic, socioeconomic, emotional, and motivational factors that may affect the loss of weight or decreased oral intake

D. Assess psychosocial responses to fear, anxiety, stress, depression, and noxious stimuli in the environment

Management (Ezeoke & Morley, 2015)

I. Interventions to monitor complications related to anorexia

A. Maintain a daily dietary intake record

B. Weigh regularly

C. Assess for signs and symptoms of electrolyte imbalances and dehydration

D. Assess for overall skin and nail condition for adverse effects of poor nutrition or intake—skin breakdown, dehiscence, or poor wound healing

II. Interventions to include patient and caregiver in care

A. Encourage caregiver to provide foods within dietary restrictions, explore necessity of dietary restrictions when nutritional requirements not being met as a result of restrictions

B. Teach caregiver methods to enhance protein-calorie content of foods and methods to enhance food intake

C. Teach patient and caregiver about the signs and symptoms of dehydration (dry skin and mucous membranes, poor skin turgor, decreased urinary output), delayed wound healing, malnutrition (wasting of skeletal mass, body fat decrease, weight loss, sepsis, reduced energy) and when to report critical symptoms to the treatment team

D. Develop strategies with patient and caregiver to increase protein-calorie intake each day

1. Provide a list of high-calorie, high-protein foods

2. Offer suggestions for supplementing nutritional value by adding protein or milk powders and supplements

3. Use of medications as ordered by licensed provider—pain medications, vitamin supplements, and medications that may stimulate appetite (e.g., corticosteroids or megestrol acetate [Megace])

4. Plan mealtimes that are relaxed, unhurried, and pleasant

5. Encourage a positive eating environment by setting table attractively, listening to music, and avoiding eating from cartons or cans

6. Use a variety of foods to avoid taste fatigue

7. Avoid fixating on intake to the point that it may become counterproductive

III. Interventions to enhance adaptation and rehabilitation

A. Provide written/audiovisual materials on nutrition at patient's level of understanding

B. Initiate early referral to a dietitian for nutritional assessment or intervention

CACHEXIA

Overview

I. Definition (Berry, Blonquist, T., Mayak, 2018; Cunningham, 2018; LeBlanc, Nipp, Rushing, et al., 2015).

A. Progressive deterioration with muscle wasting that occurs when protein and calorie requirements are not met

B. Greater than 5% involuntary weight loss over 6 months or a body mass index (BMI) of less than 20 and any degree of weight loss more than 2%, or an appendicular skeletal muscle index with sarcopenia and any degree of weight loss more than 2% (Douglas & McMillan, 2014)

C. Characterized by anorexia, weight loss, skeletal muscle atrophy, and asthenia

D. Often occurs with anorexia, which constitutes a clinical syndrome known as the cancer anorexia–cachexia syndrome (CACS)

E. Associated with poor QOL, impaired functional status, muscle wasting, inflammation, fatigue, and ultimately shortened survival

II. Sequalae of cachexia

A. Increased morbidity and mortality present in 80% with advanced cancer

B. Decreased tissue sensitivity to insulin and decreased insulin response to glucose

C. Impairment of immunocompetence—humoral, cellular, secretory, and mucosal immunity

D. Poor wound healing and increased infection rates

E. Protein-calorie malnutrition with resultant weight loss; visceral and somatic protein depletion that compromises enzymatic, structural, and mechanical functions

F. Constipation caused by lack of food and fluid intake and the effects of cancer treatments

III. Pathophysiology

A. Complex process involving anorexia, metabolic alterations, release of cytokines, and other catabolic factors that lead to skeletal muscle wasting

B. Mediated by proinflammatory cytokines, including tumor necrosis factor (TNF), IL-1, IL-6, interferon (IFN)-alpha, and IFN-beta, which may be produced by the tumor itself or by the immune system in response to the tumor

C. Metabolic alterations—include decreased gluconeogenesis; alterations in glucose metabolism; increased metabolic rate; changed lipid, protein, carbohydrate metabolism

IV. Risk factors
  A. Disease related—cancer, especially lung and pancreatic cancers and gastric carcinomas, AIDS, infections, sepsis, inflammatory diseases
  B. Treatment related—chemotherapy; biotherapy; RT; surgery of the head, neck, stomach, pancreas, and bowel
  C. Situation related
    1. Psychological aspects of nutritional intake—cancer cachexia viewed by some to be the hallmark of terminal illness; thus patients frequently "give up"
    2. Depression, inactivity, absence of an appetite, and functional losses affect the patient's QOL

Assessment (Bruggeman, Kamal, LeBlanc, Ma, Baracos, & Roeland, (2016))

I. History
  A. Previous dietary patterns, food preferences, eating habits, type and quantity of food consumed, history of anorexia discussed with patient and family
  B. Patterns of anorexia and presence of fatigue and malaise—assessment for onset, frequency, severity; associated symptoms—food intolerances, taste abnormalities, pain, dysphagia; other factors—precipitating, aggravating, alleviating factors
  C. Previous self-care strategies—ability to provide for own interventions to relieve anorexia; use of food, nutritional supplements, and other remedies
  D. Current or recent treatment for cancer and side effects experienced
  E. Associated cultural, socioeconomic, emotional, and motivational factors that may affect the loss of weight
II. Physical examination
  A. Determine present weight and amount of total and recent weight loss
  B. Assess for dehydration, electrolyte imbalances, or both
  C. Assess for muscle atrophy, loss of fat deposits, and presence of edema
  D. Anthropometric measurements or consultation with a nutritionist
  E. Review of biochemical measurements
    1. Triceps skinfolds and midarm muscle circumference
    2. Height and weight (weight loss >5% in previous 6 months significant for diagnosis of protein-calorie malnutrition)
    3. Visceral protein stores—serum albumin, prealbumin, total iron-binding capacity, transferrin, electrolytes, nitrogen balance, C-reactive protein, urine
    4. Lean body mass—computed tomography (CT) or dual energy x-ray absorptiometry (DEXA)
    5. Degree of anemia
    6. Deficiencies in trace metals and vitamins and glucose intolerance

Management

I. Medical and nursing therapies
  A. Treat underlying disease
  B. Nursing and nutritional support
    1. Five or six small meals per day
    2. High-protein snacks
    3. High-calorie, low-fat snacks
    4. Liquids that have calories, such as nutritional shakes, smoothies, or supplements
    5. Activities to increase appetite—for example, light exercise
  C. Pharmacologic interventions
    1. Megestrol acetate (Megace)—has a dose–response effect
    2. Medroxyprogesterone—increases appetite
    3. Corticosteroids—dexamethasone (Decadron), methylprednisolone (Medrol), and prednisolone (Prednisone) are effective in improving appetite
    4. Metoclopramide (Reglan)—at low doses may stimulate GI motility and decrease early satiety and nausea
    5. Metabolic inhibitors—to induce anabolism
    6. Other drugs currently being studied with uncertain efficacy—testosterone, nandrolone decanoate, and oxandrolone
    7. Enteral feedings—oral or tube feedings will help maintain normal GI flora and prevent atrophy of GI mucosa
    8. Total parenteral nutrition (TPN) to replace nutritional deficiencies during cancer treatment and according to patient goals

NUTRITION SUPPORT THERAPY
Overview

I. Definition: therapy focusing on nutritional supportive approaches that include screening, assessment, and supplemental enteral or parenteral nutritional support
II. Indications
  A. Patients who are actively receiving anticancer treatment, are malnourished, and are expected to be unable to ingest and absorb nutrients for a prolonged interval
  B. Multifactorial from treatment, tumor, and/or fluid and electrolyte disturbances
    1. Treatment
      a. Less able to tolerate therapy and receive optimal benefits from treatment
      b. More susceptible to infection, debilitation, poor wound healing, skin breakdown, weakness, fatigue, depression, and apathy; poor nutrition affects QOL
      c. Metabolic changes may occur as a result of treatment or side effects of treatment such as increased energy demands that result from fever, stress, diarrhea, vomiting, and cell division or destruction
        (1) Inability to feed oneself
        (2) Inability to masticate or swallow

   (3) Inability to move food through the stomach and bowel
   (4) Bowel diversion
   (5) Nausea and vomiting
   (6) Malabsorption of fat
   (7) Gastric hypersecretion of acid
   (8) Water and electrolyte loss
   (9) Dumping syndrome and changes in gastric motility
   (10) Xerostomia
   (11) Mucositis
   (12) Constipation
   (13) Changes in taste and smell

 2. Tumor
  a. Cancer cells compete with normal cells for nutrients needed for cellular division and growth.
  b. Exact demands of the tumor on the host are unknown; the following metabolic changes are proposed:
   (1) Cancer cells produce biochemical substances that affect the desire for food, altering taste, causing anorexia (by central mechanisms or neurotransmitters)
   (2) Malignant tumors may invade/compress structures and organs vital to the ingestion, digestion, and elimination of food and fluids, or may increase metabolic demands
   (3) Altered carbohydrate metabolism—glucose is mobilized for energy and results in glucose intolerance in selected patients
   (4) Altered protein metabolism—muscle tissue mobilized to meet increased metabolic demands and results in muscle wasting, especially in those patients with cachexia, a severe syndrome of malnutrition

 3. Fluid and electrolyte disturbances
  a. Anaerobic glycolysis—produces two adenosine triphosphate (ATP) molecules where complete oxidation of glucose yields 36 ATP molecules; thus anaerobic glycolysis used by tumors is less efficient
  b. Increased rate of gluconeogenesis—estimated 10% increase in energy expenditure for an individual with cancer
  c. Glucose intolerance—evidenced by a delayed clearing of intravenous (IV) or oral glucose, which could be caused by lack of tissue response to insulin or a defect of insulin response to hyperglycemia
  d. Prealbumin and serum albumin levels often used to measure protein status
  e. Hypoalbuminemia common in patients with cancer—normal albumin level = 4 g/dL; average albumin level in patient with cancer = 2.9 g/dL

  f. Increased uptake of amino acids by tumor
  g. Hypercalcemia—high calcium levels in blood caused by certain tumors
  h. Hyperuricemia—along with hyperphosphatemia and hyperkalemia, result of chemotherapy breakdown of cells in some leukemias and lymphomas leading to tumor lysis syndrome
  i. Hyponatremia—common presentation with bronchogenic and small cell carcinoma causing syndrome of inappropriate antidiuretic hormone (SIADH) secretion and causing persistent loss of sodium and excessive retention of water by the kidneys (see Chapter 52)
  j. Hypokalemia may be caused by chemotherapy or antifungal therapy
  k. Decreased protein synthesis
  l. Increased protein degradation; muscle protein breakdown is accelerated
  m. Protein loss by abnormal leakage or exertion, leading to depletion of protein stores and decreased muscle mass
  n. Use of protein for energy needs
   (1) Protein wasted despite intake of protein
   (2) Weight loss that is often difficult to counteract, despite aggressive feeding
   (3) Decrease in food intake, with partial starvation caused by conserving lean body mass, host depleting own muscle mass to provide amino acids needed
   (4) Loss of appetite, alteration in taste and smell, loss of appealing foods
   (5) Weakness, reduction of strength, decreased functional capacity

C. Nutrition support therapy should not be used routinely in patients undergoing major cancer operations.
 1. Perioperative nutrition support therapy may be beneficial in moderately or severely malnourished patients if administered for 7–14 days preoperatively, but the potential benefits of nutrition support must be weighed against the potential risks of the nutrition support therapy itself and of delaying the operation.
 2. Immune-enhancing enteral formulas containing mixtures of arginine, nucleic acids, and essential fatty acids may be beneficial in malnourished patients undergoing major cancer operations.

D. Nutrition support therapy should not be used routinely as an adjunct to chemotherapy.

E. Nutrition support therapy should not be used routinely in patients undergoing head and neck, abdominal, or pelvic irradiation.

F. Nutrition support therapy is appropriate in patients receiving active anticancer treatment who are malnourished and who are anticipated to be unable to ingest and/or absorb adequate nutrients for a prolonged period

G. The palliative use of nutrition support therapy in terminally ill cancer patients is rarely indicated.
H. Omega-3 fatty acid supplementation may help stabilize weight in cancer patients on oral diets experiencing progressive, unintentional weight loss.
I. Patients should not use therapeutic diets to treat cancer.

Assessment

I. Nutritional workup
  A. Nutritional screening—should be performed before therapy and at intervals during therapy (Jager-Wittenaar & Ottery, 2017)
    1. Nutrition history and dietary habits
    2. Anthropometric measurements—height, weight, midarm circumference, skinfold thickness, calculation of ideal body weight, BMI
    3. Biochemical measurements of protein status—serum albumin, transferrin, prealbumin; assessing long-term, intermediate-term, and short-term protein status
  B. Nutritional assessment—includes an evaluation of the desire and ability of the patient to ingest and process nutritional products (Jager-Wittenaar & Ottery, 2017)
    1. Ingestion, digestion, metabolism, excretion
    2. Desire to eat
    3. Patterns of dietary intake, ability of patient to prepare food and feed self
    4. Food allergies and preferences
    5. Dentition
    6. Ability of patient to moisten, chew, and swallow nutrients
    7. Ability to digest food in stomach and small intestine
    8. Ability to move stomach contents through bowel
    9. Presence of abnormal carbohydrate, fat, or protein metabolism
    10. Presence of vitamin and mineral deficiencies
    11. Fecal and urinary elimination patterns, characteristics of urine and stool
II. Nutritional assessment, including evaluation of the effects of dietary intake on the patient
  A. Physical assessment (Jager-Wittenaar & Ottery, 2017)
    1. Skin turgor
    2. Weight in comparison with ideal body weight
    3. Muscle mass as measured by the midarm circumference
    4. Fat stores as measured by triceps skinfold thickness
  B. Laboratory data
    1. Serum prealbumin, total protein, and serum transferrin to assess protein stores
    2. Nitrogen balance to assess energy balance
    3. Hemoglobin and hematocrit index
    4. Electrolyte levels

Management (Caccialanza, Pedrazzoli, Cereda, et al., 2016; Huhmann, & August, 2008; Mueller, Compher, Ellen, et al., 2011)

I. Controversies exist in nutritional support therapy for long-term management in patients with cancer
  A. Nourishing a patient with cancer may enhance tumor growth by improving its nutrient supply
  B. Beneficial effects of nutritional support are temporary
  C. Determination of calorie and protein needs
  D. Increase in weight, maintaining weight
  E. Maintaining fluid and electrolyte balance
  F. Improving sense of well-being, prolonging life
  G. Function of GI tract
  H. Severity of nutritional problem
  I. Ability of patient to masticate and swallow
  J. Length of proposed oncologic therapy and prognosis
  K. Community resources for management at home
  L. Cost
II. Types of nutritional therapy
  A. Enteral therapy—provision of nutritional replacement through the GI tract through an entry other than the mouth—for example, gastrostomy (button), jejunostomy, or nasogastric (temporary) feeding tube or combination gastrostomy and jejunostomy tube (Houston & Fuldauer, 2017).
    1. Maintenance of gut and maintenance of gut ability (including acid balance and luminal microflora) are the first line of defense against invaders into gut
    2. Enteral or parenteral therapy used only if adequate oral intake cannot be maintained
    3. Indicated if the need for nutritional support anticipated for more than 1 month, oral intake attempts unsuccessful; at least 30 cm of functioning small bowel required
    4. May require percutaneous endoscopic feeding tube placement
    5. Potential complications of enteral tube placement and feedings included in Table 43.1
    6. Selection of appropriate formula essential; different ones may need to be tried
      a. Choice of formula is based on current nutritional requirements, any abnormalities of GI absorption, motility, or diarrhea loss and other coexisting diseases; also considered are laboratory data, amount of protein needed, nitrogen balance and metabolic rate of patient; lactose tolerance or intolerance.
      b. Polymeric formulas contain nitrogen as a whole protein, carbohydrate is partially hydrolyzed starch, and fat contains long-chain triglycerides; most contain fiber.
      c. Predigested formulas contain nitrogen as short peptides or, if elemental formula, proteins are free amino acids; carbohydrates provide much of the energy content, and both long-chain and medium-chain triglycerides are present.

TABLE 43.1 Potential Complications of Enteral Tube Placement and Feedings

Complication	Nursing Intervention
Nasogastric	
Malpositioned tube	Verify proper placement via chest radiography.
	Check placement each time before using tube.
	Aspirate gastric contents.
	Observe for air bubbles by placing distal end of tube in water.
	Inject air and listen with stethoscope over stomach.
	Tape tube securely to nose.
Aspiration	Give bolus feeding rather than continuous feeding.
	Administer no more than 350–400 mL over 20 minutes every 3–4 hr while patient is awake.
	Administer initial volume of 240 mL.
	Keep head of bed elevated by 30 degrees during and 1 hr after infusion.
Contaminated equipment, clogged tube	Change feeding bag and tube daily.
	Flush nasogastric tube with 30 mL of water after each feeding.
	If tube is clogged, flush with hot water or pulsating motions.
Abdominal distention, vomiting, cramping, diarrhea	Regulate infusion accurately over 20 min.
	Give formula at room temperature; you may need to decrease volume of formula given.
	Diarrhea may be caused by formula, lactose intolerance, bacterial contamination, osmolality, antibiotics, or Clostridium difficile.
Nasoduodenal	
Aspiration	Risk of occurrence is less because tube is in the small bowel.
	Give continuous rather than bolus feeding.
	Small bowel is sensitive to osmolarity; therefore administer at initial rate of 30–50 mL/hr for isotonic formula and increase by 25 mL/hr every 12 hr until desired volume is reached.
Contaminated equipment	Do not allow amount of formula in bag to exceed that which can be administered in 4 hr.
	Change entire administration set every 24 hr, and rinse with hot water every 8 hr.

d. Disease-specific formulas are as follows:
   (1) Requires the gut to have some degree of digestive and absorptive capacity
   (2) Indicated in presence of significant malabsorption
   (3) Respiratory failure formulas contain low carbohydrate-to-fat ratio to minimize carbon dioxide production
   (4) Renal failure formulas contain modified protein, electrolytes, and volume

B. Parenteral therapy provides feeding through an IV route when the GI tract cannot be used for nutritional replacement (Fletcher, 2013)
   1. Parenteral therapy requires placement of a central venous line (CVL) or peripherally inserted central catheter (PICC) line, although peripheral parenteral nutrition (PPN) can be given with a lower glucose concentration.
   2. Mixture of amino acids, glucose, fluid, vitamins, minerals, electrolytes, and trace elements. Lipid emulsions can be added to increase calories with smaller volume.
   3. Potential complications of parenteral therapy are presented in Table 43.2.

III. Interventions to maximize patient safety ⚠️
A. Administration of nutritional therapy according to institutional protocol

B. Examination of nutritional supplement for abnormalities in color
C. Check expiration date on nutritional supplement
D. Confirm feeding tube or catheter placement before administering nutritional supplement

IV. Interventions to monitor for complications of nutritional therapy
A. Infection—fever and redness; swelling, pus, pain along feeding tube, catheter tract, or exit site
B. Respiratory complications—chest pain, dyspnea, cough, cyanosis
C. Fluid overload—weight gain, edema, shortness of breath, distended neck veins
D. Hyperglycemia—blood glucose monitoring every 6 hours, pattern of urinary elimination
E. GI—character of stool, bloating, pattern of fecal elimination
F. Electrolyte abnormalities—changes in mental status, weakness, fatigue, changes in neurologic examination (restlessness, agitation)

V. Interventions to decrease the incidence and severity of complications of nutritional support therapy (see Tables 43.1 and 43.2)

VI. Interventions to include patient and caregiver in care
A. Teach patient and caregiver procedures needed to manage the feeding tube or catheter

TABLE 43.2 Potential Complications of Parenteral or Nutritional Therapy

Complications	Nursing Intervention
Technical or Mechanical	
Pneumothorax	May occur during subclavian catheter insertion. Observe patient during insertion for chest pain, dyspnea, and cyanosis. Perform chest radiography after insertion to verify placement. Verify blood return before connecting IV tubing to catheter. Pneumothorax may occur during insertion.
Arterial puncture	Observe for bright red blood pulsating from catheter. Patient may complain of pain at site. Apply pressure to site for 15 min; you may need to apply a sandbag after this.
Malpositioned catheter	Monitor the catheter for migration from the superior vena cava to another vein. Note patient complaint of neck and shoulder pain and swelling in the surrounding area. NOTE: If unable to infuse solution through catheter and unable to obtain blood return, treat catheter occlusion according to institutional policy (see Chapter 30).
Clotted catheter	Infuse 10% dextrose in water solution peripherally or through other lumen of catheter at the same rate as with TPN to prevent hypoglycemia.
Fluid overload	Regulate infusion on a volumetric pump for accuracy. Place a time tape on infusion, checking volume infused over each hour. Obtain daily weights, monitor input/output.
Air emboli	Secure all IV tubing connections with tape to prevent disconnection. If air emboli are suspected, clamp tubing immediately and place patient on left side in the Trendelenburg position.
Metabolic	
Hyperglycemia	Increase rate of infusion gradually. Check urine for sugar, ketones, and acetone every 6 hr. Monitor serum glucose levels daily.
Hypoglycemia	Administer insulin in TPN as ordered. Monitor capillary blood glucose as ordered. Observe for signs and symptoms of hypoglycemia. Monitor serum glucose levels. If sudden cessation of TPN occurs, infuse 10% dextrose in water solution peripherally at same rate as TPN. Per physician's order, administer 50 mL of 50% dextrose intravenously.
Infections	
Contaminated solution	Do not leave unrefrigerated longer than 4 hr. Check each bottle or bag before and during infusion for color and clarity of solution.
Contaminated equipment	Change all IV tubing per institutional or agency procedure using aseptic technique. Avoid interrupting TPN for other infusions or blood collecting.
Local site infection	Change dressing, using aseptic technique and following institutional procedure. Observe site: redness, tenderness, swelling, and exudates.
Fever	Monitor vital signs every 4 hr. Obtain both peripheral and central line blood cultures to identify source of infection.

B. Teach patient/caregiver about signs and symptoms of nutritional support therapy complications
C. Encourage patient/caregiver participation in decision making about nutritional therapy

III. Patient and caregiver discuss rationale for nutritional support therapy, list signs and symptoms of complications of nutritional support therapy to report to the health care team.

Expected Patient Outcomes

I. Patient will demonstrate stable weight or progressive weight gain toward goal with normalization of laboratory values and is free of signs of malnutrition or stable for optimal QOL per goals of care.
II. Patient and caregiver will verbalize understanding of nutritional strategies to manage alterations in nutrition related to cancer and cancer treatment.

REFERENCES

Arends J, Bachmann, P., Baracos, V., Barthelemy, N., Bertz, H., Bozzetti, F… Preiser, J.C. (2016). ESPEN guidelines on nutrition in cancer patients, *Clinical Nutrition*. Retrieved from, https://doi.org/10.1016/j.clnu.2016.07.015.

Berry, D. L., Blonquist, T., Mayak, M. M., Roper, K., Hilton, N., Lombard, H., … McManus, K. (2018). Cancer anorexia and cachexia screening in an ambulatory infusion service and nutrition consultation. *Clinical Journal of Oncology Nursing, 22* (1), 63–68. https://doi.org/10.1188/18.CJON.63-68.

Bruggeman, A. R., Kamal, A. H., LeBlanc, T. W., Ma, J. D., Baracos, V. E., & Roeland, E. J. (2016). Cancer cachexia: beyond weight loss. *Journal of Oncology Practice, 12*(11), 1163–1171. https://doi.org/10.1200/JOP.2016.016832.

Caccialanza, R., Pedrazzoli, P., Cereda, E., Gavazzi, C., Pinto, C., Paccagnella, A., … Zagonel, V. (2016). Nutritional support in cancer patients: a position paper from the Italian Society of Medical Oncology (AIOM) and the Italian Society of Artificial Nutrition and Metabolism (SINPE). *Journal of Cancer, 7*(2), 131–135. https://doi.org/10.7150/jca.13818.

Douglas, E., & McMillan, D. C. (2014). Towards a simple objective framework for the investigation and treatment of cancer cachexia: the Glasgow Prognostic Score. *Cancer Treatment Reviews, 40*(6), 685–691. https://doi.org/10.1016/j.ctrv.2013.11.007.

Ezeoke, C. C., & Morley, J. E. (2015). Pathophysiology of anorexia in the cancer cachexia syndrome. *Journal of Cachexia, Sarcopenia, and Muscle, 6*(4), 287–302. https://doi.org/10.1002/jcsm.12059.

Farrell, C., Brearley, S. G., Pilling, M., & Molassiotis, A. (2013). The impact of chemotherapy-related nausea on patients' nutritional status, psychological distress and quality of life. *Supportive Care in Cancer, 21*(1), 59–66.

Fletcher, J. (2013). Parenteral nutrition: indications, risks, and nursing care. *Nursing Standard, 27*(46), 50–57. https://doi.org/10.7748/ns2013.07.27.46.50.e7508.

Houston, A. & Fuldauer, P. (2017). Enteral feeding: Indications, complications, and nursing care. *American Nurse Today, 12*(1), Retrieved from, https://www.americannursetoday.com/enteral-feeding-indications-complications-and-nursing-care/.

Huhmann, M. B., & August, D. A. (2008). Review of American Society for Parenteral and Enteral Nutrition (ASPEN) clinical guidelines for nutrition support in cancer patients: nutrition screening and assessment. *Nutrition in Clinical Practice, 23*(2), 182–188. https://doi.org/10.1177/0884533608314530.

Jager-Wittenaar, H., & Ottery, F. D. (2017). Assessing nutritional status in cancer: role of the Patient-Generated Subjective Global Assessment. *Current Opinion in Clinical Nutrition & Metabolic Care, 20*(5), 322–329. https://doi.org/10.1097/MCO.0000000000000389.

Kalaskar, A. R. (2014). Management of chemotherapy induced dysgeusia: an important step towards nutritional rehabilitation.

International Journal of Physical Medicine and Rehabilitation, 2. 198. https://doi.org/10.4172/2329-9096.1000198.

LeBlanc, T. W., Nipp, R. D., Rushing, C. N., Samsa, G. P., Locke, S. C., Kamal, A. H., … Abenethy, A. P. (2015). Correlation between the International consensus definition of the cancer anorexia-cachexia syndrome (CACS) and patient-centered outcomes in advanced non-small cell lung cancer. *Journal of Pain and Symptom Management, 49*(4), 680–689. https://doi.org/10.1016/j.jpainsymman.2014.09.008.

Mueller, C., Compher, C., Ellen, D. M., & American Society of Parenteral and Enteral Nutrition (A.S.P.E.N.) Board of Directors. (2011). A.S.P.E.N. clinical guidelines: nutrition screening, assessment, and intervention in adults. *Journal of Parenteral and Enteral Nutrition, 35*(1), 16–24. https://doi.org/10.1177/0148607110389335.

Murtaza, B., Hichami, A., Khan, A. S., Ghiringhelli, F., & Khan, N. A. (2017). Alteration in taste perception in cancer: causes and strategies of treatment. *Frontiers in Physiology, 8*(134). Retrieved from https://www.ncbi.nlm.nih.gov/pmc/articles/PMC5340755/.

Nguyen, H. M., Reyland, M. E., & Barlow, L. A. (2012). Mechanisms of taste bud cell loss after head and neck irradiation. *Journal of Neuroscience, 32*(10), 3473–3484. https://doi.org/10.1523/JNEUROSCI.4167-11.2012.

O'Leary, C. M. (2016). Gastrointestinal, genitourinary, and hepatic toxicities. In B. H. Gobel, S. Triest-Robertson, & W. H. Vogel (Eds.), *Advanced oncology nursing certification: review and resource manual* (pp. 525–576). Pittsburgh, PA: Oncology Nursing Society.

Sroussi, H. Y., Epstein, J. B., Bensadoun, R., Saunders, D. P., Lalla, R. V., Migliorati, C. A., … Zumsteg, Z. S. (2017). Common oral complications of head and neck cancer radiation therapy: mucositis, infections, saliva change, fibrosis, sensory dysfunctions, dental caries, periodontal disease, and osteoradionecrosis. *Cancer Medicine. 6*(12), 2918–2931. https://doi.org/10.1002/cam4.122.

White, J. V., Guenter, P., Jensen, G., Malone, A., & Schofield, M. (2012). Consensus statement: Academy of Nutrition and Dietetics and American Society for Parenteral and Enteral Nutrition: Characteristics Recommended for the Identification and Documentation of Adult Malnutrition (Undernutrition). *Journal of Parenteral and Enteral Nutrition, 36*(3), 275–283. https://doi.org/10.1177/0148607112440285.

44

Pain

Jeannine M. Brant

OVERVIEW

I. Definition.
   A. A sensory and emotional experience associated with actual or potential tissue damage or described in terms of such damage (IASP, 2018).
II. Characteristics of pain (Gallagher, Rogers, & Brant, 2017)
   A. Acute pain—typically lasts less than 6 months; etiology is often known; pain behaviors are more frequently exhibited.
   B. Chronic pain—typically lasts longer than 3 months; etiology of the pain is often unknown with nonmalignant chronic pain; fatigue and depression are common.
   C. Cancer pain—includes acute and chronic cancer-related pain associated with direct tumor involvement, diagnostic/therapeutic procedures, or cancer treatment; often clusters with fatigue, depression and anxiety, and sleep disturbance (Miaskowski et al., 2017).
   D. Breakthrough pain (BTP)—a flare in the pain pattern that occurs in conjunction with well-controlled background pain.
      1. Incident pain—transient pain precipitated by any movement or activity.
      2. Insidious pain—spontaneous pain that occurs without warning
III. Types of pain (Anwar, 2016)
   A. Nociceptive pain—from activation of nociceptors (pain fibers) in deep and cutaneous tissues.
      1. Somatic pain—arises from the bone, joint, or connective tissue; described as sharp, throbbing, or pressure; well localized.
      2. Visceral pain—from nociceptor activation related to distention, compression, or infiltration of the thoracic or abdominal tissue (i.e., pancreas, liver, gastrointestinal [GI] tract); characterized by a diffuse, aching, or cramping sensation; poorly localized.
   B. Neuropathic pain—results from compression, inflammation, infiltration, ischemia, or injury to the peripheral, sympathetic, or central nervous system (CNS)

   1. Peripheral neuropathic pain—caused by peripheral nerve injury, often characterized by a numbness and tingling sensation.
   2. Centrally mediated pain—characterized by radiating and shooting sensations with a background of burning and aching.
   3. Sympathetically maintained pain—centrally generated, caused by autonomic dysregulation; complex regional pain syndrome (CRPS).
IV. Physiology (Fig. 44.1) (Anwar, 2016).
   A. Transduction
      1. Initiated by mechanical, thermal, or chemical noxious stimuli.
      2. Neurotransmitters released at the time of injury include prostaglandins (PG), bradykinin (BK), serotonin (5-HT), substance P (SP), and histamine (H), which initiate an inflammatory response.
      3. An action potential/depolarization is generated along the neuron; sodium moves into the cell and potassium out; pain message begins its way to the CNS.
   B. Transmission
      1. Action potential continues to the dorsal horn where nociceptors terminate.
      2. Neurotransmittors and excitatory substances are released in the spinal cord that inhibit presynaptic and postsynaptic nociceptive transmission.
      3. Neurons relay the message to the thalamus and other centers in the brain.
      4. The thalamus transmits the message to the cerebral cortex.
   C. Perception—the cerebral cortex processes the experience of pain and responds to the noxious stimuli to reduce pain perception via descending modulating mechanisms.
   D. Modulation
      1. Neurons in the brainstem (pons and medulla) descend to the dorsal horn and release neuromediators—endogenous opioids, norepinephrine, serotonin.
      2. Neuromediators inhibit the transmission of pain impulses at the dorsal horn.

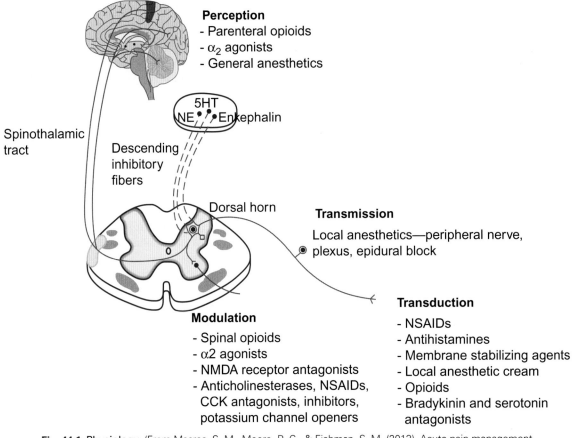

Perception
- Parenteral opioids
- α₂ agonists
- General anesthetics

5HT
NE Enkephalin

Spinothalamic
tract

Descending
inhibitory
fibers

Dorsal horn

Transmission
Local anesthetics—peripheral nerve,
plexus, epidural block

Transduction
- NSAIDs
- Antihistamines
- Membrane stabilizing agents
- Local anesthetic cream
- Opioids
- Bradykinin and serotonin
  antagonists

Modulation
- Spinal opioids
- α2 agonists
- NMDA receptor antagonists
- Anticholinesterases, NSAIDs,
  CCK antagonists, inhibitors,
  potassium channel openers

Fig. 44.1 Physiology. (From Macres, S. M., Moore, P. G., & Fishman, S. M. (2013). Acute pain management. In Barash PG, Cullen BF, Stoelting RK, et al. (Eds.), Clinical anesthesia (7th ed., pp. 1611–1642). Philadelphia: Lippincott Williams & Wilkins.)

3. Opioids work at the dorsal horn by binding to receptors and preventing transmission of the pain signal to the higher brain centers.

V. Risk factors (Paice, 2016)

A. Disease-related factors

1. Types of cancer: prevalence higher in head and neck, lung, and breast cancer

2. Advanced, metastatic, or terminal disease: prevalence 66.4%

B. Treatment-related factors

1. Prevalence

a. 55% of patients have pain during cancer treatment

b. 39.3% of patients have pain after curative treatment

2. Chemotherapy-related side effects causing pain (Oncology Nursing Society [ONS], 2018)

a. Mucositis—occurs in 40% of patients undergoing chemotherapy, 80% undergoing hematopoietic stem cell transplantation, 100% of head and neck cancer patients receiving combined chemotherapy and radiation therapy.

b. Peripheral neuropathies—occur in 10% to 100% depending on treatment; characterized by burning, numbness, tingling of hands/feet.

c. Postherpetic neuralgia—characterized by burning, aching, and shocklike pain; often occurs due to immunosuppression from chemotherapy; topical agents, such as a lidocaine patch/gel and long-acting gabapentin, are indicated for postherpetic neuralgia (Mallick-Searle, Snodgrass, & Brant, 2016).

3. Radiation therapy–related pain

a. Visceral—chest pain/tightness, dermatitis, cystitis, enteritis, proctitis, mucositis

b. Somatic—osteoporosis, osteoradionecrosis, pelvic fractures

c. Neuropathic—myelopathy, peripheral nerve entrapment, plexopathies

4. Postsurgical pain syndromes (Brant, 2014)

a. Postmastectomy—characterized by tightness in axilla, upper arm, chest; often exacerbated with movement, extending, reaching, lifting, pulling, pushing; caused by intercostobrachial nerve damage.

b. Postthoracotomy—characterized by aching, numbness, and/or burning in the incisional area. Believed to be caused by intercostal nerve damage.

c. Postsurgical head and neck cancer pain—characterized by tightness, burning, shocklike pain. Thought to be caused by injury to the accessory and superficial cervical plexus, followed by denervation and atrophy of the trapezius muscle, subsequent downward and lateral scapula displacement, and thus shoulder dysfuction and pain.

d. Postlimb amputation—phantom or stump pain; may be neuropathic.

e. Lymphedema—characterized as arm/shoulder fullness, heaviness, or tightness. Can result from any cancer surgery that affects the lymphatic system in any body part (e.g., arm, leg). Most common in breast cancer (Oncology Nursing Society, 2018).

C. Personal and psychosocial factors
1. Patient-related fears
   a. Fear of addiction.
   b. Fear that pain may be a sign of progressive disease; denial prevents patient from taking adequate analgesia.
   c. Desire to be a "good patient"; therefore pain not reported.
   d. Fear of side effects (e.g., loss of mental clarity)

TABLE 44.1 Pain Assessment Parameters

Domain	Pain Assessment Components
Physical Domain	
WILDA	• **W**ords used to describe the pain • **I**ntensity: On a scale of 0–10 what is your pain now, at rest, with movement, worst pain possible in the past 24 hours? What is your comfort/function goal? • **L**ocation: Where is your pain? • **D**uration: Is the pain constant? Does the pain come and go? Do you have both types of pain (one that is constant and one that comes and goes)? • **A**ggravating/**A**lleviating factors: What makes the pain worse? What makes the pain better?
PQRST	• **P**rovocation/Palliation: What caused it? What relieves it? • **Q**uality: What does it feel like? • **R**egion/**R**adiation: Where is the pain located? Does the pain radiate? • **S**everity: How severe is the pain on a 0–10 scale? • **T**iming: Constant or intermittent?
OLDCART	• **O**nset: When did the pain start? • **L**ocation: Where is the pain located? Is there more than one location? • **D**uration: How often does the pain occur? Is it constant or intermittent? How long does the pain last? • **C**haracteristics: How does the pain feel (intensity)? What words would you use to describe the pain? (Descriptors can aid in diagnosing the pain syndrome.) • **A**ggravating factors: What makes your pain worse? • **R**elieving factors: What makes your pain better? • **T**reatment: What treatments (pharmacologic and/or nonpharmacologic) have you tried to control the pain? How are they working? How do the treatments affect the pain intensity?
Psychological Domain	• The meaning of pain to the patient and family • History of anxiety, depression, or other psychological illness • Cognition, including confusion or delirium • Usual coping strategies in response to pain • Psychological responses to pain and illness, such as depression, anxiety, and fear • Past pain experience • Beliefs about opioids, addiction, and other concerns • Willingness to try complementary modalities such as cognitive behavioral therapy
Social Domain	• Functional assessment: interference of pain on daily living, including physical or social withdrawal from activity • Family caregiver communication and response to illness • Support system • Economic impact of the pain and its treatment (e.g., ability to afford analgesics)
Spiritual/Existential Domain	• Spiritual beliefs related to pain and illness • Presence of a spiritual community and its role related to pain and illness • Influence of religion or spirituality on coping with pain • Influence of suffering on the pain experience • Use of traditional medicine in healing

From Fink, R. M., & Brant, J. M. (2018). Complex cancer pain assessment. *Hematology/Oncology Clinics of North America, 32*(3), 353–369. https://doi.org/10.1016/j.hoc.2018.01.001.

2. Provider-related—lack of knowledge, fear of addiction, reluctance to prescribe due to regulations.

3. Culture—influences the perceptions and expression of pain.

ASSESSMENT

I. Special populations (Table 44.1) (Gallagher et al., 2017) (Fink & Brant, 2018)
   A. Older adult population
      1. Obtain a comprehensive medication history— higher risk for polypharmacy and drug interactions in populations over age 70 taking five medications or more.
      2. Start with lower doses, titrate slowly, advanced age results in a prolonged half-life and metabolism of the drug.
      3. Consider appropriateness of pain screening scale; may need to employ the use of a nonverbal pain assessment tool if the patient cannot verbally report pain.
      4. Assess for the presence of confusion and poor vision, availability of home supervision, and cost when planning analgesics for older adults.
   B. Pediatric population (Haskamp & Lafond, 2016)
      1. Assess pediatric population according to developmental age.
      2. Choose a developmentally appropriate pain scale.
         a. Pain faces are usually used in children ages 7 years and younger.
         b. The "0 to 10" scale may be used for school-aged and older children.
         c. The FLACC scale is used for children who cannot verbalize pain.
      3. Starting dosage should be calculated according to weight.
   C. Patients with substance use disorder (SUD) (Brant, 2016).
      1. Patients should be routinely assessed for presence of an SUD.
      2. Assessment to include the 5 A's: analgesic response; activities of daily living; adverse events; aberrant activities that suggest misuse, abuse, or addiction; affect.

II. Clinical pain assessment (Brant, 2017; Gallagher et al., 2017) (Fink & Brant, 2018)
   A. Physical domain—onset, location, duration, characteristics, aggravating factors, relieving factors, and treatment.
   B. Psychological domain—meaning of pain to patient/ family, how pain affects the patient's affect (e.g., depression, anxiety, hopelessness); usual coping strategies, beliefs about opioids/addiction, how medications affect cognitive functioning, willingness to try complementary modalities.
   C. Social domain—how pain/pain medications affect activities of daily living (physical/social withdrawal from activity), support system/family dynamics, and financial impact of pain (i.e., ability to afford analgesics).
   D. Spiritual/existential domain—influence of spiritual/ religious beliefs related to pain/illness, presence of spiritual support/community and its role in patient's pain/illness, use of traditional medicines.

III. History and physical examination (Brant, 2014; Fink & Brant, 2018)
   A. Medical history: current and prior oncologic treatment (e.g., chemo, radiation therapy [RT], surgery), other significant comorbidities, preexisting chronic pain.
   B. Evaluation of imaging studies (computed tomography [CT], magnetic resonance imaging [MRI], bone scan, etc.) and laboratory values (tumor markers).
   C. Physical and neurologic examination—assess pain behaviors (physical limitations, guarding), changes in muscle tone, loss of deep tendon reflexes.
   D. Assess for alterations in the following systems:
      1. Respiratory status—decreased rate and volume, increased CO_2 levels.
      2. CNS changes—sedation/lethargy, euphoria, coordination, mood.
      3. Cardiovascular system—hypotension.
      4. GI system—constipation, bowel obstruction, inability to evacuate stool, nausea.
      5. Genitourinary system—urinary retention, difficult urination.
      6. Dermatologic system— diaphoresis, facial flushing, pruritus.

IV. Evaluation and reassessment of pain (National Comprehensive Cancer Network [NCCN], 2019).
   A. Assess/screen each patient for pain at each contact (on admission to the hospital and at regular follow-up intervals, during each home visit, or at outpatient clinic visits).
   B. Comprehensive pain assessment with each new report of pain.
   C. Pain should be reassessed after appropriate intervals after pain interventions (e.g., evaluate pain approximately 1 hour after oral medication administration).

MANAGEMENT

I. Medical management (Brant, Keller, McLeod, Yeh, & Eaton, 2017; Brant, Rodgers, Gallagher, & Sundaramurthi, 2017).
   A. Tailor pain management according to the patient's individualized pain assessment.
      1. Administer long-acting analgesics around the clock when pain is constant.
      2. Distinguish and manage breakthrough pain (Brant, Rodgers, et al., 2017).

a. Use BTP analgesics with a rapid onset; consider transmucosal fentanyl.

b. Oral immediate-release opioids (e.g., morphine, oxycodone): administer 10% to 20% of the 24-hour dose; does not apply to transmucosal fentanyl; administer at intervals before anticipated painful activity for incident pain (NCCN, 2019).

3. End-of-dose failure—pain that increases before the next scheduled dose, may be managed by increasing the opioid dose or frequency.

4. Use equianalgesic conversion tables to guide opioid conversion.

5. Begin with least invasive route of administration (oral preferred, transdermal [TD]); change routes or rotate opioids if intolerable side effects or intractable pain occurs despite escalating doses.

6. Implement strategies to minimize side effects of analgesic therapy: bowel regimen that includes stool softener and stimulant, antiemetics, H2 antagonists, CNS stimulants to counteract sedation.

7. Taper and discontinue opioids when no longer needed.

B. Use the World Health Organization (WHO) analgesic ladder to manage pain (Fig. 44.2) (World Health Organization, 2018).

1. Step 1—nonopioid analgesics.

a. Use for mild pain or as adjuvants with opioid medications.

b. Examples: acetaminophen, acetylsalicylic acid (aspirin and ASA), nonsteroidal antiinflammatory drugs (NSAIDs).

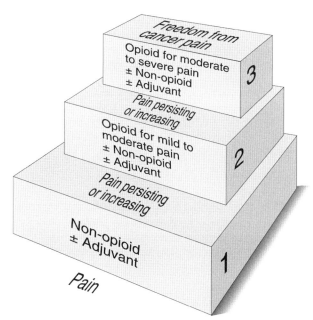

Fig. 44.2 The WHO Three-Step Analgesic Ladder. (From World Health Organization. (2018). *WHO's pain ladder*. Retrieved from http://www.who.int/cancer/palliative/painladder/en/.)

2. Step 2—opioid analgesics.

a. Opioids for mild to moderate pain.

b. Examples: hydrocodone and oxycodone in fixed combinations with acetaminophen or aspirin.

3. Step 3—opioid analgesics.

a. Opioids for severe pain.

b. Step 3 opioids are used most frequently in managing cancer-related pain (e.g., morphine, oxycodone, hydromorphone, fentanyl).

4. Analgesic adjuvant: use on each step of the WHO ladder to enhance analgesia, relieve concurrent symptoms that exacerbate pain, and/or relieve side effects.

C. Administer analgesics for safe and effective pain management (American Pain Society, 2017; Brant, Keller, et al., 2017; Brant, Rodgers, et al., 2017; Sundaramurthi, Gallagher, & Sterling, 2017).

1. Nonopioids

a. Acetaminophen should not exceed 3000 mg in 24 hours; use caution in opioid/acetaminopen combinations.

b. Carefully weigh risk/benefit ratio of NSAIDs; side effects include inhibition of platelet aggregation, renal compromise, and gastrointestinal toxicity.

2. Opioids

a. Avoid or use morphine with caution in patients with renal impairment due to potential M3G and M6G metabolite accumulation, which may cause oversedation, respiratory depression, myoclonus.

b. Consider delayed onset of TD fentanyl and administer as-needed analgesics until efficacy established.

c. Administer methadone with caution; its long half-life can lead to accumulation and oversedation.

d. TD buprenorphine is a partial mu-agonist approved for cancer pain; a ceiling dose exists; may precipitate withdrawal symptoms in patients on pure mu-agonists (e.g., morphine).

e. Tramadol and tapentadol are weak mu-opioids that block the reuptake of serotonin and norepinephrine; potential for serotonin symdrome; ceiling dose.

3. Adjuvants (Table 44.2)

a. Use adjuvants specific for individual pain syndromes (e.g., neuropathic pain).

b. Management of bone metastases.

(1) Radionuclides (e.g., strontium 89, samarium 153) for pain relief in disseminated metastatic bone cancer.

(2) Bone-modifying agents (e.g., zoledronic acid, denosumab) for pain relief in osteolytic bone metastases.

TABLE 44.2   Adjuvant Analgesics

Drug Classifications	Indications	Side Effects
Acetaminophen (Tylenol)	Mild to moderate pain, fever; maximum dose 4000 mg/day	Hepatotoxicity, increased risk with alcohol consumption, liver failure
α₂-Adrenergic agonist: clonidine hydrochloride (Catapres)	Epidural analgesia for neuropathic/postsurgical pain	Hypotension, bradycardia, central nervous system, depression, dry mouth
CNS Stimulants Caffeine Dextroamphetamine (Dexedrine) Methylphenidate (Ritalin) Modafinil (Provigil) Atomoxetine (Strattera)	Counteract psychomotor retardation, reduce sedation side effects of opioids	Nervousness, sleep disorder, hypertension, palpitations, anxiety
Anticonvulsants Gabapentin (Neurontin) Pregabalin (Lyrica) (most commonly used)	Neuropathic pain, trigeminal neuralgia, postherpetic neuralgia, peripheral neuropathy	Sedation, dizziness, ataxia, edema, fatigue, bone marrow depression, nausea, rash, impaired concentration
Antidepressants TCAs: Amitriptyline (Elavil) Desipramine (Norpramin) Nortriptyline (Pamelor) SNRIs: Venlafaxine (Effexor) Duloxetine (Cymbalta)	Neuropathic pain, postherpetic neuralgia, postsurgical neuropathies, chemoimmunotherapy-related neuropathies	Dry mouth, sedation, constipation, agitation, delirium, tachycardia, orthostatic hypotension, worsening of cardiac conduction abnormalities, more side effects with TCAs
Antispasmodics Baclofen (Lioresal)	Spastic pain, centrally mediated pain from spinal lesions	Drowsiness, slurred speech, hypotension, constipation, urinary retention
Benzodiazepines Alprazolam (Xanax) Clonazepam (Klonopin) Diazepam (Valium) Lorazepam (Ativan)	Anxiety associated with pain, panic attack, muscle spasm, procedure-related pain	Sedation, dementia, delirium, motor incoordination, hypotension, dizziness, respiratory depression
Corticosteroids Dexamethasone (Decadron) Methylprednisolone (Solu-Medrol)	Brachial and lumbosacral plexopathies, lymphedema and visceral distention, increased intracranial pressure	Euphoria/psychosis, increased appetite, hyperglycemia, weight gain, Cushing syndrome, osteoporosis, GI bleeding, gastritis
Local Anesthetics Lidocaine IV or patch (Lidoderm) Mexilitine (Mexitil) EMLA cream	Lidocaine for postherpetic neuralgia, peripheral neuropathy, postsurgical neuropathies EMLA for dermal anesthesia	Lidocaine patch may cause a mild rash at the application site
Muscle Relaxants Cyclobenzaprine (Flexeril) Carisoprodol (Soma) Metaxalone (Skelaxin) Methocarbamol (Robaxin) Tizanidine (Zanaflex)	Should be used short term for musculoskeletal pain, tetanus Tizanidine may be used for longer periods; used for headache or neuropathic pain	Sedation, lightheadedness, blurred vision, hypotension, akathisia (movement disorder characterized by a feeling of inner restlessness and an urgent need to move)
N-methyl-D-Aspartate Antagonists Ketamine Amantadine (Symmetrel) Memantine (Namenda)	Neuropathic pain, synergistic with opioids, may be helpful in preventing tolerance to opioids Note: Methadone also has NMDA activity	Psychotomimetic side effects, hallucinations, drowsiness

TABLE 44.2	Adjuvant Analgesics—cont'd	
Drug Classifications	**Indications**	**Side Effects**
NSAIDs COX-2 inhibitor: Celecoxib (Celebrex) Nonselective COX inhibitors: Ibuprofen (Advil, Motrin, Nuprin) Indomethacin (Indocin) Ketorolac (Toradol) Naproxen (Naprosyn, Aleve, Anaprox)	Bone metastases, soft tissue infiltration, tumor, fever, inflammation	COX-1 inhibitors may cause inhibition of platelet aggregation, gastric ulceration, renal toxicity, confusion in older adults COX-2 NSAIDs are more selective and cause fewer GI side effects

TCA, Tricyclic antidepressant; *SNRI,* serotonin and norepinephrine reuptake inhibitors.
Data from American Pain Society. (2017). *Principles of analgesic use in the treatment of acute pain and cancer pain* (6th ed.). Glenview, IL: APS Press.

4. Intraspinal analgesia
   a. Epidural or intrathecal route—percutaneous catheters, implantable pumps, or Ommaya reservoir.
   b. Indicated for specific pain syndromes; lower doses of opioids used, thus limiting severity and toxicity of side effects.
II. Nursing management (Eaton, Brant, McLeod, & Yeh, 2017; NCCN, 2019)
   A. Radiation therapy may alleviate painful bone metastases and reduce large, localized bulky tumors.
   B. Nerve blocks and interventional strategies for well-localized pain syndromes
      1. Head and neck—peripheral nerve block.
      2. Upper extremity—brachial plexus neurolysis.
      3. Thoracic wall—epidural, intrathecal, intercostal, dorsal root ganglion neurolysis.
      4. Abdominal—celiac plexus block, thoracic splanchnictectomy.
      5. Pevlic—superior hypogastric plexus block.
      6. Rectal—intrathecal neurolysis, midline myelotomy, superior hypogastric plexus block, ganglion impar block.
      7. Unilateral pain—cordotomy.
      8. Neurostimulation for CRPS, neuralgias, peripheral neuropathy.
   C. Minimally invasive surgical procedures.
      1. Percutaneous kyphoplasty/vertebroplasty—for treatment of osteoclastic lesions (spinal metastasis/compressions fractures) to restore spinal stability.
      2. Optimal debulking of tumor to limit pain, or improve or maintain function.
   D. Psychoeducational interventions
      1. Educate patients and families about strategies to prevent and manage pain.
      2. Discuss the importance of good pain management in attaining optimal quality of life and the impact of pain on depression, sleep disturbance, and fatigue.
      3. Educate patients and families regarding the use of pain rating scales to communicate pain and the responsiveness to interventions.
      4. Encourage the patient to take analgesics early in the pain experience to avoid severe pain; take long-acting analgesics around the clock for constant pain.
      5. Educate the patient and family about modalities available to control pain: analgesics, interventional procedures, complementary techniques.
      6. Incorporate patient's social network (family leaders, minister/spiritual leader, healer) as appropriate; manage psychological distress, which can increase pain.
      7. Differentiate among tolerance, physical dependence, and addiction (Brant, 2016).
         a. Analgesic tolerance—physiologic state of adaptation whereby the repeated exposure to a drug results in diminished effect of the drug over time and a possible need to increase the drug dose to achieve the same level of effect.
         b. Physical dependence—a physiologic state of adaptation manifested by the emergence of a withdrawal syndrome if drug use is abruptly stopped, is rapidly decreased, or an antagonist is administered.
         c. Addiction—a neurobiological disease with genetic, psychosocial, and environmental influences; characterized by psychological dependency, cravings, and compulsive use despite harm.
   E. Monitor the patient for safety.
      1. Monitor for opioid-related side effects, including respiratory depression.
      2. Educate patients who are at high risk for spinal cord compression to notify the health care team if early signs of impending compression occur.

EXPECTED PATIENT OUTCOMES

I. The patient and caregiver will understand the plethora of options available to effectively and safely manage pain.
II. The patient's pain will be managed to provide optimal quality of life.

REFERENCES

American Pain Society. (2017). *Principles of analgesic use in the treatment of acute pain and cancer pain* (6th ed.). Glenview, IL: APS Press.

Anwar, K. (2016). Pathophysiology of pain. *Disease-a-month, 62*(9), 324–329. https://doi.org/10.1016/j.disamonth.2016.05.015.

Brant, J. M. (2014). Pain. In D. W. Ch. Yarbor, & B. Holmes (Eds.), *Cancer symptom management* (pp. 69–92). Burlington, MA: Jones & Bartlett.

Brant, J. M. (2016). Patients with substance use disorder. In C. Dahlin, P. J. Coyne, & B. R. Ferrell (Eds.), *Advanced practice palliative nursing* (pp. 516–524). New York: Oxford.

Brant, J. M. (2017). Holistic total pain management in palliative care: cultural and global considerations. *Palliative Medicine and Hospice Care*: (pp. S32–S38). https://doi.org/10.17140/PMHCOJSE-1-108.

Brant, J. M., Keller, L., McLeod, K., Yeh, C., & Eaton, L. H. (2017). Chronic and refractory pain: a systematic review of pharmacologic management in oncology. *Clinical Journal of Oncology Nursing, 21*(3), 31–59. https://doi.org/10.1188/17.CJON.S3.31-53.

Brant, J. M., Rodgers, B. B., Gallagher, E., & Sundaramurthi, T. (2017). Breakthrough cancer pain: a systematic review of pharmacologic management. *Clinical Journal of Oncology Nursing, 21*(3), 71–80. https://doi.org/10.1188/17.CJON.S3.71-80.

Eaton, L. H., Brant, J. M., McLeod, K., & Yeh, C. (2017). Nonpharmacologic pain interventions: a review of evidence-based practices for reducing chronic cancer pain. *Clinical Journal of Oncology Nursing, 21*(3), 54–79. https://doi.org/10.1188/17.CJON.S3.54-70.

Fink, R. M., & Brant, J. M. (2018). Complex cancer pain assessment. *Hematology/Oncology Clinics of North America, 32*(3), 353–369. https://doi.org/10.1016/j.hoc.2018.01.001.

Gallagher, E., Rogers, B. B., & Brant, J. M. (2017). Cancer-related pain assessment: monitoring the effectiveness of interventions. *Clinical Journal of Oncology Nursing, 21*(3), 8–12. https://doi.org/10.1188/17.CJON.S3.8-12.

Haskamp, A. C., & Lafond, D. A. (2016). Pediatric oncology. In C. Dahlin, P. J. Coyne, & B. R. Ferrell (Eds.), *Advanced practice palliative nursing (pp. 575-586)*. New York, NY: Oxford University Press.

IASP (Producer). (2018). Definition of pain. IASP Taxonomy. Retrieved from http://www.iasp-pain.org/Content/NavigationMenu/GeneralResourceLinks/PainDefinitions/default.htm

Mallick-Searle, T., Snodgrass, B., & Brant, J. M. (2016). Postherpetic neuralgia: epidemiology, pathophysiology, and pain management pharmacology. *Journal of Multidisciplinary Healthcare, 9*, 447–454. https://doi.org/10.2147/JMDH.S106340.

Miaskowski, C., Barsevick, A., Berger, A., Casagrande, R., Grady, P. A., Jacobsen, P., … Marden, S. (2017). Advancing symptom science through symptom cluster research: expert panel proceedings and recommendations. *Journal of the National Cancer Institute. 109*(4)https://doi.org/10.1093/jnci/djw253.

National Comprehensive Cancer Network. (2019). *Clinical practice guidelines in oncology: Adult cancer pain v.1. NCCN*. Retrieved from http://www.nccn.org/professionals/physician_gls/PDF/pain.pdf.

Oncology Nursing Society. (2018). *Putting evidence into practice*. Retrieved from https://www.ons.org/practice-resources/pep.

Paice, J. A. (2016). Pain. In C. Dahlin, P. J. Coyne, & B. R. Ferrell (Eds.), *Advanced practice palliative nursing* (pp. 219–232). New York, NY: Oxford University Press.

Sundaramurthi, T., Gallagher, N., & Sterling, B. (2017). Cancer-related acute pain: a systematic review of evidence-based interventions for putting evidence into practice. *Clinical Journal of Oncology Nursing, 21*(3), 13–30. https://doi.org/10.1188/17.CJON.S3.13-30.

World Health Organization. (2018). *WHO's pain ladder*. Retrieved from http://www.who.int/cancer/palliative/painladder/en/.

45

Respiratory Symptoms

Leslie Matthews

ANATOMIC OR SURGICAL ALTERATIONS

Overview

I. Definition—inadequate ventilation or oxygenation resulting from anatomic or surgical alterations (Lumb, 2017; Sarkar, Niranjan, & Banyal, 2017). Alterations in respiratory or cardiovascular systems may cause ventilation/perfusion (V/Q) mismatch causing hypoxemia (Lumb, 2017).
   A. Anatomic alterations
      1. Space-occupying lesions within the lung itself or in the pleural space (e.g., from primary or metastatic cancer to the lung)
      2. Airway obstruction of the tracheobronchial tree from direct extension of primary or metastatic tumors or enlarged lymph nodes
      3. Abnormal accumulation of fluid within lung or pleural space
         a. Pneumothorax—abnormal accumulation of air within the pleural space
         b. Hemothorax—abnormal accumulation of blood within the pleural space
         c. Hydrothorax (effusion)—abnormal accumulation of fluid within the pleural space
         d. Empyema—abnormal accumulation of infected fluid or pus in the pleural space caused by recent chest surgery, immunocompromise, or lung infection
      4. Compression of tracheobronchial tree from bronchospasm, laryngeal swelling from hypersensitivity reactions related to chemotherapy and/or biotherapy treatments, or superior vena cava syndrome (SVCS) (see Chapter 53)
   B. Surgical alterations
      1. Thoracic surgery for removal of primary or metastatic cancer of the lung
         a. Pneumonectomy—surgical removal of an entire lung
         b. Lobectomy—removal of a lobe of the lung
         c. Segmental resection—removal of one or more segments of a lung lobe
         d. Wedge resection—removal of a small wedge-shaped localized area near the lung surface
      2. Tracheostomy after head and neck surgery, laryngectomy

II. Risk factors
   A. Primary or metastatic cancer of the lung
   B. Recent surgery (especially thoracic or abdominal), immobility, or situations in which hypoventilation is likely
   C. Cancers associated with SVCS (see Chapter 53)
   D. Thoracic or head and neck surgery
   E. Primary or adjuvant tracheobronchial surgeries
   F. Surgery for palliation, tumor debulking
   G. History of obstructive or restrictive pulmonary disease
   H. History of cardiovascular disease
   I. Smoking history or environmental exposure to irritants such as pollution, pesticides, chemicals, or other irritants

Assessment

I. History (Lumb, 2017)
   A. Cough
   B. Sputum production, hemoptysis
   C. Dyspnea—shortness of breath; tachypnea—rapid breathing; orthopnea—difficulty breathing when supine; paroxysmal nocturnal dyspnea—awakening from sleep with shortness of breath
   D. Wheeze, stridor, chest pain, hoarseness
   E. Ability to carry out activities of daily living (ADLs)
   F. Tobacco use—pack-year history
   G. Chronic obstructive pulmonary disease (COPD)
   H. Exercise or activity tolerance
   I. Number of pillows used for sleep and comfort
   J. Level of consciousness, mental status
   K. Anxiety and apprehension
      1. Acute—less than 2 to 3 weeks
      2. Chronic—longer than 2 months
II. Presence of risk factors
III. Diagnostic tests (Lumb, 2017)
   A. Chest radiography, computed tomography (CT), magnetic resonance imaging (MRI), and positron emission tomography (PET) to delineate anatomic extent of involvement
   B. Pulmonary function tests (PFTs) to quantify air flow limitation
   C. Arterial blood gases (ABGs)
   D. Ventilation-perfusion scans

E. Bronchoscopy for direct visualization; endobronchial ultrasound (EBUS)

F. Endobronchial thoracentesis

IV. Physical examination (Lumb, 2017)

A. Abnormal or altered breathing patterns; tachypnea, pursed-lip breathing or use of accessory muscles of respiration

B. Abnormal breath sounds—wheezes, decreased or absent breath sounds

C. Sputum—amount, color, presence of blood

D. Cyanosis

E. Vital signs and pulse oximetry; hypoxemia

F. Evaluate airway swelling, oropharyngeal swelling

G. Presence of enlarged lymph nodes or masses in the head and neck area

Management (Lumb, 2017)

I. Medical management

A. Treat the underlying disease process

1. Radiation therapy (RT), chemotherapy, biotherapy, and targeted agents for primary or metastatic cancer of the lung or to reduce obstruction of the tracheobronchial tree

2. Supplemental oxygen administration as indicated for hypoxemia

3. Incorporate measures to minimize pain, which may contribute to ineffective breathing (see Chapter 44)

4. Systemic antibiotic treatment for empyema

II. Nursing management

A. Use measures to ease and increase the effectiveness of breathing and to promote physical comfort

1. Thoracentesis to remove abnormal accumulated contents in pleural space

2. Proper positioning, use of pillows

B. Prioritize patient activity and exercise, and use of energy conservation strategies

C. Maximize safety ⚠

1. Encourage patient to use supplemental oxygen and assistive devices (e.g., cane, walker, wheelchair) as needed for ambulation to prevent hypoxia and potential falls

2. Report critical changes to the oncology provider

D. Educate patient and caregiver regarding the following:

1. Prioritize activity and energy conservation strategies

a. Frequent rest periods

b. Easy-to-prepare meals

c. Often-used items within reach

d. Emergency care, available community resources, and medication management

e. Signs and symptoms to report to the health care team

PULMONARY TOXICITY RELATED TO CANCER THERAPY

Overview

I. Definition—parenchymal pulmonary disease caused by antineoplastic therapy, radiation, chemotherapy, biological

TABLE 45.1 Chemotherapy and Biological Agents Predisposing to Radiation Pneumonitis

Chemotherapy Agents	Targeted Therapies
Bleomycin	Alemtuzumab
Busulfan	Bevacizumab
Chlorambucil	Cetuximab
Cyclophosphamide	Rituximab
Doxorubicin	Trastuzumab
Ifosfamide	Idelalisib
Methotrexate	
Mitomycin	
Vinblastine	
Vincristine	

Data from Rovirosa, A., & Valduvieco, I. (2010). Radiation pneumonitis. *Clinical Pulmonary Medicine, 17*(5), 218-222.

agents, targeted therapies (Kroschinsky et al., 2017; Postow et al., 2018)

II. Classification

A. Radiation-induced lung toxicity (RILT), pneumonitis (Kong et al., 2015)

1. Subacute inflammatory response to radiation exposure to the lung; occurs in 1% to 20% of patients receiving thoracic radiation

2. Toxic effects are proportionate to the following:

a. Total radiation dose and volume of lung tissue irradiated

b. Fractionation schedule; hyperfractionation schedules may cause less RT pneumonitis

c. Concomitant administration of chemotherapy (Table 45.1)

B. Chemotherapy-induced pulmonary toxicity (Ranchoux et al., 2015) (Table 45.2)

1. Targets rapidly proliferating cells and may impart direct injury to parenchymal endothelial cell membranes of lung, causing bilateral interstitial infiltrates or fibrosis

2. Systemic release of cytokines, hypersensitivity reaction, or immune complex–related reaction

3. Administration of immunotherapy or targeted therapy-induced pulmonary toxicity (Haanen et al., 2017; Naidoo et al., 2017; Zimmer et al., 2016)

a. May induce overwhelming inflammatory responses and autoimmunity

b. Inflammation process affects the interstitial lung parenchyma, causing infectious and noninfectious lung injury

C. Risk factors

1. Radiation, chemotherapy, or targeted therapy (Haanen et al., 2017; Naidoo et al., 2017; Zimmer et al., 2016)

a. Occurs in 5% to 15% of all patients receiving RT

b. Concurrent chemotherapy and RT or sequential RT to lungs

c. Cumulative dose of administered drug

TABLE 45.2	Chemotherapy and Targeted Therapy–Related Pulmonary Abnormalities	
Pattern of Lung Involvement	**Specific Agents**	**Radiologic Abnormality**
Acute pneumonitis	Bortezomib, cetuximab, dasatinib, erlotinib, everolimus, gefitinib, gemcitabine, idelalisib, imatinib, irinotecan, pemetrexed, piritrexim, procarbazine, rituximab, sorafenib, sunitinib, temozolomide, temsirolimus, thalidomide, trastuzumab	Diffuse, patchy, ground-glass opacities; diffuse reticular pattern
Bronchiolitis	Bortezomib, busulfan, cetuximab, panitumumab, topotecan	Hyperinflation, air trapping
Hemoptysis	Bevacizumab	Bilateral ground-glass opacities, consolidation
Hypersensitivity reactions	Alpha-interferon, cetuximab, etoposide, gemcitabine, L-asparaginase, obinutuzumab, panitumumab, rituximab, taxanes, vinca alkaloids	Air flow obstruction, airway hyperreactivity, hyperinflation
Interstitial pneumonitis	Erlotinib, everolimus, gefitinib, idelalisib, ofatumumab, rituximab, sorafenib, sunitinib, temsirolimus, thalidomide, trastuzumab	Diffuse, patchy, ground-glass opacities
Isolated acute chest pain	Bleomycin, doxorubicin, etoposide, methotrexate	Nonspecific
Isolated cough	Alpha-interferon, IL-2, methotrexate	Nonspecific
Isolated diminished diffusion capacity of lungs for carbon monoxide (DLCO)	Bischloroethylnitrosourea (BCNU; carmustine), gemcitabine, paclitaxel	Nonspecific
Mediastinal lymphadenopathy	Bleomycin, interferon, methotrexate	Hilar, mediastinal lymphadenopathy
Pleural effusion	Bleomycin, bortezomib, busulfan, dasatinib, etoposide, fludarabine, gemcitabine, imatinib, IL-2, methotrexate, procarbazine, taxanes, thalidomide, trametinib	Pleural effusion
Pneumothorax	Carmustine	Pneumothorax
Pulmonary edema	Ara-C, alpha-interferon, azathioprine, decitabine, granulocyte colony-stimulating factor (G-CSF), gemcitabine, imatinib, nitrogen mustard, paclitaxel, vinorelbine	Diffuse alveolar infiltrates, without cardiomegaly or pleural effusion
Pulmonary embolus (PE)	Axitinib, bevacizumab, dasatinib, imatinib, lenalidomide, thalidomide	Acute PE Right-sided heart enlargement, acute PE
Pulmonary hypertension	Dasatinib, Imatinib	

Adapted from Guntur, V. P., & Dhand, R. (2012). Pulmonary toxicity of chemotherapeutic agents. In Perry, M. C. (Ed.). (2012). *Perry's chemotherapy source book* (5th ed., pp. 206–213). Philadelphia: Lippincott Williams & Wilkins; Barber, N. A., & Ganti, A. K. (2011). Pulmonary toxicities from targeted therapies: a review. *Targeted Oncology, 6*(4), 235-243; Kroschinsky, F., et al. (2017). New drugs, new toxicities: severe side effects of modern targeted and immunotherapy of cancer and their management. *Critical Care, 21*, 89-100.

    d. Previous chemo or RT

    e. Biological factors/cytokines, such as transforming growth factor beta-1 (TGF-B1)

  2. Preexisting pulmonary disease, interstitial lung disease (e.g., COPD), renal dysfunction or cardiovascular disease

  3. Smoking history

  4. Poor performance status

  5. More severe in older adults and in females

  6. Age—older than 60 years

Assessment

I. History (Leger et al., 2017; Ranchoux et al., 2015)

  A. Radiation, chemotherapy, or targeted therapy-induced pulmonary toxicity

    1. Dyspnea is the cardinal symptom; also nonproductive cough, malaise, fatigue, fever

    2. Generally develops over weeks to months, but can also develop quickly (within hours) and may occur years after drug exposure

    B. Early nonspecific symptoms include nonproductive cough, mild dyspnea, low-grade temperature, pleuritic chest pain

    C. May occur 6–12 weeks after completion of RT, although symptoms can range from 1 to 6 months after RT

    D. Exclude other causes of pulmonary infiltrates—infection, recurrent tumors, thromboembolic disease, lymphangitic carcinomatosis

II. Physical examination (Kroschinsky et al., 2017)

  A. Physical examination—may be unreliable

    1. Respiratory rate, rhythm, effort

    2. Assess for signs of pulmonary toxicity—dyspnea, dry persistent cough, basilar rales, tachypnea, pleuritic pain

    3. Moist rales, pleural friction rub

    4. Evidence of pleural fluid heard over the area of irradiation

    5. Low-grade fever, congestion

    6. Tachypnea, cyanosis (late)

7. Early—diffuse haziness, ground-glass opacification
8. Late—infiltrates or dense consolidation corresponding to the region of radiation exposure

III. Radiographic changes
   A. Results may be normal, early onset, as late as 2 months, or even years after therapy
   B. Diffuse bilateral lung infiltrates
   C. Classic diffuse reticular pattern, ground-glass opacities, usually bilateral

IV. Diagnostic tests and findings.
   A. PFTs—may reveal restrictive defect or obstructive pattern
      1. Decreased lung volume
      2. Decreased restrictive ventilatory pattern, diminished diffusion capacity of the lungs for carbon monoxide (DLCO); DLCO measures the ability of the lungs to transfer gas from inhaled air to the red blood cells (RBCs) in pulmonary capillaries
   B. High-resolution CT
      1. Detection of radiation fibrosis
         a. Early—diffuse haziness, ground-glass opacification
         b. Late—infiltrates or dense consolidation corresponding to the region of radiation exposure
      2. Abnormality is generally nonspecific
   C. ABGs
      1. Hypoxia
      2. Hypocapnia, respiratory alkalosis

Management

I. Manage treatment-related pulmonary toxicity that is RT induced (Kong & Wang, 2015); chemotherapy induced (Leger et al., 2017; Ranchoux et al., 2015); targeted therapy induced (Haanen et al., 2017; Naidoo et al., 2017, Zimmer et al., 2016)
   A. Mild symptoms—cough suppressants, antipyretics, rest
   B. Severe symptoms and impaired gas exchange—glucocorticoid therapy until symptoms improve, then taper slowly; pneumonitis may flare if taper is too rapid; about 50% respond to glucocorticoid therapy
   C. Monitor baseline PFTs and limit cumulative dose
   D. Discontinue suspected agent or reduce dose for prompt resolution

II. Encourage balanced activity training to decrease or prevent adverse effects of therapy
   A. Evaluate cardiorespiratory fitness
   B. Monitor activities to minimize energy expenditure
   C. Monitor for adequate relief of symptoms

DYSPNEA

Overview

I. Definition—a subjective sensation of difficulty breathing, the feeling of inability to get enough air, and the reaction to the sensation (Baker et al., 2017)
II. Risk factors

A. Disease related
   1. Tumors that impinge on respiratory structures and decrease air flow
   2. Conditions that increase metabolic demands (e.g., fever, infection)
   3. Cerebral metastasis, which affects the respiratory center or stimulates the central and peripheral chemoreceptors
   4. Metastatic effusions in the pleural or cardiac space or abdominal cavity, which compromise lung expansion, gas exchange, or blood flow to the lungs
   5. Coexisting pulmonary, cardiac, or neuromuscular disease, which compromises lung expansion or blood flow to the lungs
   6. Advanced disease or terminal illness
B. Treatment related
   1. Incisional pain that may compromise lung expansion
   2. Immediate and long-term effects of RT to the lung fields
      a. May be acute or delayed (up to 10 years after treatment)
      b. May be dose related, reversible, or chronic
   3. Antineoplastic agents that may cause pulmonary toxicity
      a. May be acute or delayed (up to 10 years after treatment)
      b. May be dose related, reversible, or chronic
   4. Anaphylactic reactions to antineoplastic agents, biological response modifiers, or targeted therapy agents
   5. Pneumothorax related to placement of vascular access catheters, fine-needle aspiration, or thoracentesis
C. Lifestyle related
   1. Strong emotional responses, particularly anxiety or anger, contribute to the sensation of dyspnea
   2. Tobacco use or exposure to environmental toxic substances—asbestos, chromium, coal products, ionizing radiation, vinyl chloride, chloromethyl ethers
   3. Obesity

Assessment (Baker et al., 2017)

I. History
   A. Presence of risk factors such as smoking, chemical exposure
   B. Subjective reports of shortness of breath, "can't catch breath," "smothering," "air hunger," uncomfortable breathing, anxiety, or panic
   C. Pattern of dyspnea—onset, frequency, severity, associated symptoms, aggravating or alleviating factors
   D. Impact of dyspnea on ADLs, lifestyle, relationships, role responsibilities, emotional well-being, sexuality, and body image
   E. Intake and output
   F. Vascular perfusion

II. Physical findings
  A. Tachypnea, hypercapnia, increased respiratory excursion
  B. Use of accessory muscles, retraction of intercostal spaces, nostril flaring
  C. Clubbing of digits caused by chronic hypoxemia; cyanosis, pallor, jugular vein distention, upper extremity swelling, venous congestion in thorax or chest region
III. Diagnostic tests and findings
  A. Complete blood cell (CBC) count—hemoglobin deficiencies
  B. Pulse oximetry—severity of hypoxia
  C. Chest radiography and CT—structural abnormalities, PFTs
  D. Bronchoscopic examination
  E. Sputum or bronchial cultures
  F. ABGs
  G. Assessment scales such as a numeric rating scale to measure degree of patient's dyspnea (Baker et al., 2017)
IV. Psychological signs and symptoms
  A. Concentration difficulties, memory difficulties, or both; confusion
  B. Restlessness

Management

I. Manage treatment-related dyspnea (Baker et al., 2017; ONS, 2017)
  A. Supplemental oxygen, as indicated
  B. Treatment of underlying disease with thoracentesis, RT, chemotherapy, antimicrobial medications
  C. Pharmacologic agents
    1. Glucocorticoids—decrease local inflammation
    2. Opioids and anxiolytics—decrease pain and anxiety
    3. Bronchodilators—increase air flow to the lungs
    4. Diuretics—decrease fluid overload
II. Manage the discomfort of dyspnea
  A. Immediate-release oral and parenteral opioids, which decrease central respiratory drive by reducing ventilatory demand
    1. Recommended for practice
  B. Pharmacologic agents—extended-release morphine, midazolam plus morphine, nebulized opioids, furosemide, lidocaine
    1. May alleviate dyspnea in some patients
    2. Effectiveness not established—more studies needed
    3. Expert opinion—low-risk interventions
  C. Oxygen therapy for relief of hypoxia
  D. Benzodiazepines for anxiety
III. Promote comfort
  A. Increased ambient air flow directed at face or nose
  B. Cooler temperatures.
  C. Promotion of relaxation and stress reduction techniques

D. Providing educational, emotional, and psychosocial support to patient and caregiver; referral to other disciplines as appropriate
E. Further research needed for use of acupuncture and cognitive behavioral approaches
F. Avoidance of volume overload
G. Encourage positioning to facilitate breathing—upright position; forward position with elbows on knees, table, or pillows
H. Instruct patient about diaphragmatic breathing techniques with slow exhalation; may not be effective and may be harmful in patients with pulmonary restrictive disease
I. Recommend assistive devices such as wheelchair, walker, and portable oxygen as needed
J. Exercise rehabilitation
IV. Maximize safety
  A. Encourage use of assistive devices such as cane, walker, or wheelchair as needed for ambulation and ADLs
  B. Use activity limitation, conservation of energy strategies
    1. Frequent rest periods
    2. Use of ready-made meals
    3. Often-used items within reach
V. Monitor subjective reports of the changes in the pattern of dyspnea or psychological responses to dyspnea such as anxiety or distress
VI. Educate patient and caregiver
  A. Teach about activity limitation, energy conservation strategies
  B. Provide information about accessing emergency care, available community resources
VII. Decrease the sense of dyspnea and enhance psychosocial well-being
  A. Encourage use of relaxation techniques, prayer and meditation, aromatherapy
  B. Use of language that is easy to understand (e.g., shortness of breath instead of dyspnea)
  C. Use complementary and alternative therapies such as relaxation techniques and stress reduction strategies

PLEURAL EFFUSIONS

Overview

I. Definition—presence of excess fluid in the pleural space
II. Classification (Thomas, Jenkins, & Singh, 2015)
  A. Benign pleural effusion and malignant pleural effusion, the presence of malignant cells in the pleura that signifies distant spread of disease, may be caused by the following:
    1. Increased hydrostatic pressure (congestive heart failure [CHF])
    2. Increased permeability in microvascular circulation (infection, trauma)
    3. Increased negative pressure in the pleural space (atelectasis)

4. Decreased oncotic pressure in the microvasculature (nephrotic syndrome, cirrhosis, hypoalbuminemia)
5. Direct extension of primary tumor to the pleura or mediastinum or mesothelioma involving the pleura
6. Impaired lymphatic drainage from the pleural space resulting from obstruction caused by tumor
7. Increased permeability caused by inflammation or disruption of the capillary endothelium
8. Altered mucosal lung or mediastinal tissue resulting from RT

III. Risk factors (Thomas, Jenkins, & Singh, 2015)
   A. Primary tumors of lung, breast, hematopoietic system
   B. Prior pleural effusion
   C. Radiation to the chest, thorax, or abdomen
   D. Surgical modification of venous or lymphatic vessels

Assessment

I. History
   A. Presence of risk factors
   B. Symptoms—severity related to the speed of accumulation, not amount; usually caused by pulmonary compression
      1. Dyspnea, progressive, exertional
      2. Cough usually dry and nonproductive
      3. Chest pain
II. Physical examination
   A. Fever, tachypnea
   B. Restricted chest wall expansion
   C. Dullness to percussion
   D. Auscultation—diminished or absent breath sounds, egophony (an increased resonance of voice sounds heard when auscultating the lungs, often caused by lung consolidation and fibrosis), pleural friction rub
   E. General manifestations—compression atelectasis or mediastinal shift if pleural effusion severe
III. Diagnostic tests (Soni, et al., 2015).
   A. Chest radiography—effusion size, position of mediastinum and diaphragm; blunting of costophrenic angle
   B. Chest CT—to identify loculated effusion or alternative diagnosis
   C. Ultrasonography—to assess pleural fluid volume; to identify optimal site for ultrasound-guided thoracentesis (Soni et al., 2015)
   D. Gastrointestinal (GI) disease—GI abscess, pancreatic disease, postabdominal surgery
   E. Pleural biopsy—increases diagnostic yield when combined with cytologic studies
   F. Thoracentesis—pleural fluid withdrawal for cytology, chemical analysis, and culture (rule out infection); diagnostic and therapeutic
   G. Pleural fluid evaluation (lactate dehydrogenase [LDH], glucose, protein)—to determine transudative or exudative fluid
      1. Transudative—systemic factors causing effusion, such as CHF, cirrhosis, nephrotic syndrome, hypoalbuminemia

2. Exudative—local factors causing effusion
   a. Neoplastic—metastatic or primary tumor
   b. Infectious—bacterial, fungal, viral, parasitic
   c. Pulmonary embolus

Management

I. Manage pleural effusions (Fig. 45.1)
   A. Therapeutic aspiration using intrapleural chemical agent; talc most efficacious, evidence-based
      1. Obliterates the pleural space to prevent fluid reaccumulation
      2. May improve patient comfort, relieve dyspnea for palliation
      3. Reaccumulation of fluid is common
      4. Potential for hypoproteinemia, pneumothorax, empyema, fluid loculation
      5. Hydrodissection with irrigation device into the pleural space
      6. Talc pleurodesis if large effusion or recurrent
   B. Thorascopic drainage and talc poudrage
   C. Video-assisted thoracoscopic surgery (VATS)
   D. Indwelling pleural catheters (IPC)—for palliative relief
   E. Chemotherapy and mediastinal radiation—may be effective in responsive tumors (lymphoma, small cell lung cancer [SCLC])
II. Decrease symptom severity associated with pleural effusion
   A. Educate about measures to increase the ease and effectiveness of breathing
   B. Incorporate measures to minimize discomfort (e.g., opioid analgesia before chest tube insertion and as needed)
   C. Recommend the use of relaxation techniques as indicated for coping with anxiety
III. Maximize safety
   A. Encourage use of assistive devices as needed for ADLs
   B. Use activity limitation and conservation of energy strategies
   C. Instruct caregiver in use of and precautions related to oxygen therapy
   D. Instruct caregivers in the appropriate use of medications to manage disease
IV. Monitor the consequences of therapy
   A. Respiratory rate, rhythm, effort, adventitious breath sounds
   B. Characteristics of pain and relief measures
   C. Subjective response to drainage and rate of fluid reaccumulation
   D. Report critical changes to the oncology provider—chest pain, fever, change in character of respiration
V. Educate patient and caregiver regarding the following:
   A. Activity limitation, conservation of energy strategies
   B. Emergency care, available community resources
   C. Signs and symptoms to report to the health care team
   D. Procedures that may be required to alleviate pleural effusions

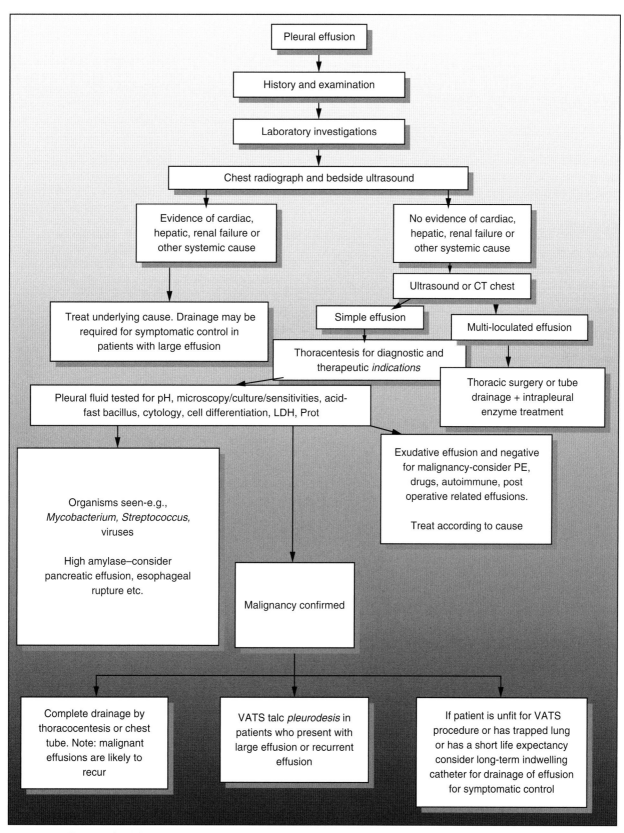

Fig. 45.1 Decision making and management of pleural effusion. (From Quinn, T., Alam, N., Aminazad, A., Marshall, M. B., & Choong, C. K. C. (2013). Decision making and algorithm for the management of pleural effusions. *Thoracic Surgery Clinics, 23*(1), 11–16.)

VI. Enhance adaptation or rehabilitation
   A. Assist the patient to maintain independence within the limitation of symptoms
   B. Encourage the patient and family to express concerns

EXPECTED PATIENT OUTCOMES

I. The patient will experience optimal oxygenation and less shortness of breath.
II. The patient will maintain optimal functional status.
III. The patient will report comfort from respiratory symptoms such as dyspnea and pleuritic pain.

REFERENCES

Baker, K. M., DeSanto-Madeya, S., & Banzett, R. B. (2017). Routine dyspnea assessment and documentation: nurses' experience yields wide acceptance. *BMC Nursing.* https://doi.org/10.1186/s12912-016-0196-9. 16-3.

Haanen, J.B.A.G., Carbonnel, F., Robert, C., Kerr, K.M., Peters, S., Larkin, J., … Jordan, K. (2017). Management of toxicities from immunotherapy: ESMO Clinical Practice Guidelines for diagnosis, treatment and follow-up. *Annals of Oncology, 28*(4), iv119-iv142. doi.org/10.1093/annonc/mdx225

Kong, F., & Wang, S. (2015). Non-dosimetric risk factors for radiation-induced lung toxicity. *Seminars in Radiation Oncology, 25*(2), 100–109.

Kroschinsky, F., Stolzel, F., vonBonin, S., Beutel, G., Kochanek, M., Kiehl, M., & Schellongowski, P. (2017). New drugs, new toxicities: severe side effects of modern targeted and immunotherapy of cancer and their management. *Critical Care, 21*, 89–100.

Leger, P., Limper, A. H., & Maldonado, F. (2017). Pulmonary complications from conventional chemotherapy. *Clinics in Chest Medicine, 38*(2), 209–222.

Lumb, A. B. (2017). *Nunn's applied physiology* (8th ed., p. 2017). Elsevier Ltd.

Naidoo, J., Wang, X., Woo, K. M., Iyriboz, T., Halpenny, D., Cunningham, J., … Hellmann, M. D. (2017). Pneumonitis in patients treated with Anti-Programmed Death-1/Programmed Death Ligand 1 therapy. *Journal of Clinical Oncology, 35*, 709–717.

Oncology Nursing Society, (2017). Dyspnea. Retrieved from: https://www.ons.org/practice-resources/pep/dyspnea

Postow, M. A., Sidlow, R., & Hellmann, M. D. (2018). Immune-related adverse events associated with immune checkpoint blockade. *New England Journal of Medicine, 378*, 158–168.

Ranchoux, B., Gunther, S., Quarck, R., Chaumais, M. C., Dorfmuller, P., Antigny, F., … Perros, F. (2015). Chemotherapy-induced pulmonary hypertension: role of alkylating agents. *American Journal of Pathology, 185*(2), 356–371.

Sarkar, M., Niranjan, N., & Banyal, P. K. (2017). Mechanisms of hypoxemia. *Lung India, 34*(1), 47–60.

Soni, N. J., Franco, R., Velez, M. I., Schnobrich, D., Dancel, R., Restrepo, M. I., & Mayo, P. H. (2015). Ultrasound in the diagnosis and management of pleural effusions. *Journal of Hospital Medicine, 10*(12), 811–816.

Thomas, R., Jenkins, S., & Singh, B. (2015). Physiology of breathlessness associated with pleural effusions. *Current Opinion in Pulmonary Medicine, 21*(4), 338–345.

Zimmer, L., Goldinger, S. M., Hofmann, L., Loquai, C., Ugurel, S., Thomas, I., … Heinzerling, L. M. (2016). Neurological, respiratory, musculoskeletal, cardiac and ocular side-effects of anti-PD-1 therapy. *European Journal of Cancer, 60*, 210–215. https://doi.org/10.1016/j.ejca.2016.02.024.

46

Sleep–Wake Disturbances

Tricia Montgomery and Jeannine M. Brant

OVERVIEW

I. Definition (Carskadon & Dement, 2011; Matthews, Carter, Page, Dean, & Berger, 2018; Otte et al., 2014)
   A. Sleep—an active biobehavioral process; includes temporary perceptual disengagement and environmental unresponsiveness
   B. Sleep–wake disturbances—actual or perceived disturbance in sleep with resulting daytime impairment
   C. Lack of consistency exists to define sleep disorders (Reynolds & O'Hara, 2013)

II. Sleep–wake disturbances—include insomnia, sleep-related breathing problems, circadian rhythm disorders, and excessive sleepiness often in combination with fatigue, anxiety, and depression (Denlinger et al., 2014; Reynolds & O'Hara, 2013)
   A. Insomnia—transient inability to initiate or maintain sleep (Howell et al., 2014)
   B. Experienced by 30%–80% of patients with cancer (Matthews et al., 2018)
   C. Often overlooked in cancer patients (Howell et al., 2014)
   D. Poor sleep could be due to one or more sleep disorders (Otte et al., 2014)
   E. Patients may not report due to thinking it's a normal reaction to the cancer diagnosis or treatment (Howell et al., 2014)

III. Physiology (National Cancer Institute, 2016)
   A. Sleep–wake cycle
      1. Consists of two phases.
         a. Rapid eye movement (REM)—phase where the brain is active
         b. Non–rapid eye movement (NREM)—quiet or restful sleep
      2. Stages repeat, with each cycle lasting approximately 90 minutes. Four to six cycles during a 7- to 8-hour sleep period.
      3. Dictated by an inherent biological clock or circadian rhythm.

IV. Risk factors—several risk factors can increase the risk of difficulty sleeping (Matthews et al., 2018; National Cancer Institute, 2016)
   A. Lifestyle
      1. Sleep hygiene practices: daytime naps, use of caffeine and/or nicotine close to bedtime, lack of daily exercise, lack of a regular bedtime routine
   B. Demographic
      1. Older patients may be experiencing sleep-related issues before diagnosis due to aging and its impact on sleep patterns
      2. Menopause, which may be treatment induced (Xu, Lang, & Rooney, 2014)
   C. Environment
      1. Frequent monitoring during hospitalization
      2. Temperature of the room—cool is preferred between 60 and 67 degrees Fahrenheit
   D. Disease related
      1. Paraneoplastic syndrome (increased steroid production), tumor invasion symptoms (pain, obstruction, fatigue, pruritis)
      2. Medications—opioids, caffeine, steroids, dietary supplements, some antidepressants, nicotine
      3. Physical/psychological—pain, loss of function, inability to care for self, cost of treatment
   E. Treatment-related factors
      1. Side effects of systemic chemotherapy (nausea, vomiting, diarrhea, use of steroids), surgery (pain, use of opioids, frequent monitoring)

ASSESSMENT

I. History and physical information (Matthews et al., 2018; National Cancer Institute, 2016)
   A. Disease-related factors—paraneoplastic syndromes (increased steroid production), tumor invasion symptoms (pain, fever, obstruction, fatigue).
   B. Treatments for disease, either current or previous—surgery (pain, opioid use), systemic chemotherapy, hormonal therapy, biological and targeted therapies, steroids.
   C. Current medications—opioids, sedatives/hypnotics, steroids, caffeine/nicotine, some antidepressants. Dietary supplements and alternative therapies should be assessed.
   D. Environmental factors—hospitalization (frequent checks, roommates, lights on/off) or at home (temperature of room, lights on/off, others living in home).

E. Physical stressors—inability to move self, pain, limited motion.

F. Psychological stressors—depression, anxiety (fear of loss of income, increased cost of health care, fear of death), delirium (side effect of medications or due to cancer itself).

G. Diet and exercise history—dietary supplement usage, alternative therapies, regular exercise routine.

II. Sleep screening (National Comprehensive Cancer Network, 2017)

A. Screen at regular intervals and with any changes in clinical status

B. Screening questions
   1. Are you having any problems falling asleep or staying asleep?
   2. Are you experiencing excessive sleepiness?
   3. Have you been told that you snore frequently or stop breathing during sleep?

C. If yes, conduct a more in-depth assessment

III. Characterization of sleep

A. Sleep patterns—usual bedtime, bedtime routine, how long it takes to fall asleep

B. Sleep duration—episodes of being awake, ability to fall back asleep, time it takes to wake up

C. How sleep changed after diagnosis; sleep changes with treatment or hospitalization

D. Family/personal history of sleep disturbances

E. Others' perceptions of patient sleep quantity and quality

IV. Physical examination and diagnostic testing

A. Polysomnography—diagnostic tool to diagnose sleep–wake disturbances such as sleep-related breathing disorders and limb movement disorders.

B. Physical signs of sleep disturbance—falling asleep during conversations, difficulty following conversations, yawning, need to support self with arm to keep head up, head lying back on wall or bed

V. Sleep–wake disturbances can change throughout the cancer journey; sleep should be continually assessed.

MANAGEMENT

I. Medical management (National Cancer Institute, 2016; Matthews et al., 2018)

A. While many agents are Food and Drug Administration (FDA) approved for sleep, most have not been well tested in patients with cancer (Matthews et al., 2018).

B. Drug classes to treat insomnia
   1. Hypnotics—may be preferred in cancer patients when a hypnotic effect is desired; next-day drowsiness is the major side effect.
   2. Benzodiazepines—higher risk for tolerance, dependence, withdrawal. May carry risk of morning sedation if the agent has long half-life. Shorter half-life preferred for difficulty falling asleep and in older adults.
   3. Antihistamines—treat only difficulty falling asleep, limited evidence for insomnia. May be preferred if

concerned about cross-dependence; anticholinergic and to be used with caution in older adults.

   4. Antidepressants and antipsychotics—first line when insomnia is associated with depression or anxiety symptoms.
   5. Melatonin receptor agonists—may be used for difficulty falling asleep or circadian sleep disorders. Less risk of other impairments/dependence but does not treat patients who have difficulty staying asleep.
   6. Melatonin—hormone produced by the pineal gland during hours of darkness, linked to circadian rhythm.
   7. Antipsychotics—sedating effects; should be considered as last resort due to serious side effect profile.
   8. Alpha-adrenergic receptor blockers—relax muscles, inhibit norepinephrine
   9. Orexin receptor antagonist—blocks orexin in the brain, which inhibits arousal; the controlled substance suvorexant is the only agent on the market.

II. Nursing management (National Cancer Institute, 2016; National Comprehensive Cancer Network, 2018; Matthews et al., 2018)

A. Promote sleep hygiene
   1. Help patient establish a routine of only going to bed when sleepy at about the same time each night and waking up at the same time each day.
   2. Educate patient on developing a bedtime routine, including trying to do something relaxing 1 to 2 hours before bed.
   3. Have patient avoid caffeine after noon and avoid heavy meals, drinking alcohol, or smoking close to bedtime.
   4. Encourage the patient to make their bedroom restful, free of distractions like computers or television, and to keep the room cool and dark.

B. Provide interventions to maximize patient comfort (National Cancer Institute, 2016; National Comprehensive Cancer Network, 2018)
   1. Treat contributing factors: pain, depression, delirium nausea
   2. Skin care
   3. Keep bedding clean and without wrinkles
   4. Coordinate bedside contacts as to not interrupt sleep if possible
   5. Minimize noise

C. Employ cognitive interventions (Matthews et al., 2018)
   1. Cognitive therapies have shown to be as effective as pharmacologic therapies, although studies with cancer patients are limited; in studies with cancer patients, shown to improve sleep with sustained benefits.
   2. Have patient set aside time to think about what may be causing them stress during the day.

D. Offer alternative suggestions to promote sleep
   1. Discuss exposure to natural light at least 20–30 minutes each day, if possible in the morning.

2. Educate patient if unable to fall asleep, leave room and try to relax in a different area that is dark and quiet. Go back to bed when sleepy.
3. Educate patient on condition and treatment options

EXPECTED PATIENT OUTCOMES

I. The patient and caregiver will identify the risk factors that put them at risk for sleep–wake disturbances.
II. The patient and caregiver will describe sleep hygiene practices and specific behavioral and cognitive interventions to promote sleep.
III. The patient and caregiver will understand the risk/benefit ratio of pharmacologic strategies to facilitate sleep.

REFERENCES

Carskadon, M. A., & Dement, W. C. (2011). Normal human sleep: an overview. In M. H. Kryger, T. Roth, & W. C. Dement (Eds.), *Principles and practice of sleep medicine* (5th ed., pp. 16–26). Philadelphia, PA: Elsevier.

Denlinger, C. S., Ligibel, J. A., Are, M., Baker, K. S., Demark-Wahnefried, W., Friedman, D. L., & Freedman-Cass, D. (2014). Survivorship: sleep disorders, version 1.2014. *Journal of the National Comprehensive Cancer Network*, 12(5), 630–642.

Howell, D., Oliver, T. K., Keller-Olaman, S., Davidson, J. R., Garland, S., Samuels, C., & Taylor, C. (2014). Sleep disturbance in adults with cancer: a systematic review of evidence for best practices in assessment and management for clinical practice.

Annals of Oncology, 25(4), 791–800. https://doi.org/10.1093/annonc/mdt506.

Matthews, E., Carter, P., Page, M., Dean, G., & Berger, A. (2018). Sleep-wake disturbance: A systematic review of evidence-based interventions for management in patients with cancer. *Clinical Journal of Oncology Nursing*, 22(1), 37–52. https://doi.org/10.1188/18.CJON.37-52.

National Cancer Institute. (2016). *Sleep disorders.* Retrieved from (2016). https://www.cancer.gov/about-cancer/treatment/side-effects/sleep-disorders-pdq.

National Comprehensive Cancer Network. (2017). *NCCN clinical practice guidelines in oncology: survivorship (v.3.2017).* Retrieved from (2017). https://www.nccn.org/professionals/physician_gls/pdf/survivorship.pdf.

National Comprehensive Cancer Network. (2018). *NCCN clinical practice guidelines in oncology: palliative care (v.1.2018).* Retrieved from (2018). http://www.nccn.org/professionals/physician_gls/pdf/palliativepdf.

Otte, J. L., Carpenter, J. S., Manchanda, S., Rand, K. L., Skaar, T. C., Weaver, M., & Landis, C. (2014). Systematic review of sleep disorders in cancer patients: can the prevalence of sleep disorders be ascertained? *Cancer Medicine.* https://doi.org/10.1002/cam4.356.

Reynolds, C. F. 3rd, & O'Hara, R. (2013). DSM-5 sleep-wake disorders classification: overview for use in clinical practice. *American Journal of Psychiatry*, 170(10), 1099-1101. doi:https://doi.org/10.1176/appi.ajp.2013.13010058.

Xu, Q., Lang, C. P., & Rooney, N. (2014). A systematic review of the longitudinal relationships between subjective sleep disturbance and menopausal stage. *Maturitas*, 79(4), 401–412. https://doi.org/10.1016/j.maturitas.2014.09.011.

47

Altered Body Image

Elizabeth Freitas

OVERVIEW

I. Altered body image (Rhoten, 2015)
   A. Self-perception related to an actual or perceived change in appearance.
   B. Decline or change in function that may be visible or internal: examples:
      1. Alopecia:
         a. Chemotherapy: total hair loss (e.g., eyelashes, nose hair, pubic hair); typically starts 2 weeks after chemotherapy, may occur over a day to weeks, and occurs later with low dose of chemotherapy. Hair regrowth usually starts 6–8 weeks after completion of treatment. Hair may come back slowly, thinner, or take up to a year.
         b. Radiation therapy will cause either temporary or permanent hair loss in treatment field.
      2. Nutrition alteration: cachexia with inadequate nutritional intake or obesity with steroids.
      3. Colostomy/ileostomy may result in leakage/odor and changes in function and appearance.
      4. Mastectomy/lymphedema results in changes in function and appearance.
      5. Moon face: high-dose corticosteroids in treatment for leukemia.
      6. Sensory change, such as neuropathic pain or numbness associated with neurotoxic chemotherapeutic agents, results in altered function and may result in altered body image.
      7. Amputations or surgical scar.
         a. Results may lead to psychological distress regarding changes in appearance and/or function.

ASSESSMENT

I. Risk factors of altered body image—reactions are individual and may be related to:
   A. Age: young individuals may be at higher risk for altered body image (Paterson et al., 2016; Teo et al., 2016). Childhood cancer survivors have similar body image issues compared with healthy controls (Lehmann et al., 2016). Parents of adolescents with cancer may have more body image issues than the adolescents themselves (Stinson et al., 2014).
   B. Sex: body image issues are a concern for both males and females—generally based upon focus of body image before alteration for females, and males tend to be more concerned with body changes that affect function (Clarke et al., 2014).
   C. Treatment type: body image issues are more significant for individuals who experience multiple treatment modalities and more radical surgeries (Teo et al., 2016).
   D. Disease: altered body image affects individuals with all types of cancer; individuals have more significant body image issues when cancer is metastatic or recurs (McClelland, Holland, Griggs, 2015).
   E. Timing of reconstruction: satisfaction varies based on the stage of reconstruction and is similar when surgery is completed (Teo et al., 2016).
   F. Time since diagnosis: body image satisfaction is not dependent on time since diagnosis (Clarke, Newell, Thompson, Harcourt, & Lindenmeyer, 2014).
   G. Less social support increases body image disturbance (Milbury Cohen, Jenkins, Skibber, & Schover, 2013).
   H. Appearance concerns at baseline are correlated with distress postsurgically (Clarke et al., 2014).

II. Physical examination
   A. Hair loss (WHO, 2009) classifications of alopecia range from grade 0 (no alopecia) to grade 4 (irreversible alopecia)
   B. Function: assess for functional limitations that may affect body image such as lymphedema, a colostomy, or presence of neuropathy.
   C. Surgical site: wound healing, scaring, or amputation.
   D. Weight: cachexia or weight gain.

III. Psychosocial assessment: many assessment tools are available to measure altered body image. There is significant variation in assessment methods resulting in a broad spectrum of responses (Clarke et al., 2014). Altered body image can result in psychological distress manifesting in changes in:

A. Quality of life (Olsson, Sandin-Bojö, Bjuresäter, & Larsson, 2016), emotional well-being (Teo et al., 2016) ranges on the spectrum from feeling upset and less attractive (Rugo et al., 2017) to distress (Alcorso & Sherman, 2016).

B. Coping often by avoidance, a decline in sexual interaction (Benedict et al., 2015), and increased distress from the reaction of others.

C. Anxiety can result from an altered body image (Alcorso & Sherman, 2016) and is less likely if the individual is less anxious at baseline (Clarke et al., 2014).

D. Depression can result from an altered body image (Alcorso & Sherman, 2016; Sherman, Woon, French & Elder, 2017) and is less likely if the individual is less depressed at baseline.

E. Role changes can result from body image changes: wife/mother, husband/father.

MANAGEMENT

I. Medical Interventions and Nursing Interventions
   A. No pharmacological interventions are approved to prevent hair loss.
   B. Antianxiety or antidepression medications may be recommended in combination with psychotherapy if body image distress is prolonged and unresponsive to nonpharmacologic management.

II. Nursing management
   A. Communication strategies for nurses (Table 47.1)
   B. Nurses should ask about individuals' body image throughout the diagnosis, treatment, and survivorship continuum
   C. Interventions to enhance adaptation and rehabilitation
      1. Educate patient, partner, and family about cancer treatment process.
      2. Concealment: wigs, hats, and clothing.
      3. Cognitive therapy: identify previous successful coping strategies and encourage self-compassion

TABLE 47.1 Communication Strategies for Nurses

	Body Image Challenge	Typical Approaches	PREFERRED APPROACHES	
			Exploratory Phrases	Empathic Phrases
Example #1	"I can't stand to look in the mirror or show my body to my husband since my mastectomy."	*Premature reassurance:* You look great! Don't worry, your swelling will continue to go down, and things will look even better in a few weeks.	What do you see when you look in the mirror? Have you discussed your concerns with your husband?	This must be a huge adjustment for you, since you used to be more comfortable in your body.
Example #2	"I rarely leave the house since my surgery. I don't like when people stare at me or talk about my appearance or garbled speech. I worry about what others think of me, especially my grandkids."	*Cheerleader:* You need to get out more, and you will feel better. Your family needs you and loves you just the way you are.	What do you think your grandkids think of you now? Do you think your friends and family miss seeing you?	You obviously love your grandkids tremendously. It must be very difficult for you to not spend time with them like you used to.
Example #3	"I had beautiful hair down to my waist before I started chemotherapy. I can't stop crying about my hair falling out."	*Cheerleader:* Don't give up! You're nearly done with chemo.	Tell me more about what this is like for you. Do you have any close friends or family you feel comfortable with talking about your concerns?	I know how much pride you take in your appearance, so this must be very difficult for you.
Example #4	"There is no way I'm getting a (colostomy) bag. Everyone will be able to see it through my clothes, and my wife will never sleep with me again."	*Premature reassurance:* Ostomy bags are easily concealable beneath your clothes. *Education, scare tactic:* If you don't get proper treatment, you will die of your cancer.	Tell me more about your concerns. Have you discussed this issue with your wife?	I can imagine the thought of a colostomy bag must be shocking and can be difficult to accept at first. I understand you have a lot of concerns.

Used with permission from Fingeret, M. C., Teo, I., & Epner, D. (2014). Managing body image difficulties of adult cancer patients: lessons from available research. *Cancer, 120*(5), 633-641. doi: 10.1002/cncr.28469

(Fingeret, Teo, & Epner, 2014; Sherman, Woon, French & Elder, 2017)

4. Hypnotic relaxation may improve body image (Cieslak et al., 2016)

D. Interventions to incorporate individual, partner (encourage communication between partners and empathy), and social support in the continuum of care (Clarke et al., 2014)

E. Lymphedema: "complete decongestive therapy, compression bandages, and compression garments are effective treatment/preventative measures. Weight management, full-body exercise, information provision, prevention, and early intervention protocols are likely to be effective" (Fu, Deng, & Armer, 2014).

F. Scalp cooling for alopecia prevention demonstrates no evidence of increase in scalp metastases (Rugo & Voigt, 2018).

1. Types: automatic (start 30–45 minutes before and 20–150 minutes after) and manual (start 30 minutes before)

2. Effectiveness based on treatment, contact with scalp, hair type, and liver function.

3. Side effect: headache can be mitigated with acetaminophen.

G. Creative psychological interventions such as art and dance have not shown to be effective (Archer, Buxton & Sheffield, 2015).

H. Mindfulness/prayer are not consistently effective in managing alterations in body image.

EXPECTED PATIENT OUTCOMES

I. The patient identifies body image changes, significance of changes, and adaptive coping strategies.

II. The patient will optimize functional status, including roles, social interactions, and sexual functioning.

III. The patient will experience decreased psychological distress and will be offered individualized support and counseling if experiencing distress.

REFERENCES

Alcorso, J., & Sherman, K. A. (2016). Factors associated with psychological distress in women with breast cancer-related lymphoedema. *Psychooncology*, 25(7), 865–872. https://doi.org/10.1002/pon.4021.

Archer, S., Buxton, S., & Sheffield, D. (2015). The effect of creative psychological interventions on psychological outcomes for adult cancer patients: a systematic review of randomised controlled trials. *Psychooncology*, 24(1), 1–10. https://doi.org/10.1002/pon.3607.

Benedict, C., Phill, E. J., Baser, R. E., Carter, J., Schuler, T. A., Jandorf, L., & Nelson, C. (2015). Body image and sexual function in women after treatment for anal and rectal cancer. *Psychooncology*, 25(3), 316–323. https://doi.org/10.1002/pon.3847.

Cieslak, A., Elkins, G., Banerjee, T., Marsack, J., Hickman, K., ... Barton, D. (2016). Developing a hypnotic relaxation intervention to improve body image: a feasibility study. *Oncology nursing forum*, 43(6), E233-E241. doi: https://doi.org/10.1188/16.ONF.E233-E241

Clarke, S. S., Newell, R., Thompson, A., Harcourt, D., & Lindenmeyer, A. (2014). Appearance concerns and psychosocial adjustment following head and neck cancer: a cross-sectional study and nine-month follow-up. *Psychol Health Med*. 19(5), 505–518. https://doi.org/10.1080/13548506.2013.855319.

Fingeret, M. C., Teo, I., & Epner, D. (2014). Managing body image difficulties of adult cancer patients: lessons from available research. *Cancer*. 120(5), 633–641. https://doi.org/10.1002/cncr.28469.

Fu, M. R., Deng, J., & Armer, J. M. (2014). Putting evidence into practice: cancer-related lymphedema: evolving evidence for treatment and management from 2009-2014. *Clinic Journal of Oncology Nursing*, 18(6), 68–79. https://doi.org/10.1188/14.CJON.S3.68-79.

Lehmann, V., Hagedoorn, M., Gerhardt, C. A., Fults, M., Olshefski, R. S., ... Tuinman, M. A. (2016). Body issues, sexual satisfaction, and relationship status satisfaction in long-term childhood cancer survivors and healthy controls. *Psychooncology*. 25(2), 210-6. doi: https://doi.org/10.1002/pon.3841.

McClelland, S. I., Holland, K. J., & Griggs, J. J. (2015). *Quality Life Research*, 24(12), 2939–2943. https://doi.org/10.1007/s11136-015-1034-3.

Milbury, K., Cohen, L., Jenkins, R., Skibber, J. M., & Schover, L. R. (2013). The association between psychosocial and medical factors with long-term sexual dysfunction after treatment for colorectal cancer. *Support Care Cancer*, 21(3), 793–802. https://doi.org/10.1007/s00520-012-1582-9.

Olsson, C., Sandin-Bojo, A. K., Bjuresater, K., & Larsson, M. (2016). Changes in Sexuality, Body Image and Health Related Quality of Life in Patients Treated for Hematologic Malignancies: A Longitudinal Study. *Sex Disabil*, 34(4), 367–388. https://doi.org/10.1007/s11195-016-9459-3.

Rhoten, (2015). Body image disturbance in adults treated for cancer - a concept analysis. *Journal Adv Nurs*, 72(5), 1001-11. https://doi.org/10.1111/jan.12892.

Rugo, H. S., & Voigt, J. (2018). Scalp hypothermia for preventing alopecia during chemotherapy. A systematic review and meta-analysis of randomized controlled trials. *Clin Breast Cancer*. 18(1), 19–28. https://doi.org/10.1016/j.clbc.2017.07.012. Epub 2017 Aug 10.

Sherman, K. A., Woon, S., French, J., & Elder, E. (2017). Body image and psychological distress in nipple-sparing mastectomy: the roles of self-compassion and appearance investment. *Psychooncology*. 26(3), 337–345. https://doi.org/10.1002/pon.4138.

Stinson, J., Jibb, L., Greenberg, M., Barrera, M., Luca, S., White, M., & Gupta, A. (2014). *Journal Adolesc Young Adult Oncology*, 4(2), 84–90. https://doi.org/10.1089/jayao.2014.0036.

Teo, I., Reece, G. P., Christie, I. C., Guindani, M., Markey, M. K., Heinberg, L. J., & Fingeret, M. C. (2016). Body image and quality of life of breast cancer patients: influence of timing and stage of breast reconstruction. *Psychooncology*. 25(9), 1106–1112. https://doi.org/10.1002/pon.3952.

WHO. (2009). *WHO Toxicity Scale*. Retrieved from http://www.oncoprof.net/Generale2000/g09_Chimiotherapie/Complements/g09-gb_comp01.htm.

48

Caregiver Burden

Geline J. Tamayo

OVERVIEW

I. Definition
  A. Caregiver: a trained or untrained spouse, family member, or friend who assumes a typically uncompensated, allied role in domestically supporting the health management and well-being of another person, involving significant amounts of time and energy for months or years, and performing tasks requiring physical, emotional, social, or financial demands (Kent, Rowland, et al., 2016)
    1. Primary caregiver: mainly provides and/or assists the care recipient with day-to-day care, activities of daily living (ADLs), facilitates health care delivery, and participates in decisions regarding care (Saria, Courchesne, et al., 2017).
    2. Secondary caregiver: assists the primary caregiver with caregiving or provides support to patients (Saria, Courchesne, et al., 2017).
  B. Caregiving: a complex and dynamic process of assisting with the continuum of health care activities for someone unable to independently care for themselves or who needs help/assistance to manage their care (Given, et al., 2012; Roth, et al. 2015).
    1. An aging and growing population has made caregiving a major public health concern (Feinberg, 2014; Haylock, 2010; Talley & Crews, 2007).
      a. Imposes time-sensitive, life-changing commitment/experience
      b. Includes shifting and evolving existing, often long-standing, relationships
    2. Caregiving is associated with significant physical, psychosocial, relationship, and economic burden (Girgis, et al. 2013; Waldrop & Kutner, 2013)
    3. Caregivers often cite positive aspects of the experience, including:
      a. The caregiver feels good about themselves, as if they are needed
      b. Gives meaning to their lives
      c. Enables them to learn new skills
      d. Strengthens their relationships with others
    4. Dependency creates an environmental stressor; caregiver and recipient at high risk for depression (Clark, Nicholas, Wassira, & Gutierrez, 2013).

      a. Change in the dynamic of close relationships
      b. Impact of the disease increases dependency, further limiting caregiver control over the caregiving situation
  C. Caregiver burden: emotional, physical, social, financial, and spiritual impact perceived by a caregiver (Halpern, et al., 2017; Zarit et al., 1980)
    1. Caregiver burden is influenced by patient comorbidities, depression, and symptoms (Johansen, Cvancarova, & Ruland, 2017)
    2. Caregiver fatigue, depression, sleep disturbance, low self-efficacy, and low social support affect caregiver burden (Johansen, Cvancarova, & Ruland, 2017)
II. Epidemiology of family caregiving and caregiver burden
III. Factors that may influence the impact of caregiving (Waldrop & Kutner, 2013)
  A. Caregiver resilience
  B. Relationship with the patient
  C. Presence of difficult-to-manage symptoms
  D. Degree of challenge (e.g., physical assistance required or the presence of dementia)
  E. Financial impact of patient and caregiver income, costs of medical care
  F. Lack of information and professional support. This may include:
    1. Quality of interface between health care team, patient, and caregiver
    2. Implementation and integration of relevant caregiver legislation
    3. Access to patient advocacy/support/respite care groups
  G. Degree to which caregivers think that they are carrying out patients' wishes
  H. Social support available to the caregiver
IV. Family caregiving legislation
  A. Recognize, Assist, Include, Support, and Engage Family Caregivers Act of 2017, or the RAISE Family Caregivers Act, provides for establishment and maintenance of a family caregiving strategy (AARP, 2018)
  B. CARE (Caregiver, Advise, Record, and Enable) Act (Kent et al., 2016)
    1. Requires hospitals to record family caregiver name with hospital admission

2. The hospital is required to notify the caregiver when the patient is discharged
3. Provides instructions of medical tasks for transitions of care
C. The Credit for Caring Act (AARP, 2018)
1. Supports family caregivers who work
2. Helps address the financial challenges of family caregiving and assists family caregivers to stay in the workforce and be more financially secure
3. Gives eligible family caregivers the opportunity to receive a tax credit for 30% of the qualified expenses above $2000 paid to help a loved one, up to a maximum credit amount of $3000

ASSESSMENT

I. Family caregivers should be assessed for their needs, especially when care plans are dependent upon them (Feinberg, 2014).
  A. Identify designated caregiver with patient; document in the electronic health record
  B. Identify problems, needs, strengths, and resources of the caregiver, and ability of the caregiver to contribute to the needs of the care recipient (Feinberg, 2008) (Table 48.1).
II. Caregiver clinical measurement tools (Table 48.2)
  A. Generalized findings are based on a wide variety of measures available to assess caregiving tasks, burden, and health outcomes (Halpern et al., 2017).

TABLE 48.1   Topics and Selected Questions for Caregiver Assessment

Category	Question
Context of care	
Caregiver relationship	What is the caregiver's relationship to the patient?
	How long has the caregiver been in this role?
Caregiver profile	What is educational background of the caregiver?
	Is the caregiver employed?
	Does the caregiver have dependents who require care as well?
Additional caregivers	Are other family members or friends involved in providing care?
	Are paid caregivers (e.g., home health aides) involved?
Living arrangements	Does the caregiver live in the same household?
	If the caregiver lives elsewhere, how far away are they and do they have access to dependable transportation?
Physical environment	Does the care recipient's home have grab bars and other adaptive devices and necessary equipment to assist with care?
	Is the care recipient homebound?
	Other concerns (i.e., laundry, grocery shopping, meal prep, medication pick-ups from the pharmacy)?
	Is there a readily accessible bathroom on same floor that care recipient spends most of the day? Stairs?
	Is the care recipient a pet owner? Can they handle pet care?
Caregiver's perception of care recipient's overall health	
Cognitive status	Is the patient cognitively impaired?
	How does this affect care provision?
Health perceptions	What medical problems does the care recipient have?
	What is the caregiver's perception of the care recipient's medical problems and prognosis and goals of care?
Caregiving needs	Is the care recipient totally dependent 24/7 or only partially?
	Is there evidence that the caregiver is providing adequate care?
Assessment of caregiver values	
Willingness	Is the caregiver willing to undertake the caregiver role?
	Is the care recipient willing to accept care provision?
Cultural norms	What care arrangements are considered culturally acceptable for family (i.e., ethnicity, personal beliefs, religion, language barriers, values, communication, decision making) (Giesbrecht, et al., 2012)?
Assessment of caregiver health	
Caregiver health	How does the caregiver assess his or her own health?
	Does the caregiver have limitations that affect ability to give care?
	Does the caregiver feel she or he is under a lot of stress?
	Is there evidence of anxiety, depression, suicidal ideation?
	How does the caregiver rate his or her quality of life?
Impact of caregiving	Is the caregiver socially isolated?
	Does the caregiver feel health has suffered because of caregiving?

Continued

TABLE 48.1 Topics and Selected Questions for Caregiver Assessment—cont'd

Category	Question
Assessment of caregiver knowledge and skills	
Caregiving confidence	How knowledgeable does the caregiver feel about care recipient's condition?
Caregiver competence	Does the caregiver have appropriate knowledge of medical tasks required to provide care (e.g., wound care, transferring patient, health literacy for administrating complex medication regimen)?
Assessment of caregiver resources	
Social support	Do friends and family assist with care so that the caregiver has time off?
	Are there additional support systems given (e.g., dates, times, and expectations for stepping in to assist)?
Coping	What does the caregiver do to relieve stress and tension?
Financial resources	Does the caregiver feel financial strain associated with caregiving?
	Does the caregiver have access to insurance coverage information?
Community resources and services	Have providers (nurses and social workers) given the caregiver information about available community resources and services (caregiver support programs, religious organizations, volunteer agencies, respite services)?

B. Selected caregiver assessment measures: https://www.caregiver.org/selected-caregiver-assessment-measures-resource-inventory-practitioners-2012

MANAGEMENT (ONCOLOGY NURSING SOCIETY, 2017)

I. Medical management
   A. Prescribe assistive devices that make caregiving less strenuous
   B. Refer to physical or occupational therapy to teach caregiver safe transfer techniques and to encourage as much self-care by the patient within the limits of the disease
II. Nursing management
   A. Incorporate needs and preferences of patients and caregiver in care planning (Table 48.2)
   B. Improve caregivers' understanding of their role; teach skills necessary
   C. Facilitate caregiver coping (Ferrall, S. M., 2018; 2017; Waldrop & Kutner, 2013)
      1. Provide written instructions for reinforcement
      2. Reinforce teaching with each interaction
      3. Ensure that caregiver knows who to call with questions
      4. Provide clear instruction on when and how to use medications and nonpharmacologic interventions for symptom control
      5. Ensure caregiver knows who to call if plan of care for symptom control is not working or a new symptom develops, whatever the time of day
      6. Provide information to clarify any misperceptions or misunderstandings
   D. Provide continuous therapeutic communication with caregivers
      1. Clarify patient and family goals, including advance care planning, to ensure plan of care is congruent with patient and family goals

TABLE 48.2 Caregiver Clinical Measurement Tools

Name of Tool	Number of Items	Domain
Zarit Burden Interview	22	Burden (health, psychological well-being, finances, social life, and relationship with impaired person)
Caregiver Reaction Assessment	24	Burden (self-esteem, lack of family support, and impact on finances, schedule, and health)
CG QOL Scale-Cancer (CQOL-C)	35	QOL (burden, disruptiveness, positive adaptation, and financial concerns)
Preparedness for Caregiving Scale	8	Needs assessment
Caregiver Strain Index	13	Burden (employment, financial, physical, social, and time aspects)
Caregiver Burden Scale	15	Burden (patient needs, caregiver tasks, and caregiver burden)

From Eaton, L.H., Tipton, J.M., & Irwin, M (Eds). (2011). *Putting Evidence into Practice: Improving oncology patient outcomes (vol. 2).* Pittsburgh, PA, Oncology Nursing Society.

2. Communicate changes in patient condition, especially signs and symptoms of imminent death, so that caregivers feel as prepared as possible
   E. Provide psychosocial support and refer to appropriate resources as needed
      1. Actively listen to fears, concerns, expressions of grief
      2. Encourage caregiver interventions, including respite options:
         a. Caregiver support services: in-person and online support groups
         b. Counseling
         c. Family meetings

F. Facilitate physical support
  1. Demonstrate physical caregiving (e.g., changing sheets on occupied bed, catheter care, dressing change); have the caregiver do a return demonstration with home health aide available for coaching and support
  2. Encourage caregivers to accept assistance so that they have time for self-care, including sleeping, eating, and other restorative activities

G. Mobilize resources
  1. Augment caregiving with home health aides, personal care assistants, home services
  2. Make referrals to social worker, chaplain, counselors, and community resources
  3. Encourage the caregiver to call on extended family members, friends, and faith community networks for assistance with direct caregiving or household tasks
  4. Increase the level of care if symptoms are not responding to usual treatment (e.g., palliative care or hospice referral, transfer to an inpatient facility, initiation of continuous hospice care at home)
  5. Family caregivers should have access to relevant information through technology

EXPECTED CAREGIVER OUTCOMES

I. Physical activity interventions will significantly decrease caregiver distress and increase well-being, quality of life, sleep quality, physical activity levels, and self-efficacy for caregiving (Lambert et al., 2016)

II. Caregivers will perceive increasing or high-stable levels of personal mastery and have positive caregiving well-being (Litzelman, Tesauro, & Ferrer, 2017)

REFERENCES

AARP Retrieved 01/28/2018 from https://www.aarp.org/caregiving.

Clark, M. C., Nicholas, J. M., Wassira, L. N., & Gutierrez, A. P. (2013). Psychosocial and biological indicators of depression in the caregiving population. *Biological Research in Nursing, 15*(1), 112–121. https://doi.org/10.1177/1099800411414872.

Feinberg, L. F. (2008). Caregiver assessment. *American Journal of Nursing, 108*(9 Suppl), 38–39. https://doi.org/10.1097/01.NAJ.0000336412.75742.6e.

Feinberg, L. F. (2014). Recognizing and supporting family caregivers: the time has come. *Public policy & Aging Report, 24*(2), 65–69. https://doi.org/10.1093/ppar/pru007.

Ferrall, S. M. (2018). Caring for the family. In N. J. Bush & L. M. Gorman, L. M. *Psychosocial nursing care along the cancer continuum.* (3rd Ed. pp 497 - 508). Pittsburgh, PA, Oncology Nursing Society.

Ge, L., & Mordiffi, S. Z. (2017). Factors associated with higher caregiver burden among family caregivers of elderly cancer patients: a systematic review. *Cancer Nursing, 40*(6), 471–478. https://doi.org/10.1097/NCC.0000000000000445.

Giesbrecht, M., Crooks, V. A., Williams, A., & Hankivsky, O. (2012). Critically examining diversity in end-of-life family caregiving: implications for equitable caregiver support and Canada's Compassionate Care Benefit. *International Journal for Equity in Health, 11*, 65.

Girgis, A., Lambert, S., Johnson, C., Waller, A., & Currow, D. (2013). Physical, psychosocial, relationship, and economic burden of caring for people with cancer: a review. *American Society of Clinical Oncology, 9*(4), 197–202. https://doi.org/10.1200/JOP.2012.000690.

Given, B. A., Given, C. W., & Sherwood, P. (2012). The challenge of quality cancer care for family caregivers. *Seminars in Oncology Nursing, 28*(4), 205–212. https://doi.org/10.1016/j.soncn.2012.09.002.

Halpern, M. T., Fiero, M. H., & Bell, M. L. (2017). Impact of caregiver activities and social supports on multidimensional caregiver burden: analyses from nationally-representative surveys of cancer patients and their caregivers. *Quality of Life Research, 26*(6), 1587–1595. https://doi.org/10.1007/s11136-017-1505-9.

Haylock, P. J. (2010). Advanced cancer. Emergence of a new survivor population. *Seminars in Oncology, 26*(3), 144–150. https://doi.org/10.1016/j.soncn.2010.05.008.

Hellman, R., Copeland, C., & Van Derhei, J. (2012). *The 2012 retirement confidence survey: job insecurity, debt weight on retirement confidence, savings.* Washington, DC: Employee Benefit Research Institute.

Hoffman, G. J., Lee, J., & Mendez-Luck, C. A. (2012). Health behaviors among baby boomer informal caregivers. *Gerontologist, 52*(2), 219–230. https://doi.org/10.1093/geront/gns003.

Johansen, S., Cvancarova, M., & Ruland, C. (2017). The effect of cancer patients' and their family caregivers' physical and emotional symptoms on caregiver burden. *Cancer Nursing.* https://doi.org/10.1097/NCC.0000000000000493.

Kamal, K. M., Covvey, J. R., Dashputre, A., Ghosh, S., Shah, S., Bhosle, M., & Zacker, C. (2017). A systematic review of the effect of cancer treatment on work productivity of patients and caregivers. *Journal of Managed Care & Specialty Pharmacy, 23*(2), 136–162. https://doi.org/10.18553/jmcp.2017.23.2.136.

Kent, E. E., Rowland, J. H., Northouse, L., Litzelman, K., Chou, W. Y. S., Shelburne, N., Timura, C., O'Mara, A., & Huss, K. (2016). Caring for caregivers and patients: research and clinical priorities for informal cancer caregiving. *Cancer, 122*(13), 1987–1995. https://doi.org/10.1002/cncr.29939.

Kim, H. H., Kim, S. Y., Kim, J. M., Kim, S. W., Shin, I. S., Shim, H. J., Hwang, J. E., Chung, I. J., & Yoon, J. S. (2016). Influence of caregiver personality on the burden of family caregivers of terminally ill cancer patients. *Palliative & Supportive Care, 14*(1), 5–12. https://doi.org/10.1017/S1478951515000073.

Lambert, S. D., Duncan, L. R., Kapellas, S., Bruson, A. M., Myrand, M., Santa Mina, D., Culos-Reed, N., & Lambrou, A. (2016). A descriptive systematic review of physical activity interventions for caregivers: effects on caregivers' and care recipients' psychosocial outcomes, physical activity levels, and physical health. *Annals of Behavioral Medicine, 50*(6), 907–919. https://doi.org/10.1007/s12160-016-9819-3.

Litzelman, K., Tesauro, G., & Ferrer, R. (2017). Internal resources among informal caregivers: trajectories and associations with well-being. *Quality of Life Research, 26*(12), 3239–3250. https://doi.org/10.1007/s11136-017-1647-9.

Litzelman, K., & Yabroff, K. R. (2015). How are spousal depressed mood, distress, and quality of life associated with risk of depressed mood in cancer survivors? Longitudinal findings from a national sample. *Cancer Epidemiology, Biomarkers &*

Prevention, 24(6), 969–977. https://doi.org/10.1158/1055-9965. Epi-14-1420.

Maltby, K. F., Sanderson, C. R., Lobb, E. A., & Phillips, J. L. (2017). Sleep disturbances in caregivers of patients with advanced cancer: a systematic review. *Palliative & Supportive Care, 15*(1), 125–140. https://doi.org/10.1017/s1478951516001024.

Nielsen, M. K., Neergaard, M. A., Jensen, A. B., Bro, F., & Guldin, M. B. (2016). Psychological distress, health, and socio-economic factors in caregivers of terminally ill patients: a nationwide population-based cohort study. *Supportive Care in Cancer, 24*(7), 3057–3067. https://doi.org/10.1007/s00520-016-3120-7.

Oncology Nursing Society (2017). Putting evidence into practice: caregiver strain and burden. Retrieved from https://www.ons.org/practice-resources/pep/caregiver-strain-and-burden.

Rodakowski, J., Skidmore, E. R., Rogers, J. C., & Schulz, R. (2012). Role of social support in predicting caregiver burden. *Archives of Physical Medicine and Rehabilitation, 93*(12), 2229–2236. https://doi.org/10.1016/j.apmr.2012.07.004.

Ross, A., Shamburek, R., Wehrlen, L., Klagholz, S. D., Yang, L., Stoops, E., Flynn, S. L., Remaley, A. T., Pacak, K., Shelburne, N., & Bevans, M. F. (2017). Cardiometabolic risk factors and health behaviors in family caregivers. *Public Library of Science One, 12*(5), e0176408. https://doi.org/10.1371/journal.pone.0176408.

Roth, D. L., Fredman, L., & Haley, W. E. (2015). Informal caregiving and its impact on health: a reappraisal from population-based studies. *The Gerontologist, 55*(2), 309–319. https://doi.org/10.1093/geront/gnu177.

Saria, M. G., Courchesne, N., Evangelista, L., Carter, J., MacManus, D. A., Gorman, M. K., Nyamathi, A. M., Phillips, L. R., Piccioni, D., Kesari, S., & Maliski, S. (2017). Cognitive dysfunction in patients with brain metastases: influences on caregiver resilience and coping. *Supportive Care in Cancer, 25*(4), 1247–1256. https://doi.org/10.1007/s00520-016-3517-3.

Saria, M. G., Nyamathi, A., Phillips, L. R., Stanton, A. L., Evangelista, L., Kesari, S., & Maliski, S. (2017). The hidden morbidity of cancer burden in caregivers of patients with brain metastases. *Nursing Clinics of North America, 52*(1), 159–+. https://doi.org/10.1016/j.cnur.2016.10.002.

Schulz, R., Beach, S. R., Cook, T. B., Martire, L. M., Tomlinson, J. M., & Monin, J. K. (2012). Predictors and consequences of perceived lack of choice in becoming an informal caregiver. *Aging & Mental Health, 16*(6), 712–721. https://doi.org/10.1080/13607863.2011.651439.

Sherwood, P. R., Price, T. J., Weimer, J., Ren, D. X., Donovan, H. S., Given, C. W., Given, B. A., Schulz, R., Prince, J., Bender, C., Boele, F. W., & Marsland, A. L. (2016). Neuro-oncology family caregivers are at risk for systemic inflammation. *Journal of Neuro-Oncology, 128*(1), 109–118. https://doi.org/10.1007/s11060-016-2083-3.

Talley, R. C., & Crews, J. E. (2007). Framing the public health of caregiving. *American Journal of Public Health, 97*(2), 224–228.

Waldrop, D., & Kutner, J. S. (2013). Caregivers. In N.E. Goldstein & R. S. Morrison *Evidence-based practice of palliative medicine* (pp. 421–435). Philadelphia, PA: Saunders/Elsevier.

Zarit, S. H., Reever, K. E., & Bach-Peterson, J. (1980). Relatives of the impaired elderly: correlates of feelings of burden. *Gerontologist, 20*(6), 649–655.

49

Cultural and Spiritual Care

Emily A. Haozous

OVERVIEW

I. Human beings are unique individuals. Each of us interacts with our world according to values, beliefs, and social norms that are influenced by our spiritual, religious, and cultural perspectives.

II. Oncology nurses should recognize the importance of spiritual, religious, and cultural diversity, and apply the nursing process to meet the unique needs of patients and caregivers with sensitivity and an understanding of interventions that support optimal outcomes.

III. Definitions—understanding diversity in health care begins with establishing a common language to ensure clear communication among different people. Cross-cultural health care delivery requires appreciation for the dynamic nature of communication, particularly language. Operationalization of terms allows for clarity, which then translates to meaningful and focused information for oncology nurses providing patient- and family-centered care.

  A. Diversity
    1. Condition of being composed of differing elements, especially the inclusion of people of different races or cultures in a group (Merriam-Webster, 2018).

  B. Culture
    1. A word with many definitions, but for the purposes of this context culture is defined as the customary beliefs, social forms, material traits, and characteristic features of everyday existence shared by people of a racial, religious, or social group in a place or time (Cain, Surbone, Elk, & Kagawa-Singer, 2018).
    2. Learned and passed from one generation to the next and, as such, responds to larger societal and environmental influences.
    3. Encompasses the religious and economic views, language use, social structure, and use of technology within a shared group: for example, youth culture is often cited as strikingly different from previous generations in their use of technology, language, spending habits, and preferred manner of interpersonal communication.

    4. Although frequently considered in the context of race or ethnicity, cultural traits are observed across diverse groups; for example, nursing culture varies from one practice area to another.

  C. Race and ethnicity: according to the U.S. Census Bureau, ethnicity and race are defined by the federal government via the Office of Management and Budget as two distinct concepts, shaping how American society and demographers conceptualize what are in practice social definitions without any biological foundations (U.S. Census Bureau Quickfacts, 2017).
    1. Race: a social construct based on expressed phenotype (observable characteristics such as skin tone and hair texture) in which people are categorized based on external, selective, and arbitrary physical features (Solar & Irwin, 2010). This contrasts with genotype, which refers to a person's overall genetic makeup. Understanding these differences is important to appreciating the arbitrary nature of race as a social construct; an example of this would be to consider three children of a mixed-race family—one child may express the phenotypes of their fair-skinned, blond, and blue-eyed parent and resemble that parent closely; one child may express the phenotypes of their dark-skinned, black hair, and brown-eyed parent and resemble that parent; and the third child may have the fair skin of one parent but the dark hair and eyes of the other. All three children have the same genotype but express very different phenotypes.
    2. Ethnicity: cultural heritage; historical, cultural, contextual, and geographic experiences of a specific community or population (Jones, 2002).
      a. Ethnic groups may comprise more than one racial group. For example, people who identify as Hispanic or Latino/a have wide racial diversity but share characteristics based on geographic, historic, contextual, and cultural group of origin (Race & Ethnicity, 2017).

  D. Sexuality: sexual diversity includes sexual preference (heterosexual, homosexual, lesbian, gay, bisexual, asexual, queer), sexual identity, and gender identity (transgender, nonbinary, cisgender, intersex), gender expression, and those who feel their sexual identity does not or should not fit into a label.

E. Spirituality
1. That which "gives meaning and purpose to a person's life"; inclusive of "belief in a higher power that may inspire hope, seek resolution, and transcend physical and conscious constraints" (Canfield et al., 2016).
2. According to the North American Nursing Diagnosis Association (NANDA), spiritual distress is indicated by suffering through an impaired inability to find meaning and purpose through connections with "self, others, the world, or a superior being" (Herdman & Kamitsuru, 2018).
3. Spiritual distress can result from a disconnect from one's community, the spirit world, and other nonreligious but still sacred ties to a higher power.

F. Religion—personal set or institutionalized system of religious attitudes, beliefs, and practices, often linked to a defined system of worship or faith-based organization (Merriam-Webster, 2018).

G. Sacred—connected with a higher power/s, creator, or God, and venerated as through this association; or regarded and revered by a particular culture, religion, group, or individual through this association (Herdman & Kamitsuru, 2018).
1. Although similar in ends to religion, what is sacred exists outside established religion; for example, in Native American traditions, knowledge about traditional medicine is considered sacred and protected knowledge but is not associated with a specific organized religious practice, nor is it typically published in any religiously oriented text.

H. Socioeconomic status (SES)—a person's position in the social hierarchy, this term typically encompasses social class, occupation, level of educational achievement, and annual income (Solar & Irwin, 2010).

I. Poverty
1. In the United States, the federal poverty guidelines refer to a single person earning $12,140 or less per year (all amounts are as of January 2018). Federal poverty guidelines vary based on household size and are adjusted to accommodate higher costs of living in Alaska and Hawaii (DHHS, 2018).
2. The culture of poverty crosses racial and ethnic groups and has a major impact on health status (Solar & Irwin, 2010).

IV. Cultural diversity
A. Health care consumers in the United States include increasingly diverse populations.
1. The U.S. Census Bureau defines the Hispanic or Latino population as "a person of Cuban, Mexican, Puerto Rican, South or Central American, or other Spanish culture or origin regardless of race" (Hispanic Origin, 2018).
2. Hispanics account for 18.1% of the U.S. population (U.S. Census Bureau Quickfacts, 2017).
3. Asians account for 5.8% of the total population.
4. Native Hawaiian and other Pacific Islanders represent 0.2% of the total population.
5. 2.7% of the U.S. population identifies itself as being of two or more races.
6. By 2044, the majority of the U.S. population is projected to identify with a race or ethnicity other than non-Hispanic white (Colby & Ortman, 2015).

B. Cultural norms influence relationships between health care practitioners and patients or caregivers.
1. Culture is intersectoral, influenced by race, ethnicity, gender, sexual orientation, age, geography, and income.
2. Although traditions and trends can emerge in various groups, generalizing across populations is inappropriate.
3. Culture affects time orientation to past, present, or future. In some cultures, time is fluid and flexible, and the process takes priority over the task at hand.

D. Cultural norms vary widely. Examples include (Dossey & Keegan, 2015):
1. Cultures hold wide-ranging beliefs about personal space and eye contact.
a. Closeness of personal space, eye contact, touching, and even shaking hands is either respectful and comforting or intrusive and violating.
b. Facial expressions have a wide range of meanings; smiling may be inviting and indicate an emotional connection or happiness, or it may be a nervous or socially accepted response to unpleasant news.
c. Winking means different things in different cultures.
   (1) As a sexual invitation
   (2) To convey a shared joke
   (3) A rude or patronizing gesture
2. Hand gestures hold meanings unique to a culture.
a. The hand signal that people in the United States use to mean "OK" is the symbol for money in some cultures, and in other cultures, it is used as an offensive gesture to indicate a bodily orifice.
b. The "thumbs up" gesture widely recognized in the United States as a congratulatory gesture has vulgar connotations in other cultures.
c. Many cultures view pointing with a single finger as rude and prefer using the entire hand or

a gesture with the face, lips, or chin to point to something or indicate direction.

3. Posture and physical position have varying significance in different cultures.
   a. Showing the bottom of the feet to others is rude in some cultures.
   b. In some cultures, it is important to be facing the person to whom you are speaking, whereas others see this as overly assertive or aggressive.
   c. In some cultures, placing hands on the hips while speaking to someone is indicative of anger or confrontation.

4. Some cultures are more modest than others.
   a. Nudity may be acceptable and even embraced in some cultures.
   b. In some cultures, it is taboo for people from the opposite gender to see or touch their body, even when coming from a health care provider.

E. Human sexuality contributes to health and well-being (WHO, 2016).
   1. Recognition of sexual diversity includes rejecting heteronormative assumptions that all people are heterosexual and/or happily conforming to the gender conventions of the dominant culture.
   2. If unsure, best practice is to ask a patient's preferred pronouns (she/her/hers, he/him/his, they/theirs).

V. Poverty and cancer
   A. Poverty negatively affects people's health status.
      1. Access to health care services is a major determinant of health status.
         a. Cancer prevention through early screening is harder to access for people without access to primary health care (NCI, 2018).
            (1) Poor people may lack access to quality health care.
            (2) Pursuit of food and shelter takes priority over seeking care for cancer diagnosis or treatment unless symptoms prohibit basic activities of daily living.
            (3) Poor people have a higher risk for illness, including cancer, due to higher exposure to poor nutrition, workplace carcinogens, and modifiable risk factors such as habitual tobacco use.
            (4) People living in poverty are more often diagnosed with cancer in advanced stages (Boscoe, Henry, Sherman, & Johnson, 2016).
      2. Cancer prevention, defined as health-seeking behaviors and regular screening, is a determinant of prevention and early diagnosis (NCI, 2018).

VI. Racial/ethnic diversity in cancer (see Chapter 1)

VII. Responses to the cancer experience
   A. The meaning of a life-threatening illness (e.g., cancer) is largely influenced by culture.

B. Cultural norms and behaviors have a major impact on all aspects of the cancer experience, including screening, seeking diagnosis, treatment options, symptom management, response to advanced cancer, hospice use, and end-of-life care (Busolo & Woodgate, 2015; Cain et al., 2018).

C. Cancer prevention behaviors.
   1. Cultures that do not trust the conventional medicine system in the United States may not participate consistently in cancer prevention, screening, or treatment.
   2. Some cultures rely heavily on traditional healers and may choose not to pursue allopathic/conventional models of health and wellness.
   3. Individuals or groups who are recent immigrants to the United States may lack knowledge about cancer screening.
   4. Some cultures may hold a fatalistic view of cancer.
      a. They may view cancer as being synonymous with certain death, and they may not believe that anything can be done to change their fate. This belief may keep them from participating in screening.

D. Response to diagnosis of cancer
   1. Diagnosis of cancer is most often considered devastating news.
      a. Depending on an individual's culture, the response may range from one of stoic acceptance to one that is highly demonstrative.
      b. Regardless of demonstrative emotional response, it is incumbent on nurses to assist all patients with positive coping strategies.

E. Participation in clinical trials
   1. Cultural influences determine the response to clinical trials as a health care option; cultural factors, such as lack of trust, present barriers to patient participation in clinical trials.
   2. Some patients resist clinical trials based on historical precedent of unethical research conducted with people from their ethnic/racial group.

F. Coping with advanced cancer and end of life
   1. Cultural and religious beliefs and norms lead to varied responses to advanced cancer and end of life.
   2. These responses range on a continuum from fearing and fighting cancer as an enemy to acceptance and integrative therapies to assist with symptom management, including psychosocial symptoms (Lichtenstein, Berger, & Cheng, 2017; Vrinten et al., 2017).

VIII. Spiritual and religious diversity
   A. *Spirituality* is the relationship or connection to the sacred, giving a broader meaning and purpose that is experienced through personal or communal devotions or through meditation, art, nature, or ceremony (Peteet & Balboni, 2013; Sun et al., 2016).

B. *Religion* describes organized systems of faith and worship that follow regulated practices intended to enhance spirituality.
   1. For this reason, religiosity is rarely discussed without spirituality being at the core of the discussion.
   2. A person may consider himself or herself a spiritual being without belonging to an organized religion.
   3. As defined in this chapter, spirituality applies to all persons, whether they consider themselves spiritual or not.
C. Spiritual care is an important component of comprehensive, patient-centered nursing care in the following ways (Canfield et al., 2016; Ferrell & Baird, 2012; Jim et al., 2015; Lichtenstein et al., 2017; Peteet & Balboni, 2013; Sun et al., 2016):
   1. Strongly influences health-related decision making
   2. May influence a person's health-seeking behaviors (e.g., cancer prevention).
   3. Delays in seeking medical care may stem from religious/spiritual (R/S) beliefs associated with fatalism or disease attribution.
   4. May have a positive impact on the patient's response to cancer and treatment.
   5. Patients may experience R/S distress associated with a cancer diagnosis, with feelings of abandonment, meaning-making, identity, and existential distress.
D. The patient with cancer may experience a heightened sense of spirituality associated with a cancer diagnosis. Patients may:
   1. Discover an intensified sense of spirituality or faith, which may include closer relationships with friends, family, and community, and a greater connection to the simple pleasures of life
   2. Experience a sense of betrayal linked to their R/S beliefs.
E. R/S and cultural beliefs may influence how people respond to cancer across the spectrum of care; for some R/S inspires active participation, yet others may feel it more appropriate to respond with a passive or fatalistic perspective on cancer treatment, seeing cancer death as "the will of God" (Bryn, 2017).
F. R/S also influences how caregivers perceive the cancer experience.
   1. As with patients, R/S may be a source of strength for caregivers; they may also feel betrayed, punished, or abandoned in their time of need.
   2. Healthy caregivers may experience guilt when their loved one is suffering.
G. R/S may have a beneficial or harmful impact on the patient's and caregiver's adjustment to cancer and their participation in treatment (NCI, 2017).
   1. Relying on faith as a coping mechanism may help patients overcome the initial shock and distress related to a new diagnosis of cancer.
   2. Acceptance of the cancer diagnosis related to a belief in a higher power in control of life and death has been shown to correlate with better adjustment to illness.
   3. Patients may transfer their faith in a higher power to faith in their physician to be able to cure their disease.
   4. Feeling punished, abandoned, or both has been shown to contribute to higher levels of distress for patients; may be a barrier to active participation in treatment.
H. R/S may have a beneficial or harmful influence on responses to end-of-life issues.
   1. Patients who believe in existence after death may find joy in prospect of afterlife.
   2. Patients whose belief system does not include an afterlife may or may not feel despondent about the finality of death.

ASSESSMENT

I. Assessment includes the cultural, spiritual, and religious beliefs of patients and caregivers, and incorporates assessment findings into their nursing diagnoses and nursing plan of care (Dossey & Keegan, 2015; Ferrell & Baird, 2012).
   A. The oncology nurse should first recognize his or her own culture, sexual orientation, spirituality, and religiosity and how this may affect his or her perception of others.
   B. The oncology nurse recognizes culture, sexual orientation, spirituality, and religiosity as part of the whole person, which are assessed in the context of the human experience.
   C. Assessment of the patient and caregivers includes but is not limited to the patient's support system and chosen community, cultural beliefs and practices, philosophical or religious belief system, sense of belonging, and love for self and others.
   D. The oncology nurse's spiritual assessment is performed without judgment and includes the following in both patient and caregiver(s) (*Clinical Practice Guidelines for Quality Palliative Care*, 2013):
      1. Identification of R/S background, preferences, beliefs, rituals, preferred practices.
      2. Identification of possible symptoms of R/S distress, such as emotional pain, guilt, resentment, despair, despondency, and hopelessness.
      3. Ways that the oncology nurse may support the patient's and caregivers' spiritual needs include deep listening, holding a presence, bearing witness, and practicing compassion (Ferrell & Baird, 2012).

MANAGEMENT

I. Provide interventions to enhance cultural comfort, R/S, and hopefulness
   A. Identify patient's cultural identity and any needs that may affect cancer care.

1. Plan treatment around cultural holidays or events when possible.
2. Ask before assuming stereotypes.
3. Make space for extended family, appreciating cultural norms regarding modesty, physical space, gestures, and contact.

B. Respect patient's R/S beliefs and plan care that honors these beliefs

1. Create time, space, and privacy, as needed, for spiritual or religious rituals
2. When appropriate (per patient request), pray with patient, caregivers, or both as a sincere, genuine gesture
3. Encourage patient and caregivers to speak with their R/S leader

C. Avoid proselytizing—the nurse does not impose his or her own spiritual or religious beliefs on patients and caregivers

D. Support the patient's use of spiritual coping

1. Refer the patient and caregiver to a hospital chaplain or group that can support coping with spiritual issues as needed

E. Assist the patient in exploring modalities to enhance spiritual well-being

1. Meditation (e.g., mindfulness meditation), yoga, prayer
2. Expressive therapies
   a. Art therapy
   b. Music therapy
   c. Journaling: gratitude or expressive journaling

EXPECTED PATIENT OUTCOMES

I. The patient and caregiver will feel respected for their cultural, spiritual, and religious beliefs.
II. The patient and caregiver will have adequate resources to support cultural, spiritual, and religious beliefs.

REFERENCES

Boscoe, F. P., Henry, K. A., Sherman, R. L., & Johnson, C. J. (2016). The relationship between cancer incidence, stage and poverty in the United States. *Int J Cancer, 139*(3), 607–612. https://doi.org/10.1002/ijc.30087.

Bryn, N. (2017). When medicine and religion do not mix. Cancer. *Cytopathology, 125*(11), 813–814. https://doi.org/10.1002/cncy.21943.

Busolo, D., & Woodgate, R. (2015). Palliative care experiences of adult cancer patients from ethnocultural groups: a qualitative systematic review protocol. *JBI Database of Systematic Reviews and Implementation Reports, 13*(1), 99–111. https://doi.org/10.11124/jbisrir-2015-1809.

Cain, C. L., Surbone, A., Elk, R., & Kagawa-Singer, M. (2018). Culture and palliative care: preferences, communication, meaning, and mutual decision making. *J Pain Symptom Manage,* 55(5), 1408–1419. https://doi.org/10.1016/j.jpainsymman.2018.01.007.

Canfield, C., Taylor, D., Nagy, K., Strauser, C., VanKerkhove, K., Wills, S., … Sorrell, J. (2016). Critical care nurses' perceived need for guidance in addressing spirituality in critically ill patients. *Am J Crit Care, 25*(3), 206–211. https://doi.org/10.4037/ajcc2016276.

Clinical Practice Guidelines for Quality Palliative Care. (2013). Retrieved from Pittsburgh, PA www.nationalconsensusproject.org.

Colby, S. L., & Ortman, J. M. (2015). *Projections of the size and composition of the U.S. population: 2014-2060.* Retrieved from Washington, D.C.:.

DHHS. (2018). *HHS Poverty Guidelines for 2018.* Retrieved from https://aspe.hhs.gov/poverty-guidelines.

Dossey, B. M., & Keegan, L. (2015). In C. C. Barrere, M. B. Helming, D. A. Shields, & K. Avino (Eds.), *Holistic nursing: a handbook for practice* (7th ed.). Burlington, MA: Jones & Bartlett Learning.ethnomed. Retrieved from http://ethnomed.org/about.

Ferrell, B. R., & Baird, P. (2012). Deriving meaning and faith in caregiving. *Semin Oncol Nurs, 28*(4), 256–261. https://doi.org/10.1016/j.soncn.2012.09.008.

Herdman, T. H., & Kamitsuru, S. (2018). *NANDA International nursing diagnoses: definitions & classifications, 2018-2020* (Eleventh ed.). Oxford: Wiley Blackwell.

Hispanic Origin. (2018). Retrieved from https://www.census.gov/topics/population/hispanic-origin/about.html.

Jim, H. S., Pustejovsky, J. E., Park, C. L., Danhauer, S. C., Sherman, A. C., Fitchett, G., … Salsman, J. M. (2015). Religion, spirituality, and physical health in cancer patients: a meta-analysis. *Cancer, 121*(21), 3760–3768. https://doi.org/10.1002/cncr.29353.

Jones, C. A. (2002). Confronting institutionalized racism. *Phylon, 50*(1), 7–22. https://doi.org/10.2307/4149999.

Lichtenstein, A. H., Berger, A., & Cheng, M. J. (2017). Definitions of healing and healing interventions across different cultures. *Ann Palliat Med, 6*(3), 248–252. https://doi.org/10.21037/apm.2017.06.16.

Merriam-Webster. (2018). Retrieved from https://www.merriam-webster.com/.

NCI. (2017). *Spirituality in cancer care (PDQ) - Health professional version.* PDQ (c) Retrieved from https://www.cancer.gov/about-cancer/coping/day-to-day/faith-and-spirituality/spirituality-hp-pdq#section/_1.

NCI. (2018). *Cancer disparities.* Retrieved from https://www.cancer.gov/about-cancer/understanding/disparities.

Peteet, J. R., & Balboni, M. J. (2013). Spirituality and religion in oncology. *CA Cancer J Clin, 63*(4), 280–289. https://doi.org/10.3322/caac.21187.

Race & Ethnicity. (2017). Retrieved from https://www.census.gov/mso/www/training/pdf/race-ethnicity-onepager.pdf.

Solar, O., & Irwin, A. (2010). *A conceptual framework for action on the social determinants of health.* Retrieved from Geneva http://www.who.int/sdhconference/resources/ConceptualframeworkforactiononSDH_eng.pdf.

Sun, V., Kim, J. Y., Irish, T. L., Borneman, T., Sidhu, R. K., Klein, L., & Ferrell, B. (2016). Palliative care and spiritual well-being in lung cancer patients and family caregivers. *Psychooncology, 25*(12), 1448–1455. https://doi.org/10.1002/pon.3987.

U.S. Census Bureau Quickfacts. (2017). *Hispanic or Latino, percent.* Retrieved from https://www.census.gov/quickfacts/fact/dashboard/US/RHI725217#viewtop.

Vrinten, C., McGregor, L. M., Heinrich, M., von Wagner, C., Waller, J., Wardle, J., & Black, G. B. (2017). What do people fear about cancer? A systematic review and meta-synthesis of cancer fears in the general population. *Psychooncology, 26*(8), 1070–1079. https://doi.org/10.1002/pon.4287.

WHO. (2016). *FAQ of health and sexual diversity: The basics.* Retrieved from http://www.who.int/gender-equity-rights/news/20160517-faq-on-health-and-sexual-diversity.pdf.

50

Psychosocial Disturbances and Coping

Kathleen Murphy-Ende

EMOTIONAL DISTRESS

Overview

I. Distress
  A. Psychosocial distress and existential concerns are common in patients with cancer
  B. A psychological (cognitive, behavioral, emotional), social, and spiritual nature may interfere with ability to cope effectively with cancer, its physical symptoms, and its treatment. Distress extends along a continuum, ranging from common normal feelings of vulnerability, sadness, and fears to problems that may become disabilities, such as depression, anxiety, panic, social isolation, and existential and spiritual crises (NCCN, 2018)
  C. Psychological, social, spiritual, physical, and financial stressors that strain the individual's and family's coping abilities
  D. Defined as "severe pressure of trouble, pain, sickness or sorrow" (Oxford University Press, 2013)
  E. Used to describe the unpleasant emotional experience associated with the stressors that patients face when living with cancer
  F. Reflects a normative response different from psychological or psychiatric diagnoses such as clinical depression, adjustment disorder, posttraumatic stress disorder (PTSD), delirium, and anxiety disorder
  G. Distress and psychiatric morbidity in cancer patients are associated with poorer outcomes, decreased quality of life (QOL), and mortality (Chan et al., 2015)

II. Risk factors
  A. All patients experience some form or level of distress related to their diagnosis or treatment, and so are faced with coping challenges (Cohen & White, 2018; National Comprehensive Cancer Network [NCCN], 2018).
    1. Disease and stage (Cohen & White, 2018)
      a. Highest level of distress reported in patients with lung cancer
      b. Higher level of distress in patients in advanced stage of disease
      c. Impact of physical symptoms such as poor pain control
    2. Situational
      a. Personal meaning of the diagnosis
      b. Resources—emotional and practical support, spiritual guidance, and financial security
      c. Changes in roles—occupation, within family, between friends, altered physical capacity, and cognitive functioning
    3. Developmental
      a. Developmental life tasks disrupted by diagnosis and treatment
      b. Personality and coping style

III. General treatment approaches
  A. Psychotherapeutic interventions that have been effective in the cancer population—individual supportive psychotherapy, cognitive behavioral therapy, and group therapy (Cope et al., 2017; https://www.ons.org/practice-resources/pep/anxiety)
  B. Family psychotherapy
  C. Psychoeducational approaches
  D. Spiritual counseling
  E. Support groups
  F. Relaxation exercises, including meditation and guided imagery (Cope et al., 2017; https://www.ons.org/intervention/cognitive-behavioral-interventionsapproach-2)

IV. Potential sequelae of emotional distress
  A. Ineffective coping—may occur in crisis and may lead to suicidal ideation (Cohen & White, 2018)
  B. Chronic emotional distress
  C. Development of major psychiatric disorders—anxiety, depression, adjustment disorder, and suicidal ideation or suicide ⚠
  D. Acute stress disorder or PTSD. Traumatic event or experience prompting responses. PT3D may occur in cancer survivors with similar experiences of those in military combat or natural disasters. Diagnostic criteria for PTSD and acute stress disorder are different. Symptoms are similar and in general include the following:
    1. Cognitive (e.g., forgetful, distracted, cannot concentrate)
    2. Behavioral (e.g., fight-or-flight response, avoidance, isolation)

3. Emotional (e.g., numbing feeling, irritable, angry outbursts)
4. Physiologic (e.g., insomnia, nightmares, agitated) (APA, 2013)
E. Somatic symptoms such as sleep disturbance, fatigue, loss of appetite, and gastrointestinal (GI) disturbances
F. Declined performance at home, school, or work
G. Nonadherence or misunderstanding of health information

Assessment

I. Screening
   A. National Comprehensive Cancer Network Guideline (NCCN, 2018)
      1. Screen patients routinely to identify the level and source of their distress so that further evaluation can be completed.
      2. Identifying and treating psychological issues is a complex process; appropriate referrals should be made to mental health specialists such as licensed clinical psychologists or psychiatrists.
      3. Psychological needs vary, depending on the individual, developmental stage, phase of disease trajectory, past coping skills, and available emotional and practical resources.
   B. Screening tools for distress
      1. Information obtained from screening checklists useful for identifying specific concerns and needs, rather than identifying a clinical diagnosis
      2. Distress Thermometer, developed in the late 1990s, is still used today (Roth et al., 1998)—a unidimensional screening tool in which the patient is asked to indicate the severity of distress in the domains of emotional, spiritual, physical, practical, and family matters
         a. Designed for rapid assessment of patient distress; well validated in patients with cancer
         b. Can be used as a one-item scale assessing the level of distress
         c. Contains a problem list; the source of distress can be identified
         d. Sensitive to changes over time; takes a few minutes to complete
         e. Not useful for identifying specific psychiatric disorders
         f. Clinical pathways for the Distress Thermometer available to guide the follow-up assessment and management of distress (NCI, 2017); can be downloaded as part of the Distress Guidelines through the website for the NCCN (NCCN, 2018)

II. History
   A. Age, diagnosis, stage of disease, and treatment regimen
   B. Presence of risk factors
   C. Distressing thoughts, feelings, and behaviors such as nervousness, worry, jitteriness, tearfulness, hopelessness, difficulty concentrating, irritability, social withdrawal, ruminating, thoughts of death, suicidal ideation, self-harm, or harm to others

III. Pattern of emotional distress
   A. Distress occurs across the disease continuum, accompanied by vulnerability, sadness, fear of disability, worry of becoming a burden to others, depression, anxiety, panic, social isolation, and existential and spiritual crises.
   B. For each specific distressing symptom, the following should be assessed: frequency and intensity of specific distress, associated symptoms, and precipitating and alleviating factors.
   C. Duration of symptoms to determine if symptoms are episodic or prolonged.
      1. Episodic symptoms often occur during disease transitions such as diagnosis or relapse.
      2. Persistent symptoms may represent a psychiatric disorder, and the patient should be referred to a psychologist or psychiatrist.

IV. Impact on functional status—physical, interpersonal, occupational, academic performance, and spiritual practices

Management

I. Nonpharmacologic
   A. Address hopelessness
      1. Identify which dimension (affective, cognitive, behavioral, affiliative, temporal, or contextual) applies to the patient; support and facilitate the individual's hope; professionals may increase cancer patients' sense of hope by being present, giving accurate information, and showing care.
      2. Assist patient to explore his or her value system, purpose, life meaning
      3. Promote goal setting
      4. Offer psychological support programs that are grounded on the construct of hope and have successfully helped cancer patients to gain hope
   B. Address PTSD
      1. Assist the patient in identifying perceived threats and providing accurate information on actual risks
      2. Provide an opportunity for patients to give a narrative of their experience with support in the form of family and friends, nursing staff, support groups, and individual psychotherapy
      3. Offer supportive and expressive group therapy
   C. Address ineffective role performance
      1. Assist the patient in identifying realistic goals based on what he or she wants to accomplish in the current role
      2. Ask the patient to list the priorities within his or her personal, professional, and social roles
      3. Refer the patient to his or her employer's human resource department to assist with job schedule and duty changes
      4. Refer to occupational rehabilitation psychologist, if indicated

ANXIETY

Overview

I. Definition—anxiety is a "mood state characterized by apprehension and somatic symptoms of tension in which an individual anticipates impending danger, catastrophe, or misfortune. The future threat may be real or imagined, internal or external. It may be an identifiable situation or a vaguer fear of the unknown" (American Psychiatric Association, 2007).

   A. Commonly associated with cancer

   B. Characterized by a high negative affect in which the patient may experience feeling distressed, fearful, hostile, jittery, nervous, and scornful.

   C. Anxiety frequently occurs with depression.

II. Risk factors

   A. Disease related

      1. Disease trajectory points—new diagnosis, treatment initiation, completion of treatment, recurrent disease, advanced phase, end of life

      2. Physical symptoms—pain, insomnia, dyspnea, urinary retention, pruritus

      3. Abnormal metabolic states—hyperthyroidism, hormone-secreting tumors, paraneoplastic syndromes, electrolyte imbalance, hypoxia, sepsis, delirium, and hypoglycemia

      4. Psychiatric disorders such as depression, delirium, paranoia, and persecution delusions, which may predispose the patient to anxiety

      5. Preexisting anxiety disorders, genetics, age, and gender influence the expression and manifestation of anxiety (Murphy-Ende, 2019)

   B. Treatment related

      1. Patients undergoing palliative chemotherapy, radiation, or phase I or II clinical trials (Fatemeh, Behboudifar, Pouresmail, & Shafiee, 2016)

      2. Prolonged treatment and hospitalization, blood and marrow transplantation, major surgery, or prolonged phase of recovery

      3. Medications—corticosteroids, neuroleptics causing akathisia, thyroxine, bronchodilators, antihistamines, decongestants, beta-adrenergic stimulants, opioids that induce hallucinations

      4. Opioid, alcohol, or benzodiazepine withdrawal

      5. Body image changes from mastectomy, orchiectomy, colostomy, alopecia, skin changes, amputation, and weight loss or gain

      6. Failure of therapy, progression of disease, or relapse

   C. Intrapersonal related

      1. Concern about future health, relationships, finances, and social or occupational roles and responsibilities

      2. Loss of independence and perceived loss of sense of control

      3. Limited coping skills

      4. Cumulative losses that contribute to social isolation

      5. Limited social resources

III. General treatment approaches

   A. Treatment should be aimed at the exact cause whenever possible.

   B. Physical symptoms such as pain, insomnia, pruritus, urinary retention, dyspnea, and infection should be treated.

   C. Psychoeducational interventions, including a focus on providing information about the medical system and treatment process and anticipatory guidance, are likely to reduce anxiety (Murphy-Ende, 2019).

      1. Orientation to the health care setting and oncology team

      2. Providing information about support groups may reduce anxiety

   D. Written or Internet education materials about specific types of cancer, treatment, and side effects should be provided.

   E. Self-care and relaxation techniques need to be taught to the patient.

   F. The patient and family should be instructed about managing and treating the side effects of chemotherapy and radiation therapy.

   G. Refer to a licensed psychologist for individual cognitive behavioral therapy, cognitive existential group psychotherapy, or family psychotherapy and counseling.

   H. Refer to cancer support groups to provide anxiety management techniques and coping skills.

   I. Pharmacologic management is accomplished with anxiolytics, azapirones, antihistamines, antidepressants, or atypical neuroleptics.

   J. Complementary therapies such as exercise, art therapy, massage, music therapy, meditation, and progressive muscle relaxation.

IV. Potential sequelae of anxiety (APA, 2013)

   A. Somatic symptoms—nausea, vomiting, headaches, change in bowel habits

   B. Behavioral issues—substance use, altered eating habits, self-harm, social dysfunction

   C. Cognitive effects—difficulty concentrating and making decisions, poor attention span, and impaired memory

   D. Anxiety disorders—may occur as a maladaptive response; include adjustment disorder with anxious mood, generalized anxiety disorder, panic attacks, phobias, obsessive-compulsive disorder, PTSD, and depression

   E. Interference with performance at home, school, or work

Assessment

I. Presence of risk factors

II. Subjective symptoms

A. Persistently tense, unable to relax, worried, easily excitable, having poor concentration or poor attention, indecisive, easily overwhelmed, and irritable; experiencing panic attacks, loss of control, insomnia, eating disturbances, palpitations, feelings of suffocation, dizziness, fatigue or exhaustion, difficulty swallowing, and a sense of impending doom; crying easily

III. Objective symptoms

A. Facial tension or flushing, pallor, tremors, twitches, pacing, restlessness, nail biting, wringing of hands, voice quivering, rapid heart rate, increased respirations, increased blood pressure, constricted pupils, and cold hands

Management

I. Pharmacologic

A. Antidepressants: serotonin reuptake inhibitors, tricyclic antidepressants (Table 50.1)

B. Anticonvulsants

C. Benzodiazepines (low dose and short term for situational anxiety)

II. Nonpharmacologic

A. Interventions to address anxiety

1. Provide a safe environment
   a. Assess the potential for self-harm
   b. Provide a subdued space with reduced stimuli
2. Use active and empathic listening skills

TABLE 50.1 Selected Antidepressants	
Tricyclic Antidepressants	• Amitriptyline (Elavil) • Clomipramine (Anafranil) • Desipramine (Norpramin) • Doxepin (Sinequan) • Imipramine (Tofranil) • Nortriptyline (Pamelor)
Selective Serotonin Reuptake Inhibitors	• Citalopram (Celexa) • Fluoxetine (Prozac) • Fluvoxamine (Luvox) • Paroxetine (Paxil) • Sertraline (Zoloft)
Monoamine Oxidase Inhibitors	• Tranylcypromine (Parnate) • Phenelzine (Nardil)
Atypical Antidepressants	• Bupropion (Wellbutrin) • Trazodone (Desyrel) • Nefazodone (Serzone) • Mirtazapine (Remeron) • Maprotiline (Ludiomil) • Venlafaxine (Effexor)

3. Use positive interpersonal skills—calm demeanor, speaking slowly with an even voice, listening, encouraging identification of the cause of anxiety, normalizing or affirming fears, assisting the patient to identify past effective coping skills

4. Assist patient to identify overwhelming feelings such as vulnerability, hopelessness, helplessness, fear, loss of control, and fear of the unknown

5. Administer medications, monitor for side effects, evaluate effectiveness
   a. Explain the rationale for medications provided, including psychopharmacology information, to patient and family

6. Provide information about psychological resources

7. Address iatrogenic causes of anxiety (medications, physical symptoms)

8. Address spiritual needs

B. Interventions to address death anxiety

1. Consider the developmental differences in conceptualizing death

2. Establish a nurturing and supportive relationship
   a. Provide continuity of care by assigning the same staff and avoiding the introduction of new staff members

3. Assist the patient to contain the anxiety associated with impending death by listening to the concerns and being present
   a. Allow patient to have discussions about fears concerning dying
   b. Facilitate open communication with family

4. Encourage family and friends to visit if the patient okay with visitors
   a. Facilitate open communication
   b. Provide privacy

5. Assist the patient to identify and address practical concerns of death

6. Assist the patient to identify finding pleasure in short-term goals
   a. Provide information about predictable physical symptoms
   b. Reassure patient that pain/symptoms will be assessed and addressed

7. Explain common emotional phases that patients may face
   a. Acknowledge defense mechanisms as denial, which is a possible adaptive response to impending death

8. Encourage the patient to identify his or her spiritual belief system that helps face the transition of death
   a. Offer to arrange for clergy services, as needed
   b. Ask how faith-based interventions can be incorporated into care

9. Refer to palliative care or a psychologist to provide short-term psychological interventions

DEPRESSION

Overview

I. Depression
   A. A mood state of feeling sad, discouraged, hopeless, and worthless
      1. May vary from mild and transient emotional distress to a major psychiatric illness
      2. Several types of depressive disorders that may affect one's physical, affective, cognitive, and social well-being
      3. Reactive depression—a normal response to a precipitating event or situation and can be a response to the cancer diagnosis, prognosis, treatment, fear of the unknown, cumulative losses, or fear of death
      4. Depression characterized by low positive affect, with symptoms of anhedonia and cognitive and motor slowing
   B. Patient evaluation by a qualified mental health practitioner such as a psychologist or psychiatrist critical for accurate diagnosis and treatment
      1. Clinicians and patients may believe depression is normal in cancer, which may be one barrier to accurate evaluation and effective treatment.
      2. Nurses may underestimate the level of depressive symptoms in patients with moderate or severe depression; nurses are key to identify patients who are at risk and make referrals for further evaluation.
      3. The *Diagnostic and Statistical Manual of Mental Disorders* (DSM-V) criteria for a diagnosis of a major depressive disorder are as follows:
         a. Depressed mood or loss of interest in pleasure in nearly all activities for at least 2 weeks
         b. Have five or more of the following symptoms—change in appetite or weight change (5% or more in a month), insomnia or hypersomnia nearly every day, psychomotor agitation or retardation nearly every day (observable by others), decreased energy, feelings of worthlessness or guilt, difficulty concentrating or making decisions, recurrent thoughts of death or suicidal ideation, or plans or attempts (APA, 2013).⚠
      4. The symptoms listed here do not meet the diagnostic criteria if they are caused by the direct physiologic effects of a substance or a general medical condition, or if the symptoms are accounted for by bereavement.
      5. It is often difficult to determine if physical symptoms are caused by the cancer and its treatment or by a mood disorder such as major depression.
         a. Many patients with cancer have physical symptoms and anxiety; psychologists should use clinical judgment and other diagnostic criteria besides the DSM-V.
      6. Depression indicators that require more focused interventions (Box 50.1)
      7. Possible medical causes of cancer-related depression (Table 50.2)
II. Mood disorder
   A. Caused by a medical condition with depressive features
   B. Defined as depression that has a cause in a medical illness or is caused by a direct biological condition and the full criteria for a major depressive episode are not met (APA, 2013)
III. Adjustment disorder with depressed mood
   A. Considered acute if lasts less than 6 months
   B. Considered chronic when symptoms last for 6 months or longer (APA, 2013)
IV. Demoralization
   A. Defined as the loss of meaning, which is a different construct from depression and should be considered a separate syndrome
   B. Characterized by loss of meaning, purpose, and hope
   C. Patient may still experience pleasure in the present (Robinson et al., 2016)
V. Risk factors
   A. History and situational
      1. Personal history of major depression
      2. Previous suicide attempt
      3. Family history of depression

BOX 50.1   Depression Indicators

Indicators of Depression Requiring More Focused or Involved Interventions
- History of depression
- Weak social support system (e.g., not married, few friends, solitary work environment)
- Evidence of persistent irrational beliefs, negativistic thinking about the diagnosis
- More serious prognosis
- Greater dysfunction related to cancer
- Depressed mood for most of the day on most days

General Symptoms for More Than 2 Weeks
- Diminished pleasure or interest in most activities
- Significant change in appetite and sleep patterns
- Psychomotor agitation or slowing
- Fatigue
- Feelings of worthlessness or excessive, inappropriate guilt
- Poor concentration
- Recurrent thoughts of death or suicide

Because suicide risk is elevated in patients with cancer, those whose screens suggest suicide risk should be asked about suicidal ideation as part of their clinical evaluation.⚠

Adapted from Cohen, M., & Bankston, S. (2011). Cancer-related distress. In C. H. Yarbro, D. Wujick, & B. H. Gobel (Eds.), *Cancer nursing: principles and practice* (7th ed., pp. 667–684). Sudbury, MA: Jones and Bartlett.

TABLE 50.2 Possible Medical Causes of Cancer-Related Depression

Mood-Affecting Treatments	• Corticosteroids • Methyldopa • Reserpine • Barbiturates • Propranolol • Antibiotics (e.g., amphotericin B)
Chemotherapy and Immunotherapy	• Procarbazine • L-asparaginase • Interferon-alpha • Aldesleukin (interleukin-2 [IL-2])
Metabolic Changes	• Hypercalcemia • Sodium or potassium imbalance • Anemia • Vitamin B_{12} or folate deficiency • Fever
Endocrine Abnormalities	• Hyperthyroidism or hypothyroidism • Adrenal insufficiency

Adapted from National Cancer Institute. (2011). *Depression (PDQ)*. www.cancer.gov/cancertopics/pdq/supportivecare/depression/ Patient; Lee, H. Y., & Jin, S. W. (2013). Older Korean cancer survivors' depression and coping: directions toward culturally competent interventions. *Journal of Psychosocial Oncology, 31*(4), 357–376. https://doi.org/10.1080/07347332.2013.798756; Boyajian, R. (2010). Depression's impact on survival in patients with cancer. *Clinical Journal of Oncology Nursing, 14*(5), 649–652. https://doi.org/10.1188/10.CJON.649-652.

4. Comorbid conditions (e.g., chronic illness, substance use disorder)
5. Sleep deprivation
6. Social isolation
7. Other unexpected life events (e.g., changes in role, relationships, occupation, or living arrangement)
8. Spouse with an illness
9. Numerous cumulative losses of friends and family members

B. Disease and treatment related
   1. Severe active disease—may lead to feelings of uncertainty about the future
   2. Pancreatic, lung, central nervous system tumors, head and neck cancer
   3. Younger adult patients with cancer (Lange et al., 2015)
   4. Poorly controlled pain, nausea, or dyspnea
   5. Physical limitations or restrictions
   6. Prolonged treatment or treatment failure
   7. Medications—use of biological agents, chemotherapy, hormone therapy (antiestrogens), corticosteroids, benzodiazepines, and opioids

C. General treatment approaches
   1. Refer patients who express thoughts of suicide or desire to hasten death for immediate psychological evaluation
   2. Treat underlying medical conditions and physical symptoms

3. Provide patient and family with education about depression, treatment, and reason for referral for further evaluation and treatment
4. Coordinate psychological or psychiatric care
5. Provide education about prescribed medications and expected effects, time for response, importance of regular dosing, and possible side effects
   a. Explain the rationale for not stopping the medication without first discussing this with the prescriber
6. Monitor the patient for side effects and assess for positive response to medication, such as improved mood, appetite, and sleep
7. Facilitate individual cognitive behavioral or psychotherapy or family therapy by a highly trained mental health specialist
8. Provide pharmacologic management of depression with selective serotonin reuptake inhibitors, tricyclic antidepressants, serotonin-norepinephrine reuptake inhibitors, atypical antipsychotics, and central nervous system stimulants

D. Potential sequelae of depression
   1. Suicide or self-harm ⚠️
   2. Altered sleep patterns
   3. Inability to maintain current role—functional disability
   4. Poor quality of life and social withdrawal
   5. Adherence issues
   6. Increased morbidity and mortality (Chan et al., 2015)

Assessment

I. History
   A. Presence of risk factors for depression
   B. Presence of either a depressed mood or loss of interest or pleasure, and at least five of the defining symptoms of depression for a period of 2 consecutive weeks or more (see Overview section earlier)
   C. Variation in cultural groups in their interpretations about the meaning of depressive symptoms and use of different terms to describe symptoms
   D. Suicidal ideation, suicide attempt, suicide plan, suicide means/motive ⚠️
   E. Past use of effective or noneffective treatment for depression
   F. Concept and meaning of depression
   G. Impact of depressive symptoms on individual role and interpersonal communications or relationships

II. Symptoms and signs (APA, 2013)
   A. Subjective symptoms—report of depressed mood or anhedonia, insomnia, social withdrawal, fatigue, sense of worthlessness or guilt, difficulty concentrating, thoughts of death, suicide ideation, irritability, and somatic complaints without cause
   B. Objective symptoms—depressed or flat affect, crying, weight loss or gain, slow speech, and psychomotor excitation or retardation

III. Laboratory or measurement findings
- A. Medical laboratory testing—cortisol level, thyroid-stimulating hormone, complete blood cell count, or chemistry panel
- B. Mental status examination—changes may indicate depression, early delirium
- C. Depression screening instruments—Geriatric Depression Scale, Zung Self-Rating Depression Scale, Beck Depression Inventory, and Hospital Anxiety and Depression Scale (HADS)
- D. Functional rating scales—Eastern Cooperative Oncology Group (ECOG Scale), Karnofsky Rating Scale, and Palliative Performance Scale (PPS)

Management

I. Pharmacologic
- A. Antidepressant therapy—serotonin reuptake inhibitors, serotonin-norepinephrine reuptake inhibitors, tricyclics, norepinephrine-dopamine reuptake inhibitors, mixed serotonin receptor agonist/antagonists, and alpha-adrenergic receptor antagonists (see Table 50.1)

II. Nonpharmacologic
- A. Address risk of suicide
- B. Stay with the patient and keep him or her safe from self-harm
- C. Obtain immediate psychological or psychiatric referral
- D. Provide the patient and family with information on suicide prevention and a contact number for a clinician who is available 24 hours a day
- E. Identify and modify patient's psychological pain by assisting to alter the stressful environment and obtain aid from significant other, family, or friends
- F. Build a trusting relationship and offer realistic support by recognizing or validating the patient's concerns and struggles
- G. Coordinate care with mental health providers

III. Interventions to address situational low self-esteem
- A. Facilitate expression of feelings by acknowledging the patient's pain and despair, and engaging in active listening
- B. Reinforce depression may be self-limiting and that effective treatment exists
- C. Assist the patient to identify his or her strengths and accomplishments
- D. Collaborate with patient to identify factors that cause low self-esteem (e.g., interpersonal deficits, role transitions, role disputes, marital conflict, grief)
- E. Assist patient to identify personal growth goals, problem-solving strategies

LOSS OF PERSONAL CONTROL

Overview

I. Loss of personal control
- A. People facing cancer often feel a loss of control over their situation, a loss of ability to cope with current and future events, or both.

1. Loss of personal control is the perception that one's own actions will not significantly affect an event or an outcome.
2. Having a perceived lack of control may influence one's level of optimism, motivation level, and goals.
3. The concept of internal-external locus of control, which is a personality trait conceptualized by Rotter (1966), considers how much an individual believes that outcomes depend on his or her own actions or on circumstances outside the individual's control.
4. Self-efficacy is the perceived ability to cope with specific situations.
5. Concept of powerlessness is generally situationally determined.
- B. People tend to be strongly motivated to gain control over their circumstances.
- C. Perception of lack of control has negative effects on well-being.
- D. Belief that an event or one's reaction can be controlled may facilitate adjustment.
- E. Personal control is correlated with better emotional well-being and health outcomes, enhanced ability to cope with stress, and improved motor and intellectual tasks in those living with a serious illness.
- F. Some patients may have a perceived sense of control to inappropriately blame themselves for negative outcomes, which may result in guilt, remorse, and emotional distress.
- G. The response to the situation and level of perceived control is influenced by the meaning of the event, comparison of similar events, patterns of coping, personality, support system, and available resources.

II. Risk factors
- A. Disease related
  1. Unexpected diagnosis; lack of understanding of disease and treatment
  2. Uncertainty of the prognosis
  3. Inability to perform usual activities or a change in routine
  4. Physical disability or cognitive impairment
  5. Frequent hospitalizations or placement in an intensive care unit
  6. Terminal phase of illness
- B. Treatment related
  1. Insufficient understanding about treatment, side effects, outcomes
  2. Lengthy treatment course, travel to treatment site, need for assistance with occupation and domestic responsibilities during treatment phase
  3. Unexpected or poorly controlled side effects of treatment
  4. Treatment failure
  5. Body image issues such as weight loss or gain, alopecia, loss of limb
- C. Situation related
  1. Dependency on others and loss of independence

2. Loss of decision-making capacity
3. Lack of privacy
D. Developmental, personality, and culture related
   1. Age-specific considerations
      a. Young children tend to be externally controlled.
      b. Adolescents tend to depend on peers for approval, test their independence.
      c. Young adults concerned about launching often conceptualize illness as a disruption of roles.
      d. Adults may be responsible for family members (children and aging parents) and conceptualize illness as a disruption of productivity in family and work.
      e. Older adults often facing retirement and comorbid illnesses; conceptualize illness and possible death as separation from family and friends.
   2. Personality—degree of internal-external locus of control and other traits such as neuroticism, extraversion, openness, agreeableness, and conscientiousness
   3. Cultural differences from health care providers or health care system may affect communication and choices—dominant language, gender roles, high-risk behaviors, spiritual concerns, basic value, belief system

III. General treatment approaches
A. Patient and family education
   1. Encouraging questions and providing time for it
   2. Explaining that education is an ongoing process
B. Assist patient/family in decision making—explain options, risks, benefits
C. Offer to arrange for individual counseling with a mental health specialist
D. For the pediatric population, provide opportunities to make choices and express concerns through play and expressive arts (e.g., art therapy)
E. Encourage verbalization of feelings, providing emotional support and assisting in basic problem-solving

IV. Potential sequelae of prolonged loss of personal control
A. Lowered self-esteem
B. Helplessness and hopelessness
C. Nonadherence or delay in treatment
D. Depression, anxiety, or both
E. Cancer fatalism with avoidance of health-promoting behaviors and cancer-screening practices

Assessment

I. History and presence of risk factors
II. Symptoms and signs
A. Subjective characteristics of loss of personal control
   1. Overt or covert statements that suggest a loss of control
   2. Expressed frustration or dissatisfaction with care
   3. Anger or criticism toward staff
B. Presence of objective characteristics of loss of personal control

1. Refusal or reluctance to participate in decision making
2. Refusal or reluctance to participate in activities of daily living (ADLs)
3. Reluctance to express emotions
4. Behavioral responses may include apathy, resignation, withdrawal, uneasiness, anxiety, and aggression
5. Responses to limitations on personal control may include attempts to circumvent limits, increased attempts to exercise control, ignore limits
6. Nonadherence with the medical treatment regimen

III. Patient's problem-solving abilities
A. Ability to identify sense of powerlessness, insight into contributing factors
B. Past coping behaviors during other uncontrollable events
C. Ability to identify aspects of care that the individual can make choices about
D. Identification of other people or events that reduce feelings of powerlessness

Management

I. Nonpharmacologic interventions
A. Provide patient and family with orientation to the health care system and health education on the diagnosis, treatment, and expected outcomes
B. Provide updated information on the current plan of care
C. Provide opportunities for the patient to control decisions
D. Assist patient to identify the factors that can be controlled
E. Reassure patient or power of attorney for health care (POAHC) that he or she has the right to make decisions regarding medical care and will be assisted in the decision-making process

II. Interventions to address impaired individual resilience
A. Assist the patient in identifying past successful coping techniques
B. Ask the patient to list his or her coping strengths
C. Provide positive reinforcement when patient demonstrates resilient behavior

LOSS AND GRIEF

Overview

I. Loss, grief, bereavement, and anticipatory grief
A. Loss involves any perceived or experienced change in function, role, relationship, or lifestyle and implies separation from the people and things that are meaningful (Kubler-Ross, 1969).
   1. Although loss is a part of normal growth and development as attachments are given up, the sudden or

cumulative losses associated with cancer are often distressing.

B. Grief is the active, adaptive process of recognizing, coping with, and reconciling loss (Kubler-Ross, 1969).
  1. The individual's reaction to the loss is often based on his or her perception of the loss.
  2. Grief response may be affected by personality, coping skills, and available supportive resources.

C. Bereavement is deprivation of something or someone, such as a relation or friend, especially by death (Oxford University Press, 2013).
  1. A bereft person is deprived of nonmaterial assets and may feel robbed of someone or something important, and future plans.

D. Anticipatory grief begins in response to the awareness of the impending loss of a loved one and acknowledgment of future losses.

II. Risk factors
  A. Disease related and treatment related
    1. Unexpected diagnosis, high risk of recurrence, advanced disease, poor prognosis
    2. Changes in body structure, function, or image (e.g., amputation, mastectomy, colostomy, alopecia, cachexia, or cognition)
    3. Poor pain control or chronic pain
    4. History of psychiatric illness
  B. Situational and social
    1. Loss of a person through death, divorce, or separation
    2. Loss of something considered valuable, such as pet, home, possessions
    3. Nature of the relationship with lost person
    4. Cumulative losses
    5. Limited social support
    6. Occupational or employment restrictions
  C. Developmental (Loney & Murphy-Ende, 2009) (Table 50.3)
  D. Risk for complicated grief
    1. Perception of death as preventable
    2. Ambivalent relationship to the deceased
    3. Coexisting medical conditions
    4. Coexisting financial or legal problems
  E. General treatment approaches
    1. Provide basic information (verbal and written) on the grief process
    2. Explore spiritual beliefs that may offer a sense of comfort and referral to spiritual care
    3. Refer to grief counselor or psychologist for individual or family counseling
    4. Refer to support groups in the community
    5. Offer music or art therapy
    6. Provide pharmacologic management of severe symptoms
  F. Potential sequelae of loss and grief
    1. Complicated grief
    2. Depression or anxiety

TABLE 50.3 Developmental Grief and Loss Responses

Age	Concept of Loss
Younger than 2 years	Self-centered and sees loss as deprivation of needs or separation
2–5 years	Concept is temporary and concrete; may express little distress of not being loved
5–9 years	Concept is concrete and logical; may see loss as fear of punishment or bodily harm
9–12 years	Concept is realistic; may perceive loss as separation
12–18 years	Concept is abstract and realistic; may perceive loss as a threat to independence
18–25 years	Impact of loss is complex, with disruption in lifestyle
25–45 years	Impact of loss may represent a threat to future
45–65 years	Loss or death represents disruption of productivity in family or work
65 to death	Concept of loss may be philosophical, with death perceived as separation

  3. Denial
  4. Self-neglect or inability to take care of others
  5. Social isolation
  6. Physical symptoms
  7. Cognitive symptoms
  8. Substance abuse
  9. Suicidal ideation or attempt

Assessment

I. History
  A. Presence of risk factors, including previous losses
  B. Nature and meaning of the loss
  C. Personality and past coping responses
  D. Family characteristics and communication style
  E. Symptoms and signs of grief
    1. Cognitive—lack of concentration, distractibility, preoccupation with loss, searching for meaning, intrusive thoughts, or psychiatric symptoms
    2. Physical—fatigue, headache, shortness of breath, GI complaints, sleep disturbance, cardiac symptoms, fatigue, or exhaustion.
    3. Psychological—shock, denial, guilt, anger, hostility, ambivalence, sadness, shame, depression, preoccupation, ruminating, anxiety, or dulled senses
    4. Social—dependency on or avoidance of others and occupational lapses
    5. Spiritual distress—searching for meaning or change in views or beliefs

II. Stage of grief (Parkes, 1987)
  A. Alarm—a physiologic response
  B. Searching—psychological pain with obtrusive wish for the lost person

C. Mitigation—feeling comfort in sensing the presence of the deceased

D. Anger and guilt—may be angry at others or self

E. Gaining a new identity—recovery of lost functions, adaptation to new roles

III. Patient and family level of understanding of their grief

IV. Meaning of the loss

V. Impact of losses and grief on routine, roles, relationships, occupation, and school

Management

I. Nonpharmacologic

A. Interventions to address grieving
1. Establish a trusting relationship and encourage the patient and family to share their grief without imposing own values or judgment
2. Validate the grief and encourage ways to express it
3. Be prepared for negative affect such as anger, increased demands, irritability, sarcasm, and blaming
4. Remain calm during patient's behavioral outbursts and set limits on inappropriate or dangerous behavior
5. Convey acceptance and empathetic concern
6. Assist patient and family in exploring coping methods
7. Provide anticipatory guidance before loss—discuss impending loss, review significance of past losses and responses to those losses, provide information on mourning process, assist in formulating coping strategies

B. Interventions to address interrupted family processes
1. Provide privacy for expression of feelings
2. Encourage family members to share their perceptions with each other and remind them that everyone grieves in unique ways
3. Validate each member's grief
4. Consider cultural, religious, and social customs of mourning
5. Refer family to professional family or individual bereavement counseling

COPING

Overview

I. Definitions

A. Coping—use of cognitive and behavioral strategies to manage demands of a situation when these are appraised as taxing or exceeding one's resources, or to reduce the negative emotions and conflict caused by stress (APA, 2007).

B. Coping mechanism—conscious or unconscious adjustment or adaptation that decreases tensions/anxiety in a stressful experience or situation (APA, 2007).

C. Coping behavior—characteristic and often automatic action(s) in dealing with stressful/threatening situations (APA, 2007); adaptive or maladaptive.

II. Types of coping

A. Problem focused—directed toward reducing or eliminating a stressor

B. Emotion focused—directed toward changing one's own emotional reaction

C. Meaning focused—deriving meaning from the stressful experience

D. Primary appraisal—coping-based beliefs, values, and goals (Folkman, 2013)

E. Secondary appraisal—coping based on one's belief and conception of being able to reduce or minimize the threat (Folkman, 2013).

F. Problem focused—directed toward reducing or eliminating the stressor

G. Situational coping—directed at the specific situational factors that are causing stress (Arnold, 2016)

H. Posttraumatic growth—positive psychological change from a traumatic life event (Tallman, 2013).

III. Adaptation

A. Ability to minimize disruptions to social roles, regulate experience of emotional distress, and maintain active engagement in meaningful life activities (Cohen & White, 2018)

B. According to Jean Piaget's theory of cognitive development, adaptation is the process of adjusting one's cognitive structures to meet environmental demands, involving the complementary process of assimilation and accommodation (APA, 2007)

IV. Factors influencing coping in oncology patients and their family members (Cohen & White, 2018; National Cancer Institute, 2017)

A. Cancer diagnosis related (Oberoi et al., 2017)—prevailing perception that diagnosis of cancer is a death sentence

B. Lack of knowledge of the disease process

C. Effects of the treatments
1. Fear of the effects of treatment
   a. Chemotherapy
   b. Biotherapy
   c. Immunotherapy
   d. Radiation therapy
   e. Surgery
   f. Clinical trials
2. Posttreatment (survivorship)
3. Psychological
4. Comorbidities—psychiatric history such as neurodevelopmental, psychotic, depressive, anxiety, obsessive-compulsive, personality, somatic symptom, eating, sleep–wake and substance use, illness anxiety disorders, sexual dysfunction, PTSD, other minor/major mental illness
5. Adjustment disorders—criteria or symptoms based on American Psychiatric Association's DSM-5 (APA, 2013)

D. Social factors
1. Roles—maintaining or changing
2. Routine health tasks, family issues, financial management, and living conditions that affect the individual's ability to cope

3. Family influences
4. Cultural factors, beliefs, values, and health practices
5. Community resources issues
6. Factors influenced by gender

V. Ineffective coping
  A. The conscious or unconscious attempt to deny the knowledge or meaning of an event to reduce anxiety or fear but leading to the detriment of health
    1. Delays seeking health care attention
    2. Displaced fears of the impact of the disease
    3. Limited perception of relevance of symptoms
  B. Risk assessment and interventions
  C. Suicidal ideation
    1. Screen for risk factors—gender (more often men), age, diagnosis, social supports, stressful life events (Cole, Bowling, Paletta, & Blazer, 2014)
  D. Denial
    1. Conscious or unconscious attempt to deny the knowledge or meaning of an event to reduce anxiety or fear but leading to the detriment of health
      a. Delays seeking health care attention
      b. Displaces fears of the impact of the disease
      c. Does not perceive personal relevance of symptoms
      d. Uses self-treatment
    2. Denial not necessarily considered dysfunctional coping
    3. Assessment of coping distress and coping status

Assessment

I. Assessment tools—interview, questionnaire, checklists, psychological tests, observation, metrics (biofeedback, psychoneuroimmunology)
II. Commonly used assessment tools
  A. NCCN Distress Thermometer (DT) (NCCN, 2018)
    1. 0 (no distress) to 10 (severe distress) measurement, with accompanying simple questions identifying source of distress
    2. Recommendation that score of 4 or more triggers further physician or nurse evaluation, referral to psychosocial services, or both
  B. HADS (Carlson, Waller, & Mitchell, 2012)
    1. 14-item scale (7 questions: anxiety; 7 questions: depression)
    2. Score from 0 to 21 (0–3 per question) to evaluate anxiety or depression levels
III. Components of assessment
  A. Assess psychosocial distress
  B. Identify psychosocial needs that affect QOL, ADLs
  C. Identify of patterns of coping
  D. Observe for contributing factors to ineffective coping (see Ineffective Coping section earlier)
    1. Anxiety, depression, insomnia
    2. Previous stressors and the coping mechanisms used
    3. Diagnosis of mental disorders
  E. Provide opportunities for patient to discuss the meaning of the situation

1. Self-described definitions of well-being and QOL
F. Identifying contributors to distress
  1. Social factors contributing to distress
  2. Presence of family and community support
  3. Management
  4. Nonpharmacologic

Management

I. Provide effective communication and emotional support.
  A. Use verbal and nonverbal therapeutic communication approaches, including empathy, active listening, and confrontation, to encourage patient and family to express emotions and solve problems
    1. Encourage the patient to express feelings and thoughts.
    2. Explore the meaning of the person's illness experience on their physical, psychological, social, and spiritual functioning and needs.
    3. Provide honest perception about symptoms and response to symptoms.
    4. Encourage the patient to explore and try adaptive behaviors to optimize functioning and accomplish ADLs
  B. Encourage the patient to identify stressors
    1. Ability to relate the facts of the contributing stress factors
    2. Ability to recognize the source of the stressors
    3. Assisting the patient to expand personal skills and knowledge
  C. Assist patient to identify strengths and positive/alternative coping behaviors
    1. Identify past methods used to self-manage distress
    2. Assist patient to set realistic expectations of emotional response to stress
    3. List strengths and identify how these can be used to cope with situation
    4. Participate in planning care and scheduled activities
      a. Support decisions regarding patient's method of integrating therapeutic regimens
      b. Validate difficulty of the situation
      c. Find a new sense of normal and routine
      d. Provide positive reinforcement on behaviors that minimize distress and maximize independence
    5. Encourage opportunities for social support
      a. Support groups
      b. Brief visits with friends or phone/social media connection
    6. Support spiritual needs
      a. Hospital chaplain services
      b. Spiritual readings or music
    7. Initiate and coordinate referrals to clinical psychologist or counselor
II. Patient and family education
  A. Provide verbal and written information to the patient and family about the disease, process, therapy, expected effects of therapy, side effects, and management. Offer instructions regarding common and simple brief coping strategies

B. Provide and explain the types of available resources

C. Provide the patient and family with a list of appropriate community-based resources (e.g., housing, home health care, hospice care, community meals)

III. Referrals or counseling

A. Coordinate referral appointments

B. Provide documentation/assessment to support counseling or therapy referral

IV. Support groups

A. Psychosocial support groups and resources are available to patients across the continuum of cancer care. Consider patient's preference for the following: disease specific (type of cancer), spiritual beliefs, cultural concerns, age specific, caregivers, and ongoing open group or time-limited group.

B. General support groups provide patients and caregivers a place to share experiences and obtain knowledge from those with similar situations.

C. Support groups may have a positive effect on an individual's coping.

D. Support groups may offer inspiration through witnessing the motivation to survive, experiencing the courage of others, and exposure to role modeling of others with similar problems.

E. Participation in online support groups may provide easy access to patients.

V. Self-care

A. Self-care skill building

1. Multifocused education programs may build coping skills (preparatory education, cognitive restructuring, building current coping skills, guided imagery) (Garssen et al., 2013; Gatson-Johansson et al., 2013).

2. Identifying strengths and recognizing and managing the source of stressors.

B. Offer complementary and alternative medicine (CAM) and treatment

1. Various strategies effective; individual preference

2. Types include but are not limited to massage, yoga, aromatherapy, exercise groups, mindfulness meditation, guided imagery, nutrition, animal-facilitated therapy, art therapy, and music therapy

3. Psychoeducational and complementary interventions—review the literature and make recommendations accordingly

Expected Patient Outcomes

I. The patient and family will progress toward overcoming hopelessness and anxiety, using positive coping.

II. The patient will remain safe and be protected from self-harm.

III. The patient will experience an improved mood and interact positively with family and friends.

IV. The patient will return to their previous or desired level of physical and psychological functioning.

V. The patient will identify a sense of control and participate in decision making.

VI. The patient's grief trajectory will be supported with acceptance of new limitations in occupational, social, physical, and psychological functioning.

REFERENCES

American Psychiatric Association (APA). (2007). *APA dictionary of psychology* (p. 63). Washington, DC: American Psychological Association.

American Psychiatric Association (APA). (2013). *Diagnostic and statistical manual of mental disorders (DSM-5)* (5th ed.). Washington, DC: American Psychiatric Association.

American Psychological Association (APA). (2007). *APA dictionary of psychology* (p. 17). Washington, DC: American Psychological Association.

Arnold, E. (2016). Empowerment oriented communications strategies to reduce stress. In E. C. Arnold & K. U. Boggs (Eds.), *Interpersonal relationships: professional communication skills for nurses* (pp. 309–332). St. Louis, MO: Elsevier.

Boyajian, R. (2010). Depression's impact on survival in patients with cancer. *Clinical Journal of Oncology Nursing, 14*(5), 649–652. https://doi.org/10.1188/10.CJON.649-652.

Carlson, L., Waller, A., & Mitchell, A. (2012). Screening for distress and unmet needs in patients with cancer; review and recommendations. *Journal of Clinical Oncology, 30,* 1160–1177. https://doi.org/10.1200/JCO.2011.39.5509.

Chan, C., Ahmad, W., Yousof, M., Ho, G., & Krupat, E. (2015). Effects of depression and anxiety on mortality in a mixed cancer group: a longitudinal approach using standardised diagnostic interviews. *Psycho-Oncology, 24*(6), 718–725. https://doi.org/10.1002/pon.3714.

Cohen, M., & Bankston, S. (2011). Cancer-related distress. In C. H. Yarbro, D. Wujick, & B. H. Gobel (Eds.), *Cancer nursing: principles and practice* (7th ed., pp. 667–684). Sudbury, MA: Jones and Bartlett.

Cohen, M. Z., & White, L. (2018). Cancer-related distress. In C. H. Yarbro, D. Wujcik, & B. H. Gobel (Eds.), *Cancer nursing: principles and practice* (8th ed., pp. 759–779). Sudbury, MA: Jones and Bartlett.

Cole, T., Bowling, J., Paletta, M., & Blazer, D. (2014). Risk factors for suicide among older adults with cancer. *Aging & Mental Health.* https://doi.org/10.1080/13607863.2014.892567.

Cope, D., Coignet, H., Conley, S., Doherty, A., Drapek, L., & Feldenzer, K. (2017). In T. Sherner, P. Patsy Smith, T. Thiruppavai Sundaramurthi, K. Deborah, & D. Walker (Eds.), *Putting evidence into practice.* ONS Press.

Fatemeh, H., Behboudifar, A., Pouresmail, Z., & Shafiee, M. (2016). Effect of pre-treatment education programs on the anxiety of patients receiving radiotherapy. An integrative literature review. *Evidenced Based Care Journal, 6*(1), 49–62. https://doi.org/10.22038/EBCJ.2016.6735.

Folkman, S. (2013). Psychological aspects of cancer: a guide to emotional and psychological consequences of cancer, their causes and management. In B. I. Carr & J. Steel (Eds.), *Stress, coping, and hope* (pp. 119–127). New York, NY: Springer.

Garssen, B., Boomsma, M., Meezenbroek, E., Porsild, T., Berkhof, J., Berbee, M., et al. (2013). Stress management training for breast cancer surgery patients. *Psycho-Oncology, 22*(3), 572–580. https://doi.org/10.1002/pon.3034.

Gatson-Johansson, F., Fall-Dickson, J., Nanda, J., Sarenmalm, E., Maria Browall, M., & Goldstein, N. (2013). Long-term effect of the self-management comprehensive coping strategy program on quality of life in patients with breast cancer treated with high-dose chemotherapy. *Psycho-Oncology, 22*, 530–539. https://doi.org/10.1002/pon.3031.

Kubler-Ross, E. (1969). *On death and dying.* New York: Macmillan.

Lang, M., David, V. & Giese-Davis, J. (2015) The age conundrum: a scoping review of younger age or adolescent and young adult as a risk factor for clinical distress, depression, or anxiety in cancer. *Journal of Adolescent and Young Adult Oncology, 4,*4. https://www.liebertpub.com/toc/jayao/4/4. https://doi.org/10.1089/jayao.2015.0005.

Lee, H. Y., & Jin, S. W. (2013). Older Korean cancer survivors' depression and coping: directions toward culturally competent interventions. *Journal of Psychosocial Oncology, 31*(4), 357–376. https://doi.org/10.1080/07347332.2013.798756.

Loney, M., & Murphy-Ende, K. (2009). Death, dying, and grief in the face of cancer. In C. Burke (Ed.), *Psychosocial dimensions of oncology nursing care* (pp. 159–185). Pittsburgh: Oncology Nursing Society.

Murphy-Ende, K. (2019). Mental health issues in cancer. In J. Payne & K. Murphy-Ende (Eds.), *Current trends in oncology nursing.* Pittsburgh: Oncology Nursing Society.

National Cancer Institute. (2011). *Depression (PDQ).* www.cancer.gov/cancertopics/pdq/supportivecare/depression/Patient.

National Cancer Institute. (2017). *Adjustment to cancer: anxiety and distress (PDQ).* www.cancer.gov/cancertopics/pdq/supportivecare/adjustment/HealthProfessional.

National Comprehensive Cancer Network (NCCN). (2018). *Distress management.* Ver 2.2018. www.nccn.org. 2.2018 - February 23

https://www.nccn.org/professionals/physician_gls/pdf/distress.pdf.

Oberoi, D. V., White, V. M., Seymour, J. F., Prince, H. M., Harrison, S., Jefford, M., & Wong Doo, N. (2017). Distress and unmet needs during treatment and quality of life in early cancer survivorship: a longitudinal study of haematological cancer patients. *European Journal of Haematology, 99*(5), 423–430. https://doi.org/10.1111/ejh.12941.

Oxford University Press (2013). Oxford English Dictionary. dictionary.oed.com.

Parkes, C. (1987). *Bereavement: studies of grief in adult life.* Madison, CT: International University Press.

Robinson, S., Kissane, D., Brooker, J. & Burney, S., (2014). A review of the construct of demoralization: history, definitions, and future directions for palliative care. *Journal of Hospice and Palliative Medicine, 49*(3). https://doi.org/10.1177/1049909114553461.

Roth, A. J., Kornblith, A. B., Batel-Copel, L., Peabody, E., Scher, H., & Holland, J. (1998). Rapid screening for psychological distress in men with prostate carcinoma: a pilot study. *Cancer, 82*(10), 1904–1908. https://doi.org/10.1002/(SICI)1097-0142(19980515)82:10<1904::AID-CNCR13>3.0.CO;2-X.

Rotter, J. (1966). Generalized expectations for internal versus external control of reinforcement. *Psychological Monographs, 80*(1), 1–28. https://doi.org/10.1037/h0092976.

Tallman, B. A. (2013). Anticipated posttraumatic growth from cancer: the roles of adaptive and maladaptive coping strategies. *Counselling Psychology Quarterly, 26*(1), 72–88. https://doi.org/10.1080/09515070.2012.728762.

Van Laarhoven, H., Schilderman, J., Bleijenberg, G., Donders, R., Vissers, K., Verhagen, C., et al. (2011). Coping, quality of life, depression and hopelessness in cancer patients in a curative and palliative care setting. *Cancer Nursing, 34*(4), 302–314.

51

Sexuality and Sexual Dysfunction

Patricia W. Nishimoto and Hana K. Choi

OVERVIEW

I. Sexuality
   A. Sexuality is a component of survivorship that can significantly affect quality of life (QOL) (Leonardi-Warren et al., 2016; Rhoten, 2017).
   B. Discussions about sexuality related to cancer/cancer treatment normalizes it as a part of routine care, opens communication (Seidler, Lawsin, Hoyt, & Dobinson, 2015), provides comfort, relieves suffering, and facilitates connections (Nelson, 2017).
   C. The Oncology Nursing Society's (ONS) Sexuality Standard of Care reinforces nursing responsibility of addressing sexuality changes (Brant & Wickham, 2013).
      1. Despite the ONS Standard, patients (Leonardi-Warren et al., 2016; Vermeer et al., 2015) frequently initiate the conversation rather than the nurse (Seske, Raheim & Gjengedal, 2015). See Boxes 51.1 and 51.2 for patient/provider hesitation.
      2. Risks of not addressing sexual concerns include blaming dysfunction on the partner, use of unsafe "home remedies," decreased QOL (Rhoten, 2017), relationship discord, isolation, emotional morbidity (Vermeer, Bakker, Kenter, Stiggelbout, & ter Kuile, 2016), perception of an unsupportive provider (Leonardi-Warren et al., 2016), and decreased sexual function (Hoyt, McCann, Savone, Saigal, & Stanton, 2015).
      3. Adolescents, the elderly, and the terminally ill are those at greatest risk if not given the opportunity to discuss their concerns about sexuality.
         a. For any age group, intimacy or self-perception as a sexual being does not end when given a terminal prognosis (Wang et al., 2017).
         b. Intimacy is identified as "very important" in those with recurrent or advanced disease (Reese & Haythornthwaite, 2016).
   D. Nurses tend to focus on the medical-technical aspects when discussing sexuality or providing psychosexual support (Vermeer et al., 2015).
      1. Sexuality is not defined to only intercourse or orgasm (Seidler et al., 2015; Seske, Raheim, & Gjengedal, 2015). It also encompasses self-concept, behavior, affect, and information processing (Dizon, 2018).
      2. Psychosexual support includes intimacy, partner concerns, and relationship satisfaction by emphasizing a sex-positive message (Vermeer et al., 2016).
   E. Basic knowledge of potential treatment-related changes is critical (Table 51.1).
      1. Chemotherapy and radiation therapy can cause long-term sexual changes in 30% to 100% of survivors (Leonardi-Warren et al., 2016) and can occur years after treatment (Dizon, 2018). Surgery can negatively affect erectile functioning and orgasm intensity (Barocas et al., 2017) and sexual confidence (Hoyt et al., 2015).
      2. Physiological changes can negatively alter self-perceptions as a sexual being. Sexual dysfunction and negative affect are often intertwined (Benedict et al., 2015).
      3. Relationship problems that existed before treatment are often exacerbated during treatment (Olsson, Sandin-Bojo, Bjeuresater, & Larsson, 2016).
      4. Alterations in nonsexual organ function can affect sexual functioning, for example, taste bud changes or fingertip tenderness due to peripheral neuropathy.
      5. For women, menopausal symptoms such as changes to the atrophic urogenital and vaginal areas, sleep, mood, body image, sense of femininity, and weight can affect sexuality (Tierney, Palesh, & Johnston, 2015). Men can experience retrograde ejaculation, infertility, diminished self-image, and orgasm changes (Barocas et al., 2017; Hoyt et al., 2015) that could negatively affect sexuality.
      6. Nurses need to balance safety without unnecessary constraints (Box 51.3).

ASSESSMENT

I. Multiple models are used to begin the conversation with patients about changes in sexual functioning due to a cancer diagnosis or treatment (Box 51.4).
II. The specific model used depends on the clinician's comfort with the topic and the chosen model.

BOX 51.1   Reasons Survivors Hesitate to Ask Questions About Sexual Functioning

- Embarrassment/avoidance
- Unaware treatment is possible
- Concern question will be considered "unimportant" or physician will view them as "ungrateful"
- Physician may not have "time" to discuss topic (Vermeer et al., 2015)
- Belief that they are the "only one" who has this concern
- Cultural/religious beliefs
- Sexual orientation
- If a minor, concern physician will tell parents that questions were asked
- Lack of a supportive partner
- Time, cost, and transportation for a separate consultation (Dizon, 2018; Falk, 2016; Vermeer et al., 2016)

BOX 51.2   Reasons Nurses/Physicians May Hesitate to Ask About Sexuality

- Unaware treatment is possible, so avoid in order to prevent increased distress for the patient
- Consider sexuality not "important" compared to "saving life" (Traa et al., 2014)
- Cultural/religious beliefs
- Biased beliefs about age, partner availability, gender (Traa et al., 2014)
- Lack of time (Leonardi-Warren et al., 2016) or privacy for counseling (Traa et al., 2014)
- Feeling it is not their responsibility (Leonardi-Warren et al., 2016; Rhoten, 2017)
- Inappropriate fear of offending (Leonardi-Warren et al., 2016; Vermeer et al., 2015)
- Lack of knowledge/education/practice
- Lack of knowledge about referrals/resources (Traa et al., 2014)

TABLE 51.1   Potential Physiological Changes Due to Cancer Treatments That Affect Sexual Function

Treatment	Possible Changes Due to Cancer Treatments
Endocrine therapy for men	Gynecomastia, feminization, erectile dysfunction (ED), decreased fertility, penile or testicular atrophy, decrease/loss of libido.
Endocrine therapy for women	Decreased vaginal lubrication, vaginal atrophy, libido changes, masculinization, amenorrhea, temporary or permanent menopause.
Immunotherapy for men or women	Fatigue, fever, and flulike symptoms can affect libido. Chest pain, shortness of breath, diarrhea, and mouth sores can affect sexual behavior.
Pelvic radiation therapy for men	Vascular or nerve damage causing temporary or permanent ED, absent or weak orgasm, painful ejaculation, decreased ejaculate volume. Brachytherapy for prostate cancer causes ED in 6%–61% of patients.
Radiation therapy to penile bulb	Destruction of nitric oxide–producing cells
Pelvic radiation therapy for women	Decreased vaginal lubrication, hardened clitoris, dyspareunia, vaginal sensation changes, vaginal atrophy/vault shortening, decreased vaginal elasticity/stenosis. It can create concern of partner of "safety" after therapy (Garcia et al., 2018).
Chemotherapy for men	Decreased/loss of libido, retarded/inhibition ejaculation, ED (Catamero et al., 2017).
Chemotherapy for women	Premature menopause, decreased libido, body image changes, decreased vaginal lubrication, dispensability and capacity, dyspareunia, vaginal stomatitis (Catamero et al., 2017).
Chemotherapy for men or women	Oral stomatitis, dry mouth, taste bud changes, nausea, fluid retention, fatigue, pain, skin changes, alopecia to include pubic hair, infertility. Taxane- and platinum-based chemotherapy regimens cause peripheral neurologic symptoms that affect sexual functioning (Westin et al., 2016).
Steroids	Hyperglycemia can result in reduced sexual function, mood dysregulation, ED, decreased desire, hypoactive arousal, dyspareunia, thinning of vaginal wall, and orgasm dysfunction (Catamero et al., 2017).
Surgery	When surgery disrupts the vascular, sympathetic nervous, or parasympathetic nervous systems, it can affect the sexual response cycle.
Prostatectomy	Retrograde ejaculation, ED if damage to autonomic nerve plexus, diminished orgasm intensity, urinary incontinence (Barocas et al., 2017). Radical prostatectomy linked to ED in 70% of men at 3 years postoperatively.
Orchiectomy	Changes in orgasm, infertility, decreased sexual confidence, decreased self-image, decreased sexual satisfaction (Hoyt et al., 2015). Unilateral may not result in infertility or sexual dysfunction if contralateral testis is normal; bilateral may decrease libido, cause penile atrophy.

BOX 51.3 Potential Risky Sexual Practices When Receiving Treatment

- Increased risk of infection with shared sex toys, anal/rectal stimulation, multiple partners
- Stoma coitus
- Laryngectomy and water play
- Nipple or penile rings when thrombocytopenic
- Vaginal stimulation without lubrication when neutropenic
- Penile ring/rubber band around penis base if experiencing neurotoxicity
- Home remedies—may interact with medication
- Potential risk to partner of shared body fluids when within 3 days of chemotherapy (Kelvin, Steed, & Jarrett, 2014)

BOX 51.5 Pharmacologic/Medical Interventions

- Penile prosthesis (Pillay et al., 2017)
- Hormone replacement (Vermeulen et al., 2017)
- Phosphodiesterase type 5 inhibitors
- Intracavernosal injection therapy or intraurethral suppository
- External devices: Penile prosthesis vacuum or constriction device at base of penis
- Penile implants: Semirigid rod, fully inflatable, or self-contained inflatable unitary
- Vaginal moisturizers and lubricants (Carter et al., 2017)/vaginal dilators
- Eros therapy

BOX 51.4 Discussion Models to Enhance Sexual Health Communication

Plissit
- Give **permission** to discuss the topic.
- Provide **limited information**.
- Provide **specific suggestions**.
- Refer for **intensive therapy**.

5 A's
- **Ask:** Bring the topic up.
- **Advise:** Normalize symptoms and acknowledge the problems.
- **Assess:** Ask about sexual functioning, and use standardized assessments if needed.
- **Assist:** Provide information and resources, and refer as needed.
- **Arrange:** Provide follow-up to check how the patient is doing.

Better
- **Bring** up the topic.
- **Explain** that sexuality is part of quality of life and that patients can talk about any concerns they have.
- **Tell** the patients about resources.
- **Time** the discussion to the patients' preferences.
- **Educate** patients about side effects that may affect sexuality.
- **Record** assessments and interventions in the medical record.

From Kelvin, J. F., Steed, R., & Jarrett, J. (2014). Discussing safe sexual practices during cancer treatment. *Clinical Journal of Oncology Nursing, 18*(4), 449-453.

BOX 51.6 Pharmacologic Interventions That Can Be Unsafe

- Intracavernous and transurethral injections for erectile dysfunction (ED)—contraindicated for men with multiple myeloma due to risk of priapism (Leonardi-Warren et al., 2016)
- Herbs—may interact with medication
- Hormone-containing agents if patient has hormone-positive malignancy (Leonardi-Warren et al., 2016).
- Medication for female sexual interest/arousal disorder (FSIAD)—can be unsafe if taken with alcohol
- Lubricants—oil based can damage latex condoms, disrupt the normal vaginal bacteria, and increase risk of bacterial vaginosis; glycerin based can increase risk of yeast infection; silicone based can irritate, as can perfumed/flavored lubricants

A. Skills-based interventions targeting use of coping skills, mobilization of social support, adaptive reappraisals of stressors (Hoyt et al., 2015), reducing emotional distress, improving communication, and learning new strategies have been shown to be beneficial (Wooten, Abbott, Farrell, Austin, & Klein, 2014) (Box 51.7).
B. Sexual functioning can be improved through interventions targeting communication and couple dynamics (Reese & Haythornthwaite, 2016; Traa, DeVries, Roukema, Rutten, & Den Oudsten, 2014). Table 51.2 provides several resources.

BOX 51.7 Nonpharmacologic Measures

- Couples counseling to include marital therapy, cognitive existential couple therapy
- Clinical focus on symptoms management
- Exercise to decrease fatigue (Westin et al., 2016) and improve libido (Hamilton, Chambers, Legg, Oliffe, & Cormie, 2015).
- Pelvic floor rehabilitation (Vermeer et al., 2016)
- Cognitive behavioral stress management intervention (Hoyt et al., 2015), either in person or on telephone
- Sensate focus with exercises focused on sexual touch
- Positioning

MANAGEMENT

I. Medical management (Box 51.5).
  A. Pharmacologic and medical management strategies are available; however, sexuality is most effectively addressed using a biopsychosocial model of care.
  B. When issues are not proactively addressed, patients may try unsafe practices (Box 51.6).
II. Nursing management

TABLE 51.2 Sexuality Resources for Cancer Survivors

American Cancer Society	Women: www.cancer.org/treatment/treatments-and-side-effects/physical-side-effects/fertility-and-sexual-side-effects/sexuality-for-women-with-cancer.html Men: www.cancer.org/treatment/treatments-and-side-effects/physical-side-effects/fertility-and-sexual-side-effects/sexuality-for-men-with-cancer.html
Will2Love	https://www.will2love.com/
Planned Parenthood	https://www.plannedparenthood.org/learn/stds-hiv-safer-sex/safer-sex
Oncolink	www.oncolink.org/oncolife
Mautner Project	www.mautnerproject.org (same-sex partners for women)
Sloan-Kettering Sexual Health Program	www.mskcc.org/mskcc/html/13814.cfm

III. Fertility preservation is a key survivorship issue and can affect QOL and sexual function (Resetkova, Hayashi, Kolp, & Christianson, 2013).
   A. Women who experience infertility report lower sexual satisfaction and functioning (Sobota & Ozakinci, 2014).
   B. When a person loses the ability to "choose" conception, it can affect personhood (Croson & Keim-Malpass, 2016) and cause existential questioning. Box 51.8 provides benefits of fertility counseling.
      1. Nurses should recognize and acknowledge grief issues of infertility (Croson & Keim-Malpass, 2016).
      2. Grieving can be interrupted when there is too much focus on medical treatment (Croson & Keim-Malpass, 2016).

BOX 51.8 Benefits of Fertility Preservation Counseling

- Decreased decisional regret (Barbour et al., 2013; Grabowski, 2017; Sobota & Ozakinci, 2014)
- Decreased decisional conflict (Sobota & Ozakinci, 2014) Decreased distrust of and resentment toward medical staff (Grabowski, 2017)
- Increased sense of control of their lives when aware of options (Sobota & Ozakinci, 2014)
- More realistic expectations about the future (Sobota & Ozakinci, 2014)
- Improved physical health (Sobota & Ozakinci, 2014) and QOL (Barbour et al., 2013: Grabowski, 2017)
- Decreased stress (de Carvalho et al., 2017; Pereira & Schattman, 2017)
- Decreased depressive symptomatology (Grabowski, 2017)

C. Risk of treatment-induced infertility affects treatment decision making in 29% of patients (Bann et al., 2015).
D. Risks to fertility are based on type and stage of cancer, drug class/cumulative dose, radiation field/cumulative dose, extent of surgery, age, gender, and genetic factors (Cardonick, 2017). Box 51.9 lists fertility resources.
E. The importance of fertility counseling is recognized by the American Society of Clinical Oncologists (ASCO), the American Society for Reproductive Medicine (ASRM), and the American Academy of Pediatrics (AAP) (Bann et al., 2015). Boxes 51.10 and 51.11 list factors to discuss.
F. Oncofertility discussion is the standard of care even if emergency treatment is needed (Massarotti et al., 2017) (Box 51.12).
   1. Ideally, patients meet with an oncofertility specialist to increase use of fertility preservation interventions (Klosky, et al., 2017). Boxes 51.13 and 51.14 provide fertility options.
   2. Lack of access to an oncofertility specialist (Abe, Kuwahara, Iwasa, Nishimura, & Irahara, 2016) can result in patients seeking information from various sources, for example, "Googling" (Barbour et al., 2013; Grabowski, 2017).
   3. Due to complexities of fertility preservation, it is recommended that donors and partners meet with legal representatives for written documentation of

BOX 51.9 Factors to Discuss With Patient Surrounding Fertility Preservation

- Cancer diagnosis and prognosis
- Treatment options and risk to fertility with each option
- Will fertility preservation delay treatment start date, and will that time affect outcome/prognosis?
- Is preservation experimental or standard procedure?
- Cost of preservation, storage, implantation fee
- Insurance reimbursement
- Applicable laws and regulations of length of storage and control if donor dies
- Success rate

BOX 51.10 Fertility Resources for Patients

Alliance for Fertility Preservation	www.allianceforfertilitypreservation.org
American Society for Reproductive Medicine	www.reproductivefacts.org
LIVESTRONG Foundation	www.livestrong.org
RESOLVE: The National Infertility Association	www.resolve.org
Save My Fertility	www.savemyfertility.org

BOX 51.11   Ethical/Legal Issues of Fertility Preservation

- Privacy/confidentiality of patient, family, and progeny of stored tissue
- Assent of minors
- Safeguards to prevent conflation of research and therapy
- Terminally ill at time of diagnosis (Barbour et al., 2013; Meyer & Farrell, 2015)
- Addressing experimental status of oncofertility strategies with unknown efficacy, low viability, or possible safety risks to survivors or progeny
- Potential conflicts of interest between patients, parents, clinicians, researchers, and institutions
- Stored tissue issues: number of children that may be conceived from stored tissue; unused tissue disposition (e.g., research or termination); desired length of viable storage (de Carvalho et al., 2017; Fournier, 2016)
- "Noncontingent biographies" (where couple may break up in the future) (Gracia & Crockin, 2016) or "biographical acceleration" (new relationship) (Barbour et al., 2013; Fournier, 2016)
- Single women may refuse sperm donation for embryo cryopreservation (Massarotti et al., 2017)

BOX 51.12   Why Is Fertility Preservation Not Done? Complex and Intricate Decision Making

- Cost (Bann et al., 2015; Woodruff, 2017)
- Lack of information—patient/provider (Bann et al., 2015; Grover, Deal, Wood, & Mersereau, 2016; Woodruff, 2017)
- Provider concerns of age—prepubertal (Resetkova et al., 2013) or over 50 years (Barbour et al., 2013; Grover et al., 2016), socioeconomic status (SES), partnership status, existing children, sexual orientation (Russell, Galvin, Harper, & Clayman, 2016), religion (Linkeviciute, Boniolo, Chiavari, & Peccatori, 2014)
- Gender disparity (males counseled more frequently than females) (Bann et al., 2015)
- Too ill to discuss option (Resetkova et al., 2013) or poor prognosis
- Sense of urgency on part of patient or provider that delay would affect prognosis
- Future risk of reseeding cancer cells with autotransplantation (Resetkova et al., 2013)
- Parental values can affect decision of adolescents (Klosky, Flynn et al., 2017; Klosky, Wang et al., 2017)

BOX 51.13   Fertility Preservation Options for Males

- Sperm banking (if unable to masturbate, use testicular sperm extraction [TESE], micro-TESE, or electroejaculation) (Saraf & Nahata, 2017)
- Single intracytoplasmic sperm injection (ICSI) (Linkeviciute et al., 2014)
- Gonadal shielding during XRT
- Spermatogonial diploid stem cells—question if could reseed malignancy (Linkeviciute et al., 2014)

BOX 51.14   Fertility Preservation Options for Females

- Embryo cryopreservation (Bortoletto et al., 2017; Oktay, Turan, Bedoschi, Pacheco, & Moy, 2015)—requires delay and partner availability (Linkevicuite et al., 2014)
- Ovarian transposition (oophoropexy) for radiation therapy to the pelvis (not effective for whole body XRT (Linkeviciute et al., 2014) (approximately 90% effective in preserving ovarian function)
- Oocyte cryopreservation—allows flexibility to fertilize with future partner/donor
- Conservative fertility-sparing surgery with early-stage gynecologic malignancies (Pereira & Schattman, 2017)
- Fertoprotective neoadjuvant therapies (Woodruff, 2017)
- Suboptimal option when hormonal stimulation undesirable (transgender) (Saraf & Nahata, 2017)
- Ovarian suppression via gonadotropin-releasing hormone agonist hormone—controversial (Del Mastro & Lambertini, 2015; Demeestere et al., 2016; Pereira & Schattman, 2017) and question of safety for lymphoma patients (Bortoletto et al., 2017)
- Ovarian stimulation/phase start techniques—wide variation in practice (Bortoletto et al., 2017)

disposition rights (Fournier, 2016) and that fertility clinics update their consent forms (Gracia & Crockin, 2016).

IV. Birth control measures while on treatment are a vital component of counseling (Box 51.15).
   A. If pregnant, patient needs to be informed of risks to the fetus from treatment or diagnostic tests.
   B. Surgery that affects the bladder, large intestine, or rectum can increase the risk of miscarriage (Waimey, Smith, Confino, Jeruss, & Pavone, 2015).
   C. Mutagenic changes in gametes and/or teratogenic effects can occur if the fetus is exposed to chemotherapy or external radiation therapy (XRT).
   D. Safety and how to decrease exposure to the fetus from diagnostic tests.
      1. The challenge is that many pregnancy symptoms can mimic symptoms of malignancy, such as bloating, weight changes, fatigue, and menstrual changes.

⚠ BOX 51.15   Risks of Birth Control Methods

Hormonal birth control (implant/pill/shot/patch) contraindicated for:
- Hormone-sensitive malignancies
- History of venous thromboembolism, migraines with aura, or cardiovascular or cerebrovascular disease
- Impaired liver function
- Women >35 years and a smoker
Increased risk of infection at time of intrauterine device (IUD) insertion and for a 20-day period after insertion

Condoms: use latex unless latex allergy (although polyurethane condom more likely to break)

> ⚠ **BOX 51.16 Factors When Considering Pregnancy After Cancer Treatment**
>
> - Optimal time depends on diagnosis, treatment, and individual patient factors
> - Length of time for repair of damaged gametes: 6–12 months usually recommended
> - When aggressive cancer or at highest risk of recurrence, consider waiting 2–3 years

2. In general, most diagnostic radiology tests expose the embryo to less than 50 mSvl with little to no risk to the fetus. Using a lead shield decreases that risk.

V. Deciding when to have children after treatment

A. If a patient highly values pregnancy as "normalizing," that may overcome the concern of the child's health, mother's health, or fear of recurrence (Sobota & Ozakinci, 2014) (Box 51.16).

B. "Window of fertility" (i.e., premature ovarian failure that is shortened due to the damage to primordial follicle pool) (Roness, Kalich-Philosoph, & Meirow, 2014) may affect decision to conceive.

C. Women on long-term hormonal therapy will weigh the risk of stopping treatment to conceive against the risk of stopping treatment (Roness et al., 2014). Part of a survivorship plan is to decide whether to stop hormonal treatment for pregnancy and then restart after giving birth (Waimey et al., 2015).

D. There may not be physical restrictions for pregnancy if the cancer is surgically resected, less aggressive, and there is low risk of recurrence, but it is still important to discuss waiting 6 to 12 months to psychologically recover from the cancer diagnosis. General guidelines recommend waiting at least 1 year after cancer treatment before attempting to conceive ("Pregnancy after cancer," 2018).The most reliable strategy to assess ovarian reserve/predict onset of menopause is the serum anti-mullerian hormone (AMH) level (Cardonick, 2017) but only in females over 25 years of age (Balachandar et al., 2015).

1. Serum AMH may not be helpful in adolescent and young adult (AYA) childhood survivors (Balachandar et al., 2015).

2. Menses can continue 10 to 15 years after onset of infertility (Pereira & Schattman, 2017).

EXPECTED PATIENT OUTCOMES

I. Respectful, open conversations about sexual changes that occur after diagnosis, treatment, or partner reactions.

II. Respectful, open conversations about risks to fertility and the options to preserve fertility, potential costs, and any risks to those options.

III. Knowledgeable staff who are comfortable discussing basic changes that can occur and available resources.

REFERENCES

Abe, A., Kuwahara, A., Iwasa, T., Nishimura, M., & Irahara, M. (2016). A survey on fertility management in young women of reproductive age treated with chemotherapy. *International Journal of Clinical Oncology, 21*(6), 1183–1990.

Balachandar, S., Dunkel, I. J., Khakoo, Y., Wolden, S., Allen, J., & Sklar, C. A. (2015). Ovarian function in survivors of childhood medulloblastoma: impact of reduced dose craniospinal irradiation and high-dose chemotherapy with autologous stem cell rescue. *Pediatric Blood Cancer, 62*(2), 317–321.

Bann, C. M., Treiman, K., Squiers, L., Tzeng, J., Nutt, S., Arvey, S., & Rechis, R. (2015). Cancer survivors' use of fertility preservation. *Journal of Women's Health, 24*(12), 1030–1037.

Barbour, R. S., Porter, M. A., Peddie, V. L., & Bhattacharya, S. (2013). Counselling in the context of fertility and cancer: some sociological insights. *Human Fertility, 16*(1), 54–58.

Barocas, D. A., Alverez, J., Resnick, M. J., Koyama, T., Hoffman, K. E., Tyson, M. D., & Penson, D. F. (2017). Association between radiation therapy, surgery, or observation for localized prostate cancer and patient-reported outcomes after 3 years. *Journal of the American Medical Association, 317*(11), 1126–1140.

Benedict, C., Philip, E. J., Baser, R. E., Carter, J., Schuler, T. A., Jandorf, L., & Nelson, C. (2015). Body image and sexual function in women after treatment for anal and rectal cancer. *Psycho-Oncology, 25*(3), 316–323.

Bortoletto, P., Confinio, R., Smitch, B. M., Woodruss, T. K., & Pavone, M. E. (2017). Practices and attitudes regarding women undergoing fertility preservation: a survey of the national physicians cooperative. *Journal of Adolescent and Young Adult Oncology, 6*(3), 444–449.

Brant, J., & Wickam, R. (Eds.). (2013). *Statement on the scope and standards of oncology nursing practice: generalist and advanced practice.* Pittsburgh, PA: Oncology Nursing Society.

Cardonick, E. H. (2017). Overview of infertility and pregnancy outcome in cancer survivors. Retrieved from https://www.uptodate.com/contents/overview-of-infertility-and-pregnancy-outcome-in-cancer-survivors

Carter, J., Stabile, C., Seidel, B., Baser, R., Goldfarb, S., & Goldfrank, D. J. (2017). Vaginal and sexual health treatment strategies within a female sexual medicine program for cancer patients and survivors. *Journal of Cancer Survivorship, 11*(2), 274–283.

Catamero, D., Noonan, K., Richards, T., Faiman, B., Manchulenko, C., Devine, H., & Gleason, C. (2017). Distress, fatigue, and sexuality: understanding and treating concerns and symptoms in patients with multiple myeloma. *Clinical Journal of Oncology Nursing, 21*(5), 7–18.

Croson, E., & Keim-Malpass, J. (2016). Grief and gracefulness regarding cancer experiences among young women. *Oncology Nursing Forum, 43*(6), 747–753.

de Carvalho, B. R., Kliemchen, J., & Woodruff, T. K. (2017). Ethical, moral and other aspects related to fertility preservation in cancer patients. *Jornal Brasileiro de Reproducao Assistida, 21*(1), 45–48.

Del Mastro, L., & Lambertini, M. (2015). Temporary ovarian suppression with gonadotropin-releasing hormone agonist during chemotherapy for fertility preservation: toward the end of the debate? *The Oncologyis, 20*(11), 1233–1235.

Demeestere, I., Brice, P., Peccatori, F. A., Kentos, A., Dupuis, J., Zachee, P., & Englert, Y. (2016). No evidence for the benefit of gonadotropin-releasing hormone agonist in preserving ovarian function and fertility in lymphoma survivors treated with chemotherapy: final long-term report of a prospective randomized trial. *Journal of Clinical Oncology, 34*(22), 2568–2574.

Dizon, D. S., Katz, A., Ganz, P. A., & Vora, S. R. (2018). Overview of sexual dysfunction in male cancer survivors. Uptodate, www.uptodate.com ©2018 UpToDate.

Falk, A. T., Chargari, C., Hannoun-Lévi, J. M., Adrados, C., Antomarchi, J., Guy, J. B., & Magné, N. (2016). Brachytherapy and fertility. *Human Fertility, 19*(2), 85–89.

Fournier, E. (2016). Oncofertility and the rights to future fertility. *JAMA Oncology, 2*(2), 249–252.

Garcia, R. M., Hanlon, A., Small, W., Jr., Strauss, J. B., Lin, L., Wells, J., & Bruner, D. W. (2018). The relationship between body mass index and sexual function in endometrial cancer. *Oncology Nursing Forum, 45*(1), 25–32.

Grabowski, M. C., Spitzer, D. A., Stutzman, S. E., & Olson, D. M. (2017). Development of an instrument to examine nursing attitudes toward fertility preservation in oncology. *Oncology Nursing Forum, 44*(4), 497–502.

Gracia, C. R., & Crockin, S. L. (2016). Legal battles over embryos after in vitro fertilization: is there a way to avoid them? *Journal of the American Medical Association, 2*(2), 182–184.

Grover, N. S., Deal, A. M., Wood, W. A., & Mersereau, J. E. (2016). Young men with cancer experience low referral rates for fertility counseling and sperm banking. *Journal of Oncology Practice, 12*(5), 465–471.

Hamilton, K., Chambers, S. K., Legg, M., Oliffe, J. L., & Cormie, P. (2015). Sexuality and exercise in men undergoing androgen deprivation therapy for prostate cancer. *Supportive Care in Cancer, 23*(1), 133–142.

Hoyt, M. A., McCann, C., Savone, M., Saigal, C. S., & Stanton, A. L. (2015). Interpersonal sensitivity and sexual functioning in young men with testicular cancer: the moderating role of coping. *International Journal of Behavioral Medicine, 22*(6), 709–716.

Kelvin, J. F., Steed, R., & Jarrrett, J. (2014). Discussing safe sexual practices during cancer treatment. *Clinical Journal of Oncology Nursing, 18*(4), 449–453.

Klosky, J. L., Flynn, J. S., Lehmann, V., Russell, K. M., Wang, F., Hardin, R. N., & Schover, L. R. (2017). Parental influences on sperm banking attempts among adolescent males newly diagnosed with cancer. *Fertility and Sterility, 108*(6), 1043–1049.

Klosky, J. L., Wang, F., Russell, K. M., Zhang, H., Flynn, J. S., Huang, L., & Schover, L. R. (2017). Prevalence and predictors of sperm banking in adolescents newly diagnosed with cancer: examination of adolescent, parent, and provider factors influencing fertility preservation outcomes. *Journal of Clinical Oncology, 35*(34), 3830–3836.

Leonardi-Warren, K., Neff, I., Mancuso, M., Wenger, B., Galbraith, M., & Fink, R. (2016). Sexual health: exploring patient needs and healthcare provider comfort and knowledge. *Clinical Journal of Oncology Nursing, 20*(6), E162–E167.

Linkeviciute, A., Boniolo, G., Chiavari, L., & Perccatori, F. A. (2014). Fertility preservation in cancer patients: the global framework. *Cancer Treatment Reviews, 40*(8), 1019–1027.

Massarotti, C., Scaruffi, P., Lambertini, M., Remorgida, V., DelMastro, L., & Anserini, P. (2017). State of the art on oocyte cryopreservation in female cancer patients: a critical review of the literature. *Cancer Treatment Reviews, 57*, 50–57.

Meyer, F., & Farrell, E. (2015). Ethical dilemmas in palliative care: a case study of fertility preservation in the context of metastatic cancer. *Journal of Palliative Medicine, 18*(8), 661.

Nelson, R. (2017). *Time to have the talk! Sex and the cancer patient.* Retrieved from https//www.medscape.com/viewarticle/888119.

Oktay, K., Turan, V., Bedoschi, G., Pacheco, F. S., & Moy, F. (2015). Fertility preservation success subsequent to concurrent aromatase inhibitor treatment and ovarian stimulation in women with breast cancer. *Journal of Clinical Oncology, 33*(22), 2424–2429.

Olsson, C., Sandin-Bojo, A. . K., Bjuresater, K., & Larsson, M. (2016). Changes in sexuality, body image and health related quality of life in patients treated for hematologic malignancies: a longitudinal study. *Sexuality and Disability, 34*(4), 367–388.

Pereira, N., & Schattman, G. L. (2017). Fertility preservation and sexual health after cancer therapy. *Journal of Oncology Practice, 13*(10), 643–651.

Pillay, B., Moon, D., Love, C., Meyer, D., Ferguson, E., Crowe, H., & Wootten, A. (2017). Quality of life, psychological functioning, and treatment satisfaction of men who have undergone penile prosthesis surgery following robot-assisted radical prostatectomy. *Journal of Sexual Medicine.* https://doi.org/10.1016/jsxm.2017.10.001.

Pregnancy after cancer. (2018). Retrieved from https://www.nccn.org/patients/resources/life_after_cancer/pregnancy.aspx.

Reese, J. B., Finan, P. H., Haythornthwaite, J. A., Kadan, M., Regan, K. R., Herman, J. M., & Azad, N. S. (2014). Gastrointestinal ostomies and sexual outcomes: a comparison of colorectal cancer patients by ostomy status. *Supportive Care in Cancer, 22*(2), 461–468.

Reese, J. B., & Haythornthwaite, J. A. (2016). Importance of sexuality in colorectal cancer: predictors, changes, and response to an intimacy enhancement intervention. *Supportive Care in Cancer, 24*(10), 4309–4317.

Resetkova, N., Hayashi, M., Kolp, L. A., & Christianson, M. S. (2013). Fertility preservation for prepubertal girls: update and current challenges. *Current Obstetrics Gynecology Reports, 2*(4), 218–225.

Rhoten, B. A. (2016). Head and neck cancer and sexuality. *Cancer Nursing, 39*(4), 313–320.

Rhoten, B. A. (2017). Conceptual issues surrounding body image for oncology nurses. *Oncology Nursing Forum, 44*(5), 534–536.

Roness, H., Kalich-Philosoph, L., & Meirow, D. (2014). Prevention of chemotherapy-induced ovarian damage: possible roles for hormonal and non-hormonal attenuating agents. *Human Reproduction Update, 20*(5), 759–774.

Russell, A. M., Galvin, K. M., Harper, M. M., & Clayman, M. L. (2016). A comparison of heterosexual and LGBTQ cancer survivors' outlooks on relationships, family building, possible infertility, and patient-doctor fertility risk communication. *Journal of Cancer Survivorship, 10*(5), 935–942.

Sanoff, H. K., Morris, W. L., Mitcheltree, A. L., Wilson, S., & Lund, J. L. (2015). Lack of support and information regarding long-term negative effects in survivors of rectal cancer. *Clinical Journal of Oncology Nursing, 19*(4), 444–448.

Saraf, A. J., & Nahata, L. (2017). Fertility counseling and preservation: considerations for the pediatric endocrinologist. *Translational Pediatrics, 6*(4), 313–322.

Seidler, Z. E., Lawsin, C. R., Hoyt, M. A., & Dobinson, K. A. (2015). Let's talk about sex after cancer: exploring barriers and facilitators to sexual communication in male cancer survivors. *Psycho-Oncology, 25*(6), 670–676.

Seske, R. J. T., Raheim, M., & Gjengedal, E. (2015). Shyness and openness-common ground for dialogue between health personnel and women about sexual and intimate issues after gynecological cancer. *Health Care for Women International*, 36(11), 1255–1269.

Sobota, A., & Ozakinci, G. (2014). Fertility and parenthood issues in young female cancer patients – a systematic review. *Journal of Cancer Survivorship*, 8(4), 707–721.

Tierney, D. K., Palesh, O., & Johnston, L. (2015). Sexuality, menopausal symptoms, and quality of life in premenopausal women in the first year following hematopoietic cell transplantation. *Oncology Nursing Forum*, 42(5), 488–497.

Traa, M. J., DeVries, J., Roukema, J. A., Rutten, H. J., & Den Oudsten, B. L. (2014). The sexual health care needs after colorectal cancer: the view of patients, partners, and health care professionals. *Supportive Care in Cancer*, 22(3), 763–772.

Vermeer, W. M., Bakker, R. M., Kenter, G. G., Stiggelbout, A. M., Creutzberg, C. L., Kenter, G. G., & ter Kuile, M. M. (2015). Psychosexual support for gynecological cancer survivors: professionals' current practices and need for assistance. *Supportive Care in Cancer*, 23(3), 831–839.

Vermeer, W. M., Bakker, R. M., Kenter, G. G., Stiggelbout, A. M., & ter Kuile, M. M. (2016). Cervical cancer survivors' and partners' experiences with sexual dysfunction and psychosexual support. *Supportive Care in Cancer*, 24, 1679–1687.

Vermeulen, R. F., Beurden, M. V., Kieffer, J. M., Bleiker, E. M., Valdimarsdottir, H. B., Massuger, L. F., & Aaronson, N. (2017). Hormone replacement therapy after risk-reducing salpingo-oophorectomy minimizes endocrine and sexual problems: a prospective study. *European Journal of Cancer*. https://doi.org/10.1016/j.ejca.2017.07.018.

Waimey, K. E., Smith, B. M., Confino, R., Jeruss, J. S., & Pavone, M. E. (2015). Understanding fertility in young female cancer patients. *Journal of Women's Health*, 24(10), 812–818.

Wang, K., Ariello, K., Choi, M., Turner, A., Wan, B. A., Yee, C., & Chow, E. (2017). Sexual healthcare for cancer patients receiving palliative care: a narrative review. *Annals of Palliative Medicine*. https://doi.org/10.21037/apm.2017.10.05.

Westin, S. N., Sun, C. C., Tung, C. S., Lacour, R. A., Meyer, L. A., Urbauer, D. L., & Bodurka, D. C. (2016). Survivors of gynecologic malignancies: impact of treatment on health and well-being. *Journal of Cancer Survivorship*, 10(2), 261–270.

Woodruff, T. K. (2017). A win-win for women's reproductive health: a nonsteroidal contraceptive and fertoprotective neoadjuvant. *Proceedings of the National Academy of Sciences of the United States of America*, 114(9), 2101–2102.

Wooten, A. C., Abbott, J. M., Farrell, A., Austin, D. W., & Klein, B. (2014). Psychosocial interventions to support partners of men with prostate cancer: a systematic and critical review of the literature. *Journal of Cancer Survivorship*, 8(3), 472–484.

52

Metabolic Emergencies

Elizabeth Delaney, Carol Nikolai, and Kristi Coe

DISSEMINATED INTRAVASCULAR COAGULATION

Overview

I. Definition—a systemic disorder of coagulation. Within disseminated intravascular coagulation (DIC) extensive intravascular thrombi cause end-organ damage and hemorrhage due to the consumption of platelets and coagulation factors (Robinson, 2017).
   A. DIC can either be acute or chronic
      1. Acute DIC develops quickly, resulting in widespread blood clots in smaller vessels and dangerous bleeding. Bleeding into organs is a common presenting factor. Blood clots in small vessels may cause dysfunction and organ failure. Examples of affected organs include lungs, kidneys, brain, heart, liver, spleen, adrenals, pancreas, and gastrointestinal (GI) tract.
      2. Chronic DIC occurs with exposure to smaller amounts of thrombin over a longer period (i.e., weeks). Consumption of platelets and coagulation factors occurs but happens more slowly, which allows the body time to compensate. Patients with chronic DIC may present with more blood-clotting complications or symptoms; cancer a common cause (Boral, Williams, & Boral, 2016; Robinson, 2017).
II. Pathophysiology of DIC
   A. An understanding of the normal physiology of clot formation is essential to understand the pathophysiology of DIC (Boral et al., 2016) (Fig. 52.1). Following is a description of normal steps in the coagulation pathway:
      1. Extrinsic pathway (factor VII) activated with damage to endothelial lining of blood vessels
      2. Intrinsic pathway (factor XII) activated with damage to subendothelial tissue
      3. Extrinsic and intrinsic pathways come together; comprise the common pathway
      4. Results in clot formation and activation of coagulation cascade
      5. With a normal coagulation system homeostasis is achieved when there is balance between clot formation and breakdown (Robinson, 2017) (Fig. 52.2)
III. Activation of DIC
   A. DIC is usually secondary to an underlying disorder that causes an activation of coagulation (Levi & van der Poll, 2013).
   B. DIC can be a complication from infection, vascular abnormalities, severe allergic reactions, trauma, severe immunologic reactions, ABO-incompatible transfusion reactions, aneurysms, liver disease, L-asparaginase use, solid tumors, and leukemia (Gatot, Pringgardini, & Suradi, 2016; Levi & van der Poll, 2013; Boral et al., 2016).
   C. Cancers associated with DIC include acute and chronic leukemias, especially acute promyelocytic, lymphomas, and solid cancers, such as prostate, lung, breast, stomach, biliary, colon, and ovarian (Robinson, 2017).

Assessment

I. Physical examination
   A. Skin symptoms—pallor, petechiae, jaundice, ecchymosis, hematomas, acral cyanosis (irregularly shaped blue or gray discolored areas on extremities), bleeding from any site of invasive procedures
      1. Purpura fulminans is a rare and serious condition that is demonstrated by widespread hemorrhagic skin necrosis and tissue thrombosis
   B. Eyes, ears, mouth, nose, and throat symptoms—visual disturbances, scleral injection, periorbital edema, subconjunctival hemorrhage, eye or ear pain, petechiae on nasal or oral mucosa, epistaxis, tenderness or bleeding from gums
   C. Cardiac symptoms—tachycardia, hypotension, diminished peripheral pulses, changes in color and temperature of extremities

455

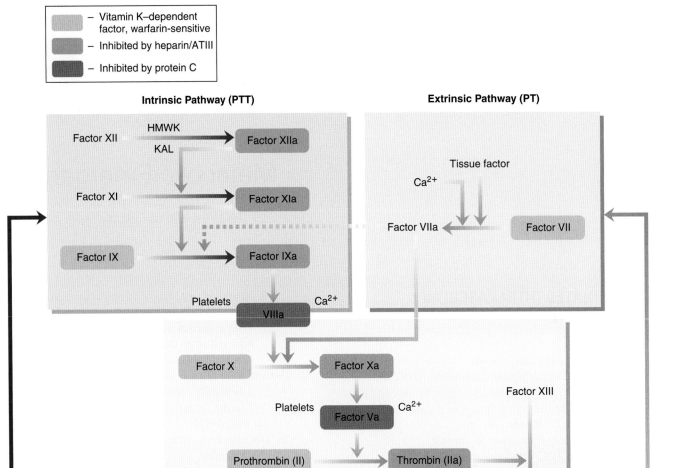

Fig. 52.1 Coagulation cascade. *PT,* Prothrombin time; *PTT,* partial thromboplastin time. (From Copstead, L., & Banasik, J. L. (2014). *Pathophysiology* (5th ed.). St. Louis, MO: Elsevier.)

D. Respiratory symptoms—dyspnea, tachypnea, hypoxia, hemoptysis, cyanosis, shortness of breath

E. GI symptoms—tarry stools, hematemesis, abdominal pain, abdominal distention, positive results of guaiac stool test

F. Genitourinary (GU) symptoms—hematuria (burning, dysuria, and frequency associated with hematuria), decreased urinary output

G. Musculoskeletal symptoms—joint pain and stiffness

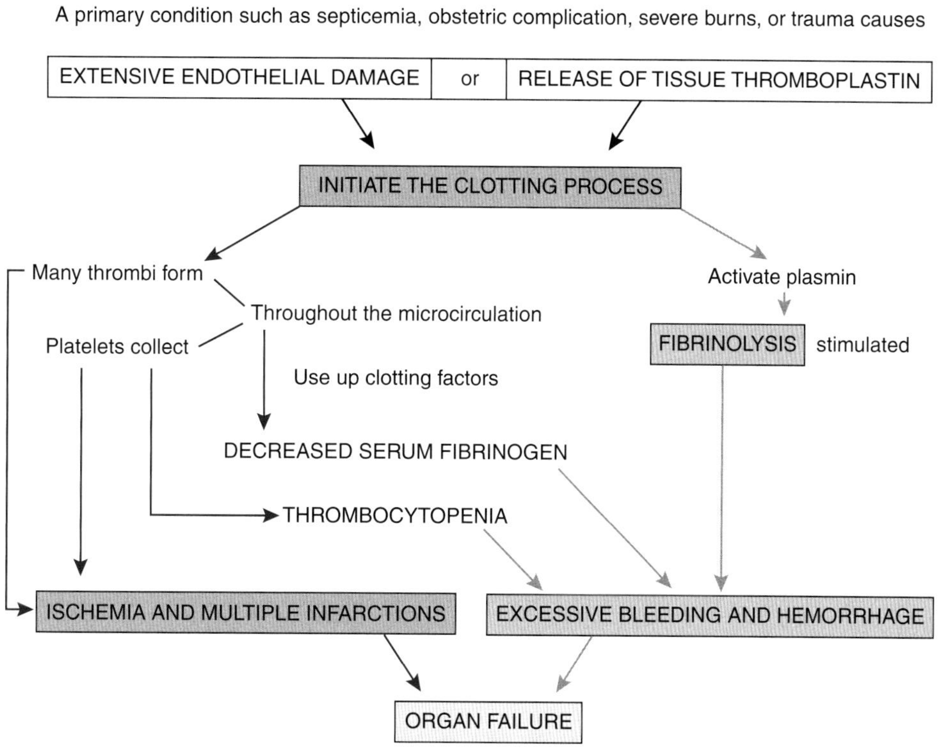

A primary condition such as septicemia, obstetric complication, severe burns, or trauma causes

Fig. 52.2 DIC cascade. (From VanMeter, K. C., & Hubert, R. J. (2018). *Gould's pathophysiology for the health professions* (6th ed.). St. Louis, MO: Elsevier.)

TABLE 52.1 Normal Laboratory Values Related to Coagulation

Laboratory Test	Results
Platelet count	150,000–400,000/mm^3
Fibrinogen	1.8–4 g/L
Thrombin time	7–12 sec
Protein C level	4 µg/mL
Protein S level	23 µg/mL
Prothrombin time	11–14 sec
Activated partial thromboplastin time	30–40 sec
International normalized ratio	1–1.2 times normal
Fibrin degradation products	<10 mg/mL
D-dimer assay	<500 ng/mL
Bilirubin level	0.1–0.2 mg/dL
Blood urea nitrogen	8–21 mg/dL

From Farinde, 2014 and adapted from Morton, P. G., Fontaine, D. K., Hudak, C. M., & Gallo, B. M. (Eds.). (2005). *Critical care nursing: A holistic approach* (8th ed.). Philadelphia: Lippincott, Williams and Wilkins.

TABLE 52.2 Laboratory Results With Disseminated Intravascular Coagulation

Increased Values	Decreased Values	Other
Thrombin time	Platelet count	Schistocytes present on peripheral smear
Prothrombin time	Fibrinogen level	
Activated partial thromboplastin time	Protein C level	
International normalized ratio	Protein S level	
Fibrin degradation products	Antithrombin III level	
D-dimer assay	Hemoglobin if anemia present	
Bilirubin level		
Blood urea nitrogen		

From Boral, B. M., Williams, D. J., & Boral, L. I. (2016). Disseminated intravascular coagulation. *American Journal of Clinical Pathology, 146* (6), 670–680. https://doi.org/10.1093/ajcp/aqw195.

H. Neurologic symptoms—headache, mental status changes (Boral et al., 2016; Robinson, 2017).

II. Diagnostic and laboratory data

A. Laboratory studies (Table 52.1 and Table 52.2)

Management

A. Treat the underlying cause; once the underlying cause is managed, DIC will likely correct itself (Robinson, 2017).

B. Laboratory data, patient condition, and underlying cause should be used to determine effective treatment strategies.

C. Pharmacologic and hematologic management

1. Avoid medications that affect platelet function

2. Transfusion of platelets, fresh frozen plasma (FFP), cryoprecipitate

3. Use of anticoagulants (e.g., heparin, low-molecular-weight heparin)—may be used in DIC when there is continued bleeding and clotting despite ongoing treatment. Anticoagulants should only be considered with the platelet count is at least 50,000/mm^3. Contraindications due to increasing risk of hemorrhage include history of acute promyelocytic leukemia, GI bleeding, central nervous system disorders, recent surgery, open wounds, or obstetrical complications that require surgery (Robinson, 2017).

4. Use of fibrinolytic agents (e.g., epsilon–aminocaproic acid, tranexamic acid)—can be used in severe cases in which bleeding does not respond to other therapies (Levi & van der Poll, 2013).

5. Anticoagulant factor concentrates (e.g., recombinant human-activated protein C)—have potential to improve DIC but not proven to reduce mortality (Levi & van der Poll, 2013).

6. Intravenous (IV) fluids, as needed, for volume repletion.

7. Oxygen therapy, as needed.

D. Nonpharmacologic management
1. Interventions to manage sites of active bleeding
   a. Application of pressure to bleeding sites via pressure dressing or sandbag
   b. Assess the role of spirituality in the patient and the impact of receiving blood products
2. Interventions for maximizing patient safety
   a. Assistance with activities of daily living (ADLs) to avoid unnecessary skin bumping or scraping, as well as heavy lifting or straining
   b. Use of electric razor instead of straight-edge razor
   c. Educate patient and caregiver
      (1) Possible risks related to injury/falls
      (2) Critical signs and symptoms to report, such as bruising; red rash; headache; black stool; blood in urine or stool; bleeding from gums, nose, eyes, vagina, rectum, wound(s) or central venous access device
      (3) Avoidance of over-the-counter medications that may interfere with normal platelet function such as aspirin and nonsteroidal anti-inflammatory drugs (NSAIDs)
   d. Provide close supervision for mobilization with appropriate device and footwear needed for ambulation
   e. If hospitalized, place bed in low locked position, two side rails up, call bell within reach, with clear pathways for ambulation
   f. If appropriate, schedule a home assessment with home nursing care and physical therapy (Robinson, 2017)
3. Interventions to assist in coping
   a. Assess available resources for patient and caregivers
   b. Provide emotional support for patient and caregivers

Expected Patient Outcomes

I. The patient will progress toward hemodynamic stability.

II. Evidence-based management strategies will be employed to prevent and manage DIC.

III. The patient and caregiver will be encouraged to verbalize and utilize coping mechanisms that are helpful in managing anxiety related to DIC.

THROMBOTIC THROMBOCYTOPENIC PURPURA

Overview

I. Definition—thrombotic thrombocytopenic purpura (TTP) is a blood disorder characterized by clotting in small blood vessels of the body (thromboses), resulting in a low platelet count. Thrombi in the small vessels may also cause thrombocytopenia, microangiopathic hemolytic anemia (MAHA), neurologic abnormalities, fever, and possibly organ damage (Saha, McDaniel, & Zheng, 2017).

II. Pathophysiology of TTP
A. Rare disease, not well understood; theories exist regarding pathophysiology
B. Von Willebrand factor (VWF) was first described in 1924 and is a carrier for factor VIII (Robinson, 2017)
C. TTP is divided into two categories: hereditary and acquired (Saha et al., 2017).
   1. The widespread microthrombi in TTP consist of little or no fibrin. The microthrombi consist of platelet aggregations and large amounts of VWF.
      ADAMTS13 (a disintegrin and metalloproteinase with thrombospondin type I motif, 13) regulates the length and binding accessibility of both VWF and ultra-large multimers of von Willebrand factor (ULVWFs) in plasma (Saha et al., 2017).
   2. With lack of ADAMTS13 in TTP, ULVWFs are not broken down and instead continue to stick to the endothelium, collecting platelets that pass by, which results in formation of thrombi in small vessels.(Saha et al., 2017).

III. Causes of TTP
A. Hereditary
   1. Hereditary TTP is an autosomal-recessive disorder and very rare
   2. Hereditary TTP is caused by a deficiency of ADAMTS13, a regulator of VWF secreted by endothelial cells, and manifests in childhood or young adulthood, typically after an event (i.e., surgery or infectious process).
   3. ADAMTS13 multiple mutations have been linked to TTP.
B. Acquired
   1. Acquired TTP is consistent with severe VWF cleaving protease deficiency and can be caused by
      a. Cancer
      b. Infection
      c. Autoimmune diseases such as systemic lupus erythematosus
      d. Drug induced (such as quinine, ticlopidine, and clopidogrel)

e. Chemotherapeutic agents (such as mitomycin-C, cisplatin, gemcitabine, bleomycin, pentostatin)

f. Anticancer agents (such as bevacizumab)

g. Pregnancy (Kuter, 2017)

Assessment

I. Physical examination

A. General—fever and overall weakness

B. Skin symptoms—jaundice, pallor, mucosal bleeding, petechiae, and ecchymosis

C. Cardiac symptoms—arrhythmia, chest pain, tachycardia

D. Respiratory symptoms—shortness of breath due to anemia

E. Head, eyes, ears, nose, throat (HEENT) symptoms—visual disturbance, aphasia, epistaxis, retinal hemorrhage

F. GI symptoms—nausea, vomiting, diarrhea, abdominal pain

G. Neurologic symptoms—headache, confusion, dizziness, seizures, paresthesia, fever, altered level of consciousness

H. Musculoskeletal symptoms—weakness (Kuter, 2017; Robinson, 2017)

II. Diagnostic and laboratory data

A. ADAMTS13 assays important in diagnosis; however, multiple versions of the assay exist, and testing takes time.

B. Laboratory studies

1. Improved reliability and timeliness of ADAMTS13 testing

2. ADAMTS13 deficiency alone not enough to determine TTP but is a valuable test (Shah & Sarode, 2013)

3. Complete blood cell count (CBC)

a. Decreased hemoglobin or hematocrit

b. Decreased platelet count (<50,000 or 50% decrease from previous count)

c. Elevated reticulocyte count (Kuter, 2017)

4. Coagulation studies

a. Normal to slightly elevated fibrin degradation products (FDPs)

b. Negative direct Coombs test (Kuter, 2017)

5. Peripheral blood smear

a. Schistocytes likely on peripheral smear

6. Metabolic panel

a. Indications of hemolysis on the metabolic panel

(1) Elevated lactate dehydrogenase (LDH)

(2) Elevated bilirubin

(3) Elevated blood urea nitrogen (BUN) and creatinine (Kuter, 2017)

7. Urinalysis

a. Presence of red blood cells (RBCs) and proteinuria in urinalysis may occur

Management

I. Medical management

A. Plasma exchange the first method to use in management of TTP

B. FFP used to replace the plasma removed in plasma exchange (plasmapheresis)

C. Other blood products as needed

D. High-dose steroids shown to be effective in treatment; need to proceed with caution with an ill cancer patient due to toxicities

E. Platelet transfusions should only be used in life-threatening emergencies in which the patient has severe bleeding or hemorrhage

F. Rituximab—used in patients with autoimmune TTP

G. Cyclosporine is a potential prophylactic treatment; can be used in conjunction with plasma exchange

H. Discontinue drugs that may prompt TTP

I. Gene therapies are under investigation

J. IV fluids as needed for volume repletion

K. Oxygen therapy as needed (Kuter, 2017; Robinson, 2017; Saha et al., 2017)

II. Nursing management

A. Determine if religion affects receipt of blood products

B. Monitor ongoing for bleeding (Kim, Park, Jung, & Kim, 2015)

1. Monitor laboratory values, specifically platelet count

2. Inspect skin, wounds, and insertion sites for bleeding

3. Apply pressure to sites of bleeding via pressure dressing or sandbag

C. Promote patient safety (see list under DIC)

D. Assist with coping

1. Assess available resources for patient and caregiver support

2. Provide education specific to TTP and its signs and symptoms

3. Assess and employ strategies for fatigue if anemia is present

4. Provide positive feedback to patients and caregivers through coaching and listening

5. Suggest resources such as psychological counseling and pastoral care services for emotional and spiritual support (Saha et al., 2017)

Expected Patient Outcomes

I. The patient progresses toward tissue and organ perfusion and hemodynamic stability.

II. The patient and caregiver will be able to articulate signs and symptoms of TTP, risk factors for bleeding, behaviors to minimize bleeding, and demonstrate behaviors for personal safety.

SYNDROME OF INAPPROPRIATE ANTIDIURETIC HORMONE

Overview

I. Definition—syndrome of inappropriate antidiuretic hormone (SIADH) is a condition in which antidiuretic hormone (ADH), in activated form called *arginine vasopressin (AVP)*, is inappropriately triggered despite the presence of normal or increased fluid balance. This results in hyponatremia and hypo-osmolality. In the oncology setting, ADH can be inappropriately produced by cancer (Maloney, 2017).

II. Pathophysiology of SIADH

A. ADH is also known as AVP in its active form. The concentration of sodium in the plasma is the major stimulant of AVP release.

B. ADH completes synthesis in the hypothalamus and is stored and released from the posterior pituitary gland; ADH is released in its activated form (AVP) when stimulated, causing renal tubules to absorb more sodium and water.

C. ADH is secreted even though the osmolality is normal, causing a dilutional hyponatremia. In addition, aldosterone secretion is decreased, and atrial natriuretic peptide (ANP) is secreted, which combine to worsen hyponatremia. Potassium loss also occurs. In addition, SIADH stimulates the thirst mechanism, which adds to the imbalance of intake and output, contributing to hyponatremia (Castillo, Vincent, & Justice, 2012; Maloney, 2017).

D. Cancer cells can cause an abnormal release AVP released in response to
1. Changes in plasma osmolality
2. Changes in plasma volume
   a. Results in an increase in free water in extracellular fluid
   b. Causes plasma hypo-osmolality and serum hyponatremia
   c. Sodium excreted from the kidneys
   d. Intracellular edema—as fluid shifts from extracellular to intracellular spaces, cerebral edema occurs

III. Causes of SIADH (Castillo et al, 2012, Jameson & Longo, 2015)

A. Nervous system disorders: include head trauma, infection, Guillain–Barré syndrome, and/or vasculitis, meningitis, hemorrhage, multiple sclerosis, epilepsy

B. Pulmonary diseases such as chronic obstructive pulmonary disease (COPD), acute respiratory failure, asthma, cystic fibrosis, sarcoidosis, pneumonia, tuberculosis.

C. Other—history of human immunodeficiency virus (HIV), acquired immunodeficiency syndrome (AIDS), giant cell arteritis, idiopathic

D. Drug induced (those that stimulate AVP release, enhance action of AVP, or have unknown mechanism of action). Numerous medications may be responsible.
1. Antidepressant agents (selective serotonin reuptake inhibitors [SSRIs], tricyclic antidepressants), carbamazepine, hydrochlorothiazide, NSAIDs, neuroleptic agents, desmopressin, oxytocin
2. Chemotherapeutic agents, including vinca alkaloids (vincristine, vinblastine), platinum compounds (cisplatin, carboplatin), alkylating agents (cyclophosphamide, ifosfamide, melphalan), methotrexate, and imatinib

E. Cancer
1. Tumors with neuroendocrine features are most commonly associated with SIADH (Jameson & Longo, 2015).
   a. Small cell lung cancer (at least 50% of patients)
   b. Carcinoid cancers
   c. SIADH may also result from other cancers, but the mechanism is unclear
      (1) Other variants of lung cancer
      (2) Central nervous system malignancy
      (3) Head and neck cancer
      (4) Genitourinary cancer
      (5) Gastrointestinal cancer
      (6) Ovarian cancer

Assessment

I. Physical examination (Castillo et al., 2012; Maloney, 2017)

A. Presentation
1. Chronic hyponatremia may produce relatively mild symptoms.
2. Acute sodium loss may produce more pronounced symptoms.

B. Signs and symptoms of SIADH—primarily neurologic and GI systems
1. Neurologic—symptoms include personality changes, headache, decreased mentation, lethargy, fatigue, weight gain, decreased urinary output, disorientation, and confusion related to osmotic shift and increased intracranial pressure. Severe neurologic symptoms: seizures and coma.
2. Cerebral edema can result from acute hyponatremia manifested by irritability, confusion, coma, seizures, and respiratory arrest.
3. GI—abdominal cramps, nausea, vomiting, diarrhea, anorexia

II. Diagnostic and laboratory data (Fenske et al., 2016; Castillo et al., 2012)

A. Basic metabolic panel
1. Sodium, decreased
2. Potassium, normal
3. Chloride, low to low-normal
4. Bicarbonate, normal

B. Plasma osmolality (<275 mOsm/kg)

C. Serum sodium (<135 mEq/L)
1. Mild: 130 to 134 mmol/L
2. Moderate: 125 to 129 mmol/L

D. Urine osmolality greater than serum osmolality

E. Urine sodium >40 mEq/L

F. Blood glucose

G. Alterations in renal function
1. Decreased creatinine
2. Decreased uric acid
3. Serum cortisol, deficiency can cause hypersecretion of ADH
4. Decreased BUN
5. Increased glomerular filtration rate (GFR)

H. Thyroid-stimulating hormone (TSH), severe hypothyroidism can cause hyponatremia
   1. Plasma AVP—decreased with hypotonic state

Management

I. Medical management (Ozsari et al., 2016)
   A. Pharmacologic management indicated for severe symptoms (seizures, obtundation). Most likely to occur in patients with serum sodium <120 mEq/L in less than 48 hours leading to potentially lethal cerebral edema.
      1. 3% hypertonic saline infusion—dosing recommendations 0.5 to 1 mL/kg body weight/hr
         a. Infused this way to prevent increase of serum sodium too rapidly and to prevent pulmonary edema, both potential side effects of hypertonic saline infusion
         b. Rapid correction of sodium may cause osmotic demyelination syndrome
      2. Demeclocycline, 600 to 100 mg/day
      3. Vasopressin receptor (V2) antagonists also approved for severe hypervolemic or euvolemic hyponatremia due to SIADH such as tolvaptan or conivaptan
      4. Employ medications to treat the underlying cause
II. Nursing management
   A. Primarily for mild symptoms
      1. Fluid restriction to 500 to 1500 mL/day; water intake should not exceed the urine output
      2. Increase salt intake
      3. Loop diuretics to increase free water excretion
   B. Place patient on seizure precautions when SIADH is severe
   C. Monitor sodium levels
   D. Weigh daily
   E. Auscultate lung sounds
   F. Maintain accurate intake and output records

Expected Patient Outcomes

I. The patient will progress toward electrolyte balance.
II. Severe symptoms related to SIADH will be prevented and appropriately managed as needed.

HYPERSENSITIVITY

Overview

I. Definition—hypersensitivity reactions in cancer care are often associated with drugs. Drug hypersensitivity is an immune-mediated reaction. Symptoms range from mild to severe. Drug hypersensitivities may occur with anticancer treatments, especially with immune and targeted therapies. The terms *drug reaction, drug allergy,* and *drug hypersensitivity* may be used interchangeably (Delves, 2018b; O'Leary, 2017).
II. Pathophysiology
   A. Hypersensitivity reactions are divided into four categories (Gell and Coombs classification):
      1. Type I—immediate immunoglobulin E (IgE)–mediated
         a. Most common type associated with antineoplastic agents
         b. Results from exposure to an antigen with formation of IgE antibodies, attached to receptors on mast cells and basophils
         c. Further exposure to the same antigen — creates a reaction with release of histamines, leukotrienes, prostaglandins, and other inflammatory mediators
      2. Type II—IgG or IgM antibody–mediated
      3. Type III—immune complex–mediated
      4. Type IV—cell-mediated or delayed
      5. Some emerging cancer treatments are not falling under the traditional classification system; therefore different classification systems are emerging (O'Leary, 2017)
   B. Severe symptoms of hypersensitivity indicate anaphylaxis (see next section).
   C. In general, hypersensitivity reactions are mediated by IgE. However, B and T cells play a significant role in the development of involved antibodies. These components initiate a cytokine cascade response. The cytokine cascade begins at the exposure of the allergen and then concludes with an immune reaction (Table 52.3).
III. Risk factors
   A. Chemotherapeutic agents have potential to induce a hypersensitivity reaction (O'Leary, 2017)
      1. Platinums (e.g., cisplatin, carboplatin, oxaliplatin)
         a. Consistent with type I reactions because most typically occur after multiple cycles of therapy
         b. Most reactions to oxaliplatin occur within the first minutes of infusion
         c. Studies on desensitization protocols for platinum agents completed
      2. Taxanes (e.g., paclitaxel, docetaxel)
         a. Paclitaxel treatment—should include premedication to prevent reactions, as well as a longer infusion time
         b. Unclear if reaction is to drug or diluent
         c. Desensitization protocols used for paclitaxel administration
         d. Most severe reactions—occur with the first or second dose within the first minutes of infusion
      3. L-Asparaginase
         a. Higher risk when given intermittently rather than daily; IV administration poses higher risk than intramuscular or subcutaneous route
         b. Intradermal skin testing performed before administration
      4. Procarbazine
         a. Corticosteroid recommended before infusion
      5. Epipodophyllotoxins (e.g., etoposide, teniposide)
         a. Reactions within first few minutes or hours after infusion; more commonly occur after multiple doses

TABLE 52.3   Classification of Drug Hypersensitivity Reactions

Type	Mechanism	Clinical Features	Timing of Reactions	Examples
Type 1 (IgE mediated)	Drug–IgE complex binds to mast cells	Urticaria, angioedema, bronchospasm, pruritus, GI symptoms, anaphylaxis	Immediate (minutes to hours after drug exposure, depending on the route of administration)	β-lactam antibiotic
Type II (cytotoxic)	Specific IgG or IgM antibodies directed at drug–hapten-coated cells	Hemolytic anemia, neutropenia, thrombocytopenia	Variable	Penicillin (hemolytic anemia), heparin (thrombocytopenia)
Type III (immune complex)	Antigen–antibody complexes	Serum sickness, vasculitis, drug fever	1–3 wk after drug exposure	Penicillin (serum sickness), sulfonamides (vasculitis), azathioprine (drug fever)
Type IV (delayed, cell mediated)	Activation and expansion of drug-specific T cell	Prominent skin findings: contact dermatitis, morbilliform eruptions	2–7 days after exposure	Topical antihistamine, penicillin, sulfonamides

From Chan, M., Rundell, K., & Aring, A. M. (2018). Drug hypersensitivity reactions. In Kellerman, R. D., & Bope, E. T. (Eds.) (2018). *Conn's current therapy 2018*. Philadelphia: Elsevier.

6. Pegylated liposomal doxorubicin—"acute infusion-related reactions consisting of, but not limited to, flushing, shortness of breath, facial swelling, headache, chills, back pain, tightness in the chest or throat, and/or hypotension occurred in 11% of patients with solid tumors treated with doxorubicin (liposomal). Serious, life-threatening and fatal infusion reactions have been reported" (Lexicomp, 2018c).

7. Cytarabine—allergic reaction and anaphylaxis are reported (Lexicomp, 2018a).

8. Monoclonal antibodies (MoABs, e.g., rituximab, cetuximab, trastuzumab, bevacizumab, obinutuzumab, ofatumumab) and checkpoint inhibitors (CIs, e.g., pembrolizumab, nivolumab, atezolizumab, avelumab, durvalumab, ipilimumab)

   a. Type of biotherapy—murine (mouse protein), chimeric (7%–9% mouse protein), humanized or fully humanized; makeup of the MoABs may lead to hypersensitivity reaction; higher content of murine protein correlates with a higher risk of reaction.

   b. Most infusion reactions occur with the first dose and are related to cytokine release rather than murine exposure

9. Ixabepilone—hypersensitivity reaction (Lexicomp, 2018b)

B. Other factors that indicate a greater risk

   1. History of other drug allergies, regardless of drug class

   2. History of hypersensitivity and history of reaction in the same drug class

   3. IV administration

   4. After several cycles of certain agents (e.g., oxaliplatin)

IV. Physical examination

A. Hypersensitivity reactions are often patient and drug dependent. Signs and symptoms of hypersensitivity may be very similar to, yet not as severe as, those of anaphylaxis.

B. Symptoms of hypersensitivity reaction (allergic reaction) may include transient flushing or rash or exanthema, fever, urticaria, bronchospasm, hypotension, edema, angioedema, hemolysis, vasculitis, nephritis, arthritis, graft rejection, contact dermatitis, formation of granulomas, or a feeling of impending doom (O'Leary, 2017)

C. There is an association of symptom onset with drug administration (Delves, 2018b)

V. Diagnostic and laboratory data

A. Test dose via skin testing (e.g., carboplatin, oxaliplatin, bleomycin)

   1. Determine if skin test is positive or negative, which could predict potential for reaction

B. Possibly drug provocation test

C. Possibly direct and indirect antiglobulin assays (Delves, 2018b)

Management

I. Medical management

A. Administer pharmacologic management used for pretherapy delivery to assist in prevention of a reaction when appropriate (Delves, 2018b; O'Leary, 2017)

   1. Corticosteroids

   2. Histamine 1 (H_1) antagonists (e.g., diphenhydramine)

   3. H_2 antagonists (e.g., ranitidine, famotidine)

   4. Antipyretics (e.g., acetaminophen)

B. Possible pharmacologic interventions in the event of a hypersensitivity reaction
  1. Epinephrine
  2. H$_1$ antagonists
  3. H$_2$ antagonists
  4. Corticosteroids
  5. Albuterol (for inhalation)
  6. Opioids (for rigors)
II. Nursing management (Delves, 2018b; O'Leary, 2017)
  A. Identify risk for allergy response
  B. Know the patient's past medical history information regarding hypersensitivity reactions
    1. Baseline knowledge of hypersensitivity risk associated with medications to be administered
    2. Awareness of the patient's current allergies
    3. Provide avoidance education for patient/significant other should hypersensitivity or anaphylaxis occur; inform patient to wear Medic-Alert bracelet if indicated
    4. Obtain baseline vital signs and additional vital signs per infusion protocol for specific medication
  C. Use premedication when appropriate
  D. Cease current infusion and be prepared for initiation of IV fluids if signs and symptoms of reaction occur
  E. Have emergency equipment easily accessible to the patient in addition to emergency drugs, oxygen, tracheostomy supplies, and automated external defibrillator (AED)/defibrillator
  F. Maintain patent airway
  G. Notify oncology care provider about signs and symptoms observed
  H. Administer supportive medications when ordered (i.e., antihistamine, epinephrine, corticosteroids, NSAID)
  I. Continue monitoring airway for potential compromise
  J. Restart infusion, potentially at a slower rate, based on orders
  K. Rechallenge or desensitize when appropriate for subsequent administrations
  L. Manage potential anxiety or fear of patient/significant other
  M. Assist patient in identifying appropriate coping strategies
    1. Encourage patient/significant other to verbalize potential signs and symptoms of hypersensitivity
    2. Provide relaxation methods as appropriate
    3. Acknowledge the patient's feelings as they are expressed
    4. Suggest resources such as psychological counseling and pastoral care services for emotional and spiritual support (Saha et al., 2017)

Expected Patient Outcomes

I. Patients will be aware of the potential for infusion reactions and immediately report potential signs and symptoms.

II. The patient will receive interventions for hypersensitivity reactions to minimize complications to maintain safety.

ANAPHYLAXIS

Overview

I. Definition—an acute, potentially fatal, multiorgan system reaction caused by the release of chemical mediators from mast cells and basophils. Involves prior sensitization to an allergen with later re-exposure, producing symptoms via an immunologic mechanism.
II. Pathophysiology
  A. IgE antibody is developed after first exposure to an antigen.
  B. At next exposure, the IgE antibody binds to mast cells and basophils.
  C. This triggers release of inflammatory mediators, including histamine, tryptase, leukotrienes, prostaglandins, and platelet-activating factor (Simons & Sheikh, 2013).
  D. The release of substances causes systemic vasodilation, increased capillary permeability, bronchoconstriction, and coronary vasoconstriction.
  E. The term *anaphylaxis* typically describes anaphylactic reactions mediated by IgE. Historically *anaphylactoid reactions* was a term used for non–IgE-mediated reactions. The World Allergy Organization (WAO) has recommended replacing this terminology with immunologic (IgE-mediated and non–IgE-mediated [e.g., IgG and immune complex complement–mediated]) and nonimmunologic anaphylaxis. Grading systems for systemic allergic reactions continue to evolve (Cox, 2017).
III. Risk factors (Delves, 2018a)
  A. Various antigens may provoke an anaphylactic response; route of administration may vary
    1. Antibiotics (most common are beta-lactams [e.g., penicillins, cephalosporins])
    2. Anesthetics or anesthetic adjuncts
    3. Antineoplastic agents (e.g., chemotherapy, biotherapy)
    4. Blood products
    5. Contrast media used for radiographic testing
    6. Foods (e.g., eggs, fish, food additives, peanuts, shellfish, milk)
    7. Insect venom
    8. Latex

Assessment

I. Physical examination
  A. Signs and symptoms (Simons & Sheikh, 2013)
    1. Dermatologic symptoms—flushing, itching, urticaria, morbilliform rash, angioedema
    2. Ophthalmologic symptoms—periorbital edema, infected conjunctiva, tears

3. Respiratory symptoms—bronchospasm, chest tightness, tachypnea, throat or nasal itching, congestion, sneezing, dysphonia, hoarseness, dry cough, stridor, cyanosis, respiratory arrest
4. Cardiovascular symptoms—chest pain, tachycardia, diaphoresis, hypotension, cyanosis, dysrhythmias, palpitations, shock
5. GI symptoms—nausea, vomiting, diarrhea, abdominal pain
6. Neurologic symptoms—headache, dizziness, uneasiness, lightheadedness, confusion, tunnel vision, loss of consciousness
7. Other symptoms—metallic taste, feeling of impending doom

II. Diagnostic and laboratory studies
   A. Test doses performed for some medications (see Hypersensitivity earlier)
   B. 24-hour urinary levels of N-methylhistamine or serum levels of tryptase may be performed (Delves, 2018a)

Management

I. Medical management
   A. Epinephrine—first-line pharmacologic therapy (Sheikh, 2013; Simons & Sheikh, 2013)
      1. Works through α- and β-adrenergic properties; increases peripheral vasoconstriction and bronchodilation, reduction of mast cells
      2. Begins working within seconds to minutes of administration
      3. Can be administered intravenously by health care provider trained in management of vasopressors; also given intramuscularly in the anterolateral aspect of the thigh
      4. Injection may be repeated after 5 minutes and up to 15 minutes
   B. Other pharmacologic treatments (Delves, 2018a)
      1. H_1 receptor antagonist—to improve cutaneous erythema and decrease itching
      2. Corticosteroids—to prevent biphasic reactions
      3. IV fluids and sometimes vasopressors for persistent hypotension
      4. Inhaled β-agonists for bronchoconstriction

II. Nursing management (Delves, 2018a)
   A. Review Hypersensitivity section
   B. Identify risk for allergy response
   C. Know the patient's past medical history information regarding hypersensitivity reactions
      1. Have baseline knowledge of hypersensitivity risk associated with medications to be administered
      2. Be aware of the patient's current allergies
      3. Educate patient/significant other regarding actions should hypersensitivity or anaphylaxis occur; encourage to wear Medic-Alert bracelet if indicated
      4. Obtain baseline vital signs and additional vital signs per infusion protocol for specific medication
      5. Use premedication when appropriate

   D. Cease current infusion and be prepared for initiation of IV fluids
   E. Use emergency equipment easily accessible to the patient in addition to emergency drugs, oxygen, tracheostomy supplies, and AED/defibrillator
   F. Maintain patent airway
   G. Notify oncology care provider about signs and symptoms observed
   H. Administer supportive medications per protocol or order (i.e., antihistamine, epinephrine, corticosteroids, NSAID)
   I. Monitor airway for potential compromise
   J. Restart infusion, potentially at a slower rate, based on orders
   K. Rechallenge or desensitize when appropriate for subsequent administrations
   L. Manage potential anxiety or fear of patient/caregiver
      1. Assist patient in identifying appropriate coping strategies
      2. Encourage patient/caregiver to verbalize potential signs and symptoms of anaphylaxis
      3. Provide relaxation methods as appropriate
      4. Acknowledge the patient's fears and feelings as they are expressed (Delves, 2018a)
      5. Suggest resources such as psychological counseling and pastoral care services for emotional and spiritual support (Saha et al., 2017)

Expected Patient Outcomes

I. The patient will know the potential for allergic reactions and report symptoms immediately.
II. The patient will receive immediate interventions to safely manage anaphylactic reactions when they occur.

SEPSIS AND SEPTIC SHOCK

Overview

I. Definitions
   A. Early sepsis—patients with infection and bacteremia are at risk for developing sepsis. No formal definition for early sepsis exists; however, early identification of those at risk is critical for prevention and to decrease mortality. Fever is an early sign (Zitella, 2014).
   B. Sepsis—life-threatening organ dysfunction caused by impaired regulation of the patient's response to infection, involving pro- and antiinflammatory responses (Singer et al, 2016).
   C. Septic shock—subset of sepsis causing profound metabolic, cellular, and circulatory compromise. Causes hypotension that requires vasopressors to maintain mean arterial pressure. Septic shock has a greater potential for mortality than sepsis, with a rate greater than 40% (Singer et al, 2016).

II. Pathophysiology
   A. Circulating bacterial, viral, or fungal products release toxins and cell components into the bloodstream (e.g., plasma cells, neutrophils, macrophages,

monocytes). Chemotherapy and radiation can cause impaired production of white blood cells (WBCs), especially neutrophils (Zitella, 2014).

B. Process begins with an infection and leads to uncontrolled, unregulated intravascular inflammation.
   1. Generalized immune response results in diffuse cellular injury and death, which leads to organ impairment or failure.
   2. Continuum of severity: infection > bacteremia > sepsis > septic shock > multiple organ dysfunction syndrome (MODS) > death (Singer et al., 2016)

C. Pathogens
   1. Gram-positive organism most common in the United States (increase in prevalence because of increased use of access devices); however, gram-negative organisms remain a substantial contributor. Most common include *Escherichia coli, Staphylococcus aureus, Klebsiella pneumoniae,* and *Streptococcus pneumoniae.* Over 50% of cases are culture negative (Savage et al, 2016).
   2. Fungal and viral infections

III. Risk factors for sepsis or septic shock (www.cdc.gov) (CDC, 2016)
   A. Compromised immune system
   B. Medical devices—central venous catheter, urinary catheter, drains
   C. Bacteremia, community acquired pneumonia
   D. Advanced age, older than 65—peripheral edema
   E. Intensive care unit (ICU) admission, previous hospitalization
   F. Diabetes, cancer
   G. Genetic factors
   H. Four types of infections most often associated with sepsis: lung, urinary tract infection (UTI), skin, gut

IV. Physical manifestations (Singer et al, 2016)
   A. Signs and symptoms of sepsis
      1. Fever >100.4°F: oncology patients are at increased risk of neutropenic fever due to chemotherapy and/or radiation.
      2. Infection-specific symptoms (i.e., cough or dyspnea suggesting pneumonia; purulent drainage from a wound suggesting abscess).
      3. Vital signs: hypotension ≤90 mm Hg; mean arterial pressure (MAP) <70 mm Hg; temperature >101°F or <96.8°F; heart rate <90 bpm; respiratory rate >20 respirations/minute or respiratory distress
      4. GI: abdominal pain, distention, firmness, guarding
      5. Genitourinary (GU): lesions or abscess, decreased urine output
      6. Skin: lesions, erythema, tenderness, breaks in skin integrity
      7. Oral mucosa: erythema, ulceration, tenderness
      8. Catheter sites: erythema, purulent drainage, inflammation, tenderness
      9. In early sepsis, skin may be warm/flushed. Progressive sepsis may result in cool skin allowing blood to be diverted to vital organs.
     10. Neurologic: confusion or disorientation
     11. Extremities: edema
     12. Extreme pain or discomfort
   B. Signs and symptoms of septic shock
      1. Patient requires vasopressors to maintain MAP ≥65 mm Hg despite adequate fluid status
      2. Elevated lactate level
   C. Organ dysfunction in sepsis/septic shock may manifest as
      1. Central nervous system—confusion, agitation, obtundation, coma
      2. Cardiovascular—tachycardia, arrhythmias, hypotension
      3. Respiratory—tachypnea, hypoxia, shortness of breath, decreased breath sounds, crackles or wheezes, pulmonary edema, acute respiratory distress syndrome (ARDS)
      4. Renal—azotemia, oliguria, or anuria. Urine output <0.5 mL/kg per hour for at least 2 hours without hypovolemia
      5. Skin—dry, warm, flushed; may progress to cold, pale, decreased perfusion, mottling
      6. Hepatic—elevated liver enzymes, jaundice
      7. GI—nausea, vomiting, ileus, GI blood loss
      8. Hematologic—neutropenia or neutrophilia, thrombocytopenia, DIC (Rhodes, 2017)
   D. Abnormal laboratory (Rhodes, 2017)
      1. Indicative of sepsis in addition to suspected or documented infection
         a. Leukocytosis or leukopenia. WBC can be normal with left shift
         b. Prolonged prothrombin time (PT) or activated partial thromboplastin time (aPTT)
         c. Arterial hypoxemia
         d. Decreased platelets
         e. Decreased fibrinogen
         f. Hyperglycemia
         g. Increased lactic acid
         h. Positive blood cultures
         i. Elevated creatinine >0.5 mg/dL
      2. Indicative of septic shock (in addition)
         a. Elevated liver functions
         b. Elevated lactate
         c. Urine output <0.5 mL/kg per hour for at least 2 hours without hypovolemia
         d. Increased creatinine >2.0 mg/dL
         e. Anemia, thrombocytopenia <100,000 cells/μL
         f. Hypoglycemia

Assessment

I. Physical exam
   A. Evaluation of mental status
   B. Capillary refill
   C. Skin changes
      1. Discoloration
      2. Mottling
      3. Bruising

4. Lymphadenopathy
5. Necrotizing fasciitis
D. Respiratory: cough, hypoxia, dyspnea, hyperventilation, rales, rhonchi, decreased breath sounds (bilateral or unilateral)
E. Cardiac: tachycardia
F. GI: abdominal rigidity, pain, distention, decreased bowel sounds, jaundice
G. GU: costovertebral angle (CVA) tenderness, pelvic pain, dysuria, hematuria, vaginal discharge
II. Laboratory and radiologic analysis
A. CBC, comprehensive metabolic panel (CMP), coagulation studies including D-dimer, serum lactate, arterial blood gas, blood cultures, wound cultures, bodily fluid cultures (sputum, urine) to look for source of infection
B. Chest x-ray, chest/abdomen computed tomography (CT)

Management

I. Medical management
A. Employ empiric antibiotic therapy with one or more antibiotics administered within first hour of presentation; additional antibiotics given if fever nonresponsive
B. Provide vasopressor therapy as ordered to maintain an MAP of 65 mm Hg and monitor for urine output of > 0.5 mL/kg per hour
C. Administer glucocorticoids, blood transfusions as indicated
II. Nursing management
A. Manage sepsis urgently.
B. Establish/maintain airway for supplemental oxygen and to address hypoxia.
C. Secure venous access and begin rapid fluid replacement.
D. Obtain cultures before giving antibiotics.
E. Monitor respiratory status. Begin oxygen therapy to maintain SpO$_2$ at >94% (e.g., nasal cannula, nonrebreather mask, or mechanical ventilation if needed)
F. Monitor clinical response
1. Vital signs
2. MAP
3. Urine output
4. Skin color
5. Pulse oximetry
6. Mental status

Expected Patient Outcomes

I. Shock is prevented as able with prompt recognition and management of infection.
II. The patient progresses toward hemodynamic stability when sepsis is managed according to current evidence.

TUMOR LYSIS SYNDROME
Overview

I. Definition—an oncologic emergency in which large numbers of tumor cells are rapidly destroyed, spilling their cellular contents into the systemic circulation, potentially resulting in serious complications, which can manifest as electrolyte abnormalities. Tumor lysis syndrome (TLS) can occur within 6 hours of cancer therapy initiation. Newer targeted treatments for cancer exhibit TLS (Howard, 2014).
II. Pathophysiology (Edeani & Shirali, 2016)
A. Antineoplastic agents induce rapid cell kill and release intracellular products into circulation: nucleic acids (which convert to uric acid), potassium, and phosphorus. Excretion of cellular contents causes acute kidney injury (AKI).
1. Hyperuricemia: uric acid crystallizes in the kidneys
2. Hyperkalemia: massive cell lysis releases potassium into circulation, manifested by muscle weakness and cardiac arrhythmia.
3. Hyperphosphatemia: may cause GI symptoms such as nausea, vomiting, and diarrhea.
4. Hypocalcemia from binding of phosphate to calcium cations. Symptoms include cramps, hypotension, tetany, and arrhythmias. Bound phosphate–calcium also accumulates in renal tissue.
B. Patients at highest risk
1. Cancers: Burkitt lymphoma, acute lymphoblastic leukemia, acute myeloid leukemia, diffuse large B-cell lymphoma, and other high-grade lymphomas
2. TLS can occur in other cancers with a rapid proliferation rate
3. Tumors with a high sensitivity to chemotherapy
4. Large volume of disease as evidenced by
a. Elevated LDH
b. WBC >50,000/mm^3
c. Significant liver metastasis
d. Involvement of the bone marrow
e. Cancer stage, proliferative rate
C. Patient comorbidities contribute to the development of TLS (Gucalp & Dutcher, 2015).
1. Chronic kidney disease (CKD)
2. Oliguria/acidic urine
3. Dehydration or insufficient fluid resuscitation
4. Exposure to nephrotoxic drugs such as vancomycin, aminoglycosides, contrast agents for diagnostic purposes
5. Splenomegaly
6. Extensive lymphadenopathy
7. Ascites
8. History of hyperuricemia or hyperphosphatemia
9. Mutations of the tumor
D. Treatments with high risk for development of TLS:
1. Chemotherapy, targeted treatments, MoABs
2. Radiation therapy
3. Hormone therapy
4. Corticosteroids

Assessment

I. Hypocalcemia
   A. Paresthesia and tetany
   B. Anxiety
   C. Bronchospasm
   D. Seizures
   E. Cardiac arrest
II. Calcium deposited in tissue may cause
   A. Itching
   B. Iritis
   C. Arthritis
III. Uremia
   A. Fatigue
   B. Weakness
   C. Nausea and vomiting
   D. Anorexia
   E. Difficulty concentrating or confusion
   F. Fluid overload
IV. Diagnosis based on laboratory studies
   A. Basic metabolic panel
   B. Liver function tests
   C. Phosphorous
   D. Urinalysis
   E. LDH

Management

I. Medical management
   A. Reduce risk of TLS (Coiffier et al, 2008)
      1. Administer IV hydration 24 to 48 hours before treatment initiation to facilitate renal perfusion and increase urine output, minimizing the risk of uric acid and calcium phosphate deposition in the renal tubules.
      2. Employ uric acid–lowering agents, (i.e., allopurinol, rasburicase, febuxostat)
   B. Promptly manage confirmed TLS—withhold treatment until resolution of TLS
   C. Manage hyperkalemia (Belay, Yirdaw, & Enawgaw, 2017)
      1. Mild
         a. Hydration
         b. Loop diuretics—promote potassium secretion
         c. Sodium polystyrene sulfonate
      2. Severe—same as mild plus the following:
         a. Hypertonic glucose, insulin—shift potassium from intracellular to extracellular space
         b. Sodium bicarbonate—shifts potassium intracellularly
   D. Manage hyperphosphatemia
      1. Administer aggressive fluid resuscitation
      2. Treat with phosphate binder
   E. Manage hyperuricemia
      1. Allopurinol, for levels of uric acid <8 mg/dL—reduces the production of new uric acid.
      2. Rasburicase—administered intravenously. Converts uric acid to an inactive and soluble metabolite of uric acid to allow excretion.

II. Nonpharmacologic management
   A. High-acuity patient requiring continuous monitoring of cardiac status, intensive monitoring of electrolytes, renal status, uric acid every 4 to 6 hours
   B. Monitor cardiac status with hyperkalemia, and review medications that contribute to elevated potassium levels
   C. Restrict dietary intake of potassium-rich foods
   D. Monitor electrocardiography (ECG) changes
   E. Monitor intake and output, daily weights
   F. Monitor indications for dialysis, and prepare patient and family for this potential (Jones et al, 2015)
      1. Severe oliguria or anuria
      2. Persistent fluid overload
      3. Intractable hyperkalemia
      4. Symptomatic hypocalcemia due to hyperphosphatemia
      5. Calcium–phosphate precipitate value $\geq 70 \text{ mg}^2/\text{dL}$

Expected Patient Outcomes

I. TLS is prevented in patients at high risk for TLS.
II. The patient will progress toward fluid and electrolyte balance.

HYPERCALCEMIA

Overview

I. Definition—abnormally high level of calcium corrected for albumin (>10.5 mg/dL); most common oncologic emergency occurring in 20% to 30% of all cancer patients
   A. Mild: calcium levels between 12 and 14 mg/dL
   B. Severe: calcium levels elevated above 14 mg/dL
II. Pathophysiology
   A. Calcium and bone metabolism regulated by parathyroid hormone (PTH), 1,25-dihydroxyvitamin D (calcitriol), and calcitonin (Mirrakhimov, 2015). These hormones influence bone, kidney, and small intestine to maintain calcium homeostasis.
   B. PTH stimulates calcium reabsorption from bones and kidneys.
   C. When the body detects low calcium levels, 1,25-dihydroxyvitamin D works on the gut and stimulates absorption of dietary calcium intake for body needs.
   D. Calcitonin works to decrease serum calcium levels by suppressing bone and renal reabsorption of calcium.
III. Causes of hypercalcemia
   A. Cancers posing a risk for hypercalcemia
      1. Solid tumors—those that commonly metastasize to the bone
         a. Breast
         b. Lung
         c. Prostate
         d. Multiple myeloma
         e. Lymphoma
         f. Hematologic malignancies

B. Hyperparathyroidism

C. Vitamin D intoxication

D. Chronic granulomatous disorders

E. Medications (e.g., diuretics, lithium)

Assessment

I. Physical examination (Maier & Levine, 2013)

A. Signs and symptoms of hypercalcemia

1. Mild hypercalcemia (<12 mg/dL) may be asymptomatic or have vague symptoms of constipation, fatigue, and depression

2. Severe hypercalcemia (12–14 mg/dL)

a. Patients with chronic elevation may not exhibit significant symptoms

b. Acute elevation may cause patient to have marked symptoms

(1) GI symptoms—anorexia, abdominal cramping, loss of appetite. Severe: nausea, vomiting, pancreatitis, peptic ulcer.

(2) Neurologic symptoms—restlessness, difficulty concentrating, lethargy, confusion. Severe: seizures, coma.

(3) Muscular symptoms—fatigue and generalized weakness. Severe: ataxia and pathologic fractures.

(4) Renal symptoms—frequent urination, nocturia, polydipsia. Severe: renal failure.

(5) Cardiovascular symptoms—orthostatic hypotension, shortened QT interval. Severe: ventricular arrhythmia, ST segment elevation.

II. Diagnosis

A. Initial testing

1. CMP (to include serum calcium). Confirm corrected calcium for albumin (Rosner, 2014).

2. Serum albumin and prealbumin. Important to adjust serum calcium for low serum albumin, as is experienced by many patients with cancer.

3. PTH level

B. Additional testing may include

1. Phosphorus, 1,25 $(OH)_2D$

2. PTH-related protein (PTHrP)

3. Alkaline phosphatase

4. Serum and urine electrophoresis

Management

I. Medical management (Rosner, 2014)

A. Reduce serum calcium with IV hydration—0.9% normal saline, 200 to 500 cc/hr, to increase renal clearance of circulating calcium (Rosner, 2014) and to produce a urine output of at least 75 mL/hour.

B. Administer loop diuretic for excessive fluid accumulation/retention; offer only after aggressive hydration, which is also beneficial in promoting urinary calcium excretion.

C. Maintain calcium in the bone/inhibit mobilization of calcium from bone.

1. Bisphosphonates: pamidronate, zoledronic acid

a. Work by inhibiting bone resorption and suppressing activity of osteoclasts.

b. May cause tubular and glomerular damage. Dose should be reduced for patients with renal compromise.

c. Zoledronic acid proven to be more effective than pamidronate.

d. Bisphosphonates can maintain calcium levels for 4 to 6 weeks

2. Denosumab

a. MoAB that decreases bone resorption.

b. Utilized in patients unable to receive bisphosphonates.

c. Not excreted through kidneys; therefore may be used in patients with renal insufficiency. Also used in patients who are refractory to bisphosphonate therapy.

d. Potential to cause severe hypocalcemia.

3. Calcitonin

a. Enhances calcium clearance in urine

b. Interferes with osteoclast function

4. Glucocorticoids

a. Reduce absorption of calcium through intestines

b. Inhibit 1,25-dihydroxyvitamin D production

D. Administer loop diuretics as needed if volume overload exists

II. Nursing management

A. Monitor intake and output closely, mental status, and symptoms related to hypercalcemia

B. Weigh daily

C. Administer IV fluids for hydration as ordered

D. Provide psychosocial support when changes in level of consciousness occur

Expected Patient Outcomes

I. The patient and caregiver will be aware of the signs and symptoms of hypercalcemia when indicated.

II. The patient will maintain a normal calcium level and electrolyte balance and safety.

REFERENCES

Belay, Y., Yirdaw, K., & Enawgaw, B. (2017). Tumor lysis syndrome in patients with hematological malignancies. *Journal of Oncology*, https://doi.org/10.1155/2017/9684909.

Boral, B. M., Williams, D. J., & Boral, L. I. (2016). Disseminated intravascular coagulation. *American Journal of Clinical Pathology*, 146(6), 670–680. https://doi.org/10.1093/ajcp/aqw195.

Castillo, J. J., Vincent, M., & Justice, E. (2012). Diagnosis and management of hyponatremia in cancer patients. *Oncologist*, 17(6), 756–765. https://doi.org/10.1634/theoncologist.2011-0400.

Centers for Disease Control and Prevention (CDC). (2016). *Making health care safer*. Retrieved from https://www.cdc.gov/vitalsigns/sepsis/index.html.

Coiffier, B., Altman, A., Pui, C. H., Younes, A., & Cairo, M. S. (2008). Guidelines for the management of pediatric and adult tumor lysis syndrome: an evidence-based review. *Journal of Clinical Oncology: Official Journal of the American Society of Clinical Oncology, 26*(16), 2767–2778. https://doi.org/10.1200/JCO.2007.15.0177 [doi].

Cox, L. S., Sanchez-Borges, M., & Lockey, R. F. (2017). World allergy organization systemic allergic reaction grading system: is a modification needed? *Journal of Allergy and Clinical Immunology Practice, 5*(1), 58–62 e55. https://doi.org/10.1016/j.jaip.2016.11.009.

Delves, P. (2018a). Anaphylaxis. Retrieved from https://www.merckmanuals.com/professional/immunology-allergic-disorders/allergic,-autoimmune,-and-other-hypersensitivity-disorders/anaphylaxis.

Delves, P. (2018b). Drug hypersensitivity. Retrieved from https://www.merckmanuals.com/professional/immunology-allergic-disorders/allergic,-autoimmune,-and-other-hypersensitivity-disorders/drug-hypersensitivity.

Edeani, A., & Shirali, A. (2016). *Tumor lysis syndrome.* Retrieved from https://www.asn-online.org/education/distancelearning/curricula/onco/Chapter4.pdf.

Fenske, W., Sandner, B., & Christ-Crain, M. (2016). A copeptin-based classification of the osmoregulatory defects in the syndrome of inappropriate antidiuresis. Best Practice & Research. *Clinical Endocrinology & Metabolism, 30*(2), 219–233. https://doi.org/10.1016/j.beem.2016.02.013 [doi].

Gatot, D., Pringgardini, K., & Suradi, R. (2016). Coagulation abnormality as a complication of L-asparaginase therapy in childhood lymphoblastic leukemia. *Paediatrica Indonesiana, 46*(1), 46–50. https://doi.org/10.14238/pi46.1.2006.46-50.

Gucalp, R., & Dutcher, J. (2015). Oncologic emergencies. *Harrison's principles of internal medicine, 19e* (19th ed.). New York, NY: McGraw-Hill Education.

Howard, S. (2014). Tumor lysis syndrome. In J. Niederhuber, J. Armitage, J. K. Doroshow M. & J. Tepper (Eds.), *Abeloff's clinical oncololgy* (5th ed., pp. 591) St. Louis: Elsevier.

Jameson, J., & Longo, D. (2015). Paraneoplastic syndromes: endocrinologic/hematologic. *Harrison's principles of internal medicine* (19e ed.). New York, NY: McGraw Hill.

Jones, G., Will, A., Jackson, G., Webb, N., & Rule, S. (2015). Guidelines for the management of tumour lysis syndrome in adults and children with haematological malignancies on behalf of the British committee for standards in haematology. *British Journal of Haematology, 169*(5), 661. https://doi.org/10.1111/bjh.13403.

Kim, W. H., Park, J. B., Jung, C. W., & Kim, G. S. (2015). Rebalanced hemostasis in patients with idiopathic thrombocytopenic purpura. *Platelets, 26*(1), 38–42. https://doi.org/10.3109/09537104.2013.869312.

Kuter, D. (2017). *Thrombotic thrombocytopenic purpura (TTP) and hemolytic-uremic syndrome (HUS).* Retrieved from https://www.merckmanuals.com/professional/hematology-and-oncology/thrombocytopenia-and-platelet-dysfunction/thrombotic-thrombocytopenic-purpura-ttp-and-hemolytic-uremic-syndrome-hus.

Levi, M., & Poll, T van d. (2013). Disseminated intravascular coagulation: a review for the internist. *Internal and Emergency Medicine, 8*(1), 23–32. https://doi.org/10.1007/s11739-012-0859-9.

Lexicomp. (2018a). *Cytarabine: Drug information.* Retrieved from https://0-www.uptodate.com.library.cedarville.edu/contents/cytarabine-drug-information?source=see_link.

Lexicomp. (2018b). *Ixabepilone: Drug information.* Retrieved from https://0-www.uptodate.com.library.cedarville.edu/contents/ixabepilone-drug-information?source=see_link.

Lexicomp. (2018c). *Pegylated liposomal doxorubicin: Drug information.* Retrieved from https://0-www.uptodate.com.library.cedarville.edu/contents/pegylated-liposomal-doxorubicin-drug-information?source=see_link.

Maloney, K. W. (2017). Metabolic emergencies. In S. Newton, M. Hickey, & J. M. Brant (Eds.), *Mosby's oncology nursing advisor* (pp. 367–376). St. Louis: Elsevier.

Mirrakhimov, A. E. (2015). Hypercalcemia of malignancy: an update on pathogenesis and management. *North American Journal of Medical Sciences, 7*(11), 483–493. https://doi.org/10.4103/1947-2714.170600 [doi].

O'Leary, C. (2017). Hypersensitivity reactions. In S. Newton, M. Hickey, & J. M. Brant (Eds.), *Mosby's oncology nursing advisor* (pp. 315–317). St. Louis: Elsevier.

Ozsari, L., Busaidy, N., & Habra, M. (2016). Endocrine and metabolic complications of cancer therapy. *The MD Anderson manual of medical oncology* (3e ed.). New York, NY: McGraw-Hill Medical.

Rhodes, A., Evans, L. E., Alhazzani, W., Levy, M. M., Antonelli, M., Ferrer, R., … Dellinger, R. P. (2017). Surviving sepsis campaign: international guidelines for management of sepsis and septic shock: 2016. *Intensive Care Medicine, 43*(3), 304–377. https://doi.org/10.1007/s00134-017-4683-6 [doi].

Robinson, J. (2017). Hematologic emergencies. In S. Newton, M. Hickey, & J. M. Brant (Eds.), *Mosby's oncology nursing advisor* (pp. 377–398). St. Louis: Elsevier.

Rosner, M. H., & Dalkin, A. C. (2014). Electrolyte disorders associated with cancer. *Advances in Chronic Kidney Disease, 21*(1), 7–17. https://doi.org/10.1053/j.ackd.2013.05.005 [doi].

Saha, M., McDaniel, J. K., & Zheng, X. L. (2017). Thrombotic thrombocytopenic purpura: pathogenesis, diagnosis and potential novel therapeutics. *Journal of Thrombosis and Haemostasis: JTH, 15*(10), 1889–1900. https://doi.org/10.1111/jth.13764.

Savage, R. D., Fowler, R. A., Rishu, A. H., Bagshaw, S. M., Cook, D., Dodek, P., … Daneman, N. (2016). Pathogens and antimicrobial susceptibility profiles in critically ill patients with bloodstream infections: a descriptive study. *Canadian Medical Association Journal Open, 4*(4), E569–E577. https://doi.org/10.9778/cmajo.20160074 [doi].

Shah, N., & Sarode, R. (2013). Thrombotic thrombocytopenic purpura-what is new? *Journal of Clinical Apheresis, 28*(1), 30–35. https://doi.org/10.1002/jca.21264.

Sheikh, A. (2013). Emergency management of anaphylaxis: current pharmacotherapy and future directions. *Expert Opinion in Pharmacotherapy, 14*(7), 827–830. https://doi.org/10.1517/14656566.2013.781583.

Simons, F. E., & Sheikh, A. (2013). Anaphylaxis: the acute episode and beyond. *BMJ (Clinical Research Ed:), 346, f602.* https://doi.org/10.1136/bmj.f602.

Singer, M., Deutschman, C. S., Seymour, C. W., Shankar-Hari, M., Annane, D., Bauer, M., … Angus, D. C. (2016). The third international consensus definitions for sepsis and septic shock (sepsis-3). *Journal of the American Medical Association, 315*(8), 801–810. https://doi.org/10.1001/jama.2016.0287 [doi].

Zitella, L. (2014). Infection. In C. Yarbro, D. Wujcik, & B. Gobel (Eds.), *Cancer symptom management (4th ed., pp. 131).* Burlington, MA: Jones and Bartlett.

53

Structural Emergencies

Wendy Vogel

INCREASED INTRACRANIAL PRESSURE

Overview

I. Definition—a potentially life-threatening neurologic event that occurs with an increase in brain tissue, blood, cerebrospinal fluid (CSF), or all of these in the intracranial cavity, resulting in nerve cell damage, permanent neurologic deficits, and death (Leinonen, Vanninen, & Rauramaa, 2017)

II. Pathophysiology
   A. The intracranial cavity is a nonexpandable chamber that contains brain tissue, blood, and CSF. An increase in intracranial pressure (ICP) (with or without displacement of intracranial structures) occurs with an increase in the volume of any of the three components or due to mass effect (Allen, 2018). An increase of pressure >20 mm Hg in adults is considered pathologic (Smith & Amin-Hanjani, 2017).
   B. Causes of ICP in the oncology setting include primary or metastatic tumors within the intracranial cavity, leptomeningeal metastases, blood clots, posterior reversible encephalopathy syndrome, infection, or a metabolic disorder (Shelton, Ferrigno, & Skinner, 2013; Smith & Amin-Hanjani, 2017).
   C. Brain injury results from brainstem compression and/or reduction in cerebral blood flow; leads to tissue necrosis (Smith & Amin-Hanjani, 2017; Witherspoon & Ashby, 2017).
      1. Displacement or edema of brain tissue
      2. Obstruction of CSF outflow
      3. Increased vascularity associated with tumor growth

Assessment

I. Identification of patients at risk
   A. Patients with cancers of the lung, breast, and kidney, as well as melanoma, who have increased risk for metastases to the brain
   B. Patients with primary tumors of the brain or spinal cord
   C. Patients with a diagnosis of leukemia, lymphoma, or neuroblastoma
   D. Oncology patients with thrombocytopenia, platelet dysfunction, or disseminated intravascular coagulation (DIC) may have bleeding that may cause increased ICP.
   E. Patients with infections such as encephalitis, meningitis, or systemic candidiasis, especially immunocompromised patients.
   F. Patients with syndrome of inappropriate antidiuretic hormone secretion (see Chapter 52).
   G. Patients with history of radiation therapy (RT) to the brain.
   H. Patients with occluded Ommaya reservoir.
   I. Patients treated with high-dose cytosine arabinoside (HiDAC) (Nurgat et al., 2017).
   J. Patients treated with drugs for risk of posterior reversible encephalopathy syndrome (PRES) (e.g., immunosuppressants, immune checkpoint inhibitors, tyrosine kinase inhibitors, certain chemotherapeutic agents) (Dhar, 2017; Hottinger, 2016; Kamiya-Matsuoka et al., 2016; Shah, 2017; Shankar & Banfield, 2017).

II. Signs and symptoms depend on volume, location, and rate of ICP
   A. Early signs and symptoms: may be subtle and include headaches (worse in the mornings, bending over, or during Valsalva maneuvers), nausea, vomiting, weakness (Allen, 2018)
   B. Later signs and symptoms (Allen, 2018; Shelton, Ferrigno, & Skinner, 2013; Smith & Amin-Hanjani, 2017)
      1. Neurologic: headaches, cranial nerve abnormalities, papilledema
         a. Headache pain may be initiated or aggravated by Valsalva maneuver, coughing, vomiting, exercise, or bending over
         b. Headache pain may be described as dull, sharp, or throbbing, and may increase in severity, frequency, and duration over time
         c. Blurred vision (diplopia), photophobia, contralateral pupillary dilation, decreased visual fields
         d. Extremity drifts, ipsilateral weakness
         e. Lethargy, apathy, confusion, restlessness
         f. Speech alterations such as slowed or delayed responses, word confusion
         g. Level of consciousness—sensitive index of the patient's neurologic status: decreased ability to concentrate, personality changes, hemiplegia, hemiparesis, seizures, pupillary changes

TABLE 53.1 Glasgow Coma Scale

	Score
Eye Opening	
Spontaneous	4
Response to verbal command	3
Response to pain	2
No eye opening	1
Best Verbal Response	
Oriented	5
Confused	4
Inappropriate words	3
Incomprehensible sounds	2
No verbal response	1
Best Motor Response	
Obeys commands	6
Localizing response to pain	5
Withdrawal response to pain	4
Flexion to pain	3
Extension to pain	2
No motor response	1

Glasgow Coma Scale score—lowest score is 3 (worst) and highest is 15 (best). Record by the three parameters: eye opening (E), verbal response (V), and motor response (M). (Example: E4V4M4 is a score of 12.) A score of 13 or higher correlates with mild brain injury, scores of 9 to 12 correlate with moderate brain injury, and a score of 8 or less correlates with severe brain injury.

        h. Papilledema (considered cardinal sign of increased ICP), which is a swelling of the optic nerve where it meets the eye (the optic disc) and usually noted bilaterally

        i. Glasgow Coma Scale score less than 8 (Table 53.1)

        j. Abnormal posturing

        k. Temperature elevations

    2. Gastrointestinal (GI)

        a. Nausea/vomiting: often worse in early morning; moderate to severe in intensity; global or localized; may be projectile, sudden, unexpected, not related to food intake

        b. Loss of appetite

    3. Cardiovascular—bradycardia, widening pulse pressure; as ICP increases, blood pressure rises

    4. Respiratory—slow, shallow respirations; tachypnea; Cheyne–Stokes respirations

    5. Cushing triad (bradycardia, respiratory depression, and hypertension)—late and poor prognostic sign ⚠

III. Diagnostic testing

  A. May include contrast-enhanced magnetic resonance imaging (MRI) (often preferred), computed tomography (CT), cerebral angiography, or positron emission tomography (PET) with CT. A negative finding does not rule out increased ICP (Smith & Amin-Hanjani, 2017).

  B. ICP monitoring—per intraventricular, intraparenchymal, subarachnoid, or epidural site (Smith & Amin-Hanjani, 2017); most reliable method to diagnose ICP; goal is to keep ICP at less than 20 mm Hg and cerebral perfusion pressure (CPP) between 60 and 75 mm Hg; risks of ICP monitoring include central nervous system (CNS) infection and intracranial hemorrhage (Czosnyka, Pickard, & Steiner, 2017; Schimph, 2012). ⚠

  C. CT- or MRI-guided stereotactic biopsy for tissue diagnosis if malignancy is suspected cause (Shelton, Ferrigno, & Skinner, 2013)

  D. CSF examination if leptomeningeal metastasis or meningitis is suspected (Shelton, Ferrigno, & Skinner, 2013)

Management

I. Medical management

  A. Surgery

    1. Remove offending cause (such as tumor or hematoma)

    2. Shunt placement: provides an alternative pathway for CSF

    3. Ommaya reservoir placement for intrathecal chemotherapy administration

  B. RT— if radiosensitive tumor is cause; however, RT should be used with caution if elevation of ICP is uncontrolled, as this may cause acute herniation and death (Giglio & Gilbert, 2010). Radiation techniques such as stereotactic radiosurgery, including Cyber-Knife, or brachytherapy could be utilized.

  C. Hyperventilation: the most rapid method to decrease ICP by causing vasoconstriction; decreases cerebral blood volume and ICP; requires patient to be sedated, intubated, and ventilated to a partial pressure of carbon dioxide (PCO_2) between 26 and 30 mm Hg; contraindicated in traumatic head injury and acute stroke (Smith & Amin-Hanjani, 2017). Effects short-lived, and prolonged hyperventilation could lead to increased ICP due to compensating metabolic alkalosis (Allen, 2018).

  D. Pharmacologic measures

    1. Discontinue offending agent as in cases of PRES

    2. Treatment of tumor with chemotherapy or targeted agents

        a. Regional drug delivery such as through the intrathecal or intraventricular (via CSF) routes, circumvents the blood–brain barrier

    3. Corticosteroids may be indicated in setting of brain tumor or CNS infection but could be contraindicated in head injuries, cerebral infarction or intracranial hemorrhage (Allen, 2018; Smith & Amin-Hanjani, 2017).

    4. Osmotherapy—to maintain euvolemia and normo-osmolality to hyperosmolality (Witherspoon & Ashby, 2017)

a. Isotonic fluids such as normal saline. Hypertonic saline expands the intravascular volume, increases blood pressure and increases cerebral blood flow. Continuous infusion or bolus may be utilized. Observe for renal failure, electrolyte disturbances, acute red blood cell (RBC) lysis, or phlebitis (Smith & Amin-Hanjani, 2017). ⚠️

b. Mannitol bolus—decreases reabsorption of water and sodium across renal tubules, creating a diuretic effect. Monitor blood pressure carefully, observe for signs of cardiac overload, and caution in patients with renal dysfunction. ⚠️

5. Anticonvulsant therapy if indicated
6. Antipyretic therapy to reduce fever
7. Sedative agents
8. Loop diuretics (e.g., furosemide) may be given with mannitol to potentiate effect; however, this may exacerbate dehydration and hypokalemia ⚠️
9. Stool softeners as ordered to prevent constipation and straining
10. Antiemetics if indicated

II. Nursing management
A. Position to reduce ICP by maximizing venous outflow from head
1. Head elevation—usually about 30 degrees
2. Avoid excessive flexion or rotation of neck and restrictive neck taping
3. Use of log-roll technique when turning patients, keeping patient passive
4. Avoid prone position or activities that exert pressure on the abdomen
5. Avoid Valsalva maneuver
B. Provide mechanical cooling
C. Minimize endotracheal suctioning
D. Avoid rectal temperatures
E. Maintain a calm environment:
1. Minimizing external stimulation—light, noise, touch, temperature extremes
2. Encouraging calm interactions between the patient and others
3. Teaching about stress reduction strategies to patient and family
4. Developing a daily schedule of activities with appropriate rest periods
F. Maintain bed rest with increasing ICP and progressive symptoms
G. Prevent injury ⚠️
1. Keep bed in lowest position with side rails elevated
2. Use assistive devices as needed
3. Use bed alarms to monitor patient activity
H. Facilitate physical mobility and prevent injury ⚠️
1. Assess skin integrity regularly; inspect pressure points and immobile extremities
2. Use pressure-distributing devices or padding as needed
3. Change position every 2 hours

4. Instruct patient about proper use of assistive devices
5. Assist patient and family to set realistic goals to maintain optimal activity and self-care levels within limitations imposed by the disease
I. Address knowledge deficit
1. Instruct patient on signs and symptoms that might indicate progressive disease
2. Include family or significant other in educational process
3. Assess readiness to learn and preferred learning method
4. Instruct patient about self-care, community resources, emergency contacts
5. Provide information about disease process, interventions, expected outcomes
J. Monitoring
1. Monitor for mental status changes
2. Monitor for changes of decreasing cardiac output (changes in vital signs, decreased urinary output, changes in mentation)
3. Monitor for sensory or motor changes—changes in visual acuity, pupil reactions, verbal expression; decrease in muscle strength, coordination, movement
4. Monitor for associated symptoms such as nausea, vomiting, and headache
5. Monitor for seizure activity
6. Any negative changes of neurologic function require immediate action (Allen, 2018).

Expected Patient Outcomes

I. Progressive perfusion deficit will be recognized early and managed properly
II. Tissue perfusion will be adequate to prevent permanent neurologic damage
III. Patient and/or family will identify signs and symptoms of increased ICP to report to health care team

SPINAL CORD COMPRESSION (SCC)

Overview

I. Definition—a neurologic emergency that occurs when the spinal cord or cauda equina is compromised by direct pressure, vertebral collapse, or both caused by metastatic spread or direct extension of a malignancy; compression results in compromised neurologic function if not treated promptly (Rucker, 2018).
II. Pathophysiology (Rucker, 2018)
A. The spinal cord is a cylindric body of nervous tissue that occupies the upper two-thirds of the vertebral canal. The spinal cord is surrounded by protective bones (vertebral bodies, lamina and pedicles, and spinous processes) (Schiff, 2016).
B. The spinal cord has motor, sensory, and autonomic functions.

C. Compression of the spinal cord may occur because of tumor invasion of the vertebrae and results from subsequent collapse of the spinal cord that causes increased pressure, or because of primary tumors of the spinal cord.

D. Compression of the spinal cord may result in minor changes in motor, sensory, and autonomic function or complete paralysis. SCC is the second most frequent neurologic complication of metastatic cancer.

E. Ambulatory status and extent of neurologic compromise at diagnosis is directly related to prognosis and quality of life.

F. SCC is a poor prognostic sign, and most patients die within a year of diagnosis (Rucker, 2018).

Assessment

I. Identification of patients at risk (Kaplan, 2013; Lo et al., 2015; Rucker, 2018; Schiff, 2016):
   A. Cancers that have a natural history for metastasizing to the bone—breast, lung, prostate, renal, melanoma, non-Hodgkin lymphoma, myeloma
   B. Cancers that metastasize to the brain and spinal cord—lymphoma, seminoma
   C. Primary cancers of the spinal cord—ependymoma, astrocytoma, glioma
   D. History of vertebral compression fractures
   E. Metastatic disease at presentation

II. History
   A. Histology of primary tumor, date of diagnosis, stage at diagnosis, treatment history, history of metastatic disease; responses to treatment and survival following treatment vary among types of cancer.
   B. Time since onset of symptoms; level and degree of compression
   C. Comprehensive pain assessment, including onset, duration, location, intensity, description, and exacerbating and relieving factors
   D. Pre-existing medical problems and current medications

III. Physical examination—presenting signs and symptoms vary, depending on the location and severity of the compression (Kaplan, 2013; Rucker, 2018)
   A. Early signs and symptoms:
      1. Localized pain is the most common initial symptom (96% of patients), often described as dull or achy. Pain may precede other symptoms by up to 2 months (Rucker, 2018).
      2. Neck or back pain—always requires prompt evaluation in cancer patients
   B. Late signs and symptoms (Kaplan, 2013; Khan, Shanholtz, & McCurdy, 2017; Rucker, 2018)—ominous; treatment must be instituted on an emergent basis. ⚠
      1. As SCC compression progresses, pain may become radiating or radicular, and may increase when supine, coughing, sneezing, or with Valsalva maneuvers.

2. Gentle percussion and palpation of the vertebral column, neck flexion, and straight-leg raises—may indicate the level of cord compression
3. Motor weakness or dysfunction is the second most common symptom and may present as heaviness, stiffness, or weakness of extremities and lead to loss of coordination and ataxia. Once patient has progressed to paraplegia, very few will regain mobility. Muscle atrophy can occur (Table 53.2).
4. Sensory loss—regarding light touch, pain, or temperature (occurs less often than motor deficits) (see Table 53.2)
   a. Loss of sensation for deep pressure, vibrations, position
   b. Changes begin distally and move proximally
5. Autonomic dysfunction
   a. Incontinence or retention of urine or stool
   b. Sexual impotence
   c. Loss of sweating below lesion
   C. Grade peripheral sensory neuropathy and motor neuropathy and document according to Common Toxicity Criteria for Adverse Events (CTCAE) criteria

IV. Diagnostic testing
   A. Laboratory testing: no diagnostic laboratory tests exist; however, calcium and serum albumin tests should be examined in patients with bone metastases due to potential hypercalcemia (Kaplan, 2013) ⚠ (see Chapter 52)

TABLE 53.2 Assessment of Motor and Sensory Function

Function	Assessment Techniques
Muscle strength	Upper extremities—ask patient to grip your finger as firmly as possible.
	Lower extremities—ask patient to resist plantar flexion of his or her feet.
Coordination of hands and feet	Ask patient to touch each finger to his or her thumb in rapid sequence.
	Ask patient to turn hand over and back as quickly as possible.
	Ask patient to tap your hand as quickly as possible with the ball of each foot.
Sensory perception	Touch patient along length of extremities and trunk with the blunt and sharp ends of a safety pin, and ask patient to identify as either sharp or dull.
	Ask patient to report the sensation of touch when touched with a wisp of cotton.
	Move one of the patient's fingers and ask if the finger is being moved up or down.
	Touch skin of patient with test tube of hot water and then cold water; ask the patient to describe the temperature.

B. Diagnostic studies (Kaplan, 2013; Khan, Shanholtz, & McCurdy, 2017; Lo et al., 2015; Rucker, 2018; Schiff, 2016)
1. MRI—diagnostic procedure of choice for evaluating SCC; entire spine should be assessed, as multiple sites of metastasis may exist.
2. CT—alternative when MRI unavailable or contraindicated; less sensitive
3. Myelography—used with or without CT when MRI and other imaging modalities are nondiagnostic
4. Spinal radiography—shows bone abnormalities or soft tissue masses; should not be used to diagnose or rule out spinal metastasis
5. PET—both sensitive and specific but less available than MRI; should not be used alone for diagnosis or treatment guidance

Management

I. Medical management (Kaplan, 2013; Lo, et al., 2015; Rucker, 2018; Schiff, Brown, & Shaffrey, 2017)
A. Radiation
1. For radiosensitive tumors such as lymphoma, myeloma, breast, prostate cancers and small cell lung cancers (SCLC)
2. Treatment of choice for most epidural metastases and cord compressions
3. Used alone when no evidence of spinal instability
4. Most common dose is 30 Gy given in 10 fractions
5. Helpful in managing pain even in patients with poor prognosis
6. Stereotactic body radiation therapy (SBRT) standard of care for areas of previous radiation
7. If performed after decompressing surgery, radiation is delayed at least a week
B. Surgery
1. Laminectomy used to decompress a vertebral body in patients with spinal instability and for tumors not responsive to RT
2. Urgency of surgery dependent on neurologic compromise
3. May be used if recurrent tumor is in an area that has received maximal safe radiation dose
C. Pharmacologic interventions
1. Corticosteroids
a. Immediate high initial dose given intravenously (IV); patients may experience a sudden, intense burning or tingling perineal discomfort; slow IV administration may lessen or eliminate this sensation. Taper corticosteroids when discontinued. ⚠
b. Monitor blood glucose and assess for other adverse events such as mania and insomnia. ⚠
c. GI prophylaxis with proton pump inhibitors
2. Analgesics
a. More than 95% of patients with SCC have pain; opioids commonly employed
b. Coanalgesics for neuropathic pain
(1) Anticonvulsants
(2) Antidepressants
c. Observe for adverse events such as constipation, nausea, somnolence, and pruritus ⚠
3. Chemotherapeutic agents
a. For chemosensitive tumors (such as lymphomas, neuroblastoma, germ cell neoplasms and breast cancers)
b. Also manages malignancy in other parts of the body
4. Anticoagulation
a. Patients with SCC have increased risk of thrombus
b. Low-molecular-weight heparin prophylaxis
5. Bowel regimen
a. Needs vary depending upon extent of SCC
6. Bone-remodeling agents to reduce the incidence of skeletal-related events
II. Nursing management
A. Treat emergently within 24 hours of signs of neurologic compromise
B. Promote physical mobility
1. Mobilize the patient based on findings of stable or unstable spine
2. Maintain neutral spine alignment by using log-roll technique until neurologically stable
3. Assist patient to maintain a safe level of independence within the limitations imposed by the cord compression
4. Encourage patient and family to express concerns about the effect of residual limitations on activities of daily living (ADLs) and lifestyle
C. Improve or maintain neurologic function (Kaplan, 2013)
1. Monitor for progression of motor or sensory deficits every 8 hours
2. Monitor bowel and urinary elimination patterns and effectiveness
a. Palpation for bladder distention if interval between voiding increases
b. Record frequency and characteristics of stool with each bowel movement
c. Conduct gentle digital rectal examination to check for impaction if no bowel movement within 3 days, unless neutropenic or thrombocytopenic
d. Record intake and output every 8 hours
3. Monitor for
a. Decrease in muscle strength and coordination
b. Decrease in perception of temperature, touch, position
c. Change in level of consciousness
4. Improve or maintain skin integrity
a. Regularly assess skin integrity and evaluating intervention
b. Institute a skin care regimen

c. Provide instructions to the patient and family about assessing the pressure and temperature of objects, contact with areas of compromised feeling or sensation

5. Increase knowledge of disease process and therapeutic interventions

a. Provide education about reporting any changes in bowel and urinary elimination patterns; pain, sensory and motor function; skin integrity; or sexual dysfunction

b. Provide education about treatment modalities, potential adverse events, self-care

Expected Patient Outcomes

I. SCC is recognized and treated promptly, avoiding permanent neurologic damage

II. Pain is regularly assessed and promptly treated

III. Patient maintains optimal level of physical mobility

SUPERIOR VENA CAVA SYNDROME (SVCS)

Overview

I. Definition: results from compromised venous drainage of the head, neck, upper extremities, and thorax through the superior vena cava (SVC) because of compression or obstruction of the vessel such as by tumor, lymph nodes, or thrombus

II. Pathophysiology (Friedman, et al., 2017; Shelton, 2013; McNally, 2018; Drews and Rabkin, 2017; Khan, Shanholtz, McCurdy, 2017)

A. The SVC is a thin-walled major vessel that carries venous drainage from the head, neck, upper extremities, and upper thorax to the heart.

B. The SVC is located in the mediastinum; surrounded by structures of the sternum, trachea, vertebrae, aorta, right bronchus, lymph nodes, and pulmonary artery.

C. The SVC is a low-pressure vessel easily compressed; compression (acute or gradual) can occur from multiple causes. Right-sided lung cancers are responsible for most cases of SVCS.

D. When obstruction of the SVC occurs, venous return to the heart from the head, neck, thorax, and upper extremities is impaired.

1. Venous pressure and congestion in head, neck, upper extremities, and upper thorax increase but eventually decreases over time as blood flow diverts to multiple smaller collaterals to the azygos vein or the inferior vena cava.

2. Rapid tumor growth often does not allow time to develop collateral flow

3. Decreased cardiac filling and output may ensue

4. Hemodynamic compromise occurs from mass effect on the heart

5. Concomitant thrombosis often occurs

Assessment

I. Identification of patients at risk (Drews & Rabkin, 2017)

A. Presence of chest malignancy, most often non–small cell lung cancer (NSCLC) and SCLC, followed by lymphoma. Other malignancies can cause SVC syndrome.

B. Presence of central venous catheters and pacemakers.

C. Previous RT to the mediastinum secondary to vascular fibrosis.

D. Associated conditions (e.g., fungal infection, benign tumors, aortic aneurysm)

E. Cardiovascular disease

II. History (Khan, Shanholtz, McCurdy, 2017; Shelton, 2013; McNally, 2018)

A. Assess for risk factors

B. Assess rapidity of symptom onset

C. Symptoms more pronounced in the morning or when bending over and improve after being upright for several hours

D. Assess for symptoms such as dyspnea (most common symptom), sensation of head fullness, headache, blurred vision, nasal stuffiness, hoarseness, dysphagia, nonproductive cough, need to sleep in an upright position, chest pain

E. Mild symptoms may disappear after patient has been upright for a few hours

III. Physical examination (Friedman et al., 2017; McNally, 2018; Shelton, 2013)

A. Redness and edema in conjunctivae and around the eyes and face

B. Swelling of the neck, arms, hands; men may have problems buttoning shirt collars (Stokes sign)

C. Neck and thoracic vein distention—with visible collateral veins

D. Hoarseness

E. Women may experience swelling of their breasts

F. Dysphagia, hoarseness, hemoptysis

G. Horner syndrome—the combination of drooping of the eyelid (ptosis) and constriction of the pupil (miosis), sometimes accompanied by decreased sweating (anhidrosis) of the face on the same side

H. Later signs:

1. Cyanosis of upper torso

2. Symptoms of increased ICP—severe headache, visual disturbances, blurred vision, dizziness, syncope, irritability, changes in mental status

3. Stridor, signs of congestive heart failure

4. Tachycardia, tachypnea, orthopnea

5. Hypotension, absence of peripheral pulses

I. Grade toxicities according to CTCAE criteria

IV. Diagnostic testing (Drews & Rabkin, 2017; Friedman et al., 2017; McNalley, 2018)

A. CT of the thorax (contrast or helical)—the preferred diagnostic test; often identifies cause of SVCS and presence of collateral vessels

B. MRI—sensitive for SVCS, beneficial in those who cannot tolerate contrast; may be complicated by inability to tolerate supine position, longer scanning time, higher cost

C. PET useful when planning the radiation field and to determine if the cause is malignant or benign

D. Contrast venography is more invasive but useful to determine the extent of thrombus formation and if stent placement or surgery is planned.

E. Chest radiography results are usually abnormal, showing mediastinal widening and pleural effusion.

F. Additional tests to determine the histologic diagnosis of the primary condition include bronchoscopy, bone marrow biopsy, mediastinoscopy, thoracentesis, sputum analysis, and needle biopsy of palpable lymph nodes.

G. Evaluation of laboratory data—comparison of available laboratory data against previous and normal values.
   1. Arterial blood gases
   2. Electrolytes, kidney function
   3. Complete blood cell count (CBC)
   4. Coagulation studies

Management

I. Medical management (Drews & Rabkin, 2017; McNally, 2018; Shelton, 2013)

A. Goals of treatment include relief of the obstruction and treatment of the underlying cause and presenting symptoms (Drews & Rabkin, 2017; Friedman et al., 2017; Khan, Shanholtz, McCurdy, 2017; Shelton, 2013)
   1. Treatment and prognosis determined by rapidity of onset and cause of obstruction.
   2. Histologic diagnosis necessary for treatment of the causes of the primary tumor, but treatment of airway obstruction or laryngeal edema should not be delayed.

B. Thrombolytic therapy or tissue plasminogen activators may be used to treat a thrombosis that is catheter induced.
   1. Systemic anticoagulation may also be indicated, especially after stent placement.
   2. Observe for complications related to stent placement, such as infection, pulmonary embolus, stent migration, hematoma at insertion site, bleeding or perforation of the SVC. ⚠

C. Corticosteroids—may reduce edema or inflammation (e.g., to prevent postradiation edema); useful in steroid-responsive malignancies. Blood glucose should be monitored closely. ⚠

D. Diuretics—may reduce edema and intravascular volume.

E. Antineoplastic therapy alone or in conjunction with radiation in patients who have chemosensitive disease such as SCLC, non-Hodgkin lymphoma, or germ cell cancer.
   1. Antineoplastic therapy may follow initial emergent treatment.
   2. Alternative sites of administration (such as femoral vein port-a-cath or dorsal foot vein) may be utilized. If vesicant agents are prescribed, great care must be taken to avoid extravasation. ⚠

F. Radiation therapy
   1. The primary treatment for SVCS if the patient has NSCLC but often used in other types of malignancies.
   2. RT also used as initial treatment if a histologic diagnosis cannot be made or the clinical status of the patient is deteriorating.

G. Percutaneous intravascular stent placement
   1. Most effective treatment modality when urgent intervention needed; restores blood flow, and symptoms rapidly resolve.
   2. Percutaneous balloon angioplasty may be necessary to enlarge the vascular lumen prior to stent placement.
   3. Stent placement will require at least short-term anticoagulation (Calsina Juscafresa et al., 2017; Khan, Shanholtz, McCurdy, 2017; Niu, Xu, Cheng, & Cao, 2017).
   4. Observe for procedure complications such as acute pulmonary edema and bleeding (Morin et al., 2017).

H. Remove the central venous catheter to avoid embolization.

I. Surgical reconstruction of SVC is rarely required because of effectiveness of stent placement. Surgical resection of the tumor is rare because of the poor prognosis in many patients with SVCS.

II. Nursing management (Drews & Rabkin, 2017; McNally, 2018; Shelton, 2013)

A. Maintain adequate gas exchange (Drews & Rabkin, 2017; Shelton, 2013)
   1. Maintain airway
   2. Position in Fowler or semi-Fowler position to decrease edema, dyspnea, and hydrostatic pressure
   3. Instruct patient to avoid Valsalva maneuver or other straining activities
   4. Assist with ADLs to conserve breathing and energy
   5. Assess for progressive respiratory distress
   6. Administer oxygen as ordered

B. Maintain adequate cardiac output (Shelton, 2013)
   1. Monitor for changes in tissue perfusion (decreased peripheral pulses, decrease in blood pressure, cyanosis)
   2. Monitor for changes of decreasing cardiac output (changes in vital signs, decreased urinary output, changes in mentation)
   3. Monitor intake, output, and weight

C. Increase knowledge of disease process and therapeutic interventions (Shelton, 2013)
 1. Provide information about critical signs and symptoms that might indicate progressive disease
 2. Include family or significant other in educational process
 3. Assess readiness to learn and preferred learning method
 4. Instruct patient in self-care measures, community resources, and emergent contacts
 5. Educate about disease process, interventions, expectations of outcome

D. Prevent injury (Drews & Rabkin, 2017; Shelton, 2013) ⚠
 1. Avoid venipunctures, IV fluid administration, intramuscular (IM) injections, or measurement of blood pressure in the upper extremities
 2. Remove jewelry (e.g., rings) and restrictive clothing
 3. Assess for changes in neurologic or mental status
 4. Monitor for signs and symptoms of adverse effects of anticoagulant therapy—petechiae; ecchymosis; bleeding—gums, nose, urinary tract, GI system
 5. Monitor for signs and symptoms of adverse effects of steroid therapy—muscle weakness, mood swings, steroid-induced glycosuria, dyspepsia, insomnia

Expected Patient Outcomes

I. Early recognition and prompt management of SVCS will provide rapid relief of symptoms.
II. The underlying cause of SVCS will be identified and treated.
III. Dyspnea will be regularly monitored; signs of cardiac compromise will be promptly managed.

CARDIAC TAMPONADE

Overview

I. Definition—a life-threatening situation of excessive accumulation of fluid in the pericardial sac exerting extrinsic pressure on the cardiac chambers, resulting in impaired intracardiac filling, decreased cardiac output, and compromised cardiac function
II. Pathophysiology (Appleton, Gillam, & Koulogiannis, 2017; Hoit, 2017; Kearns & Walley, 2017; Khan, Shanholtz, & McCurdy, 2017)
 A. The pericardium is a two-layered sac (parietal and visceral layers) surrounding the heart
 B. As intrapericardial pressure increases, the following occur:
  1. The space between the two layers is the pericardial cavity.
  2. The cavity normally is filled with 10 to 50 mL of fluid produced by the mesothelial cells of the visceral pericardium. This fluid between opposing layers of the heart allows the heart to move without friction.
  3. Recesses and sinuses may accommodate a limited increase of pericardial fluid.
  4. Fluid accumulation in the pericardial sac occurs secondary to the following:
   a. Direct or metastatic tumor invasion to the pericardial sac
   b. Fibrosis of the pericardial sac related to RT
   c. Infections causing pericardial effusions
   d. Obstruction of mediastinal lymph nodes
   e. Increased capillary permeability from chemotherapy or biotherapy
   f. Direct trauma to the chest
   g. Improper insertion of central line or pacemaker
  5. Cardiac chambers are compressed, and left ventricular filling decreases
  6. The ability of the heart to pump decreases
  7. Cardiac output decreases, and blood pressure falls
  8. Impaired systemic perfusion occurs, and cardiogenic shock may follow
III. Rate of pericardial fluid increase is more important than volume accrued because the slow accumulation allows time for the pericardium to expand. Acute increases may cause severe symptoms, even with a small amount of fluid (Khan, Shanholtz, & McCurdy, 2017)
IV. Malignant pericardial involvement has a poor prognosis

Assessment

I. Identification of patients at risk (Kearns & Walley, 2017; Story, 2013)
 A. Patients with primary tumors of the heart, including mesothelioma and sarcomas (including Kaposi sarcoma)
 B. Patients with metastatic tumors to the pericardium—lung, breast, GI tract, leukemia, Hodgkin or non-Hodgkin lymphoma, sarcoma, melanoma
 C. Patients who have received more than 4000 cGy of radiation to a field in which the heart is included
 D. Patients receiving chemotherapy or biotherapy associated with increased capillary permeability (e.g., anthracyclines, interferon, interleukin, granulocyte–macrophage colony-stimulating factor)
 E. Those with comorbidities such as heart disease, connective tissue disorders, myxedema (dry, waxy, non-pitting edema with abnormal deposits of mucin in the skin often associated with hypothyroidism), tuberculosis, aneurysms, renal failure, and history of cardiac surgery (e.g., valve surgery)
II. History
 A. Early signs and symptoms (Appleton, Gillam, & Koulogiannis, 2017; Kearns & Walley, 2017; Khan, Shanholtz, & McCurdy, 2017; Story, 2013)
  1. May be nonspecific
  2. Exertional dyspnea
  3. Tachycardia, chest pain
  4. Restlessness
  5. Fatigue, malaise
 B. Late signs and symptoms (Appleton, Gillam, & Koulogiannis, 2017; Kearns & Walley, 2017; Story, 2013)

1. Retrosternal chest pain relieved by leaning forward and intensified when lying supine or by inspiration; may radiate to neck and jaw; chest pain may be difficult to differentiate from a myocardial infarction. ⚠
2. Oliguria
3. Peripheral edema
4. Diaphoresis
5. Anxiety and agitation, mental status changes
6. Hiccups
7. Hoarseness, dysphagia
8. Chest pain—may disappear
9. Vague, right upper quadrant pain resulting from hepatic venous congestion

III. Physical examination (Appleton, Gillam, & Koulogiannis, 2017; Kearns & Walley, 2017; Khan, Shanholtz, & McCurdy, 2017; Story, 2013)
  A. Beck triad: muffled heart sounds, hypotension, and increased jugular venous pressure may be seen in about one third of patients, less common in chronic effusions
  B. Pulsus paradoxus (decrease in blood pressure of more than 10 mm Hg with inspiration) is found in over 75% of patients with tamponade (Appleton, Gillam, & Koulogiannis, 2017). An ominous finding. ⚠
  C. Decreased systolic pressure and rising diastolic pressure (narrow pulse pressure)
  D. Pericardial friction rub is common but may be absent in large pericardial effusions
  E. Jugular venous distention
  F. Tachycardia—more than 100 beats/min; a protective mechanism
  G. Weak or absent apical and peripheral pulses, heart palpitations
  H. Tachypnea, orthopnea
  I. Increased central venous pressure (CVP)
  J. Altered levels of consciousness
  K. Cyanosis, central and peripheral; mottled, cool skin
  L. Delayed capillary refill

IV. Diagnostic testing (Appleton, Gillam, & Koulogiannis, 2017; Kearns & Walley, 2017; Khan, Shanholtz, & McCurdy, 2017; Story, 2013)
  A. Chest radiography shows enlarged transverse pericardial diameter (water bottle heart) after more than 200 mL of fluid has accumulated; however, it is not a definitive diagnostic tool.
  B. CT is very useful because it can also reveal pleural effusion, masses, or pericardial thickening; however, it may overestimate the volume of effusion. It can reveal whether effusion is hemorrhagic and estimate pericardial thickness.
  C. Echocardiography is the initial and most precise diagnostic test and should be repeated frequently to monitor for progression. Effusion, collapse of right or left atrium, respiratory variation in flow velocities, and dilation of inferior vena cava may be seen.
  D. Electrocardiography (ECG) results vary, depending on the extent of the tamponade; signs similar to

pericarditis (elevation of ST segments with reciprocal ST depression in aVR. T-wave inversions may be seen with large pericardial effusions) may be seen. Typically, sinus tachycardia, low QRS voltage, and electrical alternans are present.
  E. Cardiac catheterization may demonstrate right-sided pressures and equalizations of the right atrial, right ventricular, and pulmonary capillary wedge pressures.
  F. MRI is very sensitive in the detection of effusions as small as 30 mL; however, it requires more time and involves increased cost.
  G. Evaluation of laboratory data.
    1. Arterial blood gas values if patient has respiratory distress
    2. Electrolyte values

Management

I. Medical management (Kearns & Walley, 2017; Khan, Shanholtz, & McCurdy, 2017; McCanny & Colreavy, 2017; Story, 2013)
  A. Emergent pericardiocentesis is the treatment for acute pericardial tamponade.
    1. Pericardiocentesis is the temporary removal of excess pericardial fluid.
    2. Usually performed under ultrasound.
    3. Cytology testing of fluid may be performed.
      a. Bloody fluid is associated with a positive cytology test result.
      b. Cytology testing has a significant false-negative rate.
    4. About half of malignant pericardial effusions will reaccumulate; continue to monitor for tamponade.
    5. Observe for complications such as bleeding, change in vital signs, cardiac arrhythmias, infection, and abdominal or shoulder pain. ⚠
  B. Pericardial window is a surgical opening of the pericardium to allow fluid drainage. Alternatively, an indwelling catheter may be placed.
  C. Total pericardectomy is the removal of the pericardial sac for patients with constrictive or chronic pericarditis.
  D. Percutaneous balloon pericardiotomy (an alternative to surgical pericardial window) involves a balloon being used to create a pericardial window by stretching the pericardium
  E. For surgical interventions, it is important to be aware of possible delay in scheduling the procedure and to ensure patient stability. Local anesthesia is preferred because anesthesia with endotracheal intubation may cause life-threatening hypotension and cardiac arrest. Surgical procedures may be contraindicated in thrombocytopenia and with anticoagulation therapy.
  F. RT may be performed to treat radiosensitive tumors of the pericardium. RT is contraindicated in radiation pericarditis and when area involved has previously received radiation.

G. Volume resuscitation is done to correct hypovolemia. Monitor for negative changes in hemodynamic stability due to fluid overload. ⚠

H. Pericardial sclerosis (to prevent recurrence of pericardial effusion) is an instillation through a pericardial catheter of an agent (e.g., doxycycline [Doxy 100], thiotepa [Thioplex], bleomycin [Blenoxane], mitomycin C [Mitomycin], sterile talc) that causes inflammation and subsequent fibrosis.

I. Pharmacologic interventions (Kearns & Walley, 2017; Khan, Shanholtz, & McCurdy, 2017; McCanny & Colreavy, 2017; Story, 2013)

1. Systemic antineoplastic therapy may be used for treating chemotherapy-sensitive malignancies such as lymphoma, breast cancer, or SCLC.

2. Corticosteroids may be used after drainage of the effusion but are not used in urgent treatment.

3. Analgesics as indicated.

4. Any intervention that lowers the heart rate (e.g., beta blocker or anesthesia) could cause dangerous decrease in cardiac output. ⚠

II. Nursing management

A. Conduct frequent, regular assessment of cardiovascular status, evaluating for instability (e.g., sinus tachycardia, drop in blood pressure)

B. Assess character and amount of drainage from pericardial catheter if present

C. Assess catheter site for signs and symptoms of infection

D. Conduct frequent, regular assessment of respiratory status, evaluating for changes

E. Administer oxygen therapy as ordered

F. Position with head of bed (HOB) elevated

Expected Patient Outcomes

I. Patient will maintain optimal cardiac output.

II. Patient will maintain optimal respiratory status.

III. The oncology nurse systematically and regularly evaluates the patient's responses to interventions for cardiac tamponade.

BOWEL OBSTRUCTION

Overview

I. Definition: cessation of forward movement of bowel contents

II. Pathophysiology (Obita, et al., 2016; Rami Reddy & Cappell, 2017; Shimura & Joh, 2016; Yeh & Bordeianou, 2017)

A. Mechanical obstruction—most common in end-stage cancer, may be partial or complete, and may be caused by extrinsic or intrinsic factors.

B. Functional obstructions—caused by changes to peristalsis such as by infiltration of bowel muscle by tumor; includes fecal impaction.

C. Small-intestine obstructions are more common.

D. Large-bowel obstructions (about 25% of bowel obstructions) most often at or distal to the transverse colon.

E. Bowel dilation occurs proximal to the obstruction to due intestinal stasis that increases gas from bacterial proliferation and fermentation of ingested food. Mural edema occurs, and the bowel loses its absorptive ability, leading to accumulation of fluids. This leads to bowel distention because of the stationary solids, intestinal fluids, and gas. Tension increases in the intestinal wall, and an increased risk for bowel perforation exists (see section on bowel perforation later). Transudative fluid leakage from the intestinal lumen to the peritoneal cavity may occur. Loss of fluids in addition to emesis secondary to the obstruction may lead to hypovolemia and electrolyte disturbance. If obstruction is not relieved, bowel ischemia and necrosis may result.

F. Colorectal obstruction may lead to perforation, colonic necrosis, and septic shock.

G. Causes of obstructions:

1. Cancer, most often colorectal cancer, and may be the presenting symptom

a. Malignant obstruction occurs in 8% to 29% of colorectal cancers and 10% to 50% of ovarian cancers.

b. Cholangiocarcinoma, pancreatic, and gallbladder carcinoma are the most common tumors causing duodenal obstruction.

c. Intraluminal tumors that may occlude the lumen or act as a point of intussusception.

d. Intramural tumors that may extend to the mucosa and obstruct the lumen or impair peristalsis.

e. Mesenteric and omental masses or malignant adhesions that may kink or angulate the bowel, creating an extramural obstruction.

f. Tumors that infiltrate into the mesentery bowel muscle or the enteric or celiac plexus and cause dysmotility.

2. Postoperative intra-abdominal adhesions—entrap a loop of intestine and contract, causing an obstruction and possibly strangulation; may develop a few days after surgery or many years later

3. Nonsurgical adhesions after an infection such as peritonitis or after RT; may occur at any time after the infection or completion of RT

4. Hernias with colonic incarceration

5. Miscellaneous conditions such as inflammatory bowel disease

6. Volvulus: twisting of the intestine that may cut off blood flow; most common benign cause of bowel obstruction

7. Diverticulitis—repetitive bouts causing strictures

8. Pseudo-obstruction from paraneoplastic destruction of enteric neurons in rare cases

9. Severe ileus caused by:

a. Pharmacologic agents: anticholinergic drugs, opioids, certain antineoplastic agents and antihypertensive agents, antidiarrheals/antispasmodics

b. Medical conditions: pancreatitis, gastroenteritis, spinal cord injury, hypokalemia, diabetic ketoacidosis, myocardial infarction, stroke, and other comorbid conditions

10. Objects blocking the intestinal lumen—for example, foreign bodies and fecal or barium impaction

III. Poor prognostic factor in colorectal cancer

Assessment

I. Identification of patients at risk (Yeh & Bordeianou, 2017)
  A. Disease related: cancers such as colorectal, ovarian, pancreatic most common
  B. Treatment related
    1. Prior abdominal surgery due to adhesive bowel disease (more common in small-bowel obstructions)
    2. Stricture formation from prior colorectal resection
    3. Surgical trauma to neurogenic pathways to intestines, rectum, or both
    4. RT to abdominal area
  C. Previous intestinal obstruction
  D. Frequent intestinal inflammation from diseases such as diverticulitis, colitis, inflammatory bowel disease
  E. Abdominal wall hernia
  F. Chronic constipation, fecal impaction
  G. Peritoneal carcinomatosis (Lambert & Wiseman, 2018)
II. History (Yeh & Bordeianou, 2017)
  A. Abdominal pain and intestinal colic from intestinal stretching and pressure of peristalsis as the bowel tries to push its contents past the obstruction.
    1. Assess characteristics of pain (description, timing, duration, location, intensity, associated symptoms)
    2. May describe as cramping and spasmodic in mechanical obstructions (every 20–30 minutes) or as diffuse, constant, and less intense pain (may be described as pressure or fullness) in functional obstructions
    3. In partial obstructions, pain may be described as cramping pain after eating
    4. In complete obstructions, pain intensifies and comes in waves or spasms as the bowel tries to push intestinal contents past the obstruction
    5. With strangulation pain is constant and severe pain intensified with movement
    6. A sudden relief of pain followed by more severe pain may indicate bowel perforation (see section on bowel perforation later)
  B. Nausea and vomiting
    1. Small-bowel obstructions—more severe nausea and vomiting
    2. Gastric outlet obstruction—sour emesis that is not bile-colored and often contains undigested food
    3. Proximal small-intestine obstruction—rapid-onset, bitter, bile-stained emesis that may be projectile

4. Distal small-intestine obstruction or colonic obstruction with an incompetent ileocecal valve—orange-brown, malodorous, feculent emesis
  C. Anorexia, appetite changes
  D. Change in bowel habits—constipation to obstipation
    1. May experience lack of bowel movements and flatus or may have paradoxical diarrhea (if partial blockage exists)
    2. Bowel may evacuate below an obstruction
  E. Bloating, abdominal distention
  F. Assess current medications
  G. Note endocrine and immunologic history
  H. Dietary history
III. Physical examination (Lambert & Wiseman, 2018; Rami Reddy & Cappell, 2017; Yeh & Bordeianou, 2017)
  A. Immediate assessment for signs of dehydration, shock, or abdominal compartment syndrome ⚠️
  B. Presentation will vary according to severity, location, duration, and etiology of the bowel obstruction
  C. Abdominal
    1. Distention: baseline measurement of abdominal girth should be obtained and section of measurement marked. Serial exams are needed.
    2. Abnormal bowel sounds:
      a. Mechanical obstruction: intermittent borborygmi (loud prolonged gurgles of hyperperistalsis)
      b. Nonmechanical:
        (1) Proximal to obstruction—high-pitched, tinkling, or hyperactive bowel sounds that may be heard in clusters or rushes
        (2) Distal to the obstruction—bowel sounds hypoactive or absent
        (3) Hypoactive, low-pitched gurgles or weak tinkles
        (4) Absent bowel sounds indicating a paralytic ileus
    3. Abdominal palpation:
      a. Boardlike abdomen may indicate peritonitis
      b. Abdominal tympany noted over air-filled bowel
      c. Abdominal dullness noted over fluid-filled bowel
      d. Abdominal tenderness often present but does not correlate well with location of obstruction
      e. Note surgical scars
      f. Assess for abdominal hernia, abdominal mass, hepatomegaly, lymphadenopathy
      g. Rebound tenderness, guarding may indicate ischemia or bowel perforation
    4. Rectal examination may note fecal impaction or rectal mass
  D. Vital signs:
    1. Pyrexia may indicate mucosal ischemia and sepsis
    2. Tachycardia, hypotension, and orthostasis could indicate dehydration
  E. Dry mucous membranes and poor skin turgor may indicate dehydration
  F. May appear restless and acutely ill

IV. Diagnostic testing (Ramanathan, Ojili, Vassa, & Nagar, 2017; Rami Reddy & Cappell, 2017; Yeh & Bordeianou, 2017)
  A. Abdominal radiography: less sensitive than CT
  B. CT of the abdomen: highly sensitive and specific
    1. Can identify multifocal disease, metastatic disease, ascites, or carcinomatosis
    2. Can identify ischemia, necrosis, or perforation
  C. Lower endoscopy may assist in patients with chronic symptoms or with nondiagnostic CT
  D. MRI:
    1. More time consuming and expensive
    2. Useful in persons with Crohn disease and when radiation is a concern, such as pregnant patients
  E. Abdominal ultrasound
    1. Useful in pregnancy and in children
    2. Poor diagnostic ability in early obstruction
  F. Laboratory studies: CBC with differential, electrolyte panel; carcinoembryonic antigen (CEA) if imaging shows mass consistent with colorectal malignancy

Management

I. Medical management (Lambert & Wiseman, 2018; Obita et al., 2016; Shimura & Joh, 2016; Yeh & Bordeianou, 2017)
  A. Initial management is supportive care, and subsequent management depends on etiology, location, comorbidities, prognosis, and goals of treatment (Obita et al., 2016; Rami Reddy & Cappell, 2017; Shimura & Joh, 2016; Yeh & Bordeianou, 2017)
  B. Chemotherapy/targeted therapy
    1. If surgery cannot be performed, or before surgery as neoadjuvant treatment, or after surgery as adjuvant treatment
    2. After a stent placement
  C. IV fluid therapy for dehydration and correction of electrolyte abnormalities
  D. Pharmacologic management
    1. Low-dose steroids to decreased bowel wall edema and to decrease nausea
    2. Antiemetic agents
    3. Octreotide to decrease intestinal secretions and stretching of bowel wall, thus decreasing pain
    4. Hyoscine butylbromide or scopolamine butylbromide
    5. Metoclopramide
  E. Flexible sigmoidoscopy to initially decompress colon allowing time for planning surgical intervention
  F. GI stenting allows time to plan surgical intervention or for palliation in advanced disease
  G. Surgical management:
    1. Ostomy alone for fecal diversion
    2. Colectomy with primary anastomosis with or without ostomy
    3. Hartmann procedure: resection of the rectosigmoid colon with closure of the rectal stump and formation of an end colostomy

  4. Emergent surgery has worse outcomes than elective surgery with more complications (such as sepsis and organ failure) and higher rates of local recurrence, as well as metastatic disease and lower 5-year survival rates
II. Nursing management
  A. Obtain dietary consultation for possible total parenteral nutrition
  B. Provide patient comfort measures
    1. Ensure a relaxing environment
    2. Position patient on side and support with pillows
    3. Provide frequent oral care; use of moistened sponge sticks; avoidance of lemon or glycerin swabs
  C. Provide nasogastric tube care:
    1. Assess pressure around nostrils every shift
    2. Apply a water-soluble lubricant to nasal mucosa
    3. Irrigate the tube with normal saline
    4. Elevate HOB to 45 degrees to improve ventilation and prevent aspiration
  D. Monitor for complications related to bowel obstruction
    1. Assess for signs and symptoms of dehydration—dry mouth and lips, poor skin turgor, decreased urinary output
    2. Assess for interference with deep breathing related to abdominal distention
    3. Assess for signs and symptoms of peritonitis—boardlike abdomen, increased pain on movement, shallow respirations, tachycardia
    4. Measure of abdominal girth during every shift
    5. Monitor intake and output ratio, including gastric output

Expected Patient Outcomes

I. Patient will have adequate pain control.
II. Patient has adequate fluid volume and electrolyte balance.
III. Patient receives adequate nutrition while bowel is obstructed.

BOWEL PERFORATION
Overview

I. Definition: a full-thickness injury of the bowel wall allowing bowel contents to leak out
II. Pathophysiology (Cahalane, 2017; Lee-Kong & Lisle, 2015; Li et al., 2016; Rogalski, et al., 2015)
  A. Perforation of the bowel may happen acutely or indolently. Perforation may be due to direct trauma or spontaneously.
  B. When the bowel perforates, leakage of fluids into the abdominal cavity may cause peritonitis, or the fluid may be contained, as with an abscess or fistula formation. This depends on the location of the perforation and the patient's immune response. Inflammation after perforation could lead to abdominal compartment syndrome.
  C. Clinical presentation depends on the organ affected, what is released from the bowel, and the immune response.

D. Causes:
   1. Tumor—most commonly colorectal cancers; poorer outcomes are noted in patients with colorectal cancer who present with perforation.
   2. Instrumentation—includes endoscopies, stent placement, endoscopic sclerotherapy, nasogastric intubation, and esophageal dilation.
   3. Procedures not directly related to the bowel such as chest tube insertion, peritoneal dialysis catheter insertion, paracentesis, peritoneal lavage, percutaneous drainage of fluid collections/abscesses.
   4. Surgery
   5. Blunt, penetrating injury
   6. Bowel obstruction (see earlier section)
      a. Perforation usually occurs proximal to the obstruction.
      b. Pressure increases, exceeding intestinal perfusion pressure. This leads to ischemia and then necrosis, breaking down the bowel wall.
      c. Diastatic rupture occurs when pressure increases, causing the bowel wall to split with no necrosis present.
   7. Inflammation
   8. Peptic ulcer disease
   9. Corrosive medications/agents
      a. Acetylsalicylic acid (ASA) and nonsteroidal anti-inflammatory drugs (NSAIDs)
      b. Glucocorticoids
      c. Antibiotics
      d. Potassium supplements
      e. Immunosuppression therapy
      f. Chemotherapy
      g. Iron supplementation
   10. Violent retching
   11. Hernia
   12. Inflammatory bowel disease such as Crohn disease
E. Immunosuppression increases the risk for perforation.
F. Serious complications of GI tract perforations are abdominal compartment syndrome, tension pneumothorax, tension pneumoperitoneum, subcutaneous emphysema, and peritonitis.

Assessment

I. Identification of patients at risk (Cahalane, 2017; Teixeira et al, 2015)
   A. Colorectal cancers or other abdominal cancers or metastatic disease
   B. Bowel obstruction
   C. Recent GI procedures such as endoscopy, stent placement
   D. History of diverticula
   E. Comorbid diseases such as immunosuppression, diabetes, cirrhosis, HIV, inflammatory bowel disease
   F. Recent abdominal surgery, particularly emergent surgery
   G. Certain medication use (see Causes section earlier)
   H. Severe nausea and vomiting with violent retching
   I. Hernia

II. History (Cahalane, 2017; Schmidt, et al., 2016)
   A. Carefully assess patients complaining of neck, chest, or abdominal pain.
      1. Assess characteristics of pain (description, timing, duration, location, intensity, associated symptoms)
      2. Patients may be able to pinpoint the precise time of perforation, noting a sudden relief of pain, followed by more severe pain, which may indicate bowel perforation
      3. Pain may be present in the shoulder or psoas muscles
   B. Assess for dysphagia
   C. Medication review
   D. Assess for risk factors as noted earlier
   E. Assess for history of surgery (recent or remote), procedures, prior malignancies
   F. Assess postoperative wounds for drainage

III. Physical examination (Cahalane, 2017)
   A. Abdomen
      1. Mass may be palpated
      2. Abdomen may be tender and/or distended (distention more common in small-bowel perforation)
   B. Rectal—mass or abscess may be palpable on digital rectal exam
   C. Signs of sepsis
      1. Hemodynamic instability, may or may not be febrile
      2. Mental status changes
      3. Organ dysfunction
      4. Ill appearing
      5. Initially vital signs may be normal or mildly tachycardic or hypothermic
   D. Neck and chest
      1. Assess for facial swelling
      2. Palpate/percuss/auscultate for any signs of effusion

IV. Diagnostic testing (Cahalane, 2017)
   A. Laboratory studies: CBC, electrolytes, blood urea nitrogen (BUN), creatinine, liver function tests, amylase, lipase, C-reactive protein
   B. Radiograph of the chest and abdomen—however, cannot rule out a perforation or determine location of perforation
   C. CT is the most sensitive and specific modality
   D. Endoscopy may be useful in certain situations
   E. Barium should not be used as an oral contrast agent ⚠
   F. Abdominal surgical exploration

Management

I. Medical management (Cahalane, 2017; Rogalski et al., 2015)
   A. Initial management will likely occur in intensive care unit
   B. Antibiotics—broad spectrum until known suspected site of perforation

C. Proton pump inhibitors for patients with upper GI tract perforations

D. Analgesics

E. Stent placement

F. Endoscopic procedure—closure of perforation (Li et al., 2016; Schmidt et al., 2016)

G. Surgery—immediate consult if perforation is suspected ⚠

II. Nursing management (Cahalane, 2017; Rogalski et al., 2015; Schmidt et al., 2016)

A. Monitor drainage of effusion or abscess

B. Provide nutritional support

C. Stent placement

D. Position the patient to reduce the risk of intraluminal content leakage

Expected Patient Outcomes

I. Patient will have adequate pain control.

II. Patient has adequate fluid volume and electrolyte balance.

III. Patient receives adequate nutrition during emergent treatment and after.

IV. Signs of sepsis are noted early and promptly managed.

PNEUMONITIS

Overview

I. Definition: inflammation of the interstitial lung parenchyma with interstitial and alveolar infiltrates caused by a noninfectious source such as a chemical or radiation treatment

II. Pathophysiology (King, 2017a; King, 2017b; Maldonado & Limper, 2016; Postow & Wolchok, 2018)

A. Pharmacologic treatment–induced pneumonitis pathogenesis is not well understood. It is postulated that lung injury results from direct cytotoxicity.

1. Injury to pneumocytes and alveolar epithelial cells causes release of cytokines resulting in endothelial dysfunction, capillary leak syndrome, and pulmonary edema.

2. Inflammatory cells recruited to the site of injury, causing further cellular damage.

3. Oxidative injury from free oxygen radicals and proteases may occur.

4. Certain agents that target epidermal growth factor receptor (EGFR) may impair alveolar repair mechanisms.

5. Fibroblasts proliferate, leading to the production of collagen, widening of alveolar septae, and subsequent alveolar exudate. Resolution occurs here with some patients, although others will continue to have fibrotic progression.

6. Alveolar hemorrhage may occur (Maldonado & Limper, 2017).

B. Pathophysiology of radiation pneumonitis (Bledsoe, Nath, & Decker, 2017; Kroschinsky et al., 2017)

1. Direct cytotoxic damage to type II pneumocytes and vascular endothelial cells occurs and subsequently:

a. Immediate phase—an inflammatory response that causes leukocyte infiltration, resulting in intra-alveolar edema and vascular congestion.

b. Latent phase—thick secretions are produced due to increase in goblet cells and ciliary malfunction.

c. Acute exudate phase—hyaline membrane formation, proliferation of type II pneumocytes, sloughing of epithelial and endothelium. Patient begins having symptoms of radiation pneumonitis usually within 4 to 12 weeks of completion of radiation.

d. Intermediate phase—repair of the lung begins; dissolution of hyaline membranes, migration of fibroblasts, and capillary regeneration occur.

e. Fibrotic phase—fibrosis is progressive as fibroblasts deposit collagen resulting in diminished lung volume.

2. Radiation recall pneumonitis may occur when a subsequent injury occurs, such as with cytotoxic chemotherapy (such as carmustine, doxorubicin, etoposide, gefitinib, gemcitabine, paclitaxel, and trastuzumab)

C. Several subtypes of pneumonitis have been identified:

1. Cryptogenic

2. Ground-glass opacities

3. Interstitial—most acute onset and rapidly progresses (King, 2017)

4. Hypersensitivity

5. Not otherwise specified

D. Causes:

1. Radiation to chest (Bledsoe, Nath, & Decker, 2017; Olivier & Peikert, 2017)

a. Risk varies by type of radiation given, dose, dose–time factor, use of induction or concomitant chemotherapy, and volume of lung irradiated.

2. Pharmacologic agents:

a. ALK inhibitors (Maldonado & Limper, 2017)

b. Bcr-Abl tyrosine kinase inhibitors (Maldonado & Limper, 2017)

c. Checkpoint inhibitor immunotherapy (Postow & Wolchok, 2018)

d. EGFR inhibitors (Maldonado & Limper, 2017)

e. Immunotherapeutics such as rituximab (Kroschinsky, et al., 2017)

f. MEK inhibitors (Maldonado & Limper, 2017)

g. mTOR inhibitors (Maldonado & Limper, 2017; Willemsen et al., 2015)

h. PD-1/PD-L1 immune checkpoint inhibitors (Cuellar, 2017)

i. PI3K inhibitors such as idelalisib (Kroschinsky, et al., 2017)

j. Taxanes (King, 2017b)

k. Tyrosine kinase inhibitors (Kroschinsky et al., 2017)

l. Vascular endothelial growth factor (VEGF) inhibitors (Maldonado & Limper, 2017)

Assessment

I. Identification of patients at risk (King, 2017a, King, 2017c; Postow & Wolchok, 2018)

A. Immunosuppression

B. Pre-existing autoimmune disorder

C. Prior immune-related toxicity

D. Pre-existing lung disease

E. Occupational and environmental exposures such as silicates, carbon, metals, organic or inorganic dusts

F. Those undergoing concomitant therapy or combination therapy

II. History (King, 2017a; Olivier & Peikert, 2017)

A. Review medication list.

B. Assess for risk factors noted earlier.

C. Inquire about current/past oncologic treatments.

D. Document any comorbidities.

E. Ask about dyspnea, cough, and other pulmonary symptoms—inquire whether this is an acute onset or exacerbation of a chronic problem. Patients may describe being unable to take a deep breath.

F. Assess for low-grade fever and hypoxia.

G. Assess for weight loss, anorexia, fatigue, malaise.

H. Assess timing of symptoms—early in course of therapy or later; assess time of treatments, including past treatments.

1. Radiation pneumonitis usually develops about 4 to 12 weeks after radiation completion (Olivier & Peikert, 2017).

I. Patients may complain of pleuritic or substernal chest pain.

III. Physical examination (Maldonado & Limper, 2016; Olivier & Peikert, 2017)

A. Evaluate hemodynamic status stability.

B. Vital signs: low-grade fever may be present.

C. Pulse oximetry—hypoxia may be present; oxygen saturation below 90% or more than a 4% decrease from baseline with worsening clinical status should be reported immediately. ⚠ Tachypnea and cyanosis may be present in more severe cases.

D. Pulmonary: may be normal, but bibasilar crackles or a pleural rub are often heard. Wheezing is rare.

E. Assess for rash, which could indicate a hypersensitivity reaction.

F. Grade and document pneumonitis according to CTCAE criteria.

IV. Diagnostic testing (King, 2017a; King, 2017c; Maldonado & Limper, 2016; Olivier & Peikert, 2017; Postow & Wolchok, 2018)

A. Laboratory testing: CBC, chemistry panel, liver and kidney function, arterial blood gases; consider antinuclear antibody and rheumatoid factor

B. Chest radiography—compare with previous to assess rate of change; chest radiography can be normal in 10% of patients with interstitial lung disease.

C. High-resolution CT: more accurate than chest radiography, generally preferred.

D. PET scanning is not as useful as CT scanning.

E. Pulmonary function testing, possible bronchoscopy and bronchoalveolar lavage (to rule out other causes).

F. Cardiac evaluation is useful in some patients.

G. Lung biopsy in certain situations, such as progressive or severe disease and when etiology of pneumonitis is uncertain.

H. No specific test will establish the diagnosis of anticancer drug–induced pneumonitis, as this is primarily a diagnosis of exclusion; consider rechallenging with suspected agent after patient recovers; decision is made on a case-by-case basis

I. It is important to rule out infectious causes of the pneumonitis.

Management

I. Medical management (King, 2017a; King, 2017b; Maldonado & Limper, 2016)

A. Management principles

1. Stop offending agent/therapy for any grade 3 or 4 pneumonitis

2. Prevent complications such as thromboembolism, GI bleeding, and nosocomial pneumonia

B. Glucocorticoid therapy may be considered, depending on the severity of symptoms and progressiveness of the pneumonitis. Monitor blood glucose in diabetics, and ensure infectious cause has been excluded. ⚠ Tapering of glucocorticoid will likely occur over 1 to 2 months.

C. Proton pump inhibitors may be indicated for patients on steroids.

D. Inhaled bronchodilators.

E. For severe, immunotherapy-related pneumonitis, immunosuppression with infliximab with/without cyclophosphamide may be considered (Postow & Wolchok, 2018).

F. For those patients who will be receiving steroids long term, prophylaxis for Pneumocystis pneumonia should be considered.

G. Antibiotics for any subsequent opportunistic infection.

H. Mechanical ventilation may be indicated in severe compromise.

II. Nursing management (King, 2017b; Maldonado & Limper, 2016)

A. Provide oxygen therapy

B. Provide supportive care for dyspnea, discomfort

Expected Patient Outcomes

I. Pneumonitis will be recognized early and managed promptly.

II. Patients will understand new or worsening respiratory symptoms should be reported promptly.

III. Toxicities will be graded appropriately so that treatment decisions may be made competently.

REFERENCES

Allen, D. (2018). Increased intracranial pressure. In Yarbro, C., Wujcik, D., & Gobel, B.'s *Cancer nursing: principles and practice*, 8th edition, pp 1169-1185. Jones & Bartlett Learning: Burlington, MA.

Bledsoe, T., Nath, S., & Decker, R. (2017). Radiation pneumonitis. *Clinics in Chest Medicine*, *38*(2), 201–208. https://doi.org/10.1016/j.ccm.2016.12.004.

Cahalane, M. (2017). Overview of gastrointestinal tract perforation. In Weiser, M. & Kao, L. (Eds), *UpToDate*, Waltham, MA. (Accessed on February 12, 2018.).

Calsina Juscafresa, L., Bazo, G., Grochowicz, L., Paramo Alfaro, M., Lopez-Picazo Gonzalez, J., et al. (2017). Endovascular treatment of malignant superior vena cava syndrome secondary to lung cancer. *Hospital Practice*, *45*(3), 70–75. https://doi.org/10.1080/21548331.2017.1342507.

Cuellar, S. (2017). Non-small cell lung cancer: clinical review of adverse events. *Journal for the Advanced Practitioner in Oncology*, *8*, 65–75. doi.org/10.6004/jadpro.2017.8.5.18.

Czosnyka, M., Pickard, J., & Steiner, L. (2017). Principles of intracranial pressure monitoring and treatment. *Handbook of Clinical Neurology*, *140*, 67–89. https://doi.org/10.1016/B978-0-444-63600-3.00005-2.

Dhar, R. (2017). Neurologic complications of transplantation. In: *Handbook of Clinical Neurology* (pp. 545–572). https://doi.org/10.1016/B978-0-444-63599-0.00030-2.

Drews, R. & Rabkin, D. (2017). Malignancy-related superior vena cava syndrome. In Bruera, E., Eidt, J., & Mills, J. (Ed), *UpToDate*, Waltham, MA. (Accessed on January 29, 2018.).

Friedman, T., Quencer, K., Kishore, S., Winokur, R., & Madoff, D. (2017). Malignant venous obstruction: superior vena cava syndrome and beyond. *Seminars in Interventional Radiology*, *34*, 398–408.

Giglio, P., & Gilbert, M. (2010). Neurologic complications of cancer and its treatment. *Current Oncology Reports*, *12*(1), 50–59. https://doi.org/10.1007/s11912-009-0071-x.

Hoit, B. (2017). Pathophysiology of the pericardium. *Progress in Cardiovascular Diseases*, *59*, 341–348. https://doi.org/10.1016/j.pcad.2016.11.001.

Hottinger, A. (2016). Neurologic complications of immune checkpoint inhibitors. *Current Opinion in Neurology*, *29*(6), 806–812.

How, J., Blattner, M., Fowler, S., Wang-Gillam, A., & Schindler, S. (2016). Chemotherapy-associated posterior reversible encephalopathy syndrome: a case report and review of the literature. *Neurologist*, *21*(6), 112–117.

Kamiya-Matsuoka, C., Paker, A., Chi, L., Youssef, A., Tummala, S., & Loghin, M. (2016). Posterior reversible encephalopathy syndrome in cancer patients: a single institution retrospective study. *Journal of Neurooncol*, *128*, 75–84. https://doi.org/10.1007/s11060-016-2078-0.

Kaplan, M. (2013). Spinal Cord Compression. In Kaplan, M.'s *Understanding and Managing Oncologic Emergences* (2nd ed., pp. 337–383). Pittsburgh, PA: Oncology Nursing Society.

Kearns, M., & Walley, K. (2017). Tamponade: hemodynamic and echocardiographic diagnosis. *Chest*. https://doi.org/10.1016/j.chest.2017.11.003. S0012-3692(17)33071-4.

Khan, U., Shanholtz, C., & McCurdy, M. (2017). Oncologic mechanical emergencies. *Hematology Oncology Clinics of North American*, *31*, 927–940. https://doi.org/10.1016/j.hoc.2017.08.001.

King, T. (2017a). Acute interstitial pneumonia (Hamman-Rich syndrome). In Flaherty, K. (Ed), *UpToDate*, Waltham, MA. (Accessed on March 3, 2018.).

King, T. (2017b). Taxane-induced pulmonary toxicity. In Flaherty, K. and Drews, R. (Ed), *UpToDate*, Waltham, MA. (Accessed on March 3, 2018.).

King, T. (2017c). Approach to the adult with interstitial lung disease: diagnostic testing. In Flaherty, K. (Ed), *UpToDate*, Waltham, MA. (Accessed on February 12, 2018.).

Kroschinsky, F., Stolzel, F., von Bonin, S., Beutel, G., Kochanek, M., Kiehl, M., et al. (2017). New drugs, new toxicities: severe side effects of modern targeted and immunotherapy of cancer and their management. *Critical Care*, *21*, 89. https://doi.org/10.1186/s13054-017-1678-1.

Lambert, L., & Wiseman, J. (2018). Palliative management of peritoneal metastases. *Annals of Surgical Oncology*., (Jan 30). https://doi.org/10.1245/s10434-018-6335-7.

Lee-Kong, S., & Lisle, D. (2015). Surgical management of complicated colon cancer. *Clinics in Colon and Rectal Surgery*, *28*, 228–233. https://doi.org/10.1055/s-0035-1564621.

Leinonen, V., Vanninen, R., & Rauramaa, T. (2017). Raised intracranial pressure and brain edema. *Handbook of Clinical Neurology*, *145*, 25–37. https://doi.org/10.1016/B978-0-12-802395-2.00004-3.

Li, Y., Wu, J., Meng, Y., Zhang, Q., Gong, W., & Liu, S. (2016). New devices and techniques for endoscopic closure of gastrointestinal perforations. *World Journal of Gastroenterology*, *22*(33), 7453–7462. https://doi.org/10.3748/wjg.v22.i33.7453.

Lo, S., Ryu, S., Chang, E., Galanopoulos, N., Jones, J., Kim, E., et al. (2015). ACR appropriateness criteria metastatic epidural spinal cord compression and recurrent spinal metastasis. *Journal of Palliative Medicine*, *18*(7), 573–584. https://doi.org/10.1016/B978-0-444-63599-0.00039-9.

Maldonado, F., & Limper, A. (2016a). Pulmonary toxicity associated with antineoplastic therapy: molecularly targeted agents. In Flaherty, K. (Ed), *UpToDate*, Waltham, MA. (Accessed on March 3, 2018.).

Maldonado, F., & Limper, A. (2016b). Pulmonary toxicity associated with systemic antineoplastic therapy: clinical presentation, diagnosis, and treatment. In Flaherty, K. (Ed), *UpToDate*, Waltham, MA. (Accessed on February 12, 2018.).

McCanny, P., & Colreavy, F. (2017). Echocardiographic approach to cardiac tamponade in critically ill patients. *Journal of Critical Care*, *39*, 271–277. https://doi.org/10.1016/j.jcrc.2016.12.008.

McNally, G. (2018). Superior vena cava syndrome. In C. Yarbro, D. Wujcik, & B. Gobel (Eds.), *Cancer Nursing: Principles and Practice* (8th ed., pp. 1187–1205). Burlington, MA: Jones & Bartlett Learning.

Morin, S., Grateau, A., Reuter, D., Kerviler, E., Margerie-Mellon, C., Bazelaire, C., et al. (2017). Management of superior vena cava syndrome in critically ill cancer patients. *Supportive Care in Cancer*, *26*, 521–528. https://doi.org/10.1007/s00520-017-3860-z.

Niu, S., Xu, Y., Cheng, L., & Cao, C. (2017). Stent insertion for malignant superior vena cava yndrome: effectiveness and long-term outcome. *Radiologia Medica*, *122*(8), 633–638. https://doi.org/10.1007/s11547-017-0767-1.

Nurgat, Z., Alzahrani, H., Lawrence, M., Mannan, A., Rasheed, W., & Aliurf, M. (2017). Intracranial hypertension secondary to high dose cytosine arabinoside – a case study. *Journal of Infection and Chemotherapy, 23*(5), 319–322. https://doi.org/10.1016/j.jiac.2016.11.005.

Obita, G., Boland, E., Currow, D., Johnson, M., & Boland, J. (2016). Somatostatin analogues compared with placebo and other pharmacologic agents in the management of symptoms of inoperable malignant bowel obstruction: a systematic review. *Journal of Pain and Symptom Management, 52*(6), 901–919.

Olivier, K. & Peikert, T. (2017). Radiation-induced lung injury. In Jett, J & Schild, S. (Ed), *UpToDate*, Waltham, MA. (Accessed on February 12, 2018.).

Postow, M., & Wolchok, J. (2018). Toxicities associated with checkpoint inhibitor immunotherapy. In Atkins, M. (Ed), *UpToDate*, Waltham, MA. (Accessed on February 12, 2018.).

Ramanathan, S., Ojili, V., Vassa, R., & Nagar, A. (2017). Large bowel obstruction in the emergency department: imaging spectrum for common and uncommon causes. *Journal of Clinical Imaging Science, 7*, 15.

Rami Reddy, S., & Cappell, M. (2017). A systematic review of the clinical presentation, diagnosis, and treatment of small bowel obstruction. *Current Gastroenterology Reports, 19*(28). https://doi.org/10.1007/s11894-017-0566-9.

Rogalski, P., Daniluk, J., Baniukiewicz, A., Wroblewski, E., & Dabrowski, A. (2015). *World Journal of Gastroenterology, 21*(37), 10542–10552. https://doi.org/10.3748/wjg.v21.i37.10542.

Rucker, Y. (2018). Spinal cord compression. In C. Yarbro, D. Wujcik, & B. Gobel (Eds.), *Cancer Nursing: Principles and Practice* (8th ed., pp. 1153–1167). Burlington, MA: Jones & Bartlett Learning.

Schiff, D. (2016). Clinical features and diagnosis of neoplastic spinal cord compression, including cauda equina syndrome. In Drews, R. DeAngelis, L. (Ed), *UpToDate*, Waltham, MA. (Accessed on January 29, 2018.).

Schiff, D., Brown, P., & Shaffrey, M. (2017). Treatment and prognosis of neoplastic epidural spinal cord compression, including cauda equina syndrome. In Drews, R. DeAngelis, L. (Ed), *UpToDate*, Waltham, MA. (Accessed on January 29, 2018.).

Schimpf, M. (2012). Diagnosing increased intracranial pressure. *Journal of Trauma Nursing, 19*(3), 160–167. https://doi.org/10.1097/JTN.0b013e318261cfb4.

Schmidt, A., Fuchs, K. H., Caca, K., Küllmer, A., & Meining, A. (2016). The endoscopic treatment of iatrogenic gastrointestinal perforation. *Deutsches Ärzteblatt International, 113*, 121–128. https://doi.org/10.3238/arztebl.2016.0121.

Shah, R. (2017). Anti-angiogenic tyrosine kinase inhibitors and reversible posterior leukoencephalopathy syndrome: could hypomagnesaemia be the trigger? *Drug Safety, 40*(5), 373–386. https://doi.org/10.1007/s40264-017-0508-3.

Shankar, J., & Banfield, J. (2017). Posterior reversible encephalopathy syndrome: a review. *Canadian Association of Radiologists Journal, 68*(2), 147–153. https://doi.org/10.1016/j.carj.2016.08.005.

Shelton, B. (2013). Superior vena cava syndrome. In Kaplan, M.'s *Understanding and Managing Oncologic Emergences* (2nd ed., pp. 385–410). Pittsburgh, PA Oncology Nursing Society.

Shelton, B., Ferrigno, C., & Skinner, J. (2013). Increased intracranial pressure. In Kaplan, M.'s *Understanding and Managing Oncologic Emergences* (2nd ed., pp. 157–197). Pittsburgh, PA Oncology Nursing Society.

Shimura, T., & Joh, T. (2016). Evidence-based clinical management of acute malignant colorectal obstruction. *Journal of Clinical Gastroenterology, 50*(4), 273–285.

Smith E. & Amin-Hanjani, S. (2017). Evaluation and management of elevated intracranial pressure in adults. In Aminoff, M. (Ed), *UpToDate*, Waltham, MA. (Accessed on January 26, 2018.).

Story, K. (2013). Cardiac tamponade. In Kaplan, M.'s *Understanding and Managing Oncologic Emergences, 2nd edition, pp* (pp. 43–68). Pittsburgh, PA: Oncology Nursing Society.

Teixeira, F., Skaishi, E., Ushinohama, A., Dutra, T., Netto, S., Utiyama, E. et al. (2015). Can we respect the principles of oncologic resection in an emergency surgery to treat colon cancer? *World Journal of Emergency Surgery, 10*:5. https://doi.org/10.1186/1749-7922-10-5.

Willemsen, A., Grutters, J., Gerritsen, W., vanErp, N., van Herpen, C., & Tol, J. (2015). *International Journal of Cancer, 138*, 2312–2321. https://doi.org/10.1002/ijc.29887.

Witherspoon, B., & Ashby, N. (2017). The use of mannitol and hypertonic saline therapies in patients with elevated intracranial pressure. *Nursing Clinics of North America, 52*, 249–260. https://doi.org/10.1016/j.cnur.2017.01.002.

Yeh, D. & Bordeianou, L. (2017). Overview of mechanical colorectal obstruction. In Weiser, M. (Ed), *UpToDate*, Waltham, MA. (Accessed on February, 12, 2018.).

Standards of Practice and Professional Performance

Barbara Lubejko

I. Definition of standards
   A. Nursing and other health care organizations develop standards and guidelines for practice. Standards and guidelines are not the same and are differentiated by expectations of compliance.
   B. Standards for professional nursing practice are defined as "authoritative statements of the duties that all registered nurses [RNs], regardless of role, population, or specialty, are expected to perform competently" (ANA, 2015a, p. 3).
   C. Clinical practice guidelines differ from standards and are defined as "statements that include recommendations intended to optimize patient care that are informed by a systematic review of evidence and an assessment of the benefits and harms of alternative care options" (IOM, 2011, p. 15).
II. Why published standards are needed
   A. Nursing standards of practice and professional performance (NSPPP) set expectations for competent nursing practice.
   B. NSPPP apply to all nursing roles in all settings where nurses care for patients. When implementing the standards, consideration should be given to the characteristics of the practice setting as well as current health care and nursing trends (ANA, 2015a).
   C. NSPPP serve as powerful guides for ensuring evidence-based, quality nursing care and provide direction to nurses and their employers related to expectations and development of competence.
   D. NSPPP provide the public with information about what they can expect in terms of professional competence from nurses who provide services to them.
III. Who defines nursing standards in the United States
   A. It is the responsibility of professional organizations to determine what standards should apply to those nurses whose practice falls within their profession or specialty area.
   B. American Nurses Association (ANA): ANA represents RNs in the United States. They develop general

NSPPP that apply to all RNs, no matter the role, educational preparation, practice setting or specialty area. Key NSPPP include:
   1. Nursing: Scope and Standards of Practice (ANA, 2015a)
   2. Code of Ethics for Nurses with Interpretive Statements (ANA, 2015b)
   C. Oncology Nursing Society (ONS): Defines standards for oncology nursing practice across settings, patient populations and subspecialties.
   D. Standards for oncology nursing focus on helping people at risk for or with a cancer diagnosis achieve the best quality of life and outcomes. ONS publishes a variety of standards based upon the best available evidence to guide oncology nursing practice.
   E. Oncology Nursing Scope and Standards of Practice
      1. ONS first released NSPPP in 1979, which have been periodically updated. The latest version was released in 2013 (Brant & Wickham, 2013), and an updated version is expected to be released in 2019.
      2. Scope of oncology nursing practice
         a. The scope addresses "the 'who,' 'what,' 'where,' 'when,' 'why,' and 'how' of nursing practice" (ANA, 2015a).
         b. The scope of oncology nursing practice defines the practice of nursing as it is performed within the specialty area of oncology.
         c. The scope addresses all levels of oncology nursing from the generalist RN to graduate-level prepared and advanced practice RNs.
         d. Concepts addressed within an oncology scope of practice include (ANA, 2015a):
            (1) History of cancer care and oncology nursing
            (2) Populations and practice settings that are the focus of oncology nursing
            (3) Qualifications for oncology nurses, including educational background, professional development and certification

(4) Code of ethics as applied to oncology nursing
(5) Trends in oncology and nursing practice affecting the oncology nurse

3. Standards of Oncology Nursing Practice and Professional Performance
   a. Describe the expectations for oncology nursing practice across care settings.
   b. Include standards of practice and standards of professional performance (Table 54.1).
   c. For each standard, criteria for demonstrating competence are provided at the RN level that apply to all nurses who provide care to patients with cancer or practice in an oncology setting. Additional standards that apply to graduate-level prepared nurses and advanced practice RNs are included for some standards.

4. Application in practice: the Oncology Nursing Scope and Standards of Practice can be used to define oncology nursing roles, develop individual competence, and highlight the contribution oncology nurses make to quality cancer care, such as:
   a. Development of job descriptions, performance appraisals, evaluation instruments, and peer review

TABLE 54.1	Standards of Oncology Nursing Practice and Professional Performance
Standards of Practice	**Description**
Assessment	The oncology nurse systematically and continually collects data regarding the physical, psychological, social, spiritual, and cultural health status of the patient, including in-depth data specific to the disease and treatment experience of the patient with cancer.
Diagnosis	The oncology nurse analyzes assessment data to determine nursing diagnoses, problems, and issues related to health concerns of people with cancer.
Outcomes Identification	The oncology nurse identifies expected outcomes individualized to the patient, caregiver, or both with a focus on symptom management, survivorship, or a comfortable death.
Planning	The oncology nurse develops an individualized and holistic plan of care that prescribes interventions to attain expected outcomes.
Implementation	The oncology nurse implements the plan of care to achieve the identified expected outcomes for the patient.
Coordination of Care	The oncology nurse ensures that care is coordinated throughout the cancer care continuum.
Health Teaching and Health Promotion	The oncology nurse uses evidence-based strategies to engage patients in learning to promote health and safety.
Evaluation	The oncology nurse systematically and regularly evaluates the patient's response to interventions to determine progress toward achievement of expected outcomes.
Standards of Professional Performance	**Description**
Ethics	The oncology nurse uses ethical principles as a basis for decision making and patient advocacy.
Culturally Congruent Care	The oncology nurse considers cultural diversity and inclusion principles with planning and providing care.
Communication	The oncology nurse uses evidence-based strategies to foster mutual respect and shared decision making that enhance clinical outcomes and patient satisfaction in all practice settings.
Collaboration	The oncology nurse partners with the patient and family, the interprofessional team, and community resources to optimize cancer care.
Leadership	The oncology nurse demonstrates leadership in the practice setting and in the nursing profession by acknowledging the dynamic nature of cancer care and the necessity to prepare for evolving technologies, modalities of treatment, and supportive care.
Education	The oncology nurse seeks and expands personal knowledge and competence that reflect the current evidence-based state of cancer care and oncology nursing, and contributes to the professional development of peers, assistive personnel, and interprofessional colleagues.
Evidence-Based Practice and Research	The oncology nurse integrates relevant research into clinical practice and identifies clinical dilemmas and problems appropriate for study while supporting research efforts.
Quality of Practice	The oncology nurse systematically evaluates the quality, safety, and effectiveness of oncology nursing practice within all practice settings and across the continuum of cancer care.
Professional Practice Evaluation	The oncology nurse consistently evaluates their own nursing practice and that of their peers and other health care providers.
Resource Utilization	The oncology nurse considers factors related to safety, efficiency, effectiveness, and cost in planning and delivering care to patients.
Environmental Health	The oncology nurse practices in an environmentally safe and healthy manner.

Adapted from Brant, J. M., & Wickham, R. (2013). *Statement on the scope and standards of oncology nursing practice: generalist and advanced practice.* Pittsburgh, PA: Oncology Nursing Society; and American Nurses Association (ANA). (2015a). *Nursing: scope and standards of practice* (3rd ed.) Silver Spring. MD: American Nurses Association.

b. Self-assessment to identify professional development needs

c. Basis for organizational policies, procedures, and protocols

d. Inform patients, public, legislators and regulatory bodies about the impact of oncology nursing on safe, high-quality cancer care

e. Inform quality assessment and quality improvement projects and initiatives

f. Reveal organizational, regional, or national evidence gaps that provide appropriate questions for nursing research

g. Identify quality outcomes that can be used to demonstrate the impact of oncology nursing on patient outcomes.

h. Promote ways oncology nursing can contribute to evolving health care delivery and reimbursement models

i. Develop curriculum to prepare nursing students and practicing nurses for oncology nursing–specific role responsibilities (ANA, 2015a; Brant & Wickham, 2013).

F. Standards of Oncology Nursing Education: generalist and advanced practice levels

1. Developed to provide guidance to educators in schools of nursing and clinical settings about preparing students and practicing nurses to meet the care needs of cancer survivors across care settings.

2. Addresses educational structure, process, and outcomes at the generalist and advanced practice levels, including faculty qualifications, clinical and educational resources, relevant curriculum, teaching-learning process and expectations.

3. Application in practice: can be used by individuals and organizations when:

   a. Planning, updating, and evaluating education offered in prelicensure and graduate-level nursing programs.

   b. Planning and evaluating cancer-related continuing education for nurses at all levels of practice (Jacobs & Mayer, 2015).

G. Standards of Oncology Education: Patient/Significant Other and Public

1. Defines expectations for the oncology nurse, resources, curriculum, the teaching-learning process, and different types of learners.

2. The intended outcomes for these standards are to set expectations for quality education for patients and caregivers in all phases of cancer care and to engage the public to promote healthy behaviors (Blecher et al., 2016).

3. Application in practice: can be used by individuals and organizations to:

   a. Develop education for nurses new to oncology about the needs and evidence-based interventions recommended for teaching patients, caregivers, and the public about cancer-related topics.

b. Develop, implement, and evaluate education plans for individual patients or populations.

c. Provide direction when developing, implementing, and evaluating educational programs for patients, caregivers, and the public.

d. Perform a self-evaluation of the educational content, techniques, and outcomes provided to patients, caregivers, and the public.

e. Identify areas for personal professional development related to educating patients, caregivers, and the public about cancer-related topics.

H. ONS Nursing Documentation Standards for Cancer Treatment (Wiley, Galioto, Matey, & Wyant, 2017)

1. Detail nursing documentation requirements for people with cancer undergoing treatment and requiring supportive care.

2. Using terms that further standardize health terminology, these standards are intended to reflect the minimal elements to include in documentation about people undergoing treatment for cancer. Nurses should build upon and individualize the required elements based upon individual patient assessment and plan of care.

3. Sections of these standards address the following:

   a. Chemotherapy and biotherapy administration

   b. Radiation therapy

   c. Blood and marrow transplantation

   d. Surgery

   e. Treatment with a central venous access device

   f. Blood product transfusion

   g. Extravasation management (Wiley, Galioto, Matey & Wyant, 2017)

4. Application in practice:

   a. Evaluate current and develop new organizational policies and procedures related to documentation requirements for oncology nursing care.

   b. Develop orientation and professional development programs related to documentation in oncology settings.

   c. Compare standards to current documentation processes and platforms to identify gaps.

   d. Evaluate the adequacy of one's own documentation in relation to the criteria addressed in the standards.

   e. Provide structure for documentation audits to identify areas for improvement.

I. Access Device Standards of Practice for Oncology Nursing

1. Provide guidance on best practices in the care of people with cancer who have access devices.

2. Practices are categorized according to the strength of the evidence.

   a. Practice standard: strong evidence to accept practice.

b. Practice recommendation: evidence less strong, but use suggested based on expert opinion, common practice, and nursing judgment.

c. No definitive recommendation can be made: adequate evidence is lacking.

3. Includes standards and recommendations for venous and specialty access devices.

4. Application in practice: can be used by individuals and organizations to:

    a. Evaluate current and develop new organizational policies and procedures related to use and management of access devices in people with cancer.

    b. Develop didactic and clinical educational programs for nurses who care for people with access devices.

    c. Evaluate initial and ongoing competence of nurses caring for people with access devices.

    d. Evaluate own knowledge and skills related to access devices and identify needs for professional development.

    e. Guide quality assessment and improvement projects to identify, address, and reevaluate gaps in practice. (Camp-Sorrell & Matey, 2017)

J. ASCO/ONS Chemotherapy Administration Safety Standards

1. Interprofessional standards that outline best practices to reduce the risk of error during the process of chemotherapy provision.

2. Detailed standards address

    a. Appropriate staff and policies

    b. Planning, consent, and education for patients and caregivers

    c. Ordering, preparing, and administering by parenteral and oral routes and documentation

    d. Monitoring adherence, side effects, and complications (Neuss et al., 2016)

3. Application in practice: can be used by organizations and individuals to:

    a. Evaluate current and develop new organizational policies and procedures related to the process surrounding treatment with chemotherapy.

    b. Develop didactic and clinical educational programs for health care professionals involved in the administration of chemotherapy.

    c. Evaluate initial and ongoing competence of health care professionals involved in the process of treatment with chemotherapy.

    d. Evaluate own knowledge and skills related to the process of treatment with chemotherapy and identify needs for professional development.

    e. Guide quality assessment and improvement projects to identify, address, and reevaluate gaps in practice.

    f. Provide evidence required for reporting of quality outcomes metrics and identify topics for quality outcomes research.

REFERENCES

American Nurses Association (ANA). (2015a). *Nursing: scope and standards of practice* (3rd ed.) Silver Spring. MD: American Nurses Association.

American Nurses Association (ANA). (2015b). *Code of ethics for nurses with interpretive statements.* Silver Spring, MD: Nursesbook.org.

Blecher, C. S., Ireland, A. M., & Watson, J. L. (2016). *Standards of oncology education: patient/significant other and public* (4th Ed.). Pittsburgh, PA: Oncology Nursing Society.

Brant, J. M., & Wickham, R. (2013). *Statement on the scope and standards of oncology nursing practice: generalist and advanced practice.* Pittsburgh, PA: Oncology Nursing Society.

Camp-Sorrell, D., & Matey, L. (2017). *Access device standards of practice for oncology nursing.* Pittsburgh, PA: Oncology Nursing Society.

IOM (Institute of Medicine). (2011). *Clinical practice guidelines we can trust.* Washington, DC: The National Academies Press.

Jacobs, L. A., & Mayer, D. K. (2015). *Standards of oncology nursing education: generalist and advanced practice levels.* Pittsburgh, PA: Oncology Nursing Society.

Neuss, M., Gilmore, T. R., Belderson, K. M., Billett, A. L., Conti-Kalchik, T., Harvey, B. E., Hendricks, C., LeFebvre, K. B., Mangu, P. B., McNiff, K., Olsen, M., Schulmeister, L., Von Gehr, A., & Polovich, M. (2016). 2016 Updated American Society of Clinical Oncology/Oncology Nursing Society Chemotherapy Administration Safety Standards, including Standards for Pediatric Oncology. *Oncology Nursing Forum, 44,* 31–43. https://doi.org/10.1188/17.ONF.31-43.

Wiley, K., Galioto, M., Matey, L., & Wyant, T. (2017). *Oncology nursing society documentation standards for cancer treatment.* Pittsburgh, PA: Oncology Nursing Society.

55

Evidence-Based Practice

Jennifer Shamai, Tia Wheatley, and Allison Winacoo

EVIDENCE-BASED PRACTICE

I. Overview: evidence-based practice (EBP)
   A. Key to delivering high-quality health care, achieving improved patient outcomes, and decreasing health care costs (Melnyk & Fineout-Overholt, 2015).
   B. First developed as a method for clinical learning in evidence-based medicine in the 1980s at McMaster University in Hamilton, Ontario, Canada.
   C. Goal is to guide oncology nursing interventions that are demonstrated to enhance the quality and outcomes of cancer care.
      1. Quality and Safety Education for Nurses (QSEN) established EBP as a quality and safety competency necessary to prepare nurses to deliver safe and high-quality care (QSEN, 2018).
      2. The oncology nursing profession has mandated the inclusion of EBP in its standards—a component of each of the six Standards of Care and five of the Standards of Professional Practice (Brant & Wickham, 2013).
      3. A professional obligation and ethical imperative exist for nurses to deliver evidence-based patient care (Cleary-Holdforth, 2017).
   D. Definitions and components of EBP include the following:
      1. Integration of the best possible research evidence with clinical expertise and patient needs.
      2. A paradigm and lifelong problem-solving approach to clinical practice that integrates the best evidence from well-designed studies with a patient's preferences and values and a clinician's expertise to improve outcomes for individuals, groups, communities, and systems (Melnyk & Fineout-Overholt, 2015).
      3. A systematic approach to practice that emphasizes using best evidence in combination with clinical experience and patient preferences and values to make decisions about care and treatment.
      4. Essential components—a systematic review and synthesis of research that results in a systematic process for change, including systematic and rigorous assessment, implementation, and evaluation of outcomes.

II. Need for EBP based on the following:
   A. The Institute of Medicine has mandated that 90% of all health care decisions in the United States will be evidence based by 2020.
   B. Evidence continues to evolve on a continual basis, and without EBP can take decades to transition into practice (Melnyk & Fineout-Overholt, 2015).
   C. An EBP culture can increase nurse satisfaction and retention and decrease turnover (Fridman & Frederickson, 2014).
   D. Pay-for-performance programs, nonpayment for complications when evidence-based guidelines are not followed, and patients and family members seeking the latest evidence online are increasing (Melynk & Fineout-Overholt, 2015).
   E. EBP is not consistently implemented at health care institutions throughout the United States and globally (Melynk & Fineout-Overholt, 2015).

III. EBP Registered Nurse Professional Competencies (Melnyk, Gallagher-Ford, Long, & Fineout-Overholt, 2014)
   A. To promote an EBP culture and provide high-quality health care, the registered nurse is expected to maintain the following knowledge, skills, and attitude:
      1. Question clinical practice for improving health care quality
      2. Use internal evidence to describe clinical problems (assessment data, quality indicators)
      3. Use the PICOT format to ask clinical questions (see Section IV)
      4. Search external evidence to answer clinical questions
      5. Critically appraise evidence using practice guidelines and literature synthesis
      6. Critically appraise research studies; determine applicability to clinical practice
      7. Evaluate evidence and consider applicability to clinical practice
      8. Collect data for decision making in the care of individuals, groups, or populations
      9. Use internal and external evidence to plan EBP changes

10. Implement practice change based on evidence, clinical expertise, and patient preference to improve quality of care and patient outcomes
11. Evaluate outcomes of EBP to determine best practice
12. Disseminate best practice to improve quality of care and patient outcomes
13. Sustain and promote an EBP culture

IV. Using evidence to support clinical practice change is a multistep process (Melnyk & Fineout-Overholt, 2015; Brown, 2014):
   A. Cultivate a sense of inquiry and create an EBP culture
      1. Question current practice
      2. Journal clubs, ongoing EBP education, access to key databases
      3. National Nursing Standards & Recommendations for Best Practice (National Cancer Institute, National Comprehensive Cancer Network, Oncology Nursing Society, Agency for Healthcare Research & Quality, American Nurses Association)
      4. Organizational and/or unit-based shared governance
      5. Collaborate with other health care professionals who have in-depth knowledge of EBP
      6. Administrative and leadership support and mentorship
      7. Regular recognition of EBP values and implementation
   B. Identify a problem or trigger
      1. Problem-focused: existing data which show an opportunity for improvement (financial data, quality data, benchmark data, clinical problems [e.g., patient falls])
      2. Knowledge-focused: new research or practice guidelines that warrant practice change
      3. Problems with higher volume or cost association will have higher organizational priority
   C. Identification of information and stakeholders needed to solve the problem
   D. Stakeholders develop, implement, and evaluate change with other disciplines
   E. Search and critique of the literature for relevant studies
      1. Use a clinical question to develop a list of keywords
         a. Using the PICOT format for clinical questions will yield the most relevant evidence:
            (1) P – Patient Population of Interest
            (2) I – Intervention or Issue of Interest
            (3) C – Comparison Intervention or Control Group
            (4) O – Outcomes
            (5) T – Time Frame
      2. Data sources for EBP include but are not limited to the following:
         a. Electronic health records
         b. Benchmark data

c. Textbooks
d. Nursing theories
e. Journals
   (1) Systematic reviews
   (2) Research articles (randomized control trials [RCTs])
   (3) Expert opinion/editorials
   (4) Case studies, case reports
   (5) Clinical practice guidelines
f. Databases
   (1) MEDLINE, CINAHL, PsychINFO, Cochrane Database, UpToDate, ClinicalKey for Nursing, PubMed, Embase, Ovid, National Guideline Clearinghouse
   F. Critically appraise the evidence
      1. Quantitative evidence (numerical data with statistical analysis)
         a. Does the evidence answer the clinical question?
         b. Are the measures/tools valid and reliable? How was the data analyzed?
         c. What was the sample size?
         d. Determine the strength of the evidence
            (1) Level 1: systematic review of RCTs—highest level of evidence on which to base practice change
            (2) Level 2: single-site RCT studies
            (3) Level 3: quasi-experimental studies
            (4) Level 4: case or cohort studies
            (5) Level 5: systematic review of descriptive or qualitative studies
            (6) Level 6: single descriptive or qualitative study
            (7) Level 7: expert opinion—lowest level on which to base practice change
      2. Qualitative evidence (non-numeric data)
         a. Are the results of the study valid/credible?
         b. What are the results/outcomes?
         c. How will the results help address the clinical problem?
      3. Develop an evidence table to organize data, compare results, and identify themes
      4. Critical appraisal of the evidence should occur before piloting a practice change
      5. Evidence should be integrated with clinical expertise and patient preferences/values
   G. Pilot a practice change in the clinical setting
      1. Practice changes should first be implemented in one or two practice areas to ensure feasibility, sustainability, and outcomes
      2. If the implementation is successful, it can be implemented across the organization
   H. Evaluate practice change and outcomes
      1. Evaluation of practice changes is an important step to determine if impact on health care quality, cost, or patient outcomes was achieved in the clinical setting due to EBP

2. Consider using existing data sources for demonstrating improvement in outcomes
   a. Quality indicators (nurse-sensitive indicators, incident reports, sentinel events, patient satisfaction)
   b. Financial/cost–benefit analysis
   c. Electronic health records, dashboards, and/or scorecards
   d. Survey of staff, patients and family, and/or environment
3. Evaluation tools should be validated and reliable to ensure accuracy of results
4. Determine if practice change should be implemented across the organization based on reported outcomes or results
5. Monitor for any deviations in practice or changes in outcomes

I. Disseminate outcomes and results
   1. EBP is most valuable when clinical practice changes and impact on patient outcomes are communicated effectively and adopted into the current literature
   2. Information gained from EBP should be shared with colleagues through, but not limited to, the following methods:
      a. Oral and poster presentations at national, regional, or local conferences
      b. Panel presentations
      c. Roundtable discussions
      d. EBP grand rounds
      e. Nursing journal publications
      f. Institutional or national health care policies
      g. News conferences

J. An EBP model can assist nurses with designing, implementing, and sustaining an EBP change
   1. Stetler Model of Evidence-Based Practice (www.nccmt.ca/knowledge-repositories/search/83)
   2. The Iowa Model of Evidence-Based Practice (Brown, 2014)
   3. Model for Evidence-Based Practice Change (Rosswurm & Larrabee, 1999)
   4. The Evidence-Based Advancing Research & Clinical Practice Through Close Collaboration (ACRR) Model (Melnyk, Fineout-Overholt, Giggleman, & Choy, 2017)
   5. Promoting Action on Research Implementation in Health Services Framework
   6. Clinical Scholar Model (Honess, Gallant, & Keane, 2009)
   7. The Johns Hopkins Evidence-Based Practice Model (https://www.hopkinsmedicine.org/evidence-based-practice/ijhn_2017_ebp.html)
   8. ACE Star Model of Knowledge Transformation (http://nursing.uthscsa.edu/onrs/starmodel/institute/su08/starmodel.html)

V. Potential roles of the oncology nurse generalist that can facilitate EBP:
   A. Identify practice problems by observing patient populations and quality improvement activities. Examples of practice problems include the following:
      1. Develop and evaluate nurse-led intervention to enhance medication knowledge of and adherence to oral chemotherapy (Boucher et al. 2015)
      2. Develop, implement, and evaluate a sepsis bundle to improve timeliness and adherence to sepsis practice guidelines in a population of ambulatory patients with hematologic malignancies (Shelton et al., 2016)
   B. Participate in evaluation of existing research or clinical evidence
      1. Use identified measurement criteria to outline staff nurse roles and responsibilities in oncology nursing research (Ness & Royce, 2017).
         a. American Nursing Association Scope and Standards of Practice and Code of Ethics
         b. Nursing practice act of state in which staff nurse is practicing
         c. 2016 Oncology Nursing Society Oncology Clinical Trials Nurse Competencies (ONS, 2016)
         d. EBP Competencies for Practicing Registered Nurses & Advanced Practice Nurses (Melnyk, Gallagher-Ford, et al., 2014)
      2. Assist in studies related to high-incidence problem areas or oncology nursing priorities
         a. Consider which nursing interventions promote excellence in oncology nursing and quality cancer care
         b. Assist in studies in high-priority research areas and cross-cutting themes in oncology nursing research (Knobf et al., 2015):
            (1) Symptom management
            (2) Late effects of cancer treatment and survivorship care
            (3) Palliative and end-of-life care
            (4) Self-management
            (5) Aging
            (6) Family and caregivers
            (7) Health care systems improvement and risk reduction
            (8) Cross-cutting themes (biomarkers, bioinformatics, comparative effectiveness research, and dissemination and implementation science)
         c. Use of standards to identify possible oncology nursing–related research questions:
            (1) Evaluate team-based-approach models of communication on patient and family outcomes in palliative and end-of-life care
            (2) Develop, test, and implement interventions to improve the care of older adult patients (Knobf et al., 2015)

C. Collaborate with other health care providers or nurse researchers to identify and implement a potential solution to a specific clinical problem

D. Participate in research activities or research training programs under the guidance of qualified nursing researchers and/or advanced practice nurses that may lead to practice changes and add to EBP (Black, Balneaves, & Garossino, 2015).

1. Conceptualization and design of a research study
   a. Establish that the problem is clinically significant and that a gap exists in the current literature
   b. Assess the feasibility of the methods and procedures for the proposed study
2. Implementation of a nursing research study
   a. Identify and enroll patients
   b. Implement protocol-specific orders
   c. Collect study data
   d. Educate patients, caregivers, and other health care team members about the study

E. Role of oncology nurses in clinical trials (see Chapter 11)

VI. Critiquing research reports for applicability to EBP

A. Guidelines and exact questions for completing a critique vary, depending on the study methodology, and include evaluation of the following:

1. Research problem or purpose
   a. What clinical question does the study address? Are the purpose, study variables, and population to be studied explicitly stated (Greenhalgh, 2014)?
   b. Does the problem have significance for nursing?
2. Are there formally stated hypotheses or research questions that directly relate to the research problem?
3. Theoretic framework (most common in nursing research)
   a. Is a theoretic framework identified?
   b. Does the framework support the hypothesis, research statement, or question?
4. Design or method
   a. What is the study design, and is it well suited to the research problem?
      (1) Qualitative research to describe or explore phenomena, gain understanding.
         (a) Characteristics—process focused, subjective, and not generalizable
         (b) Types—descriptive, survey, phenomenology, content analysis
      (2) Quantitative research to describe relationships between variables, examine cause and effect, and identify facts.
         (a) Characteristics—outcome focused, objective, may be generalizable
         (b) Types—quasi-experimental, experimental, correlational
   b. Is the method adequate to answer the research question or phenomenon studied?
5. Sampling
   a. Are criteria for participant selection clearly identified? For a qualitative study, was purposive sampling done?
   b. Is participant selection appropriate for the research purpose and method?
   c. Is the sample representative of a larger population?
6. Data collection
   a. Are data collection criteria and procedures clearly identified?
   b. Do data collection tools seem appropriate for the research question and methodology?
   c. Are the tools valid and reliable, and is information about this clear?
   d. Is protection of human subjects (e.g., informed consent, protected health information) clearly addressed?
   e. For qualitative research, is data saturation described?
7. Data analysis—differs depending on qualitative or quantitative methodology used
   a. Qualitative
      (1) Is the data analysis strategy compatible with the study purpose?
      (2) Are the findings presented in a manner that allows the reader to verify the researcher's theoretic conclusions?
      (3) Do conclusions, implications, and recommendations reflect the findings of the study?
      (4) Would a quantitative approach be more appropriate?
   b. Quantitative
      (1) Does the report include the appropriate statistics?
      (2) Were results of any statistical tests significant, and was this information adequately reported?
      (3) Could the study have been strengthened by including qualitative data?
8. Findings, implications, and recommendations
   a. Are important results presented; is their interpretation consistent with the results?
   b. Are specific limitations of the study presented?
   c. Are identified implications appropriate as related to specified study limitations?
   d. Are implications for nursing practice discussed?
   e. Are specific recommendations for future research discussed?

VII. Questions to ask before implementing research findings into nursing practice:

A. Are the results clinically significant and can they be generalized?

B. Are implementation strategies discussed by the researcher desirable/feasible in practice?

C. Are institutional support and resources adequate to implement the study findings?

D. Can the outcome of implementing study findings be measured?

REFERENCES

Black, A. T., Balneaves, L. G., & Garossino, C. (2015). Promoting evidence-based practice through a research training program for point-of-care clinicians. *Journal of Nursing Administration, 45*(1), 14–20.

Boucher, J., Lucca, J., Hooper, C., Pedulla, L., & Berry, D. L. (2015). A structured nursing intervention to address oral chemotherapy adherence in patients with non-small cell lung cancer. *Oncology Nursing Forum, 42*(4), 383–389. https://doi.org/10.1188/15. ONF.383-389.

Brant, J. M., & Wickham, R. S. (Eds.), (2013). *Statement on the scope and standards of oncology nursing practice* (2nd ed.). Pittsburgh: Oncology Nursing Society.

Brown, C. G. (2014). The Iowa model of evidence-based practice to promote quality care: an illustrated example in oncology nursing. *Clinical Journal of Oncology Nursing, 18*, 157–159.

Cleary-Holdforth, J. (2017). Evidence-based practice: an ethical perspective. *Worldview on Evidence-Based Nursing, 14*(6), 429–431.

Fridman, M., & Frederickson, K. (2014). Oncology nurses and the experience of participation in an evidence-based practice project. *Oncology Nursing Forum, 41*(4), 382–388.

Greenhalgh, T. (2014). *How to read a paper: the basics of evidence based medicine.* London: BMJ.

Honess, C., Gallant, P., & Keane, K. (2009). The clinical scholar model: evidence-based practice at the bedside. *Nursing Clinics of North America, 44*(1), 116–130.

Knobf, M. T., Cooley, M. E., Duffy, S., Doorenbos, A., Eaton, L., Given, B., Mayer, D. K., McCorkle, R., Miaskowski, C.,

Mitchell, S., Sherwood, P., Bender, C., Cataldo, J., Hershey, D., Katapodi, M., Menon, U., Schumacher, K., Sun, V., Von Ah, D., LoBiondo-Wood, G., & Mallory, G. (2015). The 2014-2018 Oncology Nursing Society Research Agenda. *Oncology Nursing Forum, 42*(5), 450–465.

Melnyk, B. M., & Fineout-Overholt, E. (2015). *Evidence-based practice in nursing & healthcare: a guide to best practice (3rd Ed.).* Philadelphia: Wolters Kluwer.

Melnyk, B. M., Fineout-Overholt, E., Giggleman, M., & Choy, K. (2017). A test of the ARCC model improves implementation of evidence-based practice, healthcare culture, and patient outcomes. *Worldviews on Evidence Based Practice Nursing, 14*(1), 5–9.

Melnyk, B. M., Gallagher-Ford, L., Long, L. E., & Fineout-Overholt, E. (2014). The establishment of evidence-based practice competencies for practicing registered nurses and advanced practice nurses in real-world clinical settings: proficiencies to improve healthcare quality, reliability, patient outcomes, and costs. *Worldviews on Evidence-Based Nursing, 11*, 5–15.

Ness, E. A., & Royce, C. (2017). Clinical trials & the role of the oncology clinical trials nurse. *Nursing Clinics of North America, 52*(1), 133–148.

Oncology Nursing Society [ONS]. (2016). *2016 oncology clinical trials nurse competencies.* Retrieved from: https://www.ons.org/sites/default/files/OCTN_Competencies_FINAL.PDF.

Rosswurm, M. A., & Larrabee, J. H. (1999). A model for change to evidence-based practice. *Image: Journal of Nursing Scholarship, 31*(4), 317–322.

Quality and Safety Education for Nurses. (2018). *QSEN competencies.* Retrieved from http://qsen.org/competencies/pre-licensure-ksas/#evidence-based_practice.

Shelton, B. K., Stanik-Hutt, J., Kane, J., & Jones, R. J. (2016). Implementing the surviving sepsis campaign in an ambulatory clinic for patients with hematologic malignancies. *Clinical Journal of Oncology Nursing, 20*(3), 281–288. https://doi.org/10.1188/16.CJON.281-288.

56

Principles of Education and Learning

Diane Cope

I. Educational theory provides the foundation for any formal and informal educational interventions, whether aimed at an individual patient, staff, nurse, or community. Learning theories can be useful for formulating teaching strategies in clinical practice (Table 56.1) (Miller & Stoeckel, 2019).

II. Patient education
   A. Needs assessment (Kitchie, 2019; Miller & Stoeckel, 2019)
      1. What does the patient know and from what source? The patient needs to be asked what he or she understands about the diagnosis, tests, treatment, needed self-care, and follow-up.
      2. What does the patient want to know? This may be different from what the nurse thinks the patient wants to know.
      3. Will any cultural or religious beliefs or practices affect the teaching or learning process (Miller & Stoeckel, 2019)? For example, alternative supplements may be a traditional and important part of the patient's belief system, but these supplements may interfere with chemotherapy drugs.
      4. What language does the patient speak? If the nurse does not speak the same language, what is the alternative teaching plan (Miller & Stoeckel, 2019)? The availability of translators on site should be explored.
      5. Does the patient have a physical (e.g., hearing, vision, mobility, dexterity) or cognitive (e.g., stroke, confusion, somnolence) impairment that might impede learning?
      6. Does the patient have a preferred learning style (e.g., visual, aural, or kinesthetic—seeing, hearing, doing; global or analytic—big picture, component parts)?
      7. What is the patient's educational background and level of literacy?
      8. Individual assessment involves specific questions such as the following: What is the most important thing you want to learn now? Do you have concerns about continuing your normal activities during chemotherapy treatments?
      9. Caregiver assessment. Are you able to assist the patient? What information do you want to learn to assist in your care?
      10. Community assessment before development of targeted patient education program or materials (Miller & Stoeckel, 2019)
         a. Survey or checklist
         b. Interested party analysis
         c. Interview and key informant
         d. Focus group
   B. Goals and objectives (also called *outcome criteria* or *outcome objectives*) (Bastable & Quigley, 2019; Miller & Stoeckel, 2019)
      1. Objectives: specific assessment criteria; for example, ability to state four foods with high iron content after reading information regarding foods with high iron content
      2. SMART: providing a global view of intended outcomes—for example, ability for self-care after discharge
         a. S—specific
         b. M—measurable
         c. A—attainable
         d. R—realistic
         e. T—timely
      3. ABCD: "who" will do "what" by "when" and "to what extent":
         a. A—audience (who the learner is)
         b. B—behavior (what the learner is to do)
         c. C—condition (under what circumstances)
         d. D—degree (how much; to what extent the learner is to perform)
   C. Teaching plan: decisions about the content (Miller & Stoeckel, 2019)
      1. Who will do the teaching (e.g., staff nurse, patient educator, patient-to-patient volunteer)?
      2. How it will be taught based on patient's preference, health literacy, and availability of alternative methods (e.g., one-on-one, group, demonstration and return demonstration, self-instruction activities, video, computer, print, combination)?
      3. Preparing for teaching by reviewing evidence-based teaching practices in the literature

TABLE 56.1 Learning Theories

Learning Theory	Description
Behavioral learning theory (operant conditioning, classical conditioning) (Aliakbari, Parvin, Heidari, & Haghani, 2015; Omrod, 2016; Miller & Stoeckel, 2019).	Learning based on observable behaviors that are reinforced to increase the strength of the behavior. Behavioral intervention examples: relaxation techniques, biofeedback, and visual imagery. Often used to help pediatric patients with cancer cope with painful procedures; adult patients with cancer can use them to reduce stress, pain, and anxiety, and to increase coping ability.
Cognitive learning theory (Miller & Stoeckel, 2019; Omrod, 2016).	Internal process that leads to learning that requires attention, thought, and reasoning for information to be retrieved and applied. An example of cognitive learning is the creation of a mnemonic for symptoms that should trigger a phone call to the physician or other health care provider. A patient's ability to differentiate systemic from local treatment demonstrates cognitive learning.
Social learning theory (Bandura, 1977; McLeod, 2016).	Learning takes place based on watching and imitating others. Core concepts of social learning theory include attention, retention, reproduction, and motivation.
Motivational learning theory (Cook & Artino, 2016).	Concerned with the processes that describe why and how human behavior is activated and directed. Motivation can result from internal cues or drive (e.g., "I want to be here for my children, so I've got to stop smoking") or environmental (external) cues (e.g., "I have to stop smoking because my workplace has a nonsmoking policy and I hate sneaking out for a cigarette") that activate behavior.
Humanistic learning theory (Aliakbari, Parvin, Heidari, & Haghani, 2015).	Everyone is unique, and all individuals have a desire to learn and grow in a positive manner. It is a learner-directed approach and is based on spontaneity, the importance of emotions and feelings, the right of individuals to make their own choices, and human creativity.
Adult learning theory (andragogy) (Knowles, Holton, & Swanson, 2015).	The adult learner is described as someone who is self-directed, independent, and problem centered. Learning is based on past experience. An example of an adult learning experience would be an independent Internet search for information related to a new cancer diagnosis.

(professional journal articles or recent textbooks), standards of care, and hospital procedure manuals and consulting experts (e.g., advanced practice nurses, physicians)

4. Organizing and practicing all teaching sessions before the actual teaching
5. Planning the teaching to coincide with a teachable moment when the learner might be most likely to be receptive to the message (e.g., smoking cessation in caregivers when a patient is diagnosed with lung cancer; self-care skills before discharge; cancer screening to coincide with a public awareness campaign)
6. Determination of ways to measure learning (e.g., learner explains in own words, return demonstration, quiz, behavior change)
7. Documentation of learning outcomes (e.g., patient can state the side effects of the medication; patient can demonstrate correct catheter care technique) on care plan, documentation form, or nursing notes
8. Reassessment and reinforcement of teaching and learning at next available opportunity

D. Evaluation (Kitchie, 2019; Miller & Stoeckel, 2019; Worral, 2019)
   1. Assessing knowledge can be done through testing in a variety of ways such as multiple choice, essay, or short answer.
   2. Skills can be assessed through case studies, case presentations, discussion, and written questions.
   3. Knowledge application can be assessed through simulation and observation in a variety of settings.
III. Caregiver education—caregivers may have the same or different learning needs; addressing these learning needs is especially important if the caregiver has a role in caring for the patient at home (Miller & Stoeckel, 2019)
   A. Needs assessment with, or independent of, the patient
   B. Identification of overlapping and separate needs
   C. Obtaining patient's permission to include caregiver in teaching (Health Insurance Portability and Accountability Act [HIPAA])
   D. Scheduling teaching sessions when caregiver can be available
   E. Assessment of learning; reinforcement as necessary

F. Documentation as indicated by needs and relationship with patient (e.g., caregiver)

IV. Staff education (Bastable & Gonzalez, 2019)

A. Assessment: identifying staff learning needs, learning styles, readiness to learn

1. Targeted needs assessment for learning objectives, such as those related to critical events, new or revised policies or procedures, and new treatment or orientation of new staff nurses

2. Institution (e.g., new staff nurses must understand hospital policies and sign off on learning; staff nurses must be informed when nursing policies or procedures change)

3. Self-assessment (e.g., nurses evaluate their own learning needs based on the type of patient for whom they will provide care; nurses identify learning needs based on interest)

4. Diagnostic methods (e.g., nurses are tested for competence in specific areas; nurses are observed in practice)

B. Determination of objectives of teaching (e.g., nurse will demonstrate venipuncture technique; nurse will identify components of a patient's admission assessment)

C. Teaching plan development

1. Use principles of adult learning (Knowles, Holton, & Swanson, 2015).

2. Adults should understand why they must learn something and be self-directed.

3. Teaching plan should consider prior learning and experience.

4. Educators can create a learning environment by giving staff opportunities to learn.

5. Determine teaching method (e.g., class, one-on-one, print or computer, self-directed or teacher-directed, games and simulations, grand rounds, panels and seminars, case studies, webinars).

6. Determine specific content.

7. Establish evaluation criteria (e.g., test, observation, dialogue, learner satisfaction, performance improvement, patient satisfaction).

D. Evaluation

1. Performance analysis (e.g., information is obtained from quality improvement and incident reports; infection control data are analyzed)

V. Community education/community health nursing (Lundy, Janes, & Hartman, 2016)

A. Community can be defined geographically (e.g., New York City, state of Missouri), by ethnic or religious group (e.g., African Americans, evangelical Christians), and by interest or characteristics (e.g., sexual orientation, occupation), among many others.

B. The role of the nurse in community health is defined by many organizations, including the American Nurses Association (http://www.ana.org), the American Public Health Association (http://www.apha.org),

and state and local departments of health. Many definitions include the word "populations" as the target of nursing interventions.

C. Healthy People 2020—national priorities established by the U.S. Department of Health and Human Services (DHHS, 2010) to improve health and reduce health disparity

D. Community assessment (Lundy & Barton, 2016)

1. Analyze data such as descriptive data (e.g., demographics, history, ethnicity, values and beliefs, physical environment, health and social services) and illness prevalence data

2. Assess health learning needs (e.g., human immunodeficiency virus [HIV] and acquired immunodeficiency syndrome [AIDS] prevention, smoking prevention in teens)

3. Identify common health problems (e.g., high incidence of heart disease, tuberculosis)

4. Develop a community health diagnosis; e.g., senior citizens at risk for social isolation due to lack of public transportation—generally aimed at primary, secondary, and tertiary prevention

E. Intervention

1. Working with community (e.g., key informants, leaders, health care community, schools) to prioritize and develop interventions to meet health needs identified in assessment

2. Plan implemented using community resources, advocates, and agencies

F. Evaluation

1. Intervention is evaluated for impact on identified health need.

2. Intervention may be modified for ongoing health needs. Is it cost-effective? Were objectives met? What are the long-term implications of continuing or not continuing the intervention?

REFERENCES

Aliakbari, F., Parvin, N., Heidari, M., & Haghani, F. (2015). Learning theories application in nursing education. *Journal of Education and Health Promotion*, 4(2). https://doi.org/10.4103/2277-9531.151867. Retrieved from https://www.ncbi.nlm.nih.gov/pmc/articles/PMC4355834/.

Bandura, A. (1977). *Social learning theory*. Englewood Cliffs, NJ: Prentice Hall.

Bastable, S. B., & Gonzalez, K. M. (2019). Overview of education in health care. In S. B. Bastable (Ed.), *Nurse as educator: principles of teaching and learning* (5th ed., pp. 2–33). Burlington, MA: Jones and Bartlett.

Bastable, S. B., & Quigley, L. G. (2019). Behavioral objectives and teaching plans. In S. B. Bastable (Ed.), *Nurse as educator: principles of teaching and learning* (5th ed., pp. 421–457). Burlington, MA: Jones and Bartlett.

Cook, D. A., & Artino, A. R. (2016). Motivation to learn: an overview of contemporary theories. *Medical Education, 50*, 997–1014. https://doi.org/10.1111/medu.13074.

Kitchie, S. (2019). Determinants of learning. In S. B. Bastable (Ed.), *Nurse as educator: principles of teaching and learning* (5th ed., pp. 114–167). Burlington, MA: Jones and Bartlett.

Knowles, M. S., Holton, E. F., & Swanson, R. A. (2015). *The adult learner.* New York, NY: Routledge.

Lundy, K. S., & Barton, J. A. (2016). Community and population health: assessment and intervention. In K. S. Lundy & S. Janes (Eds.), *Community health nursing: caring for the public's health* (pp. 33–68). Burlington, MA: Jones and Bartlett.

Lundy, K. S., Janes, S., & Hartman, S. (2016). Opening the door to healthcare in the community. In K. S. Lundy & S. Janes (Eds.), *Community health nursing: caring for the public's health* (pp. 3–32). Burlington, MA: Jones and Bartlett.

McLeod, S. A. (2016). *Bandura - social learning theory.* www.simplypsychology.org/bandura.html. Retrieved from.

Miller, M. A., & Stoeckel, P. R. (2019). *Client education: theory and practice* (3rd ed.). Burlington, MA: Jones and Bartlett.

Omrod, J. E. (2016). Human learning (7th ed.). Englewood Cliffs, NJ: Pearson Education.

Worral, P. S. (2019). Evaluation in healthcare education. In S. B. Bastable (Ed.), *Nurse as educator: principles of teaching and learning* (5th ed., pp. 594–631). Burlington, MA: Jones and Bartlett.

57

Legal Issues

Julie Ponto

I. Nurses care for and interact with individuals who are possibly at the most vulnerable point in their lives and yet are among the most trusted professionals
   A. Legal, regulatory, and practice standards exist to help ensure well-prepared, competent nurses
   B. Adhering to legal principles and standards can help mitigate risks and unintended negative outcomes
   C. Nurses are individually licensed and are consequently responsible for their nursing actions

II. Regulation of nursing practice
   A. State boards of nursing (BoNs)—provide oversight of nursing practice by enforcing the state nurse practice act to protect the health, welfare, and safety of the public
      1. State BoNs typically have employed staff (e.g., executive officer, attorney, administrative staff) and appointed or elected representatives of various nursing groups (e.g., registered nurses, licensed practical or vocational nurses, advanced practice registered nurses).
      2. Membership, selection, and length of term of appointed or elected members are determined by the state and vary by state.
      3. Nurses can influence practice and policy by being active in the state BoN (e.g., appointed or elected member; attend public meetings of the BoN; communicate with BoN regarding issues important to cancer care and cancer nursing).
   B. National Council of State Boards of Nursing (NCSBN)—develops the National Council Licensure for Registered Nurses (NCLEX-RN) examination, encourages consistency among state BoNs (e.g., provides model language for nurse practice acts) (NCSBN, 2018a)
   C. Nursing licensure compact—allows nurses to practice (physically, electronically, telephonically) in multiple states without obtaining multiple nursing licenses (NCSBN, 2018b)
      1. Approximately 30 states currently have this legislation, with additional states pursuing compact membership

      2. Helpful for traveling nurses, nurses who live near state lines, nurses who move, large health care organizations with sites in multiple states, distance and online nursing education students/programs
   D. Nurse practice acts—define nursing roles, titles, and scopes of practice; define educational program standards, requirements for licensure, and grounds for disciplinary action
   E. Definitions of regulatory terms (McTeigue, 2015a)
      1. Sources of law—laws governing practice come from a variety of sources
         a. Statute—"written law passed by Congress or state legislature and signed into law by the president or state governor" (NOLO, 2018)
         b. Common law—law based on court decisions and custom compared with legislative actions; often serves as the basis for malpractice litigation
      2. Administrative rule or regulation—a statement adopted by a government-sanctioned agency (e.g., BoN) intended to make the law (e.g., nurse practice act) more specific or to explain the agency's organization or procedures
         a. Relate to specific statutes and undergo a process allowing for public comment
         b. Have the force and effect of law once they are enacted
   F. BoN disciplinary cases in nursing practice (McTeigue, 2015b; NCSBN, 2018c)
      1. Practice related—failure to uphold standard of care (e.g., failure to assess patients or document care, practicing outside scope of practice or without a license)
      2. Substance abuse (e.g., impairment related to controlled substances or alcohol)
      3. Diversion of controlled substances—misuse of controlled substances intended for patients (e.g., stealing pain medications from work for own personal use, to give to others, or for financial gain)
      4. Professional boundary violations—extending therapeutic relationship for personal benefit

(e.g., flirting, showing favoritism, keeping secrets with patients)

5. Sexual misconduct—inappropriate sexual contact between nurse and patient (e.g., behaviors considered seductive, sexually demeaning, harassing)

6. Abuse—physical, mental, or emotional maltreatment of patients/clients

7. Fraud—misrepresenting the truth (e.g., overstating own credentials or experience, falsely documenting care, submitting/authorizing inaccurate records for billing)

8. Positive criminal background checks—rules vary according to the extent of past criminal activity and potential future risk to patients (e.g., the more severe the past criminal activity, the more extensive potential consequences on licensure)

9. Improper social media use—unethical, unprofessional, insensitive use of social media (e.g., posting disparaging comments about patients even without using the patient name, posting photos of work settings, breaching patient privacy or confidentiality, texting information about patients to coworkers)

G. Potential disciplinary actions by BoNs (NCSBN, 2018d)

1. Fine or civil penalty
2. Referral to alternative-to-discipline program
3. Public reprimand or censure
4. Requirements for monitoring, remediation, education
5. Limitation or restriction of practice
6. Separation from practice (e.g., suspension, loss of license)

III. Patient's bill of rights in health care

A. A variety of documents from national organizations and health care institutions outline what consumers can expect from the health care environment.

B. The Affordable Care Act legislated a new set of patient's rights in the health care environment (U.S. Department of Health & Human Services, 2017).

1. Provides coverage to Americans with preexisting conditions
2. Mandates insurers to offer dependent coverage for children to age 26
3. Prohibits annual and lifetime limits on coverage
4. Prohibits preexisting condition exclusions for children
5. Prohibits arbitrary withdrawals of insurance coverage
6. Mandates essential health services (e.g., screening, vaccination)
7. Provides four tiers of benefit coverage (e.g., low to high monthly premiums and out-of-pocket costs)
8. Established individual mandate for insurance coverage (later repealed)

C. Individuals who are hospitalized have the right to the following (American Hospital Association, 2003):

1. High-quality hospital care
2. A clean and safe environment
3. Involvement in their care
4. Protection of their privacy
5. Help when leaving the hospital
6. Help with billing claims

IV. Standards of practice—outline nationally determined practice expectations for individuals or organizations; provide guidance for nurses, employers, and educators and often used in legal situations to determine whether an individual or organization met what is regarded as the standard of care

A. Nursing professional practice standards

1. Nursing—scope and standards of practice (American Nurses Association [ANA], 2015a)
2. Code of ethics for nurses—with interpretative statements (ANA, 2015b)
3. Nursing's social policy statement—the essence of the profession (ANA, 2010)

B. Oncology nursing practice standards (Table 57.1)—practice standards can be used by individual nurses, health care organizations, and educational programs to promote and support high-quality cancer care

C. Accreditation and certification agencies or programs for health care institutions

1. The Joint Commission (www.jointcommission.org)
2. National Patient Safety Goals (NPSG) (https://www.jointcommission.org/standards_information/npsgs.aspx)
3. Magnet Recognition Program (https://www.nursingworld.org/organizational-programs/magnet/)
4. Occupational Safety and Health Administration (OSHA) (www.osha.gov)
5. Centers for Disease Control and Prevention (CDC) (www.cdc.gov)
6. Department of Health and Human Services (DHHS) (www.hhs.gov)
7. National Institutes of Health (NIH) (www.nih.gov)
8. Centers for Medicare and Medicaid (CMS) (www.cms.gov)
9. National Institute for Occupational Safety and Health (NIOSH) (https://www.cdc.gov/niosh/index.htm)

D. Oncology-specific accreditation and certification agencies and programs

1. Oncology Nursing Certification Corporation (ONCC) (www.oncc.org)
2. American College of Surgeons – Commission on Cancer (ACS-COC) (https://www.facs.org/quality-programs/cancer/coc)

TABLE 57.1 Oncology Nursing Society Standards for Practice

Standard Title	Standard Description
Access Device Standards of Practice for Oncology Nursing (Camp-Sorrell & Matey, 2017)	Provides an overview of literature and standards of practice related to device selection, care, optimal use, and legal implications in oncology care.
ONS Nursing Documentation Standards for Cancer Treatment (Wiley, Galioto, Matey, & Wyant, 2017)	Provides a comprehensive overview of documentation standards for multiple cancer treatments, use of vascular access devices, blood product transfusion, and chemotherapy extravasation.
ONS Standard for Educating Nurses Who Administer Chemotherapy and Biotherapy (ONS, n.d.a)	Describes pathways for chemotherapy/biotherapy course and/or certificate completion based on administration volume or number of chemotherapy and/or biotherapy agents.
Statement on the Scope and Standards of Oncology Nursing Practice Generalist and Advanced Practice (Brant & Wickham, 2013)	Describes scope of oncology nursing practice, standards of care for RNs and advanced practice RNs, and professional performance issues.
Standards of Oncology Education: Patient/ Significant Other and Public (4th ed.) (Blecher, Ireland, & Watson, 2016)	Describes formal and informal education standards that oncology nurses can use for planning and evaluating education for patients and significant others.
Standards of Oncology Nursing Education: Generalist and Advanced Practice Levels (4th ed.) (Jacobs & Mayer, 2015)	Addresses standards of oncology nursing academic and clinical education for faculty and/or clinical educators.
Survivorship Care Standards for Accreditation (ONS, n.d.b)	Describes the Commission on Cancer (CoC) and National Accreditation Program for Breast Centers (NAPBC) survivorship care plans requirements, including documentation, implementation, and key elements of the care plan.
2016 Updated American Society of Clinical Oncology/Oncology Nursing Society chemotherapy administration safety standards, including standards for pediatric oncology (Neuss et al., 2017)	This paper describes the recommended components of safe administration of enteral and parenteral chemotherapy, including policies and procedures outlining staff training and continuing education, chemotherapy preparation, chemotherapy administration, and patient education and management guidelines.

3. Quality Oncology Practice Initiative (QOPI) (https://practice.asco.org/quality-improvement/quality-programs/quality-oncology-practice-initiative)

V. Legal issues for individuals with cancer (Cancer Legal Resource Center [CLRC], 2012; Ponto, 2018; Retkin, Antoniadis, Pepitone, & Duval, 2013; Schulmeister, 2018)
   A. Advance care planning (e.g., advance directives, orders for life-sustaining treatment)
   B. Bankruptcy—3% of cancer survivors file for bankruptcy (Banegas et al., 2016)
   C. Competence for decision making
   D. Disability insurance
   E. Employment discrimination
   F. Genetic testing and discrimination
   G. Health insurance
   H. Hospital-acquired conditions (HACs) (Kirkland-Walsh, 2016; Rawson, 2014)
   I. Human subjects research
   J. Informed consent for chemotherapy (oral and parenteral)
   K. Lesbian, gay, bisexual, transgender (LGBT) discrimination (Cahill, 2018)
   L. Medical errors
   M. Organ and tissue donation
   N. Privacy and confidentiality
   O. Survivorship care planning
   P. Time off from work (Family & Medical Leave Act [FMLA])
   Q. Withdrawing treatment—right to receive or discontinue treatment

VI. Practice issues in oncology nursing with legal implications (Polovich, Olsen, & LeFebvre, 2014; Ponto, 2018; Schulmeister, 2018)
   A. Patient-related issues
     1. Adverse drug events
     2. Iatrogenic/HACs (e.g., falls, infection)
     3. Inadequate patient/family education
     4. Proper use of telephone triage
     5. Treatment-related errors (e.g., chemotherapy administration errors)
     6. Vesicant administration
     7. Withholding and withdrawing life support
   B. Professional practice/nursing issues
     1. Drug or substance diversion
     2. Documentation errors/omissions (e.g., inadequate/nonexistent informed consent, patient/family education, or telephone triage documentation)
     3. Exposure to occupational and environmental hazards

4. Improper risk evaluation and mitigation strategies (REMS) reporting
5. Lack of competency/lack of competency documentation (e.g., chemotherapy administration, patient safety, preventing iatrogenic conditions)
6. Malpractice
7. Mandatory reporting (state regulations requiring nurses and other health care providers to report certain conditions or events, e.g., suspected child, sexual, domestic, or elder abuse; communicable diseases; death)
8. Misuse of social media (National Council of State Boards of Nursing [NCSBN], 2015)
9. Off-label drug or device use (Saiyed, Ong, & Chew, 2017)
10. Practicing outside of authorized scope of practice
11. Workplace behavior and performance issues—lateral violence, bullying, verbal intimidation (U.S. Department of Labor, 2016)
    a. Can range in severity from disruptive behaviors to assault
    b. Currently no national workplace laws governing workplace bullying, but some state laws have established penalties
    c. OSHA—requires employers to provide a workplace free from hazards and recommends policies and procedures that reflect "zero-tolerance for all forms of violence from all sources" (U.S. Department of Labor, 2016)
    d. Need for all staff to receive education and training to ensure a clear understanding of their role in situations involving lateral violence, bullying, and intimidation

VII. Legislative policy issues affecting oncology care (ONS, n.d.c.)
A. Quality cancer care
B. Patient/staff safety
C. Workforce/education
D. Value of oncology nurses
E. Scope of practice (National Academies of Science, 2010)

VIII. Legal liability terms and definitions (https://dictionary.law.com/)
A. Negligence—deviation from the acceptable standard of care that a reasonable person would use in a specific situation
B. Malpractice—deviation from a professional standard of care
C. Duty—care relationship between patient and provider
D. Breach of duty—failure to meet an acceptable standard of care
E. Defamation—the act of harming the reputation of another by making false statements to a third person

F. False imprisonment—a restraint of a person in a bounded area without justification or consent
G. Slander—a defamatory statement expressed in a transitory form, especially speech
H. Proximate cause—the cause that directly produces an event and without which the event would not have occurred
I. Civil—of or pertaining to private rights and remedies that are sought by action or suit but distinct from criminal proceedings
J. Assault—the threat of, or use of, force on another that causes that person to have a reasonable apprehension of imminent harmful or offensive contact

IX. Common causes of litigation against nurses (Watson, 2014)
A. Lack of informed consent
B. Improper medical device use
C. Not following standards of care
D. Failure to communicate effectively/appropriately
E. Inadequate or inappropriate patient assessment, monitoring, or teaching
F. Lack of patient advocacy
G. Failure to communicate/report changes in patient condition
H. Inadequate or inappropriate treatment or care
I. Medication errors
J. Inappropriate delegation or supervision—lack of consideration for delegating the right task, to the right person, at the right time, under the right circumstances, and providing the right supervision
K. Inadequate documentation
L. Working while impaired (substance use, fatigue)

X. Strategies for minimizing risk of malpractice or disciplinary action (Brous, 2012; Watson, 2014)
A. Development of skills in interpersonal communication—positive relationships with patients and families reduce the likelihood of a patient or family complaint.
    1. Communicating clearly when educating patients and families
    2. Listening carefully to family member questions and concerns
B. Maintaining knowledge and skills
    1. Attending relevant continuing education programs
    2. Obtaining specialty certification
    3. Obtaining an advanced or graduate degree
    4. Joining relevant professional associations (e.g., Oncology Nursing Society, Hospice and Palliative Nurses Association, American Society for Pain Management Nursing)
    5. Becoming involved in advocacy initiatives with nursing professional organizations
C. Verifying that job description fits within state-defined scope of practice

D. Maintaining individual professional liability insurance—can protect a nurse beyond what employer policies may cover

E. Maintaining a "job well done" file—keeping letters of commendation, thank-you notes or cards from patients and family members, colleagues, and supervisors

F. Keeping a list of community service activities which demonstrate civic-mindedness (e.g., participation in cancer screening activities; teaching community basic life support classes; leading cancer support groups)

G. Maintaining positive relationship with supervisor—demonstrating willingness to contribute to the professional environment (e.g., serving on unit or institutional committees; leading journal club)
1. Demonstrating effective follower behaviors (e.g., offering constructive feedback; participating in workplace decision making; offering creative solutions to problems in the workplace)

H. Keeping abreast of current regulatory and practice issues through state BoN

I. Maintaining professional boundaries with patients

J. Respecting physical limitations (e.g., fatigue related to rotating shifts, overtime)

XI. Role of documentation in reducing legal risks
A. Reflects the quality of care
B. Can be used in legal disputes to determine whether a standard of care was met
1. Nurses may be deposed and questioned about own or others' documentation
C. Seven essentials of quality nursing documentation revealed by a meta-analysis (Jefferies, Johnson, & Griffiths, 2010):
1. Patient centered
2. Contained the actual work of nurses, including education and psychosocial support
3. Written to reflect the objective clinical judgment of the nurse
4. Presented in logical and sequential manner
5. Written as events occur
6. Reflected variances in the patient's condition (e.g., changes in patient response or nursing interventions)
7. Fulfilled legal requirements

XII. Resources
A. American Association of Legal Nurse Consultants—www.aalnc.org
B. American Hospital Association—www.aha.org
C. American Nurses Association—https://www.nursingworld.org/
D. Cancer Legal Resource Center—http://cancerlegalresources.org/
E. National Cancer Legal Services Network—www.nclsn.org
F. National Council of State Board of Nursing—www.ncsbn.org

G. Oncology Nursing Society—www.ons.org
H. Oncology Nursing Certification Corporation—www.oncc.org
I. Quality Oncology Practice Initiative—https://practice.asco.org/quality-improvement/quality-programs/quality-oncology-practice-initiative

REFERENCES

American Hospital Association. (2003). *The patient care partnership: understanding expectations, rights and responsibilities.* Retrieved from the AHA website https://www.aha.org/system/files/2018-01/aha-patient-care-partnership.pdf.

American Nurses Association. (2010). *Nursing's social policy statement: the essence of the profession.* Silver Spring, MD: American Nurses Association.

American Nurses Association. (2015a). *Nursing: scope and standards of practice* (3rd ed.). Silver Spring, MD: American Nurses Association.

American Nurses Association. (2015b). *Code of ethics for nurses with interpretive statements.* Silver Spring, MD: American Nurses Association.

Banegas, M.P., Guy, G.P., de Moor, J.S., Ekwueme, D.U., Virgo, K.S., et al. (2016). For working-age cancer survivors, medical debt and bankruptcy create financial hardships. *Health Affairs, 35*(1), 54-61L.

Blecher, C. S., Ireland, A. M., & Watson, J. L. (Eds.), (2016). *Standards of oncology education: patient/significant other and public* (4th ed.). Pittsburgh, PA: Oncology Nursing Society.

Brant, J., & Wickham, R. (Eds.), (2013). *Statement on the scope and standards of oncology nursing practice generalist and advanced practice.* Pittsburgh, PA: Oncology Nursing Society.

Brous, E. (2012). Professional licensure protection strategies. *American Journal of Nursing, 112,* 43–47.

Cahill, S. R. (2018). Legal and policy issues for LGBT patients with cancer or at elevated risk of cancer. *Seminars in Oncology Nursing, 34*(1), 90–98.

Camp-Sorrell, D., & Matey, L. (2017). *Access device standards of practice for oncology nursing.* Pittsburgh, PA: Oncology Nursing Society.

Cancer Legal Resource Center (CLRC). (2012). *The HCP manual: a legal resource guide for oncology health care professionals.* Los Angeles: Cancer Legal Resource Center. http://cancerlegalresources.org/wp-content/uploads/sites/3/2017/09/HCPManual-3rdEdition1-23-12withforms.pdf.

Jacobs, L. A., & Mayer, D. K. (2015). *Standards of oncology nursing education: generalist and advanced practice levels* (4th ed.). Pittsburgh, PA: Oncology Nursing Society.

Jefferies, D., Johnson, M., & Griffiths, R. (2010). A meta-study of the essentials of quality nursing documentation. *International Journal of Nursing Practice, 16,* 112–124. https://doi.org/10.1111/j.1440-172X.2009.01815.x.

Kirkland-Walsh, H. (2016). Legal perspectives: transparency, QI mitigate HAPU lawsuit risk. *Nursing Management, 47*(6), 10–12.

McTeigue, J. (2015a). *The U.S. legal system.* In Elsevier, *Legal and ethical issues for health professions* (3rd ed.). St. Louis, MO: Elsevier Saunders.

McTeigue, J. (2015b). *Code and standards infractions.* In Elsevier, *Legal and ethical issues for health professions* (3rd ed.). St. Louis, MO: Elsevier Saunders.

National Academies of Science. (2010). The future of nursing: leading change, advancing health. Committee on the Robert Wood Johnson Foundation Initiative on the Future of Nursing, at the Institute of Medicine. Retrieved from National Academies Press: https://www.nap.edu/catalog/12956/the-future-of-nursing-leading-change-advancing-healthfile:///Z:/02_ed/05_Resupply/ons/Ref/0002218519.html - sLink18ir0140.

National Council of State Boards of Nursing (NCSBN). (2015). *Social media in nursing: understand the benefits and the risks.* Chicago, IL: National Council of State Boards of Nursing.

National Council of State Boards of Nursing (NCSBN). (2018a). NCLEX and other exams. Retrieved from NCSBN website: https://www.ncsbn.org/nclex.htm.

National Council of State Boards of Nursing (NCSBN). (2018b). Enhanced nurse licensure compact (eNLC) implementation. Retrieved from NCSBN website: https://www.ncsbn.org/enhanced-nlc-implementation.htm.

National Council of State Boards of Nursing (NCSBN). (2018c). Initials Review of Complaint. Retrieved from NCSBN website: https://www.ncsbn.org/1616.htm.

National Council of State Boards of Nursing (NCSBN). (2018d). Board Action. Retrieved from NCSBN website: https://www.ncsbn.org/673.htm.

Neuss, M. N., Gilmore, T. R., Belderson, K. M., Billett, A. L., Conti-Kalchik, T., Harvey, B. E., Hendricks, C., LeFebvre, K. B., Mangu, P. B., McNiff, K., Olsen, M., Schulmeister, L., Von Gehr, A., & Polovich, M. (2017). 2016 Updated American Society of Clinical Oncology/Oncology Nursing Society chemotherapy administration safety standards including standards for pediatric oncology. *Oncology Nursing Forum, 44,* 31–43. https://doi.org/10.1188/17.ONF.31-43.

NOLO. (2018). Nolo's plain-English law dictionary: Statute. Retrieved from NOLO website: https://www.nolo.com/dictionary/statute-term.htmlfile:///Z:/02_ed/05_Resupply/ons/Ref/0002218519.html.

Oncology Nursing Society. (n.d.a). *ONS standard for educating nurses who administer chemotherapy and biotherapy.* Pittsburgh, PA: Oncology Nursing Society.

Oncology Nursing Society. (n.d.b). *Survivorship care standards for accreditation.* Pittsburgh, PA: Oncology Nursing Society.

Oncology Nursing Society (n.d.c). *Legislative and regulatory health policy agenda 115th Congress, 1st Session.* Retrieved from https://www.ons.org/sites/default/files/ONS_HP_Agenda_115th_1st_Session_012317.pdf.

Polovich, M., Olsen, M., & LeFebvre, K. (Eds.), (2014). *Chemotherapy and biotherapy guidelines and recommendations for practice* (4th ed.). Pittsburgh, PA: Oncology Nursing Society.

Ponto, J. (2018). Legal issues in cancer care. In M. M. Gullatte (Ed.), *Clinical guide to antineoplastic therapy: a chemotherapy handbook* (4th ed.). Pittsburgh, PA: Oncology Nursing Society.

Rawson, E. L. (2014). Hospital-acquired infections: Alfred Nel v Guy's & St. Thomas' NHS Foundation Trust. *Clinical Risk, 20*(4), 95–99.

Retkin, R., Antoniadis, D., Pepitone, D. F., & Duval, D. (2013). Legal services: a necessary component of patient navigation. *Seminars in Oncology Nursing, 29,* 149–155.

Saiyed, M. M., Ong, P. S., & Chew, L. (2017). Off-label drug use in oncology: a systematic review of literature. *Journal of Clinical Pharmacy and Therapeutics, 42*(3), 251–258. https://doi.org/10.1111/jcpt.12507.

Schulmeister, L. C. (2018). Legal and safety issues. In C. H. Yarbro, D. Wujcik, & B. H. Gobel (Eds.), *Cancer nursing: principles and practice* (8th ed.). Burlington, MA: Jones and Bartlett.

U.S. Department of Health & Human Services (DHHS) (2017). About the affordable care act. Retrieved from https://www.hhs.gov/healthcare/about-the-aca/index.html.

U.S. Department of Labor Occupational Safety and Health Administration (2016). Guidelines for preventing workplace violence for healthcare and social service workers. Retrieved from https://www.osha.gov/Publications/osha3148.pdf.

Watson, E. (2014). Nursing malpractice: costs, trends, and issues. *Journal of Legal Nurse Consulting, 25*(1), 26–31.

Wiley, K., Galioto, M., Matey, L., & Wyant, T. (2017). *Oncology Nursing Society Documentation standards for cancer treatment.* Pittsburgh, PA: Oncology Nursing Society.

58

Ethical Issues

Jeanne Marie Erickson and Joshua Hardin

I. Ethics and oncology nursing
   A. Ethics is the study about what is morally good, whether actions are judged to be right or wrong, and how people and institutions make and implement ethical choices. Ethics pervades every nursing interaction and does not exist in isolated or sporadic dilemmas (Moore, Engel, & Prentice, 2014).
   B. Oncology nurses frequently experience ethical issues due to the life-threatening nature of cancer and difficult decisions around complex treatments (Rushton, Batcheller, Schroeder, & Donohue, 2015).
   C. Individuals perceive ethical issues differently, based on their individual values, knowledge, reflective thinking, and reasoning.
   D. Ethics constantly evolves due to changes in professional roles, codes, and legislation, as well as changes in society and culture (Kangasniemi, Pakkanen, & Korhonen, 2015).
II. American Nurses Association (ANA) Code of Ethics
   A. Understanding and using nursing's Code of Ethics
      1. The *Code of Ethics for Nurses with Interpretive Statements* (ANA, 2015), referred to here as *the code*, may be accessed free online via the ANA's website (www.nursingworld.org) or purchased through most book distributors.
      2. The code (ANA, 2015) articulates nursing's core values to the public and the discipline. The ANA's (2015) ethical code outlines general provisions followed by interpretive statements to help nurses better understand the deeper meaning underlying each provision and how each nurse might best embody the code.
   B. Provisions
      1. Winland-Brown, Lachman, and Swanson (2015) observe that the first four provisions of the code present nursing's core values, duties, and accountabilities, and include:
         a. *The nurse practices with compassion and respect for the inherent dignity, worth, and unique attributes of every person.*
         b. *The nurse's primary commitment is to the patient whether an individual, family, group, community, or population.*
         c. *The nurse promotes, advocates for, and protects the rights, health, and safety of the patient.*
         d. *The nurse has authority, accountability, and responsibility for nursing practice; makes decisions; and takes action consistent with the obligation to promote health and to provide optimal care.*
      2. Provisions five through nine of the code establish boundaries of duty and loyalty, and delineate nursing's responsibilities toward social justice, health policy, and advancement of nursing as a science and profession, and include (Lachman, Swanson, & Winland-Brown, 2015):
         a. *The nurse owes the same duties to self as to others, including the responsibility to promote health and safety, preserve wholeness of character and integrity, maintain competence, and continue personal and professional growth.*
         b. *The nurse, through individual and collective effort, establishes, maintains, and improves the ethical environment of the work setting and conditions of employment that are conducive to safe, quality health care.*
         c. *The nurse, in all roles and settings, advances the profession through research and scholarly inquiry, professional standards development, and the generation of both nursing and health policy.*
         d. *The nurse collaborates with other health professionals and the public to protect human rights, promote health diplomacy, and reduce health disparities.*
         e. *The profession of nursing, collectively through its professional organizations, must articulate nursing values, maintain integrity of the profession, and integrate principles of social justice into nursing and health policy.*
III. Ethical theories and approaches
   A. Philosophical underpinnings
      1. Ethical theories provide a common frame of reference that facilitates ethical discourse. Some commonly encountered ethical theories are:
         a. Utilitarianism. This theory identifies what is good as what will result in the most good for

the most people. Proponents of utilitarianism choose actions based on what will generate the most good or, as is often the case, the least harm (Haddad, 2016).

    b. Deontology. This theory argues that an action's goodness is derived from intention. From this perspective, certain actions are *intrinsically* right or wrong.

B. Approaches to health care ethics

  1. Currently, the dominant approach to health care ethics is the bioethical model (Haddad, 2016; Moore et al., 2014).

    a. The bioethical model is strongly associated with medicine as a discipline and principlist approaches to ethics.

    b. A principlist ethical approach entails determining the salient ethical principles related to an ethical dilemma and balancing those principles to achieve a justifiable resolution that maximizes good.

    c. Beauchamp and Childress (2012) propose that the ethical principles of nonmaleficence, beneficence, autonomy, and justice are universally applicable to health care. These principles are summarized in Box 58.1.

  2. Virtue- and care-based ethics provide alternative approaches to health care ethics (Haddad, 2016; Moore et al., 2014).

    a. Virtue-based approaches arise from the notion that dynamic character traits motivate actions. If nurses acquire qualities like courage, fidelity, and veracity, they will make ethically sound decisions (Haddad, 2016).

    b. Care-based ethical approaches centralize the relationship between nurse and patient/family as the locus of moral decision making. This approach suggests that nurses form connections with patients that allow them to interpret

IV. Selected areas in oncology nursing where ethical issues commonly arise:

A. Communication with patients and families

  1. Effective communication between nurses and patients is essential for the development of a trusting relationship that shows compassion and respect.

  2. Truth-telling and ensuring the patient has adequate information are critical to support patient autonomy.

  3. Ineffective communication leads to increased distress and poorer outcomes in patients, and increased stress and burnout in oncology nurses. Oncology nurses report the communication challenges that may raise ethical concerns (Banerjee et al., 2016):

    a. Nurses may be aware of bad news before the patient is told; may observe the patient did not accurately grasp bad news or bad news was not honestly delivered.

    b. Nurses may feel they lack skills to communicate with empathy—not knowing the best thing to provide comfort. Nurses can be troubled by some patients and families who are angry or disrespectful and do not welcome empathy.

    c. Differences in age, culture, and personality may create challenges in communication between nurses and patients in difficult situations.

B. Confidentiality and privacy

  1. Privacy and confidentiality are issues of autonomy; respecting confidentiality and privacy is part of respecting human dignity.

    a. Privacy is an expectation and a right codified by law, while confidentiality is a professional and personal duty to keep certain types of information private.

    b. In the United States, confidentiality and privacy as they relate to protected health information are defined by the Health Insurance Portability and Accountability Act (HIPAA, 1996; Morris, 2013).

    c. For health care providers, HIPAA requires that only the minimum amount of Protected Health Information (PHI) required to care for patients be accessed or shared; the law requires that (PHI) be kept private and held in confidence by health care providers (HIPAA, 1996; Morris, 2013).

  2. Genomics, personalized medicine, and genetically-developed pharmacotherapeutics are rapidly evolving fields, creating new ethical challenges involving autonomy, beneficence, veracity, and justice.

    a. Helping patients understand risks and benefits of genetic tests, and genomic data collection are

---

BOX 58.1   Ethical Principles

Beneficence—The duty to do good or do what is of benefit. However, the duty is more complex than the simple definition implies. What is good for one patient may not be for another patient, and the options available for doing good may be scarce (Haddad, 2016). Compassion is a defining quality of beneficence.

Nonmaleficence—The duty to not harm others. Sometimes, this means ensuring that the benefits of a treatment outweigh the harm. Exemplified by the Hippocratic admonition, "First, do no harm."

Autonomy—The respect for another person's right to choose, or self-determination (Haddad, 2016). Autonomy stems from the core value of dignity (ANA, 2015).

Justice—In relation to health care ethics, justice refers to the fair allocation of resources. This concept is referred to as distributive justice (Beauchamp & Childress, 2012).

poised to take greater importance as a nursing function in the future (Lea, 2016).

    b. Confidentiality of genetic information protected by law, but risks include discrimination and unequal treatment related to sharing of genetic test results (Blix, 2014).

3. Social media and social networking sites are commonly encountered and used by consumers in health care today.

    a. Social media may be used positively. Patients can research their conditions, interact with other people in similar situations, become better informed health care consumers.

    b. Social media may be used negatively. For nurses, the clearest risks are associated with privacy and confidentiality breaches since it is difficult to completely deidentify data (Henderson & Dahnke, 2015).

    c. Social media can blur professional boundaries; ethically questionable to connect with patients on social media outside nurse-patient relationship (Henderson & Dahnke, 2015).

    d. Posting deidentified information about a patient encounter may erode patients' trust in nursing as a discipline, places patients at risk of identification (Henderson & Dahnke, 2015).

C. The ethical climate of the practice environment

1. Characteristics of the practice environment may create ethical problems for nurses if behaviors are present that demonstrate a lack of respect for other people.

    a. Intimidating behavior ranges from incivility and disruptive conduct to bullying and to physical and emotional assault (Lachman, 2014).

    b. Horizontal/lateral violence is rude or derogatory remarks or condescending behavior toward (or about) a coworker. If the coworker is at a comparable level within the organization, the violence is lateral. If the behavior is directed at someone above or below the aggressor's organizational level, the conduct is horizontal.

2. Nurses may perceive inadequate resources and support in their setting that prevents them from practicing according to their values and fulfilling their professional duties.

    a. Nurses who carry a higher caseload of patients, who work in acute care settings, and who report unsafe staffing levels may have higher moral distress (deVeer et al., 2013; Whitehead, Herbertson, Hamric, Epstein, & Fisher, 2015).

    b. A poor ethical climate for nurses reflects lack of support from peers and managers, lack of respect between colleagues, lack of involvement in decision making, and poor nurse–physician collaboration (Lamiani, Borghi, & Argentero, 2017).

D. Clinically challenging patient care situations

1. Oncology nurses may experience ethical concerns in situations when they feel they are not able to deliver optimal care that is in the best interest of the patient.

    a. Nurses describe situations where they report "feeling torn between competing obligations" and situations where different moral views are not discussed (Pavlish, Brown-Saltzman, Jakel, & Fine, 2014).

    b. Nurses report moral distress watching patients suffer due to lack of communication by and between providers, aggressive and prolonged care that is not in the best interest of patients, and a lack of continuity of care (Ameri & Safavibayatneed, 2016; de Veer et al., 2013; Whitehead et al., 2015).

2. Situations that triggered ethics consultations by oncology nurses required mediation in disagreements and decisions about the appropriate level of care, informed consent, code status, and difficult discharges of patients (Gallagher, Neel, & Sotomayor, 2018).

E. End-of-life care

1. End-of-life situations commonly raise ethical issues for nurses and cause moral distress (Gallagher et al., 2018; Cheon, Coyle, Wiegand, & Welsh, 2015).

    a. Increased technology and availability of life support measures increase the likelihood of aggressive care longer, contributing to concerns about overtreatment, inappropriate treatment, and prolonging the dying process (Cheon et al., 2015).

    b. Advance directives may improve the likelihood that patients receive their preferred end-of-life care, but nurses report a lack of knowledge and a lack of time to help patients with advance directives and situations that threaten patient autonomy (Cheon et al., 2015).

    c. Despite advances in symptom management, nurses report concerns over patient suffering related to unrelieved pain, other symptoms, and undermedication and overmedication (Cheon et al., 2015).

2. Nurses may encounter patients at the end of life who express a desire to die and who make requests related to assisted dying, assisted suicide, and euthanasia.

    a. Nurses should assess for any mental disorder, such as depression, or for psychological or physical suffering in patients who express a desire to die (Wilson et al., 2014).

    b. Although controversial, assisted dying is legal in several countries and in several U.S. states. Nurses need to be prepared to discuss options and resources with patients who desire death (Lehto, Olsen, & Chan, 2016).

3. Nurses have increased moral distress when they learn best practices in end-of-life care but are unable to implement them in their settings (Whitehead, 2015).

4. End-of-life care is more difficult when patients are from different cultures, when language barriers require translation, and when providers lack cultural training (Pavlish et al., 2014).

F. Issues related to decision making

1. Shared decision making is the contemporary model where patients choose treatment options based on guidance from health care professionals (Jones & Campbell, 2016) (see Chapter 6).

2. Informed consent process ensures the patient has adequate understanding of risks, benefits, alternatives, and consequences of treatment (Rock & Hoebeke, 2014); supports autonomy and human dignity; touches on issues of beneficence, justice, and veracity.

3. Decision-making capacity determined by health care providers, including nurses. Competency is a legal term, determined by courts of law (Rock and Hoebeke, 2014).

   a. Optimally, the decisionmaker is the patient, but this may not be possible due to the nature of the illness or physiopsychological status.

   b. Patients may voluntarily imbue another person with the power to make decisions for them as their power of attorney (POA). If no POA is available, the patient's next of kin is the decisionmaker. Courts may select a guardian or proxy to make decisions on the patient's behalf.

4. Pediatric patients younger than 18 years of age cannot legally consent to treatments or procedures. Therefore their parents or guardians make decisions on the child's behalf.

   a. Assent for procedures should be sought from pediatric patients as young as 7 years of age. Assent is expression of approval or agreement relating to the planned intervention (Webster, Lewis, & Brown, 2014).

V. Resources for addressing ethical issues

A. Importance of addressing ethical issues

1. Moral distress in nurses is associated with burnout, lower job satisfaction, and intention to leave a position (deVeer et al., 2013; Rushton et al., 2015).

2. Emotional responses to ethical issues can accumulate and cloud thinking, creating a crescendo effect over time that leads to providers having stronger emotional reactions and ultimately emotional exhaustion (Hamric, 2012).

3. When providers are focused on their own moral struggles or interprofessional conflicts, they may miss the needs of patients and families (Pavlish et al., 2014).

4. Some degree of moral tension is inevitable in the clinical setting and may even be desirable as it reflects providers' sensitivity to moral issues, which will always be present (DeVeer et al., 2013).

B. Everyday professional comportment

1. Nurses can take responsibility and ownership for their professional behaviors, words, and practice. This type of conduct is exemplified by the concept of *everyday professional comportment* and includes attributes of mutual respect, harmony in beliefs and actions, commitment to colleagues and patients, and collaboration (Clickner & Shirey, 2013).

C. Creating an ethical community

1. Moral communities are characterized by respectful team relationships, open and honest communication, ethics-minded leadership, and readily available ethics resources that are used by providers (Pavlish et al., 2014).

2. Leaders with management styles that focus on people and relationships rather than policies may reduce moral distress in staff (deVeer et al., 2013).

D. Framework for ethical decision making

1. Doherty and Purtilo (2015) outline one process to address ethical concerns and facilitate a decision or resolution to the problem; process can be used by individual nurses, advanced practice nurses who act as resources in clinical settings, and ethics consultants in the organization (Box 58.2).

E. Education

1. Ethical formation in nursing is a career-long process developed by the intersection of philosophical and applied ethical theory with discipline-specific norms and experience. Reflection, mentoring, and communication are critical.

BOX 58.2 **Identifying Ethical Concerns**

Step 1. Gather information from key participants and obtain facts to understand the multiple complex perspectives of the ethical problem.

Step 2. Identify the type of ethical problem that exists. Define what makes this an ethical problem.

Step 3. Analyze the problem using ethical theories or approaches. Discuss what principles, codes, laws, or perspectives are relevant.

Step 4. Explore practical alternatives. Discuss possible courses of action, with the goal of an action that is ethically reasonable and most likely to achieve the desired outcome with the least harm.

Step 5. Evaluate the process and outcome. Debriefing sessions with those involved are critical for exploring whether the problem was adequately resolved, for addressing emotions and distress, and for discussing implications for future similar situations.

2. Continuing education in ethics available by participation in ethics committees, conferences, and educational programs (Catlin, 2014). Professional journals offer sections related to ethical issues in nursing or are dedicated to ethics, such as *Nursing Ethics*.

F. Ethics consultation/committees

1. All hospitals should have access to ethics consultation services.

2. Ethics committees should be open to anyone within the health care system who is experiencing moral uncertainty or distress, regardless of position (Catlin, 2014).

3. Functions of hospital ethics committees are education, policy development, and case consultation (Catlin, 2014). Additional functions include difficult situation debriefing, organization and operational ethics leadership, and risk management related to ethics.

REFERENCES

Ameri, M. & Safavibayatneed, Z. (2016). Moral distress of oncology nurses and morally distressing situations in oncology units. *Australian Journal of Advanced Nursing, 33*(3), 6–14.

American Nurses Association (ANA). (2015). *Code of ethics for nurses with interpretive statements.* Silver Spring, MD: American Nurses Association.

Banerjee, S. C., Manna, R., Coyle, N., Shen, M. J., Pehrson, C., Zaider, T., & Bylund, C. L. (2016). Oncology nurses' communication challenges with patients and families: a qualitative study. *Nurse Education in Practice, 16*(1), 193–201. (2016). https://doi.org/10.1016/j.nepr.2015.07.007.

Beauchamp, T. L. & Childress, J. F. (2012). *Principles of biomedical ethics* (7th ed.). New York: Oxford University Press.

Blix, A. (2014). Personalized medicine, genomics, and pharmacogenomics: a primer for nurses. *Clinical Journal of Oncology Nursing, 18*(4), 437–441. https://doi.org/10.1188/14.CJON.437-441.

Catlin, A. (2014). The hospital ethics committee and the nurse. *Advances in Neonatal Care, 14*(6), 398–402. https://doi.org/10.1097/ANC.0000000000000151.

Cheon, J., Coyle, N., Wiegand, D. L., & Welsh, S. (2015). Ethical issues experienced by hospice and palliative nurses. *Journal of Hospice and Palliative Nursing, 17*, 7–13. https://doi.org/10.1097/NJH.0000000000000129.

Clickner, D. A. & Shirey, M. R. (2013). Professional comportment: the missing element in nursing practice. *Nursing Forum, 48*, 106–113. ISSN: 0029-6473.

de Veer, A., Francke, A. L., Struijs, A., & Willems, D. L. (2013). Determinants of moral distress in daily nursing practice: a cross sectional correlational questionnaire survey. *International Journal of Nursing Studies, 50*, 100–108. https://doi.org/10.1016/j.ijnurstu.2012.08.017.

Doherty, R. F. & Purtilo, R. B. (2015). *Ethical dimensions in the health professions-e-book.* Elsevier Health Sciences. St. Louis: Elsevier.

Gallagher, C. M., Neel, M. B., & Sotomayor, C. R. (2018). A retrospective review of clinical ethics consultations requested by nurses for oncology patients. *Journal of Nursing, 7*(1), 1–7. https://doi.org/10.18686/jn.v7i1.137.

Haddad, A. M. (2016). Principles of ethics. In J. M. Erickson & K. Payne (Eds.), *Ethics in oncology nursing* (pp. 1–18). Pittsburgh, PA: Oncology Nursing Society.

Hamric, A. B. (2012). Empirical research on moral distress: issues, challenges, and opportunities. *HEC Forum, 24*(1), 39–49. https://doi.org/10.1007/s10730-012-9177-x.

Health Insurance Portability and Accountability Act (HIPAA). (1996). Public Law No. 104-191. Retrieved from https://www.gpo.gov/fdsys/pkg/PLAW-104publ191/content-detail.html.

Henderson, M. & Dahnke, M. D. (2015). The ethical use of social media in nursing practice. *Medsurg Nursing, 24*(1), 62. Retrieved from http://www.ncbi.nlm.nih.gov/pubmed/26306360.

Jones, R. A. & Campbell, C. (2016). Treatment decision making. Principles of ethics. In J. M. Erickson & K. Payne (Eds.), *Ethics in oncology nursing* (pp. 41–54). Pittsburgh, PA: Oncology Nursing Society.

Kangasniemi, M., Pakkanen, P., & Korhonen, A. (2015). Professional ethics in nursing: an integrative review. *Journal of Advanced Nursing, 71*(8), 1744–1757. 10.1111/jan.12619.

Lachman, V. D. (2014). Ethical issues in the disruptive behaviors of incivility, bullying, and horizontal/lateral violence. *Medsurg Nursing, 23*(1), 56–60.

Lachman, V. D., Swanson, E. O., & Winland-Brown, J. (2015). The new 'code of ethics for nurses with interpretative statements' (2015): practical clinical application, part II. *Medsurg Nursing, 24*(5), 363.

Lamiani, G., Borghi, L., & Argentero, P. (2017). When healthcare professionals cannot do the right thing: a systematic review of moral distress and its correlates. *Journal of Health Psychology, 22*(1), 51–67. https://doi.org/10.1177/1359105315595120.

Lea, D. H. (2016). Genetics and genomics. In J. M. Erickson & K. Payne (Eds.), *Ethics in oncology nursing* (pp. 123–134). Pittsburgh, PA: Oncology Nursing Society.

Lehto, R. H., Olsen, D. P., & Chan, R. R. (2016). When a patient discusses assisted dying: nursing practice implications. *Journal of Hospice & Palliative Nursing, 18*(3), 184–191. https://doi.org/10.1097/NJH.0000000000000246.

Moore, J., Engel, J., & Prentice, D. (2014). Relational ethics in everyday practice. *Canadian Oncology Nursing Journal, 24*(1), 31–34. https://doi.org/10.5737/1181912x24.

Morris, K. (2013). Sing a song of HIPAA. *Ohio Nurses Review, 88*(2), 12–14.

Pavlish, C., Brown-Saltzman, K., Jakel, P., & Fine, A. (2014). The nature of ethical conflicts and the meaning of moral community in oncology practice. *Oncology Nursing Forum, 41*(2), 130–140. https://doi.org/10.1188/14.ONF.130-140.

Rock, M. J. & Hoebeke, R. (2014). Informed consent: whose duty to inform? *Medsurg Nursing, 23*(3), 189–194.

Rushton, C. H., Batcheller, J., Schroeder, K., & Donohue, P. (2015). Burnout and resilience among nurses practicing in high-intensity settings. *American Journal of Critical Care, 24*(5), 412–420. (2015). https://doi.org/10.4037/ajcc2015291.

Webster, S., Lewis, J., & Brown, A. (2014). Ethical considerations in qualitative research. In J. Ritchie, J. Lewis, C. M. Nicholls, & R. Ormston (Eds.), *Qualitative research practice: a guide for social science students & researchers* (pp. 77–110). Los Angeles, CA: Sage.

Whitehead, P. B., Herbertson, R. K., Hamric, A. B., Epstein, E. G., & Fisher, J. M. (2015). Moral distress among healthcare professionals: report of an institution-wide survey. *Journal of Nursing Scholarship, 47*(2), 117–125. 10.1111.jnu.12115.

Wilson, K. G., Dalgleish, T. L., Chochinov, H. M., Chary, S., Gagnon, P. R., Macmillan, K., & Fainsinger, R. L. (2014). Mental disorders and the desire for death in patients receiving palliative care for cancer. *BMJ Supportive & Palliative Care, 6,* 170–177. https://doi.org/10.1136/bmjspcare-2013-000604.

Winland-Brown, J., Lachman, V. D., & Swanson, E. O. (2015). The new 'code of ethics for nurses with interpretive statements' (2015): practical clinical application, part I. *Medsurg Nursing, 24*(4), 268.

59

Professional Issues

Lani Kai Clinton

QUALITY IMPROVEMENT

I. Impact of medical errors
  A. Approximately 200,000 people die in hospitals each year because of preventable medical errors (Andel, Davidow, Hollwander, & Moreno, 2012).
  B. 770,000 patient injuries and deaths are due to adverse drug events (U.S. Department of Health and Human Services, 2001) resulting in longer hospital stays, increased medical costs, permanent disability, and death (Du et al., 2012)
  C. Financial cost of medical errors is estimated to be $19.5 billion annually from expenses of additional care, lost income, and disability
  D. Nonfinancial costs of medical errors include loss of trust in the health care system, low hospital employee morale, and lower levels of health in the general population

II. Types of errors
  A. Diagnostic—error or delay in diagnosis
  B. Treatment—error in administering or an avoidable delay in treatment
  C. Preventive—inadequate risk assessment (falls, suicide, infection, etc.)
  D. Other—communication or equipment failure

III. Several strategies for improvement provided by the Institute of Medicine (IOM) report, *To Err Is Human: Building a Safer Health System* (IOM, 1999)
  A. National focus to increase the knowledge about safety—creation of Center for Patient Safety tasked with setting national safety goals and tracking their progress
  B. Improved identification of errors—both mandated and confidential voluntary reporting systems to improve participation
  C. Implementing safety systems and development of a "culture of safety" where safety is an explicit organizational goal

IV. IOM report, *Delivering High-Quality Cancer Care: Charting a New Course for a System in Crisis* (IOM, 2013; Ferrell, McCabe, & Levit, 2013)
  A. Conceptual framework for high-quality cancer care delivery system with six key elements of the model (IOM, 2013)
    1. Engaged patients
    2. Optimally trained and coordinated workforce for team-based cancer care
    3. Evidence-based cancer care
    4. A health care information technology (IT) system for cancer care that meets "meaningful use" criteria
    5. Translation of evidence into clinical practice, quality measurement, and performance improvement
    6. Accessible, affordable cancer care to reduce disparities and reform traditional fee-for-service payment reimbursements to new payment models
      a. The Affordable Care Act (ACA or "Obamacare") 2010 made significant advancements in this area with an estimated 30% of traditional Medicare payments flowing through alternative payment models like bundled payments or accountable care organizations (Obama, 2016)
      b. The individual mandate, stating that individuals must sign up for health insurance or face a tax penalty, was repealed in late 2017
        (1) Without a higher number of healthy members to stabilize risk pools, premiums will go up as the balance shifts toward less healthy, higher-cost beneficiaries
  B. Implementing and sustaining improvements in health care can be accomplished with a systematic approach (Mate and Rakover, 2016) in four proposed steps:
    1. Choose a pilot unit within the organization
    2. Start with the immediate supervisor at the point of care
    3. Use early wins to build momentum
    4. Motivate front-line clinical managers by tracking what irks them

V. Model for quality improvement
  A. Plan-Do-Study-Act (PDSA) model (Langley, Nolan, Nolan, Norman, & Provost, 2009) developed by Associates in Process Improvement
    1. Three fundamental questions:
      a. What is our goal?
      b. How will we know that a change is an improvement?
      c. What changes can we make that will result in improvement?

2. Alternate between the PDSA cycle and asking the three fundamental questions
3. Applying the PDSA model in a pragmatic research example (pragmatic clinical trials occur in real-world settings where everyday care occurs)
   a. Strategies and Opportunities to STOP Colon Cancer in Priority Populations (STOP CRC) used PDSA to optimize the research implementation of an automated colon cancer screening program and provided a structure for staff to focus on improving the program and allowed staff to test the change they wanted to see (Coury et al., 2017)

INTERDISCIPLINARY COLLABORATION

I. Oncology Nursing Society (ONS) *Statement on the Scope and Standards of Oncology Nursing Practice: Generalist and Advanced Practice* (Brant & Wickham, 2013). Collaboration involves a partnership between the oncology nurse and the patients, families, interdisciplinary team, and community resources to provide optimal care for complex cancer patients.
II. Barriers to the development of collaborative relationships
   A. Lack of clearly defined, distinct domain of influence
   B. Lack of understanding regarding scope of practice (Schadewaldt, McInnes, Hiller, & Gardner, 2013)
   C. Overlapping and changing domains of practice that produce competition
   D. Lack of recognition for knowledge and expertise
   E. Legal responsibility (Schadewaldt et al., 2013)
III. Opportunities for collaboration
   A. Potential for collaboration among health care providers and agencies exists whenever and with whomever the patient and family have contact.
      1. Although emphasis is often placed on physician–nurse collaboration, nurses have the opportunity for collaborative relationships with any member of the multidisciplinary health care team.
   B. During interdisciplinary tumor boards, some information (e.g., biomedical factors) dominates other information, such as patient comorbidities and psychosocial factors
      1. A recent study showed that inputs from surgeons, radiologists, pathologists, and oncologists positively affected the team's ability to make a decision; patient comorbidity information and nursing inputs were negative predictors (Soukup et al., 2016)
      2. Perhaps the cases with more patient comorbidities as well as those with more nursing input should be flags that categorize these cases as highly complex, perhaps requiring more detailed review to assess unique patient needs

C. There are many opportunities for nurse-to-nurse collaboration within different domains of responsibility, shifts, subspecialty, and practice settings
   1. Day, evening, night shift nurses collaborate to develop change-of-shift report guidelines.
   2. Collaboration among nurses in different subspecialties may lead to the development of educational cancer care materials
D. The future of oncology nursing depends on critical collaborative partnerships being formed within the clinical practice arenas and with other organizations.

PATIENT ADVOCACY

I. For 16 consecutive years, Americans rated nurses the highest on honesty and ethical standards in the Gallup survey (Brenan, 2017); thus nurses are in an excellent position to advocate for patients
II. Definition
   A. In the broadest terms, advocacy is support for a particular cause.
   B. Nurses are natural advocates as they are on the front lines of patient care
   C. Advocacy involves the use of ethical principles (see Chapter 58)
   D. Advocacy is a core value of many professional organizations such as the ONS.
      1. ONS promotes advocating for patients.
         a. Maximizing quality of life
         b. Optimizing patient access to excellent care
         c. Advocating for public policy, especially with respect to health issues
      2. ONS promotes advocating for nurses.
         a. Supporting and respecting oncology nurses
         b. Promoting access to continuing education
         c. Emphasizing a safe work environment and fair compensation
II. Types of advocacy
   A. Simplistic advocacy—one person pleading the cause of another
   B. Paternalistic advocacy—doing something for or to another without that person's consent on the premise that it serves the person's own good
   C. Consumer advocacy—ensuring that patients have adequate information
   D. Consumer-centric advocacy—providing information, supporting the patient's decision
   E. Existential advocacy—acknowledging that various experiences in health care such as the definition of health versus illness, pain versus suffering, and the experience of dying are highly personal; ensuring the patient's beliefs are accepted and supported

F. Human advocacy—as a personal extension of self, disclosing one's own views on health issues and life as a means to connect more deeply with the patient

III. Risks of advocacy

A. Nurses may lack autonomy to take moral actions.

B. Conflicting demands of different patients may create ethical conflicts.

C. Independent action may be restricted by conflicting accountability to public, employer, and patients.

D. Supporting ideas or well-being of another person may lead to personal difficulty and sacrifice.

E. Oncology nurses often must deal with very difficult and controversial issues such as pain management, end-of-life care, and ethical decision making.

IV. Avenues to be advocates

A. Within one's own work setting
1. By listening and speaking out for the needs expressed by patients and their families, thereby empowering patients and their families
2. By keeping current on clinical trials, newly available evidence-based treatments, health legislation that affects practice and health care delivery, hospice, and other resources that can benefit patients and families under their care

B. Within one's own community
1. By volunteering or practicing in minority, underserved, medically disadvantaged, or vulnerable populations to decrease health disparities in cancer and other areas that affect health and well-being
2. By becoming active politically to ensure that legislation protects the health of his or her community, state, and nation

C. Within professional organizations
1. By becoming actively involved in organizational legislative committees advocating for nurses, cancer care, and patients
2. By using avenues available to ONS, American Nurses Association (ANA), and other professional organizations to provide testimony or letters to state legislators, congressional representatives, or both groups to support health care and health care initiatives and reform

EDUCATIONAL AND PROFESSIONAL DEVELOPMENT

I. Synopsis

A. Nursing training evolves to keep pace with our health care system, patient needs and expectations, technological advances, and increasing specialization.

B. Key recommendations of the IOM report, *The Future of Nursing: Leading Change, Advancing Health* (IOM, 2011), are as follows:
1. Nurses practice to the full potential of their education and training.

2. Nurses achieve higher levels of education and training through improved education systems.

3. Nurses engage as full partners with physicians and health care professionals in redesigning health care.

4. Nurses develop effective workforce planning and policy making through better data collection and information infrastructure.

D. Barriers to practice
1. Variability in educational pathways leading to entry-level registered nurse (RN) licensure
2. State variability in licensure requirements of advanced practice RNs (APRNs)
3. Variability in advanced certification requirements across specialties

II. Educational development

A. Need for the proportion of nurses with a bachelor of science degree in nursing (BSN) to increase to 80% by 2020 (IOM, 2011)
1. Strategies include the following:
a. RN to BSN or Master of Science in nursing (MSN) degree programs—some nursing schools offer these programs to provide an efficient bridge for nurses with an associate degree (AD) to obtain their BSN or MSN degree.
b. BSN at community colleges—some community colleges offer AD students a streamlined, automatic transition to universities to obtain BSN degrees.

B. Participation in organizational, local, and national educational and professional seminars, webinars, workshops, and conferences to expand knowledge base in oncology and to obtain continuing education credits for relicensure

C. Graduate education
1. Formalized university or college education to increase depth of professional knowledge and skills
2. Formalized university/college education to redirect career path or fulfill career development plan

D. Implementation of oncology nurse practitioner fellowships at academic centers is a potential solution for those seeking training in managing patients with cancer (Alencar et al., 2018)

III. Professional development

A. Obtaining certification in oncology nursing
1. Certification—assures public that the certified nurse has the knowledge and qualifications needed to practice in his or her clinical area of nursing (Summers, 2013); provided by the Oncology Nursing Certification Corporation (ONCC)
2. Six certifications available in oncology nursing (ONCC, 2013a)—Oncology Certified Nurse (OCN), Advanced Oncology Certified Nurse Practitioner (AOCNP), Advanced Oncology Certified Clinical Nurse Specialist (AOCNS), Certified Pediatric Hematology Oncology Nurse (CPHON),

Certified Breast Care Nurse (CBCN), and the Blood and Marrow Transplant Certified Nurse (BMTCN)

3. Initial certifications in Certified Pediatric Oncology Nurse (CPON) and Advanced Oncology Certified Nurse (AOCN) no longer available, but renewals are available for nurses who currently hold these credentials

4. Requirements for OCN, CPON, CPHON, CBCN, and BMTCN certifications (ONCC, 2013b)
   a. Current, active, unrestricted RN license at time of application and examination
   b. Minimum of 1 year of experience as an RN within 3 years prior to application
   c. Minimum of 1000 hours of practice in the area of certification applying for within the 2½ years (30 months) prior to application
   d. Completion of a minimum of 10 contact hours in the area of certification applying for within the 3 years (36 months) prior to application

5. Requirements for AOCNS and AOCNP certifications (ONCC, 2013b)
   a. Current, active, unrestricted RN license at time of application and examination
   b. Graduate degree from an accredited APRN program
   c. Practice hours
      (1) If graduated from an accredited nurse practitioner (NP) or clinical nurse specialist (CNS) program with concentration in adult oncology, 500 hours supervised clinical practice as adult CNS or NP obtained within or following the graduate program, or both
      (2) If graduated from an accredited NP or CNS program with non-oncology concentration, 1000 hours supervised clinical practice as adult CNS or NP obtained within and/or following the graduate program
   d. One graduate-level oncology course of at least 2 credits or 30 hours oncology continuing education units

B. Membership and participation in local, state, national, and international professional organizations such as the ONS, ANA, American Society of Clinical Oncology (ASCO), and American Society of Hematology (ASH)

REFERENCES

Alencar, M. C., Butler, E., MacIntyre, J., & Wempe, E. P. (2018). Nurse practitioner fellowship: developing a program to address gaps in practice. *Clin J Oncol Nurs*, 22(2), 142–145. https://doi.org/10.1188/18.CJON.142-145.

Andel, C., Davidow, S. L., Hollander, M., & Moreno, D. A. (2012). The economics of health care quality and medical errors. *Journal of Health Care Finance*, 39(1), 38–50.

Brant, J. M., & Wickham, R. (Eds.), (2013). *Statement on the scope and standards of oncology nursing practice: generalist and advanced practice*. Pittsburgh: Oncology Nursing Society.

Brenan, M. (2017). *Nurses keep healthy lead as most honest, ethical profession*. http://news.gallup.com/poll/224639/nurses-keep-healthy-lead-honest-ethical-profession.aspx?g_source=CATEGORY_SOCIAL_POLICY_ISSUES&g_medium=topic&g_campaign=tiles. Accessed 20 April 2018.

Coury, J., Schneider, J. L., Rivelli, J. S., Petrik, A. F., Seibel, E., D'Agostini, B., & Coronado, G. D. (2017). Applying the Plan-Do-Study-Act (PDSA) approach to a large pragmatic study involving safety net clinics. *BMC Health Serv Res*, 17(1), 411. https://doi.org/10.1186/s12913-017-2364-3.

Du, D., Goldsmith, J., Aikin, K. J., Encinosa, W. E., & Nardinelli, C. (2012). Despite 2007 law requiring FDA hotline to be included in print drug ads, reporting of adverse events by consumers still low. *Health Aff (Millwood)*, 31(5), 1022–1029. https://doi.org/10.1377/hlthaff.2010.1004.

Ferrell, B., McCabe, M. S., & Levit, L. (2013). The Institute of Medicine report on high-quality cancer care: implications for oncology nursing. *Oncology Nursing Forum*, 40(6), 603–609. https://doi.org/10.1188/13.ONF.603-609.

Institute of Medicine. (1999). *To err is human: building a safer health system*. Washington, DC: National Academies Press.

Institute of Medicine. (2011). *The future of nursing: leading change, advancing health*. Washington, DC: National Academies Press.

Institute of Medicine. (2013). *Delivering high-quality cancer care: charting a new course for a system in crisis*. Washington, DC: National Academies Press.

Langley, G. L., Nolan, K. M., Nolan, T. W., Norman, C. L., & Provost, L. P. (2009). *The improvement guide: a practical approach to enhancing organizational performance*. San Francisco: Jossey-Bass.

Mate, K. S., & Rakover, J. (2016). 4 steps to sustaining improvement in healthcare. *Harvard Business Review Operations Management, Retrieved from* https://hbr.org/2016/11/4-steps-to-sustaining-improvement-in-health-care. Accessed 5/4/2018.

Obama, B. (2016). United States health care reform: progress to date and next steps. *Journal of the American Medical Association, 316*(5), 525–532.

Oncology Nursing Certification Corporation. (2013a). General information. www.oncc.org/TakeTest.

Oncology Nursing Certification Corporation. (2013b). Eligibility. www.oncc.org/Eligibility.

Schadewaldt, V., McInnes, E., Hiller, J. E., & Gardner, A. (2013). Views and experiences of nurse practitioners and medical practitioners with collaborative practice in primary health care—an integrative review. *BMC Fam Pract*, 14. https://doi.org/10.1186/1471-2296-14-132.

Soukup, T., Lamb, B. W., Sarkar, S., Arora, S., Shah, S., Darzi, A., & Sevdalis, N. (2016). Predictors of treatment decisions in multidisciplinary oncology meetings: a quantitative observational study. *Ann Surg Oncol*, 23(13), 4410–4417. https://doi.org/10.1245/s10434-016-5347-4.

Summers, B. L. (2013). Scope of practice. In J. M. Brant, & R. Wickham (Eds.), *Statement on the scope and standards of oncology nursing practice: generalist and advanced practice.* Pittsburgh: Oncology Nursing Society.

US Department of Health and Human Services, Agency for Healthcare Research and Quality. (2001). Reducing and preventing adverse drug events to decrease hospital costs. Research in Action, no. 1. Rockville, MD: Agency for Healthcare Research and Quality, March 2001. Retrieved from, http://www. ahrq.gov/research/findings/factsheets/errors-safety/aderia/ index.html (accessed April 15, 2018).

60

Compassion Fatigue

Susie Newton

OVERVIEW

I. People who are attracted to professions that involve caring for others such as nursing are prone to compassion fatigue by the nature of their tendency to put other's needs ahead of their own.

II. Oncology nurses are even more likely to experience compassion fatigue because they care for patients who may be facing a terminal disease.

III. Compassion fatigue is often correlated with burnout, but there are differences between the two phenomena.

IV. Job stress and burnout occur in approximately 40% of nurses (Duarte & Pinto-Gouveia, 2017)

V. It is beneficial to invest in strategies to reduce compassion fatigue and burnout in nurses, as it has been shown to reduce turnover, increase job satisfaction, increase the ability to provide quality care, and decrease overall health care expenditures (Anderson, & Gustavson, 2016).

VI. Definitions

    A. Compassion fatigue is defined as a state of physical/emotional distress that results from caring for those experiencing pain (Mooney et al., 2017). It is also defined as fatigue, emotional distress, or apathy resulting from the constant demands of caring for others (Denigris, Fisher, Maley, & Nolan, 2016). Compassion fatigue is often referred to as *secondary traumatic stress.*

    B. Burnout is a syndrome involving exhaustion, cynicism, and inefficacy that arises in response to chronic stressors on the job and evolves slowly over a prolonged period of stress (Valcour, 2016).

        1. Exhaustion: including physical, emotional, and cognitive fatigue. Tends to occur over an extended period as opposed to after one long day.

        2. Cynicism: feelings of detachment, depersonalization, and a lack of engagement. Distancing from work or from personal interactions.

        3. Inefficacy: feelings of incompetence, feeling overwhelmed, and a lack of achievement and productivity.

    C. Compassion satisfaction is the positive feelings derived from helping others, whether it be from direct contribution or for the betterment of society (Stamm, 2010). This concept explains the pleasure derived from work.

ASSESSMENT

I. Assessment tools

    A. Professional Quality of Life Scale (ProQOL) (Stamm, 2010)

        1. Most common tool used for assessing and measuring compassion fatigue and is easy to use and score. Includes three subscales:

          a. Secondary traumatic stress

          b. Burnout

          c. Compassion satisfaction.

    B. Maslach Burnout Inventory–Human Services Survey MBI-HSS (Russell, 2016)

    C. Modified Abendroth Demographic Questionnaire (Wu, Singh-Carlson, Odell, Reynolds, & Su, 2016)

    D. Self-Care Assessment

II. Risk factors for compassion fatigue (Ko & Kiser-Larson, 2016; Smart et al., 2014).

    A. Younger age (under 40)

    B. Single

    C. Less than 10 years of work experience

    D. High job expectations: corporate or self-imposed

    E. Work setting issues such as an inpatient setting, a heavy caseload, high stress levels, and prolonged periods of working with high-acuity patients

    F. Predictors of compassion fatigue and burnout (Duarte & Pinto-Gouveia, 2017).

        1. Personal distress

        2. Psychological inflexibility

        3. High level of being self-judgmental

        4. Empathy-based guilt feelings

        5. Two major work stressors are feeling overworked and poor communication between nurses and physicians

    G. Symptoms of compassion fatigue: physical, behavioral or emotional, and work related (Lanier, 2017).

        1. Physical: frequent headaches, digestive problems such as constipation or diarrhea, muscle tension, sleep disturbances, fatigue, cardiac issues such as chest pain, tachycardia or palpitations, and experiencing frequent illness.

        2. Behavioral/emotional: mood swings/irritability; anxiety; abuse of alcohol, food, illicit drugs, or

nicotine; lack of joyfulness; memory issues; poor judgement; overextension issues; poor concentration; and anger or resentment.

3. Work related: dread of going to work, frequent use of sick days, decreased ability to empathize with patients or families, and avoiding working with certain patients.

MANAGEMENT

I. Emphasize self-care (Ko & Kiser-Larson, 2016; Valcour, 2016)
   A. Good sleep habits
   B. Exercise (recommend three to four times weekly for 20–30 minutes)
   C. Nutrition/eating well
   D. Massage
   E. Enjoying a hobby, listening to music, humor, and enjoying nature
   F. Schedule preventive and medical care appointments
   G. Set aside time each day to do something for self
   H. Keep a self-care journal

II. Grief support and counseling (Zajac, Moran, & Groh, 2017)
   A. Verbalization with others such as family members, friends, and other nurses (Ko & Kiser-Larson, 2016). Many nursing units involve the use of social workers or chaplains to assist in this area.
   B. Mindfulness-based interventions (Duarte & Pinto-Gouveia, 2016).
   C. Activities that focus a person's attention on the present experience, becoming more aware of one's physical, mental, and emotional condition, in a way that is nonjudgmental. Mindfulness has been shown to be effective at reducing stress. The interventions can be offered individually or in a group setting.
   D. Healthy and supportive work environments that promote teamwork and cohesiveness and engaged leadership styles (Wu et al., 2016).
   E. Recognition is first step with support from management (Ko & Kiser-Larson, 2016):
      1. Increased staffing
      2. Providing and encouraging frequent breaks
      3. Grief meeting or huddle after the loss of a patient
      4. Fun gatherings outside of work
      5. Mentoring novice nurses
      6. Encouraging verbalization of feelings and grief support

III. Self-reflection exercises (Houck, 2014)
   A. Keep a journal
   B. Make time for prayer and meditation
   C. Take pride in personal accomplishments
   D. Send cards to the family, reminisce about time spent with patients, sometimes attend the funeral of patients with whom there has been a close bond

REFERENCES

Anderson, L., & Gustavson, C. (2016). The impact of a knitting intervention of compassion fatigue in oncology nurses. *Clinical Journal of Oncology Nursing, 20*(1), 102–104. https://doi.org/10.1188/16.

Denigris, J., Fisher, K., Maley, M., & Nolan, E. (2016). Perceived quality of work life and risk for compassion fatigue among oncology nurses: a mixed-methods study. *Oncology Nursing Forum, 43*(3), E121–E131. https://doi.org/10.1188/16.ONF.E121-E131.

Duarte, J., & Pinto-Gouveia, J. (2016). Effectiveness of a mindfulness-based intervention on oncology nurses' burnout and compassion fatigue symptoms: a non-randomized study. *International Journal of Nursing Studies, 64*, 98–107. https://doi.org/10.1016/j.ijnurstu.2016.10.002.

Duarte, J., & Pinto-Gouveia, J. (2017a). Empathy and feelings of guilt experienced by nurses: a cross-sectional study of their role in burnout and compassion fatigue symptoms. *Applied Nursing Research, 35*, 42–47. https://doi.org/10.1016/j.apnr.2017.02.006.

Duarte, J., & Pinto-Gouveia, J. (2017b). The role of psychological factors in oncology nurses' burnout and compassion fatigue symptoms. *European Journal of Oncology Nursing, 28*, 114–121. https://doi.org/10.1016/j.ejon.2017.04.002.

Houck, D. (2014). Helping nurses cope with grief and compassion fatigue: an educational intervention. *Clinical Journal of Oncology Nursing, 18*(4), 454–458. https://doi.org/10.1188/14.CJON.454-458.

Ko, W., & Kiser-Larson, N. (2016). Stress levels of nurses in oncology outpatient units. *Clinical Journal of Oncology Nursing, 20*(2), 158–164. https://doi.org/10.1188/16.

Lanier, J. (2017). Running on empty: compassion fatigue in nurses and non-professional caregivers. *Ohio Nurses Review.* Nov./Dec. 21-26.

Mooney, C., Fetter, K., Gross, B., Rinehart, C., Lynch, C., & Rogers, F. (2017). A preliminary analysis of compassion satisfaction and compassion fatigue with considerations for nursing unit specialization and demographic factors. *Journal of Trauma Nursing, 24*(3), 158–163. https://doi.org/10.1097/JTN.0000000000000284.

Russell, K. (2016). Perceptions of burnout, its prevention, and its effect on patient care as described by oncology nurses in the hospital setting. *Oncology Nursing Forum, 43*(1), 103–109. https://doi.org/10.1188/16.ONF.103-109.

Smart, D., English, A., James, J., Wilson, M., Daratha, K., Childers, B., & Magera, C. (2014). Compassion fatigue and satisfaction: a cross-sectional survey among US healthcare workers. *Nursing and Health Sciences, 16*, 3–10. https://doi.org/10.1111/nhs.12068.

Stamm, B. H. (2010). *The ProQOL concise manual* (2nd ed.). Retrieved from http://www.proqol.org/ProQOl_Test_Manuals.html.

Valcour, M. (2016). Beating burnout: How to tell if you have it and what to do about it. *Harvard Business Review* (pp. 98–101).

Wu, S., Singh-Carlson, S., Odell, A., Reynolds, G., & Su, Y. (2016). Compassion fatigue, burnout, and compassion satisfaction among oncology nurses in the United States and Canada. *Oncol Nursing Forum, 43*(4), E161–E169. https://doi.org/10.1188/16.ONF.E161-E169.

Zajac, L., Moran, K., & Groh, C. (2017). Confronting compassion fatigue: assessment and intervention in inpatient oncology. *Clinical Journal of Oncology Nursing, 21*(4), 446–453. https://doi.org/10.1188/17.

Note: Page numbers followed by *f* indicate figures, *t* indicate tables, and *b* indicate boxes.